Handbook of
Drug Abuse Prevention

Handbooks of Sociology and Social Research

Series Editor:
Howard B. Kaplan, *Texas A&M University, College Station, Texas*

A Continuation Order Plan is available for this series. A continuation order will bring delivery of each new volume immediately upon publication. Volumes are billed only upon actual shipment. For further information please contact the publisher.

Handbook of
Drug Abuse Prevention
Theory, Science, and Practice

Edited by

Zili Sloboda

University of Akron
Akron, Ohio

and

William J. Bukoski

National Institute on Drug Abuse
Bethesda, Maryland

Kluwer Academic/Plenum Publishers
New York   Boston   Dordrecht   London   Moscow

Library of Congress Cataloging-in-Publication Data

Handbook of drug abuse prevention: theory, science, and practice/edited by Zili
Sloboda and William J. Bukoski.
    p. cm. — (Handbooks of sociology and social research)
    Includes bibliographical references and index.
    ISBN 0-306-47342-9
    I. Drug abuse—Prevention. 2. Drug abuse—Prevention—Research. 3. Drug
abuse—United States—Prevention. I. Sloboda, Zili. II. Bukoski, William J. III. Series.

HV5801 .H282 2002
362.29′17—dc21

2002072682

ISBN: 0-306-47342-9

© 2003 Kluwer Academic / Plenum Publishers, New York
233 Spring Street, New York, New York 10013

http://www.wkap.nl/

10 9 8 7 6 5 4 3 2 1

A C.I.P. record for this book is available from the Library of Congress

Printed in the United States of America

Contributors

Sergio Aguilar-Gaxiola, Department of Psychology, California State University at Fresno, Fresno, California 93740

Steve Alder, Department of Family and Preventive Medicine, University of Utah, Salt Lake City, Utah 84112

Laura Andrade, Instituto de Psiquiatria, Universidate de Sao Paulo, Sao Paulo, Brazil

Michael W. Arthur, Social Development Research Group, University of Washington, Seattle, Washington, 98115

Charles D. Ayers, Social Development Research Group, University of Washington, Seattle, Washington 98115

Michael T. Bardo, Department of Psychology, University of Kentucky, Lexington, Kentucky 40506

Fred Beauvais, Tri-Ethnic Center for Prevention Research, Colorado State University, Fort Collins, Colorado 80523

Audrey L. Begun, Department of Psychology, University of Wisconsin at Milwaukee, Milwaukee, Wisconsin 53211

Marvin W. Berkowitz, College of Education, University of Missouri at St. Louis, St. Louis, Missouri 63121

Rob Bijl, Epidemiology, Netherlands Institute of Mental Health, Utrecht, Netherlands

Luiz Guilherme Borges, Departamento de Investigaciones en Servicios de Salud, Instituto Nacional de Psiquiatria & Universidad Autonoma Metropolitana-Xochimilco, Calzada, Mexico

Kris Bosworth, College of Education, University of Arizona, Tucson, Arizona 85721

Gilbert J. Botvin, Institute for Prevention Research, Weill Medical College of Cornell University, New York, New York 10021

David W. Brook, Department of Community and Preventive Medicine, Mount Sinai School of Medicine, New York, New York 10029

Judith S. Brook, Department of Community and Preventive Medicine, Mount Sinai School of Medicine, New York, New York 10029

C. Hendricks Brown, Department of Epidemiology and Biostatistics, University of South Florida, Tampa, Florida 33612

William J. Bukoski, National Institute on Drug Abuse, National Institutes of Health, Bethesda, Maryland 20892

Bert Burraston, Oregon Social Learning Center, Eugene, Oregon 97403

Jorge J. Caraveo-Anduaga, Instituto Mexicano de Psiquiatria, Calzada, Mexico

Richard F. Catalano, Social Development Research Group, University of Washington, Seattle, Washington 98115

W. William Chen, Department of Health Science Education, University of Florida, Gainesville 32611

Kristin Cole, School of Social Work, Columbia University, New York, New York 10025

Linda M. Collins, Methodology Center, The Pennsylvania State University, University Park, Pennsylvania 16802

Royer F. Cook, The ISA Group, Alexandria, Virginia 22314

David S. DeGarmo, Oregon Social Learning Center, Eugene, Oregon 97401

David J. DeWit, Addiction Research Foundation, London, Ontario, Canada N6G 4X8

Thomas J. Dishion, Child and Family Center, Department of Psychology, University of Oregon, Eugene, Oregon 97403

Lewis Donohew, Department of Communication, University of Kentucky, Lexington, Kentucky 40506

Susan C. Duncan, Oregon Research Institute, Eugene, Oregon 97403

Terry E. Duncan, Oregon Research Institute, Eugene, Oregon 97403

Robert L. DuPont, Institute for Behavior and Health, Inc.; Bensinger, DuPont & Associates, Rockville, Maryland 20852

James H. Dwyer, UCLA Medical School, University of Southern California, Los Angeles, California 90089

J. Mark Eddy, Oregon Social Learning Center, Eugene, Oregon 97401

Leona L. Eggert, School of Nursing, University of Washington, Seattle, Washington 98195

Brian P. Flaherty, Methodology Center, The Pennsylvania State University, University Park, Pennsylvania 16802

Brian R. Flay, Preventive Research Center, University of Illinois at Chicago, Chicago, Illinois 60680

Randy R. Gainey, Department of Sociology and Criminal Justice, Old Dominion University, Norfolk, VA 23529

Kelly A. Graham, Social Development Research Group, University of Washington, Seattle, Washington 98115

Kenneth W. Griffin, Institute for Prevention Research, Weill Medical College of Cornell University, New York, New York 10021

Kevin P. Haggerty, Social Development Research Group, University of Washington, Seattle, Washington 98115

J. David Hawkins, Social Development Research Group, University of Washington, Seattle, Washington 98115

Gale Held, MPA. Independent Consultant, Kensington, Maryland, 20895-3823

Michael J. Hench, Department of Family Studies, University of Kentucky, Lexington, Kentucky 40506

Harold D. Holder, Pacific Institute for Research and Evaluation, Berkeley, California, 94704

Thomas Kelly, Department of Psychology, University of Kentucky, Lexington, Kentucky 40506

Ronald C. Kessler, Department of Health Care Policy, Harvard Medical School, Boston, Massachusetts 02115

Barry M. Kibel, Pacific Institute for Research and Evaluation, Chapel Hill, North Carolina 27514

Bo Kolody, Sociology Department, San Diego State University, San Diego, California 92182

Karol L. Kumpfer, Department of Family and Preventive Medicine, University of Utah, Salt Lake City, Utah 84112

Fuzhong Li, Oregon Social Learning Center and Oregon Research Institute, Eugene, Oregon 97403

John E. Lochman, Department of Psychology, University of Alabama, Tuscaloosa, Alabama 35487

Donald R. Lynam, Department of Psychology, University of Kentucky, Lexington, Kentucky 40506

R. S. Lynch, Tri-Ethnic Center for Prevention Research, Colorado State University, Fort Collins, Colorado 80523

David P. MacKinnon, Department of Psychology, Arizona State University, Tempe, Arizona 85287-1104

Charles R. Martinez, Jr., Oregon Social Learning Center, Eugene, Oregon 97401

Kathleen R. Merikangas, National Institute of Mental Health, Bethesda, Maryland 20892-2670

Joel Milam, Institute for Health Promotion and Disease Prevention Research, University of Southern California, Los Angeles, California

Richard Milich, Department of Psychology, University of Kentucky, Lexington, Kentucky 40506

Beth E. Molnar, Harvard School of Public Health, Harvard University, Boston, Massachusetts 02115

Howard Moss, Department of Psychiatry, University of Pennsylvania, Philadelphia, Pennsylvania 19104

E. R. Oetting, Tri-Ethnic Center for Prevention Research, Colorado State University, Fort Collins, Colorado 80523

Philip Palmgreen, Department of Communication, University of Kentucky, Lexington, Kentucky 40506

Mary Ann Pentz, Department of Preventive Medicine, University of Southern California, Alhambra, California 91803

John Petraitis, Department of Psychology, University of Alaska, Anchorage, Alaska 99508

Brooke P. Randell, School of Nursing, University of Washington, Seattle, Washington 98195

Linda Richter, The National Center on Addiction and Substance Abuse, Columbia University, New York, New York 10029

Louise Ann Rohrbach, Institute for Health Promotion and Disease Prevention Research, University of Southern California, Alhambra, California 91803

Keith E. Saylor, NeuroScience, Inc., Bethesda, Maryland 20814

Steven Schinke, School of Social Work, Columbia University, New York 10025

Zili Sloboda, Department of Sociology and Institute for Health and Social Policy, The University of Akron, Akron, Ohio 44325

Ralph E. Tarter, School of Pharmacy, University of Pittsburgh, Pittsburgh, Pennsylvania 15260

Joseph E. Trimble, Center for Cross-Cultural Research, Department of Psychology, Western Washington University, Bellingham, Washington 98226

William L. Turner, Department of Family Social Science, University of Minnesota-Twin Cities, St. Paul, Minnesota 55108

Michael Vanyukov, School of Pharmacy, University of Pittsburgh, Pittsburgh, Pennsylvania 15260

William A. Vega, Institute for Quality Research and Training, Robert Wood Johnson Medical School, New Brunswick, New Jersey 08901

Ellen E. Walters, Department of Health Care Policy, Harvard Medical School, Boston, Massachusetts 02115

Hans-Ulrich Wittchen, Clinical Psychology and Epidemiology, Max Planck Institute of Psychiatry, Muenchen, Germany 80804

Martin Whiteman, Department of Community and Preventive Medicine, Mount Sinai School of Medicine, New York, New York 10029

Preface

There are a number of reasons why this book is important. First, there is no one source that summarizes what we know about the prevention of substance abuse from the research field, so the book serves as a repository of accumulated knowledge on prevention theory, intervention design, and development and prevention research methodology. Second, as an evolving field, prevention science has only begun to assert itself in both the arenas of practice and policy. The formation of the Society for Prevention Research in 1991 was the first recognition that a science of prevention existed and required a separate forum to present the rapidly growing content of the field for discussion and review. Finally, there is a need to establish a baseline, a reference point against which progress in the field of prevention science can be assessed. This book serves all of these purposes.

The idea for this book grew from the observation in the early 1990s that after decades of attempts to develop effective interventions to prevent drug use among children and adolescents in the United States that we were finally having success, particularly in addressing the initiation of use. These successes are the result of research that has provided a better understanding of the factors and processes associated with the onset of substance use. The convergence of accumulating and consistent epidemiologic information regarding trends in substance use, sequential use patterns and vulnerability and protection and the progress being made in developing behavior theory and research on curriculum design have influenced this achievement. These accomplishments however, should not be viewed as final. The work completed to date only lays a foundation on which the whole field of drug use prevention is built. There remain many gaps in our knowledge base: gaps that unless filled, can greatly diminish the impact of what we have learned so far. Among the most prominent gaps are the development of interventions that target children and adolescents at high risk to substance use; understanding the differential response to interventions by gender, age and ethnicity; and understanding the impact of multiple interventions within the community context. Furthermore, drug abuse prevention programming must also be flexible to reflect changing trends in types of drugs being used and the growing knowledge regarding the biological processes and implications of drug use.

Given the previous, this *Handbook* had been conceived as documentation of the current knowledge in the field of drug use prevention and addresses specifically the gap areas. It is seen as a "work in progress" and as a snapshot of prevention science at the beginning of the 21st century. The book is designed to cover a broad range of subjects from theory to practice. It is written to respond to the needs of researchers, practitioners, policymakers, students, and the lay public. It can be used in academic institutions as a text in courses on drug abuse and drug abuse prevention and as a reference source for both practitioners and policymakers.

The book is organized around eight major areas: Historical Overview, Social Contexts of Prevention, Prevention as Social Control, Theoretical and Empirical Foundations, Special Populations, Interactions between Biology and Social Context—Risks for Multiple Behavioral and Mental Disorders, Research Design, Measurement, and Data Analytic Issues, and Drug Abuse Prevention: A Look into the Future. The authors of each chapter were specifically invited to review each of their areas of interest and to reflect on implications for future prevention planning.

The first chapter by Bukoski provides an historical framework for the content of the book, setting a base against which the progress of the field of prevention and prevention science can be assessed. In this chapter Bukoski talks about the struggling science and the first glimmerings of success. He then takes the reader to explore how findings from emergent biological and neuroscience research may impact the future of prevention. The next section of the book, Social Contexts of Prevention, presents eight chapters discussing a variety of settings in which prevention takes place. The discussions within each of these chapters presents the special attributes of each context and presents the findings from research with demonstrated impact on precursors to substance abuse or to substance abuse behaviors themselves. Palmgreen and Donohew discuss the role of the media both as a vehicle for prevention messages and as an intervention per se. The school is one of the most prevalent contexts for prevention interventions. Botvin and Griffith present findings from this body of drug abuse prevention research in their chapter. Kumpfer and Alder provide a view of the family as an important means to address the needs of children at risk for substance use. Oetting and Lynch explore peer networks or clusters as major sources of influence on substance using patterns and also as major avenues for reaching adolescents with prevention messages and establishing antisubstance use norms. Both Arthur and his associates and Kibel and Holder look to the community for support of prevention efforts. Arthur et al. discuss the organic and rich nature of communities to plan for prevention programming that meets the specific needs of each community. One of the major ways to use available resources within the community is to establish and strategically implement policies that curtail the sale and use of substances such as alcohol and tobacco. Cook and Catalano et al. write about two novel contexts for prevention programming, the work place and drug abuse treatment facilities.

At the time of the writing of these chapters, only drug testing and "no-use" policies had been researched for the section, Prevention as Social Control. Dupont and Saylor and Pentz present excellent discussions of these two under-researched areas. However, there are other areas such as law enforcement that are even less researched or understood that will be explored in the future and included in later editions of either this or other handbooks on prevention.

It was mentioned earlier that the progress made in the last decade was heavily dependent on understanding the various pathways to drug use and abuse. The section, Theoretical and Empirical Foundations, presents this knowledge base. Sloboda provides a picture of how epidemiologic findings have served and continue to serve prevention. Brook and her colleagues focus on risk and protective factors examining how these relate to drug use over time. Flay and Petraitis discuss the important role theory has played and continues to play in the development of effective prevention programming. The importance of childhood aggression, lack of social competence in children, and certain negative parenting practices have been found to be related to substance abuse in adolescence. Lochman discusses this research and the types of effective preventive strategies that intervene to disrupt the trajectory to substance abuse from childhood behavioral disorders. The final chapter in this section by Berkowitz and Begun puts prevention programming within a developmental framework. Although the emphasis is on childhood and adolescence, the entire lifespan is addressed. Each period in development has its challenges, and these authors draw from the research literature to address the design of appropriate and relevant prevention interventions.

Much of the research in the development of effective preventive interventions either has focused on Whites, or the majority population, or has failed to specifically explore prevention strategies for specific cultural and social groups. The next section, Special Populations, discusses the epidemiology of drug use and abuse among several of these populations and, where such research exists, presents the findings from studies of prevention programs. More often, the research that has examined the impact of prevention programs on these groups is sparse. In each chapter the authors recommend how the particular needs of these groups can be more effectively incorporated into prevention strategies. Rohrbach and Milam review the differences in drug use patterns by gender and in response to both drug abuse prevention and treatment programs. They conclude by discussing the implications of these findings for prevention design and practice. The next chapters in this section take a similar approach in examining prevention. Martinez and his colleagues review the problem as it relates to Latino youth; Turner and Hench discuss substance abuse and prevention for African-Americans; Beauvais and Trimble address the needs of American Indian Youth; and, Chen, Asian- and Pacific Islander-Americans.

Some of the most challenging issues that confront prevention researchers and practitioners today are coming out of the biological and epidemiologic research. These include new knowledge regarding the relationship between drugs and the brain and between drug use and other problem behaviors. These issues are covered in the next section, Interaction between Biology and Social Context—Risks for Multiple Behavioral and Mental Disorders. Bardo et al. focus on drug abuse and its biologic basis. They discuss how the results of basic biological research impacts prevention for those at high risk to drug abuse. The next chapter by Kessler et al. presents the findings from surveys conducted through the International Consortium in Psychiatric Epidemiology specifically examining the relationship between substance use disorders and mental disorders. Implications for prevention are discussed. These chapters lead to Tarter and his associates' discussion of the role of genetics and the family as underlying contributors to drug abuse. The need for specialized prevention approaches for those at particular high risk to substance abuse had been recognized, but few effective programs have been developed. The final chapter in this section by Eggert and Randell present their experience in reaching youth at high risk and discuss their programs and outcome studies.

Along with the advances in prevention theory development and in forming a strong research foundation for prevention programming, research, and statistical methodologies also have progressed greatly over the past 10 to 15 years. This accumulated knowledge is presented in the next section, Research Design, Measurement, and Data Analytic Issues. The section begins with a chapter by Brown, who provides a conceptual framework for addressing key concerns in the design of prevention research field trials. MacKinnon and Dwyer next discuss the major data analysis issues that face prevention researchers in the "real" world. Collins and Flaherty in their chapter, Methodological Considerations in Prevention Research, conceptually take the reader from theory and modeling to the important process of developing measurements from the theory and finally the exploration of the relationships among multiple measures that form the theory. Schinke and Cole discuss research design issues related to the dissemination of prevention practices in the real world. The chapter by Dishion and associates demonstrates the importance of multiple measures using their family management practice prevention program as an example. Duncan and his colleagues in their chapter then discuss power analysis models and methods appropriate for preventive intervention field trials.

Where do we go from here? In the section, Drug Abuse Prevention: A Look into the Future, the chapters by Bosworth and Held take on two timely but difficult topics. Bosworth explores the use of computers in prevention, presenting how computers are used in education to heighten the learning experience and how they can serve to improve prevention delivery. Finally, in her chapter, Held focuses on the dissemination of the findings from prevention research and on the diffusion of effective prevention programming from the controlled setting of the research study to the community. At a time when the field has evidence of success and when this evidence has been made available to practitioners and policymakers through a number of information channels and professional networks, the widespread implementation of programs with demonstrated positive long-term outcomes has not been achieved. A number of barriers to diffusion and potential solutions to overcome them are discussed.

The editors and contributors to this book want to share their knowledge with several communities; other researchers both in the field of drug abuse prevention and in the broader areas of health promotion and education, practitioners who translate this research for the special needs of their communities, and for policymakers who may be skeptical about the progress being made in the field of drug abuse prevention. The field has formed its own professional group, the Society for Prevention Research. This group has become a major forum for establishing dialogues among researchers and has become an impetus for the development of the science of prevention. The future for progress in understanding drug abuse processes and to advance our strategies for preventing drug abuse is bright. Key areas with potential for the field include understanding the structures of communities so they can support prevention programming, linking the growing knowledge about the biological and genetic bases of drug abuse to prevention approaches and creating statistical methodologies that are more sensitive and specific to the needs of prevention researchers.

ZILI SLOBODA

Acknowledgments

The editors of this book wish to express their profound thanks to the many contributors who devoted their precious professional time, energy, and wisdom to develop their excellent cha

We wish to recognize the valuable talents of Mr. Robert Trotter, who provided his perc and highly accomplished copy-editing skills to the development of each chapter. Thanks ar extended to Sylvia Jarrett-Coker for her very helpful administrative and electronic proc support. Special recognition goes to Dr. Minda Lynch, National Institute on Drug Abus collaborating with one of the editors in helping to craft the concept of "bridging neurobiolc behavioral, and prevention sciences" in the drug abuse arena, a vision that is advanced t book.

Special thanks are extended to Mr. Richard Millstein and Dr. Peter Delany, both National Institute on Drug Abuse, for their untiring support for this book project.

Finally, a hearty thank you is offered to the excellent editorial staff at Kluwer Acac Plenum Publishers for their astute guidance, unyielding patience, and productive comm provided throughout the entire course of this wonderful and challenging book project.

Contents

VII. RESEARCH DESIGN, MEASUREMENT, AND DATA ANALYTIC ISSUES

PART I

HISTORICAL OVERVIEW

CHAPTER 1

The Emerging Science of Drug Abuse Prevention

WILLIAM J. BUKOSKI

INTRODUCTION

Over the past 15 years, prevention science has emerged as a formal biopsychosocial discipline focused upon knowledge development and the application of research findings to the improvement of practice (NIH, 1998). Basic and behavioral scientific studies funded by the National Institutes of Health (NIH) have identified highly promising prevention theories and interventions focused upon a variety of public health problems to include smoking, drug abuse, alcohol abuse, HIV/AIDS, child abuse, physical inactivity and the management of chronic conditions such as asthma, arthritis, and heart disease. However, the continued progress of drug abuse prevention science depends upon future integration with basic neurobiological, genetic, and behavioral research in order to better identify specific underlying biopsychosocial pathways to substance use disorders and to develop scientifically tested and highly efficacious targeted preventive interventions to reduce liability to and the incidence and prevalence of substance use disorders in the general population and in subgroups at heightened risk.

WILLIAM J. BUKOSKI • National Institute on Drug Abuse, National Institutes of Health, Bethesda, Maryland 20892

LANDMARKS OF DRUG ABUSE
PREVENTION SCIENCE

Given over 25 years of etiological and epidemiological research, several appropriate frameworks and models for drug abuse prevention have been identified to include the public health model, the communicable disease model, and the risk and protective factor model (Bukoski, 1991). Common to these models is the tenet that scientific knowledge of the etiology and progression of disease across the life span offers the key to the development of effective prevention interventions.

A landmark study of risk and protective factors research for alcohol and drug abuse in adolescence and early adulthood by Hawkins et al. (1992) firmly established the scientific validity of prevention science. Seventeen clusters of risk and protective factors were identified by these researchers in their review of hundreds of etiologic studies. These included laws and norms, availability, extreme economic deprivation, neighborhood disorganization, physiological factors (biochemical, genetic, and personality traits such as sensation seeking), family drug behavior, family management practices, family conflict, low bonding to family, early and persistent problem behaviors, academic failure, low bonding to school, peer rejection in elementary grades, association with drug-using peers, alienation and rebelliousness, attitudes favorable to drug use, and early onset of drug use.

In addition, this study identified separate and distinct protective factors that mediate or moderate the effects of exposure to multiple risk processes. For example, protective factors for children exposed to stressful life events include a child's positive temperament, supportive family systems, reinforcement of adaptive coping, and inculcation of positive values (Garmezy, 1985). According to emerging research, protective factors may produce an enduring shield or level of resilience against a variety of risk factors that may be reflected in resilient children's display of social problem-solving skills and belief in their own self-efficacy (Rutter, 1985). Recently, Glantz and Johnson (1999) expanded the discussion by exploring the implications for prevention science of current developmental research related to protective factors, resilience, and positive life adaptations.

Hawkins et al. (1992) concluded that theory-based drug and alcohol prevention interventions should have dual goals. The first is to reduce or eliminate the effects of risk exposure. The second is to enhance protective processes and thereby promote the synergism necessary to potentiate the effects of multiple risks.

Additional landmark events have advanced prevention science. For example, in a significant paper titled the "Science of Prevention," Coie et al. (1993) articulated that one of the major goals of prevention research is to test specific theories of risk and protective factors by first specifying the chain of events that then become the targets of the intervention and then to conduct controlled field trials to assess the underlying etiology and efficacy of the preventive intervention to alter the trajectory of risk and the emerging dysfunctional behavior, such as drug abuse. Second, these authors argue for prevention research trials that target those at high risk of the disorder. They recommend that prevention researchers conduct prospective, longitudinal studies to assess the efficacy of prevention interventions to alter the course of developmental psychopathology; that prevention researchers study transactional processes reflected by "person $\times$ environmental interactions"; that prevention research focus upon the powerful role played by cultural beliefs, norms, and behaviors; that prevention research adopt general systems theory by exploring prevention effects resulting from the interactions between multiple developmental influences to include family, school, peer, work place, community, and biology; and that prevention research carefully address the interaction of social influences and biology across the development life course.

Another landmark event for prevention science occurred with the publication of the Institute of Medicine's (IOM) report on "Reducing Risks for Mental Disorders." This systematic review (Mrazek & Haggerty, 1994) revealed that there is a substantial knowledge base of biological and psychosocial risk and protective factors associated with a variety of serious health problems to include Alzheimer's disease, schizophrenia, alcohol abuse and dependence, depressive disorders, and conduct disorders. In addition, the report identified a number of well-controlled prevention intervention research trials that demonstrated the scientific efficacy of prevention to reduce the risks for a variety of health problems related to physical health, parenting and family functioning, family preservation, prenatal and infant care, enhancing child development, promoting social competence, academic achievement, school reorganization, substance abuse, conduct disorder, social environments, violence prevention, marital relationships, challenges to childbearing and childrearing, occupational stress and job loss, depressive disorders associated with poverty and minority status, stress on family care providers of the chronically ill, coping with widowhood and bereavement, and co-morbidity of multiple disorders.

Mrazek and Haggerty also advanced the conceptual basis of prevention by their introduction of the mental health spectrum. According to these authors, the medical prevention model (primary, secondary, and tertiary prevention) was best suited to medical disorders and was not well suited to mental health problems. For example, they suggested that it is very difficult to establish a "case" of mental disorder as is done with medical disorders. There is disagreement as to what constitutes a case of mental disorder, in that symptoms may exist even though a disorder does not meet all conditions of DSM-III-R. Finally, the mental disorders of children (birth to age of 5) are difficult to diagnose as a psychiatric case because the problems relate more to impairment in psychosocial development or cognitive functioning.

As a result, the authors proposed an alternative to the medical model and called that model "the mental health intervention spectrum." Under this model, the term "prevention" includes three levels of intervention: "universal, selective, and indicated." Prevention interventions are implemented prior to the initial onset of a diagnosed disorder. Once the diagnostic threshold is reached by satisfying the requirements of a nosology such as DSM-III-R or DSM-IV, then "treatment" programs are appropriate. These would include case identification and standard treatment for known disorders. The final level is "maintenance," which includes interventions that assist with compliance to treatment regimens and to the reduction of relapse and recurrence of the disorder and after care to include rehabilitation.

An important feature of this model is the recommendation that ALL three levels of prevention interventions should be implemented in a practice setting. Mrazek and Haggerty acknowledge that "universal preventive interventions" should be targeted to the general population, e.g., prenatal care, childhood immunizations. Subgroups of the population that present greater than normal biological, psychological, or social risk associated with developing a disorder would also receive an appropriate "selective preventive intervention." Examples would include home visitation for low-birth-weight babies, preschool for disadvantaged children, and support groups for elderly widows. Finally, an "indicated preventive intervention" would be implemented for those with detectible signs or symptoms of developing the disorder. One example is parent–child interaction training for families with a child presenting behavioral problems, but whose behaviors are not sufficiently severe to warrant a clinical diagnosis.

This publication coalesced the scientific importance of the risk and protective factor model for prevention, demonstrated that prevention science had already designed and tested a number of theory-based interventions that demonstrated their efficacy to reduce the risk of a variety of mental disorders, and highlighted the importance of assessing a series of preventive interventions along a program continuum from universal through selective to indicated in order to address the range of early biological and behavioral indications of increased vulnerability to the subsequent emergence of the disorder at a clinically diagnosable level.

This IOM report increased the importance in prevention science of developing a series of "targeted interventions" that best address the biopsychosocial risk profiles of individuals at a specific developmental stage, thereby increasing the chances of producing positive and enduring preventive effects over time. The report also reinforced the importance of studying both proximal and distal variables. In the language of prevention, proximal variables are hypothesized to mediate the effects of the "distal" outcomes targeted by the intervention (Buchner and Cain, 1998).

Another landmark event in prevention science was the release of NIDA's publication titled "Preventing Drug Use Among Children and Adolescents: A Research-Based Guide (1997). This publication clearly established the beginning of the evidence-based drug abuse prevention movement that has emerged across the country over the past 5 years.

Based upon numerous well-designed, randomized controlled trials of theory-based drug abuse prevention interventions in schools, with families, in the workplace, and in the community, NIDA's research led to the formulation of clearly stated evidence-based drug abuse prevention principles that could be applied at the community level.

These principles articulate in practical terms the cumulative research evidence that supports the premise that adolescent drug abuse can be prevented by the implementation of tested prevention programs and policies that target the reduction or amelioration of individual, family, peer, school, and community risk factors, and that enhance protective factors and processes salient to adolescent drug abuse onset and progression.

Even though this publication has been widely disseminated to the prevention practice and research communities, a restatement of these seminal drug abuse prevention principles is warranted.

- "Prevention programs should be designed to enhance 'protective factors' and move toward reversing or reducing known 'risk factors.'"
- Prevention programs should target all forms of drug abuse, including the use of tobacco, alcohol, marijuana, and inhalants.
- Prevention programs should include skills to resist drugs when offered, strengthen personal commitments against drug use, and increase social competency (e.g., in communications, peer relationships, self-efficacy, and assertiveness), in conjunction with reinforcement of attitudes against drug use.
- Prevention programs for adolescents should include interactive methods, such as peer discussion groups, rather than didactic teaching techniques alone.
- Prevention programs should include a parents' or caregivers' component that reinforces what the children are learning—such as facts about drugs and their harmful effects—and that opens opportunities for family discussions about the use of legal and illegal substances and family policies about their use.
- Prevention programs should be long term, over the school career with repeat interventions to reinforce the original prevention goals. For example, school-based efforts directed at elementary and middle school students should include booster sessions to help with critical transitions from middle to high school.
- Family-focused prevention efforts have a greater impact than strategies that focus on parents only or children only.
- Community programs that include media campaigns and policy changes, such as new regulations that restrict access to alcohol, tobacco, or other drugs, are more effective when school and family interventions accompany them.

- Community programs need to strengthen norms against drug use in all drug abuse prevention settings, including the family, the school, and the community.
- Schools offer opportunities to reach all populations and also serve as important settings for specific subpopulations at risk for drug abuse, such as children with behavior problems or learning disabilities and those who are potential dropouts.
- Prevention programming should be adapted to address the specific nature of the drug abuse problem in the local community.
- The higher the level of risk of the target population, the more intensive the prevention effort must be and the earlier it must begin.
- Prevention programs should be age specific, developmentally appropriate, and culturally sensitive.
- Effective prevention programs are cost-effective. For every dollar spent on drug use prevention, communities can save 4 to 5 dollars in costs for drug abuse treatment and counseling."

Since the publication of NIDA's drug abuse prevention principles, numerous Federal agencies have launched special programs to identify and disseminate evidence-based drug abuse prevention programs and policies that have been thoroughly tested and shown to be efficacious. Frequently, these federal efforts expanded the search of evidence-based prevention programs beyond substance abuse to those targeting youth violence and juvenile delinquency.

For example, the U.S. Department of Education has developed an expert panel process to identify exemplary and promising drug prevention programs that could be used as part of their Safe and Drug-Free Schools national program (http://www.ed.gov/offices/OESE/ SDFS/ model_programs.html).

To receive an exemplary rating, a prevention program must have at least one study demonstrating its efficacy to prevent substance abuse, school violence, or other conduct problems, and to receive a strong or adequate rating on the evaluation criteria established by the committee. A promising program also would have had at least one efficacy study demonstrating positive outcomes or an efficacy study that indicated a positive program effect on one or more risk or protective factor. A promising program would have received a minimally acceptable or adequate rating on the evaluation criteria used by the committee.

As a result of this extensive review process, the Department of Education identified nine exemplary programs with advanced research evidence to support their claim, e.g., Athletes Training and Learning To Avoid Steroids (ATLAS), Life Skills Training, Project TNT (Towards No Tobacco Use), The National Center on Addiction and Substance Abuse at Columbia University's Striving Together to Achieve Rewarding Tomorrows (CASASTART), OSLC Treatment Foster Care, Project Alert, Project Northland, Second Step: A Violence Prevention Curriculum, and the Strengthening Families Program: For Parents and Youth 10–14. On their list are also 33 promising programs that have good scientific evidence to support their claims of efficacy, e.g., All Stars, Child Development Project, Lion's-Quest Skills for Adolescence, Preparing for the Drug-Free Years, Project STAR, etc. Further information on review criteria and program descriptions are available at the previously cited home page.

The Center for Substance Abuse Prevention (CSAP), Substance Abuse and Mental Health Services Administration (SAMSHA) established a "National Registry of Effective Prevention Programs." In this system, reviewers rate program research on 15 criteria to include theory, outcomes, measures, data analysis, and program integrity (http://www.samhsa.gov/centers/csap/ modelprograms/programs.cfm).

CSAP has identified 44 model programs as of April 11, 2002, and includes drug abuse prevention programs such as All-Stars, Athletes Training and Learning To Avoid Steroids (ATLAS), Brief

Strategic Family Therapy, Bullying Prevention Program, Child Development Project, Communities Mobilizing for Change on Alcohol, Incredible Years, Multisystemic Therapy, Project Toward No Drug Use (TND), and Life Skills Training. Details on the review criteria and programs were selected to include target population, setting, strategies, outcomes, and cost estimates are available on the previously cited home page. CSAP also identifies the type of prevention program—universal, selective, indicated, consistent with the IOM report mentioned earlier.

The Office of Juvenile Justice and Delinquency Prevention (OJJDP) has also identified 11 model evidence-based drug abuse and violence prevention programs and another 19 promising prevention programs in its "Blueprints" project (Mihalic et al., 2001). Key review criteria included prevention outcomes measured under a rigorous research design, evidence that prevention effects were sustained for at least a year after the end of the "treatment," and positive effects in multiple and diverse site replications. Model programs scored highest across all review major criteria to include evidence of program effects on mediating factors and a positive cost-benefit analysis. Blueprints model prevention programs include: The Midwestern Prevention Project, Big Brothers Big Sisters of America, Functional Family Therapy, The Quantum Opportunities Program, Life Skills Training, Multisystemic Therapy, Prenatal and Infancy Home Visitation by Nurses, Multidimensional Treatment Foster Care, Bullying Prevention Program, Promoting Alternative Thinking Strategies, and the Incredible Years. Program descriptions, contact information, research findings, and cost-benefit analysis of selected blueprint model programs are provided by the authors.

A final significant federal effort to identify evidence-based drug abuse and violence prevention programs was conducted by the U.S. Office of the Surgeon General (USDHHS, 2001). This report thoroughly and thoughtfully reviewed the theoretical underpinnings leading to youth violence and identified 27 substance abuse and violence prevention programs for youth that are both efficacious, based upon research findings, and cost-effective. Programs are identified by type: universal, selective, and indicated.

Four criteria were employed in the review of the research literature to identify promising programs: rigorous experimental research design, demonstrated significant deterrent effects, sustainability of effects over time, and replication of effective models in diverse settings. The report identified by name both effective and ineffective prevention strategies. Brief program descriptions are included, and, for effective strategies, the report provides detailed cost-benefit information on 10 effective prevention programs.

Using data from the Washington State Institute for Public Policy, the report identified the benefits of prevention programs for taxpayers. For example, for every dollar spent on prevention programs for adolescent juvenile offenders, the Multidimensional Treatment Foster Care Program would return $14.07; Multisystemic Therapy would return $8.38 for every dollar spent; Functional Family Therapy would return $6.85 for every dollar spent on this program. Relevant to prevention programs targeting early or middle childhood or programs for nonoffending adolescents, such as the Perry School Program, Prenatal and Infancy Home Visitation Program by Nurses, Seattle Social Development Project, and Big Brothers Big Sisters of America, taxpayers would receive back on average $.50 over and above each dollar spent on these programs.

Despite these encouraging findings, the Surgeon General's report indicates that little is known about the efficacy of hundreds of youth violence prevention programs implemented in communities across the country. That is, youth violence programs that are used nationwide have little or no evaluative data to support their adoption.

Relevant to drug prevention programs in schools, this same conclusion was reached in a survey of school-based prevention programs nationwide sponsored by the U.S. Department of Education (Silvia, Thorne, & Tashjian, 1997). This evaluation of the Drug-Free Schools and

Communities Act found that the vast majority of the 19 school districts included in the study did not implement evidence-based prevention programs, that program delivery varied substantially from classroom to classroom, and that while some of the nation's school prevention programs did produce positive outcomes, these effects were small in magnitude.

These two reports indicate that while scientific evidence on the efficacy of drug abuse and youth violence prevention programs has substantially increased over the past 10 years, the process of taking evidence-based prevention programs to scale has not yet happened and may face numerous technical, financial, and infrastructure barriers that will need to be addressed by future research and programmatic initiatives at the federal, state, and community level.

The future of going to scale with evidence-based drug abuse prevention programming and policy may depend upon the success and research evidence generated by emerging community-based performance management activities such as the Communities That Care project (Hawkins and Catalano, 1992). According to these researchers, effective community-based drug abuse prevention begins with a community specific survey of risk and protective factors for adolescent substance abuse followed by a series of system building steps that acknowledges and empowers community leadership to mobilize community action planning in order to implement evidence-based drug prevention strategies to meet the unique needs of that community risk and protective factor profile.

Action planning consists of selecting for implementation the most appropriate evidence-based drug abuse prevention strategy from a menu of potential programs. Currently, Communities That Care (Posey et al., 2000) has identified over 96 evidence-based drug prevention programs across a variety of program categories and types to include marital therapy, prenatal and infancy programs, early childhood education, parent training, family therapy, organizational change in schools, classroom management and instructional strategies, school programs for social and emotional competence, and community-based youth programs, such as after-school recreation, mentoring, youth employment, community mobilization, community policing, and community/school policies.

Another landmark event in prevention science was the establishment of the White House Office of National Drug Control Policy (ONDCP) by the Anti-Drug Abuse Act of 1988 (ONDCP, 1999a). The U.S. Congress created this office to develop and coordinate a national, comprehensive, research-based federal program to reduce drug abuse, trafficking, and related health and safety consequences. This office has the mandate to develop national drug abuse policy and program priorities, create and implement a national strategy, and coordinate federal anti-drug-abuse budgets.

In its efforts to effectively prevent and treat drug abuse and drug addiction, the Office of National Drug Control Policy has crafted a research-based policy and national strategy. According to ONDCP, the current national drug control strategy consists of five goals and related objectives that are based upon research, technology, and intelligence (ONDCP, 2001). The goals of the National Strategy are to: (1) "Educate and enable America's youth to reject illegal drugs as well as alcohol and tobacco; (2) increase the safety of America's citizens by substantially reducing drug-related crime and violence; (3) Reduce health and social costs to the public of illegal drug use by reducing the treatment gap; (4) shield America's air, land, and sea frontiers from the drug threat; and (5) break foreign and domestic drug sources of supply." (ONDCP, 2001, pp. 6–7)

To support the national strategy, ONDCP also coordinates federal anti-drug-abuse budgets. For example, according to ONDCP, total federal investments in drug abuse prevention research continued to increase from 1990 through 2000; From $127.7 million in FY1990 to 157.5 million in FY 1992 to $174.8 million in FY 1994 to $212.2 million in FY 1996 to $286.3 million in FY 1999 and to a requested amount of $294.2 million in FY 2000 (ONDCP, 1999b).

According to ONDCP the future success of the national drug abuse strategy depends upon the application of emerging research findings from basic and applied disciplines in order to improve prevention science. This includes gaining a better understanding of how to improve prevention interventions by focusing on salient genetic and environmental risk and protective factors related to drug abuse and addiction; providing communities with research-based tools to assess drug problems at the local level; translating evidence-based prevention principles to meet the needs of local communities; and, reducing the devastating effects of the linkage between drug abuse and addiction, HIV-AIDS, and hepatitis (ONDCP, 2001).

THE FUTURE DIRECTION OF DRUG ABUSE PREVENTION SCIENCE: BRIDGING NEUROBIOLOGICAL, BEHAVIORAL, AND PREVENTION SCIENCES

ONDCP's vision to broaden the future scientific base of drug abuse prevention science to include a range of basic and applied scientific disciplines has a logical appeal, yet it raises a number of important questions as to how drug abuse prevention can become a more integrated interdisciplinary science in the near future.

Several reasons justify bridging neurobiological, behavioral, and prevention sciences. While significant scientific advances have been made to identify risk and protective factors and to develop and test theory-based drug abuse prevention interventions, the majority of etiological and prevention research has neither focused upon nor sought to ameliorate through targeted preventive interventions the differences in risk and protective processes that may under lie the stages of transition from drug use to drug addiction.

For example, Glantz and Pickens (1992) hypothesized nearly 10 years ago that different factors might be associated with initial drug use onset (social and peer factors) and subsequent drug abuse behaviors (biological and psychological factors). According to these researchers drug abuse or the escalation to regular or compulsive use of illicit drugs appears to be related to several biological and psychological risk processes, such as early age of onset, frequent/intense use of drugs, family history of drug use disorders or antisocial behaviors, personality traits dealing with self-regulation (acting out, aggressivity, impulsivity, sensation seeking, etc.), and some forms of underlying psychopathology (childhood conduct disorder, antisocial behavior, hyperactivity/attention deficit disorder).

However, progress in understanding liability to substance use disorders from this perspective has proven to be elusive. Recently, in order to advance a broader array of drug abuse etiologic research that includes biological and environmental processes, NIDA launched a special research initiative to better understand the role played by the interaction between genes and environment in fostering vulnerability to drug abuse and addiction (Leshner, 1999a). This effort acknowledged that more exacting research was needed across the biopsychosocial domain given the complexity of drug abuse behaviors. It was viewed that research findings resulting from this initiative could have significant implications for the development of more effective drug abuse prevention and treatment programs.

Another reason for bridging neurobiological, behavioral, and drug abuse prevention sciences is the paucity of scientifically tested and efficacious drug abuse prevention programs targeting those youth at high risk to substance use disorders. Meta-analytic reviews of the prevention research literature (Bangert-Drowns, 1988; Tobler et al., 2000) indicate that the vast majority of promising school-based drug abuse prevention strategies for youth are universal programs rather than indicated or selective prevention programs that target high-risk populations or subpopulations already exhibiting drug use behaviors at a subclinical threshold.

A third reason for bridging neurobiological, behavioral, and prevention sciences is the need to use the resulting findings to improve the level of effectiveness of prevention programs delivered to children and adolescents. Research shows that even the most effective drug abuse prevention strategies tested to date have relatively small effect sizes, indicating that much more needs to be learned about the underlying mechanisms to substance use disorders in order to improve the efficacy of the next generation of drug abuse prevention programs (Bukoski, 1997). For example, Tobler et al.'s (2000) meta-analysis of over 207 drug abuse prevention research studies reported that the most effective type of school-based drug abuse prevention programs for youth employed interactive learning strategies that promote role-play, drug refusal activities, and interpersonal skills development. Her meta-analysis research showed that interactive drug abuse prevention programs yielded a weighted mean effect size of only 0.15 in comparison to a weighted mean effect size of approximately 0.03 for noninteractive or didactic drug abuse prevention programs.

However, related research suggests that school-based prevention interventions can be more effective if the programs target high-risk children and adolescents screened for possible subclinical problems before the manifestation of a full-blown disorder. For example, Durlak's and Well's (1998) meta-analysis of 130 research studies of indicated prevention intervention programs in mental health for children and adolescents at risk of developing a range of mental health disorders reported that behavioral and cognitive–behavioral programs yield on-average effect sizes of 0.50 and that the behavioral improvements achieved by participants in these programs exceeded 70% of the youth in the control groups.

These findings suggest that an integrated program of research across basic neurobiological, behavioral, and prevention sciences may lead to the identification of salient biological, genetic, and psychology risk factors for substance use disorders and to the development of more effective targeted drug abuse prevention interventions that demonstrate more robust effect sizes for youth in the general population and for those in subpopulations at heightened risk to substance use disorders.

One possible starting point for the discussion to bridge neurobiological, behavioral, and prevention sciences is provided by a perspective on interdisciplinary research that addresses the complex relationship between behavior and health as recently advanced in a report from the Institute of Medicine (Pellmar & Eisenberg, 2000). In that report, the scientific community recognized the complexity of drug abuse and addiction and suggested that effective problem solving requires interdisciplinary research that bridges a variety of scientific disciplines.

"The breadth of expertise needed in many fields of research—such as mental illness, drug abuse and addiction, and aging—spans many disciplines, including behavioral sciences, neuroscience, pharmacology, genetics, epidemiology, computer science, engineering, medicine, social structures, law enforcement, and the mass media. Through interdisciplinary investigations, behavior and responses to environmental conditions can be usefully linked to neurobiological process and brain structures." (Pellmar & Eisenberg, 2000, p. 19).

According to the report "interdisciplinary research" encompasses other related terms such as multidisciplinary, transdisciplinary, and translational research and represents a cooperative effort between scientists from different disciplines who have organized a program of research in order to study a challenging and complex health problem.

The report recommends that the National Institutes of Health (NIH) and the scientific community develop interdisciplinary research activities and research training programs that will bridge the behavioral and medical sciences in order to advance prevention, diagnosis, and treatment of a variety of complex diseases, and to further basic understanding of the underlying mechanisms of brain and behavior.

THE PUBLIC HEALTH MODEL AND
GENETIC EPIDEMIOLOGY

A useful paradigm for advancing interdisciplinary drug abuse prevention science is the "public health model" (Figure 1.1) that depicts the interactions between the host (individual), the environment, and the agent (drug) (Wilner, Walkley, & O'Neil, 1978).

As shown in Figure 1.1, the host includes a variety of factors or processes specific to individuals to include genetics, psychological traits, age, sex, etc. The environment includes prenatal experiences, family influences, neighborhood conditions, etc. The agent is the specific drug or drugs under investigation, such as alcohol, tobacco, marijuana.

From a prevention perspective, the public health model suggests a number of possible strategies to deter drug use onset and progression to addiction (Arnold, Kuller, & Greenlick, 1981). For example, prevention efforts could be implemented to increase individual resistance to the agent(s) through preventive interventions such as social skills training, social norms marketing, peer resistance training, or persuasive communications media campaigns. One could also promote prevention by enhancing environmental influences through enactment and enforcement of effective drug abuse policies and programs, such as those focused upon underage drinking and driving, reducing blood alcohol levels indicative of legal intoxication, effective roadside sobriety check points by law enforcement officials, enhancement of family and parent education classes, and the implementation of community watch programs. Likewise, reduction of the availability of drugs in the community could be enhanced through drug interdiction through community policing activities and law enforcement actions at national borders and internationally.

While the public health model has had a long and distinguished history, Merikangas and Avenevoli (2000) suggest that this approach is also extremely useful today to advance genetic epidemiology as a framework to look more carefully at gene–environment interactions. According to these researchers, the study of the expression of genetic influences only in the presence of specific environmental influences, i.e., gene–environment interactions, has important implications for the prevention of substance abuse disorders.

Using the methods of genetic epidemiology (controlled family studies, twin studies, adoption studies), these researchers suggest that prevention scientists could gain a better understanding

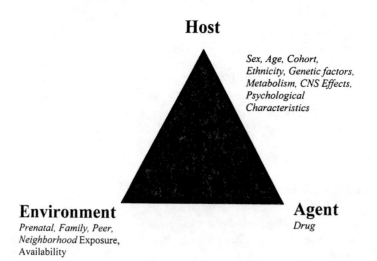

Host

*Sex, Age, Cohort,
Ethnicity, Genetic factors,
Metabolism, CNS Effects,
Psychological
Characteristics*

Environment
*Prenatal, Family, Peer,
Neighborhood* Exposure,
Availability

Agent
Drug

FIGURE 1.1. Public health model.

of how "host" characteristics under certain environmental conditions may determine individual liability to the onset of drug abuse and progression to drug addiction and dependence. For example, genetic epidemiology applied to the field of alcoholism and drug abuse has identified the key role played by having a positive family history in genetic transmission of risk of substance abuse disorders (Merikangas, Dierker, et al., 1998; Merikangas, Stolar, et al., 1998; McGue, 1994).

Results of the Yale Family Study conducted by Merikangas and Avenevoli (2000) indicate that children of adult probands with substance abuse dependence have a twofold increased rate of substance use disorders in comparison to psychiatric controls or population controls. In addition, children of adults with substance abuse dependence begin experimenting with alcohol and cannabis at an earlier age in comparison to children of parents who were in the psychiatric comparison group or normal control group.

Genetic epidemiological studies indicate that having a family history of substance abuse is a potent predictor of risk of substance abuse for children in those families. For example, research indicates a 55% "attributable risk" of substance abuse in the offspring of parents with a substance abuse disorder (Merikangas & Avenevoli, 2000).

As a result, these researchers suggest that family-based prevention interventions should be targeting the offspring of these families identified either in treatment settings or in the general population. They suggest that in time genetic epidemiological studies will lead to more effective assessments of the influence on individual vulnerability from family, community, and drug exposure on the transmission of drug abuse across multiple generations. Finally they indicate that this knowledge will lead to the future development of more effective early identification techniques and more precisely targeted prevention interventions for those at heightened risk to substance abuse.

PREVENTION RESEARCH ON GENE–ENVIRONMENT INTERACTIONS

The study of gene–environment interactions appears to have important implications for drug abuse prevention science. Research suggests that drug abuse is a complex behavior that reflects the interaction between genetics, neurobiology, learned behaviors, and environmental influences (Reiss et al., 1995). Genetic research is beginning to demonstrate that genetic expression is malleable and responsive to influences in the social environment and that future research will illuminate the mechanisms that explain how social environment may influence genetic expression of a range of behaviors such as social responsibility and how environment may directly affect behavioral outcomes (Reiss & Neiderhiser, 2000). Research tools have recently become available to study gene by environment interactions at the molecular level, such as microarray analyses, although this research methodology is still in its infancy (Sokolowski & Wahlstein, 2001).

A landmark paper by Kandel (1998) proposed a practical framework for understanding the integration of biology and psychiatry and for study of gene–environment interactions. Kandel articulated five principles to guide the blending of genetics, neurobiology, behavior, and environmental influences to include behavioral, psychopharmacology, and talk therapy employed for the prevention and treatment of mental and behavioral disorders.

Kandel (1998) provides the following five science-based principles for blending neuroscience and psychiatry and related behavioral disciplines:

1. "All mental processes, even the most complex psychological processes, derive from operations of the brain. The central tenet of this view is that what we commonly call mind is a range of functions carried out by the brain. The actions of the brain underlie not only relatively simple motor functions, such as walking and eating, but all of the complex

cognitive actions, conscious and unconscious, that we associate with specifically human behavior, such as thinking, speaking, and creating works of literature, music, and art. As a corollary, behavioral disorders that characterize psychiatric illness are disturbances of brain function, even in those cases where the causes of the disturbances are clearly environmental in origin.

2. Genes and their protein products are important determinants of the pattern of interconnection between neurons in the brain and the details of their functioning. Genes, and specifically combination of genes, therefore exert a significant control over behavior. As a corollary, one component contributing to the development of major mental illnesses is genetic.

3. Altered genes do not, by themselves, explain all of the variance of a given major mental illness. Social or developmental factors also contribute very importantly. Just as a combination of genes contribute to behavior, including social behavior, so can behavior and social factors exert actions on the brain by feeding back upon it to modify the expression of genes and thus the function of nerve cells. Learning, including learning that results in dysfunctional behavior, produces alterations in gene expression. Thus all of 'nurture' is ultimately expressed as 'nature.'

4. Alterations in gene expression induced by learning give rise to changes in patterns of neuronal connections. These changes not only contribute to the biological basis of individuality but presumably are responsible for initiating and maintaining abnormalities of behavior that are induced by social contingencies.

5. Insofar as psychotherapy or counseling is effective and produces long-term changes in behavior, it presumably does so through learning, by producing changes in gene expression that alter the strength of synaptic connections and structural changes that alter the anatomical pattern of interconnections between nerve cells of the brain. As the resolution of brain imaging increases, it should eventually permit quantitative evaluation of the outcome of psychotherapy." (pp. 6–7)

Given this framework, Kandel argues that it is important to recognize that in psychiatry (and related behavioral sciences) normal development, stressful events, life experiences, and targeted interventions such as psychotherapy or counseling through the healing words expressed by a therapist may affect processes that can trigger gene expression by altering the transcriptional regulation of genes leading to possible improvements in mental health outcomes.

As expressed in a recent National Research Council report (Singer & Ryff, 2001), the importance of environmentally induced gene expression is well researched, indicating that vulnerability and resistance to disease is dependent upon the interaction of genetic endowment and environmental influences across the life span.

For example, at the prenatal level, a mother's life experiences to include extreme stress, smoking, serious infection, drug abuse, and excessive alcohol consumption are transmitted to the fetus through several physiological signals to include endocrine functions which can result in short- and long-term changes in fetal gene expression (Roberts & Redman, 1993) and can result in fetal health difficulties such as intrauterine growth retardation (Sattar et al., 1999). The associated changes in gene expression in low-birth-weight babies with this condition leads to impaired development, elevated levels of stress hormones, increased infant's sensitivity to stress later in life, and vulnerability to later health problems such as diabetes (Ladd, Owens, & Nemcroff, 1996).

Animal research indicates that mother–child interactions within the first 2 weeks of development of rat pups can affect gene expression related to hypothalamic–pituitary–adrenal (HPA) response to stress in adult life of the rat pup (Lui et al., 1997; Plotsky & Meaney, 1993). Pups reared by mothers with high levels of licking and grooming and arched-back nursing in comparison to pups raised by mothers low in these maternal behaviors responded more effectively and with less fearfulness later in adult life to experimenter induced stress events because of better programming of genetic expression of neuroendocrine responses that resulted from maternal nurturing behaviors (Caldji et al., 1998; Francis et al., 1999).

Relevant to drug abuse in humans, True and Xian (1999) demonstrated the important interplay between genetics and environmental influences in their twin study of genetic and environmental influences on smoking and alcohol dependence. By comparing 3,356 male identical twins who share the same genes and fraternal twins who share half of the same genes, these researchers found that genetic factors explain 61% of nicotine dependence, while environment explains 39%. In the case of alcohol, these researchers found that genetic factors explain 55% of alcohol dependence, while environmental influences explain 45% of alcohol dependence.

Kendler and colleagues (1999) found in their study of female twins that genetics explain 78% of smoking initiation while environmental factors explain 22%. They also report that genetic factors explain 72% of smoking dependence and environmental factors explain 28%.

THE IMPORTANCE OF BASIC
NEUROBIOLOGICAL RESEARCH
FOR PREVENTION SCIENCE

Basic research has advanced our understanding of how genetics and environmental influences play a direct role to increase or to reduce an individual's vulnerability or liability to drugs of abuse. Major scientific discoveries in basic research focused upon neurobiology, genetics, and behavior indicate that all drugs of abuse act on normal functioning of the brain and alter thinking, emotions, and behavior (NIDA, 1999). For example, basic drug abuse research has significant implications for prevention theory by indicating that drug addiction is a chronic, compulsive, and relapsing disorder that results from the effects of drugs on brain structure and function (Leshner, 1997).

Neurobiology suggests that a variety of addictive drugs appear to act on part of the brain (nucleus accumbens, prefrontal cortex, amygdala) that regulates the effects of natural rewards such as food, sexual activity, and social interaction, and that the chronic use of drugs may hijack these reward circuits and disrupt normal functioning and our sense of pleasure and well-being (Nestler & Aghajanian, 1997; Nestler & Landsman, 2001).

This dopamine-releasing pathway within the brain may affect more than the sense of pleasure, but may more importantly affect the learning process by increasing attention to external events or stimuli which may help explain why drug consumption may continue even in the absence of the feelings of pleasure and why environmental stimuli that are associated with drug use prompt craving and possible relapse (Wickelgren, 1997).

Basic research provides critical and practical insights as to why a person may take a drug in the first place or continues to use drugs in the face of possible social and legal consequences. The key is to understand the motivation for taking drugs that could then help guide the development of more effective preventive interventions and medications. For example, Leshner (1999b) postulates that there may be two primary motives for drug abuse and addiction. The first category is sensation or novelty seeking. This category includes individuals who use drugs either to gain a sense of pleasure or to be accepted by their peers. The second category postulated by Leshner includes individuals who use drugs to self-medicate or regulate their mood in order to deal with negative feelings that may result from life's problems. The implications for prevention science seem clear.

In order to be effective, future drug interventions will need to include biological, behavioral, and social-context components (Leshner, 1997).

THE INTERACTION BETWEEN BIOLOGY AND ENVIRONMENT: IMPLICATIONS FOR ADVANCING PREVENTION SCIENCE

Prevention science is beginning to give more attention to recognizing and addressing the interaction between biology and environment. Fishbein (2000) explains that the relationship between biology and environment as related to drug abuse liability is interactive and dynamic. Research indicates that individual development along the life course results from the interplay between genetic expression and a variety of environmental processes to include environmental stimulation, social experiences, and maternal interaction (Fleming, O'Day & Kraemer, 1999; Kempermann, Kuhn & Gage, 1998; Kuhn & Schanberg, 1998; Meaney et al., 1991; Pham et al., 1997); prenatal events resulting from maternal stress or anxiety (Allen, Lewinshon, & Seeley, 1998; Glover, 1997; Kaufer et al., 1998; Lou et al., 1994; Senba & Ueyama, 1997); prenatal exposure to alcohol (Guerra, 1998), to smoking tobacco (Brook, Brook, & Whiteman, 2000; Wakschlag et al., 1997) and to the use of other drugs (Brooks-Gunn, McCarton, & Hawley, 1994; Smeriglio & Wilcox, 1999); mother–child interactions related to depression (Cicchetti et al., 1997; Goodman & Gotlib, 1999); and, maltreatment as a child or adolescent (Ito et al., 1998; Lewis, 1992).

From the perspective of prevention, Fishbein (2000) presents research to support the premise that brain functioning is now believed to be malleable and that management of the environment through appropriate behavioral interventions may decrease the liability for psychopathology and drug abuse behaviors. She suggests that prevention programs that reduce or eliminate salient adverse environmental stressors could moderate resulting neurobiological and behavioral effects.

Although prevention research has yet to establish that exposure to a drug abuse prevention intervention can directly alter related brain functioning, behavioral intervention research targeting dyslexia and employing advanced brain imaging techniques to measure the effects of the program has produced very interesting preliminary findings in support of that premise.

For example, Fletcher (2001) and Simos et al. (2002) have reported that children diagnosed as dyslexic readers in comparison to normal controls when exposed to an intensive reading program to improve decoding skills resulted in clinically significant improvements of reading scores (into the normal range) on standardized measures and dramatic changes in neural processing of the decoding task as measured by neuroimaging techniques. Using a methodology called magnetic source imaging, these researchers found that children (ranging in ages from 7 to 17 years of age) exposed to an 80-hour (2 hours per day for 8 weeks) behavioral reading intervention dramatically increased neural processing of the phonological decoding tasks from the right hemisphere to the left superior temporal region (left posterior superior temporal gyrus and the left inferior parietal region), an area of the brain that prior neuroimaging research has shown to be activated by normal subjects conducting word decoding tasks.

According to Fletcher, the study suggests that children with severe reading deficiencies can be reversed and brought up to normal levels of reading through a targeted environmental behavioral intervention as evidenced by positive changes in reading scores and brain functioning as demonstrated by neural imaging techniques. More information on this research is available on the web site for the University of Texas—Houston Health Science Center (http://www.uth.tmc.edu/clinicalneuro/dyslexia.htm).

If the future of drug abuse prevention science is toward more interdisciplinary studies that bridge neurobiological, behavioral, and prevention sciences, then what content areas need to be considered for further research?

Advancing interdisciplinary prevention science that bridges neurobiological, behavioral, and prevention sciences offers the potential to develop more effective tools to identify those in the population that are at heightened risk to substance abuse and implementation of precisely targeted interventions that would modify and forestall a probable life trajectory leading to drug use onset and progression to substance use disorders. The objective would be to develop more effective methods of early identification, screening, and referral to targeted preventive interventions that address the unique combination of genetic, biological, psychosocial, and other environmental influences that interactively determine risk liability to substance use disorders.

A variety of interdisciplinary research questions that bridge neurobiology and drug abuse prevention science could be addressed in future studies. Fishbein (2000) suggests that studies are needed to identify the neural substrates related to behavior and temperament; assess the role of environmental stress on neural substrates related to drug abuse and related psychopathologies; identify the stages of development linked to risk of drug abuse and the role played by maturation; design and test under controlled conditions preventive interventions that target critical points in development where interactions between environment and biology increase risk for substance abuse; assess how environmental influences promote the expression of genetic endowment (e.g., a family history of substance abuse) and increase subsequent liability to substance abuse; assess the psychometrics and the predictive validity of an integrated test battery that includes a combination of social, psychological, neurobiological, and genetic measures of drug abuse risk; and to create studies that explore the malleability of promising neural substrates that may be positively affected by targeted preventive interventions.

Toward this end, prevention science needs to increase its sophistication and utilization of a range of biopsychosocial measures that better assess the dynamic interactive relationship that appears to exists between the host, environment, and agent as suggested by the public health model.

For example, Fletcher's research on dyslexia suggests the potential value of employing advanced neuroimaging techniques in future laboratory-based studies of the efficacy of drug prevention strategies. One potential future drug abuse prevention intervention study might employ neuroimaging techniques to assess changes in neurological functioning that may result from exposing high sensation seekers to targeted persuasive media messages designed to increase attention, recall, and cognitive processing of anti-drug-prevention education messages.

Prevention research studies are needed in the future to include a range of neuropsychological measures (Lezak, 1995) to assess the effects of targeted drug abuse prevention interventions. For example, measures of saliva cortisol have shown to be valuable in drug use risk assessment of prepubertal boys (Moss et al., 1999) and for evaluating the efficacy of a prevention intervention for maltreated children in foster care (Fisher et al., 2000).

Deficits in executive cognitive functioning (ECF) have been associated with increased risk to substance use disorders (Giancola & Tarter, 1999). Giancola and Moss (1998) report that alcoholics, particularly those with a co-morbid diagnosis of antisocial behavior, conduct disorder, or attention deficit hyperactivity disorder, and those at high risk to alcoholism, i.e., children with a family history of alcoholism, demonstrate deficiencies on neuropsychological test batteries that assess executive cognitive function. According to these researchers, the neural substrate governing executive cognitive functioning is the prefrontal cortex with alcoholics evidencing cognitive deficiencies, e.g., long- and short-term memory, abstract reasoning, verbal skills, etc.

Laboratory-based prevention research studies are needed to study the link between substance abuse liability and deficits in ECF and to test targeted prevention interventions that may reduce, ameliorate, or prevent ECF deficiencies from increasing substance abuse liability (Fishbein, 2000).

A second area needing further research is the development of drug abuse screening measures of risk and protection that capture the richness and complexity of interactions between biology and environment. Currently, assessments of risk and protection are statistically complex in that they identify a large number of factors correlated to drug abuse across broad domains, such as culture and society, interpersonal, psychobehavioral, and biogenetic (Newcomb, 1997). Analyses involve complex statistical modeling techniques to identify possible causal pathways and mediating or moderating effects of a variety of risk and protective factors (Griffin, Botvin, et al., 2000; Griffin, Scheier, et al., 2000; Scheier et al., 1999, 2000).

While these sophisticated studies are extremely valuable for advancing our knowledge of the potential predictive value of a variety of risk and protective factors to drug abuse in a person's life history, they do not as yet provide an assessment of how certain risk processes or sets of risk processes may negatively impact an individual's health status, how a particularly risk factor may be offset or moderated by the presence of one or more protective factors to reduce overall risk of drug abuse onset and progression, or how scientific/medical knowledge of a person's risk and protection profile may be used to refer an individual to a targeted prevention intervention that best matches a person's needs and strengths.

Research is needed to better assess the potential negative (and positive) effects of the interactions between biology and environment to estimate individual risks for subsequent substance use disorders. For example, Moss et al. (1999) found that high-risk preadolescent sons (between the ages of 10 and 12) of fathers with current substance use disorder (SUD) or who were substance abusers when the child was between 3 to 6 years of age had a hyporeactive response to anticipatory stress in comparison to controls as measured by saliva cortisol. In addition, Moss reported that this lower cortisol response was associated with increased levels of monthly cigarette and marijuana use. These researchers conclude that chronic stress during childhood may be related to familial transmission of the liability to subsequent substance abuse for children of substance abusers and that hyporeactivity may indicate the underlying biological mechanism for high-risk status for substance use disorders.

The question raised is how can researchers develop drug abuse preventive interventions to address and ameliorate the risk to substance abuse for children who are characterized by lower levels of physiological arousal to life events resulting from prior stress events.

One potential line of investigation that may help to advance the application of risk and protective research may evolve from research focused upon the application of the concept of "predisease pathways" (Singer & Ryff, 2001).

Fundamental to the notion of "predisease pathways" is the concept of "allostatic load" (McEwen, 1998), which states that the many physiological systems involved in basic human homeostasis and health are challenged over the course of development by a variety of factors to include genetic endowment, adverse early life experiences, nutritional patterns, and stressful environmental conditions that produce wear and tear on the organism as it attempts to adjust and accommodate. This accumulation of physiological risk measured from all sources (biological, behavioral, environmental) across all biological systems is called allostatic load and over time could produce adverse interactions between genetic predispositions and environmental influences leading to physical disease and mental disorders.

The concept of allostatic load integrates the measurement of risk and protection across biology and environment and offers the opportunity to systematically explore "co-occurring" risk and protective processes that may prove to be common across related behavioral health disorders (substance abuse, delinquency, school failure, youth violence) and across potentially related physical disorders.

Research is needed to further the operational development and measurement of allostatic load in order to define valid and reliable interactive and developmentally relevant "predisease pathways" or health trajectories that dynamically represent the interaction of biology and environment over the life course (Singer & Ryff, 2001).

A third area in need of further research is the design and testing of targeted preventive interventions, specifically for subpopulations at risk to substance use disorders. With a better understanding of the interaction between biology and health behaviors such as substance abuse, researchers should be better able to describe the specific links between a wide range of risk and protective factors, identify subgroups within the population with the prevailing risk and protective factor profiles, and develop targeted preventive interventions to address potential predisease pathways that are appropriate across the developmental life course (Fishbein, 2000).

Using the public health model as a compass, future research is needed on targeted drug abuse prevention interventions that are multilevel and address the interactions between host, environment, and agent. Preventive interventions need to be integrated and target individuals, social settings, organizations, and communities (Singer & Ryff, 2001). Targeted prevention interventions are needed at the individual level to improve behavioral health skills and motivations, at the social level to enhance support from an individual's family, friends, or work associates, at the organization level, such as the school or workplace to increase opportunities to learn positive health behaviors in a normative setting and at the community level where health policies regarding substance abuse behaviors, e.g., drinking and driving regulations and enforcement practices, under-age drinking and smoking regulations, community policing of open-air drug markets, scheduling of substances and precursor chemicals, etc., may exert a "braking" effect on an individual's potential drug consumption behavior.

According to the National Research Council report (Singer and Ryff, 2001), there needs to be a research strategy at the National Institutes of Health (NIH) that "integrates behavioral, psychosocial, and biomedical approaches and spans multiple levels, from the individual to the societal . . . " (p. 160).

A basic question to be addressed by future drug abuse prevention intervention research is which subgroups receive the most benefit from which drug abuse prevention interventions? A working hypotheses offered by Fishbein (2000) is that the most effective preventive outcomes will result when interventions are tailor-made and matched to address individual risk levels (genetic, psychosocial, and behavioral) to drug abuse. While this type of drug abuse prevention research has yet to be developed, discussion of a prototypical example of such a research approach utilized in a related science area would be helpful.

Fisher et al. (2000) studied the impact of a prevention intervention for maltreated children to improve the child's adaptive behaviors, neuroendocrine functioning, and the child-care practices of foster parents.

The research tested the efficacy of the "Early Intervention Foster Care Program" (EFIC) to provide foster parents with parenting strategies that are consistent, nonabusive, highly reinforcing, and that lead to high levels of monitoring and supervision of the child. A goal of the intervention was to reduce parental stress when attempting to manage the behavior of their child. A second level of the intervention assisted the child through behavioral skills training to successfully adjust to their new foster care placement, particularly during the first 3 to 4 months. A third facet of the program was to assess if behavioral changes in the foster child resulting from the program produced comparable changes in the limbic–hypothalamic–pituitary adrenal axis that previous research has shown to be negatively affected by child maltreatment, thus making the child less able to adjust to stress and to regulate emotional responses. Salivary cortisol was used to measure the functioning of the neuroendocrine system.

Three groups of 10 youths each were employed in the study: youths referred to EIFC by the state's welfare system, youths referred to regular foster care, and a comparison group of nonmaltreated youth living with their own parents.

The EIFC program is a team-delivered strategy and provides to foster parents preservice training, daily telephone contacts from program staff to provide support and supervision, weekly home visits by a program staff consultant, weekly support group meetings, and a crisis intervention hotline providing round-the-clock assistance to the parent. The foster children receive direct behavioral training, counseling, and small group play therapy from a family behavioral specialist.

Over the 12 weeks of the data collection period for the study, repeated measures on parenting scales indicated that EFIC parents improved their skills to become comparable to control parents and significantly more effective than the regular foster parents group in providing consistent discipline, positive reinforcement, and monitoring. In addition, parent stress was reduced in the EFIC group, while it increased in the regular foster parents group.

Repeated measures of the behavioral adjustment of the children indicated that the number of reported problems decreased for the EFIC group and increased for the children in the regular foster parent group.

Assessment of weekly basal cortisol levels and circadian release patterns suggests exposure to the EFIC intervention reduced stress and physiological arousal over the course of the study and that these changes correlated with positive behavioral changes in the foster children.

Analyses of the circadian release patterns data suggest that unlike normal children whose cortisol levels are highest first thing in morning with a steady decline over the day, the children in the EIFC group with their history of prior maltreatment demonstrated a decrease in cortisol from waking up to midmorning and then a gradual increase in cortisol levels throughout the day. Other research indicates that this type of cortisol release may be related to sleeping disturbances and affective disorders in children and adolescence. Of interest is that after receiving the prevention intervention the circadian release pattern of the EIFC group had changed to normal when measured at the final data collection point in the study; the lowest cortisol levels were now at evening time.

SUMMARY

In summary, the field of drug abuse prevention has emerged over the past 15 years as a credible scientific discipline that has produced significant understanding of the underlying psychosocial risks and protective factors associated with drug use onset and progression to abuse. In addition, evidence from randomized controlled trials and quasi-experimental studies of theory-based drug abuse prevention interventions indicates that a growing number of drug abuse prevention programs and policies have demonstrated efficacy in reducing risks and moderating drug abuse behaviors of youths provided the programs in comparison to controls. Based upon this body of research, drug abuse prevention principles have been developed and applied in the practice community. Finally, the field of prevention science is beginning to address the important research questions associated with taking evidence-based drug abuse prevention programs and policies to scale in the prevention practice system at the state and community level.

However, numerous barriers to the continued advance of drug abuse prevention science need to be addressed and resolved. Research indicates that the vast majority of schools still use un-evaluated drug abuse prevention programs or use prevention programs that do not have strong research evidence to support their efficacy. In addition, it is clear from the research that current evidence-based drug abuse prevention programs are not targeting the youth and adolescents at high risk to drug use onset and progression to abuse. To address this problem and to substantially increase the effectiveness (effect sizes) of prevention intervention programs, it is recommended by several national research reports that a new generation of prevention interventions to address a number of behavioral health problems need to be designed and tested and that these interventions integrate our scientific knowledge across multiple disciplines to include neurobiological, behavioral, and prevention sciences. Through a better understanding of the interactions between genetic, neurobiological, and psychosocial risk and protective factors, it is proposed that more effective "targeted" prevention interventions can be developed to reach our hardest to reach groups nationwide. Several examples of how this new generation of drug abuse prevention research could be developed have been provided in this chapter to guide future thinking and planning activities.

REFERENCES

Allen, N. B., Lewinshon, P. M., & Seeley, J. R. (1998). Prenatal and perinatal influences on risk for psychopathology in childhood and adolescence. *Developmental Psychopathology, 10,* 513–529.

Arnold, C., Kuller, L., & Greenlick, M. (1981). *Advances in disease prevention.* New York: Springer.

Bangert-Drowns, R. (1988). The effects of school-based substance abuse education—A meta-analysis. *Journal of Drug Education, 18*(3), 243–264.

Brook, J. S., Brook, D. W., & Whiteman, M. (2000). The influence of maternal smoking during pregnancy on the toddlers negativity. *Archives of Pediatric and Adolescent Medicine, 154*(4), 381–385.

Brooks-Gunn, J., McCarton, C., & Hawley, T. (1994). Effects of in utero drug exposure on children's development: Review and recommendations. *Archives of Pediatric and Adolescent Medicine, 148,* 33–39.

Buchner, J. C., & Cain, A. C. (1998). Prevention science research with children, adolescents, and families: Introduction. *American Journal of Orthopsychiatry, 68*(4), 508–511.

Bukoski, W. J. (1991). A definition of drug abuse prevention research. In L. Donohew, H. E. Sypher, & W. J. Bukoski (Eds.), *Persuasive communication and drug abuse prevention* (pp. 3–21). NJ: Lawrence Erlbaum Associates.

Bukoski, W. J. (1997). *Meta-analysis of drug abuse prevention programs.* NIDA Research Monograph 170. No. 97-4146. Bethesda, MD: National Institute on Drug Abuse.

Caldji, C., Tannenbaum, B., Sharma, S., Francis, D., Plotsky, P. M., & Meaney, M. J. (1998). Maternal care during infancy regulates the development of neural systems mediating the expression of fearfulness in the rat. *Proceedings of the National Academy of Sciences, 95,* 3752–3757.

Cicchetti, D., Rogosch, F. A., Toth, S. L., & Spagnola, M. (1997). Affect, cognition, and the emergence of self-knowledge in the toddler offspring of depressed mothers. *Journal of Experimental Child Psychology, 67,* 338–362.

Coie, J. D., Watt, N. F., West, S. G., Hawkins, J. D., Asarnow, J. R., Markman, H. J., Ramey, S. L., Shure, M. B., & Long, B. (1993). The science of prevention: A conceptual framework and some directions for a national research program. *American Psychologist, 48*(10), 1013–1022.

Durlak, J. A., & Wells, A. (1998). Evaluation of indicated prevention intervention (secondary prevention) mental health programs for children and adolescents. *American Journal of Community Psychology, 26*(5), 775–802.

Fishbein, D. (2000). The importance of neurobiological research to the prevention of psychopathology. *Prevention Science, 2,* 89–106.

Fisher, P. A., Gunnar, M. R., Chamberlain, P., & Reid, J. B. (2000). Preventive intervention for maltreated preschoolers: Impact on children's behavior, neuroendrocrine activity, and foster parent functioning. *Journal of the American Academy of Child and Adolescent Psychiatry, 39*(11), 1356–1364.

Fleming, A. S., O'Day, D. H., & Kraemer, G. W. (1999). Neurobiology of mother-infant interactions: Experiences and central nervous system plasticity across development and generations. *Neuroscience Biobehavior Review, 23,* 673–685.

Fletcher, J. M. (2001). Prevention of reading disabilities. Proceedings from the 9th Annual Meeting, Society for Prevention Research. Washington, DC, May 31–June 2.

Francis, D., Diorio, J., Liu, D., & Meaney, M. J. (1999). Nongenetic Transmission across generations of maternal behavior and stress response in the rat. *Science, 286,* 1155–1158.

Garmezy, N. (1985). Stress-resistant children: The search for protective factors. In J. E. Stevenson (Ed.), *Recent research in developmental psychopathology* (pp. 213–233). *Journal of Child Psychology and Psychiatry, 4* (Book supplement).

Giancola, P. R., & Moss, H. B. (1998). Executive cognitive functioning in alcohol use disorder. In M. Galanter (Ed.), *Recent Developments in Alcoholism* (14) (pp. 227–251). New York: Plenum Press.

Giancola, P. R., & Tarter, R. E. (1999). Executive cognitive functioning and risk for substance abuse. *Psychological Science, 10*(3), 203–205.

Glantz, M. D., & Johnson, J. L. (1999). *Resilience and development—Positive life adaptations.* New York: Kluwer Academic/Plenum Publishers.

Glantz, M. D., & Pickens, R. W. (Eds., 1992). *Vulnerability to drug abuse.* Washington, DC: American Psychological Association.

Glover, V. (1997). Maternal stress or anxiety in pregnancy and emotional development of the child. *British Journal of Psychiatry, 171,* 105–106.

Goodman, S. H., & Gotlib, I. H. (1999). Risk for psychopathology in the children of depressed mothers: A developmental model for understanding mechanisms of transmission. *Psychology Review, 106,* 458–490.

Griffin, K. W., Botvin, G. J., Scheier, L. M., Diaz, T., & Miller, N. (2000b). Parenting practices as predictors of substance use, delinquency, and aggression among urban minority youth: Moderating effects of family structure and gender. *Psychology of Addictive Behaviors, 14*(2), 174–184.

Griffin, K. W., Scheier, L. M., Botvin, G. J., & Diaz, T. (2000a). Ethnic and gender differences in psychosocial risk, protection, and adolescent alcohol use. *Prevention Science, 1*(4), 199–212.

Guerra, C. (1998). Neuroanatomical and neurophysiological mechanisms involved in central nervous system dysfunctions induced by prenatal alcohol exposure. *Alcohol Clinical and Experimental Research, 22,* 304–312.

Hawkins, J. D., & Catalano, R. F. (1992). *Communities that care.* San Francisco: Jossey-Bass.

Hawkins, J. D., Catalano, R. F., & Miller, J. Y. (1992). Risk and protective factors for alcohol and other drug problems in adolescence and early adulthood: Implications for substance abuse prevention. *Psychological Bulletin, 112*(1), 64–105.

Ito, Y., Teicher, M. H., Glod, C. A., & Ackerman, E. (1998). Preliminary evidence for aberrant cortical development in abused children: A quantitative EEG study. *Journal of Neuropsychiatry and Clinical Neuroscience, 10*(3), 298–307.

Kandel, E. R. (1998). A new intellectual framework for psychiatry. *The American Journal of Psychiatry, 155*(4), 457–469.

Kaufer, D., Friedman, A., Seidman, S., & Soreq, H. (1998). Acute stress facilitates long-lasting changes in cholinergic gene expression. *Nature, 393,* 373–377.

Kempermann, G., Kuhn, H. G., & Gage, F. H. (1998). Experience-induced neurogenesis in the senescent dentate gyrus. *Journal of Neuroscience, 18*(9), 3206–3212.

Kendler, K. S., Neale, M. C., Sullivan, P., Corey, L. A., Gardner, C. O., & Prescott, C. A. (1999). A population-based twin study in women of smoking initiation and nicotine dependence. *Psychological Medicine, 29*(2), 299–308.

Kuhn, C. M., & Schanberg, S. M. (1998). Responses to maternal separation: Mechanisms and mediators. *International Journal of Developmental Neuroscience, 16,* 261–270.

Ladd, C. O., Owens, M. J., & Nemcroff, C. B. (1996). Persistent changes in corticotropin-releasing factor neural systems induced by maternal deprivation. *Endocrinology, 137*(4), 1212–1218.

Lewis, D. O. (1992). From abuse to violence: Psychophysiological consequences of maltreatment. *Journal of the American Academy of Child and Adolescent Psychiatry, 31,* 383–391.

Leshner, A. I. (1997). Addiction is a brain disease, and it matters. *Science, 278* (October 3), 45–47.

Leshner, A. I. (1999a). Institute will expand research into the interaction of genetics and environment in vulnerability to drug abuse and addiction. NIH Publication No. 99-3478. *NIDA Notes, 13*(6), 3–4, 12.

Leshner, A. I. (1999b). Science-based views of drug addiction and its treatment. *The Journal of the American Medical Association, 282* (October 13), 1314–1316.

Lezak, M. (1995). *Neuropsychological assessment.* New York: Oxford University Press.

Lou, H. C., Hansen, D., Nordenfoft, M, Pryds, O., Jensen, F., Nim, J., & Hemmingsen, R. (1994). Prenatal stressors of human life affect fetal brain development. *Developmental Medicine and Child Neurology, 36,* 826–832.

Lui, D., Diorio, J., Tannenbaum, B., Caldji, C., Francis, D., Freedman, A., Sharma, S., Pearson, D., Plotsky, P. M., & Meaney, M. J. (1997). Maternal care, hippocampal glucocorticoid receptors, and hypothalamic-pituitary-adrenal response to stress. *Science, 277,* 1659–1662.

McEwen, B. S. (1998). Protective and damaging effects of mediators of stress. *New England Journal of Medicine, 338,* 171–179.

McGue, M. (1994). Genes, environment, and the etiology of alcoholism. In R. Zucker, G. Boyd, & J. Howard (Eds.), *The development of alcohol problems: Exploring the biopsychosocial matrix* (pp. 1–39). Research Monograph No. 26. Rockville, MD: National Institute of Alcohol Abuse and Alcoholism, U.S. Department of Health, Human Services.

Meaney, M. J., Mitchell, J. B., Aitken, D. H., Bhatnagar, S, Bodnoff, S. R., Iny, L. J., & Sarrieau, A. (1991). The effects of neonatal handling on the development of the adrenocortical response to stress: Implications for neuropathology and cognitive deficits in later life. *Psychoneuroendocrinology, 16,* 85–103.

Merikangas, K. R., & Avenevoli, S. (2000). Implications of genetic epidemiology for the prevention of substance use disorders. *Addictive Behaviors, 25*(6), 807–820.

Merikangas, K. R., Dierker, L. C., & Szatmari, P. (1998). Psychopathology among offspring of parents with substance abuse and/or anxiety: A high risk study. *Journal of Child Psychology and Psychiatry and Allied Disciplines, 39,* 711–720.

Merikangas, K. R., Stolar, D. E., Stevens, D. E., Goulet, J., Preisig, M., Fenton, B., O'Malley, S., & Rounsaville, B. J. (1998). Familial transmission of substance use disorders. *Archives of General Psychiatry, 55,* 973–979.

Mihalic, S., Irwin, K., Elliot, D., Fagan, A., & Hansen, D. (2001). *Blueprints for violence prevention.* Juvenile Justice Bulletin. Washington, DC: Office of Juvenile Justice and Delinquency Prevention.

Moss, H. B., Vanyukov, M., Yao, J. K., & Kirillova, G. P. (1999). *Biological Psychiatry, 45*(10), 1293–1299.

Mrazek, P. J., & Haggerty, R. J. (1994). *Reducing risks for mental disorders.* Washington, DC: National Academy Press.

National Institute on Drug Abuse (1997). Preventing drug use among children and adolescents: A research-based guide. NIH Publication No. 97-4212. Bethesda, MD: National Institute on Drug Abuse.

National Institute on Drug Abuse (1999). *Drug abuse and addiction research: The sixth triennial report to congress from the secretary of health and human services.* Bethesda, MD: National Institute on Drug Abuse.

National Institutes of Health (1998). *Preventive intervention research at the crossroads: Contributions and opportunities from the behavioral and social sciences—Conference proceedings.* Bethesda, MD: National Institutes of Health.

Nestler, E. J., & Aghajanian, G. K. (1997). Molecular and cellular basis of addiction. *Science, 278* (October 3), 58–63.

Nestler, E. J., & Landsman, D. (2001). Learning about addiction from the genome. *Nature, 409* (February), 834–835.

Newcomb, M.D. (1997). Psychosocial predictors and consequences of drug use: A developmental perspective within a prospective study. *Journal of Addictive Disease, 16*(1), 51–89.

Office of National Drug Control Policy (1999a). *The national drug control strategy: 1999.* Washington, DC: Superintendent of Documents, U.S. Government Printing Office.

Office of National Drug Control Policy (1999b). *The national drug control strategy, 1999 budget summary.* Washington, DC: Superintendent of Documents, U.S. Government Printing Office.

Office of National Drug Control Policy (2001). *The national drug control strategy: 2001 annual report.* Washington, DC: Superintendent of Documents, U.S. Government Printing Office.

Pellmar, T. C., & Eisenberg, L. (2000). *Bridging disciplines in the brain, behavioral, and clinical sciences.* Institute of Medicine, Washington, DC: National Academy Press.

Pham, T. M., Doderstrom, S., Henriksson, B. G., & Mohammed, A. H. (1997). Effects of neonatal stimulation on later cognitive function and hippocampal nerve growth factor. *Behavioral Brain Research, 86,* 113–120.

Plotsky, P. M., & Meaney, M. J. (1993). Early, postnatal experience alters hypothalamic corticotropin-releasing factor (CRF) mRNA, median eminence CRF content and stress-induced release in adult rats. *Molecular Brain Research, 18,* 195–200.

Posey, S., Wong, S. C., Catalano, R. F., Hawkins, J. D., Dusenbury, L., & Chappell, P. J. (2000). *Communities that care prevention strategies: A research guide to what works.* Seattle, WA: Developmental Research and Programs.

Reiss, D., Hetherinton, E. M., Plomin, R., Howe, G. W., Simmens, S. J., Henderson, S. H., O'Connor, T. J., Bussell, D. A., Anderson, E. R., & Law, T. (1995). Genetic questions for environmental studies: Differential parenting and psychopathology in adolescence. *Archives of General Psychiatry, 52,* 925–936.

Reiss, D., & Neiderhiser, J. M. (2000). The interplay of genetic influences and social processes in developmental theory: Specific mechanisms are coming into view. *Development and Psychopathology, 12*(3), 357–374.

Roberts, J. M., & Redman, C. W. (1993). Pre-eclampsia: More than pregnancy-induced hypertension. *Lancet, 341,* 1447–1451.

Rutter, M. (1985). Resilience in the face of adversity: Protective factors and resistance to psychiatric disorder. *British Journal of Psychiatry, 147,* 598–611.

Sattar, N., Greer, I. A., Galloway, P. J., Packard, C. J., Shephard, J., Kelly, T., & Mathers, A. (1999). Lipid and lipoprotein concentration in pregnancies complicated by intrauterine growth restriction. *Journal of Clinical Endocrinology and Metabolism, 84,* 128–130.

Scheier, L. M., Botvin, G. J., Diaz, T., & Griffin, K. (1999). Social skills, competence, and drug refusal efficacy as predictors of adolescent alcohol use. *Journal of Drug Education, 29*(3), 251–278.

Scheier, L. M., Botvin, G. J., Griffin, K. W., & Diaz, T. (2000). Dynamic growth models of self-esteem and adolescent alcohol use. *Journal of Early Adolescence, 20*(2), 178–209.

Senba, E., & Ueyama, T. (1997). Stress-induced expression of immediate early genes in the brain and peripheral organs of the rat. *Neuroscience Research, 29,* 183–207.

Silvia, E. S., Thorne, J., & Tashjian, C. A. (1997). *School-based drug prevention programs: A longitudinal study in selected school districts.* Final report (Contract No. LC 90070001). Washington, DC: U.S. Department of Education.

Simos, P. G., Fletcher, J. M., Bergman, E., Breier, J. I., Foorman, B. R., Castillo, E. M. Davis, R. N., Fitzgerald, M., & Pananicolaou, A. C. (2002). Dyslexia-specific brain activation profile becomes normal following successful remedial training. *Neurology, 58,* 1203–1213.

Singer, B. H., & Ryff, C. D. (Eds., 2001). *New horizons in health: An integrative approach.* National Research Council, Washington, DC: National Academy Press.

Smeriglio, V. L., & Wilcox, H. C. (1999). Prenatal drug exposure and child outcome. *Clinics in Perinatology, 26*(1), 1–16.

Sokolowski, M. B., & Wahlstein, D. (2001). Gene-environment interaction and complex behavior. In H. R. Chin & S. O. Moldin (Eds.), *Methods in genomic neuroscience.* Boca Raton, FL: CRC Press.

Tobler, N. S., Roona, M. R., Ochshorn, P., Marshall, D. G., Streke, A. V., & Stackpole, K. M. (2000). School-based adolescent drug prevention programs: 1998 meta-analysis. *The Journal of Primary Prevention, 20*(4), 275–336.

True, W., & Xian, H. (1999). Common genetic vulnerability for nicotine and alcohol dependence in men. *Archives of General Psychiatry, 56*(7), 655–661.

U.S. Department of Health and Human Services (2001). *Youth violence: A report of the surgeon general.* Rockville, MD: U.S. Department of Health and Human Services.

Wakschlag, L. S., Lahey, B. B., Loeber, R., Green, S. M. Gordon, J. R., & Leventhal, B. L. (1997). Maternal smoking during pregnancy and the risk of conduct disorder in boys. *Archives of General Psychiatry, 54*(7), 670–676.

Wickelgren, I. (1997). Getting the brain's attention. *Science, 278* (October 3), 35–37.

Wilner, D., Walkley, R., & O'Neil, E. (1978). *Introduction to public health* (7th ed.), New York: MacMillan.

PART II

SOCIAL CONTEXTS OF PREVENTION

CHAPTER 2

Effective Mass Media Strategies for Drug Abuse Prevention Campaigns

PHILIP PALMGREEN

LEWIS DONOHEW

INTRODUCTION

Mass communication holds substantial promise as a tool for reaching and persuading people to adopt new and healthier lifestyles. This has long been recognized by those interested in prevention of drug abuse and in other unhealthy behaviors (Flay & Sobel, 1983; Rogers & Storey, 1987; Schilling & McAlister, 1990; Wallack, 1989). Prevention efforts, such as the National Institute on Drug Abuse's "Cocaine: The Big Lie" campaign and the Partnership for a Drug-Free America anti-drug campaign, have heavily relied on the promise. It is also reflected in the launching in 1998 of a historic $2 billion, 5-year, media-based campaign directed at reducing illicit drug use among 9- to 18-year-olds. This campaign, directed by the Office of National Drug Control Policy (ONDCP), has many facets but relies primarily on televised anti-drug public service ads (PSAs) and is by far the largest federally funded drug abuse prevention effort in history.

This strong dependence on the mass media in prevention efforts is not unusual—the mass media are the primary or leading components in a variety of public health campaigns and frequently are the only component (Backer, Rogers, & Sopory, 1992; Flay, 1987; Rice & Atkin, 1989). As Bauman et al. (1991) note, "This is the most common and practical application of mass media in public health and, unlike multiple-component approaches, is capable of ready distribution on a

PHILIP PALMGREEN AND LEWIS DONOHEW • Department of Communication, University of Kentucky, Lexington, Kentucky 40506

national level" (p. 602). At the very least, as Romer (1994) observes, "mass-media communication campaigns to alter risky behavior are seen increasingly as a critical adjunct to school-based programs and community-wide interventions" (p. 1073). To what extent is this widespread faith in the power of the media justified?

Although the early history of mass-media campaigns, particularly those involving health, was largely one of failure (Flay & Sobel, 1983; Rogers & Storey, 1987), the promise of reaching large audiences has led to continued efforts, a sharpening of design methodologies, and more realistic campaign expectations. These more sophisticated efforts, combined with more powerful evaluation methodologies, provide evidence that media health campaigns can be effective in changing beliefs, attitudes, intentions, and even behaviors, when properly designed (Backer, 1990; Perloff, 1993; Rogers & Storey, 1987).

Design elements that have contributed to successful campaigns include sophisticated audience segmentation and targeting, the use of formative research in message creation, the development of professional-quality messages that compete effectively with product ads and other features of the communication environment for the attention of the audience, the use of appropriate channels of communication, and the incorporation of more sophisticated theories of persuasion in campaign design (Backer, 1990; Perloff, 1993; Rogers & Storey, 1987). More rigorous techniques of formative, process, and summative evaluation, coupled with more powerful statistical tools, have detected a variety of campaign effects. Such research generally shows that coupling media with other kinds of interventions is more successful than either media or nonmedia efforts alone (Flora, Maibach, & Maccoby, 1989; Rogers & Storey, 1987). There is growing evidence, however, that, when used correctly, media alone can have significant positive impacts on health-related attitudes, beliefs, and behaviors (Beck et al., 1990; Flay, 1987; Flora, Maccoby, & Farquhar, 1989; Zastowny et al., 1993).

So much research has been compiled on successful public health campaigns, either media-only or media supplemented by other channels, that a series of generalizations on the most effective ways to use the media has disseminated widely through the literature for use by communication practitioners (see Backer et al., 1992; Flay, 1987; Flay & Sobel, 1983; Perloff, 1993; Rogers & Storey, 1987). This chapter highlights three of the most important principles—ones that we have found to be highly useful in our own approach to media interventions.

1. Design a campaign that will achieve widespread, frequent, and prolonged exposure to a message.

In traditional advertising terms this means that the media campaign messages must have high reach (the proportion of target audience members exposed to a message at least once) and frequency (the average number of exposures per audience member reached). These goals are much easier to state than to achieve. To accomplish them means that campaign practitioners must develop messages that can elicit high levels of attention from the target audience and disseminate the message through media channels actually used by audience members. It also means that (1) sufficient financial resources must be available to purchase adequate amounts of time or space in desired media vehicles (such as TV and radio, newspapers, magazines), or (2) considerable salesmanship and marketing skill must be used to persuade media gatekeepers to donate these precious resources in times or locations that are likely to be seen by the target audiences, or (3) a combination of both purchased and donated time and/or space should be used. More campaigns are turning to option 3, with an emphasis on purchasing, to achieve campaign goals. These include successful anti-smoking initiatives in California and Massachusetts (Hu, Sung, & Keeler, 1995; Siegel & Biener, 2000) and the ONDCP antidrug campaign. Still, paid media schedules in health campaigns are in the minority, and more research is needed to compare the effectiveness of paid versus donated schedules (Murry, Stam, & Lastovicka, 1996). One recent field experiment investigating this found no difference in effectiveness; however, the donated campaign in this study emulated the paid campaign closely, something that is rare in practice (Murry et al., 1996). The targeting advantages of paid campaigns ordinarily are substantial, so we would expect the trend toward paid media schedules to continue.

2. Use audience segmentation strategies to target messages to at-risk audiences.

This is the cornerstone of the social marketing approach. Segmentation or targeting can lead to much more efficient and effective dissemination of campaign messages to those most in need of prevention information. While demographic data can provide a rudimentary beginning, any targeting scheme should also be based on psychographic variables (such as attitudes, values, beliefs, and personality characteristics) linked both to the behavior of interest (marijuana or other substance use) and to the communication channels and message styles most preferred by target audience members (Backer et al., 1992; Slater, 1996).

3. Use formative research throughout the audience segmentation, message design, and channel selection phases.

Such research, both qualitative and quantitative, is essential in determining the relevant needs, beliefs, behaviors, and attitudes of the target audience; in designing messages to attract the attention of and persuade audience members; and in determining the media channels and vehicles most used by the audience (Atkin & Freimuth, 1989; Backer et al., 1992; Rogers & Storey, 1987). The research should involve careful pretesting of prevention message ideas at the concept stage, the "storyboard" or "rough-cut" stages, and the final production stage. Ideally, this testing should be done with members of the target audience, media professionals, and behavioral scientists knowledgeable in both the behavior of interest and theory-based approaches to message design.

Despite encouraging growth in the use of these and other principles, many important questions remain. A number of techniques have been found to be successful, for example, but little is known about the process by which media messages begin to change attitudes and behaviors. What are the causal lag periods involved? Are there more effective ways of designing and placing prevention messages? What amounts of expensive media time and space are needed to bring about the desired change? And one of the most important and vexing questions concerns the effectiveness of different channels in the media mix. Many public communications campaigns, in an effort to maximize effects, have used a variety of media simultaneously, including television, radio, newspapers, magazines, and billboards, as well as nonmedia interventions. This makes it difficult to evaluate the separate contributions of these different channels on observed changes in outcome variables.

EFFECTS OF TELEVISED PUBLIC
SERVICE ADS

The effects of television are of particular interest to those involved in drug abuse prevention because of this medium's ability to reach a variety of populations, including adolescents (Klein et al., 1993; Romer, 1994). Television is by far the most widely used means of disseminating prevention messages, usually in the form of PSAs (Backer, 1990). Understanding television's potential effects on at-risk populations, whether when used alone or in conjunction with institutional or other media channels, is vital to campaign designers; so the confounding of television's effects with those of other channels in many otherwise well-designed campaigns is unfortunate. Studies involving the use of televised anti-drug PSAs alone, on the other hand, generally suffer from mistakes in campaign execution, including violating two of the principles discussed previously: (1) lack of widespread, frequent, and prolonged exposure to messages–in several campaigns, PSAs were aired outside prime time and/or on noncommercial stations, and then only infrequently; and (2) lack of appropriate segmentation or targeting—many anti-drug PSA campaigns have been directed at nonidentifiable audience segments (Flay & Sobel, 1983).

Evaluations of such campaigns tell us little about the potential persuasive effects of well-executed PSA campaigns that use more recently developed and proven techniques. Many of these campaigns, too, have had the limited, and perhaps appropriate, primary objective of increasing knowledge levels or raising the salience of a health-related issue and have not been directly concerned with changing attitudes or behaviors. In addition, when campaigns have been correctly designed and carried out, they are not always evaluated correctly. PSA recall and campaign-issue salience have been the primary measures of effectiveness in many campaigns (especially informational ones). Simple cross-sectional post-test surveys have been used frequently. Longitudinal or panel studies often have involved simple pre- and post-test designs that fail to account for pre- and postcampaign trends in criterion variables. When such longitudinal trends, which yield potentially valuable information about change processes, have been reported, the data usually have been subjected to "eyeball" inspection rather than to appropriate statistical tests of intervention effectiveness, such as time-series analysis (Beck et al., 1990; Hammond, Freimuth, & Morrison, 1987; Krishnamurthi, Narayan, & Raj, 1986; Murry, Stam, & Lastovicka, 1993; Pierce et al., 1986, 1992; Ross & Scott, 1993; Shelley et al., 1991).

Another problem is the failure of most studies of PSA effectiveness to use control communities that are free of confounds from other mass-media efforts. A major exception is a well-controlled, 4-year longitudinal study on the prevention of cigarette smoking in adolescents that compared the impact of mass-media-plus-school interventions in two communities versus school-only interventions in two matched communities (Flynn et al., 1992, 1995). The media intervention, which took the form of four approximately 6-month-long campaigns spaced over 4 years, used a combination of television and radio spots in purchased and donated time in popular teen programming to ensure high saturation. There were significant reductions (which increased annually) in reported smoking, with related effects on smoking attitudes and beliefs, in the media-plus-school compared to the school-only communities. These reductions could be attributed directly to the addition of the PSA components, although it was not possible to distinguish between the effects of television and radio.

Despite this research, it is still an open question whether televised anti-drug PSA campaigns using more advanced principles of campaign design can go beyond well-designed and acknowledged informational or agenda-setting effects to produce significant changes in drug-related attitudes, beliefs, and ultimately behaviors. Reviews concluding that televised PSAs have effects only on knowledge or awareness are based primarily on evaluation of either information-only campaigns, campaigns that were not designed to isolate the effects of televised PSAs, or campaigns that contained flaws in execution or evaluation (Gantz, Fitzmaurice, & Yoo, 1990).

Research on the large, long-term, and well-designed Partnership for a Drug-Free America television campaign (supported by more than $3 billion in donated air time and print space since 1987) provides some evidence of such effects (Black, 1991; Zastowny et al., 1993). Published evaluations of this campaign, however, have been criticized for being based on a series of annual cross-sectional samples that used a controversial mall-intercept design for several years. No satisfactory control population exists for this national campaign. Complicating the assessment of the campaign's effects is the fact that a number of drugs (such as marijuana, cocaine, and amphetamines) were already exhibiting downward trends in use prior to the start of the campaign in 1987. Other history and maturational factors, such as media coverage of drugs, are also uncontrolled in the evaluations.

Still, areas receiving greater partnership PSA saturation have shown much larger changes in annual cross-sectional surveys (compared to less-saturated areas) in drug-related attitudes, beliefs, reported use of a variety of illicit drugs, and intentions to use such drugs (Black, 1991; Block, Morwitz, & Sen, 1996). While these latter findings should be interpreted cautiously because of their cross-sectional nature, they provide the strongest nonlaboratory evidence available that the mass media (at least televised PSAs) can successfully discourage the use of illicit drugs.

WHAT WORKS AND WHY

Despite limited empirical evidence on the effectiveness of the mass media in preventing use of illicit drugs, practitioners can take heart (and guidance) from the much larger body of research literature dealing with the impact of media-based interventions on health-related behaviors in general (Perloff, 1993; Rogers & Storey, 1987) and on the use of licit substances, such as cigarettes (Burns, 1994; Flay, 1987; Flynn et al., 1995; Hu et al., 1995; Siegel & Biener, 2000). This more general literature, as noted earlier, provides ample evidence that well-planned media campaigns can influence a wide variety of health-related attitudes, norms, and behaviors. These studies also address an issue on which the sparse media drug abuse prevention literature (with the exception of the SENTAR approach discussed in the following) is largely silent—what kinds of campaign strategies, persuasive arguments, and other message characteristics work best and why? We have already discussed three important principles for campaign design that have emerged from the public communications campaign literature. We should add, however, one very important empirical finding from this literature—that theory-based media interventions have been much more likely to be successful. Ample evidence exists of successful campaigns that used such guiding frameworks as social learning theory, diffusion of innovations, the theory of reasoned action, the health belief model, the elaboration likelihood model, and protection motivation theory (Flora et al., 1989; Maibach & Parrott, 1995; McAlister et al., 1989; Petty, Baker, & Gleicher, 1991; Rogers, 1995; Rosenstock, 1990; Schilling & McAlister, 1990; Zimmerman & Vernberg, 1994). Other theoretical perspectives, such as peer cluster theory (Oetting & Beauvais, 1987), can be drawn from school- or community-based prevention efforts.

While principles from a number of these theories have been applied, at least implicitly, in drug abuse prevention media campaigns, there has been no systematic evaluation of their relative (or combined) efficacy in such interventions. Still, their success in other health contexts strongly suggests that they can be applied effectively to drug abuse prevention. Schilling and McAlister (1990) offer a number of cogent and detailed suggestions for applying several of the more widely used theories to anti-drug campaigns. The strategic communication plan developed by Porter Novelli for the ONDCP media drug abuse prevention campaign relies heavily on principles derived from social learning theory, peer-cluster theory, and the theory of reasoned action, as well as on empirical findings from a host of media and nonmedia interventions. Evaluation of the campaign's impact will, in effect, be the first major evaluation of the explicit application of these theories in a media-based illicit-drug-abuse prevention campaign.

A SENSATION-SEEKING APPROACH TO DRUG ABUSE PREVENTION

Another theoretical approach represented in the ONDCP campaign's strategic communications plan is one we have been developing over the past 15 years at the University of Kentucky with the support of a series of grants from the National Institute on Drug Abuse. This approach is, to our knowledge, the only theory-driven approach to media-based illicit-drug-abuse prevention developed specifically for, and tested in, that important context. It revolves around sensation seeking, a particularly potent risk factor for drug use, which can be used at three critical stages in media campaign design: (1) segmenting or targeting the at-risk audience, (2) designing messages that are effective with this audience; and (3) placing these messages in program contexts that are attractive to the target audience. The result is a coherent, parsimonious, and powerful theoretical framework that guides intervention strategies from inception to delivery and meshes well with a number of other theoretical approaches to prevention.

Sensation Seeking

Sensation seeking is a personality trait associated with the need for novel, complex, ambiguous, and emotionally intense stimuli (Zuckerman, 1979, 1994). As measured by Zuckerman's sensation-seeking scale, the concept has four dimensions:

1. Thrill and Adventure Seeking: A desire to seek sensation through physically risky activities that provide unusual situations and novel experiences, such as parachuting and scuba diving.
2. Experience Seeking: A desire to seek sensation through a nonconforming lifestyle, travel, music, art, drugs, and unconventional friends.
3. Disinhibition: A desire to seek sensation through social stimulation, parties, social drinking, and a variety of sex partners.
4. Boredom Susceptibility: An aversion to boredom produced by unchanging conditions or persons and great restlessness when things are the same for any period of time.

Describing differences between high and low sensation seekers, Zuckerman (1988) has observed that:

> The high sensation seeker is receptive to novel stimuli; the low tends to reject them, preferring the more familiar and less complex. The high sensation seeker's optimal level of stimulation may depend on the levels set by the characteristic level of arousal produced by novel stimuli. Anything producing lower arousal levels may be considered 'boring.' . . . Apart from the voluntary avoidance of high intensities of stimulation, the low sensation seeker may have a type of nervous system that rejects such stimulation or inhibits cortical reactivity to high intensity stimuli. (pp. 181–182).

Sensation Seeking and Substance Use

Sensation seeking is a consistent predictor of use of a variety of drugs and earlier onset of use (Kilpatrick et al., 1976; Segal, Huba, & Singer, 1980; Zuckerman, 1979, 1983, 1994). In data from our recent study of prevention of adolescent marijuana use (Palmgreen et al., 2001), sensation seeking also correlates positively with the other five risk factors measured (deviance and lack of opportunity, and peer, family, and community use of marijuana) and negatively with all six protective factors (self-acceptance, absence of depression, quality of home life, law abidance, religiosity, perceived sanctions against marijuana use). As such, the concept of sensation seeking offers an important avenue for targeting at-risk groups and designing messages to reach them. The construct is based on psychobiological theory and has been shown to have a high heritability factor (Fulker, Eysenck, & Zuckerman, 1980; Zuckerman, 1990, 1994). It has a number of biochemical correlates, including testosterone, monoamines and their metabolites (particularly monoamine oxidase), and endorphins (Zuckerman, 1979, 1986, 1994). Research by Bardo and his colleagues (Bardo, Nieswander, & Pierce, 1989; Bardo & Mueller, 1991; Bardo, Donohew, & Harrington, 1996) strongly suggests that novelty-seeking behavior and self-administration of drugs in animals may involve a common dopamine system in the brain.

A moderate to strong association of sensation seeking with alcohol and illicit drug use has been demonstrated in a large number of studies in a variety of populations (e.g., Kilpatrick et al., 1976; Pederson, 1991; Segal et al., 1980; Zuckerman, 1979, 1994). Strong evidence has emerged in the past decade that the relationship also holds with adolescents (Barnea, Teichman, & Rahav, 1992; Clayton, Cattarello, & Walden, 1991; Huba, Newcomb, & Bentler, 1981; Newcomb & McGee, 1989; Pederson, 1991; Teichman, Barnea, & Rahav, 1989; Thombs et al., 1994), including those from different cultures (Barnea et al., 1992; Pederson, 1991; Teichman et al., 1989). In a study of junior and senior high school students in Fayette County, Kentucky, high-sensation seekers (HSS), as defined by median splits, were twice as likely as low-sensation seekers (LSS) to report use of beer and alcohol during the prior 30 days and up to 10 times as likely to report use of other drugs (Donohew, 1988, 1990). Similar patterns of HSS versus LSS differences in drug use were found among a cohort of Fayette County students measured at four timepoints from the sixth to the eighth grades as part of an evaluation of Drug Abuse Resistance Education (DARE) (Clayton et al., 1991). In addition, HSS adolescents in our most recent study (Palmgreen, et al., 2001) were up to four times as likely to exhibit past 30-day use of marijuana. Sensation seeking has been related to adolescent alcohol use in several recent studies (Huba et al., 1981; Newcomb & McGee, 1989; Pederson, 1991; Thombs et al., 1994; Webb et al., 1991); and in a cross-sectional study of 1,900 Israeli high school students, it was strongly associated with use of a number of licit and illicit drugs (Barnea et al., 1992; Teichman et al., 1989). A California study of 1,068 adolescents found moderate relationships between various sensation-seeking dimensions and a number of illicit and licit substances (Huba, et al., 1981).

In a 20-month Norwegian longitudinal study of 553 adolescents, sensation seeking was characterized by a relatively high degree of temporal stability and was a consistent and important predictor of use of cannabis, alcohol, benzodiazepine, and cigarettes (Pederson, 1991). Longitudinal studies of variables closely related to the dimensions of the sensation-seeking scale also offer strong evidence of the ability of a sensation-seeking "superfactor" to predict risk-related behaviors across long developmental time spans. A study of 1,034 boys measured at ages 6 and 10 years showed that those high on novelty seeking and low on harm avoidance at age 6 (as measured by Cloninger's personality scale) exhibited earlier onset of substance use (Masse & Tremblay, 1997). A study in New Zealand followed a cohort from age 3 ($n = 1,037$) to age 21 ($n = 961$) (Caspi et al., 1997). At age 3, study participants were rated on 22 behavioral characteristics. At age 18 they were administered the Multidimensional Personality Questionnaire (MPQ; Tellegen, 1982), and at age 21 they were measured on four different health-risk behaviors: alcohol dependence, violent crime, risky sexual behavior, and dangerous driving habits. It was found that those who exhibited each of these risky behaviors scored much lower (in comparison to those not exhibiting) on the MPQ scales of Harm Avoidance (the inverse of Thrill and Adventure Seeking), Control (roughly the inverse of Experience Seeking), and Traditionalism (in many ways the inverse of Disinhibition), and higher on Aggression (and, in some cases, on Alienation). The greatest differences on these traits were displayed by those involved in multiple risky behaviors. Moreover, those possessing this "risky personality" configuration at age 18 had displayed similar temperament qualities at age 3 (Caspi & Silva, 1995). Drawing upon other data gathered on the cohort at ages 5, 7, 9, 11, and 13 years, Caspi et al. (1997) suggest that "the origins of a personality type at risk for health-risk behaviors may be found early in life and . . . the type stabilizes during adolescence." (p. 1061).

They go on to say that, in public health interventions:

> Individual differences in personality may influence (different) steps in the persuasion process (Cacioppo, 1986). Thus, different types of individuals may attend to, comprehend, accept, and retain different types of messages. Our research shows that young adults who engage in health-risk behaviors are different psychologically from their peers. If we know the personality characteristics of a target audience, it may be possible to tailor campaigns to zero-in on the characteristic motivations, attitudes, and feelings of that audience (Plant & Plant, 1992). Knowledge of the psychological characteristics that motivate youth to engage in health-risk behaviors may thus help public health officials choose more effective campaigns that would motivate risk takers to minimize harm. (p. 1061)

Message Sensation Value and SENTAR

We have followed the path described previously in designing our own approach to drug abuse prevention—SENTAR (for SENsation-seeking TARgeting). It is well established that high-sensation seekers, including the important target group of HSS adolescents, are particularly drawn to the stimulation and/or mood-altering effects of a variety of drugs. What is especially important from a prevention perspective, however, is that they also have distinct and consistent preferences for particular kinds of messages based on their needs for the novel, the unusual, and the intense (Donohew, Lorch, & Palmgreen, 1991; Zuckerman, 1979, 1990, 1994). High-sensation seekers (usually defined as those above the median on the sensation-seeking scale) strongly prefer messages that are high in sensation value, that is, the degree to which the content and formal features of a message elicit sensory, affective, and arousal responses. These same individuals dislike messages low in sensation value; low-sensation seekers generally display the opposite pattern of message preferences. Our own extensive program of focus-group research involving HSS and LSS adolescents and young adults has confirmed that these preferences extend to televised commercials and PSAs (Donohew et al., 1991). This research shows that HSS prefer messages that have higher levels of the following attributes: (1) novel, creative, or unusual; (2) complex; (3) intense stimuli that are emotionally powerful or physically arousing; (4) graphic or explicit; (5) somewhat ambiguous; (6) unconventional; (7) fast paced; and (8) suspenseful. Of course, it is not necessary for a message to have all of these characteristics at high levels to be attractive to high-sensation seekers; but we can say with some confidence that the greater the number of these characteristics a message has, the more attractive it will be to high-sensation seekers. If any one of these characteristics is of primary importance though, it is high levels of novelty. Zuckerman (1990) has reviewed research showing that HSS "tend to give stronger physiological orienting responses than lows to novel stimuli of moderate intensity, particularly when such stimuli are of specific interest" (p. 313).

High-sensation-value messages thus may elicit more favorable evaluations and greater attention from HSS, but are they more persuasive? In one laboratory experiment we designed and produced two versions of a televised antidrug PSA—one high in sensation value (HSV) and one low in sensation value (LSV). With high-sensation-seeking young adults, the HSV message produced greater intent to call a hotline featured in each PSA than did an otherwise comparable LSV message. The opposite pattern was observed for LSS (Donohew et al., 1991; Palmgreen et al., 1991). In another experiment a perceived message sensation value scale was developed and used to classify (based on the responses of 50 subjects in a pilot study) 13 existing TV anticocaine PSAs as either HSV or LSV PSAs. The HSV PSAs were much more effective than the LSV spots with high-sensation-seeking young adults on the dependent variables of free and cued recall of message content, attitude toward cocaine, and behavioral intention to use cocaine. Low-sensation seekers displayed the opposite pattern for both free and cued recall but showed no significant HSV versus LSV difference on the attitude and behavioral intention measures (Everett & Palmgreen, 1995). The amount of variance accounted for by these interactions was high, particularly for free and cued recall.

Evidence for the persuasive impact of high-sensation-value anti-drug PSAs was also found in a field study involving an actual televised PSA campaign conducted in Lexington, Kentucky (Palmgreen et al., 1995). The campaign targeted young adults and older teens and included five PSAs developed through formative research with focus groups consisting of high-sensation seekers. The high-sensation-value spots concluded with an appeal to call a hotline for more information about exciting alternatives to drug use. The PSAs were the sole source of information about the hotline. More than 2,100 calls to the hotline were received over the course of the 5-month campaign, with 98% calling to get information for themselves (as opposed to calling to get information for friends, children, etc.). This is a relatively large number of calls from a small market and a narrowly defined target audience. More than 73% of the callers were above the population median on the sensation-seeking scale, as determined by a survey of hotline callers and by a probability survey of the general population of 18- to 25-year-olds in Lexington (the age range in which most of the callers fell). Within-campaign surveys indicated that high-sensation seekers were indeed reached frequently by the PSAs, more so than low-sensation seekers. A postcampaign probability survey also revealed the combined influence of sensation seeking and drug use on exposure to the two most-aired PSAs. Both PSAs displayed the same recall pattern, with HSS users of illicit drugs in the past 30 days displaying the highest recall certainty, followed closely by the small group of LSS users (whose use status apparently rendered the PSAs salient to them). Close behind this group were the HSS nonusers, another very important group to reach in a prevention campaign. Trailing these groups by a substantial margin (but still manifesting good recall certainty levels) was the large group of LSS nonusers, the segment least at-risk for use of illicit substances. Reported frequency of exposure was related to sensation seeking and drug use in a similar fashion.

Evidence for the impact of a SENTAR campaign on actual illicit drug use stems from a recent study (Palmgreen et al., 2001) that involved an innovative controlled interrupted time-series design to evaluate the effectiveness of televised antimarijuana PSA campaigns targeted at high-sensation-seeking adolescents in two matched cities: Lexington (Fayette County), Kentucky, and Knoxville (Knox County), Tennessee. Specifically, televised antimarijuana PSAs, designed and developed through formative research, were shown (using a combination of paid and donated time) from January through April 1997 in Lexington. Similar campaigns were conducted from January through April 1998 in both Lexington and Knoxville (see Figure 2.1). Beginning 8 months prior to the first Lexington campaign and ending 8 months after the 1998 campaigns, personal interviews (computer assisted, self-administered) were conducted with 100 randomly selected (without replacement) students in each county during each month (total $n = 6,400$). The

Fayette County	baseline $O_1 \ldots O_8$	campaign 1 $O_9 \ldots O_{12}$	post-campaign $O_{13} \ldots O_{20}$	campaign 2 $O_{21} \ldots O_{24}$	post-campaign $O_{25} \ldots O_{32}$
Knox County	baseline $O_1 \ldots O_8$	baseline $O_9 \ldots O_{12}$	baseline $O_{13} \ldots O_{20}$	campaign 1 $O_{21} \ldots O_{24}$	post-campaign $O_{25} \ldots O_{32}$

Note: O_i corresponds to the *i*th observation. Observations are separated by one month and are based on means of 100 participants each. Total $\underline{N}$ = 3,200 per county.

FIGURE 2.1. Overview of Controlled Interrupted Time-Series Design with Switching Replications.

population cohort followed was in the 7th through 10th grades initially and in the 10th grade through 9 months after high school graduation upon completion.

During the first 8 months of the study (O_1 to O_8), participants provided data on marijuana use patterns in each county prior to the first Lexington campaign. During the next 4 months, students in Fayette County were exposed to a televised anti-drug ad campaign employing high-sensation value messages developed by the research team. Data collection continued in the two counties (O_9 to O_{12}), permitting comparisons of marijuana use with and without a campaign. Data gathered over the next 8 months (O_{13} to O_{20}) established marijuana use trends after the first campaign in Lexington and extended the baseline trend in Knox County prior to that county's first campaign. During the ensuing 4 months (O_{21} to O_{24}), students in both counties were exposed to campaigns identical to the first Fayette campaign, except a few new PSAs were introduced in both counties to add novelty in Fayette. Data collection then continued (O_{24} to O_{32}) to measure postcampaign trends.

The design controlled for trends in marijuana use prior to the campaigns and allowed estimation of postcampaign trajectories. It also partially controlled for history, because any national events affecting drug use should have affected both counties. In addition, contacts with school drug prevention staff and daily monitoring of the major newspapers in each county revealed no local or regional events or prevention efforts threatening comparability.

Because the cohorts in each county aged as the study progressed, marijuana use tended to increase due to sociodevelopmental or maturational factors. However, because teens in both counties reflected this secular trend, each county served as an appropriate control for the other. Because each monthly sample was independent, sensitization, testing, and attrition were minimized. External validity was enhanced by campaign replication at different sites and times, and the design allowed both within- and between-county evaluations of campaign impact.

Full sample medians were used to separate the Knox and Fayette monthly samples into groups of high- and low-sensation seekers. Time-series regression analyses indicated that all three campaigns not only arrested but also actually reversed upward changes in 30-day marijuana use among HSS adolescents. For example, 30-day use among Knoxville HSS rose in linear fashion from 16.6% initially to 33% over the 20-month precampaign period, then fell to 24% from the start of the campaign to the completion of data gathering 12 months later. The drop in the proportion of HSS using marijuana was 26.7%. The Lexington campaign results were similar. The first campaign also reversed a strong upward trend in 30-day use among HSS. Perhaps because Lexington HSS were higher than their Knoxville counterparts on most risk factors and lower on most protective factors, the effects of the first campaign appeared to wear off about 6 months after the campaign, as indicated by the resumption of an upward trend. This trend, however, was also reversed by the second or "booster" Lexington campaign, and marijuana use continued to fall until the completion of data gathering. The time-series regression models indicated that all changes in slopes were statistically significant ($p < .003$).

Thirty-day use levels among LSS in both cities were less than one-third of HSS levels. LSS also exhibited no upward trends in use during the 32 months of the study in either community. Because of the "floor effect" of low use levels, and because LSS were not targeted by the campaign, LSS displayed no indication of campaign effects. These patterns give further emphasis to the importance of targeting high-sensation seekers with prevention messages and illustrate the strengths of an interrupted time-series design with a control community in detecting campaign effects.

PROGRAM CONTEXT.   We also applied the concept of message sensation value to the TV program context of antidrug messages. Viewers ordinarily tune in to watch programs, not commercials and PSAs. It follows that to reach high-sensation seekers at risk for drug use, PSAs should be placed, if at all possible, in programs preferred by high-sensation seekers. Our research shows that such programs have characteristics associated with high sensation value PSAs and commercials (Lorch et al., 1994). In a large laboratory experiment involving 328 young adults, we found that antidrug PSAs embedded in HSV programming received considerably higher attention levels from high-sensation seekers than did those placed in LSV programming. Exposure to the programming and ads took place with subjects placed individually in a naturalistic living room setting with various reading options available if they chose not to watch television. Results from this experiment were applied in the two campaign studies described previously by purchasing PSA time in programming preferred by HSS audience members in precampaign audience surveys. This use of HSV program contexts undoubtedly contributed to the success of these campaigns in reaching the target audience of high-sensation seekers.

Summary of SENTAR Principles

The SENTAR approach to the prevention of substance use and abuse (as well as risky sex, reckless driving, and other risk behaviors) can be summarized in the following principles.

1. *Use the sensation-seeking trait as one major segmentation variable.* While sensation seeking certainly is not the only risk factor in substance use and abuse, it is positively correlated with most other risk factors identified in the literature and is moderately to strongly related to use of a wide variety of substances. It also is longitudinally stable and predictive of drug initiation and use over long developmental time spans. While the trait should not be the only segmentation variable, it should play a major role in any psychographic/demographic or other multivariate targeting scheme.

2. *Design prevention messages high in sensation value to reach high-sensation seekers.* Designing messages that have as many high-sensation-value characteristics as possible (especially novelty) is essential to gain the attention of at-risk audience members in the highly cluttered context in which most media exposure takes place. Messages too low in sensation value are very likely to be ignored by those whom prevention practitioners would most like to reach, especially when such messages run counter to audience attitudes and behavior patterns. Breaking through the clutter is critical, and HSV messages are most likely to accomplish this and go on to effect desired changes in attitudes, beliefs, and behaviors.

3. *Use formative research with high- (and sometimes low-) sensation-seeking members of the target audience.* Such research is invaluable in determining the informational, social, and other needs of the target audience regarding the behavior of interest, in designing effective messages, and in choosing appropriate media channels and program contexts. Such research at the message-design stage is especially important since there are many ways to blend HSV message characteristics in novel and effective (or ineffective) ways. The SENTAR approach offers no rigid prescriptions for message design, but rather is an overarching theoretical framework in which there is much room for creative talent to operate. Such freedom is essential if one is to succeed at the task of constantly generating novel messages for an easily bored or habituated audience.

4. *Place prevention messages in high-sensation-value contexts.* The most elegant message consigned to a media channel or program context that no one in the target audience pays attention to is like the beautiful hemlock falling in the forest—except that in a prevention campaign it clearly makes no sound of consequence, nor is anyone there to appreciate its

beauty. Social marketers, of course, have long been aware of this important but often over-looked maxim. Our research, however, has identified clear differences in the TV channel and program preferences of high- and low-sensation seekers, based on the presence or absence of HSV attributes. Because this research also indicates that HSS older teens and young adults watch considerably less television than do LSS (as much as 45 minutes less per day), information about HSS program preferences obtained through audience surveys prior to (and during) a campaign provides valuable guidance for placement decisions. Such HSS versus LSS media consumption differences probably also extend to media channels other than television, although research has not addressed this issue.

Sensation seeking, then, can be extremely useful in drug abuse prevention campaigns from the social-marketing perspective of audience segmentation. As Slater (1996) observed in a highly sophisticated treatment of health-audience segmentation, "It is essential that segments be predictive of the targeted behavior—if there is no association between segment membership and the behavior of interest, the segment will have little or no value to the campaign designer or health educator." (p. 272). But "to better guide channel selection and intervention decisions, the segments should also be predictive of distinctive patterns of media use or reliance on different organizational, community, or interpersonal channels." (Slater, 1996, p. 272). In other words, the ideal segmentation variable should also predict use of communication channels through which the target audience might be reached. We would add one more provision: that it also specify the characteristics of messages most preferred by target audience members. Most risk and protective factors associated with drug use can satisfy criterion No. 1— they singly or multiply predict use of a variety of illicit substances. Most, however, can provide little theoretical guidance in fulfilling criterion No. 2—use of communication channels (although formative research can describe the channels used by those high or low on a particular factor). And almost none can also meet the third criterion of specifying characteristics of effective messages. Sensation seeking, on the other hand, satisfies all three criteria defining an ideal segmentation variable for drug abuse prevention. Moreover, the SENTAR approach provides both a theoretical basis and empirical evidence for the connections between sensation seeking and each segmentation criterion.

The Flexibility of SENTAR

The SENTAR approach to media drug abuse prevention does not compete with other successful theoretically based approaches, such as social cognitive theory, the theory of reasoned action, or peer cluster theory. Rather, it can and should be used in conjunction with one or more of these established approaches. For example, the televised PSAs we developed for our recent anti-marijuana campaign study primarily follow a theory of reasoned action approach in presenting a number of negatively valued social, physical, and aspirational consequences of adolescent marijuana use. Certain positively valued consequences of nonuse also portrayed, particularly by drawing upon principles from social-learning and peer cluster theories. One PSA, which used principles from all three theories, shows a group of five White and African-American teenage girls interacting socially in a family room with a television on in the background. On the screen is a white male authority figure ranting (in "Reefer Madness" style) about the evils of marijuana. One girl, in exasperation, clicks off the television with the remote and says, "Are they still trying to feed us that junk about weed?" She then proceeds to roll a joint. One of her friends replies, "Maybe you need to listen, girl. Maybe you won't become an addict on the streets; but like my cousin Derek, he sure got hung up on it." She goes on to say that "you can stop caring about things—like school, like your friends." Another friend chimes in with "and girls let me tell ya—it can sure mess up your lungs." This is followed by a pregnant pause in which the first girl stops rolling the joint, then huffs, "Well, I can see I'm in the wrong place," and gets up and leaves the room. During a closing message board containing the words, "When you know more about marijuana, you learn not to use it," we hear a buzz of conversation from the remaining members of the group, unintelligible except for "She's headed for a whole lot of trouble."

This spot combines theory of reasoned action and peer cluster theory perspectives by presenting certain negatively valued consequences, such as physical and psychological dependence, loss of focus on schoolwork, and the social consequences of coming under fire from your peer group (including social isolation). Social learning theory is incorporated as the members of the group model ways in which to argue against marijuana use with peers. From a SENTAR perspective, the PSA also contributes novelty and creativity (through the bizarre and attention-getting "Reefer Madness" harangue by the authority figure on the TV screen, the rarely portrayed frank peer-group discussion of marijuana, and unusual camera angles and movement); drama (in the realistic "slice-of-life" social interaction); complexity (there is a great deal going on visually and auditorily in the room); ambiguity/suspense (concerning what action the girl rolling the joint will take at the end of the PSA, after the suspenseful pause); and stimulus intensity (through amplified natural sounds from the room—dropped remote control striking the coffee table, the rustle of paper as the joint is rolled, and other distinctive sounds—in the absence of a music track).

As this spot shows, incorporating HSV characteristics into a prevention message often has more to do with how message arguments are presented rather than with the content of the persuasive elements themselves (although content can also be involved, as in depicting graphic physical consequences of heroin use). The important principle here is that the drug prevention practitioner should use those theoretical schemes deemed most appropriate and effective for a particular audience when developing persuasive messages, but should target the messages at high-sensation seekers using the principles we have described. In other words, we should pay attention to the communication needs of our audiences, particularly when those needs are tied so closely to the behaviors we wish to prevent.

Extensions to Nonmedia Settings

Although our primary focus here is on media campaigns, the flexibility of the SENTAR approach allows it to be extended to nonmedia settings as well, such as school-based prevention programs or to multiple-modality interventions involving media, school, and community channels. It may be extended as well to risky behaviors other than drug use. An example is provided by a SENTAR school-based intervention project directed at HIV prevention and alcohol abuse among adolescents, currently being conducted in two midwestern cities with funding from the National Institute on Alcohol Abuse and Alcoholism. This study draws on theory and data from our media research on sensation seeking and message design to adapt a nationally respected classroom-based curriculum, Reducing the Risk, to make it more appealing to higher sensation seekers and impulsive decision makers.

Although the content of the curriculum was left essentially unchanged, its format was altered to add trigger films to enhance interest in topics for discussion. Talk-show formats were used for other discussions, with video cameras placed in the hands of student participants and proceedings videotaped and played back for further discussion. Contests were held for best role-plays, and small prizes were awarded. The intervention also included greater participation in instruction by group leaders chosen from the classroom and trained for their roles and training of teachers for the revised format of classroom instruction. All programs used formative research in their development, with focus and reaction groups chosen from students similar to those in the intervention classes participating in development and testing of the classroom programs. In one of the cities, a radio campaign was developed following SENTAR principles and used to prime audiences for the classroom instruction. The radio campaign used paid and unpaid spots placed in programs popular with high sensation seekers. Results showed significantly greater gains in knowledge and on a number of the efficacy variables and significantly lower onset of sexual activity among members of the primary target group (high-sensation seekers) receiving the curriculum than in groups receiving other or no organized curricula.

This offers further evidence that it is vital in any prevention intervention aimed at risky behaviors to pay close attention to the sensation-related communication needs and preferences of the target population, no matter what delivery channels are used. The design of the HIV study also illustrates how a prevention framework based on these sensation needs can be used to integrate both media and nonmedia strategies in a theoretically coherent fashion. Such coherence, rarely achieved in prevention practice, is greatly facilitated on one very important level by following the approaches we have recommended in this chapter.

REFERENCES

Atkin, C. K., & Freimuth, V. (1989). Formative evaluation research in campaign design. In R. E. Rice & C. K. Atkin (Eds.), *Public communication campaigns* (pp. 131–150). Newberry Park, CA: Sage.

Backer, T. E. (1990). Comparative synthesis of mass media health behavior campaigns. *Knowledge: Creation, Diffusion, Utilization, 11*(3), 315–329.

Backer, T. E., Rogers, E. M., & Sopory, P. (1992). *Designing health communication campaigns: What works?* Newbury Park, CA: Sage.

Bardo, M. T., Donohew, R. L., & Harrington, N. G., (1996). Psychobiology of novelty seeking and drug seeking behavior. *Behavioural Brain Research, 77,* 23–43.

Bardo, M. T., & Mueller, C. W. (1991). Sensation seeking and drug abuse prevention from a biological perspective. In L. Donohew, H. E. Sypher, & W. J. Bukoski (Eds.), *Persuasive communication and drug abuse prevention* (pp. 209–226). Hillsdale, NJ: Lawrence Erlbaum.

Bardo, M. T., Nieswander, J. L., & Pierce, R. C. (1989). Novelty-induced place preference behavior in rats: Effects of opiate and dopaminergic drugs. *Pharmacology, Biochemistry, and Behavior, 32,* 683–689.

Barnea, Z., Teichman, M., & Rahav, G. (1992). Personality, cognitive, and interpersonal factors in adolescent substance use: A longitudinal test of an integrative model. *Journal of Youth and Adolescence, 21*(2), 187–201.

Bauman, K. E., LaPrelle, J., Brown, J. D., Koch, G. C., & Padgett, C. A. (1991). The influence of three mass media campaigns on variables related to adolescent cigarette smoking: Results of a field experiment. *American Journal of Public Health, 81*(5), 597–604.

Beck, E. J., Donegan, C., Kenny, C., Cohen, C. S., Moss, V., Terry, P., Underhill, G S., Jefferies, D. J., Pinching, A. J., Miller, D. L., Harris, J. R. W., & Cunningham, D. G. (1990). Update on HIV-testing at a London sexually transmitted disease clinic: Long-term impact of the AIDS media campaigns. *Genitourinary Medicine, 66,* 142–147.

Black, G. S. (1991). Changing attitudes toward drug use: The effects of advertising. In L. Donohew, H. E. Sypher, & W. J. Bukoski (Eds.), *Persuasive communication and drug abuse prevention* (pp. 157–191). Hillsdale, NJ: Lawrence Erlbaum.

Block, L. G., Morwitz, V. G., & Sen, S. K. (1996). Does anti-drug advertising work? *Proceedings of the marketing and public policy conference,* Washington, DC.

Burns, D. M. (1994). Use of media in tobacco control programs. *American Journal of Preventive Medicine, 10*(Suppl. 1), 3–7.

Cacioppo, J. T., Petty, R. E., Kao, C. F., & Rodriguez, R. (1986). Central and peripheral routes to persuasion: An individual difference perspective. *Journal of personality and social psychology, 51,* 1032–1043.

Caspi, A., Dickson, D., Dickson, N., Harrington, H., Langley, J., Moffitt, T. E., & Silva, P. A. (1997). Personality differences predict health-risk behaviors in young adulthood: Evidence from a longitudinal study. *Journal of Personality and Social Psychology, 73,* 1052–1063.

Caspi, A., & Silva, P. A. (1995). Temperamental qualities at age 3 predict personality traits in young adulthood: Longitudinal evidence from a birth cohort. *Child Development, 66,* 486–498.

Clayton, R. R., Cattarello, A., & Walden, K. P. (1991). Sensation seeking as a potential mediating variable for school-based prevention intervention: A two-year follow-up of DARE. *Health Communication, 3*(4), 229–239.

Donohew, L. (1988). *Effects of drug abuse message styles: Final report.* (Grant DA03462). Rockville, MD: National Institute on Drug Abuse.

Donohew, L. (1990). Public health campaigns: Individual message strategies and a model. In E. B. Ray & L. Donohew (Eds.), *Communication and health: Systems and applications.* Hillsdale, NJ: Lawrence Erlbaum.

Donohew, L., Lorch, E. P., & Palmgreen, P. (1991). Sensation seeking and targeting of televised anti-drug PSAS. In L. Donohew, H. E. Sypher, & W. J. Bukoski (Eds.), *Persuasive communication and drug abuse prevention* (pp. 209–226). Hillsdale, NJ: Lawrence Erlbaum.

Everett, M. W., & Palmgreen, P. (1995). Influences of sensation seeking, message sensation value, and program context on effectiveness of anticocaine public service announcements. *Health Communication, 1,* 225–248.

Flay, B. R. (1987). Mass media and smoking cessation: A critical review. *American Journal of Public Health, 77*(2), 153–160.

Flay, B. R., & Sobel, J. L. (1983). The role of mass media in preventing adolescent substance abuse. NIDA Research Monograph 47. In T. J. Glynn, C. G. Leukefeld, & J. P. Ludford (Eds.), *Preventing adolescent drug abuse: Intervention strategies* (pp. 5–35). Rockville, MD: National Institute on Drug Abuse.

Flora, J. A., Maccoby, N., & Farquhar, J. W. (1989). Communication campaigns to prevent cardiovascular disease: The Stanford community studies. In R. E. Rice & C. K. Atkins (Eds.), *Public communication campaigns* (pp. 233–252). Newbury Park, CA: Sage.

Flora, J. A., Maibach, E. W., & Maccoby, N. (1989). The role of media across four levels of health promotion intervention. *Annual Review of Public Health, 10,* 181–201.

Flynn, B. S., Worden, J. K., Secker-Walker, R. H., Badger, M. S., Geller, B. M., & Costanza, M. C. (1992). Prevention of cigarette smoking through mass media intervention and school programs. *American Journal of Public Health, 82*(6), 827–834.

Flynn, B. S., Worden, J. K., Secker-Walker, R. H., Badger, G. J., & Geller, B. M. (1995). Cigarette smoking prevention effects of mass media and school interventions targeted to gender and age groups. *Journal of Health Education, 26,* 45–51.

Fulker, D. W., Eysenck, H. J., & Zuckerman, M. (1980). A genetic and environmental analysis of sensation seeking. *Journal of Research on Personality, 14,* 261–281.

Gantz, W., Fitzmaurice, M., & Yoo, E. (1990). Seat belt campaigns and buckling up: Do the media make a difference? *Health Communication, 2,* 1–12.

Hammond, S. L., Freimuth, V. S., & Morrison, W. (1987). The gatekeeping funnel: Tracking a major PSA campaign from distribution through gatekeepers to target audience. *Health Education Quarterly, 14*(2), 153–166.

Hu, T., Sung, H., & Keeler, T. E. (1995). Reducing cigarette consumption in California: Tobacco taxes vs. an anti-smoking media campaign. *American Journal of Public Health, 85,* 1218–1222.

Huba, G. J., Newcomb, M. D., & Bentler, P. M. (1981). Comparison of canonical correlation and interbattery factor analysis on sensation seeking and drug use domains. *Applied Psychological Measurement, 5,* 291–306.

Kilpatrick, D. G., Sutker, P. B., & Smith, A. D. (1976). Deviant drug and alcohol use: The role of anxiety, sensation seeking, and other personality variables. In M. Zuckerman & C. D. Spielberger (Eds.), *Emotions and anxiety: New concepts, methods, and applications* (pp. 247–278). Hillsdale, NJ: Lawrence Erlbaum.

Klein, J. D., Brown, J. D., Walsh-Childers, K., Oliveri, J., Porter, C., & Dykers, C. (1993). Adolescents' risky behavior and mass media use. *Pediatrics, 92*(1), 24–31.

Krishnamurthi, L., Narayan, J., & Raj, S. P. (1986). Intervention analysis of a field experiment to assess the buildup effect of advertising. *Journal of Marketing Research, 23,* 337–45.

Lorch, E. P., Palmgreen, P., Donohew, L., Helm, D., Baer, S. A., & Dsilva, M. U. (1994). Program context, sensation seeking, and attention to televised anti-drug public service announcements. *Human Communication Research, 20*(3), 390–412.

Maibach, E., & Parrott, R. L. (1995). *Designing health messages: Approaches from communication theory and public health practice.* Thousand Oaks, CA: Sage.

Masse, L. C., & Tremblay, R. E. (1997). Behavior of boys in kindergarten and the onset of substance abuse during adolescence. *Archives of General Psychiatry, 54,* 62–68.

McAlister, A., Ramirez, A. G., Galavotti, C., & Gallion, K. J. (1989). Anti-smoking campaigns: Progress in the application of social learning theory. In R. E. Rice & C. K. Atkin (Eds.), *Public communication campaigns* (pp. 291–307), Newbury Park, CA: Sage.

Murry, J. P., Jr., Stam, A., & Lastovicka, J. L. (1993). Evaluating an anti-drinking and driving advertising campaign with a sample survey and time series intervention analysis. *Journal of the American Statistical Association, 88,* 50–56.

Murry, J. P., Jr., Stam A., & Lastovicka, J. L. (1996). Paid-versus donated-media strategies for public service announcement campaigns. *Public Opinion Quarterly, 60,* 1–29.

Newcomb, M. D., & McGee, L. (1989). Adolescent alcohol use and other delinquent behaviors. *Criminal Justice and Behavior, 16*(3), 345–369.

Oetting, E. R., & Beauvais, R. (1987). Peer cluster theory, socialization characteristics, and adolescent drug use: A path analysis. *Journal of Consulting Psychology, 34,* 205–213.

Palmgreen, P., Donohew, L., Lorch, E. P., Hoyle, R. H., & Stephenson, M. T. (2001). Television campaigns and adolescent marijuana use: Tests of sensation seeking targeting. *American Journal of Public Health, 91,* 292–296.

Palmgreen, P., Donohew, L., Lorch, E. P., Rogus, M., Helm, D., & Grant N. (1991). Sensation seeking, message sensation value, and drug use as mediators of PSA effectiveness. *Health Communication, 3*(4), 217–227.

Palmgreen, P., Lorch, E. P., Donohew, R. L., Harrington, N. G., Dsilva, M., & Helm, D. (1995). Reaching at-risk populations in a mass media drug abuse prevention campaign: Sensation seeking as a targeting variable. Co-published simultaneously in *Drugs and Society, 8,* 29–45, and in C. G. Leukefeld & R. R. Clayton (Eds.), *Prevention practice in substance abuse* (pp. 29–45). Binghamton, NY: The Haworth Press.

Pedersen, W. (1991). Mental health, sensation seeking and drug use patterns: A longitudinal study. *British Journal of Addiction, 86,* 195–204.

Perloff, R. M. (1993). *The dynamics of persuasion.* Hillsdale, NJ: Lawrence Erlbaum.

Petty, R. E., Baker, S. M., & Gleicher, F. (1991). Attitudes and drug abuse prevention: Implications of the elaboration likelihood model of persuasion. In L. Donohew, H. E. Sypher, and W. J. Bukoski (Eds.), *Persuasive Communication and Drug Abuse Prevention* (pp. 71–90). Hillsdale, NJ: Lawrence Erlbaum.

Pierce, J. P., Anderson, D. M., Romano, R. M., Meissner, H. I., & Odenkirchen, J. C. (1992). Promoting smoking cessation in the United States: Effect of public service announcements on the cancer information service telephone line. *Journal of the National Cancer Institute, 84*(9), 677–683.

Pierce, J. P., Dwyer, T., Frape, G., Chapman, S., Chamberlain, A., & Burke, N. (1986). Evaluation of the Sydney "Quit for Life" anti-smoking campaign. *The Medical Journal of Australia, 144,* 341–347.

Plant, M., & Plant, M. X. (1992). *Risk-takers: Alcohol, drugs, sex and youth.* London: Tavistock/Routledge.

Rice, R. E., & Atkin, C. K. (Eds., 1989). *Public communication campaigns* (2nd ed.) Newbury Park, CA: Sage.

Rogers, E. M. (1995). *Diffusion of innovations.* New York: Free Press.

Rogers, E. M., & Storey, J. D. (1987). Communication campaigns. In C. R. Berger & S. H. Chaffee (Eds.), *Handbook of communication science* (pp. 817–846). Newbury Park, CA: Sage.

Romer, D. (1994). Using mass media to reduce adolescent involvement in drug trafficking. *Pediatrics, 93,* 1073–1077.

Rosenstock, I. M. (1990). The health belief model: Explaining health behavior through expectancies. In K. Glanz, F. M. Lewis, & B. K. Rimer (Eds.), *Health behavior and health education: Theory, research, and practice* (pp. 39–62). San Francisco: Jossey-Bass.

Ross, J. D. C., & Scott, G. R. (1993). The association between HIV media campaigns and number of patients coming forward for HIV antibody testing. *Genitourinary Medicine, 69,* 193–195.

Schilling, R. F., & McAlister, A. L. (1990). Preventing drug use in adolescents through media interventions. *Journal of Consulting and Clinical Psychology, 58,* 416–424.

Segal, B., Huba, G. J., & Singer, J. L. (1980). *Drugs, daydreaming, and personality: A study of college youth.* Hillsdale, NJ: Lawrence Erlbaum.

Shelley, J. M., Irwig, L. M., Simpson, J. M., & Macaskill, P. (1991). Evaluation of a mass-media-led campaign to increase Pap smear screening. *Health Education Research, 6*(3), 267–277.

Siegel, M., & Biener, L. (2000). The impact of an antismoking media campaign on progression to established smoking: Results of a longitudinal youth study. *American Journal of Public Health, 90*(3), 380–86.

Slater, M. D. (1996). Theory and method in health audience segmentation. *Journal of Health Communication, 1,* 267–283.

Teichman, M., Barnea, Z., & Rahav, G. (1989). Sensation seeking, state and trait anxiety, and depressive mood in adolescent substance users. *The International Journal of the Addictions, 24*(2), 87–99.

Tellegen, A. (1982). *Brief manual for the Multidimensional Personality Questionnaire.* University of Minnesota.

Thombs, D. L., Beck, K. H., Mahoney, C. A., Bromley, M. D., & Bezon, K. M. (1994). Social context, sensation seeking, and teen-age alcohol abuse. *Journal of School Health, 64,* 73–79.

Wallack, L. (1989). Mass communication and health promotion: A critical perspective. In R. E. Rice & C. K. Atkin (Eds.), *Public communications campaigns* (pp. 353–367). Newbury Park, CA: Sage.

Webb, J. A., Baer, P. E., McLaughlin, R. J., McKelvey, R. S., & Caid, C. D. (1991). Risk factors and their relation to initiation of alcohol use among early adolescents. *Journal of the American Academy of Child and Adolescent Psychiatry, 30*(4), 563–568.

Zastowny, T. R., Adams, E. H., Black, G. S., Lawton, K. B., & Wilder, A. L. (1993). Sociodemographic and attitudinal correlates of alcohol and other drug use among children and adolescents: Analysis of a large-scale attitude tracking study. *Journal of Psychoactive Drugs, 25*(3), 223–237.

Zimmerman, R. S., & Vernberg, D. (1994). Models of preventive health behavior: Comparison, critique, and meta-analysis. *Advances in Medical Sociology, 4,* 45–67.

Zuckerman, M. (1979). *Sensation seeking: Beyond the optimal level of arousal.* Hillsdale, NJ: Lawrence Erlbaum.

Zuckerman, M. (Ed., 1983). *Biological bases of sensation seeking, impulsivity, and anxiety.* Hillsdale, NJ: Lawrence Erlbaum.

Zuckerman, M. (1986). *Sensation seeking and the endogenous deficit theory of drug abuse.* Monograph 74 NIDA Research Monograph Series (pp. 59–70). Rockville, MD: National Institute on Drug Abuse.

Zuckerman, M. (1988). Behavior and biology: research in sensation seeking and reactions to the media. In L. Donohew, H. Sypher, & T. Higgins (Eds.), *Communication, social cognition, and affect* (pp. 173–194). Hillsdale, NJ: Lawrence Erlbaum.

Zuckerman, M. (1990). The psychobiology of sensation seeking. *Journal of Personality, 58*(1), 313–345.

Zuckerman, M. (1994). *Behavioral expression and biosocial bases of sensation seeking.* New York: Cambridge University Press.

CHAPTER 3

Drug Abuse Prevention Curricula in Schools

GILBERT J. BOTVIN
KENNETH W. GRIFFIN

INTRODUCTION

Schools are the focus of most attempts to develop effective approaches to drug abuse prevention. In addition to their traditional educational mission, schools often assume responsibility for addressing a variety of social and health problems, such as health education that targets tobacco, alcohol, and drug abuse, as well as teenage pregnancy and AIDS. Although there is some debate about whether schools should provide such programming, particularly with renewed concerns about academic standards, schools offer the most efficient access to large numbers of children and adolescents. Moreover, many educators now recognize that certain problems, such as drug abuse, are a significant barrier to the achievement of educational objectives. The U.S. Department of Education, for example, has included "drug-free schools" as one of its goals for improving the quality of education.

The first school-based approaches to drug abuse prevention were based on intuitive notions of how to prevent drug abuse. They included information dissemination, affective education, and alternatives programming. More recent approaches to prevention are grounded in psychological theories of human behavior and include social resistance skills training and competence-enhancement approaches. This chapter will first describe the traditional prevention approaches and then the newer psychosocial approaches. Finally, it will look at important issues regarding the development, implementation, evaluation, and dissemination of school-based drug abuse

GILBERT J. BOTVIN AND KENNETH W. GRIFFIN • Institute for Prevention Research, Weill Medical College of Cornell University, New York, New York 10021

TABLE 3.1. Overview of Major Prevention Approaches

Approach	Focus	Methods
Information dissemination	Increase knowledge of drugs and consequences of use; promote anti-drug use attitudes	Didactic instruction, discussion, audio/video presentations, displays of substances, posters, pamphlets, school assembly programs
Affective education	Increase self-esteem, responsible decision making, interpersonal growth; generally includes little or no information about drugs	Didactic instruction, discussion, experiential activities, group problem-solving exercises
Alternatives	Increase self-esteem, self-reliance; provide viable alternatives to drug use; reduce boredom and sense of alienation	Organization of youth centers, recreational activities; participation in community service projects; vocational training
Social resistance skills	Increase awareness of social influence to smoke, drink, or use drugs; develop skills for resisting substance use influences; increase knowledge of immediate negative consequences; establish non-substance-use norms	Class discussion; resistance skills training; behavioral rehearsal; extended practice via behavioral "homework"; use of same-age or older peer leaders
Competence enhancement	Increase decision making, personal behavior change, anxiety reduction, communication, social and assertive skills; application of generic skills to resist substance use influences	Class discussion; cognitive–behavioral skills training (instruction, demonstration, practice, feedback, reinforcement)

prevention programs. Table 3.1 summarizes the focus and methods of each major type of prevention approach. Tables 3.2 through 3.5 review research evidence on the effectiveness of each approach.

TRADITIONAL PREVENTION APPROACHES

Information Dissemination and Fear Arousal

Providing students with factual information about drugs and drug abuse is the most common approach to prevention. Typically, students are taught about the dangers of tobacco, alcohol, or drug use in terms of the adverse health, social, and legal consequences. Information programs also define various patterns of drug use, the pharmacology of drugs, and the process of becoming a drug abuser. Many of these programs describe the pros and cons of drug use or have students participate in debates in order to lead them to conclude that they should not use drugs. Some programs have police officers come into the classroom and discuss law enforcement issues, including drug-related crime and penalties for buying or possessing illegal drugs. Others use doctors or other health professionals to talk about the adverse health effects of using drugs or invite former drug addicts into the classroom to discuss the problems they encountered as the result of drug abuse. More recently, there has been an emphasis on using same-age or older peers to discuss drug abuse.

TABLE 3.2. Selected Studies Testing Informational Approaches[a]

Investigator(s)	Participants	Intervention approach	Evaluation design	Results
Degnan (1972)	9th-grade students	10 weeks, information based	Pre–post	No significant attitude changes
O'Rourke & Barr (1974)	High school students	6-month course using NY state curriculum guide	Post-test only	Significant attitude changes for males only
Rosenblitt & Nagey (1973)	7th-grade students	Six 45-min sessions; information based presented as reasons for use and nonuse	Pre–post; no control group	Increased knowledge; trend toward increased usage of alcohol and tobacco

[a] Adapted from Kinder, Pape, & Walfish (1980).

Programs that rely exclusively on providing students with facts about drugs and drug abuse are based conceptually on a cognitive model of drug use and abuse. This model assumes that people make a more or less rational decision to either use or not use drugs and that those who use drugs do so because they are unaware of the adverse consequences of drug abuse. From this perspective, the solution to the problem of drug abuse is to educate students about the negative consequences of drug abuse and increase their knowledge about drugs and drug abuse. Frequently, in an effort to present information in a fair and balanced way, both positive and negative information about drug use is provided. The danger in this, of course, is that the reasons for not using drugs may not necessarily be seen by all students as outweighing the reasons for using drugs. In fact, some studies suggest that informational approaches may lead to increased drug use because they can stimulate curiosity (Stuart, 1974; Swisher et al., 1971). Table 3.2 summarizes a representative sample of studies evaluating traditional information–dissemination approaches.

In an effort to dramatize the dangers of using drugs, some programs also use fear-arousal techniques designed to scare individuals into not using drugs. The underlying assumption is that evoking fear is more effective than a simple exposition of facts. These approaches go beyond a balanced and dispassionate presentation of information and provide a clear and unambiguous message that using drugs is dangerous. Finally, some informational approaches are combined with moral appeals to not use drugs because of the fundamentally debased nature of drug abuse. In these programs providers not only offer factual information about drugs but also preach to students about the evils of smoking, drinking, or using drugs, and exhort them to avoid such behaviors on religious or moral grounds.

EFFECTIVENESS. One problem that has plagued the field of prevention is that, until recently, there were few high-quality evaluation studies. In fact, most of the published reports on drug abuse prevention programs in the 1970s and early 1980s either did not have evaluation components or used evaluation methodologies that were seriously flawed (Schaps et al., 1981). Most of the evaluation studies that were conducted focused on knowledge and attitudes instead of on actual drug use. Evaluation studies of informational approaches to prevention tended to show some impact on knowledge and anti-drug attitudes but consistently failed to show any impact on tobacco, alcohol, or drug use or intentions to use drugs. Several meta-analytic studies confirmed this overall lack of behavioral effects. In a meta-analysis of 143 adolescent drug education programs, Tobler (1986) reported that information-based programs had an impact on drug knowledge but had no effect on other outcome measures, including drug use. In a separate meta-analysis of 33 school-based drug education programs, Bangert-Drowns (1988) found positive effects on knowledge and attitudes but no effects on drug use. Consequently, the existing literature calls into question the basic assumption of the information–dissemination model—that increased knowledge will result in attitude and behavior change. In summary, while it is likely that an awareness of the hazards of using drugs does play some role in deterring drug use, it is increasingly clear that the causes of drug abuse are complex and that prevention strategies that rely either solely or primarily on information dissemination are simply not effective.

Affective Education

Another common approach to drug abuse prevention is known as "affective education." Rather than focusing on cognitive factors, affective education approaches assume that promoting personal affective development in students will directly reduce the likelihood of drug abuse. Affective education approaches often include content on decision making, effective communication, and assertiveness, and many include content on norm-setting messages. For example, the affective approaches sometimes include material showing that most people who smoke or use alcohol do so in a responsible manner.

   EFFECTIVENESS.   Like informational approaches, affective education has produced disappointing results. Although affective education approaches can have an impact on one or more of the correlates of drug use, they have not demonstrated an impact on drug use (Kearney & Hines, 1980; Kim, 1988). Rather than focusing on skills training, these programs typically emphasized experiential games and classroom activities designed to target personal growth, self-understanding, and self-acceptance. However, there is no evidence that these exercises actually improved decision making, assertiveness, or communication skills. Furthermore, it now seems likely that responsible-use messages may have been counterproductive by conveying the message that drug use is acceptable as long as it is done in a responsible fashion. Other limitations of the affective education approach are the failure to link program content to drug-specific situations and failure to acknowledge the role of social influences and peer pressure in adolescent experimentation with drugs. In summary, while more comprehensive than information–dissemination approaches, the affective education approach to drug abuse prevention has several major weaknesses, including a narrow and incomplete focus on the causes of drug abuse and the use of ineffective methods to achieve program goals. Table 3.3 summarizes a representative sample of studies that evaluated affective education approaches.

Alternatives Programming

The idea behind alternatives programming is to provide adolescents with activities that can serve as alternatives to drug use. The original model for this prevention approach included the establishment of youth centers that provided a set of activities, such as sports, hobbies, community service, or academic tutoring. It was assumed that if adolescents were provided with real-life experiences that were as appealing as drug use, these activities would take the place of involvement with drugs. Outward Bound and similar programs represent a second type of alternatives approach. They were developed in the hope that they would alter the affective–cognitive state of participants and improve the way they feel about themselves, others, and the world. These programs provide typically healthy, outdoor activities designed to promote teamwork, self-confidence, and

TABLE 3.3. Selected Studies Testing Affective and Alternative Approaches

Investigator(s)	Participants	Intervention approach	Evaluation design	Results
Moskowitz et al. (1982)	3rd–4th-graders	42 sessions over 2 years; Magic Circle technique designed to increase opportunities to communicate in small groups; implemented by teachers	Pre–post; follow-up (1 year)	No difference between those in Magic Circle and controls on variables relating to drug use and variables measuring drug use
Schaps et al. (1984)	4th–6th-graders	Effective Classroom Management (ECM) focuses on general teaching style; incorporation of communication and nonpunitive discipline skills with self-esteem enhancement by teacher; implemented by teachers	Pre–post; follow-up (1 and 2 years)	No pattern of effects for ECM was observed for either elementary or junior high school students
Malvin et al. (1985)	7th–8th-graders	12-session training by teachers of peer tutors (cross-age peer tutoring); tutors help younger children 4 times per week for a semester	Pre–post; follow-up (1 and 2 years)	Students liked tutoring but disliked weekly meetings; no effects on outcome variables such as self-esteem and school liking
Malvin et al. (1985)	7th–8th-graders	1 period per day for a semester; students work in a "school store" 2–3 times per week	Pretest; follow-up (1 and 2 years)	Students liked daily class sessions and working in store; no effects on outcome variables such as self-esteem and school liking
Schaps et al. (1982)	7th–8th-graders	12 sessions; decision making, goal setting, assertiveness, advertising, social influences, knowledge of drugs; implemented by teachers	Pre–post; follow-up (1 year)	Effects only on 7th-grade girls' drug knowledge, perception of poor attitudes; but results disappeared at follow-up; no effects for 8th grade girls or boys

self-esteem. A third alternatives approach was designed to meet the kind of needs or expectancies that are often said to underlie drug use. For example, the need for relaxation or more energy might be satisfied by exercise programs, sports, or hiking; the desire for sensory stimulation might be satisfied by activities that enhance sensory awareness (such as learning to appreciate the sensory aspects of music, art, and nature); or the need for peer acceptance might be satisfied through participation in sensitivity training or encounter groups. None of the evaluations of alternatives approaches have found any impact on drug use (Schaps et al., 1981, 1986). Table 3.3 summarizes a representative sample of studies evaluating alternatives approaches to drug abuse prevention.

SOCIAL-INFLUENCE APPROACHES

Toward the end of the 1970s, a major shift in drug abuse prevention research began. This shift occurred partly out of both a growing disappointment with traditional prevention approaches and a recognition of the importance of psychosocial factors in promoting the initiation of drug use. Unlike previous prevention approaches, the intervention strategies that were the focus of prevention research during the 1980s and 1990s had a stronger grounding in psychological theories of human behavior. Richard Evans and his colleagues at the University of Houston are credited with launching this line of prevention research (Evans, 1976; Evans et al., 1978). Evans's work emphasized the importance of social and psychological factors in promoting the onset of cigarette smoking and used a prevention approach based on McGuire's persuasive communications theory (McGuire, 1964, 1968). From this perspective, adolescent cigarette smoking is the result of social influences from peers and the media to smoke cigarettes, persuasive advertising appeals, or exposure to smokers who serve as role models for students.

Psychological Inoculation

A major component of Evans's prevention approach was based on a concept in McGuire's work called "psychological inoculation." As applied by Evans to cigarette smoking, adolescent non-smokers were "inoculated" against the kind of pro-smoking messages they would be likely to encounter in real-life situations. This was accomplished by exposing students to pro-smoking messages first in a relatively weak form and then in progressively stronger forms. In addition to preparing adolescents for pro-smoking influences, this prevention approach attempted to teach them how to deal with such influences. For example, a common situation for adolescents is that they are offered a cigarette by a peer and called "chicken" if they refuse to smoke. Students are taught to handle this type of situation by having responses ready, such as, "If I smoke to prove to you that I'm not chicken, all I'm showing is that I'm afraid of *not* doing what you want me to do. I don't want to smoke, I'm not going to." Or, since adolescents are likely to see peers posturing and acting "tough" by smoking, they can be taught to think to themselves: "If they were really tough, they wouldn't have to smoke to prove it."

Correcting Normative Expectations

The prevention approach developed by Evans included periodic surveys of smoking among students along with collection of saliva samples as objective confirmation of smoking behavior. After each survey, actual smoking prevalence rates in each classroom were announced to students. Since adolescents have a general tendency to overestimate the prevalence of tobacco, alcohol, and drug use (Fishbein, 1977), many students learned that actual classroom smoking rates were lower than they had expected. This assessment and feedback procedure helped correct the common misperception that cigarette smoking is a highly normative behavior engaged in by most adolescents. A seminal research paper by Evans and colleagues (1978) demonstrated the importance of correcting such expectations. In this study, classrooms were randomized to one of three conditions: (1) students receiving assessment and feedback concerning classroom smoking rates, (2) students receiving assessment and feedback plus the inoculation intervention, and (3) a control group. The results of this study showed that students in the two prevention conditions had smoking onset rates that were about half those observed in the control group. This was the first research to show that prevention could work—that individuals receiving a prevention program would have significantly lower rates of use than would those not receiving the program.

An interesting aspect of this study is that the inoculation intervention did not produce any incremental reduction in smoking onset over that produced by the assessment/feedback procedures. In fact, in retrospect it is evident that the prevention effect generally attributed to the inoculation component of the intervention was actually the result of providing students with feedback concerning the actual levels of smoking in their classroom. That is, an important "active ingredient" in the prevention approach developed by Evans and his colleagues was the process of correcting expectations that nearly everybody smokes cigarettes. Although the importance of correcting such expectations was originally overlooked, the success of the Evans smoking prevention study led to a dramatic increase in prevention research that transformed the entire prevention field. This research initially targeted cigarette smoking but later began to address the use of alcohol and other drugs.

Social Resistance Skills Training

Over the years several variations on the prevention strategy described previously have been developed and tested. In general, these approaches placed little emphasis on the psychological inoculation procedures developed by Evans and focused extensively on teaching students how to recognize and deal with social influences from peers and the media to use drugs. An assumption is that many adolescents do not want to smoke, drink, or use drugs but lack the confidence or skills to refuse offers to engage in these behaviors. Based on this, one of the most important aspects of the approach is an increased emphasis on skills training to help students resist social influences. This approach is called "social influence" (because it targets social influences that promote drug use), "refusal skills" (because they teach students how to refuse drugs), and "social resistance skills" (or simply "resistance skills," because they teach students skills for resisting social influences to use drugs). These terms are used interchangeably in the literature, and any one of them is an appropriate descriptor for this class of prevention approaches. The term "resistance skills" is used in this chapter because it captures two central and distinctive aspects of these prevention approaches: (1) the focus on increasing student resistance to negative social influences to engage in drug use and (2) the focus on skills training. As a class of preventive interventions, these approaches are similar in that they are based on social-learning theory (Bandura, 1977) and on a conceptual model that stresses the fundamental importance of social factors in promoting the initiation of adolescent drug use. Although this model includes social influences coming from the family, peers, and the media, the focus of most preventive interventions is on the last two, with the primary emphasis on peer influences.

METHODS. A major emphasis in resistance skills training approaches is on teaching students how to recognize situations in which they are likely to experience peer pressure to smoke, drink, or use drugs. The goal is to teach students ways to avoid these high-risk situations and give them the knowledge, confidence, and skills needed to handle peer pressure in such situations. These programs also frequently include a component that is intended to make students aware of prosmoking influences from the media, with an emphasis on the techniques used by advertisers to influence consumer behavior. Students are taught to recognize advertising appeals designed to sell tobacco products or alcoholic beverages as well as how to formulate counter-arguments to those appeals. Other methods commonly used in resistance skills training include having students make a public commitment not to smoke, drink, or use drugs. However, one study (Hurd et al., 1980) suggests that this component may not contribute to any real prevention effects. Finally, following the original model developed by Evans, prevention approaches began to include a component to correct normative expectations that the majority of adolescents smoke, drink, or use drugs.This has been accomplished in various ways. In addition to the classroom survey and feedback procedure developed by Evans, students may be asked to conduct their own surveys and provide the results to the class. Alternatively, students may be asked to estimate how many teenagers and how many adults smoke, drink, or use drugs, and then are provided with the correct statistical information from national or regional survey data. Recently, it has been proposed that resistance skills training may be ineffective in the absence of conservative social norms against drug use since, if the norm is to use drugs, adolescents will be less likely to resist offers of drugs (Donaldson, et al., 1996). This suggests that correcting normative expectations and attempting to create or reinforce conservative beliefs about the prevalence and acceptability of drug use is of central importance to the success of resistance skills training programs.

EFFECTIVENESS. A growing number of studies have documented the effectiveness of prevention approaches that use resistance skills training (Arkin et al., 1981; Donaldson et al., 1994; Hurd et al., 1980; Luepker et al., 1983; Perry et al., 1983; Snow et al., 1992; Sussman et al., 1993; Telch et al., 1982). The focus of the majority of these studies has been on smoking prevention, with studies typically examining rates of smoking onset, overall smoking prevalence, or scores on an index of smoking involvement. For the most part, studies indicate that the resistance skills prevention approach is capable of reducing smoking by 30 to 50% after the initial intervention, based on a comparison of the proportion of smokers in the experimental group to the proportion of smokers in the control group (Arkin et al., 1981; Donaldson et al., 1994; Sussman et al., 1993); Studies reporting results in terms of smoking incidence have shown reductions ranging from approximately 30 to 40%, when comparing the proportion of new smokers in the experimental group to the proportion of new smokers in the control group. Several studies have demonstrated reductions in the overall prevalence of cigarette smoking in terms of both occasional smoking (one or more cigarettes per month) and regular smoking (one or more cigarettes per week).

Although there are fewer studies of the impact of resistance skills training approaches on alcohol or marijuana use than on tobacco use, the magnitude of the reductions that have been reported in many cases is similar to that found for tobacco use (e.g., McAlister et al., 1980; Shope et al., 1992). However, one meta-analysis of resistance skills programs found fewer behavioral effects for alcohol interventions relative to smoking interventions (Rundall and Bruvold, 1988). Nevertheless, resistance skills programs as a whole have generally been successful. A comprehensive review of resistance skills studies published from 1980 to 1990 reported that the majority of prevention studies (63%) had positive effects on drug use behavior, with fewer studies

TABLE 3.4. Selected Studies Testing Social and Resistance-Skills Approaches

Investigator(s)	Participants	Intervention approach	Evaluation design	Results
Evans et al. (1978)	7th-graders	4-session social pressures curriculum using videotapes, small-group discussion, and feedback on smoking rates; peers used in videotapes	Pre–post	Smoking onset rates for initial nonsmokers exposed to the social pressures curriculum did not differ from onset rates for subjects exposed to repeated testing and a film on physiological effects of smoking
McAlister, Perry, & Maccoby (1979)	7th-graders	7-session social pressures curriculum using discussion and role playing; slightly older peers implemented curriculum	Pre–post; follow-up (2 years)	Intervention group reported substantially less smoking following treatment and 1 and 2 years thereafter; substantially lower rates of alcohol and marijuana use were also found 1 year following treatment
Perry et al. (1983)	10th-graders	3-session social pressures curriculum; implementation by regular classroom teachers versus college students	Pre–post	Intervention was no more effective than two comparison treatments in reducing smoking; no significant differences were found between the two types of instructors
Hurd et al. (1980), Minnesota Team	7th-graders	5-session social pressures curriculum; conducted by college students; utilized videotapes, discussion, and role playing; compared personalized videotapes where role models were known to students with nonpersonalized videotapes	Pre–post; follow-up (2 years)	Immediately following treatments, the personalized and nonpersonalized groups reported significantly lower smoking rates than the no-treatment control groups, with no significant difference between the two experimental groups; two years following treatment, smoking rates for the personalized group were significantly less than the nonpersonalized and control groups, and smoking rates for the latter two groups did not differ

(cont.)

TABLE 3.4. (*Continued*)

Investigator(s)	Participants	Intervention approach	Evaluation design	Results
Arkin et al. (1981), Minnesota Team	7th-graders	4 intervention conditions included (1) social pressures curriculum led by professional health educator with media supplement, (2) friendly pressures led by same-age peers with media supplement, (3) social pressures led by peers without media, and (4) long-term health consequences	Pre–post; follow-up (1-year)	Among initial nonsmokers, the long-term consequences curriculum had the most favorable initial results, but 1 year later the peer-led social pressures conditions had lower smoking rates; no differences were found for initial smokers
Murray et al. (1984), Minnesota Team	7th-graders	Same as above except regular classroom teachers replaced professional health educators	Pre–post; follow-up (1 year)	Among initial nonsmokers, no differences were found among the 4 treatment conditions following treatment; smoking rates for all groups combined were lower than a comparison group receiving standard health curriculum; differences among groups for initial smokers were not significant, although there was a tendency toward higher smoking levels for the teacher-led social pressures curriculum
Best et al. (1984)	6th-graders	8-session social influence approach, plus decision making; 2 boosters in 7th grade; 1 booster session in 8th grade; health educators	Pre–post; follow-up (2-1/2 years)	Significant effects on cross-sectional prevalence; significant reductions in experimental smokers; significant impact on "high-risk" students for experimental to regular smoking
Pentz et al. (1989); Midwestern Prevention Project	6th- and 7th-graders	10-session intervention program includes school, parent, mass-media components; school-based intervention includes resistance training, normative education, and health education; reinforced by role-play, problem solving, discussion and practice; taught by classroom teachers, using peer leaders; includes booster sessions	Pre–post; follow-up (2 years)	Proportion of smokers lower in intervention group for recent smoking and having smoked within 1 month; intervention group marginally lower in number of students who had ever smoked

Study	Population	Description	Design	Results
Johnson et al. (1990); Midwestern Prevention Project	6th- and 7th-graders; high and low risk	10-session school-based social influences curriculum mentioned above	Pre–post; follow-up (3 years)	Reductions in tobacco and marijuana use; equivalent reductions across risk levels; with marginal effect for lifetime smoking
MacKinnon et al. (1991); Midwestern Prevention Project	6th- and 7th-graders	10-session school-based social influences curriculum mentioned above	Pre–post; follow-up (1 year)	Reductions in cigarette smoking, drinking, and marijuana use; positive effects on mediating variables, such as communication skills, and beliefs about friends' tolerance of drug use
Rohrbach et al. (1994); Midwestern Prevention Project	6th-graders	13-session social influence school prevention curriculum similar to Pentz et al. (above), plus parent curriculum consisting of parent–child homework, parent training workshops, and community activities.	Pre–post; follow-up (18 month)	73% of parents participated in at least one of the components; parent participation in program resulted in less cigarette use, and marginally associated with less alcohol use at follow-up.
Donaldson et al. (1994, 1995); Adolescent Alcohol Prevention Trial	5th-graders	9-session school-based program assessing the effectiveness of Resistance-Skills Training, Normative Education, and drug education; 7th-grade booster sessions; includes discussion, homework, and video	Pre–post; follow-up (3-years); tested information only, resistance training, normative education and combined curricula	Resistance training and normative education significantly increased the skills they targeted; only normative education positively effected substance use into 8th grade; resistance training-only condition increased levels of substance abuse
Shope et al. (1992); Alcohol Misuse Prevention Study	5th- and 6th-graders	4-session resistance training curriculum, with three booster sessions; involves health education, coping strategies; uses positive reinforcement, roleplay, homework, and video	Pre–post; follow-up (26 months); compared intervention, intervention plus boosters, and control	No treatment effect as a whole for alcohol use, or misuse; program effects found for alcohol misuse in the subgroups who had experienced drinking prior to implementation
Ellickson & Bell (1990); Project ALERT	7th-graders; urban, suburban, and rural	8-session social influence and resistance skills training curriculum; three 8th-grade booster sessions; utilized role-play and discussion; conducted by classroom teachers, and older teenagers	Pre–post; follow-up (3-, 12-, and 15-month); program tested on students in three levels of risk	Initial reductions in drinking for different risk levels; intervention effects for marijuana and cigarette initiation for all risk levels; reductions in drinking not sustained after 7th grade

(cont.)

TABLE 3.4. (*Continued*)

Investigator(s)	Participants	Intervention approach	Evaluation design	Results
Bell et al. (1993); Project ALERT	7th-graders	Same as above	Pre–post; follow-up (2 years)	Effects on cognitive risk factors persist through 9th grade in teen-led condition; all effects on actual use decay after 2 years
Ellickson et al. (1993); Project ALERT	7th-graders	Same as above	Pre–post; follow-up (6 years)	Effects on substance use decay after intervention; some effects on cognitive risk factors persist until 10th grade
Flynn et al. (1992)	4th-, 5th-, and 6th-graders	4-year mass media and school-based educational intervention; 4 sessions/year in grades 5–8, and 3 sessions/year in grades 9 and 10; includes decision making, resistance training, and health information; mass-media program included health information and resistance skills components	Pre–post; follow-up (4 years annually); compared school-only and media-plus-school interventions	Reductions in smoking and targeted mediating variables for media-plus-school condition
Perry et al. (1992), Minnesota Team	7th grade	5-year behavioral health and community education program; school-based component focuses on health education, resistance skills, normative beliefs, and peer and media influences; includes role-play, discussion, and a public commitment to abstain; community smoking prevention in 7th grade	Pre–post; follow-up (7-year, annually)	Significant reductions in smoking prevalence and intensity at all subsequent test points through high school
Graham et al. (1990); Project SMART	7th-graders	12-session social skills and drug resistance curriculum, and a 12-session affective education curriculum; utilized role-play and discussion; conducted by health educators, with peer assistants	Pre–post; comparison of 2 program types within 6 subgroups (males, females, Asians, Blacks, Hispanics, and Whites); 1-year follow-up of 3 cohorts	Positive effects for females in both programs for cigarette smoking and alcohol consumption, significant sex by program interactions for cigarettes and marijuana use

TABLE 3.5. Selected Studies Testing Competence Enhancement Approaches

Investigator(s)	Subjects	Intervention approach	Evaluation design	Results
Schinke & Gilchrist (1983)	6th-graders	8-session social skills curriculum focusing on problem solving, decision making, and social pressures resistance	Pre–post	Substantially lower smoking rates 6 months following treatment for experimental vs. no-treatment control group
Gilchrist & Schinke (1983)	6th-graders	8-session social skills training	Pre–post; follow-up (15 months)	Substantially lower smoking rates 3 and 15 months following treatment for experimental group versus a comparison discussion group and a no-treatment control group
Botvin & Eng (1980); Botvin et al. (1980); Life Skills Training	8th–10th graders	10-session life skills training focusing on communication, decision making, assertion, and social pressures resistance; adult educational specialists as implementers	Pre–post; follow-up (3 months)	Substantially lower onset rates among initial nonsmokers immediately after and 3 months following treatment compared with no-treatment control group
Botvin & Eng (1982); Life Skills Training	7th-graders	12-session life skills training using slightly older peer leaders	Pre–post; follow-up (1 year)	Lower smoking rates among initial nonsmokers immediately after and 1 year following treatment
Botvin, Renick, & Baker (1983); Life Skills Training	7th-graders	15-session life skills training using regular classroom teachers; comparisons were made between intensive (daily session) and prolonged (weekly sessions) format	Pre–post; follow-up (1 year)	Among initial nonsmokers, both experimental groups had lower smoking rates immediately after and 1 year following treatment. No differences were found between the two scheduling formats immediately following treatment, but smoking rates were lower for the intensive format 1 year later. Among initial smokers, no differences were found
Botvin, Baker, Renick et al. (1984); Life Skills Training	7th-graders	20-session life skills training; implementation by older peers versus classroom teachers	Pre–post	Substantially lower substance use rates immediately following treatment for the peer-led group compared with the teacher-led group and no-treatment control group. Rates for the teacher-led group did not differ from the control group
Botvin, Baker, Botvin et al. (1984); Life Skills Training	7th-graders	20-session life skills training targeting alcohol misuse using classroom teachers	Pre–post; follow-up (6 months)	Significantly lower rates of alcohol use, misuse, and drunkenness at 6 months follow-up compared to no-treatment control group

(cont.)

TABLE 3.5. (*Continued*)

Investigator(s)	Subjects	Intervention approach	Evaluation design	Results
Botvin, Dusenbury et al. (1989); Life Skills Training	7th-graders (urban, Hispanic)	15-session life skills training using classroom teachers	Pre–post	Significantly lower experimental smoking among life skills training group than no-treatment controls
Botvin, Batson et al. (1989); Life Skills Training	7th-graders (urban, Black)	12-session life skills training using classroom teachers	Pre–post	Reduced tobacco use; increased knowledge of smoking consequences; decreased normative expectations regarding smoking
Botvin, Baker, Dusenbury et al. (1990); Life Skills Training	7th-graders	15-session life skills training using classroom teachers; 10 boosters in 8th grade, 5 boosters in 9th grade; Sessions include decision making, assertiveness, self-esteem, stress management, media influences, drug knowledge, social skills, and communication skills; utilized discussion, homework, video, role-play, behavioral rehearsal, and reinforcement	Pre–post; follow-up (3 years)	Reduced cigarette, alcohol, and marijuana use; decreased normative expectations; increased substance use knowledge; increased interpersonal and communication skills
Botvin, Baker, Filazzola et al. (1990); Life Skills Training	7th-graders	20-session life skills training using classroom teachers versus peers; 10 boosters in 8th grade;	Pre–post; follow-up (1 year)	Reduced tobacco, alcohol, and marijuana use in peer-led sessions with boosters and for females in teacher-led condition; increased tobacco knowledge and anti-smoking attitudes
Botvin et al. (1992); Life Skills Training	7th-graders (urban, Hispanic)	15-session life skills training using classroom teachers	Pre–post	Reduced cigarette use, decreased normative expectations regarding peer and adult smoking; increased smoking knowledge
Caplan et al. (1992); Positive Youth Development Program	6th- & 7th-graders	20 sessions focusing on stress management, self-esteem, problem solving, substance and health information, assertiveness and social networks; involves discussion, role-play, diaries, and video tapes; conducted by classroom teachers and health educators	Pre–post	Increased social adjustment and coping skills; intentions to use substances remained same for intervention students, but increased for controls; program effects on alcohol use but not reported drug use

58

Reference; Program	Population	Intervention	Design	Outcomes
Botvin et al. (1994); Life Skills Training	7th-graders (urban, minority)	15-session life skills training using classroom teachers; 10 boosters in 8th grade; comparisons were made between generic skills training versus culturally focused condition that utilized multicultural myths and stories to model various skills	Pre–post; follow-up (1 year)	Both programs reduced intentions to drink alcohol; generic program reduced intentions to use illicit drugs; increased anti-drug attitudes; decreased risk-taking
Botvin, Baker et al. (1995); Life Skills Training	7th-graders	15-session life skills training using classroom teachers; 10 boosters in 8th grade; 5 boosters in 9th grade (same as Botvin et al., 1990)	Pre–post; follow-up (6 years)	Reduced drug and polydrug use; strongest effects for those receiving a more complete version of the program
Botvin, Schinke et al. (1995); Life Skills Training	7th-graders (urban, minority)	15-session life skills training using classroom teachers; 10 boosters in 8th grade (same as Botvin et al., 1994)	Pre–post; follow-up (2 years)	Reduced current alcohol use and intentions to drink alcohol; increased drug refusal skills
Botvin et al. (1997); Life Skills Training	7th-graders (urban, minority)	15-session life skills training using classroom teachers	Pre–post	Reduced smoking, alcohol, marijuana use, and polydrug use; increased smoking knowledge; decreased normative expectations
Botvin et al. (1999); Life Skills Training	7th-graders (urban, minority girls)	15-session life skills training using classroom teachers; 10 boosters in 8th grade	Pre–post; follow-up (1 year)	Reduced initiation of smoking and reduced escalation to monthly smoking
Botvin et al. (2000); Life Skills Training	7th-graders	15-session life skills training using classroom teachers; 10 boosters in 8th grade; 5 boosters in 9th grade (same as Botvin et al., 1990)	Pre–post; follow-up (6.5 years)	Reduced overall illicit drug use; reduced use of hallucinogens, heroin, and other narcotics

having neutral (26%) or negative effects on behavior (11%)—with several in the neutral category having inadequate statistical power to detect program effects (Hansen, 1992). Furthermore, several follow-up studies of resistance skills interventions reported positive behavioral effects lasting up to 3 years (Luepker et al., 1983; McAlister et al., 1980; Telch et al., 1982). However, data from several longer term follow-up studies indicate that these effects gradually decay over time (Murray et al., 1988; Flay et al., 1989), suggesting the need for ongoing intervention or booster sessions. Table 3.4 summarizes several studies evaluating social influence approaches to drug abuse prevention.

The most popular and visible school-based drug education program based on the social-influence model is Drug Abuse Resistance Education, or Project DARE. The core DARE curriculum, typically provided to children in the fifth or sixth grades, contains elements of information dissemination, affective education, and social-influence approaches to drug abuse prevention. DARE is distinguished by its use of trained, uniformed police officers in the classroom to teach the drug prevention curriculum. Despite the popularity of DARE, its effectiveness has been called into question over the past several years. Some evaluation studies of DARE reported a short-term positive impact on drug-related knowledge, attitudes, or behavior (e.g., Becker, Agopian, & Yeh, 1992). However, many outcome studies have limited scientific value because of weak research designs (such as post-test only), poor sampling and data collection procedures, inadequate measurement strategies, and problems in data analysis approaches (Rosenbaum & Hanson, 1998). Several recent evaluations of DARE, using more scientifically rigorous designs (such as large samples, random assignment, and longitudinal follow-up), indicate that DARE has little or no impact on drug use behaviors, particularly beyond the initial post-test assessment (Clayton, Cattarello, & Johnstone, 1996; Dukes, Ullman, & Stein, 1996; Ennett, Rosenbaum, et al., 1994; Ennett, Tobler, et al., 1994; Rosenbaum et al., 1994; Rosenbaum and Hanson, 1998). Regarding the history of DARE evaluation studies, Rosenbaum and Hanson (1998) point out that the stronger the research design, the less impact researchers reported in terms of effects of DARE on drug use measures. Although the reasons for DARE's lack of impact are unclear, some possibilities are that DARE targets the wrong mediating processes (Hansen & McNeal, 1997), that the instructional methods are less interactive than those of more successful prevention programs, and that teenagers may simply tune out what may be perceived as an expected message from an ultimate authority figure.

COMPETENCE-ENHANCEMENT APPROACHES

Beyond Social Influences

An implicit assumption of both the psychological inoculation and resistance skills approaches is that adolescents do not want to smoke, drink, or use drugs. That is, they begin to use one or more of these substances either because they succumb to the persuasive messages targeted at them or because they lack sufficient skills to resist social influences to use drugs. A limitation of the social-influence approach is that it does not consider the possibility that some adolescents may actually *want* to use drugs. For some adolescents, using drugs is not a matter of yielding to peer pressure but has an instrumental value. Drugs, for example, may help them deal with anxiety, low self-esteem, or discomfort in social situations. In fact, the etiology literature indicates that drug use and abuse have a complex set of determinants, including a variety of cognitive, attitudinal, social, personality, pharmacological, and developmental factors (Baumrind & Moselle, 1985; Blum & Richards, 1979; Jessor & Jessor, 1977; Jones & Battjes, 1985; Kandel, 1978; Meyer & Mirin, 1979; Newcomb & Bentler, 1988; Wechsler, 1976). Given this, it seems logical that the most effective prevention strategy would be one that is comprehensive, targeting a broad array of etiologic determinants.

Toward Generic Skills Training Approaches

Among the more comprehensive approaches to drug abuse prevention are competence-enhancement approaches that emphasize generic personal and social skills in combination with resistance skills. This strategy is more comprehensive than the resistance skills training approaches and earlier cognitive/affective approaches and has been used for nearly 2 decades (Botvin, Baker, Botvin, et al., 1984; Botvin, Baker, Dusenbury et al., 1995; Botvin, Baker, Filazzola, & Botvin, 1990; Botvin, Baker, Renick et al., 1984; Botvin, Dusenbury, Baker, James-Ortiz, Botvin, & Kerner, 1992; Botvin, Epstein, Baker, Diaz, & Williams, 1997; Botvin, Eng, & Williams, 1980; Botvin, Renick, & Baker, 1983; Pentz, 1983; Botvin, Schinke, Epstein, & Diaz, 1994; Botvin, Schinke et al., 1995; Gilchrist & Schinke, 1983; Kreutter, Gewirtz, Davenny, & Love, 1991; Schinke, 1984; Schinke & Gilchrist, 1983, 1984). The theoretical foundations for the competence-enhancement approach are Bandura's social learning theory (Bandura, 1977) and Jessor's problem behavior theory (Jessor & Jessor, 1977). According to this approach, drug abuse is conceptualized as a socially learned and functional behavior that is the result of an interplay between social (interpersonal) and personal (intrapersonal) factors. Drug use behavior is learned through a process of modeling, imitation, and reinforcement and is influenced by an adolescent's pro-drug attitudes and beliefs. These factors, in combination with poor personal and social skills, are believed to increase an adolescent's susceptibility to social influences in favor of drug use.

METHODS. Although these approaches share several features with resistance skills training approaches, a distinctive aspect of competence-enhancement approaches is an emphasis on generic personal self-management skills and social skills. These skills are taught using a combination of proven cognitive–behavioral skills training methods: instruction and demonstration, group feedback and reinforcement, behavioral rehearsal (in-class practice), and extended (out-of-class) practice through behavioral homework assignments. Examples of the kind of generic personal and social skills typically included in this prevention approach are decision-making and problem-solving skills; cognitive skills for resisting interpersonal and media influences; skills for enhancing self-esteem (goal-setting and self-directed behavior-change techniques); adaptive coping strategies for dealing with stress and anxiety; general social skills (complimenting, conversational skills, and skills for forming new friendships); and general assertiveness skills. This prevention approach teaches both these general skills and their application to situations directly related to tobacco, alcohol, and drug use. An added benefit of this type of program is that it teaches adolescents a repertoire of skills they can use to deal with many of the challenges confronting them in their everyday lives, including but not limited to drug use. By teaching generic coping skills that will have broad application, this approach contrasts markedly with resistance skills training approaches designed to give students information and skills relating solely to drug use. However, the most effective approaches appear to integrate features of both generic coping skills and drug-specific resistance skills. In fact, there is some evidence that generic skills training approaches are only effective if they also contain drug-specific material (Caplan et al., 1992).

EFFECTIVENESS. Over the years, a number of evaluation studies have tested the efficacy of competence-enhancement approaches to drug abuse prevention. These studies consistently demonstrated behavioral effects as well as effects on hypothesized mediating variables. Importantly, the magnitude of the effects of these approaches has been relatively large, with studies reporting reductions in drug use behavior in the range of 40 to 80%. A criticism of contemporary prevention programs is that even though they produce impressive reductions in the incidence and prevalence of drug use behavior, these reductions generally occur with respect to experimental or occasional use. However, in addition to demonstrating reductions in the early stages of drug use, it is important to demonstrate reductions in more frequent levels of use, such as the kind of regular use that leads to addictive or compulsive patterns of use.

Findings from two studies of a competence-enhancement prevention program called Life Skills Training (Botvin, 1996) deal directly with this issue by demonstrating reductions in rates of regular cigarette smoking. Two studies have shown reductions of 56 to 67% in the proportion of pretest nonsmokers becoming regular smokers 1 year after the conclusion of the program without any additional booster sessions (Botvin & Eng, 1982; Botvin, Renick, & Baker, 1983). For those students receiving booster sessions, the reductions have been as high as 87% (Botvin et al., 1983). Results of studies using competence-enhancement approaches like Life Skills Training have also demonstrated an impact on other forms of drug use, including alcohol use (Botvin Baker, Botvin, et al., 1984; Botvin, et al., 1990; Botvin, Baker, Renick, et al., 1984; Botvin, Schinke, Epstein et al., 1995; Pentz, 1983); marijuana use (Botvin, Baker, Botvin, et al., 1984; Botvin, Baker, Dusenbury et al., 1990, 1995), and poly-drug use (Botvin, Baker, Dusenbury et al., 1995, Botvin, Epstein, Baker, et al., 1997). These reductions have generally been of a magnitude equal to that found with cigarette smoking. Finally, long-term follow-up data indicate that the prevention effects of these approaches can last for up to 6 years (Botvin Baker, Dusenbury et al., 1995; Botvin et al., 2002). In summary, drug abuse prevention programs that emphasize resistance skills and general life skills (such as competence-enhancement approaches) appear to show the most promise of all school-based prevention approaches. Table 3.5 summarizes several studies evaluating competence enhancement approaches to drug abuse prevention.

ISSUES IN SCHOOL-BASED PREVENTION

Despite the substantial gains in school-based drug abuse prevention over the past couple of decades, a number of important issues remain with regard to the development, implementation, evaluation, and dissemination of prevention interventions in schools.

Program Development

TIMING OF INTERVENTIONS.   Research on the age of onset and developmental progression of drug use indicates that the initiation of drug use tends to follow a logical and predictable sequence (Hamburg, Braemer, & Jahnke, 1975; Kandel, 1975). Most youths begin by experimenting with alcohol and cigarette smoking, followed later by the use of marijuana. A subset of these individuals will progress to the use of depressants, stimulants, hallucinogens, and other dependency-producing drugs. This progression of drug use initiation suggests that the focus of early-prevention interventions should be on drugs early in the developmental progression (cigarettes, alcohol, and marijuana), which typically begin to be used during the middle/junior high school years. Not surprisingly, the majority of published studies have involved students in junior high, with students typically in the seventh grade during the first year of intervention.

However, a criticism of school-based drug abuse prevention programs is that they typically do not acknowledge that different individuals may have different levels of programmatic needs (Institute of Medicine, 1996) and that one school prevention program may not be adequate for all children and adolescents. To address this concern, three types of prevention "tiers" have been used in categorizing prevention interventions since the early 1990s: universal, selective, and indicated programs. Universal interventions are delivered to the general population, selective interventions are targeted to "at-risk" youths who show signs of potential drug involvement, and indicated interventions are targeted to those who are already involved in drugs. Universal (or primary) prevention programs should target the use of substances at the beginning of the drug-use progression, not only because these are the most widely used substances in our society but also because preventing the use of these gateway substances may, in turn, reduce or eliminate the risk of using drugs later in this progression (illicit or dependency-producing drugs).

In high school, however, selective and indicated prevention programs are likely to be most appropriate for students already at risk for drug use, poor school performance, and school dropout, and for those who have already begun using drugs. Programs for such youths typically address the intrapersonal motivational variables (such as affect regulation) that play a role in maintaining or escalating drug use or abuse and place little emphasis on resistance skills training. For example, these programs may target specific motives for using drugs by emphasizing social network development and group support, skills training (decision making, interpersonal communication), and emotional well-being, and may take the form of a semester-long "personal-growth" class (Eggert et al., 1994; Eggert, Seyl, & Nicholas, 1990; Thompson et al., 1997). For those at highest risk, such as students unable to remain in the regular school system and attending continuation high schools, indicated prevention programming that provides drug counseling in addition to addressing motivational factors through support and skills training may be optimal (e.g., Sussman, 1996). Notably, interactive program delivery methods appear to be both more effective and better received than more didactic approaches for high school-age youths as well as for younger students (Sussman et al., 1995).

Much less research has been conducted with younger populations, although anti-drug curricula have been developed for third-graders (Rollins et al., 1994) and even for children in the preschool years (Hall & Zigler, 1997). More studies, although still limited in number, have been conducted with fifth- and sixth-graders (Campanelli et al., 1989; O'Donnell et al., 1995; Schope et al., 1992, 1996). One reason for the relative lack of attention to younger children is that rates of drug use are typically very low during elementary school, making it extremely difficult to demonstrate statistically significant behavioral effects among these children. However, several of the existing programs for young children have shown an impact on drug knowledge and anti-drug attitudes.

Program Implementation

PEER VERSUS ADULT PROVIDERS. Many school-based prevention programs use same-age or slightly older peer leaders as program providers. A number of advantages have been proposed to support the use of peer providers, although there appear to be disadvantages as well. A common argument in support of using peer providers is that they have greater credibility with junior-high-school-age students than do adults with respect to lifestyle issues, since adolescence is a time characterized by some degree of rebellion against parents and other adult authority figures. Another potentially powerful benefit of peer leaders is that they may serve as influential role models who help to alter school norms regarding drug use and its social acceptability. In this way, peer-led prevention programs may have an important impact on normative beliefs in favor of non-drug use. However, there are a number of problems inherent in using peer leaders. Peer providers may lack the teaching skills, motivation, competence in the skill being taught, and classroom management skills necessary for program success. Another problem is that, in their zeal to prevent drug use, peer leaders sometimes have a tendency to lecture or preach to students in ways reminiscent of fear-arousal prevention programs, which runs the risk of turning students off to the material being taught.

Several studies have attempted to determine the effectiveness of peer leaders relative to other program providers. By and large, the evidence supports the use of peer leaders, particularly for resistance skills prevention programs (Arkin et al., 1981; Perry et al., 1983). However, there is some evidence that the use of peer leaders may not benefit all students equally; with one study showing that girls may be more influenced by peer-led resistance skills interventions than are boys (Fisher, Armstrong, & deKler, 1983). Overall, it is not altogether clear that peer leaders are either necessary or better than other providers. In fact, a point that is often overlooked is that peer leaders nearly always function as assistants to adult program providers (teachers, program staff) who have primary responsibility for implementing the prevention program. Furthermore, while peer leaders appear to be well suited to the goals of social-influence approaches, they may not be as central to the goals of competence-enhancement prevention approaches. Adults or other authority figures may be considerably more effective than peer leaders in teaching students the kind fo "life skills" taught in these programs in much the same way that an adult music teacher, drama coach, or athletic coach would be most appropriate for teaching students skills in these areas. In summary, if peer leaders are monitored by teachers, project staff, or other adults, and have well-defined and clearly delineated responsibilities, they can have an important adjunctive value, particularly in resistance skills training programs. However, peer leaders are, in most cases, not necessarily better than other providers.

INTERACTIVE VERSUS DIDACTIC DELIVERY. One of the lessons learned about the implementation of school-based prevention programs is that the delivery method is an important ingredient of program success. In particular, prevention programs that use interactive methods and group processes (such as peer discussions, role-playing, and interactive games) are clearly more effective for adolescents than are those that use more didactic formats (such as lectures, films, and videotapes). In a recent meta-analytic study of school-based drug programs (Tobler & Stratton, 1997), the largest effect size difference among types of prevention programs was found between interactive and noninteractive programs, with interactive programs (those using group processes and classroom dynamics to deliver program content) proving to be much more effective. One of the conclusions of this meta-analysis was that drug abuse prevention programs that foster interaction among peers and use interactive technique to stimulate the active participation of students (in classroom discussion or in practicing new behaviors) were the most successful. Structured small-group activities were found to be an optimal way to introduce program content and promote the acquisition of skills.

TARGETING MULTIPLE SUBSTANCES. Another important issue in the implementation of prevention programs is whether programs should address a single substance (such as tobacco) or multiple substances (tobacco, alcohol, marijuna, and other drugs). There appear to be a variety of arguments both for and against programs that target multiple rather than single substances, and these arguments are based on behavioral as well as policy objectives. As discussed by Johnson, MacKinnon, and Pentz (1996), the behavioral arguments in favor of targeting multiple substances include the fact that many risk behaviors are intercorrelated, with the occurrence of one increasing the probability of others. In addition, an individual's motivation for either using drugs (e.g., social influences or individual vulnerability) or not using drugs (e.g., health concerns) is usually not substance specific.

Policy arguments in favor of multiple-substance prevention programs include the fact that they are more efficient and less expensive than multiple-single-substance programs, since only a limited number of programs can be cost-effectively administered in a single school setting. Arguments supporting single-substance programs, such as smoking prevention programs, include the fact that too much information can be overwhelming to students, and since the use of different drugs usually occurs in stages, it may be developmentally inappropriate to focus on drugs that are initiated later in the sequence (Johnson et al., 1996). However, in a comparison of several single-substance, multiple-substance, and general lifestyle/health promotion programs, one study concluded that multiple-purpose programs were at least as effective as single-substance programs (Johnson et al., 1996).

Prevention programs that target multiple substances usually focus on drugs used at earlier ages—tobacco, alcohol, and marijuana. Of these, alcohol has proved to be the most difficult to impact in terms of achieving behavioral changes. For example, in a meta-analysis of 47 smoking and 29 alcohol school-based prevention programs, Rundall and Bruvold (1988) concluded that smoking interventions are clearly more successful in changing student behavior than are alcohol interventions. Several factors might be responsible for the greater difficulty in demonstrating significant program effects on alcohol use. First, the near ubiquity of alcohol use in our society and generally positive attitudes toward moderate alcohol use make alcohol a much more difficult target for prevention programs. By comparison, attitudes toward the use of marijuana or tobacco are considerably more negative. Also, the goals of prevention programs that target alcohol use are sometimes unclear: Should prevention programs take a "zero tolerance" position with respect to alcohol, attempting to prevent any level of alcohol use; or should the goal be to prevent excessive alcohol use or alcohol-related problems? This is likely to depend on the target population. Abstinence may be the most appropriate goal for universal prevention programs aimed at younger students (those in elementary and middle/junior high school), while preventing alcohol abuse and alcohol-related problems are more appropriate goals for selective and indicated prevention programs targeting older students.

Despite the difficulties in achieving alcohol prevention effects that have sometimes been observed, an important advantage of competence-enhancement approaches to prevention is that they are inherently applicable to multiple substances and multiple problem behaviors. This is because they are designed to teach life skills and enhance general competence, teaching the kind of skills for coping with life that will have a relatively broad application. These skills are taught with direct application to drug use and abuse but can also be used for dealing with the many challenges that confront adolescents in their everyday lives. Accordingly, competence-enhancement programs can expand the focus of intervention to a variety of problem behaviors.

TARGETING MINORITY POPULATIONS. A general weakness of the prevention literature is that most studies have focused primarily on white, middle-class populations. As a consequence, less is known about the impact of these interventions on minority, inner-city, disadvantaged populations. However, several studies indicate that there is substantial overlap in the etiological factors that lead to the initiation and maintenance of drug use among different populations (Bettes, Dusenbury, Kerner, James-Ortiz, & Botvin, 1990; Botvin, Epstein, Schinke, & Diaz, 1994; Botvin et al., 1993; Catalano et al., 1993). This suggests that prevention approaches effective in one population should also be effective in others. Several studies conducted during the past several years have tested this hypothesis, and this gap in the literature is beginning to be filled. These studies provide preliminary evidence that competence-enhancement approaches can be generalized to minority adolescents.

For example, several studies testing the efficacy of Botvin's Life Skills Training program in minority populations have shown that it is effective in decreasing drug use, intentions to use drugs, and risk factors associated with drug use. Among African-American and Hispanic populations, parents, teachers, and students report high levels of acceptance and perceived utility for the pre-vention approach. Where appropriate, the language, examples, and behavioral rehearsal scenarios are modified to increase cultural sensitivity and relevance to each of the target populations; but no modifications are made to the underlying prevention approach. Most of this research with minority youths has involved cigarette smoking, and studies have found significant program effects with pre-dominately Hispanic (Botvin, Dusenbury et al., 1989; Botvin et al., 1992) and African-American youths (Botvin, Batson et al., 1989; Botvin & Cardwell, 1992; Botvin et al., 1999). Follow-up data with Hispanic youths have shown continued lower levels of smoking up to the 10th grade (Botvin, Schinke, Epstein et al., 1994). Several studies also show that drug abuse prevention approaches, such as Life Skills Training, can reduce alcohol and marijuana use among minority populations (Botvin, Schinke, Epstein et al., 1994, 1995; Botvin, et al., 2001a, 2001b); that they can prevent use of multiple substances (Botvin et al., 1997); and that tailoring the intervention to the culture of the target population can enhance its effectiveness (Botvin, Schinke, Epstein et al., 1995).

IMPLEMENTATION FIDELITY.   Early-prevention approaches, such as information dis-semination and affective education, failed largely because their underlying theoretical assump-tions were false. For resistance skills and competence-enhancement approaches, however, there is substantial evidence and agreement among researchers that the theoretical underpinnings are sound. When theoretically proven approaches fail, it may be due to problems in implementation. Regardless of how effective a prevention program may be, it is not likely to produce the desired results unless it is implemented with sufficient fidelity. Nevertheless, a major flaw in the eval-uation of most prevention programs is the failure to examine the extent to which the program was implemented in a manner consistent with the intervention protocol. Unless it is determined that the program was implemented correctly and that most of the target group received the full program, one cannot confidently conclude that the program is ineffective; rather, it may well be that the prevention strategy is effective but was simply not adequately implemented.

The importance of considering implementation fidelity is demonstrated in several studies showing that students who receive higher amounts of programming are more likely to show behavior changes in drug use (Botvin, Baker, Dusenbury et al., 1990, 1995; Pentz et al., 1990). For example, in one study with inner-city minority youths (Botvin, Dusenbury et al., 1989), the prevention condition was divided into low- and high-implementation fidelity groups. No significant prevention effects were found for the low-implementation group, whereas significant effects were found for the high-implementation group. Examination of post-test smoking patterns indicated that the control group had the highest smoking levels, the high-implementation treatment group had the lowest levels, and the low-implementation group fell in the middle. In summary, program implementation is an important but frequently overlooked factor that plays a crucial role in prevention program effectiveness. While there are many reasons why a prevention program might be poorly implemented, such as poorly motivated classroom teachers (Hansen et al., 1988) or lack of teacher training, further research is needed to identify and address these factors.

Program Evaluation

DURABILITY OF PREVENTION EFFECTS.   The initial challenge to the prevention field was to demonstrate that it is possible to reduce tobacco, alcohol, or drug use. Following the publication of a growing number of reports showing reductions in drug use, a logical next question concerned the durability of these prevention effects. However, considerable variability seems to exist in both the magnitude of initial program effects and their durability. Different studies testing essentially the same intervention strategy have produced different results. For example, researchers at RAND (Ellickson & Bell, 1990) tested a social-influence approach, including the teaching of resistance skills, which was similar to that used by researchers at the University of Minnesota (Murray et al., 1989). Yet, while the study by Murray and his colleagues produced prevention effects that were present for 4 years, the RAND study found effects that eroded by the time of the 3-year follow-up that took place at the end of the ninth grade. Furthermore, several longer term follow-up studies (Ellickson, Bell, & McGuigan, 1993; Flay et al., 1989; Murray et al., 1989) indicate that prevention effects produced during junior high school erode by the end of high school. There are several possible explanations for why prevention effects typically deteriorate, including (1) the length of the intervention may have been inadequate; (2) booster sessions were either not included or were inadequate; (3) the intervention was not implemented with sufficient fidelity to the intervention model; and (4) the intervention model was based on faulty assumptions, was incomplete, or was otherwise deficient (Resnicow & Botvin, 1993).

It has been suggested (Dryfoos, 1993) that the results of these follow-up studies indicate that school-based interventions are not powerful enough to produce lasting prevention effects and that multicomponent prevention approaches that target the family and the larger community are needed. Recent research suggests that school-based programming combined with community or parent interventions can lead to greater behavioral effects over time. Flynn and colleagues (Flynn et al., 1994) recently reported that school-based smoking prevention programming led to less smoking over 2 years of follow-up when it was combined with communitywide radio and TV announcements and that the media-plus-school intervention was more effective than the school-only intervention. Furthermore, in the Midwestern Prevention Project (Pentz et al., 1989), a multicomponent program that combined school-based curricula with parental involvement and a communitywide media campaign, parental participation in addition to the school-based component was shown to be associated with decreased use of alcohol and cigarettes among adolescents (Rohrbach et al., 1994). This program produced behavioral effects on drug use up to 6 years after the initial intervention (Pentz et al., 1989). Additional research is needed to investigate whether school-based prevention programs that use media, community, and family education strategies can increase public awareness and support, change school and community norms, and otherwise reinforce the anti-drug prevention message for students, parents, and communities.

However, there is also evidence that school-based interventions are by themselves capable of producing lasting effects. A large-scale randomized prevention trial involving nearly 6,000 students from 56 schools in New York state demonstrated preventive effects for tobacco, alcohol, and marijuana use after 3 years (Botvin, Baker et al., 1990) and after 6 years (Botvin et al., 1995). More importantly, poly-drug use (tobacco, alcohol, and marijuana in the previous week) was 66% lower for the intervention students relative to control students. Attrition rates were equivalent for treatment and control conditions, as were pretest levels of drug use for the final analysis sample, which support the argument that prevention effects were not the result of differential attrition or the pretest nonequivalence of the conditions. Furthermore, data from 454 individuals who were contacted after the end of the 12th grade (6.5 years from the initial baseline) has significantly lower levels of illicit drug involvement relative to control students (Botvin et al., in press), with intervention students scoring lower than control students on the combined measure of illicit drug use and illicit drug use other than marijuana. Significantly lower levels of use were also found for hallucinogens, heroin, and other narcotics in the intervention group relative to the control group.

IMPACT ON HYPOTHESIZED MEDIATORS. There is a growing awareness among drug abuse prevention researchers of the need to examine the extent to which prevention programs lead to changes in hypothesized mediating constructs, and the extent to which changes in these variables lead to changes in drug use (Botvin et al., 1992; Donaldson et al., 1994, 1996; Hansen & McNeal, 1977). Several recent papers have examined the impact of such variables using the more focused resistance skills training approach (MacKinnon et al., 1991; MacKinnon & Dwyer, 1993). These studies raise some interesting questions about the active ingredients in these intervention strategies. For example, the MacKinnon and Dwyer study did not provide evidence of an impact on resistance skills, although the results of this study did suggest the importance of modifying normative expectations concerning cigarette smoking among adolescents. A major strength of the evaluation studies conducted with the broader competence-enhancement approach is that many examined the impact of variables hypothesized to mediate the effect of the prevention programs, and studies have documented program effects on mediators in a direction consistent with non-drug use. These include significant changes in knowledge and attitudes, assertiveness, locus of control, social anxiety, self-satisfaction, decision making, and problem solving. Further research is needed to demonstrate how interventions affect the various skill domains targeted and how changes in skill level are related to reductions in drug use.

Program Dissemination

In the final analysis, research-based prevention programs shown to be successful are unlikely to have any real public health impact unless they are used in a large number of schools. However, programs with proven effectiveness, such as many of those reviewed in this chapter, are not widely used. Instead, drug prevention programs most commonly used in real-world settings are those that have not shown evidence of effectiveness or have not been evaluated properly (Silvia & Thorne, 1997). Regarding the research-based programs shown to be effective, it is unclear to what extent schools continue to use them after the research studies (and federal support) have ended. Although schools may be willing and able to implement prevention programs of this kind during the time they are participating in a federally sponsored prevention trial, they may not have the motivation or resources to continue such programs after conclusion of the studies.

Thus, an important area that deserves further attention is how effective school-based drug abuse prevention programs can be widely disseminated, adopted, and institutionalized. There are a number of challenges that interfere with the widespread implementation of effective school-based prevention programs, including the lack of appropriate infrastructures at the school and school district levels (Elias, 1997). A recent U.S. Department of Education study evaluated a sample of school-based prevention programs provided to more than 10,000 students in 19 school districts that received funding under the drug-free-schools act (Silvia & Thorne, 1997). In this study several factors were identified that appeared to facilitate the implementation of a prevention program. These included (1) the level of commitment of the program implementers, (2) the leadership provided by the prevention program coordinator and the presence of staff to assist the coordinator, (3) the level of community involvement in the program, and (4) recognition at the district level of the importance of reinforcing a school-level commitment to prevention through prevention coordinators and adequate staff training.

Furthermore, even if the distribution channels and organizational supports are present, schools must be willing to wholeheartedly embrace these programs as their own. For this to happen, prevention programs must be "user friendly" and appealing to schools, teachers, students, and even parents. Prevention programs developed by researchers, while more effective and better evaluated than commercial drug abuse prevention programs, are rarely packaged in a way that is competitive with commercial programs. Research-based prevention programs generally take the form of relatively crude intervention protocols and student handout materials. Because the emphasis is on evaluation, the bulk of the money spent is on evaluation, while commercial drug abuse prevention curricula typically invest their money in packaging their prevention materials in the most appealing and sophisticated way possible to most effectively market these prevention products. If the most effective prevention programs are to be successfully disseminated, adopted, and institutionalized by schools across the country, it will be necessary to invest more resources in the "look" of prevention materials; and increased emphasis will need to be put on the dissemination of research-based prevention approaches.

CONCLUSION

It has become clear over the past 20 years that some of the most widely used, school-based prevention approaches are either ineffective or of unproven effectiveness. Notable among these are prevention approaches that rely on provision of information concerning the adverse consequences of drug abuse, affective education, or alternatives to drug use. Now, research has demonstrated the efficacy of prevention approaches that focus on psychosocial factors associated with drug use initiation and/or drug abuse. These approaches emphasize teaching social resistance skills, either alone or in combination with generic personal and social skills. A small number of studies testing the efficacy of these approaches have shown that they are capable of reducing drug use for up to several years, including until the end of high school. Although most of this research has been conducted with cigarette smoking, prevention effects have also been demonstrated for alcohol and marijuana use. Several recent studies have also begun to elucidate the mechanism through which these prevention approaches work by assessing the impact on hypothesized mediating variables. Although research with these prevention approaches has been tested primarily with predominantly white, middle-class populations, a small number of studies have also provided evidence of the utility of these approaches with inner-city minority populations. However, while research has demonstrated that school-based drug abuse prevention programs can work, further research is needed to examine how to maximize their effects and make them last. Furthermore, proven prevention programs are unlikely to have a large public health impact unless they are more widely used. Therefore, an important goal of future research is to identify and overcome the barriers to the dissemination and adoption of proven prevention programs.

REFERENCES

Arkin, R. M., Roemhild, H. J., Johnson, C. A., Luepker, R. V., & Murray, D. M. (1981). The Minnesota smoking prevention program: A seventh grade health curriculum supplement. *Journal of School Health, 51,* 616–661.

Bandura, A. (1977). *Social learning theory.* Englewood Cliffs, NJ: Prentice-Hall.

Bangert-Drowns, R. L. (1988). The effects of school-based substance abuse education: A meta-analysis. *Journal of Drug Education, 18,* 243–264.

Baumrind, D., & Moselle, K. A. (1985). A developmental perspective on adolescent drug abuse. *Alcohol and Substance Use in Adolescence,* 45–65.

Becker, H. R., Agopian, M. E., & Yeh, S. (1992). Impact evaluation of Drug Abuse Resistance Education (DARE). *Journal of Drug Education, 22,* 283–291.

Bell, R. M., Ellickson, P. L., & Harrison, E. R. (1993). Do drug prevention effects persist into high school? *Preventive Medicine, 22,* 463–483.

Best, J. A. (1984). Smoking prevention and the concept of risk. *Journal of Applied Social Psychology, 14,* 257–273.

Bettes, B. A., Dusenbury, L., Kerner, J., James-Ortiz, S., & Botvin, G. J. (1990). Ethnicity and psychosocial factors in alcohol and tobacco use in adolescence. *Child Development, 61,* 557–656.

Blum, R., & Richards, L. (1979). Youthful drug use. In R. I. Dupont, A. Goldstein, & J. O'Donnell (Eds.), *Handbook on drug abuse* (National Institute on Drug Abuse) (pp. 257–267). Washington, DC: Government Printing Office.

Botvin, G. J. (1996). Substance abuse prevention through life skills training. In R. D. Peters & R. J. McMahon (Eds.), *Preventing childhood disorders, substance abuse, and delinquency* (pp. 215–240). Thousand Oaks, CA: Sage.

Botvin, G. J., Baker, E., Botvin, E. M., Dusenbury, L., Cardwell, J., & Diaz, T. (1993). Factors promoting cigarette smoking among black youth: A causal modeling approach. *Addictive Behaviors, 18,* 397–405.

Botvin, G. J., Baker, E., Botvin, E. M., Filazzola, A. D., & Millman, R. B. (1984). Alcohol abuse prevention through the development of personal and social competence: A pilot study. *Journal of Studies on Alcohol, 45,* 550–552.

Botvin, G. J., Baker, E., Dusenbury, L., Botvin, E. M., & Diaz, T. (1995). Long-term follow-up results of a randomized drug abuse prevention trial in a White middle-class population. *Journal of the American Medical Association, 273,* 1106–1112.

Botvin, G. J., Baker, E., Dusenbury, L., Tortu, S., & Botvin, E. M. (1990). Preventing adolescent drug abuse through a multimodal cognitive-behavioral approach: Results of a three-year study. *Journal of Consulting & Clinical Psychology, 58,* 437–446.

Botvin, G. J., Baker, E., Filazzola, A., & Botvin, E. M. (1990). A cognitive-behavioral approach to substance abuse prevention: A one-year follow-up. *Addictive Behaviors, 15,* 47–63.

Botvin, G. J., Baker, E., Renick, N., Filazzola, A. D., & Botvin, E. M. (1984). A cognitive-behavioral approach to substance abuse prevention. *Addictive Behaviors, 9,* 137–147.

Botvin, G. J., Dusenbury, L., Baker, E., James-Ortiz, S., & Kerner, J. (1989). A skills training approach to smoking prevention among Hispanic youth. *Journal of Behavioral Medicine, 12,* 279–296.

Botvin, G. J., & Cardwell, J. (1992). Primary prevention (smoking) of cancer in black populations. Grant contract number N01-CN-6508. *Final Report to National Cancer Institute* (NCI). Cornell University Medical College.

Botvin, G. J., Batson, H., Witts-Vitale, S., Bess, V., Baker, E., & Dusenbury, L. (1989). A psychosocial approach to smoking prevention for urban black youth. *Public Health Reports, 104,* 573–582.

Botvin, G. J., Dusenbury, L., Baker, E., James-Ortiz, S., Botvin, E. M., & Kerner, J. (1992). Smoking prevention among urban minority youth: Assessing effects on outcome and mediating variables. *Health Psychology, 11,* 290–299.

Botvin, G. J., Dusenbury, L., Baker, E., James-Ortiz, S., & Kerner, J. (1989). A skills training approach to smoking prevention among Hispanic youth. *Journal of Behavioral Medicine, 12,* 279–296.

Botvin, G. J., & Eng, A. (1980). A comprehensive school-based smoking prevention program. *Journal of School Health, 50,* 209–213.

Botvin, G. J., & Eng, A. (1982). The efficacy of a multicomponent approach to the prevention of cigarette smoking. *Preventive Medicine, 11,* 199–211.

Botvin, G. J., Eng, A., & Williams, C. L. (1980). Preventing the onset of cigarette smoking through life skills training. *Preventive Medicine, 9,* 135–143.

Botvin, G. J., Epstein, J. A., Baker, E., Diaz, T., & Williams, M. I. (1997). School-based drug abuse prevention with inner-city minority youth. *Journal of Child & Adolescent Substance Abuse, 6,* 5–19.

Botvin, G. J., Epstein, J. A., Schinke, S. P., & Diaz, T. (1994). Predictors of cigarette smoking among inner-city minority youth. *Developmental & Behavioral Pediatrics, 15,* 67–73.

Botvin, G. J., Griffin, K. W., Diaz, T., Miller, N., & Ifill-Williams, M. (1999). Smoking initiation and escalation in early adolescent girls: One-year follow-up of a school-based prevention intervention for minority youth. *Journal of the American Medical Women's Association, 54,* 139–143.

Botvin, G. J., Griffin, K. W., Diaz, T., Scheier, L. M., Williams, C., & Epstein, J. A. (2000). Preventing illicit drug use in adolescents: Long-term follow-up data from a randomized control trial of a school population. *Addictive Behaviors, 5,* 769–774.

Botvin, G. J., Griffin, K. W., Diaz, T., & Ifill-Williams, M. (2001a). Drug abuse prevention among minority adolescents: One-year follow-up of a school-based preventive intervention. *Prevention Science, 2,* 1–13.

Botvin, G. J., Griffin, K. W., Diaz, T., & Ifill-Williams, M. (2001b). Preventing binge drinking during early adolescence: One-and two-year follow-up of a school-based preventive intervention. *Psychology of Addictive Behaviors, 15,* 360–365.

Botvin, G. J., Renick, N., & Baker, E. (1983). The effects of scheduling format and booster sessions on a broad-spectrum psychosocial approach to smoking prevention. *Journal of Behavioral Medicine, 6,* 359–379.

Botvin, G. J., Schinke, S. P., Epstein, J. A., & Diaz, T. (1994). Effectiveness of culturally-focused and generic skills training approaches to alcohol and drug abuse prevention among minority youths. *Psychology of Addictive Behaviors, 8,* 116–127.

Botvin, G. J., Schinke, S. P., Epstein, J. A., Diaz T., & Botvin, E. M. (1995). Effectiveness of culturally-focused and generic skills training approaches to alcohol and drug abuse prevention among minority adolescents: Two-Year follow-up results. *Psychology of Addictive Behaviors, 9,* 183–194.

Campanelli, P. C., Dielman, T. E., Shope, J. T., Butchart, A. T., & Renner, D.S. (1989). Pretest and treatment effects in an elementary school-based alcohol misuse prevention program. *Health Education Quarterly, 16,* 113–130.

Caplan, M., Weissberg, R. P., Grober, J. S., Sivo, P., Grady, K., & Jacoby, C. (1992). Social competence promotion with inner-city and suburban young adolescents: Effects of social adjustment and alcohol use. *Journal of Consulting & Clinical Psychology, 60,* 56–63.

Catalano, R. F., Hawkins, J. D., Krenz, C., Gillmore, M., Morrison, D., Wells, E., & Abbott, R. (1993). Using research to guide culturally appropriate drug abuse prevention. *Journal of Consulting & Clinical Psychology, 61,* 804–811.

Clayton, R. R., Cattarello, A. M., & Johnstone, B. M., (1996). The effectiveness of Drug Abuse Resistance Education (Project DARE): Five-year follow-up results. *Preventive Medicine, 25,* 307–318.

Degnan, E. J. (1972). An exploration into the relationship between depression and positive attitude toward drugs in young adolescents and an evaluation of a drug education program. *Dissertation Abstracts, 32,* 6614–6615.

Donaldson, S. I., Graham, J. W., & Hansen, W. B. (1994). Testing the generalizability of intervening mechanism theories: Understanding the effects of adolescent drug use prevention interventions. *Journal of Behavioral Medicine, 17,* 195–216.

Donaldson, S. I., Graham, J. W., Piccinin, A. M., & Hansen, W. B. (1995). Resistance-skills training and onset of alcohol use: Evidence for beneficial and potentially harmful effects in public schools and in private catholic schools. *Health Psychology, 14,* 291–300.

Donaldson, S. I., Sussman, S., MacKinnon, D. P., Severson, H. H., Glynn, T., Murray, D. M., & Stone, E. J., (1996). Drug abuse prevention programming: Do we know what content works? *American Behavioral Scientist, 39,* 868–883.

Dryfoos, J. G. (1993). Preventing substance use: Rethinking strategies. *American Journal of Public Health, 83,* 793–795.

Dukes, R. L., Ullman, J. B., & Stein, J. A. (1996). Three-year follow-up of drug abuse resistance education (DARE). *Evaluation Review, 20,* 49–66.

Eggert, L. L., Seyl, C. D., & Nicholas, L. J. (1990). Effects of a school-based prevention program for potential high school dropouts and drug abusers. *International Journal of the Addictions, 25,* 773–801.

Eggert, L. L., Thompson, E. A., Herting, J. R., Nicholas, L. J., & Dicker, BG. (1994). Preventing adolescent drug abuse and high school dropout through an intensive school-based social network development program. *American Journal of Health Promotion, 8,* 202–215.

Elias, M. J. (1997). Reinterpreting dissemination of prevention programs as widespread implementation with effectiveness and fidelity. In R. P. Weissberg, T. P. Gullotta, R. L. Hampton, B. A. Ryan, & G. R. Adams. (Eds.), *Healthy children 2010: Establishing preventive services. Issues in children's and families' lives* (pp. 253–289). Thousand Oaks, CA: Sage.

Ellickson, P. L., & Bell, R. M. (1990). Drug prevention in junior high: A multi-site longitudinal test. *Science, 247,* 1299–1305.

Ellickson, P. L. & Bell, R. M. (1990). Prospects for preventing drug abuse among young adolescents. *Science, 247,* 1299–1305.

Ellickson, P. L., Bell, R. M., & McGuigan, K. (1993). Preventing adolescent drug use: Long term results of a junior high program. *American Journal of Public Health, 83,* 856–861.

Ennett, S. T., Rosenbaum, D. P., Flewelling, R. L., Bieler, G. S., Ringwalt, C. L., & Bailey, S. L. (1994). Long-term evaluation of Drug Abuse Resistance Education. *Addictive Behaviors, 19,* 113–125.

Ennett, S. T., Tobler, N. S., Ringwalt, C. L., & Flewelling, R. L. (1994). How effective is Drug Abuse Resistance Education? A meta-analysis of Project DARE outcome evaluations. *American Journal of Public Health, 84,* 1394–1401.

Evans, R. I. (1976). Smoking in children: Developing a social psychological strategy of deterrence. *Preventive Medicine, 5,* 122–127.

Evans, R. I., Rozelle, R. M., Mittlemark, M. B., Hansen, W. B., Bane, A. L., & Havis, J. (1978). Deterring the onset of smoking in children: Knowledge of immediate physiological effects and coping with peer pressure, media pressure, and parent modelling. *Journal of Applied Social Psychology, 8,* 126–135.

Fishbein, M. (1977). Consumer beliefs and behavior with respect to cigarette smoking: A critical analysis of the public literature. In Federal Trade Commission Report to Congress pursuant to the Public Health Cigarette Smoking Act of 1976. Washington, DC: U.S. Government Printing Office.

Fisher, D. A., Armstrong, B. K., & DeKler, N. H. (1983). A randomized-controlled trial of education for prevention of smoking in 12-year-old children. In paper presented at the fifth World Conference on Smoking and Health. Winnipeg, Canada.

Flay, B. R., Keopke, D., Thomson, S. J., Santi, S., Best, J. A., & Brown, K. S. (1989). Long-term follow-up of the first Waterloo smoking prevention trial. *American Journal of Public Health, 79,* 1371–1376.

Flynn, B. S., Worden, J. K., Secker-Walker, R. H., Pirie, P. L., Badger, G. J., Carpenter, J. H., & Geller, B. M. (1994). Mass media and school interventions for cigarette smoking prevention: Effects 2 years after completion. *American Journal of Public Health, 84,* 1148–1150.

Flynn, B. S., Worden, J. K., Secker-Walker, S., Badger, G. J., Geller, B. M., & Costanza, M. C. (1992). Prevention of cigarette smoking through mass media intervention and school programs. *American Journal of Public Health, 82,* 827–834.

Gilchrist, L. D., & Schinke, S. P. (1983). Self-control skills for smoking prevention. In P. F. Engstrom & P. Anderson (Eds.). *Advances in Cancer Control.* New York: Alan R. Liss.

Graham, J. W., Johnson, C. A., Hansen, W. B., Flay, B. R., & Gee, M. (1990). Drug use prevention programs, gender, and ethnicity: Evaluation of three seventh-grade project SMART cohorts. *Preventive Medicine, 19,* 305–313.

Hall, N.,W., & Zigler, E. (1997). Drug abuse prevention efforts for young children: A review and critique of existing programs. *American Journal of Orthopsychiatry, 67,* 134–143.

Hamburg, B. A., Braemer, H. C., & Jahnke, W. A. (1975). Hierarchy of drug use in adolescence: Behavioral and attitudinal correlates of substantial drug use. *American Journal of Psychiatry, 132,* 1155–1167.

Hansen, W. B. (1992). School-based substance abuse prevention: A review of the state of the art in curriculum, 1980–1990. *Health Education Research: Theory & Practice, 7,* 403–430.

Hansen, W. B., Malotte, C. K., & Fielding, J. E. (1988). Evaluation of a tobacco and alcohol abuse prevention curriculum for adolescents. *Health Education Quarterly, 15,* 93–114.

Hansen, W. B., & McNeal, R. B. (1997). How DARE Works: An examination of program effects on mediating variables. *Health Education & Behavior, 24,* 165–176.

Hurd, P., Johnson, C. A., Pechacek, T., Bast, C. P., Jacobs, D., & Luepker, R. (1980). Prevention of cigarette smoking in 7th grade students. *Journal of Behavioral Medicine, 3,* 15–28.

Institute of Medicine, (1996). Prevention. *In Pathways of addiction: Opportunities in drug abuse research* (pp. 139–158). Washington, DC: National Academy Press.

Jessor, R., & Jessor, S. L. (1977). *Problem behavior and psychosocial development: A longitudinal study of youth.* New York: Academic Press.

Johnson, C. A., MacKinnon, D. P., & Pentz, M. A. (1996). Breadth of program and outcome effectiveness in drug abuse prevention. *American Behavioral Scientist, 39,* 884–896.

Johnson, C. A., Pentz, M. A., Weber, M. D., Dwyer, J. H., Baer, N., MacKinnon, D. P., & Hansen, W. B. (1990). Relative effectiveness of comprehensive community programming for drug abuse prevention with high-risk and low-risk adolescents. *Journal of Consulting & Clinical Psychology, 58,* 447–456.

Jones, C. L., & Battjes, R. J. (1985). *Etiology of drug abuse: Implications for prevention.* National Institute on Drug Abuse (Research Monograph No. 56). Washington, DC: Government Printing Office.

Kandel, D. (1975). Stages in adolescent involvement in drug use. *Science, 190,* 912–914.

Kandel, D. B. (1978). Convergences in prospective longitudinal surveys of drug use in normal populations. In D. B. Kandel (Ed.), *Longitudinal research on drug use: Empirical findings and methodological issues* (pp. 3–38). Washington, DC: Hemisphere (Halsted-Wiley).

Kearney, A. L., & Hines, M. H. (1980). Evaluation of the effectiveness of a drug prevention education program. *Journal of Drug Education, 10,* 127–134.

Kim, S. (1988). A short-and long-term evaluation of 'here's looking at you.'*II. Journal of Drug Education, 18,* 235–242.

Kinder, B. N., Pape, N. E., & Walfish, S. (1980). Drug and alcohol educational programs: A review of outcome studies. *International Journal of the Addictions, 15,* 1035–1054.

Kreutter, K. J., Gewirtz, J., Davenny, J. E., & Love, C. (1991). Drug and alcohol prevention project for sixth graders: First-year findings. *Adolescence, 26,* 287–292.

Luepker, R. V., Johnson, C. A., Murray, D. M., & Pechacek, T. F. (1983). Prevention of cigarette smoking: Three year follow-up of educational programs for youth. *Journal of Behavioral Medicine, 6,* 53–61.

MacKinnon, D. P., & Dwyer, J. D. (1993). Estimating mediating effects in prevention studies. *Evaluation Review, 17,* 144–158.

MacKinnon, D. P., Johnson, C. A., Pentz, M. A., Dwyer, J. H., Hansen, W. B., Flay, B. R., & Wang, E. Y. (1991). Mediating mechanisms in a school-based drug prevention program: First year effects of the Midwestern Prevention Project. *Health Psychology, 10,* 164–172.

Malvin, J. H., Moskowitz, J. M., Schaps, E., & Schaeffer, G. A. (1985). Evaluation of two school-based alternative programs. *Journal of Alcohol & Drug Education, 30,* 98–108.

McAlister, A., Perry, C. L., Killen, J., Slinkard, L. A., & Maccoby, N. (1980). Pilot study of smoking, alcohol, and drug abuse prevention. *American Journal of Public Health, 70,* 719–721.

McAlister, A., Perry, C. L., & Maccoby, N. (1979). Adolescent smoking: Onset and prevention. *Pediatrics, 63,* 650–658.

McGuire, W. J. (1964). Inducing resistance to persuasion: Some contemporary approaches. In L. Berkowitz (Ed.), *Advances in experimental social psychology* (pp. 192–227). New York: Academic Press.

McGuire, W. J. (1968). The nature of attitudes and attitude change. In G. Lindzey & E. Aronson (Eds.), *Handbook of social psychology* (pp. 136–314). Reading, MA: Addison-Wesley.

Meyer, R. E., & Mirin, S. M. (1979). *The heroin stimulus: Implications for a theory of addiction.* New York: Plenum Medical Book Co.

Moskowitz, J. M., Schaps, E., & Malvin, J. H. (1982). Process and outcome evaluation in primary prevention: The Magic Circle program. Evaluation Review, 6, 775–788.

Murray, D. M., Davis-Hearn, M., Goldman, A. I., Pirie, P., & Luepker, R. V. (1988). Four and five year follow-up results from four seventh-grade smoking prevention strategies. *Journal of Behavioral Medicine, 11,* 395–405.

Murray, D. M. Luepker, R. V., Johnson, C. A., Mittelmark, M. B. (1984). The prevention of cigarette smoking in children: A comparison of four strategies. *Journal of Applied Social Psychology, 14,* 274–288.

Murray, D. M., Pirie, P., Luepker, R. V., & Pallonen, U. (1989). Five and six-year follow-up results from four seventh-grade smoking prevention strategies. *Journal of Behavioral Medicine, 12,* 207–218.

Newcomb, M. D., & Bentler, P. M. (1988). *Consequences of adolescent drug use: Impact on the lives of young adults.* New York: Sage.

O'Donnell, J. H., Hawkins, J. D., Catalano, R. F., Abbott, R. D., & Day, L. E. (1995). Preventing school failure, drug use, and delinquency among low-income children: Long-term intervention in elementary school. *American Journal of Orthopsychiatry, 65,* 87–100.

O'Rourke, T. W., & Barr, S. L. (1974). Assessment of the effectiveness of the New York state drug curriculum guide with respect to drug attitudes. *Journal of Drug Education, 4,* 347–356.

Pentz, M. A. (1983). Prevention of adolescent substance abuse through social skill development. In T.J. Glynn, C. G. Leukefeld, & J. B. Ludford (Eds.), *Preventing adolescent drug abuse: Intervention strategies* (47th ed.) (pp. 195–232). Washington, DC: NIDA Research Monograph.

Pentz, M. A., Dwyer, J., MacKinnon, D., Flay, B. R., Hansen, W. B., Wang, E. Y., & Johnson, C. A. (1989). A multicommunity trial for primary prevention of adolescent drug abuse. *Journal of the American Medical Association, 261,* 3259–3266.

Pentz, M. A., Dwyer, J. H., MacKinnon, D. P., et al. (1989). A multicommunity trial for primary prevention of adolescent drug abuse: Effects on drug prevalence. *Journal of the American Medical Association, 261,* 3259–3266.

Pentz, M. A., Trebow, E. A., Hansen, W. B., MacKinnon, D. P., Dwyer, J. H., Flay, B. R., Daniels, S., Cormack, C., & Johnson, C. A. (1990). Effects of program implementation on adolescent drug use behavior: The Midwestern Prevention Project (MPP). *Evaluation Review, 14,* 264–289.

Perry, C., Killen, J., Slinkard, L. A., & McAlister, A. L. (1983). Peer teaching and smoking prevention among junior high students. *Adolescence, 9,* 277–281.

Perry, C. L., Kelder, S. H., Murray, D. M., & Klepp, K. I. (1992). Community-wide smoking prevention: Long-term outcomes of the Minnesota heart health program and the class of 1989 study. *American Journal of Public Health, 82,* 1210–1216.

Resnicow, K., & Botvin, G. J. (1993). School-based substance use prevention programs: Why do effects decay? *Preventive Medicine, 22,* 484–490.

Richardson, D. W., Nader, P. R., Rochman, K. J., & Friedman, S. B. (1972). Attitudes of fifth grade students to illicit psychoactive drugs. *Journal of School Health, 42,* 389–391.

Rohrbach, L. A., Hodgson, C. S., Broder, B. I., Montgomery, S. B. et al. (1994). Parental participation in drug abuse prevention: Results from the Midwestern Prevention Project. *Journal of Research on Adolescence, 4,* 295–317.

Rohrbach, L. A., Hodgson, C. S., Broder, B. I., & Montogomery, S. B. (1994). Parental participation in drug abuse prevention: Results from the Midwestern Prevention Project. Special Issue: Preventive alcohol abuse among adolescents: Preintervention and intervention research. *Journal of Research on Adolescence, 4,* 295–317.

Rollins, S. A., Rubin, R., Hardy-Blake, B. Allen, P., Marcil, R., Groomes, E., & Winningham, K. (1994). Project K.I.C.K., a school-based drug education research project: Peers, parents, and kids. *Journal of Alcohol & Drug Education, 39,* 75–86.

Rosenbaum, D. P., & Hanson, G. S. (1998). Assessing the effects of school-based drug education: A six-year multilevel analysis of Project D.A.R.E. *Journal of Research in Crime & Delinquency, 35,* 381–412.

Rosenbaum, D. P., Flewelling, R. L., Bailey, S. L., Ringwalt, C. L., & Wilkinson, D. L. (1994). Cops in the classroom: A longitudinal evaluation of drug abuse resistance education (DARE). *Journal of Research in Crime & Delinquency, 31,* 3–31.

Rosenblitt, D. L., & Nagey, D. A. (1973). The use of medical manpower in a seventh grade drug education program. *Journal of Drug Education, 3,* 39–56.

Rundall, T. G., & Bruvold, W. H. (1988). A meta-analysis of school-based smoking and alcohol use prevention programs. *Health Education Quarterly, 15,* 317–334.

Schaps, E., Bartolo, R. D., Moskowitz, J., Palley, C. S., & Churgin, S. (1981). A review of 127 drug abuse prevention program evaluations. *Journal of Drug Issues, 11,* 17–43.

Schaps, E., Moskowitz, J. M., Malvin, J. H., & Scheffer, G. H. (1986). Evaluation of seven school-based prevention programs: A final report on the Napa Project. *International Journal of the Addictions, 21,* 1081–1112.

Schaps, E., Moskowitz, J. M., Condon, J. W., & Malvin, J. H. (1982). Process and outcome evaluation of a drug education course. *Journal of Drug Education, 12,* 353–364.

Schaps, E., Moskowitz, J. M. Condon, J. W., & Malvin, J. H. (1984). A process and outcome evaluation of an effective teacher training primary prevention program. *Journal of Alcohol & Drug Education, 29,* 35–64.

Schinke, S. P. (1984). Preventing teenage pregnancy. In M. Hersen, R. M. Eisler, & P. M. Miller (Eds.), *Progress in behavior modification* (16th ed.) (pp. 31–63). New York: Academic Press.

Schinke, S. P., & Gilchrist, L. D. (1983). Primary prevention of tobacco smoking. *Journal of School Health, 53,* 416–419.

Schinke, S. P., & Gilchrist, L. D. (1984). Preventing cigarette smoking with youth. *Journal of Primary Prevention, 5,* 48–56.

Shope, J. T., Copeland, L. A., Marcoux, B. C., & Kamp, M. E. (1996). Effectiveness of a school-based substance abuse prevention program. *Journal of Drug Education, 26,* 323–337.

Shope, J. T., Dielman, T. E., Butchart, A. T., Campanelli, P. C., & Kloska, D. D. (1992). An elementary school-based alcohol misuse prevention program: A follow-up evaluation. *Journal of Studies on Alcohol, 53,* 106–121.

Silvia, E. S., & Thorne, J. (1997). School-based drug prevention programs: A longitudinal study in selected school districts. *Final report to U.S. Department of Education.* Research Triangle Institute.

Snow, D. L., Tebes, J. K., Arthur, M. W., & Tapasak, R. C. (1992). Two-year follow-up of a social-cognitive intervention to prevent substance use. *Journal of Drug Education, 22,* 101–114.

Stuart, J. (1974). Teaching facts about drugs: Pushing or preventing? *Journal of Educational Psychology, 66,* 189–201.

Sussman, S. (1996). Development of a school-based drug abuse prevention curriculum for high-risk youth. *Journal of Psychoactive Drugs, 28,* 169–182.

Sussman, S., Dent, C. W., Simon, T. R., Stacy, A. W., Galaif, E. R., Moss, M. A., Craig, S., & Johnson, C. A. (1995). Immediate impact of social influence-oriented substance abuse prevention curricula in traditional and continuation high schools. *Drugs & Society, 8,* 65–81.

Sussman, S., Dent, C. W., Stacy, A. W., & Sun, P. (1993). Project Towards No Tobacco Use: 1-year behavior outcomes. *American Journal of Public Health, 83,* 1245–1250.

Swisher, J. D., Crawford, J. L., Goldstein, R., & Yura, M. (1971). Drug education: Pushing or preventing? *Peabody Journal of Education, 49,* 68–75.

Telch, M. J. Killen, J. D., McAlister, A. L., Perry, C. L., & Maccoby, N. (1982). Long-term follow-up of a pilot project on smoking prevention with adolescents. *Journal of Behavioral Medicine, 5,* 1–8.

Thompson, E. A., Horn, M., Herting, J. R., & Eggert, L. L. (1997). Enhancing outcomes in an indicated drug prevention program for high-risk youth. *Journal of Drug Education, 27,* 19–41.

Tobler, N. S. (1986). Meta-analysis of 143 adolescent drug prevention programs: Quantitative outcome results of program participants compared to a control or comparison group. *Journal of Drug Issues, 16,* 537–567.

Tobler, N. S., & Stratton, H. H. (1997). Effectiveness of school-based drug prevention programs: A meta-analysis of the research. *Journal of Primary Prevention, 18,* 71–128.

Wechsler, H. (1976). Alcohol intoxication and drug use among teenagers. *Journal of Studies on Alcohol, 37,* 1672–1677.

CHAPTER 4

Dissemination of Research-Based Family Interventions for the Prevention of Substance Abuse

Karol L. Kumpfer
Steve Alder

INTRODUCTION

Drug abuse and associated adolescent problem behaviors, such as delinquency, unwanted pregnancy, and school failure, are weakening this country economically, socially, and spiritually. This chapter discusses the current status of drug abuse among adolescents and research suggesting that parents and other family members are more influential than previously thought in positively influencing adolescent behaviors. However, despite their best intentions, some parents have had little chance to learn how to be effective parents. And although more than 25 model family-strengthening programs have been shown to be effective in reducing substance abuse and its childhood precursors (such as conduct disorders, violence and aggression, depression and shyness, lack of social competencies, and school failure), these programs are not being implemented as often as are untested, commercially marketed parenting programs. This chapter stresses the need for increased investment by the federal government and its state and private-sector partners in learning how to improve the dissemination and adoption of science-based models of family-strengthening interventions.

KAROL L. KUMPFER AND STEVE ALDER • Department of Family and Preventive Medicine, University of Utah, Salt Lake City, Utah 84112

ADOLESCENT DRUG ABUSE

Despite 12 years of success in reducing drug use among youth, from an all-time high in 1979, adolescent substance use increased in the United States for 7 years beginning in 1991 before declining slightly in the past few years (Johnston, O'Malley, & Bachman, 2000). The National Household Survey (DHHS, 1998) verified staggeringly high rates of increase in substance abuse among adolescents, particularly in the youngest group of teenagers. For instance, although the regular use (30-day use) of illicit drugs increased only 7% in the total population, it increased 27% between 1996 and 1997 among 12- to 17-year-olds and 73% among 12- to 13-year-olds. Regular marijuana use increased 32% in 12- to 17-year-olds. In addition, there was a 53% increase in new adolescent users of marijuana. Today we have a greater number of 12- to 17-year-olds initiating marijuana use than at the peak of the marijuana epidemic in 1979. The percentage of regular marijuana users in high school seniors more than doubled from a low point of 11.9% in 1992 to a high of 23.1% by 1999 (Johnston et al., 2000). The percentage of high school seniors reporting regular tobacco use increased in the 1990s to 34.6%, but decreased last year to 31.4%. Being drunk on alcohol has remained relatively stable at about one-third in the past 10 years among high school seniors; but adolescents have dramatically increased their use of methamphetamine, club drugs, and heroin. Worldwide heroin use increased fivefold in 5 years in the mid-1990s among youth and adults, from 68 million to 325 million users. The bulk of the 171 million new users of heroin were adolescents and young adults, who appeared to believe that either smoking or snorting heroin is not dangerous. This study also finds that drug-abusing youth are also engaging in aggressive, violent, and delinquent behaviors (SAMHSA, 1998).

What can be done to reduce this high rate of illicit drug use among adolescents? In the past 20 years, prevention researchers have discovered a number of effective strategies, including family-strengthening approaches, to reduce alcohol and drug abuse in youth (Falco, 1992; Kumpfer, 1997; Sloboda & David, 1997; Tobler & Stratton, 1997). Unfortunately, less effective prevention strategies—such as Drug Abuse Resistance Education (DARE)—have been widely implemented in schools (Ennett et al., 1994; Harrington et al., 2000), instead of coordinated, comprehensive prevention programs that can reduce risk and increase protective factors and drug resilience (NIDA/Kumpfer, 2001; Kumpfer & Hunter, in press. These alarming drug abuse statistics should be a wake-up call urging Americans to invest more heavily in drug prevention research and wide-scale dissemination of effective prevention programs. We also need more basic and applied research to determine the best substance abuse prevention programs for diverse populations (ethnic and cultural groups, rural youth) and for girls as well as for boys. Although few prevention interventions have been found to be effective for girls, family interventions are quite effective among girls of all ages and levels of family dysfunction in reducing a wide range of risk factors related to drug use and delinquency (Ashery, Robertson, & Kumpfer, 1997; Bry et al., 1997; CSAP, 1998; Kazdin, 1993; Kumpfer, 1997; Kumpfer and Alvarado, 1995, 1998, in press).

WHY FAMILY-STRENGTHENING
INTERVENTIONS ARE NEEDED

The effectiveness of family interventions should come as no surprise, since many people blame the weakening of the American family for increases in substance abuse and delinquency. The DHHS America's Children 2001 report finds that more children than ever—26%—are living in single-parent homes, most headed by females. While only 8% of children from married-couple families experienced poverty in 1999, forty-two percent of children in single-mother families suffered poverty during the same year. The number of children being reared in high-income homes (at least $68,116 for a family of four) doubled to 29% in the past 20 years. But this is not necessarily good news because these parents are working more, making it harder to spend time with their children. Parents today spend about 4.6 hours more a week working than they did in 1989, which results in less time devoted to parenting. The average amount of time per day spent talking with children has dropped to only about 7 minutes per day. In fact, most public opinion surveys show that Americans believe that faulty parenting is the primary reason for the increase in the past decade in drug use and delinquency. Recent research by Resnick and associates (1997), through their National Longitudinal Adolescent Health Survey, suggests that parents have a greater impact on their adolescents' behaviors than previously thought. Tests of the Social Ecology Model of Adolescent Drug Use (Kumpfer & Turner, 1990/1991; Turner, Sales, & Springer, 1998) suggest that parents have an early influence on the developmental pathways that lead to drug use. Although peer influence is the major reason adolescents initiate negative behaviors (Kumpfer & Turner, 1990/1991; Newcomb, 1992, 1995; Oetting, 1992; Oetting & Beauvais, 1987), positive parent–child relationships, parental monitoring, and disapproval of inappropriate behaviors and of drug use are the major reasons youngsters do not use drugs or engage in delinquent or unhealthy behaviors (Ary et al., Smolkowski, 1999; Coombs, Paulson, & Richardson, 1991; Turner, Sales, & Springer, 1998).

NEED TO IMPROVE THE DISSEMINATION
OF EFFECTIVE INTERVENTIONS

While researchers have identified effective family intervention programs, these scientifically tested prevention programs are not being implemented to the same extent as are many untested, commercially marketed programs. About 60% of all prevention programs are practitioner-developed, and 30% are commercially marketed. Less than 10% of all prevention programs implemented in schools or communities are scientifically validated, and only about a quarter of them (or 2.5% of all prevention programs) are implemented with enough fidelity to produce successful outcomes (Kumpfer & Hunter, in press). As stressed by Schorr (1988), research has identified effective programs; but policymakers appear to lack the political will to bring these programs to scale and promote their widespread adoption. Researchers are frustrated that their science-based programs are not being adopted rapidly enough to reduce problem behaviors among youth (Biglan et al., in press). Current dissemination infrastructures are insufficient to support the delivery of successful prevention programs that meet community needs (Backer & Rogers, 1999; Biglan & Taylor, 2000). The components required for such an infrastructure are not well defined. Furthermore, what is needed to effectively move programs from a research to a community setting is not easily specified. However, principles of effective dissemination have been distilled from more than 10,000 studies in the past 75 years (Backer, 1991; Backer, David, & Soucy, 1995). These principles include (1) *user-friendly and easily accessible communication,* such as newsletters or website decision support systems rather than academic research journals; (2) *user-friendly evaluations* demonstrating that innovation works better than alternatives; (3) *sufficient resources* to implement the new innovation; and (4) *systems rewarding and facilitating change* to new innovation.

    One of the most effective dissemination systems for putting scientific information into practice in this country is probably the U.S. Department of Agriculture's system of land-grant colleges and Cooperative Extension Service that spends a dollar on dissemination for every dollar spent on research (Backer, 2000; Rogers, 1995). Hence, adequate funding for dissemination is clearly needed. It is also clear that policymakers need to fund applied research (Phase 4 studies) and applications of research (Phase 5 studies) either to support the translation of research into practice (Jansen, Glynn, & Howard, 1996) or to bridge the gap between research and practice. Unless federal and state agencies fund this "bridge," providers will continue to adopt glossy but untested programs (Kumpfer & Kaftarian, 2000). In addition, we must invest in research on how to effectively disseminate prevention programs known to work. Beyond research, we must increase funding to states and communities that will implement science-based programs and policies and invest in a nationwide training and technical assistance system to get effective practices adopted with fidelity by states, communities, schools, religious communities, businesses, and families.

Scientific reviews of the research and practice literature (CSAP, 1998; Kumpfer & Alvarado, 1995, 1998) suggest that many of the commercially marketed programs do not have effectiveness results and that some can actually be counterproductive (Norman & Turner, 1993). According to Norman and Turner (1993), approaches that have the potential to be counterproductive include interventions based on information-only models and a few of the alternative activities that involve youth with adults or peers with pro-drug-use norms (Swisher & Hu, 1983). Prevention programs that group high-risk youth in youth-only groups without experienced adult leadership can also have serious negative effects (Dishion & Andrews, 1995). Additionally, child psychodynamic interventions, compared to structural family interventions, can result in deterioration of family functioning (Szapocznik et al., 1989). According to Szapocznik (1996, 1997), interventions that do not work with the total family system have the potential to weaken the family and lead to increased drug use. Because child-only interventions, so popular in drug abuse prevention, have the potential to bring about negative effects on family protective factors for drug use, prevention experts are calling for increased funding of family-focused prevention interventions.

THE POWERFUL INFLUENCE OF FAMILIES ON YOUTH

According to Bry and associates (1997): "The critical role of family factors is acknowledged in virtually every psychological theory of substance abuse" (Brook, 1990; Bry, 1983; Catalano & Hawkins, 1996; Dembo et al., 1979; Dishion, Reid, & Patterson, 1988; Elliot, Huizinga, & Menard, 1989; Hawkins, Catalano, Jr., & Associates, 1992; Jessor, 1993; Kandel & Davies, 1992; Kaplan & Johnson, 1992; Kellam et al., 1983; Kumpfer, 1987; Newcomb & Bentler, 1989; Oetting & Lynch, 1993; Wills, Vaccaro, & McNamara, 1992). Family variables are a consistently strong predictor of antisocial and delinquent behaviors (Loeber & Stouthamer-Loeber, 1986; McCord, 1991; Tolan & Loeber, 1993; Tolan, Guerra, & Kendall, 1995a,b). In fact, parental support is one of the most powerful predictors of reduced substance use among minority youth (King et al., 1992). Dishion, French, and Patterson (1995) and Hansen and associates (1987) have also found that increased parental supervision is a major mediator of peer influences. Models testing the aspects of family dynamics related to problem behaviors among youth (antisocial behavior, substance abuse, high-risk sex, and academic failure) find that family conflict is associated with reduced family involvement. Reduced involvement in turn predicts later inadequate parental supervision and possible association with peers who are involved in deviance. Ary and associates (1999) found direct paths from inadequate parental supervision and having deviant peers to problem behaviors, suggesting that not all family risk processes are mediated by deviant peer involvement.

The strongest pathway to drug use in high-risk youth involves family risk or lack of family protective factors, according to data analyzed on 8,500 youth participating in a Center for

Substance Abuse Prevention (CSAP) cross-site study of interventions directed to youth at risk for substance abuse (Turner et al., 1998). Positive family relations were related to improved family supervision and monitoring that led to anti-drug family and peer norms. In the final pathway to drug use, such norms were found to be associated with reduced or no drug use. These studies indicate that parenting and family interventions that decrease family conflict, enhance family involvement, and increase parental monitoring should reduce problem behaviors, including substance abuse (Mayer, 1995).

Family Protective and Resilience Factors

The probability of youngsters having developmental problems increases rapidly as risk factors outnumber protective factors (Dunst & Trivette, 1994; Rutter, 1990, 1993). Accordingly, the objective of family-focused prevention programs should be to decrease risk factors while increasing ongoing protective mechanisms. According to Bry and associates (1998), the five major types of protective family factors are (1) supportive parent–child relationships (Dishion et al., 1988; Werner & Smith, 1992), (2) positive discipline methods (Catalano et al., 1993; Dishion et al., 1988; Kellam et al., 1983), (3) monitoring and supervision (Ary et al., 1999; Chilcoat, Dishion, & Antony, 1995; Loeber & Stouthamer-Loeber, 1986), (4) family advocacy for the children (Brunswick, Messeri, & Titus, 1992; Kandel & Davies, 1992; Krohn & Thornberry, 1993), and (5) seeking information and support for the benefit of the children (Nye, Zucker, & Fitzgerald, 1995).

Resilience researchers (Glantz & Johnson, 1999; Kumpfer, 1999; Luthar, 1993; Werner, 1986) and those who focus on family strengths (Gary, 1996; Dunst & Trivette, 1994) identified similar protective mechanisms that help children from very high-risk families of alcohol or drug abusers to successfully avoid drug use and develop positive life adaptations (Johnson & Leff, 1999; Walker et al., in press). For instance, the characteristics of strongly resilient African-American families have been found to be (1) a strong economic base, (2) achievement orientation, (3) role adaptability, (4) spirituality, (5) extended family bonds, (6) racial pride, (7) respect and love, (8) resourcefulness, (9) community involvement, and (10) family unity (Gary et al., 1983). The challenge to family intervention researchers is to develop and test interventions that effectively address this broad range of protective factors.

LITERATURE AND PRACTICE SEARCHES FOR EFFECTIVE FAMILY INTERVENTIONS

Researchers have identified and provided empirical evidence for the effectiveness of family-based programs for the prevention of drug use and other adolescent problem behaviors, such as delinquency, teen pregnancy, and school failure (Alexander, Holtzworth-Munroe, & Jameson, 1994; Kaftarian & Kumpfer, 2000; Kumpfer & Alvarado, in press; Liddle & Dakof, 1995; Lochman, 2000; Serketich & Dumas, 1996; Szapocznik, 1996; Taylor & Biglan, 1998). Etiological research (Ary et al., 1999) suggests that common family and peer factors influence all of these problem behaviors; hence it is not surprising that family interventions effective in improving family relations, parental monitoring and supervision, and parent–child attachment should impact drug use, delinquency, and teen pregnancy.

These findings suggest that there are no simple, short-term solutions, such as teaching youngsters to "Just Say No." The most effective prevention programs involve complex and multicomponent approaches that address the early precursors of drug use and problem behaviors, with the most effective approaches often being those that change the family, school, or community environment in long-lasting and positive ways. Skills training programs, for example, are more effective than didactic, lecture-style programs (Tobler & Stratton, 1997). Information alone has not been found to have an impact on behavior change unless it is combined with time for discussion, experiential practice, role playing, and homework to solidify behavioral changes.

Other findings show that comprehensive family programs that combine social and life skills training for children and youth (to improve their social and academic competencies) with parent skills training programs (to improve supervision and nurturing) are the most effective in influencing a broad range of family risk and protective factors for drug use (Kumpfer, 1996a). Programs that ignore context and work only with youth have been found in some cases to damage family relationships (Szapocznik, 1997; Szapocznik, Rio et al., 1989). Such programs often group high-risk youth and can have negative contagion effects (Dishion & Andrews, 1995) unless skillful adult leaders are used to control group norms and acting-out behaviors (Eggerts, personal communication, November 1996).

The CSAP Prevention Enhancement Protocol System (PEPS) was developed by Prakash Grover to determine whether there is sufficient scientific evidence that a particular approach (not a specific program) is effective for drug abuse prevention. To date, scientific reviews have been conducted for tobacco-control approaches, alcohol-control approaches, family-based prevention approaches, and workplace approaches, with a school-based PEPS currently under development. The family-based PEPS (CSAP/Family PEPS, 1998) involved a national expert panel, co-chaired by Karol Kumpfer at the University of Utah and Jose Szapocznik at the University of Miami. After an extensive review of all published research articles on family approaches, categorization of programs into different types of family approaches, and application of effectiveness criteria, the panel determined that there was sufficient evidence to conclude that only four family approaches meet the National Institute of Cancer standard for "strong level of evidence of effectiveness." The four family intervention strategies effective in reducing risk factors and increasing protective factors for drug use include the following.

Behavioral Parent Training

This highly structured universal, or selective, prevention approach (Mrazek & Haggerty, 1994) includes parents only, generally in small groups led by a skilled trainer or clinician following a curriculum guide over at least twelve 1- to 2-hour sessions. Sessions include review of homework, video presentations of good and bad ways of parenting, short lectures and discussions to extract parenting principles, interactive exercises, role-playing of the parenting behavior to be changed, charting and monitoring of parenting and children's behaviors, and assignment of homework. Most behavioral parenting programs begin with improving the parent–child relationship by increasing rewards for good behavior and ignoring unwanted behavior, increased therapeutic play time, improving parent monitoring of the child's behaviors, chore charts, reward systems, improved communications with clearer requests and consequences, and ending with several sessions on effective discipline through time-outs or removal of privileges. Gerald Patterson and associates (Patterson, 1974; Patterson & Reid, 1973; Patterson, Chamberlain, & Reid, 1982) pioneered and disseminated behavioral parent training. Webster-Stratton (1981, 1982, 1990a,b) has developed very effective video-based versions for preschool and elementary school children that has been replicated with positive results by Taylor and associates (1998). Culturally appropriate versions of parent training have also been developed by various researchers for implementation in schools or communities (Kumpfer et al., in press). Dumas (1989) reviewed parent training program research and concludes, on the basis of Patterson and Fleishman's (1979) research, that such programs are clearly effective in reducing children's negative behaviors and improving parenting practices, but only if they are longer than 31 hours for average families and 100 hours for low-income, crisis-prone families. A meta-analysis of 26 behavioral parent training studies found the effect sizes for children's outcomes were very high, averaging 0.84 for parental report, 0.85 for observer report, 0.73 for teacher report, and 0.44 for parents' reports on their own behavioral and emotional changes (Serketich & Dumas, 1996).

To increase effectiveness in changing children's behaviors, most program developers are now combining behavioral parent training with children's social skills training, such as the Preventive Treatment Program for 7- to 9-year-old boys assessed as having disruptive behaviors in school (Tremblay et al., 1996). A true experimental evaluation by Kazdin, Siegel, and Bass (1992) of a combined approach compared with parent-training-only or children's-skills-training-only demonstrated, at a 1-year follow-up, an increased reduction in aggression and antisocial and delinquent behaviors in 7- to 13-year-old girls and boys, and reduced stress and overall dysfunction in the parents.

Family Skills Training or Behavioral Family Therapy

This universal, selective, or indicated multicomponent prevention approach combines (1) behavioral parent training, (2) children's social and life skills training, and (3) family-relationship-enhancement and communication practice sessions. Typically, the format involves the family coming to a community center, school, or church, and then for the first hour splitting into the parent's and children's groups. In the second hour, the parents and children are reunited in two multifamily groups. Each group is led by one of the children's trainers and one of the parent trainers. The parents and children practice together what they learned in the first hour. Family meetings are implemented and practiced. Parents are taught special therapeutic play during "Child's Game" to improve their child-play skills. Using intervention strategies developed by Forehand and McMahon (1981), the parents learn through observation, direct practice with immediate feedback by trainers and videotape, and trainer reinforcement on how to improve positive play by following the child's lead and not correcting, bossing, criticizing, or directing. Teaching parents therapeutic play has been found to improve parent–child attachment and improve child behaviors in psychiatrically disturbed and behaviorally disordered children (Egeland & Erickson, 1987; 1990; Kumpfer, Molgaard, & Spoth, 1996). After the parents master special play, they begin family communication sessions and finally practice effective discipline and request techniques to improve compliance.

Contents of the children's skills training program often include identification of feelings, anger and emotional management, accepting and giving feedback and criticism or praise, problem solving, decision making, assertion and peer-resistance skills, communication skills, and how to make and keep positive friends. Recruitment and retention are sometimes better with this approach. The children encourage the parents to sign up or stay in the program because they do not want to miss their friends. Food, transportation, and childcare are often provided to reduce barriers to attendance.

Family skills training is one type of family support currently gaining popularity. Examples include the Strengthening Families Program (Kumpfer, DeMarsh, & Child, 1989; Kumpfer et al., 2002) with versions for substance-abusing parents, African-American (Aktan, Kumpfer, & Turner, 1996), Hispanic families of 6- to 12-year-olds, and rural families of preteens and teens

(Kumpfer et al., 1996; Kumpfer, Williams, & Baxley, 1997; Spoth, Redmond, & Lepper, 1999); Focus on Families (Haggerty, Mills, & Catalano, 1991) for methadone maintenance parents; the Nurturing Program (Bavolek, Comstock, & McLaughlin, 1983) for physically and sexually abusive parents; Families and Schools Together (McDonald, 1993; McDonald et al., 1991) for high-risk students; and the Family Effectiveness Training (Szapocznik et al., 1985) for Hispanic adolescents. See Kumpfer (1993) and Kumpfer and Alvarado (1995, 1998) for reviews of these promising family programs.

Other researchers are using these broad-based family skills programs as part of even more comprehensive school-based, intervention strategies. The FAST TRACK program (Bierman, Greenberg, & the Conduct Problems Prevention Research Group (CPPRG), 1996; McMahon, Slough, & the CPPRG, 1996), one of the largest prevention intervention research projects ever funded by the National Institute of Mental Health, is one example. This selective prevention program, used with high-risk kindergartners nominated by their teachers because of such risk factors as conduct disorders, is being implemented at several different sites with a large team of nationally recognized prevention specialists. FAST TRACK includes McMahon's behavioral parent training, which is also incorporated in the Strengthening Families Program. Greenberg (1998) reported finding moderate effectiveness of FAST TRACK's multiple components on risk and protective factors.

Family Therapy

This indicated prevention approach is typically implemented for youth diagnosed with emotional or behavioral problems, such as conduct disorder, depression, and school or social problems, that if not treated can lead to more severe problems, such as delinquency or drug use (Liddle & Dakof, 1995). These programs are sometimes called "family-based, empirically supported treatments." They have been found to have preventive value for younger siblings because of positive changes made in the maladaptive family processes (Alexander, Robbins, & Sexton, 2000). These clinical interventions are conducted by trained clinicians or interns under supervision in a clinic. In the CSAP review, only four family therapy models were found to be effective for the prevention of substance abuse, namely, Jose Szapocznik's *Structural Family Therapy,* James Alexander and Bruce Parson's *Functional Family Therapy* (1982), and Don Gordon's computer interactive version used in juvenile courts called *Parenting Adolescents Wisely* (Gordon et al., 1998), and Howard Liddle's *Family Therapy* (Liddle et al., 2001).

In-Home Family Support

The CSAP Family PEPS (1998) concluded that there was only a moderate amount of evidence for in-home family support programs that often provide in-home case managers or parenting help from home visitors. While there was sufficient evidence of moderate effectiveness of family support programs with families of children from birth to 5 years of age (Yoshikawa, 1994), there does not appear to be enough evidence of effectiveness with older children, since most of these programs are tailored for working with new parents of infants and toddlers. A more recent meta-analysis (Tobler & Kumpfer, 2000) found that the effect sizes for 14 in-home family support programs were very large, averaging a 1.62 effect size (ES). This is a much larger effect size than the other types of family strengthening programs, possibly because of the intensity, dosage, and high cost of these programs.

Interventions with insufficient evidence of effectiveness for school-aged youth (5 years and up) include parent education characterized by didactic knowledge-only approaches and affect-based parent training (CSAP/Family PEPS, 1998). Programs that involve parents in supporting their children in completing in-home school homework assignments on drug prevention have recently been finding positive results for little cost (about $140 per family) (Bauman et al., 2001). The objectives of these programs are to increase parent and child communication and sharing of family substance use norms. In-school programs are only able to attract about one-third of parents even with incentives (Grady, Gersick, & Boratynski, 1985). If parents are only requested to complete homework assignments at home with their children, researchers find about 66 to 94% of parents are willing to participate (Flay et al., 1987; Perry et al., 1989, 1990; Rohrbach et al., in press). Bauman and associates (2001) found that 84% of families completed at least one of four Family Matters booklets at home. With phone support (averaging eight calls) by health educators, 62% of families completed all four booklets after devoting about 1 hour to each.

FAMILY INTERVENTIONS THAT ADDRESS RISK AND PROTECTIVE FACTORS

An analysis of the different types of parenting and family programs (Kumpfer, 1996a) found that outcomes differed by type of intervention. For instance, parenting skills training programs that stress effective discipline techniques and ignore disruptive or coercive child behaviors are effective in reducing coercive family dynamics (Webster-Stratton, 1981, 1982, 1990a, 1996; Webster-Stratton, Kolpacoff, & Hollingsworth, 1988). Behavior parenting programs that stress improved parental monitoring do, in fact, improve parental monitoring (Dishion & Andrews, 1995; Dishion, Kavanagh, & Kiesner, 1996; Dishion, Li, et al., 1996). Behavioral parent training programs, if of sufficient dosage (45 hours for high-risk families), are generally effective in reducing children's conduct disorder (Kumpfer, 1996a). Family therapy and family skills training programs are generally most effective in improving family communications, family control imbalances, and family relationships (CSAP/PEPS, 1998). In-home family-support or parent-support programs improve social support (Yoshikawa, 1994). In-home or office-based case management family services are effective in increasing a family's access to needed services. Parent education programs are effective in improving parental knowledge and awareness of parenting issues but do not necessarily change parental or children's behaviors—the most important test of an effective program (Falco, 1992). Children's social skills training added to parenting and family programs improves children's pro-social skills (Kumpfer, Williams, & Baxley, 1997) but can have a detrimental effect on acting-out behaviors when high-risk youth are aggregated together (Kumpfer, Gottfredson, & Alvarado, 2001).

PRINCIPLES OF EFFECTIVE FAMILY-FOCUSED INTERVENTIONS

Because these reviews suggest there is no one best family intervention program, providers in the field must carefully select the best program for their target population. This means they must have guidelines for determining the most effective program from a larger number of programs. NIDA has specified a number of prevention principles that can be used to guide that selection process (Sloboda & David, 1997). Parenting and family interventions must also be tailored to the developmental stage of the child and the types of risk factors in the families served. However, many ultimately fail to have long-term impact on negative outcomes, such as delinquency and drug use, in special high-risk populations, because they are not strong enough to impact the large number of risk and protective factors affecting these children. Some general principles for best practices in family programs to have maximum impact on improving parenting, family relationships, and youth functioning are as follows:

1. *Comprehensive* interventions are most effective at modifying a broad range of risk and protective factors in children.

Interventions that focus on the entire range of developmental outcomes of the child (cognitive, behavioral, social, emotional, physical, and spiritual) by fostering improvements in all environmental domains (society/culture, community/neighborhood, school, peer group, and family/extended family) demonstrate increased effectiveness in bringing about positive developmental changes. Our research reviews (Kumpfer, 1996a; Kumpfer, 1997) suggest that many programs are effective in the areas they target for changes in youth, parents, or families, but that many focus too narrowly and hence have limited results. As mentioned previously, programs combining parent training and children's skills training are more comprehensive in addressing more risk and protective factors and thus have been found in experimental designs to have increased effectiveness (Kazdin et al., 1992; Kumpfer et al., 1996).

2. *Family-focused* programs are more effective than programs that focus only on parents or children.

The first wave of child development interventions taught therapists, teachers, prevention specialists, and others to provide enrichment or therapeutic experiences for children of deficient parents. In order to maximize dosage and reduce cost, the second phase of child development interventions focused on training the parent or caretaker to better nurture and care for the child's needs. As the concept of comprehensive prevention or treatment interventions dealing with many different precursor domains emerged, interventions addressing the child, parent, and interactive family system became more popular. Research comparing the effectiveness of these three types of programs on the broader range of children's antisocial and pro-social behaviors finds the combined approach of all three programs to be most effective (DeMarsh & Kumpfer, 1985; Kumpfer, Gottfredson, & Alvarado, 2001). A number of early-childhood education program reviews (Yoshikawa, 1994) also concluded that comprehensive, holistic, family-focused programs show great potential and should be the central target of future research (Mitchell, Weiss, & Schultz, 1995).

3. *Sufficient dosage* or intensity is critical for effectiveness.

The needier the family in terms of number of risk factors, the more time will be needed to modify dysfunctional family processes. Time must be allowed for developing trust, determining the family's needs, providing or locating support services for basic needs, and comprehensively addressing deficit areas (CSAP, 1993). Research (Patterson & Fleishman, 1979) suggests that to produce longitudinal effectiveness, the family intervention must be of sufficient dosage (at least 31 hours with average families, 45 hours for high-risk families, and up to 100 hours for low-income, crisis-prone families). Kazdin (1987, 1995) estimates that at least 30 to 40 contact hours are needed to bring about a positive and lasting impact for family programs, particularly because high-risk families frequently miss sessions and have difficulty implementing the skills they have been taught (Kumpfer & Alvarado, 1995; Kumpfer & DeMarsh, 1985). Some parent and family programs fail to have much impact because they do not spend enough time teaching each skill or principle. Skills training interventions need to build on prior learned skills and require demonstration of those skills while simultaneously teaching new skills. Many parent education or training interventions fail with high-risk families because they are too short to really reduce risk-producing processes and behaviors and increase protective processes and behaviors. Short-term parent education programs are essentially for normal families. These short-term programs often stress that they must be short to get parents to attend. While this assumption may be true for very busy working parents of children with few problems, it is not as true of high-risk or in-crisis families who want help.

    4. Family programs should be *long term* and enduring.

While a few tips on improving parent–child interactions can be effective in general populations of functional families, short-term interventions have little effect on high-risk or in-crisis families. Such efforts provide only a temporary reduction of symptoms rather than long-term solutions (CSAP/Family PEPS, 1998). Although recruiting for long-term programs can be difficult, once high-risk families are involved in an intervention they often want to stay involved (Aktan, Kumpfer, & Turner, 1996). One way to improve the duration of the intervention is to encourage parents to hold weekly family meetings. This produces an enduring intervention, with parents and children planning family activities, discussing family issues, and monitoring and rewarding good behavior. Another way to improve the duration of a family program is to add booster sessions every 6 months to review parenting principles and add new, developmentally appropriate, material.

    5. Tailoring the intervention to the *cultural traditions* of the families improves recruitment, retention, and effectiveness.

Understanding the parenting assumptions of different ethnic groups participating in parenting or family programs improves program success (Catalano et al., 1993; Kumpfer & Alvarado, 1995). Many traditional cultures, for example, believe in physical punishment, downward parent-to-child communication, frequent verbal chastising, and have extremely high expectations for children's performance. Understanding why parents hold these values can help the program developers and group leaders improve program effectiveness (Turner, 2000). For instance, interviews with Pacific Islander parents participating in the Utah Strengthening Families Program (SFP) revealed that they believe Pacific Islander children have "stronger blood" than do White children and need more physical punishment (Harrison, Proskauer, & Kumpfer, 1995). Interviews with African-American parents participating in the Detroit SFP Safehaven program found that they believe their children must be more obedient because of the potentially lethal dangers of the inner-city streets. Because of differences in cultural understandings and lack of background in the psychological principles underlying many parent education programs, many so-called high-risk or dysfunctional parents may actively reject the underlying assumptions of intervention efforts or may take more time to understand and accept them.

    Ethnic families want parenting and family programs developed specifically for their parenting issues, family needs, and cultural values (Kumpfer et al., 2002). Kazdin (1993) recommends deriving culturally relevant principles to guide modifications of existing programs rather than developing separate models for each diverse ethnic group. Unfortunately, few existing model family programs (those developed and tested within NIDA/NIMH clinical research trials aimed at preventing drug use and delinquency) have been modified for ethnic families to the degree that they include culturally appropriate training and parent/child handbooks, videotapes, films, or evaluation instruments translated into different languages. Research-based exceptions include

Szapocznik's individual structural family therapy model (Szapocznik et al., 1990) and Family Effectiveness Training or Bicultural Effectiveness Training Program (Szapocznik et al., 1986, 1989) for high-risk preadolescents and adolescents; Alvy's Confident Parenting Program for parent training models for African-American and Hispanic families (Alvy et al., 1980); and Kumpfer's Strengthening Families Program for rural and urban African-American, Hispanic, Asian, Pacific Islanders, English or French Canadian families, and Australian families (Kumpfer et al., 1996). In any case, cultural modification of proven programs for ethnic families requires an organized, culturally sensitive, theoretical framework to guide program changes (Ho, 1992).

6. *Developmentally appropriate* risk and protective factors should be addressed when participants are receptive to change.

Tailoring the intervention to specific family needs can be done on an individual family assessment basis (L'Abate, 1977) or based on focus or research assessment data from similar families. Occasionally, a very short-term program can have a high impact on some participants if the material covered exactly addresses a major need of the parent or child. In addition, research demonstrates that interventions are most effective if the participants are ready for change (Spoth & Redmond, 1996a,b). Parents in the Iowa Project Family were targeted for a family intervention when children were in the sixth grade, because this is an age when even well-adjusted youth begin having behavioral and emotional adjustment problems. Parents are "ready" to participate and change because they are already beginning to see signs of oppositional behavior. Outcome results suggest that the Strengthening Families Program for 10- to 14-Year-Olds (Molgaard et al., 1994) was effective in reducing risk factors for drug use (Spoth, Redmond, & Shin, 1998). The 1- and 2-year longitudinal follow-up results show significant reductions in alcohol initiation, which only increases by the fourth year (Spoth, Redmond, & Lepper, 1999).

Different types of parenting interventions have been developed with an eye to the cognitive and developmental competencies of children at different ages. For instance, in-home parent support and cognitive/language development exercises are most effective with children from birth to 3 years (Yoshikawa, 1994). Professional medical support from home visits by a nurse is most often used with high-risk families from conception to age three (Olds & Pettitt, 1996). Behavioral parent training programs, family skills training programs, or behavioral family therapy (involving the parent and child in structured skills training activities) are most effective with children 3 to 12 years of age (CSAP/PEPS, 1998). Family therapy, or family skills training combined with behavioral parenting stressing parental monitoring, is most effective with young adolescents and adolescents (Kumpfer, 1996a).

7. Family programs are most enduring in effectiveness if they produce changes in the ongoing *family dynamics* and environment.

There is suggestive evidence that family programs that encourage families to hold weekly family meetings after the program ends have the longest effectiveness because they change the internal family organization and communication patterns in positive and lasting ways (Catalano et al., 1996; Kumpfer, 1996a). Improving parenting skills produces an ongoing intervention that is more effective over time than are short-term interventions with children or adolescents only (McMahon, 1996). The effectiveness of family interventions decays gradually with time (Harrison & Proskauer, 1995) but probably can be strengthened with new, developmentally appropriate booster sessions as recommended by Botvin (1995).

8. If parents are very dysfunctional, interventions *beginning early* in the life cycle (prenatally or in early childhood) are most effective.

For every family program we have implemented and evaluated for children from the highest risk families, we have wished that the intervention had begun earlier, before poor parenting had caused significant damage to the parent–child relationship. After the initial NIDA SFP clinical trials, the Project Reality methadone maintenance clinic began targeting pregnant drug-abusing women for improved parenting skills. Since pregnancy is generally a time when many women are willing to decrease drug use and sign up for classes to improve their parenting, many federal and state drug abuse programs for women (CSAP, CSAT, NIDA, and NIAAA) target pregnancy as a time for recruitment and family interventions. Improved pregnancy outcomes and increased services have been documented so far, but long-term improvements on the children have not been documented (Rahdert, 1996). Olds's Nurse Home Visitation Program (Olds & Pettitt, 1996) produced significant improvements in parent and child outcomes by addressing the parent–child relationship and access to needed health and social services early in the child's life. The time between repeat pregnancies was lengthened and the mother's education level improved compared to that of women in control groups.

CSAP also funded a multisite research study, called Starting Early/Starting Smart, to provide comprehensive, coordinated health, mental health, and substance abuse services for high-risk families of children from birth to 5 years of age. Many of these services are coordinated with Head Start or preschool programs and include special training for teachers and parents to help children reduce their aggression and problem behaviors. Additionally, the CSAP Developmental Predictor Variable 10-site research study includes two sites serving 3- to 5-year-old children through Head Start centers—Carolyn Webster-Stratton's project in Washington state and Ruth Kaminski's project in Oregon state (Tarter, Tolan, & Sambrano, in press).

9. Components of effective parent and family programs include strategies for improving *family relations, communication, and parental monitoring.*

Although research has shown that the final pathway to delinquency and drug use is through peer influence (Kumpfer & Turner, 1991; Swaim et al., 1989), the major family precursor is lack of parental monitoring (Ary et al., 1999; Brook et al., 1984, 1990). Because this can be moderated by increased parental caring and positive parent–child relationships, effective programs start with improving the parent–child relationship and then focusing on family communications, parent monitoring, and style of discipline (Kumpfer, 1996b; Kumpfer et al., 1997). The more effective behavioral skills training programs are distinguished from parent education because they include a structured and sequenced series of parenting skills that are role played and practiced in the group or in homework assignments, which results in increased success in the implementation of such skills.

10. *Videos* of families demonstrating good and bad parenting skills help with program effectiveness and client satisfaction.

Videotape vignettes and video-based programs enhance long-term program effectiveness (Webster-Stratton, 1990a, 1996), even when self-administered (Webster-Stratton, 1990b; Webster-Stratton, Kolpacoff, & Hollingsworth, 1988). Families generally want to see videos that address local issues and include families of their own racial group. Having the children watch the parenting videos or the parents watch the children's videos improves generalization and implementation of the video's content. Computer interactive videos, allowing self-pacing, self-testing, and selection of major content areas based on needs may be even more effective (Gordon, 1996, 1997).

DISSEMINATION OF EFFECTIVE
FAMILY-FOCUSED INTERVENTIONS

Like other family intervention researchers (Bry et al., 1991; Szapocznik et al., 1988; Szapocznik, 1997), we believe that improving parenting practices is the most effective strategy for reducing adolescent substance abuse and associated problems and could significantly reduce adolescent drug use and delinquency. And now that effective family prevention programs have been identified, researchers are focusing on how to most effectively disseminate and have them implemented with fidelity. A few technology-transfer models in science-based programs, such as the Texas Commission on Alcohol and Drugs, have been implemented by federal agencies and states, but too few to address the tremendous need for capacity building. The Center for Substance Abuse Prevention (CSAP), the primary federal agency that should be responsible for field testing research-based models and implementing effective approaches, had funding for its National Training System eliminated several years ago. As a consequence, states that have been awarded CSAP State Incentive Grants to implement science-based prevention programs are having difficulty disseminating funds to local practitioners because their proposals are too weak and not based on scientifically credible approaches. In addition, there is very little research on effective ways to promote the adoption of effective practices to guide policy decisions on whether to invest primarily in publications and conferences, in training and technical assistance systems, or in small grants.

Through a cooperative agreement between the U.S. Department of Justice's Office for Juvenile Justice and Juvenile Delinquency Prevention (OJJJDP) and the University of Utah, Kumpfer and her associates, Rose Alvarado and Connie Tait, have disseminated information on model family approaches through a five-phase technology transfer or dissemination process:

- Phase One: Dissemination of information on model programs through an internet web site (www.strengtheningfamilies.org), 14 OJJJDP bulletins on individual family programs (Kumpfer & Alvarado, 1998), and faxed fact sheets
- Phase Two: Regional conferences that showcase 34 model family programs with effectiveness results
- Phase Three: Free regional 2- to 4-day training workshops for conference attendees
- Phase Four: Free technical assistance (for 1 year) in faithfully implementing model programs and support in process and outcome evaluations
- Phase Five: $5,000 minigrants to defray the cost of recruitment incentives, manuals, food, child care, transportation, and evaluation

More than 600 participants have attended the past two regional conferences and indicated their preferences for programs in which they wanted to be trained. Twelve trainings of trainers were offered in different areas of the country. Small grants were offered in the spring of 1998 to agencies trained in model programs when it was discovered that they were having trouble locating the extra resources needed to implement research-based models with fidelity. The evaluation results of each phase suggest that all five phases are needed for effective adoption of science-based models (Kumpfer & Alvarado, 1998).

Identification of effective delivery systems is also needed, such as those developed by police departments for the Drug Awareness and Resistance Education Program (DARE). Opportunities for using the Department of Agriculture's Extension Service Network for the dissemination of family-based prevention programs were explored at two conferences held in 1998. The first, held in May, was cosponsored by NIMH and Iowa State University and focused on the NIMH/NIDA-funded Iowa Strengthening Families Program, which had been delivered successfully in schools in 20 counties in southern Iowa (Kumpfer et al., 1996; Spoth et al., 1999). Virginia Molgaard (Molgaard, 1997) presented suggestions for working with extension faculty in implementing prevention programs. In a later conference of the National Prevention Network (September 1998), Richard Spoth and a representative of the Extension Service Network presented a workshop on promoting practitioner–researcher collaboration on effectiveness and dissemination research.

Two important issues that arise in any discussion regarding dissemination of family-based programs are recruitment and retention of families and training expertise. Although many family intervention providers have a very poor turnout for their first attempts at implementing family programs, retention rates can generally be significantly improved if barriers to attendance are addressed. An 80 to 85% retention rate is possible for most programs if transportation, meals or snacks, and childcare are provided (Aktan, 1995). The intervention should be located in a nonthreatening environment and be provided by sensitive, trained, and caring professionals. Recruitment rates will vary with the type of program, incentives, types of clients targeted, and time of day offered (Spoth & Redmond, 1996b). However, the length of the program is not generally an issue in retention of high-risk families, because many such parents do not want the program to end once they have attended more than three or four sessions. Ongoing parent support group and booster sessions can help address the need for continuation of the program.

Although little data exist on how much of the effectiveness of a family program is due to the trainer versus the curriculum, estimates range from 50 to 80%. Qualitative evaluations of trainer effectiveness, participant satisfaction ratings, and long-term follow-up interviews with participants (Harrison, Proschauer, & Kumpfer, 1995) found nine important staff characteristics related to program effectiveness: (1) communication skills in presenting and listening; (2) warmth, genuineness, and empathy (Carkhuff & Truax, 1969); (3) openness and willingness to share; (4) sensitivity to family and group processes; (5) dedication, care, and concern for families; (6) flexibility; (7) humor; (8) credibility; and (9) personal experience with children as a parent or child-care provider.

Parent trainers who share the same general philosophy as that of the program being implemented are the most effective. Personal, caring, empathetic, and experienced staff members are rated the highest by the program participants, retain families longer, and produce better results. The best family and parenting programs are only as effective as the quality of the staff delivering the program. See Aktan (1995) for some guidelines for hiring high-quality staff for family programs.

RECOMMENDED FUTURE FAMILY INTERVENTION RESEARCH

Research on Effective Dissemination Strategies of Science-Based Family Programs

Clearly, many researchers are frustrated that science-based programs are not being adopted rapidly enough to help reduce the increase in drug use in this country. As evidenced by the topic of the June 1998 Annual Society for Prevention Research Conference on "Bridging the Gap Between Research and Practice" in Park City, Utah, researchers are now focusing on how to better bridge this gap and bring effective science-based models up to scale. This bridge from research to practice has been examined and found to be weak (Jansen et al., 1996).

Research on applications of research is needed to determine the best methods of getting providers to faithfully adopt model family programs. More health services research on dissemination strategies is to determine why science-based models are not being implemented by local practitioners and to find the most effective ways to get these programs brought up to scale. Since there is a dearth of research in the substance abuse prevention field on this topic, research from other fields, such as the diffusion of innovations in education, should be examined.

Applied Research on the Effectiveness of Science-Based Programs with Diverse Populations

Also needed in bridging the gap from research to practice is field testing of program models found effective under "laboratory conditions" with diverse populations in real-world situations. Such studies are needed to determine whether research-based programs work with different ethnic and cultural groups, older or younger youth, females as well as males, and families from different geographic areas (rural versus urban). New tailored curricula and videotapes need to be developed to make these science-based models more effective and culturally acceptable by the five major ethnic groups.

Research on the Relative Effects of Family-Focused versus Child-Focused Interventions

Major questions still exist (Kumpfer et al., in press) concerning whether to focus scarce prevention resources on child-only, parent-only, or total-family models. Many providers prefer to work only with children in schools or community programs. Family intervention researchers strongly believe that to have a lasting positive effect on the developmental outcomes it is essential to improve the family ecology or context by creating more nurturing and supportive parent–child interactions. Parental support and guidance by pro-social, well-adjusted parents provide a sustaining positive influence on children's developmental trajectories and risk status for drug use.

As previously discussed, there is suggestive evidence that bringing a group of at-risk youth together in a child-only group can have a negative effect (Gottfredson, 1987). Dishion and Andrews (1995) randomly assigned 119 at-risk families with 11- to 14-year-olds to one of four intervention conditions: (1) parent-focus-only, (2) teen-focus-only, (3) parent and teen focus, and (4) self-directed change. The results showed positive longitudinal trends in tobacco use in the parent-focus-only group, but suggestive evidence of negative effects in the teen-focus-only condition. Results for alcohol, marijuana, and other drugs have not yet been reported. These results stress the importance of involving parents and reevaluating strategies that aggregate high-risk youth, particularly in groups where insufficiently trained staff can't control and improve group norms. Social learning theory (Bandura, 1986) suggests that youth need exposure to positive adult role models, such as parents and group leaders, who can provide opportunities for learning behavior skills, social competencies, and higher levels of moral thinking (Levine, Kohlberg, & Hewer, 1985).

Additionally, the original 1982 to 1985 SFP research (DeMarsh & Kumpfer, 1985; Kumpfer & DeMarsh, 1985; Kumpfer, 1987) suggested that increased exposure to high-risk peers in the children's skills training groups reduces the positive gains in conduct disorders among youth from the SFP parent training only. However, the children in the children's social skills training group increase their social competencies more than among those children only enrolled in the children skills training component. The true experimental design included random assignment of experimental families to Group No. 1: parent training (PT) only, Group No. 2: PT plus children's skills training (CT), Group No. 3: PT + CT + FT (family training), and Group No. 4: a no-treatment control. Unfortunately, there was no children's skills-training-only group in the prior research on SFP cultural modifications (reviewed in Kumpfer et al. (1996)). Hence, the critical question about the effects of increased exposure to high-risk peers has not been addressed with children younger than 11 years of age (Dishion's study included 11- to 14-year-olds).

Longitudinal Studies of Family Intervention Effectiveness

Few family intervention studies have been funded for longitudinal follow-up, so critically needed to determine the actual impact on drug use rates, particularly with family studies beginning with young children. A 5-year follow-up (Harrison, Proschauer, & Kumpfer, 1995) of the Strengthening Families Program (Kumpfer, DeMarsh, & Child, 1989) was implemented in three counties in Utah. While the data collected suggest longevity of positive family functioning and maintenance of principles and behaviors taught in this family skills training program, a full parent and youth outcome assessment battery was not conducted to determine the long-term impact on drug use. With parents working more hours, increased youth isolation from positive adult role models, and increased latch-key status related to increased substance use (Richardson et al., 1989), it is worth testing whether parent training or family skills training can significantly modify this negative family environmental trend longitudinally.

Cost-Benefit and Cost-Effectiveness Analyses

Drug abuse is preventable, and effective prevention programs are cost-effective (Leshner, 1997). Few drug abuse prevention programs have calculated their costs and benefits; but those programs that have show cost-benefit ratios in the range of 8:1 (Kim et al., 1995).

Continued funding of prevention research and prevention programs will be influenced by the ability of prevention researchers to calculate cost-benefit ratios. Including comparative cost-benefit analyses on the major prevention interventions will help providers make better decisions about where to allocate scarce resources (Werthamer-Larsson et al., 1996). Unfortunately, few drug prevention studies include cost-benefit or cost-effectiveness analyses. More prospective cost-benefit studies are needed. By comparing the cost-benefit results of child-only, parent-only, and family skills training, we will gain insight into how to best use limited resources.

CONCLUSION

After 20 years of research in parenting and family interventions, we now have proven solutions. The next step is to get prevention providers to select, culturally adapt, faithfully implement, and evaluate these research-based models with diverse populations. Failure to bring these effective family programs up to scale nationwide will result in increased problems among young people because of more difficult environmental circumstances. Failure to support families of high-risk children in rearing productive, competent, non-drug-abusing youth will make the United States less competitive in the 21st century. Unfortunately, economic circumstances, cultural norms, and federal legislation over the past 2 decades have created an environment that is less supportive of strong, stable families.

We must support the dissemination and adoption of effective model strategies in lieu of ineffective, but glitzy, "fun-and-games" approaches currently being marketed by commercial companies. Few of the highly marketed parenting and family programs (except Bavolek's *Nurturing Program,* Hawkins and Catalano's *Preparing for the Drug-free Years,* and Alvy's *Effective Black Parenting Program*) were found to have effectiveness results in high-quality research designs. Although many social scientists feel that marketing their programs is selling out to commercialism, those researchers willing to risk their own personal finances to stake the up-front costs of developing marketable products are doing the prevention field a major service. Through such efforts, high-quality prevention products are getting to the practitioners. These efforts are helping bridge the gap between science and practice so needed to reduce drug use.

While it is good that funders are requesting proof of effectiveness before funding programs, additional work is needed to develop consistent criteria by which to determine whether a program is really science based and effective. Currently, different federal agencies and nongovernment foundations have overlapping but somewhat different lists of science-based models because they are using different criteria to judge effectiveness. Some criteria, like the work of the authors, allow for three levels of effectiveness: (1) exemplary programs based on randomized control trials, (2) model programs based on several quasiexperimental trials, and (3) promising programs that are in the process of being tested but have most of the same components and content as exemplary models. Many of these are culturally, gender, or locally adapted versions of science-based programs. However, the development of a consistent vocabulary by which to judge and classify these programs is needed to help advance the dissemination process.

To promote the dissemination of these effective science-based prevention programs, policymakers and funders must refuse to support any prevention interventions that do not have evidence of effectiveness. Hence, funders must know what works in prevention and demand outcome evaluation reports to improve accountability and field trials of promising programs. Additionally, in selecting the best programs, funders and program providers must begin asking hard questions about the evaluation, including (1) what type of experimental design was used (true experimental, quasiexperimental, or a nonexperimental design); (2) what control groups were used; and (3) whether actual drug use behaviors changed or whether precursors related to risk, protective, and resiliency factors changed, rather than just knowledge or client satisfaction.

In conclusion, a major investment is needed if we are to learn how to better disseminate and market effective research-based programs and reduce children's emotional, behavioral, and drug abuse problems. At this point, drug dealers appear to be better marketers than prevention specialists. Drug dealers use one of the fastest growing entrepreneurial marketing methods around: multilevel marketing. Multilevel marketing allows people to be self-employed and to have dealers working under them for a cut of the profits. The marketers go to the clients, to their homes and their cars. There is low overhead with no stores or furnishings. Parties are held to demonstrate the wares and the benefits of being a dealer and to encourage others to become dealers. Changing to a discussion of the need to compete against this type of marketing for promoting validated means of preventing substance abuse would be beneficial. Further, funding is needed to allow these programs to compete against the lucrative drug-dealing marketplace. Collaborations with marketing and technology transfer specialists in fields like medicine, agriculture, and the pharmaceutical industry, where innovations are rapidly disseminated, could help the drug prevention field be more successful in disseminating research-based family interventions.

REFERENCES

Aktan, G. (1995). Organizational framework for a substance use prevention program. *International Journal of Addictions, 30,* 185–201.

Aktan, G., Kumpfer, K. L., & Turner, C. (1996). Effectiveness of a family skills training program for substance abusing families in inner city African-American families. *Substance Use and Misuse, 31,* 157–175.

Alexander, J. F., Holtzworth-Munroe, A., & Jameson, P. B. (1994). The process and outcome of marital and family therapy: Research review and evaluation. In A. E. Bergin & S. L. Garfield (Eds.), *Handbook of psychotherapy and behavior change.* New York: Wiley.

Alexander, J. F., Robbins, M. S., & Sexton, T. L. (2000). Family-based interventions with older, at-risk youth: From promise to proof to practice. *Journal of Primary Prevention, 21*(2), 185–205.

Alvy, K. T., Fuentes, E. G., Harrison, D. S., & Rosen, L. D. (1980). *The culturally-adapted parent training project: Original grant proposal and first progress report.* Studio City, CA: Center for the Improvement of Child Caring.

Ary, D., Duncan, T. E., Biglan, A., Metzler, C. W., Noell, J. W., & Smolkowski, K. (1999). Developmental model of adolescent problem behavior. *Journal of Abnormal Child Psychology, 27*(2), 141–150.

Ashery, R., Robertson, E., & Kumpfer, K. L. (1997). *Drug Abuse Prevention Through Family Interventions,* NIDA Research Monograph #177. DHHS, National Institute on Drug Abuse, Rockville, MD, NIH Publication No. 97-4135.

Backer, T. E. (1991). *Drug abuse technology transfer.* Rockville, MD: National Institute on Drug Abuse.

Backer, T. E. (2000). The failure of success: Challenges of disseminating effective substance abuse prevention programs. *Journal of Community Psychology, 28*(3), 363–373.

Backer, T. E., David, S. L., & Soucy, G. (1995). *Reviewing the behavioral science knowledge base on technology transfer.* Rockville, MD: National Institute on Drug Abuse.

Backer, T., & Rogers, E. (1999). *Dissemination best practices workshop briefing paper: State-of-the-art review on dissemination research and dissemination partnership.* Encino, CA: NCAP.

Bandura, A. (1986). *Social foundations of thought and action: A social cognitive theory.* Englewood Cliffs, NJ: Prentice-Hall.

Bauman, K. E., Foshee, V. A., Ennett, S. T., Hicks, K., & Pemberton, M. (2001). Family matters: A family-directed program designed to prevent adolescent tobacco and alcohol use. *Health Promotion and Practice, 2*(1), 81–96.

Bavolek, S. J., Comstock, C. M., & McLaughlin, J. A. (1983). *The Nurturing Program: A validated approach to reducing dysfunctional family interactions.* Final report, No. 1R01MH34862. Rockville, MD: National Institute of Mental Health.

Bierman, K. L., Greenberg, M. T., & the Conduct Problems Prevention Research Group (1996). Social skill training in the FAST TRACK program. In R. DeV. Peters & R. J. McMahon (Eds.), *Prevention and early intervention: Childhood disorders, substance abuse and delinquency.* Thousand Oaks, CA: Sage.

Biglan, A., Mrazek, P. J., Carnine, D., & Flay, B. R. (in press). The integration of research and practice in the prevention of youth problem behaviors. *American Psychologist.*

Biglan, A., & Taylor, T. K. (2000). Increasing the use of science to improve child-rearing. The *Journal of Primary Prevention, 21*(2), 207–226.

Botvin, G. J. (1995). Drug abuse prevention in school settings. In G. J. Botvin, S. Schinke & M. A. Orlandi (Eds.), *Drug Abuse Prevention with Multiethnic Youth* (pp. 169–192). Thousand Oaks, CA: Sage.

Brook, J. S., Whiteman, M., Gordon, A. S., & Brook, D. W. (1984). Paternal determinants of female adolescents marijuana use. *Developmental Psychology, 20,* 1032–1043.

Brook, J. S., Whiteman, M., Gordon, A. S., Brook, D. W., & Cohen, P. (1990, May). The psychosocial etiology of adolescent drug use: A family interactional approach. *Genetic, Social & General Psychology Monographs, 116*(2), 111–267.

Brunswick, A., Messeri, P., & Titus, S. (1992). Predictive factors in adult substance abuse: A prospective study of African-American adolescents. In M. Glantz & R. Pickens, (Eds.), *Vulnerability to drug abuse* (pp. 419–464). Washington, DC: American Psychological Association.

Bry, B. H. (1983). Predicting drug abuse: Review and reformulation. *International Journal of Addictions, 18,* 223–233.

Bry, B. H., Catalano, R. F., Kumpfer, K. L., Lochman, J. E., & Szapocznik, J. (1997). Scientific findings from family prevention intervention research. In R. Ashery, S. David & K. L. Kumpfer (Eds.), *Family-focused preventions of drug abuse: research and interventions,* NIDA Research Monograph, 177. DHHS, National Institute on Drug Abuse, Rockville, MD, NIH Publication No. 97-4135.

Bry, B. H., Greene, D. M., Schutte, C., & Fishman, C. (1991). Targeted family intervention: Procedures Manual. Unpublished document.

Catalano, R. F., & Hawkins, J. D. (1996). The social development model: A theory of antisocial behavior. In J. D. Hawkins (Ed.), *Delinquency and crime: Current theories* (pp. 149–197). New York: Cambridge University Press.

Catalano, R. F., Haggerty, K. P., Flemming, C., & Brewer, D. (1996). Focus on families: Scientific findings from family prevention intervention research. Paper presented at the NIDA conference: 'Drug Abuse Prevention Through Family Intervention,' Gaithersburg, MD, January 1996.

Catalano, R. F., Hawkins, J. D., Krenz, C., Gillmore, M., Morrison, D., Wells, E., & Abbot, R. (1993). Using research to guide culturally appropriated drug abuse prevention. *Journal of Consulting and Clinical Psychology, 61,* 804–811.

Center for Substance Abuse Prevention (1993). *Signs of effectiveness in preventing alcohol and other drug problems* (Contract No. ADM-SA-88-005). Washington, DC: Superintendent of Documents, U.S. Government Printing Office.

Center for Substance Abuse Prevention (1998). *Family-centered approaches to prevent substance abuse among children and adolescents: A guideline.* Prevention Enhancement Protocol System (PEPS). Contract Number 277-92-1011. Washington, DC: Superintendent of Documents, U.S. Government Printing Office.

Chilcoat, H. D., Dishion, T. J., & Antony, J. C. (1995). Parent monitoring and the incidence of drug sampling in urban elementary school children. *American Journal of Epidemiology, 141,* 25–31.

Coombs, R. H., Paulson, M. J., & Richardson, M. A. (1991). Peer vs. parental influence in substance use among Hispanic and Anglo children and adolescents. *Journal of Youth and Adolescence, 20,* 73–88.

DeMarsh, J. K., & Kumpfer, K. L. (1985). Family environmental and genetic influences on children's future chemical dependency. *Journal of Children in Contemporary Society: Advances in Theory and Applied Research, 18*(1/2), 117–152.

Dembo, R., Farrow, D., Scheidler, J., & Burgos, W. (1979). Testing a causal model of environmental influences on the early drug involvement of inner city junior high school youth. *American Journal of Alcohol Abuse, 6,* 313–336.

DHHS (1998). Results of the National Household Survey. Press release, Friday, August 1998.

DHHS (2001). American's Children's Report, 2001. Department of Health and Human Services. Washington, DC: U.S. Government Printing Office.

Dishion, T. J., & Andrews, D. W. (1995). Preventing escalation in problem behaviors with high-risk young adolescents: Immediate and 1-year outcomes. *Journal of Consulting and Clinical Psychology, 63,* 538–548.

Dishion, T. J., French, D., & Patterson, G. R. (1995). The development and ecology of antisocial behavior. In D. Cicchetti & D. Cohen (Eds.), *Manual of developmental psycho pathology* (pp. 421–471). New York: Wiley.

Dishion, T. J., Kavanagh, K., & Kiesner, J. (1996). Prevention of early adolescent substance use among high-risk youth: A multiple gating approach to parent intervention. Paper presented at the NIDA conference: 'Drug Abuse Prevention Through Family Intervention,' Gaithersburg, MD, January 1996.

Dishion, T. J., Reid, J. B., & Patterson, G. R. (1988). Empirical guidelines for a family intervention for adolescent drug use. *Journal of Chemical Dependency Treatment, 1,* 189–224.

Dishion, T. J., Li, F., Spracklen, K., Brown, G., & Haas, E. (1996). The measurement of parenting practices in research on adolescent problem behavior: A multi method and multi trait analysis. Paper presented at the NIDA conference: 'Drug Abuse Prevention Through Family Intervention,' Gaithersburg, MD, January 1996.

Dumas, J. E. (1989). Treating antisocial behavior in children: Child and family approaches. *Clinical Psychology Review, 9,* 197–222.

Dunst, C. J., & Trivette, C. M. (1994). Methodological considerations and strategies for studying the long-term follow-up of early intervention. In S. Friedman & H. C. Haywood (Eds.), *Developmental follow-up: Concepts, domains and methods* (pp. 277–313). San Diego, CA.

Egeland, B., & Erickson, M. F. (1987). Psychologically unavailable care giving: The effects on development of young children and the implications for intervention. In M. Brassard, S. Hart & B. Germain (Eds.), *Psychological maltreatment of children and youth* (pp. 110–120). New York: Pergamon Press.

Egeland, B., & Erickson, M. F. (1990). Rising above the past: Strategies for helping new mothers break the cycle of abuse and neglect. *Zero to Three, 11*(2), 29–35.

Elliot, D., Huizinga, D., & Menard, S. (1989). *Multiple problem youth: delinquency, substance use, and mental health problems.* New York: Springer-Verlag.

Ennett, S. T., Tobler, N. S., Ringwalt, C., & Flewelling, R. (1994). How effective is Drug Abuse Resistance Education? A meta-analysis of Project DARE evaluations. *American Journal of Health, 84*(9), 1394–1401.

Falco, M. (1992). *The making of a drug-free America: Programs that work.* New York: Times Books.

Flay, B. R., Hansen, W. B., Johnson, C. A., Collins, L. M., Dent, C. W., Dwyer, K. M., Grossman, L., Hockstein, G., Rauch, J., Sobel, J., Sobol, D. F., Sussman, S., & Ulene, A. (1987). Implementation effectiveness trial of a social influences smoking prevention program using schools and television. *Health Education Research, 2,* 385–400.

Forehand, R. L., & McMahon, R. J. (1981). *Helping the noncompliant child. A clinician's guide to parent training.* New York: Guilford Press.

Gary, L. E. (1986). Family life events, depression, and Black men. In: R. A. Lewis & R. E. Salt (Eds.), *Men in Families*, 215–231. Beverly Hills, CA: Sage.

Gary, L. E., Beatty, L. A., Berry, G. L., & Price, M. D. (1983). *Stable Black families: Final report.* Washington, DC: Institute for Urban Affairs and Research, Howard University.

Glantz, M., & Johnson, J. (1999). *Resiliency in the face of adversity.* New York: Plenum Press.

Gordon, D. (1996). *Parenting adolescents wisely.* Workshop presented at 2nd National Training Conference on Strengthening America's Families. Snowbird Ski Resort, Salt Lake City, Utah, October 12–14, 1996.

Gordon, D. (1997). *Parenting adolescents wisely.* Workshop presented at 3rd National Training Conference on Strengthening America's Families. Westin City Center, Washington DC, March 23–25, 1997.

Gordon, D. A., Arbruthnot, J., Gustafson, K. A., & McGreen, P. (1998). Home based behavioral-systems family therapy with disadvantaged juvenile delinquents. *American Journal of Family Therapy, 16*(3), 243–255.

Gottfredson, G. D. (1987). Peer group interventions to reduce the risk of delinquent behavior: A selective review and a new evaluation. *Criminology, 25*(3), 671–714.

Grady, K., Gersick, K. E., & Boratynski, M. (1985). Preparing parents for teenagers: A step in the prevention of adolescent substance abuse. *Family Relations, 34,* 541–549.

Greenberg, M. (1998). Results of Project FAST TRACK. Panel on Effective School-based Prevention Programs. Annual Conference of the American Psychological Association, San Francisco, CA, August 15, 1998.

Haggerty, K. P., Mills, E., & Catalano, R. F. (1991). *Focus on Families: Parent training curriculum (unpublished).* Social Development Research Group, Seattle, WA.

Hansen, W. B., Graham, J. W., Sobel, J. L., Shelton, D. R., Flay, B. R., & Johnson, C. A. (1987). The consistency of peer and parent influences on tobacco, alcohol, and marijuana use among young adolescents. *Journal of Behavioral Medicine, 10,* 559–579.

Harrington, N., Hoyle, R., Giles, S. M., & Hansen, W. B. (2000). The All-Stars prevention program. In W. B. Hansen, S. M. Giles, & M. D. Fearnow-Kenney (Eds.), *Improving prevention effectiveness* (pp. 203–212). Greensboro, NC: Tanglewood Research Inc.

Harrison, R. S., & Proskauer, S. (1995). The impact of family skills training on children at risk for substance abuse and their families: A five-year evaluation. Social Research Institute, Graduate School of Social Work, University of Utah, Salt Lake City, Utah, 84112. Manuscript submitted as final report to CSAP.

Harrison, S., Proskauer, S., & Kumpfer, K. L. (1995). *Final evaluation report on Utah CSAP/CYAP project.* Submitted to the Utah State Division of Substance Abuse. Social Research Institute, University of Utah, Salt Lake City, Utah 84112.

Hawkins, J. D., Catalano, R. F., Jr., & Associates (1992). *Communities that care.* San Francisco, CA: Jossey-Bass.

Ho, M. K. (1992). Differential application of treatment modalities with Asian American youth. In L. A. Vargas & Koss-Chioino (Eds.), *Working with culture: Psychotherapeutic interventions with ethnic minority children and adolescents* (pp. 182–203). San Francisco: Jossey-Bass.

Jansen, M. A., Glynn, T., & Howard, J. (1996). Prevention of alcohol, tobacco, and other drugs abuse: Federal efforts to stimulate prevention research. *American Behavioral Scientist, 39*(7), 790–801.

Jessor, R. (1993). Successful adolescent development among youth in high-risk settings. *American Psychology, 48,* 117–126.

Johnson, J. L., & Left, M. (1999). Children of substance abusers: Overview of research findings. *Pediatrics, 103*(5), 1085–1100.

Johnston, L. D., O'Malley, P. M., & Bachman, J. G. (1998). Drug use rises again in 1995 among American teens. News release. University of Michigan Monitoring the Future Study of American Youth, December 1996.

Johnston, L. D., O'Malley, P. M., & Bachman, J. G. (2000). National survey results on drug use from the Monitoring the Future study, 1975–2000 Volume I: Secondary school students (NIH Publication No. 2000). Rockville, MD: National Institute on Drug Abuse, c. 420 pp.

Kaftarian, S. J., & Kumpfer, K. L. (Guest Eds., 2000). Special Issue: Family-focused research and primary prevention practice. *The Journal of Primary Prevention, 21*(2), New York: Kluwer Academic/Human Sciences Press.

Kandel, D. B., & Davies, M. (1992). Progression to regular marijuana involvement: Phenomenology and risk factors for near-daily use. In M. Glantz & R. Pickens (Eds.), *Vulnerability to Drug Abuse* (pp. 211–242). Washington, DC: American Psychological Association.

Kaplan, H. B., & Johnson, R. J. (1992). Relationships between circumstances surrounding initial illicit drug use and escalation of drug use: Moderating effects of gender and early adolescent experiences. In M. Glantz & R. Pickens (Eds.), *Vulnerability to Drug Abuse* (pp. 299–352). Washington, DC: American Psychological Association.

Kazdin, A. E. (1987). Treatment of antisocial behavior in children: Current status and future directions. *Psychological Bulletin, 102,* 187–203.

Kazdin, A. E. (1993). Adolescent mental health: Prevention and treatment programs. *American Psychologist, 48*(2), 127–140.

Kazdin, A. E. (1995). *Conduct disorders in childhood and adolescence* (2nd ed.). Thousand Oaks, CA: Sage.

Kazdin, A. E., Siegel, T. C., & Bass, D. (1992). Cognitive problem-solving skills training and parent management training in treatment of antisocial behavior in children. *Journal of Consulting and Clinical Psychology,16,* 733–747.

Kellam, S. G., Brown, C. H., Rubin, B. R., & Ensminger, M. E. (1983). Paths leading to teenage psychiatric symptoms and substance use: Developmental epidemiological studies in Woodlawn. In S. B. Guze, F. J. Earls & J. E. Barrett (Eds.), *Childhood psychopathology and development* (pp. 17–51). New York: Raven Press.

Kim, S. W., Coletti, S. D., Crutchfield, C. C., Williams, C., & Howard, J. (1995). Benefit-cost analysis of drug abuse prevention programs: A macroscopic approach. *Journal of Drug Education, 25*(2), 111–127.

King, J., Beals, J., Manson, S. M., & Trimble, J. E. (1992). A structural equation model of factors related to substance use among American Indian adolescents. *Drugs & Society, 6*(3–4), 253–268.

Krohn, M. D., & Thornberry, T. P. (1993). Network theory: A model for understanding drug abuse among African-American and Hispanic youth. In M. R. De La Rosa & J-L. R. Adrados (Eds.), *Drug abuse among minority youth: Advances in research and methodology* (pp. 102–128). National Institute in Drug Abuse Research Monograph 130. NIH Pub. No. 93–3479. Washington, DC: Superintendent of Documents, U.S. Government Printing Office.

Kumpfer, K. L. (1987). Special populations: Etiology and prevention of vulnerability to chemical dependency in children of substance abusers. In B. S. Brown & A. R. Mills, (Eds.), *Youth at high risk for substance abuse* (pp. 1–71). National Institute on Drug Abuse Monograph, DHHS Publication Number (ADM) 90-1537. Washington, DC: Superintendent of Documents, U.S. Government Printing Office.

Kumpfer, K. L. (1993). *Strengthening America's families: Promising parenting and family strategies for delinquency prevention.* A User's Guide, prepared for the U.S. Department of Justice under Grant No. 87-JS-CX-K495 from the Office of Juvenile Justice and Delinquency Prevention, Office of Juvenile Programs, U.S. Department of Justice.

Kumpfer, K. L. (1996a). Principles of effective family-focused parent programs. Paper presented at the NIDA conference: 'Drug Abuse Prevention Through Family Intervention,' Gaithersburg, MD, January 1996.

Kumpfer, K. L. (1996b). Selective prevention approaches for drug abuse prevention: The Strengthening Families Program. Paper presented at the NIDA conference: 'Drug Abuse Prevention Through Family Intervention,' Gaithersburg, MD, January 1996.

Kumpfer, K. L. (1997). What works in the prevention of drug abuse: Individual, school and family approaches. DHHS, Center for Substance Abuse Prevention. *Secretary's Youth Substance Abuse Prevention Initiative: Resource Paper* (pp. 69–105). March 1997.

Kumpfer, K. L. (1999). Factors and processes contributing to resilience: The resilience framework. In M. D. Glantz & J. L. Johnson (Eds.), *Resilience and development: Positive life adaptions* (pp. 179–224). New York: Kluwer Academic/Plenum Publishers.

Kumpfer, K. L., & Alvarado, R. (1995). Strengthening families to prevent drug use in multi-ethnic youth. In G. Botvin, S. Schinke & M. Orlandi (Eds.), *Drug abuse prevention with multi-ethnic youth* (pp. 253–292). Newbury Park, CA: Sage.

Kumpfer, K. L., & Alvarado, R. (1998). Effective Family Strengthening Interventions. Juvenile Justice Bulletin, Family Strengthening Series, OJJDP, November 1998.

Kumpfer, K. L., & Alvarado, R. (in press). Family strengthening approaches for the prevention of youth problems. In R. Weissberg & K. L. Kumpfer (Eds.), *American Psychologist.*

Kumpfer, K. L., Alvarado, R., Smith, R., & Bellamy, N. (2002). Cultural issues in universal family strengthening prevention programs. *Prevention Science, 3*(3), September, 239–244.

Kumpfer, K. L., Alvarado, R., Tait, C., & Toledo, S. (in press). Effectiveness of school-based family and children's skills training for substance abuse prevention among 6–8 year old rural children. In R. Tarter, P. Tolan & S. Sambrano (Guest Eds.), *American Psychologist.*

Kumpfer, K. L., & DeMarsh, J. P. (1985). Prevention of chemical dependency in children of alcohol and drug abusers. *NIDA Notes, 5,* 2–3.

Kumpfer, K. L., DeMarsh, J. P., & Child, W. (1989). *Strengthening families program: Children's skills training curriculum manual, parent training manual, children's skill training manual, and family skills training manual* (Prevention Services to Children of Substance-abusing Parents). University of Utah: Social Research Institute, Graduate School of Social Work.

Kumpfer, K., Gottfredson, D., & Alvarado, R. (2001). Strengthening Washington, DC, families: Annual third year progress report. University of Utah, Department of Health Promotion and Education, SLC, Utah, 84112, unpublished document.

Kumpfer, K. L., & Hunter, L. (2002). *Prevention of alcohol and drug abuse: What works?* AMERSA.

Kumpfer, K. L., & Kaftarian, S. J. (2000). Bridging the gap between family-focused research and substance abuse prevention practice: Preface. *Journal of Primary Prevention, 21*(2), 169–183.

Kumpfer, K. L., Molgaard, V., & Spoth, R. (1996). The Strengthening Families Program for prevention of delinquency and drug use in special populations. In R. DeV. Peters & R.J. McMahon (Eds.), *Childhood disorders, substance abuse, and delinquency: Prevention and early intervention approaches.* Thousand Oaks, CA: Sage.

Kumpfer, K. L., & Turner, C. W. (1990/1991). The social ecology model of adolescent substance abuse: Implications for prevention. *The International Journal of the Addictions 25*(4A), 435–463.

Kumpfer, K. L., Turner, C., Sales, L., & Springer, F. (1998). Welcome (including results of CSAP High Risk Youth Survey). National Prevention Network Annual Research Conference. San Antonio, TX, Sept. 2, 1998.

Kumpfer, K. L., Williams, M. K., & Baxley, G. (1997). Selective prevention for children of substance abusing parents: The Strengthening Families Program. Resource Manual, National Institute on Drug Abuse, Technology Transfer Program, Silver Springs, MD.

L'Abate, L. (1977). *Enrichment: Structured interventions with couples, Families and groups.* Washington, DC: University Press of America.

Leshner, A. (1997). Drug abuse and addiction treatment research. *Archives of General Psychiatry, 54*(8), 691–694.

Levine, C., Kohlberg, L., & Hewer, A. (1985). The current formulation of Kohlberg's theory and a response to critics. *Human Development 28*(2), 94–100.

Liddle, H. A., & Dakof, G. A. (1995). Efficacy of family therapy for drug abuse: Promising but not definitive. *Journal of Marital and Family Therapy, 21*(4), 511–543.

Lochman, J. E. (2000). Parent and family skills training in targeted prevention programs for at-risk youth. *Journal of Primary Prevention, 21*(2), 253–265.

Loeber, R., & Stouthamer-Loeber, M. (1986). Family factors as correlates and predictors of juvenile conduct problems and delinquency. In N. Morris & M. Tonry (Eds.), *Crime and justice: An annual review of research* (vol. 7, pp. 29–149), Chicago: University of Chicago Press.

Luthar, S. S. (1993). Annotation: Methodological and conceptual issues in research on childhood resilience. *Journal of Child Psychology and Psychiatry, 34,* 441–453.

Mayer, G. R. (1995). Preventing antisocial behavior in the schools. *Journal of Applied Behavioral Analysis, 28*(4), 467–478.

McCord, J. (1991, July). *A thirty-year follow-up of treatment effects.* Paper presented at the annual meeting of the William T. Grant Faculty Scholars, Durham, NC.

McDonald, L. (1993). Families Together with Schools. In *Promising programs for safe schools.* Washington, DC: American Psychological Association.

McDonald, L., Billingham, S., Dibble, N., Rice, C., & Coe-Braddish, D. (1991). F.A.S.T.: An innovative substance abuse prevention program. *Social Work in Education, 13*(2), 118–12.

McMahon, R. (1996). Helping the Non-compliant Child. Workshop presented at 2nd National Training Conference on Strengthening America's Families. Snowbird Ski Resort, Salt Lake City, Utah, October 12–14, 1996.

McMahon, R. J., Slough, N. M., & the Conduct Problems Prevention Research Group (1996). In R. DeV. Peters & R. J. McMahon (Eds.), *Prevention and early intervention: Childhood disorders, substance abuse and delinquency.* Thousand Oaks, CA: Sage.

Mitchell, A., Weiss, H., & Schultz, T. (1995). *Evaluating education reform: Early childhood education. A review of research on early education, family support and parent education, and collaboration.* OERI, U.S. Department of Education.

Molgaard, V. K. (1997). The Extension Service as key mechanism for research and services delivery for prevention of mental health disorders in rural areas. *American Journal of Community Psychology, 25*(4), 515–544.

Molgaard, V., Kumpfer, K. L., & Spoth, R. (1994). *The Iowa Strengthening Families Program for pre- and early teens.* Ames, IA: Iowa State University.

Mrazek, P. J., & Haggerty, R. J. (1994). *Reducing risks for mental disorders: Frontiers for preventive intervention research.* Washington, DC: National Academy Press for the Institute of Medicine, Committee on Prevention of Mental Disorders.

Newcomb, M. D. (1992). Understanding the multidimensional nature of drug use and abuse: The role of consumption, risk factors, and protective factors. In M. D. Glantz & R. Pickens, (Eds.), *Vulnerability to drug abuse* (pp. 255–297). Washington DC: American Psychological Association.

Newcomb, M. D. (1995). Drug use etiology among ethnic minority adolescents: Risk and protective factors. In G. Botvin, S. Schinke & M. Orlandi (Eds.), *Drug abuse prevention with multi-ethnic youth* (pp. 253–292). Newbury Park, CA: Sage.

Newcomb, M. D., & Bentler, P. M. (1989). Substance use and abuse among children and teenagers. *American Psychologist, 44,* 242–248.

NIDA/Kumpfer, K. L. (2001). Literature review: Identification of drug abuse prevention programs. Published on NIDA web site: www.nida.nih.gov.

Norman, E., & Turner, S. (1993). Adolescent substance abuse prevention programs: Theories, models, and research in the encouraging 80's. *Journal of Primary Prevention 14*(1), 3–20.

Nye, C., Zucker, R., & Fitzgerald, H. (1995). Early intervention in the path to alcohol problems through conduct problems: Treatment involvement and child behavior change. *Journal of Consulting and Clinical Psychology, 63,* 831–840.

Oetting, E. (1992). Planning programs for prevention of deviant behavior: A psychosocial model. In J. E. Trimble, C. E. Bolek & S. J. Niemcryk (Eds.), *Ethnic and Multi cultural drug use: Perspectives on current research.* New York: Haworth Press.

Oetting, E., & Beauvais, F. (1987). Peer cluster theory, socialization characteristics and adolescent drug use: A path analysis. *Journal of Counseling Psychology, 34*(2), 205–213.

Oetting, E. R., & Lynch, R. S. (1993). Peers and the prevention of adolescent drug use. Fort Collins, CO: Department of Psychology, Colorado State University.

Olds, D., & Pettitt, L. (1996). Reducing Risks for Substance Abuse with a Program of Prenatal and Early Childhood Home Visitation. Paper presented at NIDA Family Intervention Symposium, WDC, January 1996.

Patterson, G. (1974). Intervention for boys with conduct problems: Multiple settings, treatments, and criteria, *Journal of Consulting and Clinical Psychology, 42,* 471–481.

Patterson, G. R., Chamberlain, P., & Reid, J. D. (1982). A comparative evaluation of a parent training program. *Behavior Therapy, 13,* 638–650.

Patterson, G., & Fleishman, M. J. (1979). Maintenance of treatment effects: Some considerations concerning family systems and follow-up data. *Behavior Therapy, 10,* 168–185.

Patterson, G., & Reid, J. B. (1973). Intervention for families of aggressive boys: A replication study. *Behavior Therapy Research, 11,* 383–394.

Perry, C. L., Grant, M., Ernberg, G., Florenzano, R. U., Langdon, M. C., Myeni, A. D., Waahlberg, R., Berg, S., Andersson, K., & Fisher, K. J. (1989). WHO collaborative study on alcohol education and young people: Outcomes of a four-country pilot study. *International Journal of the Addictions, 24,* 1145–1171.

Perry, C. L., Pirie, P., Holder, W., Halper, A., & Dudovitz, B. (1990). Parent involvement in cigarette smoking prevention: Two pilot evaluations of the 'Unpuffables Program.' *Journal of School Health, 60*(9), 443–447.

Rahdert, E. R. (1996). Introduction to the Perinatal-20 Treatment Research Demonstration Program. In E. R. Rahdert (Ed.), *Treatment for drug-exposed women and their children: Advances in research methodology* (pp. 1–4). NIDA Research Monograph 166. Washington DC: Superintendent of Documents, U.S. Government Printing Office.

Resnik, M., Bearman, P. S., Blum, R. W., Bauman, K. E., Harris, K. M., Jones, J., Tabor, J., Beuhring, L. H., Sleving, R. E., Shaw, M., Ireland, M., Bearinger, L. H., & Udry, R. I. (1997). Protecting adolescents from harm. *Journal of the American Medical Association, 278*(10), 823–832.

Richardson, J. L., Dwyer, K., McGuigan, K., Hansen, W. B., Dent, C., Johnson, C. A., Sussman, S. Y., Brannon, B., & Flay, B. (1989). Substance use among eighth-grade students who take care of themselves after school. *Pediatrics 84*(3), 556–566.

Rogers, E. M. (1995). *Diffusion of innovations* (4th ed.). New York: Free Press.

Rohrbach, L. A., Hodgson, C. S., Broder, B. I., Montgomery, S. B., Flay, B. R., Hansen, W. B., & Pentz, M. A. (1994). Parental participation in drug abuse prevention: Results from the Midwestern prevention project. *The Journal of Research on Adolescence, 4*(2), 295–317.

Rutter, M. (1990). Psychosocial resilience and protective mechanisms. *American Orthopsychiatric Association,* 316–331.

Rutter, M. (1993). Resilience: Some conceptual considerations. *Journal of Adolescent Health, 14,* 626–631.

Schorr, L. B. (1988). *Within our reach: Breaking the cycle of disadvantage.* New York: Doubleday.

Serketich, W. J., & Dumas, J. E. (1996). The effectiveness of behavioral parent training to modify antisocial behavior in children: A meta-analysis. *Behavior Therapy, 27*(2), 171–186.

Sloboda, Z., & David, S. National Institute on Drug Abuse (1997). *Preventing drug use among children and adolescents.* NIH Publication No. 97-4212. Washington, DC: U.S. Government Printing Office.

Spoth, R., & Redmond, C. (1996a). Illustrating a framework for prevention research: Project Family studies of rural family participation and outcomes. In R.DeV. Peter & R. J. McMahon (Eds.), *Childhood disorders, substance abuse, and delinquency: Prevention and early intervention approaches.* Newbury Park, CA: Sage.

Spoth, R., & Redmond, C. (1996b). Study of participation barrier in family-focused prevention: Research issues and preliminary results. *International Journal of Community Health Education, 13,* 365–388.

Spoth, R., Redmond, C., & Lepper, H. (1999). Alcohol initiation outcomes of universal family-focused preventive interventions: One- and two-year follow-ups of a controlled study. *Journal of Studies on Alcohol,* Special NIAAA Issue, Supplement 13, 103–111.

Spoth, R., Redmond, C., & Shin, C. Y. (1998). Direct and indirect latent variable parenting outcomes of two universal family-focused prevention: Extending a public health-oriented research base. *Journal of Consulting and Clinical Psychology, 66*(2), 385–399.

Swaim, R. C., Oetting, E. R., Edwards, R. W., & Beauvais, F. (1989). Links from emotional distress to adolescent drug use: A path model. *Journal of Consulting and Clinical Psychology, 57*(2), 227–231.

Swisher, J. D., & Hu, T. W. (1983). Alternatives to drug abuse: Some are and some are not. In T. J. Glynn, C. G. Leukefeld & J. P. Ludford (Eds.), *Preventing adolescent drug abuse: intervention strategies* (Research monograph 47). Washington, DC: Office for Substance Abuse Prevention.

Szapocznik, J. (1996). Scientific findings that have emerged from family intervention research at the Spanish Family Guidance Center and the Center for Family Studies. Paper presented at the NIDA conference: 'Drug Abuse Prevention Through Family Intervention,' Gaithersburg, MD, January 1996.

Szapocznik, J. (1997). Cultural competency and family program implementation. Plenary session presented at 3rd National Training Conference on Strengthening America's Families. Westin City Center, Washington DC, March 23–25, 1997.

Szapocznik, J., Kurtines, W., Santisteban, D. A., & Rio, A. T. (1990). The interplay of advances among theory, research and application in treatment interventions aimed at behavior problem children and adolescents. *Journal of Consulting and Clinical Psychology, 58*(6), 696–703.

Szapocznik, J., Perez-Vidal, A., Brickman, A., Foote, F. H., Santisteban, D., Hervis, O., & Kurtines, W. H. (1988). Engaging adolescent drug abusers and their families into treatment: A Strategic Structural Systems approach. *Journal of Consulting and Clinical Psychology,* 552–557.

Szapocznik, J., Rio, A., Murray, E., Cohen, R., Scopetta, M. A., Rivas-Vasquez, A., Hervis, O. E., & Poseda, V. (1989). Structural family versus psychodynamic child therapy for problematic Hispanic boys. *Journal of Consulting and Clinical Psychology, 57*(5), 571–578.

Szapocznik, J., Santisteban, D., Rio, A., Perez-Vidal, A., & Kurtines, W.M. (1985). Family effectiveness training (FET) for Hispanic families: Strategic structural systems intervention for the prevention of drug abuse. In H. P. Lefley & P. B. Pedersen (Eds.), *Cross cultural training for mental professionals.* Springfield, IL: Charles C Thomas.

Szapocznik, J., Santisteban, D., Rio, A., Perez-Vidal, A., & Kurtines, W. M. (1989). Family effectiveness training: An intervention to prevent drug abuse and problem behaviors in Hispanic adolescents. *Hispanic Journal of Behavioral Sciences, 6*(4), 303–330.

Szapocznik, J., Santisteban, D., Rio, A., Perez-Vidal, A., Kurtines, W. M., & Hervis, O. (1986). Bicultural effectiveness training (BET): An intervention modality for families experiencing intergenerational/intercultural conflict. *Hispanic Journal of Behavioral Sciences, 6*(4), 303–330.

Tarter, R., Tolan, P., & Sambrano, S. (Guest Eds.) (in press). Psychology of addictive behaviors. *American Psychologist.* Special Issue on the CSAP Predictor Variable Cross-site Study.

Taylor, T. K., & Biglan, A. (1998). Behavioral family interventions for improving child-rearing: A review for clinicians and policy makers. *Clinical Child and Family Psychological Review, 1*(1), 41–60.

Taylor, T. K., Schmidt, F., Pepler, D., & Hodgins, C. (1998). A comparison of eclectic treatment with Webster-Stratton's parents and children series in a children's mental health center: A randomized controlled trial. *Behavior Therapy, 29*(2), 221–240.

Tobler, N. S., & Kumpfer, K. L. (2000). Meta-analysis of family based strengthening programs. Report to CSAP.

Tobler, N. S., & Stratton, H. H. (1997). Effectiveness of school-based prevention programs: A meta-analysis of the research. *Journal of Primary Prevention, 18*(1), 71–128.

Tolan, P. H., Guerra, N. G., & Kendall, P. C. (1995a). A developmental-ecological perspective on antisocial behavior in children and adolescents: Toward a unified risk and intervention framework. *Journal of Consulting and Clinical Psychology, 63,* 579–584.

Tolan, P. H., Guerra, N. G., & Kendall, P. C. (1995b). Introduction to special section: Prediction and prevention of antisocial behavior in children and adolescents. *Journal of Consulting and Clinical Psychology, 63,* 515–517.

Tolan, P. H., & Loeber, R. L. (1993). Antisocial behavior. In P. H. Tolan & B. J. Cohler (Eds.), *Handbook of Clinical Research and Clinical Practice with Adolescents* (pp. 307–331). New York: Wiley.

Traux, C. B., & Carkhuff, R. R. (1965). Experimental manipulation of therapeutic conditions. *Journal of Consulting and Clinical Psychology, 29*(2), 119–124.

Tremblay, R. E., Masse, L., Pagani, L., & Vitaro, F. (1996). From childhood physical aggression to adolescent maladjustment: The Montreal Prevention Experiment. In R. DeV. Peters & R. J. McMahon (Eds.), *Childhood disorders, substance abuse, and delinquency: Prevention and early intervention approaches.* Thousand Oaks, CA: Sage.

Turner, W. (2000). Cultural considerations in family-based primary prevention programs in drug abuse. In S. Kaftarian & K. L. Kumpfer (Guest Eds.), Special Section: Family-focused research and primary prevention practice. *Journal of Primary Prevention, 21*(3), 285–303.

Turner, C., Sales, L., & Springer, F. (1998). Analysis of the High Risk Youth Grantee Program: Pathways to substance use. Paper presented at the 3rd Annual CSAP High Risk Youth Conference, Cincinnati, OH, July 23, 1998.

Walker, R., Kumpfer, K. L., Alder, S. C., & Richardson, G. (in press). Resilience in adult children of alcoholics: Empirical model of spirit, mind, and body precursors of healthy life adaptation. *Substance Use and Misuse.*

Webster-Stratton, C. (1981). Videotape modeling: A method of parent education. *Journal of Clinical Child Psychology, 10,* 93–97.

Webster-Stratton, C. (1982). Long term effects of a videotape modeling parent education program: Comparison of immediate and 1-year-followup results. *Behavior Therapy, 13,* 702–714.

Webster-Stratton, C. (1990a). Long-term follow-up of families with young conduct-problem children: From preschool to grade school. *Journal of Clinical Child Psychology, 19*(2), 114–149.

Webster-Stratton, C. (1990b). Enhancing the effectiveness of self-administered videotape parent training for families with conduct-problem children. *Journal of Abnormal Child Psychology, 18*(5), 479–492.

Webster-Stratton, C. (1996). Video-based Parent Training Program. Workshop presented at 2nd National Training Conference on Strengthening America's Families. Snowbird Ski Resort, Salt Lake City, Utah, October 12–14, 1996.

Webster-Stratton, C., Kolpacoff, M., & Hollingsworth, T. (1988). Self-administered videotape therapy for families with conduct-problem children: Comparison with two cost-effective treatments and a control group. *Journal of Consulting and Clinical Psychology, 56*(4), 558–566.

Werner, E. E. (1986). Resilient offspring of alcoholics: A longitudinal study from birth to age 18. *Journal of Studies on Alcoholism, 47*, 34–40.

Werner, E. E., & Smith, R. S. (1992). *Overcoming the odds: High risk children from birth to adulthood.* Ithaca, NY: Cornell University Press.

Werthamer-Larsson, L., Lillie-Blanton, M., Chatterji, P., Fienson, C., & Caffrey, C. (1996). Methods for investigating costs and benefits of drug abuse prevention. Paper presented at the NIDA conference: 'Drug Abuse Prevention Through Family Intervention,' Gaithersburg, MD, January 1996.

Wills, T. A., Vaccaro, D., & McNamara, G. (1992). The role of life events, family support, and competence in adolescent substance use: A test of vulnerability and protective factors. *American Journal of Community Psychology, 20*, 349–374.

Yoshikawa, H. (1994). Prevention as cumulative protection: Effects of early family support and education on chronic delinquency and its risks. *Psychological Bulletin, 115*(1), 28–54.

CHAPTER 5

Peers and the Prevention
of Adolescent Drug Use

E. R. OETTING

R. S. LYNCH

INTRODUCTION

Adolescent drug use has changed dramatically over the past 50 years, but the strong relationship between drug use and drug use by one's friends has remained a constant. In 1950, only a few adolescents used marijuana; but even then, Becker (1953) pointed out that teenagers who did use marijuana had friends who used marijuana; that friends taught them how and when to smoke it and even how they were supposed to react to the drug. Twenty years later, in the early 1970s, adolescent use of marijuana was increasing rapidly. It became a form of recreation for college students and moved from the realm of jazz musicians and artists to the affluent suburbs, high schools, and to the nation's servicemen in Vietnam. Newspaper reports of the ultimate "pot party" at Woodstock in August 1969 brought national attention to the increasingly widespread use of drugs (Anonymous, 1997); and marijuana became, for many adults, a primary symbol of youthful protest. As drug use among adolescents and young adults increased during the 1970s, scientists continued to point out that drug-using youth had drug-using friends (Adler & Lotecka, 1973; Huba, Wingard, & Bentler, 1979; Lawrence & Velleman, 1974; Tolone & Dermott, 1975; Wechsler & Thum, 1973).

In the early 1980s, when drug use was at its peak, there were major changes in the drugs used. There were new drugs, such as ecstasy, and new forms of older drugs, such as crack cocaine. Public TV ads were increasingly directed towards the evils of drugs. The famous fried-egg ad, "This is your brain on drugs," was but one dramatic example of a national media campaign that may

E. R. OETTING AND R. S. LYNCH • Tri-Ethnic Center for Prevention Research, Colorado State University, Fort Collins, Colorado 80523

have prevented some youths from using drugs. However, exaggerations in these media campaigns also allowed drug-using youths to discount their abstinence-promoting messages. For example, friends started asking each other if they wanted to "go fry an egg" (Cotts, 1997). In the late 1980s adolescent drug use declined throughout the decade; and, despite major changes in the prevalence of anti-drug media messages, articles continued to report the same strong links between peers and drug use (Battistich & Zucker, 1980; Brook, Lukoff, & Whiteman, 1980; Brook, Whiteman, & Scovell-Gordon, 1982, 1983; Kandel, 1985; Lopez, Redondo, & Martin, 1989).

Then, in the 1990s, drug use began to go up again. There is no clear explanation for this, but there are some possible reasons. Perhaps because the drug problem seemed to be going away, American society became complacent. Along with societal apathy, the internet may have had some effect. Whole sites gave computer-literate youths a way of researching the drugs they wanted to use and often glamorized the use of drugs. Major movies about early rock stars showed heavy drug use as part of an "exciting" lifestyle. But even during this recent period of increasing drug use, the fundamental finding—that drug users have drug-using friends—continued to appear in research studies (Ary et al., 1993; Brook et al., 1992; Clapper, Martin, & Clifford, 1994; Cousineau, Savard, & Allard, 1993; Dishion et al., 1995; Duncan, Duncan et al., 1995; Duncan, Tildesley et al., 1995; Iannotti & Bush, 1992; Khavari, 1993; Swaim et al., 1993).

The consistency of these findings, occurring despite major historical changes in drug use and in society, makes it clear that peer drug involvement is a critical factor in adolescent drug use. In fact, while many different psychosocial characteristics are related to drug use, up to half of the variance in adolescent drug use can be predicted by a combination of peer drug use, peer encouragement to use drugs, and peer sanctions against using drugs (Oetting & Beauvais, 1987). These and other research results led to the development of peer cluster theory (Oetting & Beauvais, 1986), which states that ". . . social and psychological variables interact to form a substrate that can make an individual susceptible to drug use. . . . When a young person uses drugs, however, it is almost always a direct reflection of the peer group. Friends, acquaintances, and siblings provide drugs and teach the young person to use them. Peers shape attitudes about drugs, provide the social contexts for drug use, and, when young people share their ideas, help form the rationales and excuses that the youth uses to explain and excuse drug use." (p. 19).

Primary socialization theory (Oetting & Donnermeyer, 1998) is a more recently developed general theory of deviant behavior that incorporates peer cluster theory. Primary socialization theory proposes that normative and deviant behaviors, including drug use, are learned social behaviors; they are products of the interaction of social, psychological, and cultural characteristics. The norms for social behaviors are learned predominantly in the context of interactions with these primary socialization sources.

Primary socialization theory states that every society or culture, at a given historical period, will establish specific primary sources for socialization. In different cultures, and at different times, these sources will vary, but there will always be identifiable primary socialization sources. The society's culture and subcultures are transmitted mainly through these primary sources. Secondary socialization sources are important, but their effects are strongly mediated by or moderated by the influence of the primary socialization sources. These primary socialization sources change developmentally, but at each stage of development there must be, and will be, appropriate and effective primary socialization sources that provide opportunities for bonding and that serve as sources for transmission of that society's cultural skills and norms. The youth will then bond with those sources and the culture's norms for attitudes and behaviors will be communicated through the primary socialization process.

During infancy and early childhood, the primary socialization source is the family. When the child enters school, the teachers and other school personnel become primary socialization sources. Later, peer clusters emerge as additional primary socialization sources (peer clusters are

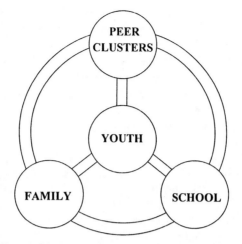

FIGURE 5.1. Primary socialization during adolescence.

small groups of close friends, best friends, or couples). By the time a youth is an adolescent, the three primary socialization sources are the family, the school, and peer clusters. Figure 5.1 shows the interactions between the dominant socialization forces in an adolescent's life (Oetting & Beauvais, 1987; Oetting, 1992; Oetting & Donnermeyer, 1998). This model indicates that youths are enmeshed in a social network, and that the three most important elements in that network are the family, the school, and peer clusters. In the ideal situation, an adolescent is connected to each of these, and they are connected to each other; the total forms a solid, strong figure, a wheel or circle that supports and maintains the youth. This model provides a useful tool for envisioning the most important factors influencing the child and for considering how to mount effective prevention programs. The circle is a firm figure, resistant to distortion or damage, but only when it is intact. If even one of the elements is strained, the whole structure is weakened and in danger. The child, family, school, and peer clusters all need to be "healthy" and strong. In addition, the parts that connect these systems, that link the child to family, school, and peers, and that connect these primary socialization forces to each other need to be strong. There must be strong bonds of caring and respect, and these bonds must be used to communicate norms for socially acceptable behaviors.

In this model, the family is usually a source of pro-social norms. Most families do their best to teach their children to do the right thing and try to prevent them from going astray. There are, sadly, parents who are exceptions to the rule. They beat their children, engage in incest, fight constantly, or even teach their children to use drugs. Even though these severely dysfunctional families constantly appear in the news, they are rare; most families try hard to do their best for their children. The school is also usually a positive force. Children do not usually learn deviant attitudes and behaviors directly from teachers or from other school staff. When the school itself is the source of a problem, it is likely to involve systemic factors that prevent or limit bonding of the child to the school; examples include punitive teachers, prejudice against minority students, or merely lack of resources that could provide children with successful learning experiences and reward them for being in school. However, as with families, most schools communicate pro-social norms. On the other hand, while families and the schools are usually sources of socially appropriate norms, there is no guarantee about peers. Peers can be either a positive or a negative force. Peers can become the dominant social influence in the lives of adolescents. If peers hold positive values and communicate pro-social norms, all will be well. If not, the chances are great that the child will be caught up in deviant behaviors, including drug use.

Although, among adolescents, drug-using norms are usually transmitted through involvement in peer clusters, the youth's links to the family and school are critically important; because they are major factors that determine whether a youth is likely to select and bond with friends who will transmit drug-using norms. When the bonds between the child and the family, as well as between the child and the school, are weakened, then the only strong connections left are likely to be with peers. It is possible, when that happens, that the resulting peer clusters could share positive norms. However, it is not likely. Most of the time the adolescents who are caught in this situation will seek out or be attracted to other youths who are also having some kind of problem. The resulting peer clusters are likely to be engaged in deviant behaviors, including drug use.

The rim of the wheel is formed by the bonds between the youth's primary socialization sources. When the family has strong bonds to the school, the family is more likely to support the child's education and help the child build strong bonds to the school. When the family is not linked to the school or to school goals, the child may still bond with the school; but the task may be more difficult. Bonds between peers and school are also highly important. Young people who form peer clusters with others who have poor school adjustment are likely to have their negative attitudes toward school reinforced. Poor family–school and peer–school bonds can also interact. For example, family–school bonds are often a problem for ethnic minority youths when the parents do not communicate well in the majority language or when the parents themselves had negative experiences with school (Alexander, Entwisle, & Bedinger, 1994; Curiel, 1991; Entwisle & Hayduck, 1982; Fernandez & Velez, 1989; Hare, 1988; Robledo, 1989; Wehlage et al., 1989). One effect may be increased dropout rates for some ethnic minority groups. Since potential dropouts are more likely to form peer clusters with other dropouts, and since dropouts have high rates of drug use (Swaim, 1997), the end result may be involvement in drug-using peer clusters and the use of drugs.

The bonds between the family and peers may also be important. When the family knows and likes a child's friends, and when those friends know and like the family, the peer clusters are more likely to consist of "good kids" and to have a positive influence on the child. These family–peer bonds may even be a valuable adjunct in treatment. Selekman (1991) interviewed families with drug-using children whose peers were involved in treatment. He recommended against involving highly deviant peers in family treatment; but when a youth was able to identify peers who "might be helpful" in reducing involvement with drugs, those peers often proved to be an asset to family treatment. Parents were sometimes able to build bonds with these peers, and the peers could improve communication between parents and their children. These peers were also useful in tertiary prevention, the prevention of relapse. They were able to help the youths identify and avoid drug use situations and could be on call during parent–child conflicts.

In general, when things go right, it is a result of strong bonds with the family, the school, and pro-social peers. When things go wrong, it can usually be linked to the formation of deviant peer clusters and can often be traced back to earlier problems, such as dysfunctional relationships with parents, poor school adjustment, and/or earlier problems in peer relationships.

THE PATHS TO DRUG ABUSE

Getting involved in a drug-using peer cluster can be a Kafkaesque experience because life-changing events that lead to association with deviant peers can be random. For example, an accidental choice of a seat on a school bus can lead to a friendship with a drug-involved youth; or "Dirty Eddie" moves in next door just at a time when a child needs a friend. However, involvement in a drug-using peer cluster does not usually occur randomly. There are strong selection factors in

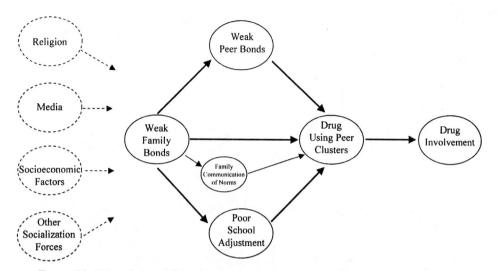

FIGURE 5.2. Theoretical model showing socialization influences on adolescent drug involvement.

the formation of peer clusters. Some are external, such as age, ethnicity, proximity—living in the same neighborhood or sitting next to someone in class (Hallinan & Williams, 1989; Kandel, 1978, 1985; Maccoby, 1990; Rubin, 1980). Other major factors are similarity of attitudes, social skills, interests, and abilities (Burleson & Lucchetti, 1990; Duck, Miell, & Gaebler, 1980; Insko et al., 1973; Mohan, Sehgal, & Bhandari, 1982; Tesser, Campbell, & Smith, 1984). Above all, the most important factor in formation of deviant peer clusters may be deviant norms. Adolescents who have good basic attitudes and values and who want to be "good" do not readily make friends with deviant youths. On the other hand, adolescents who have problems have a penchant for finding each other. When they do, the resulting peer clusters have a high potential for deviance.

The problems that create the potential for identifying with deviant peers are likely to be rooted in family problems, in school adjustment difficulties, in early peer relationships, and in personal characteristics that produce problems in bonding with the primary socialization sources. Elliot and Voss (1974) and Kandel (1978) were among the first to note that strong bonds with the school and the family are very likely to prevent formation of bonds with deviant peers. Wills and Cleary (1996) found that strong parental support is associated with improved academic competence, low tolerance of deviance, and a sense of control, and that these factors reduce the chances of involvement with drug-using peers. Hawkins and his colleagues also point out the critical importance of families, schools, and peers in determining drug use, and that the family and school may influence drug use through their effect on selection of friends (Gillmore et al., 1990; Hawkins, Catalano, & Wells, 1986; Hawkins, Lishner et al., 1986; Hawkins et al., 1991; Wells et al., 1992; Jenson et al., 1993; Catalano et al., 1992).

Figure 5.2 shows a theoretical path model indicating that problems with the family, school, and peers are likely to lead to association with drug-using peers and that the influence of these peer clusters, in turn, leads to drug use.

The path model in Figure 5.2 indicates that drug involvement is predominantly a function of involvement in drug-using peer clusters. The primary socialization sources (the family, school, peers) determine the probability that a youth will get involved in a drug-using peer cluster. When the bonds are strong between the individual and the primary socialization sources and when those sources communicate pro-social norms, involvement with drug-using peers is likely to be minimal. Any breakdown in bonds with the primary socialization sources or the communication of deviant norms from those sources is likely to lead to association with deviant and drug-using peers. Figure 5.2 also shows that there is a wide range of community and societal characteristics that can influence drug use, but that those characteristics must first influence the primary socialization process.

The model in Figure 5.2 is theoretical and does not include path coefficients. Both the fit of the model and the path coefficients need to be established in future research. The basic hypothesis is that, since the model describes the basic primary socialization process, the general model will fit quite well for different drugs, for both males and females, and for different ethnic groups in our society. However, the size of the actual path coefficients will differ for different drugs as well as by gender and ethnicity. Further, although the major source of variance in drug use is likely to be concurrent use by members of peer clusters, there may also be residual direct paths from family and/or school for some drugs and in some specific groups. We know, for example, that family communication of norms through modeling of marijuana use has more effect on young girls than on boys (Duncan et al., 1995). Kaplan (1996) notes that females with problems may be more attracted to deviant peers. Molina and Chassin (1996) found complex and curvilinear ethnic differences in the changes in family support that occur during puberty, and research has shown that family influence may be stronger, and peer influence weaker, in some U.S. ethnic minority groups and that these differences may interact with gender (Barnes & Welte, 1986; Beauvais, 1992; Brinson, 1991; Catalano et al., 1992; Rodriguez, 1996; Swaim, Oetting, & Casas, 1996). There are also differences in the influence of specific socialization sources at different ages or developmental stages.

The size of the path coefficients and the existence of residual paths will also be related to the measures used to assess the relevant constructs. For example, Wills and Cleary (1996) show, in general agreement with primary socialization theory, that most of the variance associated with adolescent substance use is mediated by association with drug-using peers; but they find small residual direct paths from tolerance for deviance and negative life events. In another study, Wills, Windle, and Cleary (1998) find that most of the substance use variance is mediated by links to drug-using peers, but that there are residual direct paths from poor control and harm avoidance. In both of these studies, the measure of peer substance use consists of only three items asking whether the youth had friends who used beer or wine, smoked cigarettes, or used marijuana. This measure places severe limits on the possible correlation with drug use because, while young people who use drugs have friends who use those same drugs, they also have friends who use other drugs. Dinges and Oetting (1993) found that for about 90% of the time drug users had friends using the drugs they were using; while two-thirds of the adolescents who got drunk but used no drugs had friends who used marijuana, and almost a third of those who used marijuana had friends who used cocaine. If the measure of peer drug involvement had specified drug use within peer clusters or had included items assessing peer encouragement to use and peer sanctions against use, the correlation between peer drug use and drug use may have been higher and the residual paths may not have been present. Further research is needed to explore this question.

Developmental Stages in the Evolution of Drug Use

Although nearly all drug use starts during pre-adolescence and adolescence, early experiences can establish the risk factors that lead to involvement with drug-using peers. Primary socialization theory suggests that, as a youth ages, the sources of pro-social and deviant norms change (Oetting, Donnermeyer, Trimble et al., 1998). During the preschool years, the family is the dominant source for socialization. The most important developmental task during these early years is parent/child bonding. When there are problems in family bonding and/or failure to communicate pro-social norms, a negative path toward later deviance can be established that is difficult to change. On the other hand, strong family–child bonding, transmission of pro-social norms, and adequate development of behavioral, cognitive, and social skills can provide a positive base for building the future, including the next stage, the early grade-school years, when creation of a positive school adjustment also becomes important. School adjustment then shares in importance with family influences. The grade-school child may have characteristics, such as hyperactivity, that interfere with school adjustment, or there may be problems on the school side of the equation, such as inadequate teaching or negative teacher attitudes toward lower social class or ethnic minority students. Whatever its source, poor school adjustment during these years greatly increases the probability of bonding with deviant peers. During the early grade-school years, peers are not yet a strong source for norms, but the ability to build good relationships with peers is critical, since weak peer bonding can lead to later association with deviant peers.

Quite often, today, there will be articles or references claiming either that psychologists no longer blame parents for a child's problems or that children do not learn from their parents, they learn from their friends. These articles are reporting on the point of view that has been presented by Judith Harris (1995). She challenges the standard belief that "it is all the parent's fault." In fact, she believes that children, even very young children, learn almost entirely from their peers.

Harris's position is probably too extreme. There is plenty of evidence that parents are a major factor in a child's development and evidence that children learn from and emulate their parent's behavior and attitudes. In fact, parents have a crucial influence on children, an influence that starts before birth and continues all the way through adolescence and beyond. The foundation of the protective shield starts with parents, and parent–child bonds continue, throughout the years, to be an important part of the protective shield. In fact, children who do not learn from their parents are more likely to be in trouble.

Children do learn from other children, but in these early preschool years, parents are the real underlying influence on the child. The child plays with other children, but parents (or substitutes for parents, such as extended family, babysitters or daycare staff) supervise that play. The attitudes picked up from other children are likely to be similar to those expressed by the parents, since the children's parents are likely to be the parent's friends or neighbors. Those neighbors whose children are selected as playmates are likely to be similar to the parents in many ways. They are involved in the same culture as the parents and are, therefore, likely to have about the same attitudes and beliefs as the child's parents. So what children learn from other children is likely to be an extension of and consistent with what they learn from their parents. Parents also monitor and correct what children learn. When children do pick up something bad from another child, when they learn a bad word, a behavior, or an attitude that is inconsistent with the parent's values, the parents try to stop it and, if necessary, isolate the child from that influence. Parents are the real controlling influence during the preschool years: the real influence of peers, independent of that of the family, appears later.

During the next stage of development, the early grade-school years, the creation of a positive school adjustment also becomes important. However, the family not only sets the stage for good school adjustment but also continues to be important in creating strong child–school bonds. When the school and family communicate the same attitudes, values and beliefs, it provides consistency and support for the development of the child's attitudes and behaviors. When parents express strong educational values and encourage and support the child's school work, it helps build liking for school and helps the child succeed in school. When parents can be involved in school and with the child's teachers, it not only provides further support for the child but also builds communication between the school and parents so any problems can be identified and resolved. On the other hand, if parents denigrate education, criticize the child's schoolwork, or simply fail to support the child's efforts, it can produce problems in school–child bonding. There is also an opportunity for the school to provide support where parents have not been able to do so. Many children with family problems have reported that their saving grace was an elementary school teacher who cared for them and supported them through these difficult years.

There are other factors that can produce problems in school–child bonding. The grade-school child may have characteristics, such as hyperactivity, that interfere with school adjustment, or there may be problems on the school-side of the equation, such as inadequate teaching or negative teacher attitudes toward lower social class or ethnic minority students. Whatever its source, poor school adjustment during these years greatly increases the probability that the child will, later on, bond with deviant peers.

As the child matures into pre-adolescence and adolescence, peers play an increasing role in communicating both pro-social and deviant norms. After adolescence, the patterns of primary socialization become much more complex as young adults get jobs, go to college, marry, and form sometimes complicated sets of new associations that serve as primary sources for social norms (for further discussion, see Oetting (1999)).

The effects of primary socialization are determined by the interaction between the individual's attitudes, behaviors, and needs, and the environment's reinforcement of attitudes and behaviors and whether it meets those needs. To completely understand the process at any given age or in a specific group, it is probably necessary to know the child's characteristics, the child's developmental status (as described by Piaget, Bronfenbrenner, Erickson, Gilligan, Kohlberg, Loevinger, or other developmental theorists), the child's attitudes and behaviors, and the response of the primary socialization environment (whether the interactions produce strong bonding and whether they reinforce pro-social or deviant norms). For example, children who possess a difficult temperament are going to be hard for parents to deal with, but those personality traits create really serious problems when the father also has certain types of personality problems or is involved with drugs and when the parent–child interaction leads to family dysfunction and child abuse (Blackson et al., 1994, 1996). Different factors may be more important at some stages of development than at others. (For a discussion of these risk factors, see Hawkins et al., (1986) and Swaim (1991).) However, in general terms, the socialization process leading to pro-social or deviant norms can be grasped by examining the three major and continuing sources of primary socialization—the family, the school, and peers.

The Family

The earliest influences on a child are from the family, and the family continues to provide a base for the child's experiences, even during adolescence when many youths are rebellious and/or are separating themselves from their families. Generally, when the primary socialization model in Figure 5.1 is intact, the family, along with peers and school, will continue to have an influence on normative behaviors. When the pro-social bonds are weakened, family influence is weakened, and peer clusters are likely to be the sole remaining influence. Research has consistently shown that problems in the family are likely to be related to drug use (Adler & Lotecka, 1973; Blackson et al., 1994; Blumenfield et al., 1972; Brook, Lukoff, & Whiteman, 1977; Duncan, Duncan, & Hops, 1994; Frumkin, Cowan, & Davis, 1969; Galli & Stone, 1975; Green, Blake, & Zehaysem, 1973; Oetting & Goldstein, 1979; Pandina & Scheule, 1983; Peterson et al., 1994; Streit, Halsted, & Pascale, 1974; Tec, 1974; Tolone & Dermott, 1975). Early parent–child bonding problems can have persistent effects. Weak family–child bonds in infancy have been linked to aggression in preschool children (Brook & Tseng, 1996; Brook et al., 1996; Troy & Sroufe, 1987); and Shedler and Block (1990) found that having nonresponsive and cold mothers at 5 years of age predicts adolescent drug use.

The definition of family can be relatively broad; it consists of those adults who take care of the child and monitor, reinforce, or punish the child's behavior. A single parent, foster parents, daycare providers, or members of the extended family can play these roles; but the rules remain the same: to prevent deviance, the family must provide strong adult–child bonding and communicate pro-social norms through those bonds.

The path model in Figure 5.2 also shows that it is not enough for a family to care. A strong family–child bond still needs to communicate appropriate norms; caring has to translate into communication of strong family sanctions against using drugs. When parents do not strongly discourage drug use, children are likely to end up developing bonds with drug-using peers and using drugs themselves. A few will take an opposite route and reject their parents' substance use, but many studies have shown that parental substance use is related to substance use of the child. Children of parents who use a specific substance are more likely to use that substance (Andrews et al., 1993; Brook et al., 1985; Chassin et al., 1991, 1994; Fisher et al., 1987; Gfroerer, 1987; Kandel & Andrews, 1987; Lau, Quadrel, & Hartman, 1990; Needle et al., 1986). Recent studies reviewing this literature include those of Andrews et al. (1993), Bennet and Wolin (1990), and Lau et al. (1990).

Strong family sanctions against drug use require more than simply not using drugs. Andrews et al. (1993) found that adolescent drug involvement is related to parent modeling, expression of negative attitudes toward drugs, communication about the dangers of drug use, and disciplining children who use drugs. Family communication of norms includes supervision and monitoring; studies have shown that the family can use monitoring to protect against association with deviant peers and reduce the chances of substance use (Brook et al., 1990; Loeber & Stouthamer-Loeber, 1986; Patterson & Dishion, 1985; Patterson & Stouthamer-Loeber, 1984). Weak parent monitoring is associated with parent drug use and is related to forming associations with drug-using peers (Dishion, Patterson, & Reed, 1988; Chassin et al., 1993, 1996). The interactions among these factors may be complex. Curran and Chassin (1996) found that monitoring, consistency of discipline, and parental support are strongly related to whether a child will use drugs, but only concurrently and not prospectively, and that better parenting by the mother could not compensate for the father's alcoholism. The effects of weak family sanctions can show up even in very young children. Asian-American and White-American fifth-graders who saw their parents as more tolerant of drug use stated that they were more likely to use drugs (Gillmore et al., 1990).

The School

Poor school adjustment involves doing poorly in school and/or not liking school, and in essentially every study where school adjustment has been assessed, it has been found to be related to substance use (Annis & Watson, 1975; Bakal, Milstein, & Rootman, 1975; Brook et al., 1977; Clayton & Voss, 1982; Frumkin et al., 1969; Galli, 1974; Jessor, 1976; Kandel, 1975; Svobodny, 1982). Young people who like school and are doing well in school tend to share positive values and attitudes that make it easier for them to become friends. They are likely to form peer clusters that oppose deviance. School policies and procedures may assist in this process of forming pro-social peer clusters. For example, schools tend to put good students and students who are active in school affairs together in the same advanced classes. Peer clusters formed in these classes are more likely to find involvement in school rewarding. On the other hand, school policies sometimes force together students who are doing poorly. The school puts these students together in remedial classes, pushes them into vocational courses, or places them together in detention. These policies can bring together at-risk students, encouraging the formation of deviant peer clusters. Even if these environmental factors were not involved, poor school adjustment would increase the chances of involvement in a deviant peer cluster. Youths who are doing poorly in school are very likely to find each other and build friendships in which they can share their anger and hostility toward the teachers and administrators they feel are punishing them.

Peers

Family and school problems may help set the stage, but an adolescent's peer clusters actually determine drug use. Voss and Clayton (1984) list a number of studies showing transmission of drug use by friends and associates; they also provide further supportive data for this argument. White (1972) was among the first to note that the merging of attitudes and characteristics when friendships are formed is a primary basis for building common drug attitudes and behaviors within peer clusters. Curran, Stice, & Chassin (1997) were able to show that there are mutual interactions over time between an adolescent and his or her peers that eventually determine alcohol use.

Several longitudinal studies appear to contradict this principle; however, these studies show weak or no relationships between early and later peer drug use (Farrell, 1994; Farrell & Danish, 1993). However, there is a fundamental technical reason why longitudinal studies across the junior high school and high school years will almost always show only a weak correlation from prior peer influence to later drug use. The huge increase in drug use across these developmental years must, mathematically, lead to large numbers of false positives and, therefore, to weak longitudinal correlations. The vast majority of very young children are not using drugs, and, in accord with peer cluster and primary socialization theory, their friends are also not using drugs. But, because of the increase in drug use during adolescence, many of these nonusing children will use drugs in later adolescence, and, in accord with the theory, their peers will also use drugs. Longitudinal correlations have to be low, however, because, while longitudinal false positives will be rare (e.g., Curran et al. (1997) found only 5 out of 442 students whose substance use declined precipitously), false negatives in very large numbers must occur as children who were not using drugs when they were young are using drugs in late adolescence. Using weak longitudinal relationships across adolescence as evidence against the potency of peer influence is, therefore, an egregious error. Actually, at any given age throughout this developmental period, nearly 90% of youths who are using drugs will have friends who are using those same drugs (Dinges & Oetting, 1993). Since false positives are rare (i.e., those young children with drug-using friends will continue to use drugs, and many children who do not use drugs and, therefore, have nonusing friends, will continue to avoid drugs), carefully conducted longitudinal studies will show this peer influence.

Early friendships do have an influence on drug use. Early formation of bonds with other deviant youth is likely to lead to continuous and long-term problems. Weak bonding with peers by young children can also be a problem that can lead to identification with deviant peer clusters. Young children who are aggressive, who are antisocial, or who express deviant attitudes are often rejected by their peers (Coie, Belding, & Underwood, 1988; Dodge & Frame, 1982). This rejection can make them susceptible to forming peer clusters with other youths who have a high potential for deviance and drug use (Dishion et al., 1995, 1996; Egeland, Carleson, & Sroufe, 1993).

Although peer cluster theory insists that the major influence on adolescent drug use is from peers, there is some question as to the strength of the bonds between deviant peers. Delinquent adolescents spend large amounts of time together and engage in delinquency together, but they may not feel close to their deviant friends (Pabon, Rodriguez, & Gurin, 1992). Bonding between deviant peers needs further study. It may be that if bonding is assessed by time spent together, by communication of deviant norms, or by sharing of deviant attitudes and beliefs, deviant peer clusters would appear to have strong peer bonds. On the other hand, if bonding were assessed by mutual affection and mutual trust, deviant peer clusters may appear to have weak peer bonds, since deviant youths may have problems in sharing affection that relate all the way back to early problems with parents and peers. Thus, they may not be able to trust each other.

Other Socialization Factors

The model shows that other social factors can have an influence on substance use; but the effects of many of these factors are likely to occur because they alter family relationships, school adjustment, and/or peer clusters. Figure 5.2 shows only three examples: religion, socioeconomic factors, and the media; but there are many other factors that could be considered. For example, social structures of communities can influence substance use (physical characteristics, rurality, ethnicity, heterogeneity, occupational type, occupational mobility, and age distribution). Other influences could come from the extended family, from associated groups, or from the general peer environment. Oetting, Donnermeyer, and Deffenbacher (1998) discuss the impact of most of these secondary socialization sources on the primary socialization process. The three examples included in Figure 5.2 illustrate the general principle: that secondary socialization sources have an effect because they influence the primary socialization sources and the communication of norms through those sources.

RELIGION.   Religion is a source of pro-social values in most societies. Drug use is almost always negatively related to religious identification (Bogg & Hughes, 1973; Brook et al., 1977; Burkett & Ward, 1993; Jessor, 1976; Jessor, Jessor, & Finney, 1973; Tittle & Welch, 1983; Turner & Willis, 1984). Where the religion disapproves of use of a particular substance, use of that substance will be lower (Adlaf & Smart, 1985; Burkett & Ward, 1993). Religion, therefore, influences adolescent drug use, but the model shows that it does so primarily through its influence on the primary socialization process. Major effects occur through the family; a strong religious identification increases the chances of family bonding (Oetting & Beauvais, 1987) and provides norms for non-substance-use that are transmitted to youths. Religious identification also tends to enhance school bonding (Oetting & Beauvais, 1987), possibly because conformity to religious norms is correlated with the ability to conform to school norms. Religious identification also influences peer clusters, both directly and indirectly; indirect influence occurs because it enhances family and school bonding, which improve the chances of forming pro-social peer clusters; direct influence occurs because youths with high religious identification are more likely to form peer clusters with others who are also religious (Newcomb, Mahaddian, & Butler, 1986; Tittle & Welch, 1983). Oetting, Donnermeyer, and Deffenbacher (1998) provide a further discussion of religion and primary socialization; and Oetting (1999) discusses spirituality.

SOCIOECONOMIC STATUS.   Studies of the relationship between socioeconomic status and drug use have sometimes found weak and inconsistent relationships (Davis et al., 1996; Jessor & Jessor, 1977; Penning & Bames, 1982), but when groups with serious social and economic problems are studied, drug use is often very high (Beauvais, 1992; Brunswick, 1979; Padilla et al., & Olmedo, 1979). These results suggest that the effects of poverty and inadequate opportunity may only occur when they are relatively extreme, or that socioeconomic factors are more important when many families in a neighborhood or community are suffering from the same kinds of economic problems, and when those problems are associated with other characteristics of neighborhoods that encourage deviance, such as living on reservations, in ghettos, or in barrios. In either case, primary socialization theory suggests that if socioeconomic factors are going to influence substance use, that influence is likely to be indirect, occurring because poverty and lack of opportunity affect the family, school adjustment, and peers. It is likely that poverty and little economic opportunity stress and weaken some families. Families, therefore, have less ability to form strong bonds with children and less ability to communicate pro-social norms. These children may also find it more difficult to adjust to school. In neighborhoods with endemic poverty, schools are likely to be poor and have limited resources, producing students with school adjustment problems. Family and school problems, in turn, increase the chances that an adolescent will become involved with a substance-using peer cluster. Economic problems are particularly likely to produce family problems that may lead to association with substance-using peers (Conger et al., 1990; Takeuchi, Williams, & Adair, 1991; Wills, McNamara, & Vaccaro, 1995; Wills, Pierce, & Evans, 1996). When impoverished families are isolated in a ghetto, barrio, or on a reservation, the effects of these problems are that there are many more children who are not attending school and there is high unemployment, so youths have large amounts of free time to interact with other unemployed peers. The result is more opportunity to form peer clusters with a high potential for deviance.

THE MEDIA.   The media represent another socialization force in our society that might influence drug use, but the influence of media probably occurs primarily because of its influence on the primary socialization process. Television provides an excellent example of how other socialization influences can be mediated by family and peers. Young people spend a lot of time watching television, and an assumption is sometimes made that this exposure directly determines their attitudes and behaviors and that televised exposure to drug use leads directly to experimenting with drugs. The influence of television on adolescents, however, is likely to be strongly mediated by other socialization factors, particularly peers. The programs adolescents watch are determined, for example, by the programs their friends watch. Their perceptions of what they are seeing are also influenced by their friends and by already existing attitudes and beliefs that have been formed in association with family and friends. They tend to see what they expect to see, and they tend to remember only what can be tied to what they already know or believe. Bogart (1967) and Gerbner (1990) point out that multiple media messages are being presented all the time, so selection plays a critical role in determining exposure. Arnett (1995) points out that adolescents are not blank slates; they have already learned principles and ideals that influence their media choices and how they interpret media messages. A show that has an impact of any kind is usually discussed within peer clusters, and mutual decisions are made about the meaning of the show—whether the expressed attitudes, clothing, or behaviors should be emulated or avoided. Television can foster adolescent drug use norms or anti-drug-use norms, but its actual influence is likely to be strongly mediated by interactions within peer clusters. The effects of media on the primary socialization process are discussed in more detail by Oetting, Deffenbacher, and Donnermeyer (1998).

PERSONALITY AND THE FORMATION
OF DEVIANT PEER CLUSTERS

The basic premise of personality theory is that there are deep-seated and persistent personal characteristics that determine motivation and behavior. Some theorists propose that personality traits are proximal causes of drug use and deviance (Petraitus et al., 1995; Russell & Mehrabian,

1977; Spotts & Shontz, 1980, 1984a,b). In contrast, primary socialization theory agrees with the basic idea that personality traits can influence drug use but suggests that the effects of personality are indirect—personality characteristics influence the primary socialization process and that, in turn, determines drug use (Oetting, Deffenbacher, & Donnermeyer, 1998).

Two types of theories attempt to link personality traits directly to adolescent drug use, but research does not provide particularly strong support for either. One theory views drug use as an attempt to alleviate chronic emotional distress caused by personality traits, such as depression, anxiety, and low self-esteem. In other words, the drug taken makes you feel better when you are suffering (Russell & Mehrabian, 1977). However, research has yielded, at best, only mixed support for this hypothesis. For example, when correlations are found between adolescent drug use and emotional distress, the relationships are likely to be small and may be in different directions (Dielman et al., 1987; Fisher, 1975; Mirin et al., 1971; Riggs, 1973; Sorosiak, Thomas, & Balet, 1976; Wingard, Huba, & Bentler, 1979; Green et al., 1973; Jones, 1973; Miranne, 1981; O'Malley, 1975; Schoolar, White, & Cohen, 1972; Simon et al., 1974; Spevack & Pihl, 1976). Adolescents apparently do not take drugs primarily because they are chronically anxious, depressed, or to compensate for low self-esteem. However, Oetting, Donnermeyer, and Deffenbacher (1998) point out that it is likely that emotional distress does play a role in establishing and maintaining drug dependence.

Another theory, psychodynamic theory, proposes that the action of the drug meets a deep-seated need derived from problems in emotional development (Khantzian, 1980). These psychodynamic theories have been somewhat more successful than self-medication theories, but only when describing drug use of very special and very small groups of people. Spotts and Shontz (1980, 1984a,b), for example, have shown that people who chronically and consistently use only one drug often choose a drug that compensates for developmental problems and that helps them maintain the illusion that life is tolerable. But most adolescents do not fit this model. Those who use drugs heavily almost never use only one drug; they use several different drugs and often use drugs that are available and have very different physiological and emotional effects. Except in the case of addiction, adolescent drug use is driven by social interactions, not by drugs. Psychodynamic theories do not predict adolescent drug use; but social and lifestyle theories, such as peer cluster theory and primary socialization theory, do predict the style of adolescent drug use quite well.

Primary socialization theory points out that personality traits play an important role in adolescent drug use, but this role is an indirect influence; personality traits influence the primary socialization process and that, in turn, influences drug use. Developmentally, personality traits can have a strong influence on the early primary socialization process, either enhancing or detracting from bonding with the family, school, or peers. Early psychopathology, for example, can interfere with the ability of parents to bond with their children and teach them attitudes and behaviors. Serious emotional problems can also interfere with school adjustment, and aggressive behaviors can interfere with early peer relationships. Externalizing disorders, such as oppositional disorder and conduct disorder, are particularly likely to produce family and school adjustment problems, leading to bonding with deviant and drug-using peers. Although anxiety and depression also cause personal problems, they are less likely to interfere with the socialization process (except when extreme) and are, therefore, less likely to lead to drug use. Kessler et al. (1996) confirm this point. They found that conduct disorders and antisocial behavior are more strongly linked to drug use than are anxiety or affective disorders.

Traits other than psychopathology also influence drug use. Socialization is influenced by the bonding between an individual and the primary socialization sources. However, bonding is not a one-way street determined solely by the primary socialization sources. Bonding is an interaction, and the characteristics of the child play an important role in that interaction. In normal circumstances, the parents and children interact, and if there are problems, they may originate with the child. The child may have traits that make parent–child bonding difficult. Or the problem may lie entirely with the parents. Dysfunctional, abusive, and drug-using parents can form unhealthy bonds with their children, and even when these bonds are strong, they are pathological and result in communication of deviant norms to the child. Blackson et al. (1994, 1996) provide seminal studies that examine the interaction between paternal history of substance use, father and son temperament, parental abuse, family dysfunction, and drug use. Their results suggest that the father's tendency to abuse substances and the temperaments of both the fathers and sons can interact to produce family dysfunction, possibly resulting in "... the premature disengagement of the son from the parental sphere of influence to a deviant peer network or toward social withdrawal that is antecendant to early-age onset of substance abuse. ..."

Interactions between personal characteristics and parent–child bonding show up in other circumstances as well. Although twin studies tend to view children in the same families as having the same environment, Reiss (1997) points out that the relationships between parents and different adolescent siblings can differ greatly. His analyses of genetic versus environmental contributions suggest that when they do differ it is probably because of fundamental differences in the children, not in the parenting. A difficult child is treated more harshly by the parents. It is possible that exceptional parenting skills can compensate for those traits that make a child difficult to handle, but it is important to recognize that the characteristics of the adolescent play an important role in the parent–child interaction.

While many personality traits of adolescents do not show strong links to drug use, there are relatively strong links between drug use and three traits—anger, deviant norms, and sensation seeking. Figure 5.3 shows how these variables are probably related to substance use. The figure shows that each of these traits is related to the formation of drug-using peer clusters. Involvement in those peer clusters then leads to drug use.

Due to the importance that has been placed on some other emotional distress characteristics, four such emotional distress characteristics are included in the model. The model shows that

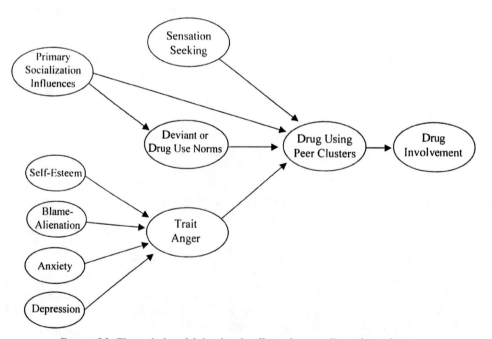

FIGURE 5.3. Theoretical model showing the effects of personality traits on drug use.

emotional distress traits, such as low self-esteem, anger, alienation, and depression, do not directly relate to drug use or to the formation of drug-using peer clusters; whatever correlation with drug use they do have is accounted for by their relationship to trait anger (Evans, Weinberg, & Jackson, 1992; Swaim et al., 1989; Oetting et al., 1989). A further discussion of the role played by self-esteem in the etiology of drug use can be found in Oetting, Deffenbacher, and Donnermeyer (1998), and a later section of this paper shows that while anxiety and depression are not strongly related to adolescent drug use, they may directly influence the consequences of that drug use.

ANGER.   High-trait anger, including chronic tendencies to be aggressive, is correlated with substance use, particularly alcohol use (Brennan, Walfish, & AuBochon, 1986; Brooks et al., 1981; Liebsohn, Oetting, & Deffenbacher, 1994; Moos et al., 1977). There are probably a number of reasons why anger increases the chances that youth get involved with drug-using peers. Angry youths are more likely to have acted aggressively in earlier peer interactions, which led to problems in bonding with pro-social peers. Angry youths are also more likely to have conflicts with parents and school officials, damaging bonding with parents and school. Anger, in effect, increases the chances of bonding with deviant peers. The problem is exacerbated within the peer cluster. When a peer cluster includes angry youths, the members of that peer cluster are likely to reinforce each other's expressions of anger and deviant behaviors. Drug use may grow out of these shared feelings, particularly if drug use is viewed by the group as a rebellious or authority-challenging behavior. Walters's (1980) "rowdies" used drugs in just this way.

Deviant Norms

Constructs that reflect deviant norms appear in different models under different names, but they are always strongly related to drug use. Tolerance of deviance was found to be a correlate of drug use in early studies by Jessor et al. (1968) and by Jessor Jessor, (1977, 1978). Oetting and Beauvais (1989) used a different scale to assess tolerance of deviance but found the same strong relationship to drug use in samples of Native-American youths. Brook and her colleagues have consistently shown that "unconventionality," a trait that incorporates Jessor's measure of tolerance of deviance, is an important predictor of drug use (Brook, Gordon, & Whiteman, 1985; Brook, Lukoff, & Whiteman, 1980; Brook et al., 1984, 1990, 1992). Newcomb and Bentler (1988) found that the latent construct of social conformity is negatively related to later drug use. Their measure of social conformity involves both law abidance and religious commitment, suggesting nondeviant norms.

Deviant or drug use norms (norms related to tolerance of deviance and unconventionality) emerge as an outcome of the primary socialization process; these norms are learned through interactions with the primary socialization sources, most often deviant peers. So, the deviant norms held by adolescents are a product of earlier experiences. Once present, however, these norms increase the chances of further involvement in drug-using peer clusters. The alternative also holds true: Youths holding nondeviant norms are not likely to be attracted to deviant friends and are more likely to form peer clusters with other nondeviant youths.

Sensation Seeking

Sensation seeking is related to drug use (Donohew, 1988, 1990; Donohew et al., 1990; Donohew, Lorch, & Palmgreen, 1991; Segal & Singer, 1976; Spotts & Schontz, 1984c; Zuckerman, Eysenck, & Eysenck, 1978; Zuckerman, 1988). It is correlated with risk taking and a need for excitement. Sensation seeking has at least a partial biological basis (Benjamin et al., 1996; Ebstein et al., 1996), although if chromosomal differences exist, they only account for about 10% of the variance in sensation seeking. Sensation seekers appear to have some physiological characteristics that make them more sensitive to the effects of drugs (Bardo & Mueller, 1991), finding drugs to be more rewarding (Carrol, Zuckerman, & Vogel, 1982). A theory that sensation seekers use drugs for their physiological and emotional effects is, therefore, attractive. (But the model presented in Figure 5.3 suggests that the effects of sensation seeking, as with other personality traits, occur mainly because of its influence on peer clusters.) The high-sensation seeker finds others who also need a high level of stimulation and excitement and forms peer clusters with them. The norms of these peer clusters then determine whether the "exciting" activities they choose will involve drug use. Donohew et al. (1990, 1991) found confirming evidence that sensation seekers are more likely to form bonds with other sensation seekers. They also found that the high correlation between sensation seeking and drug use is mediated by peer influences. Wills, Windle, and Cleary (1998) also found that novelty seeking is related indirectly to drug use through its links to drug-using peers.

Further research on the movement of sensation seekers toward drug use is needed. Primary socialization theory suggests that the same risk factors that influence the movement toward drug use in other youths also influence sensation seekers. The theory suggests that, where there is a solid foundation from earlier primary socialization, sensation seekers will identify with pro-social peers, and the resulting peer clusters will find pro-social means for meeting their needs. On the other hand, the effects of early problems in family, school, or peer bonding may be exacerbated by sensation seeking. When the at-risk sensation seeker forms peer clusters with deviant peers, those peers are more likely to be sensation seekers as well. The result for these individuals may be drug use and high-risk drug-using behaviors.

Summary: Personality Traits and Deviance

Primary socialization theory points out that while anger, tolerance of deviance, and sensation seeking are all correlated with drug use, they do not directly cause drug use. Adolescents do not take drugs primarily to change internal feelings and emotions or because a personality characteristic directly increases the need for drugs. They take drugs because drug use is part of their interactions with their peers. Angry youths, for instance, may be more likely to seek out friends who support their anger, much of which may be focused on parents, the school, or other authorities. The resulting peer clusters have a high potential for getting involved in deviant behaviors, including drug use. Sensation-seeking youths want and need excitement in their lives. For adolescents, this usually means doing exciting things with friends. Unfortunately, these "exciting" activities can include drug use. The most important factor in the formation of a peer cluster that has a high tendency for substance use is probably deviant norms. While deviant norms are likely to have been produced by prior interactions with peers, once present, they become very important. A youngster who has a high tolerance for deviance and who is willing to engage in deviant behaviors is likely to find friends who also have a high potential for deviance. Within the peer cluster, that youth is also a source for communication of deviant norms. These peer clusters then provide further reinforcement for maintaining deviant norms and have a high potential for deviant behavior, including drug use.

PREVENTION AND PEERS

There are two general approaches to prevention: supply reduction and demand reduction. Supply reduction usually focuses on legal and political efforts, such as destruction of crops, changing of laws, increasing law enforcement, and reducing children's access to tobacco and alcohol. But drugs are actually distributed among adolescents through peer networks and peer clusters. It would take some imaginative effort to find ways to disrupt this distribution and reduce supply, but interfering with the peer distribution network might be more effective than many other ways used to reduce supply. There may be a major research opportunity in studying peer distribution networks and developing methods for interfering with peer distribution of drugs.

Demand reduction prevention programs have had moderate success in reducing drug use. Treatment of drug users is reasonably successful and reduces demand in a group at very high risk. Programs to reduce initiation and exacerbation of adolescent drug use have also been somewhat successful. They do not stop drug use, but they do stop some adolescents from initiating drug use and reduce the overall level of use. The National Institute on Drug Abuse points out that prevention programs have five targets: the individual, the school, the family, the community, and the peer group (Drug Abuse Prevention: What Works, 1997). The role played by each of these targets has already been discussed. However, the models that are presented all emphasize the critical role played by peers in substance use. Prevention efforts should always keep this fact in focus; drug use is not likely to change unless peer clusters change. Every prevention program should consider how it will influence selection of drug-using peers or how it will influence the communication of drug use norms through peer clusters. Regardless of the target, unless there is a basis for believing that a prevention program will lead to change in this immediate peer influence, a prevention program is not likely to be successful.

How do we change the influence of peer clusters? Peer clusters can change in many ways, all of which offer opportunities for prevention: (1) a program can lead individuals to identify with "healthier" peer clusters and reject deviant peers; (2) a prevention effort can be aimed at influencing peer clusters to provide less encouragement of drug use and stronger sanctions against drug use; (3) another prevention program might attempt to help peer clusters find ways other than drugs to meet the individual and social needs of their members; (4) prevention programs could target opportunity by reducing the time that peer clusters are unsupervised and thereby reduce the opportunities for drug use; and (5) if psychoactive substances are used, harm-reduction programs can be aimed at changing peer behaviors to encourage lower levels of use or reduce dangerous methods of use, such as needle sharing.

Prevention programs aimed at changing attitudes toward drugs may actually influence drug use because the youths involved in the program carry anti-drug norms to their present and future peer clusters. The transmission of those anti-drug attitudes within peer clusters can then influence drug use of the peer cluster. Prevention programs aimed at refusal skills can help adolescents avoid drug use, but only if they lead to refusal of association with drug-using peers or if they are potent enough that the youth can refuse drug use within the peer cluster. The latter is difficult, since it often leads to rejection by other members of the peer cluster.

Prevention programs offered in schools will be effective if they can reduce selection of drug-using peer clusters or change transmission of drug use norms within peer clusters. School programs that use peers are more effective because they have a greater chance of influencing peer clusters. Naginey and Swisher (1990) found that the higher the drug use, the more students would seek advice from peers and the less they would seek advice from teachers or administrators. Peers may, therefore, be more effective in presenting anti-drug programs to at-risk youths than are teachers. In other studies peer-led groups with booster sessions were more effective than teacher-led programs. Botvin et al. (1990) and Perry (1989), in a major international study, found that peer presenters were effective while teacher-led groups were not. But other studies of peer-led programs have found only small amounts of effectiveness, although their effectiveness is still better than when teachers led the programs (Johnson et al., 1986; Murray et al., 1987). Wiist and Snider (1991) developed a program that used peers to identify presenters and found that the approach might be effective, but the study had too few subjects to confirm the findings as significant.

There are also potential dangers in interventions that involve peers. There is always the possibility that a prevention program will create opportunities for adolescents to form new peer clusters with deviant youths. If that happens, drug use can be increased by the prevention program. Palinkas et al., (1996) report on a drug abuse prevention program that brought together young female adolescents who were at risk for drug use and unwanted pregnancy to teach them refusal skills. The treated group was almost three times more likely to use marijuana as the control group. The researchers state that the prevention program "...led to improved social relations with drug-using peers, thereby increasing exposure to peer pressure to use drugs...."

Prevention programs could also be aimed at other characteristics that can change the behavior of peer clusters. There may be two general approaches toward prevention that have somewhat different goals and require different methods: (1) changing general social norms and (2) changing risk factors.

Changing Social Norms

Although not aimed directly at peers, prevention efforts should probably continue to be aimed at changing social norms so that substance use is perceived as deviant, particularly the more dangerous forms of use. Despite the independence/dependence conflicts of adolescents, the majority want to do what is right. Nevertheless, some of these basically "good" youths become involved in peer clusters that use drugs, and many are in groups that use alcohol to excess. If society's attitudes toward these behaviors becomes more negative, the behaviors would become socially unacceptable and would be much less likely to be reinforced in peer clusters. For these pro-social youths, the wheel is intact. The child is bonded to family, school, and peers, and the bonds are used to communicate positive social norms. If those norms change to strong disapproval of drug use, drug use will decline in the group. Cultural factors are important in establishing norms for pro-social behaviors. For example, Rodriguez points out that traditional beliefs about gender roles may lead to a greater tendency for Hispanic adolescent males than females to engage in antisocial behaviors; but the effects of cultural identification are not simple. These effects depend on cultural knowledge and social context (Guarnaccia & Rodriguez, 1996). Oetting, Donnermeyer, Trimble et al. (1998) provide a detailed description of ethnicity and culture and their influence on drug use.

Despite the fact that early prevention programs that only talked about the dangers of drugs proved to have little influence on drug use, one way of changing social norms may be to continue, in public forums and the media, to emphasize the dangers and risks of drug use. Johnston, O'Malley, and Bachman (1992) found that as perceived danger from drugs increased, drug use decreased. This effect might be simply due to personal decision making; but peer cluster theory suggests the result might occur because perceived danger was a factor in changing peer cluster norms, decreasing peer encouragement to use drugs, and increasing peer sanctions against using drugs. If so, the reduction in drug use that we have seen over the past decade would be among those peer clusters that are more susceptible to changes in social norms, not those at high risk because they include youths who espouse deviant norms. Researchers should explore this issue.

Changing social norms may not be enough. The changes may need to occur along with provision of alternatives. Adults might be happy if all children stayed childish and never engaged in any adult behaviors until they reached the magical age of 21. Adults might be even more satisfied if children always followed good advice, never made mistakes, always had good judgment, and never did anything dangerous. But unless adolescents are in a culture where they are constantly observed and monitored, this is not going to happen. We have, instead, the "adolescent conspiracy"; youths will meet their perceived needs but will mutually hide the deviant behavior, including drug and alcohol use, from adults. If there were more formal opportunities for youths to meet personal and social needs, including a need to do something stimulating and exciting, there might be less of a need to seek out informal associations (not open to adult observation) that are, therefore, potential opportunities for drug use. But most communities do not provide enough alternatives for youths, particularly acceptable alternatives that meet the needs of high sensation-seeking peer clusters.

Changing Risk Factors

Changing social norms and providing alternatives, however, will only influence those youths who already identify positively with the culture. It will have minimal influence on those who form peer clusters that not only tolerate but also encourage deviance. The wheel, presented in Figure 5.1, illustrates the most important risk factors that can lead to association with deviant peers. Each part of the wheel presents its own challenge, from improving a child's capacity to bond with the family, to altering the interaction between parents and the school. The youths identified as having weaknesses in one or more areas of this wheel are considered to be most at risk for substance use.

Prevention programs can take many forms, depending on the pattern of risk factors identified and the developmental stage of the children involved. Very early prevention must identify breakdowns in child–family bonds and weaknesses in family-to-child transmission of pro-social norms. In elementary school, prevention may have to target both the family and the school adjustment. Still later, the bonds among peer clusters, school, and the family may come into play. To be fully effective, however, any prevention program will eventually need to influence peer clusters. When, and if, peer clusters change, drug use will change.

Children and adolescents who have suffered breakdowns in their primary socialization process, who have family, school, or peer bonding problems, will be the hardest to reach and to change. Unless a prevention program effectively changes either the strength of the peer bonds or the use of those bonds to communicate nondeviant norms, there will be no change in drug use. The difficulty and the costs of interventions aimed at altering risk factors for high-risk youths are likely to be great, but the benefits from success will also be great. Deviant youths create immense costs for society and for themselves.

CONCLUSION

The premise of this chapter is that adolescent substance use is a social behavior that is determined primarily by social norms, particularly the norms developed within peer clusters. When a particular form of substance use is generally tolerated by society (for example, alcohol use), it is likely to be reinforced and encouraged within most adolescent peer clusters. Most drug use and some forms of alcohol use, however, are deviant behaviors not tolerated by society, and young people who engage in these behaviors are likely to do so in the social context of peer clusters involving deviant youths.

The major socialization forces in a youth's life consist of the family, the school, and peer clusters. The family and school usually transmit positive social norms. Peers, however, can transmit either healthy or deviant norms. When a youth has strong bonds with the family and school, and when the youth's friends are also bonded to the family and school, the youth's peer clusters are likely to be a source of positive norms. When there are breakdowns in these links, however, the chances that a youth will identify with peer clusters possessing deviant norms are greatly increased.

Primary socialization theory indicates that there are three possible sources for drug use norms. Parents can, either directly or by example, encourage drug use. The family, however, is nearly always a source of pro-social norms; and nearly all parents try to prevent their children from using drugs. Although a few teachers use drugs, and occasionally a teacher will victimize a student, schools are also usually sources for pro-social norms. Peers, on the other hand, can be sources for either pro-social or antisocial norms. Ultimately, the youth's membership in peer clusters will determine whether that youth initiates and maintains drug use. If the peer clusters transmit pro-social and anti-drug norms, drug use is not likely. If a youth's peer clusters transmit norms that encourage use of a particular substance, use of that drug will almost invariably occur. A prevention program would be highly successful if young people could be steered away from drug-using peer clusters. Prevention would also be successful if peer clusters did not transmit norms for drug use. Understanding the formation of peer clusters and their effects is, therefore, important when planning and implementing prevention programs.

Prevention programs need to establish general social norms against substance use and against risky forms of substance use. These changes will reduce the chances that peer clusters consisting of reasonably "healthy" youths will get involved with drugs. Prevention also needs to target high-risk peer clusters—those whose members have suffered from breakdowns in the links to family, school, and peers. Reducing the chances that adolescents will get involved in deviant peer clusters by improving family and school bonds may require early and intense effort, but the payoff for that effort could be great.

REFERENCES

Adlaf, E. M., & Smart, R. C. (1985). Drug use and religious affiliates, feelings and behavior. *Br. J. Addict. 80*(2), 163–171.

Adler, P. T., & Lotecka, L. (1973). Drug use among high school students: Patterns and correlates. *The International Journal of the Addictions, 8,* 537–548.

Alexander, K. L., Entwisle, D. R., & Bedinger, S. D. (1994). When expectations work: Race and socioeconomic differences in school performance. *Social Psychological Quarterly, 57,* 283–299.

Andrews, J. A., Hops, H., Ary, D., Tildesley, E., & Harris, J. (1993). Parental influences on early adolescent substance use: Specific and nonspecific effects. *Journal of Early Adolescence, 13*(3), 285–310.

Annis, H. M., & Watson, C. (1975). Drug use and school dropout: A longitudinal Study. *Canadian Counselor, 9,* 155–162.

Anonymous. (1997). 1969 Woodstock Festival & Concert [online]. http://www.woodstock69.com.

Arnett, J. J. (1995). Adolescents' uses of media for self-socialization. *Journal of Youth and Adolescents, 24*(5), 519–533.

Ary, D. V., Tildesley, E., Hops, H., & Andrews, J. (1993). The influence of parent, sibling, and peer modeling attitudes on adolescent use of alcohol. *The International Journal of the Addictions, 28*(9), 853–880.

Bakal, D., Milstein, S. L., & Rootman, I. (1975). Trends in drug use among rural students in Alberta: 1971–1974. *Canadian Mental Health, 23,* 8–9.

Bardo, M. T., & Mueller, C. W. (1991). Sensation seeking and drug abuse prevention from a biological perspective. *Persuasive communication and drug abuse prevention.* Hillsdale, NJ: Lawrence Erlbaum Associates.

Barnes, G. M., & Welte, J. W. (1986) Patterns and predictors of early alcohol use among 7–12th grade students in New York State. *J. Stud. Alcohol, 47,* 53–62.

Battistich, V. A., & Zucker, R. A. (1980). A multivariate social-psychological approach to the prediction of psychoactive drug use in young adults. *The International Journal of the Addictions, 15*(4), 569–583.

Beauvais, F. (1992). Comparison of drug use rates for reservation Indian, non-reservation Indian and Anglo youth. *American Indian and Alaska Native Mental Health Research, 5,* 13–31.

Becker, H. S. (1953). Becoming a marijuana user. *The American Journal of Sociology, 49,* 235–242.

Benjamin, J., Li, L., Patterson, C., Greenberg, B. D., Murphy, D. L., & Hamer, D. H. (1996). Population and familial association between the D4 dopamine receptor gene and measures of novelty seeking. *Nature Genetics, 12*(1), 81–84.

Bennett, L. A., & Wolin, S. J. (1990). Family culture and alcoholism transmission. In R. L. Collins, K. E. Leonard, & J. S. Searles (Eds.), *Alcohol and the family: Research and clinical perspectives* (pp. 194–219). New York: Guilford.

Blackson, T. C., Tarter, R. E., Loeber, R., Ammerman, R. T., & Windle, M. (1996). The influence of paternal substance abuse and difficult temperament in fathers and sons on sons' disengagement from family to deviant peers. *Journal of Youth and Adolescence, 25*(3), 389–411.

Blackson, T. C., Tarter, R. E., Martin, C., & Moss H. (1994). Temperament induced father-son family dysfunction: Etiological implications for child behavior problems and substance abuse. *American Journal of Orthopsychiatry, 64*(2), 280–292.

Blumenfield, M., Riester, A. E., Serrano, A. C., & Adams, R. L. (1972). Marijuana use in high school students. *Diseases of the Nervous System, 33*(9).

Bogart, L. (1967). *Strategy in advertising.* New York: Harcourt.

Bogg, R. A., & Hughes, J. (1973). Correlates of marijuana usage at a Canadian Technological Institute. *International Journal of the Addictions, 8,* 489–504.

Botvin, G. J., Baker, E., Filazzola, A. D., & Botvin, E. M. (1990). A cognitive behavioral approach to substance abuse prevention: One-year follow-up. *Addictive Behaviors, 15,* 47–63.

Brennan, A. F., Walfish, S., & AuBochon, P. (1986). Alcohol use and abuse in college students. I. A review of individual and personality correlates. *International Journal of the Addictions, 21,* 449–474.

Brinson, J. (1991). A comparison of the family environment of black male and female adolescent alcohol users. *Adolescence 26,* 877–884.

Brook, J. S., Brook, D. W., Gordon, A. S., Whiteman, M., & Cohen, P. (1990). The psychosocial etiology of adolescent drug use: A family interactional approach. *Genetic, Social, and General Psychology Monograph, 116*(2).

Brook, J. S., Gordon, A. S., & Whiteman, M. (1985). Stability of personality during adolescence and its relationship to stage of drug use. *Genetic, Social, and General Psychology Monographs, 111,* 317–330.

Brook, J. S., Lukoff, I. F., & Whiteman, M. (1977). Correlates of marijuana use as related to age, sex, and ethnicity. *Yale Journal of Biological Medicine, 50,* 383–390.

Brook, J. S., Lukoff, I. F., & Whiteman, M. (1980). Initiation into adolescent marijuana use. *Journal of Genetic Psychology, 137,* 133–142.

Brook, J. S., & Tseng, L. J. (1996). Influence of parental drug use, personality, and child-rearing on toddler's anger and negativity. *Genetic, Social, and General Psychology Monograph, 122*(1), 107–128.

Brook, J. S., Whiteman, M., Cohen, P., & Tanaka, J. S. (1992). Childhood precursors of adolescent drug use: A longitudinal analysis. *Genetic, Social and General Psychology Monographs, 118*(2), 195–213.

Brook, J. S., Whiteman, M., & Scovell-Gordon, A. (1982). Qualitative and quantitative aspects of adolescent drug use: Interplay of personality, family, and peer correlates. *Psychological Reports, 51,* 1151–1163.

Brook, J. S., Whiteman, M., Gordon, A. S., & Brook, D. W. (1990). The role of older brothers in younger brothers' drug use viewed in the context of parent and peer influences. *The Journal of Genetic Psychology, 151*(l), 59–75.

Brook, J. S., Whiteman, M., & Scovell-Gordon, A. (1983). Stages of drug use in adolescence: Personality, peer, and family correlates. *Developmental Psychology, 19,* 269–277.

Brook, J. S., Whiteman, M., Gordon, A. S., & Brook, D. W. (1984). Paternal determinants of female adolescent marijuana use. *Developmental Psychology, 20,* 1032–1043.

Brook, J. S., Whiteman, M., Gordon, A. S., & Brook, D. W. (1985). Father's influence on his daughter's marijuana use viewed in a mother and peer context. *Advances in Alcohol & Substance Abuse, 3*(3–4), 165–190.

Brooks, M., Walfish, S., Stenmark, D., & Canger, J. (1981). Personality variables in alcohol abuse in college students. *Journal of Drug Education, 11,* 185–189.

Brinson, J. (1991). A comparison of the family environment of black male and female adolescent alcohol users. *Adolescence, 26,* 877–884.

Brunswick, A. (1979). Black youths and drug-use behavior. In G. M. Beschner & A. S. Friedman, (Eds.), *Youth Drug Abuse: Problems, Issues and Treatment.* Toronto: D. C. Heath.

Burkett, S. R., & Ward, D. A. (1993). A note of perceptual deterrence, religiously based moral condemnation, and social control. *Criminology, 31*(1), 119–134.

Burleson, B. R., & Lucchetti, A. E. (1990). *Similarity-attraction revisited: Similarity in social cognition, communication skills, and communication values as predictors of friendship choices in two age groups.* Paper presented at the Fifth International Conference on Personal Relationships, Oxford University, Oxford, England.

Carrol, E. N., Zuckerman, M., & Vogel, W. H. (1982). A test of the optimal level of arousal theory of sensation seeking. *Journal of Personality and Social Psychology, 42,* 572–575.

Catalano, R. F., Morrison, D. M., Wells, E. A., Gillmore, M. R., Iritani, B., & Hawkins, J. D. (1992). Ethnic differences in family factors related to early drug initiation. *Journal of Studies on Alcohol, 53*(3).

Chassin, L., Curran, P. J., Hussong, A. M., & Colder, C. R. (1996). The relation of parent alcoholism to adolescent substance use: A longitudinal follow-up study. *Journal of Abnormal Psychology, 105*(1), 70–80.

Chassin, L., Pillow, D., Curran, P., Molina, B., & Barrera, M. (1993). The relation of parental alcoholism to early adolescent substance use: A test of three mediating mechanisms. *Journal of Abnormal Psychology, 102*(1), 449–463.

Chassin, L., Presson, C. C., Sherman, S. J., & Edwards, D. A. (1991). Four pathways to young adult smoking status: Adolescent social psychological antecedents in a Midwestern community sample. *Health Psychology, 10,* 409–416.

Chassin, L., Presson, C. C., Sherman, S. J., & Mulvenon, S. (1994). Family history of smoking and young adult smoking behavior. *Psychology of Addictive Behaviors, 8,* 102–110.

Clapper, R. L., Martin, C. S., & Clifford, P. R. (1994). Personality, social environment, and past behavior as predictors of late adolescent alcohol use. *Journal of Substance Abuse, 6,* 305–313.

Clayton, R. R., & Voss, H. R. (1982). *Technical review on drug abuse and dropouts.* Report on a National Institute on Drug Abuse technical review meeting. Rockville, NM: National Institute on Drug Abuse.

Coie, J. D., Belding, M., & Underwood, M. (1988). Aggression and peer rejection in childhood. In B. B. Lahey & A. E. Kazdin (Eds.), *Advances in Clinical Child Psychology, Vol. 11* (pp. 125–158). New York: Plenum Press.

Conger, R. D., Elder Jr., G. H., Lorenz, F. O., Conger, K. J., Simons, R. L., Whitbeck, L. B., Huck, S., & Melby, J. N. (1990). Linking economic hardship to marital quality and instability. *Journal of Marriage and the Family, 52,* 643–656.

Cotts, C. (1997). The partnership: Hard sell in the drug war. *The Nation Magazine* [online]. http://www.drugtext. http://www/think/pdfacott/.htm.

Cousineau, D., Savard, M., & Allard, D. (1993). Illicit drug use among adolescent students: A peer phenomenon? *Canadian Family Physician, 39,* 523–527.

Curiel, H. (1991). Strengthening family and school bonds in promoting Hispanic children's school performance. In M. Sotomayer (Ed.), *Empowering Hispanic families: A critical issue for the 90s.* Milwaukee, WI: Family Service America.

Curran, P. J., & Chassin, L. (1996). A longitudinal study of parenting as a protective factor for children of alcoholics. *Journal of Studies on Alcohol, 57,* 305–313.

Curran, P. J., Stice, E., & Chassin, L. (1997). The relation between adolescent alcohol use and peer alcohol use: A longitudinal random coefficients model. *Journal of Consulting and Clinical Psychology, 65,* 130–140.

Davis, N., Moss, H., Kirisci, L., & Tarter, R. (1996). Neighborhood crime rates among drug abusing and non-drug abusing families. *Journal of Child and Adolescent Substance Abuse, 5*(4), 1–14.

Dielman, T. E., Campanelli, P. C., Shope, J. T., & Butchart, A. T. (1987). Susceptibility to peer pressure, self-esteem and health locus of control as correlates of adolescent substance abuse. *Health Education Quarterly, 14,* 207–221.

Dinges, M. M., & Oetting, E. R. (1993). Similarity in drug use patterns between adolescents and their friends. *Adolescence, 28*(110), 253–266.

Dishion, T. J., Andrews, D. W., Spracklen, K. M., & Patterson, G. R. (1996). Deviancy training in male adolescent friendships. *Behavior Therapy, 27*(3), 373–390.

Dishion, T. J., Capaldi, D., Spracklen, K. M., & Li, F. (1995). Peer ecology of male adolescent drug use. Special Issue: Developmental processes in peer relations and psychopathology. *Development & Psychopathology, 7*(4), 803–824.

Dishion, T. J., Patterson, G. R., & Reid, J. R. (1988). *Parent and peer factors associated with drug sampling in early adolescence: Implications for treatment.* National Institute on Drug Abuse: Research Monograph Series. No. 77, 69–93.

Dodge, K. A., & Frame, C. L. (1982). Social cognitive biases and deficits in aggressive boys. *Child Development, 53*(3), 620–635.

Donnermeyer, J. F., & Huang, T. C. (1991). Age and alcohol, marijuana and hard drug use. *Journal of Drug Education, 21*(3), 255–268.

Donohew, L. (1988). Effects of drugs abuse message styles: Final report. A report of a study conducted under a grant from the National Institute on Drug Abuse.

Donohew, L. (1990). Public health campaigns: Targeting strategies and a model. In E. B. Ray & L. Donohew (Eds.), *Communication and health: Systems, processes, and applications.* Hillsdale, NJ: Lawrence Erlbaum Associates.

Donohew, L., Helm, D., Lawrence, P., & Shatzer, M. (1990). Sensation seeking, marijuana use, and responses to drug abuse prevention messages. In R. Watson (Ed.), *Prevention and treatment of drug and alcohol abuse.* Clifton, NJ: Humana.

Donohew, L., Lorch, E., & Palmgreen, P. (1991). Sensation seeking and targeting of televised Anti-Drug PSAS. *Persuasive communication and drug abuse prevention.* Hillsdale, NJ: Lawrence Erlbaum Associates.

Drug Abuse Prevention: What Works (1997). National Institutue on Drug Abuse, National Institutes on Health, Publication #97-4110. Rockville, MD: U.S. Government.

Duck, S. W., Miell, D. K., & Gaebler, H. C. (1980). Attraction and communication in children's interaction. In H. C. Foot, A. J. Chapman, and J. R. Smith (Eds.), *Friendship and social relations in children.* Chichester: Wiley.

Duncan, T. E., Duncan, S. C., & Hops, H. (1994). The effects of family cohesiveness and peer encouragement on the development of adolescent alcohol use: A cohort-sequential approach to the analysis of longitudinal data. *Journal of Studies on Alcohol, 55,* 588–599.

Duncan, T. E., Duncan, S. C., Hops, H., & Stoolmiller, M. (1995). An analysis of the relationship between parent and adolescent marijuana use via generalized estimating equation methodology. *Multivariate Behavioral Research, 30*(3), 317–339.

Duncan, T. E., Tildesley, E., Duncan, S. C., & Hops, H. (1995). The consistency of family and peer influences on the development of substance use in adolescence. *Addiction, 90,* 1647–1660.

Ebstein, R. P., Novick, O., Umansky, R., Priel, B., Osher, Y., Blaine, D., Bennett, E. R., Nemanov, L., Katz, M., & Belmaker, R. H. (1996). Dopamine D4 receptor (D4DR exon III) polymorphism associated with the human personality trait of novelty seeking. *Nature Genetics, 12*(1), 78–80.

Egeland, B., Carlson, E., & Sroufe, L. A. (1993). Resilience as process. *Development and Psychopathology, 5,* 517–528.

Elliot, D. S., & Voss, H. L. (1974). *Delinquency and Dropout.* Lexington, D.C. Heath and Company.

Entwisle, D. R., & Hayduck, L. A. (1982). *Early schooling: Cognitive and affective outcomes.* Baltimore: The John Hopkins University Press.

Evans, M., Weinberg, R., & Jackson, A. (1992). Psychological factors related to drug use in college students. *The Sport Psychologist, 6,* 24–41.

Farrell, A. D. (1994). Structural equation modeling with longitudinal data: Strategies for examining group differences and reciprocal relationships. *Journal of Consulting and Clinical Psychology, 62,* 477–487.

Farrell, A. D., & Danish, S. (1993). Peer drug associations and emotional restraint: Causes or consequences of adolescent's drug use? *Journal of Consulting and Clinical Psychology, 43,* 522–527.

Fernandez, R., & Velez, W. (1989). *Who stays? Who leaves? Findings from the ASPIRA Five Cities High School Dropout Study.* Washington, DC: ASPIRA Institute for Policy Research.

Fisher, S. (1975). The quest for predictors of marijuana abuse in adolescents. In D. J. Lettieti (Ed.), *Predicting adolescent drug abuse: A review of issues, methods and correlates.* DHEW Publication No. ADM 76-299. Rockville, NM: National Institute on Drug Abuse.

Fisher, D. G., MacKinnon, D. P., Angling, M. D., & Thompson, J. P. (1987). Parental influences on substance use: Gender differences and stage theory. *Journal of Drug Education, 17,* 69–85.

Frumkin, R. M., Cowan, R. A., & Davis, J. R. (1969). Drug Use in a Midwest Sample of Metropolitan Hinterland High School Students. *Corrective Psychology, 15,* 8–13.

Galli, N. (1974). Patterns of Student Drug Use. *Journal of Drug Education, 4,* 237–248.

Galli, N., & Stone, D. B. (1975). Psychological status of student drug users. *Journal of Drug Education, 5,* 327–333.

Gerbner, G. (1990). Stories that hurt: Tobacco, alcohol, and other drugs in the mass media. In H. Resnik, S. Gardner, R. Lorian, & C. Marcus (Eds.), *Youth and drugs: Society's mixed messages,* (pp. 53–128). Rockville, MD: Office for Substance Abuse Prevention, U.S. Department of Health and Human Services.

Gfroerer, J. (1987). Correlation between drug use by teenagers and drug use by older family members. *American Journal of Drug and Alcohol Abuse, 13*(1–2), 95–108.

Gillmore, M. R., Catalano, R. F., Morrison, D. M., Wells, E. A., Iritani, B., & Hawkins, J. D. (1990). Racial differences in acceptability and availability of drugs and early initiation of substance use. *American Journal of Drug and Alcohol Abuse, 16*(3, 4), 185–206.

Green, M. G., Blake, B. F., & Zehaysem, R. T. (1973). Some implications of marijuana usage by middle-class high school students. *Proceedings of the 81st Annual Convention of the American Psychological Association, 8,* 679–680.

Guarnaccia, P. J., & Rodriguez, O., (1996). Concepts of culture and their role in the development of culturally competent mental health services. *Hispanic Journal of Behavioral Sciences, 18*(4), 419–443.

Hallinan, M. T., & Williams, R. A. (1989). Interracial friendship choices in secondary schools. *American Sociological Review, 54,* 67–78.

Hare, B. (1988). Black youth at-risk. In *The state of Black America* (pp. 81–92). New York: National Urban League.

Harris, J. R. (1995). Where is the child's environment? A group socialization theory of development. *Psychological Review, 102*(3), 458–489.

Hawkins, J. D., Catalano, R. F., & Wells, E. A. (1986). Measuring effects of a skills training intervention for drug abusers. *Journal of Consulting Clinical Psychology, 54,* 661–664.

Hawkins, J. D., Jenson, J. M., Catalano, R. F., & Wells, E. A. (1991). Effects of a skills training intervention with juvenile delinquents. *Resource Social Work Practice, 1,* 107–121.

Hawkins, J. D., Lishner, D. M., Catalano, R. F., & Howard, M. O. (1986). Childhood predictors of adolescent substance abuse. *Toward an empirically grounded theory.* New York: Haworth Press.

Hirshman, R. S., Leventhal, H., & Glynn, K. (1984). The development of smoking behavior: Cross-sectional survey data. *Journal of Applied Social Psychology, 14,* 184–206.

Huba, G. J., Wingard, J. A., & Bentler, P. M. (1979). Beginning adolescent drug use and peer and adult interaction patterns. *Journal of Consulting and Clinical Psychology, 47*(2), 265–276.

Ionnatti, R. J., & Bush, P. J. (1992). Perceived vs. actual friends' use of alcohol, cigarettes, marijuana, and cocaine: Which has the most influence? *J. Youth Adolescence 21,* 375–389.

Insko, C. A., Thompson, V. D., Stroebe, W., Shaud, K. F., Pinner, B. E., & Layton, B. D. (1973). Implied evaluation and the similarity-attraction effect. *Journal of Personality and Social Psychology, 25,* 297–308.

Jenson, J. M., Wells, E. A., Plotnick, R. D., Hawkins, J. D., & Catalano, R. F. (1993). The effects of skills and intentions to use drugs on post treatment drug use of adolescents. *American Journal of Drug & Alcohol Abuse, 19*(1), 1–18.

Jessor, R. (1976). Predicting time of onset of marijuana use: A Developmental study of high school youth. *Journal of Consulting and Clinical Psychology, 44*, 125–134.

Jessor, R., Graves, T. D., Hanson, R. C., & Jessor, S. L. (1968). *Society, personality, and deviant behavior: A study of a tri-ethnic community.* New York: Holt, Rinehart, & Winston.

Jessor, R., & Jessor S. L. (1977). *Problem behavior and psychosocial development: A longitudinal study of youth.* New York: Academic Press.

Jessor, R., & Jessor, S. L. (1978). Theory testing in longitudinal research on marijuana use. In D. B. Kandel (Ed.), *Longitudinal research on drug use: Empirical findings and methodological issues* (pp. 41–71). Washington, DC: Hemisphere.

Jessor, R., Jessor, S. L., & Finney, J. (1973). A social psychology of marijuana use: longitudinal studies of high school and college youth. *Journal of Personality and Social Psychology, 26*, 1–15.

Johnson, C. A., Hansen, W. B., Collins, L. M., & Graham, J. W. (1986). High school smoking prevention: Results of a three-year longitudinal study. *Journal of Behavioral Medicine, 9*(5), 439–542.

Johnston, L. D., O'Malley, P. M., & Bachman, J. G. (1992). *Smoking, drinking, and illicit drug use among American secondary school students, college students, and young adults, 1975–1991.* Rockville, NM: National Institute on Drug Abuse.

Jones, A. P. (1973). Personality and value differences related to use of LSD-25. *International Journal of the Addictions, 8*, 549–557.

Kandel, D. B. (1975). Reaching the hard-to-reach: Illicit drug use among high school absentees. *Addictive Diseases: An International Journal, 1*, 465–480.

Kandel, D. B. (1978). Convergences in prospective longitudinal surveys of drug use in normal populations. In D. Kandel (Ed.), *Longitudinal research in drug use: Empirical findings and methodological issues.* Washington, DC: Hemisphere-John Witen.

Kandel, D. B. (1985). On processes of peer influences in adolescent drug use: A developmental perspective. *Advances in Alcohol & Substance Abuse, 4*(3, 4), 139–163.

Kandel, D. B., & Andrews, K. (1987). Processes of adolescent socialization by parents and peers. *International Journal of the Addictions, 22*(4), 319–342.

Kaplan, H. B. (1996). Empirical validation of the applicability of an integrative theory of deviant behavior to the study of drug use. *Journal of Drug Issues, 26*, 345–377.

Kessler, R. C., Nelson, C. B., McGonagle, K. A., Edlund, M. J., Frank, R. G., & Leaf, P. J. (1996). The epidemiology of co-occurring addictive and mental disorders in the National Comorbidity Survey: Implications for prevention and service utilization. *American Journal of Orthopsychiatry, 66*(1), 17–31.

Khantzian, E. J. (1980). An ego/self theory of substance dependence: A contemporary psychoanalytic perspective. In D. J. Lettieri, M. Sayers, & H. W. Pearson (Eds.), *Theories on drug abuse: Selected contemporary perspectives.* NIDA Research Monograph 30. Rockville, NM: National Institute on Drug Abuse.

Khavari, K. A. (1993). Interpersonal influences in college students' initial use of alcohol and drugs—The role of friends, self, parents, doctors, and dealers. *The International Journal of the Addictions, 28*(4), 377–388.

Lau, R. R., Quadrel, M. J., & Hartman, K. A. (1990). Development and change of young adults' preventive health beliefs and behavior: Influence from parents and peers. *Journal of Health and Social Behavior, 31*, 240–259.

Lawrence, T. S., & Velleman, D. J. (1974). Correlates of student drug use in a suburban high school. *Psychiatry, 37*, 129–136.

Liebsohn, M. T., Oetting, E. R., & Deffenbacher, J. L. (1994). Effects of trait anger on alcohol consumption and consequences. *Journal of Child & Adolescent Substance Abuse, 3*(3), 17–32.

Loeber, R., & Stouthamer-Loeber, M. (1986). Family factors as correlates and predictors of juvenile conduct problems and delinquency. In M. Tonry & N. Morris (Eds.), *Crime and justice: A review of research, Vol. 12* (pp. 29–149). Chicago: University of Chicago Press.

Lopez, J. M. O., Redondo, L. M., & Martin, A. L. (1989). Influence of family and peer group on the use of drugs by adolescents. *The International Journal of the Addictions, 24*(11), 537–548.

Maccoby, E. E. (1990). Gender and relationships: A developmental account. *American Psychologist, 45*(4), 513–520.

Miranne, A. C. (1981) Marijuana use and alienation: A multivariate analysis. *International Journal of the Addictions, 16*, 697–707.

Mirin, S. M., Shapiro, L. M., Meyer, R. E., Pillard, R. C., & Fisher, S. (1971). Casual versus heavy use of marijuana: A redefinition of the marijuana problem. *American Journal of Psychiatry, 127*, 1134–1140.

Mohan, J., Sehgal, M., & Bhandari, A. (1982). Sociometric status, personality, academic achievement and personal problems. *Indian Psychological Review, 22*, 20–29.

Molina, B. S. G., & Chassin, L. (1996). The parent-adolescent relationship at puberty: Hispanic ethnicity and parent alcoholism as moderators. *Developmental Psychology, 32*, 675–686.

Moos, R., Moos, B., & Kulik, J. (1977). Behavioral and self-concept antecedents and correlates of college student drinking patterns. *International Journal of the Addictions, 12,* 603–615.

Murray, D. M., Richards, P. S., Luepker, R. V., & Johnson, C. A. (1987). The prevention of cigarette smoking in children: Two and three-year follow-up comparison of four prevention strategies. *Journal of Behavioral Medicine, 10*(6), 595–611.

Naginey, J. L., & Swisher, J. D. (1990). To whom would adolescents turn with drug problems? Implications for school professionals. *The High School Journal, 73,* 80–85.

Needle, R., McCubbin, H., Wilson, M., Reineck, R., Lazar, A., & Mederer, H. (1986). Interpersonal influences in adolescent drug use—The role of older siblings, parents, and peers. 1. *The International Journal of the Addictions, 21*(7), 739–766.

Newcomb, M. D., & Bentler, P. M. (1988). *Consequences of adolescent drug use: Impact on the lives of young adults.* Newbury Park, Beverly Hills, London, New Delhi: Sage.

Newcomb, M. D., Maddahian, E., & Bentler, P. M. (1986). Risk factors for drug use among adolescents: Concurrent and longitudinal analyses. *American Journal of Public Health, 76*(5), 525–531.

O'Malley, P. M. (1975). Correlates and consequences of illicit drug use. *Dissertation Abstracts International, 36,* 3011B (University Microfilms No. 75-29, 302).

Oetting, E. R. (1992). Planning programs for prevention of deviant behavior: A psychosocial model. In J. E. Trimble, C. E. Bolek, & S. J. Niemcryk (Eds.), *Ethnic and multicultural drug abuse: Perspectives on current research.* New York: Haworth Press.

Oetting, E. R. (1999). Comments on primary socialization theory: Developmental stages, spirituality, government institutions, sensation seeking, and theoretical implications: Part V. *Substance use and misuse, 34*(7), 947–982.

Oetting, E. R., & Beauvais, F. (1986). Peer cluster theory: Drugs and the adolescent. *Journal of Counseling and Development, 65*(1), 17–22.

Oetting, E. R., & Beauvais, F. (1987). Peer cluster theory, socialization characteristics, and adolescent drug use: A path analysis. *Journal of Counseling Psychology, 34*(2): 205–213.

Oetting, E. R., & Beauvais, F. (1989). Epidemiology and correlates of alcohol use among Indian adolescents living on reservations. In D. L. Spiegler, D. A. Tate, S. S. Aitken, & C. M. Christian (Eds.), *Alcohol use among U.S. ethnic minorities* (pp. 239–269). NIAAA Research Monograph No. 18, DHHS Pub. No. (ADM) 89-143 5. Washington, DC: U.S. Government Printing Office.

Oetting, E. R., & Donnermeyer, J. F. (1998). Primary socialization theory: The etiology of drug use and deviance. Part I. *Substance Use & Misuse, 33*(4).

Oetting, E. R., Donnermeyer, J. F., Trimble, J., & Beauvais, F. (1998). Culture, ethnicity, cultural identification and primary socialization theory: The links between culture and substance use. *Substance Use and Misuse, 33*(10), 2075–2107.

Oetting, E. R., Donnermeyer, J. T., & Deffenbacher, J. (1998). Primary socialization theory: The influence of the community on drug use and deviance. *Substance Use & Misuse, 33*(8), 1629–1665.

Oetting, E. R., & Goldstein, G. S. (1979). Drug use among Native American adolescents. In G. Beschner & A. Freidman (Eds.), *Youth drug abuse.* Lexington, MA: Lexington Books.

Oetting, E. R., Swaim, R. C., Edwards, R. W., & Beauvais, F. (1989). Indian and Anglo adolescent alcohol use and emotional distress: Path models. *American Journal of Alcohol and Drug Abuse, 15*(2), 153–172.

Pabon, E., Rodriguez, O., & Gurin, G. (1992). Clarifying peer relations and delinquency. *Youth and Society, 24*(2) 149–165.

Padilla, E. R., Padilla, A. M., Morales, A., & Olmedo, E. L. (1979). Inhalant, marijuana, and alcohol abuse among Barrio children and adolescents. *International Journal of the Addictions, 714,* 943–964.

Palinkas, L. A., Atkins, C. J., Miller, C. M., & Ferreira, D. (1996). Social skills training for drug prevention in high-risk female adolescents. *Preventive Medicine, 25,* 692–701.

Pandina, R. T., & Scheule, J. A. (1983). Psychosocial correlates of alcohol and drug use of adolescent students and adolescents in treatment. *Journal of Studies on Alcohol, 44,* 950–973.

Patterson, G. R., & Dishion, T. J. (1985). Contributions of families and peers to delinquency. *Criminology, 23,* 63–79.

Patterson, G. R., & Stouthamer-Loeber, M. (1984). The correlation of family management practices and delinquency. *Child Development, 55*(4), 1299–1307.

Peele, S. (1985). *The meaning of addiction.* Lexington, NM: Lexington Books.

Penning, M., & Bames, G. E. (1982). Adolescent marijuana use: A review. *International Journal of the Addictions, 17,* 749–791.

Perry, C. L. (1989). Prevention of alcohol use and abuse in adolescence: Teacher vs. peer-led intervention. *Crisis, 10,* 52–61.

Peterson, P. L., Hawkins, J. D., Abbott, R. D., & Catalano, R. F. (1994). Disentangling the effects of parental drinking, family management, and parental alcohol norms on current drinking by Black and White adolescents. *Journal of Research on Adolescence, 4*(2), 203–227.

Petraitus, J., Flay, B. R., and Miller, T. Q. (1995). Reviewing theories of adolescent substance use: Organizing pieces in the puzzle. *Psychol. Bull. 117*(1), 67–86.

Reiss, D. (1997). Mechanisms linking genetic and social influences in adolescent development: Beginning a collaborative search. *Current Directions in Psychological Science, 6*(4), 100–105.

Riggs, D. E. (1973). Students and Drug Use: A study of personality characteristics and extent of drug using behavior. *Canadian Counselor, 7,* 9–15.

Robledo, M. (1989). The prevention and recovery of dropouts: An action agenda. In *Valued Youth Anthology* (pp. 1–4). San Antonio, TX: Intercultural Development Research Association.

Rodriguez, O. (1996). The new immigrant Hispanic population: An integrated approach to preventing delinquency and crime. *National Institute of Justice research preview.* U.S. Department of Justice, NIJ. 1–2.

Rubin, Z. (1980). *Children's friendships.* London: Fontana.

Russell, J. A., & Mehrabian, A. (1977). Environmental effects on drug use. *Environmental Psychology and Nonverbal Behavior, 2,* 109–123.

Schoolar, J. C., White, E. H., & Cohen, C. P. (1972). Drug abusers and their clinic-patient counterparts: A comparison of personality dimensions. *Journal of Consulting and Clinical Psychology, 39,* 9–14.

Segal, B., & Singer, J. L. (1976). Daydreaming, drug and alcohol use in college students: A factor analytic study. *Addictive Behaviors,* 227–235.

Selekman, M. (1991). 'With a little help from my friends': The use of peers in the family therapy of adolescent substance abusers. *Family Dynamics Addiction Questions, 1*(1), 69–76.

Shedler, J., & Block, J. (1990). Adolescent drug use and psychological health: A longitudinal inquiry. *American Psychologist, 45,* 612–630.

Simon, W. E., Primavera, L. H., Simon, M. G., & Omdoff, R. K. (1974). A comparison of marijuana users and nonusers on a number of personality variables. *Journal of Consulting and Clinical Psychology, 42,* 917–918.

Sorosiak, F. M., Thomas, L. E., & Balet, F. N. (1976). Adolescent drug use: An analysis. *Psychological Reports, 38,* 211–221.

Spevack, M., & Phil, R. O. (1976). Nonmedical drug use by high school students: A three-year survey study. *International Journal of the Addictions, 11,* 755–792.

Spotts, J. V., & Shontz, F. C. (1980). A Life Theme Theory of Chronic Drug Abuse. In D. J. Lettieri, M. Sayers, & H. W. Pearson (Eds.), *Theories on drug abuse: Selected contemporary perspectives.* NIDA Research Monograph No. 30, Rockville, NM: National Institute on Drug Abuse.

Spotts, J. V., & Shontz, F. C. (1984a). Drug induced ego states. I. Cocaine: Phenomenology and implications. *International Journal of the Addictions, 19,* 119–152.

Spotts, J. V., & Shontz, F. C. (1984b). The phenomenological structure of drug induced states. II. Barbiturates and Sedative Hypnotics. *International Journal of the Addictions, 19,* 295–326.

Spotts, J. V., & Shontz, F. C. (1984c). Correlates of sensation seeking by heavy, chronic drug-users. *Perceptual and Motor Skills, 58,* 427–435.

Streit, F., Halsted, D. L., & Pascale, P. J. (1974). Differences among youth users and nonusers of drugs based on their perceptions of parental behavior. *International Journal of the Addictions, 9,* 749–755.

Svobodny, L. A. (1982). Biographical, self concept and educational factors among chemically dependent adolescents. *Adolescence, 17,* 847–853.

Swaim, R. C., (1991). Childhood risk factors and adolescent drug and alcohol use. *Educational Psychology Review, 3*(4), 363–398.

Swaim, R. C., Beauvais, F., Chavez, E. L., & Oetting, E. R. (1997). The effect of school dropout rates on estimates of adolescent substance use among three ethnic groups. *American Journal of Public Health, 87*(1), 5–55.

Swaim, R. C., Oetting, E. R., & Casas, J. M., (1996). Cigarette use among migrant and non-migrant Mexican-American youth. A socialization latent variable model. *Health Psychology, 15*(4), 269–281.

Swaim, R. C., Oetting, E. R., Edwards, R. W., & Beauvais, F. (1989). The links from emotional distress to adolescent drug use: A path model. *Journal of Consulting and Clinical Psychology, 57*(2), 227–231.

Swaim, R. C., Oetting, E. R., Thurman, P. J., Beauvais, F., & Edwards, R. (1993). American Indian adolescent drug use and socialization characteristics: A cross-cultural comparison. *Journal of Cross Cultural Psychology, 24*(1), 42–52.

Takeuchi, D. T., Williams, D. R., & Adair, R. K. (1991). Economic stress in the family and children's emotional and behavioral problems. *Journal of Marriage and the Family, 53,* 1031–1041.

Tec, N. (1974). Parent-child drug abuse: Generational continuity of adolescent deviancy? *Adolescence, 9,* 350–364.

Tesser, A., Campbell, J., & Smith, M. (1984). Friendship choice and performance: Self evaluation maintenance in children. *Journal of Personality and Social Psychology, 46,* 561–574.

Tittle, D. R., & Welch, M. R. (1983). Religiosity and deviance: Toward a contingency theory of constraining effects. *Social Forces, 61*(3), 653–682.

Tolone, W. L., & Dermott, D. (1975). Some correlates of drug use among high school youth in a Midwestern rural community. *The International Journal of the Addictions, 10*(5), 761–777.

Troy, M., & Sroufe, L. A. (1987). Victimization among preschoolers: Role of attachment relationship history. *Journal of the American Academy of Child & Adolescent Psychiatry, 26*(2), 166–172.

Turner, C. J., & Willis, R. J. (1984). The relationship between self-reported religiosity and drug use by college students. In S. Eiseman, J. Wingar, & G. Huba (Eds.), Drug abuse: *Foundation for a psychosocial approach.* Farmingdale, NY: Baywood.

Voss, H. L., & Clayton, R. R. (1984). 'Turning on' other persons to drugs. *International Journal of the Addictions, 19,* 633–652.

Walters, J. M. (1980). Buzzin': PCP Use in Philadelphia. In H. W. Feldman, M. H. Aga, & G. Beschener, (Eds.), *Angel Dust,* Lexington, MA: D.C. Heath.

Wechsler, H., & Thum, D. (1973). Drug use among teenagers: Patterns of present and anticipated use. *The International Journal of the Addictions, 8*(6), 909–920.

Wehlage, G., Rutter, R., Smith, G., Lesko, N., & Fernandez, R. (1989). *Reducing Risk.* Philadelphia, PA: Falmer Press.

Wells, E. A., Morrison, D. M., Gillmore, M. R., Catalano, R. F., Iritani, B., & Hawkins, J. D. (1992). Race differences in antisocial behaviors and attitudes and early initiation of substance use. *Journal of Drug Education, 22*(2), 115–130.

White, R. W. (1972). *The enterprise of living: Growth and organization in personality.* New York: Holt, Rinehart and Winston.

Wiist, W. H., & Snider, G., (1991). Peer education in friendship cliques: Prevention of adolescent smoking. *Health and Education Research, 6*(1), 101–108.

Wills, T. A., & Cleary, S. D. (1996). How are social support effects mediated? A test with parental support and adolescent substance use. *Journal of Personality and Social Psychology, 71*(5), 937–952.

Wills, T. A., McNamara, G., & Vaccaro, D. (1995). Parental education related to adolescent stress-coping and substance use. *Health Psychology, 14,* 464–478.

Wills, T. A., Pierce, J. P., & Evans, R. I. (1996). Large-scale environmental risk factors for substance use. *American Behavioral Scientist, 39,* 808–822.

Wills, T. A., Windle, M., & Cleary, S. D. (1998). Temperament and novelty seeking in adolescent substance use: Convergence of dimensions of temperaments with constructs from Cloninger's theory. *Journal of Personality and Social Psychology, 74*(2), 387–406.

Wingard, J. A., Huba, G. J., & Bentler, P. M. (1979). The relationship of personality structure to patterns of adolescent substance use. *Multivariate Behavioral Research, 14,* 131–143.

Zuckerman, M. (1988). Behavior and biology: Research on sensation seeking and reactions to the media. In L. Donohew, H. Sypher, & T. Higgins (Eds.), *Communication, social cognition, and affect* (pp. 173–194). Hillsdale, NJ: Lawrence Erlbaum Associates.

Zuckerman, M., Eysenck, S. B., & Eysenck, H. J. (1978). Sensation seeking in England and America: Cross-cultural, age, and sex comparisons. *Journal of Consulting and Clinical Psychology, 46,* 139–149.

CHAPTER 6

Mobilizing Communities To Reduce Risk for Drug Abuse: A Comparison of Two Strategies

MICHAEL W. ARTHUR
CHARLES D. AYERS
KELLY A. GRAHAM
J. DAVID HAWKINS

INTRODUCTION

The abuse of alcohol and other drugs is one of the most significant and costly public health problems in this country. Recent estimates put the social costs of drug and alcohol abuse at $277 billion in 1995 (National Institute on Drug Abuse, 1998). Although the increases in adolescent drug use seen in the early 1990s have leveled off in recent years, use of drugs remains at unacceptably high levels (Johnston, O'Malley, & Bachman, 1998; Office of National Drug Control Policy, 1999). Moreover, use of alcohol and other drugs by adolescents is often related to problems such as delinquency, school failure and dropout, teen pregnancy, and high-risk sexual behavior, all of which pose significant long-term threats to the health and development of adolescents (Dryfoos, 1990; Resnick et al., 1997).

Prevention research suggests that a public health model for prevention, based on reducing risk factors and promoting processes that protect or buffer against risk, offers a promising

MICHAEL W. ARTHUR, CHARLES D. AYERS, KELLY A. GRAHAM, AND J. DAVID HAWKINS • Social Development Research Group, University of Washington, Seattle, Washington 98115

strategy for prevention of alcohol and other drug abuse (e.g., Coie et al., 1993; Hawkins, Arthur, & Catalano, 1995; Mrazek & Haggerty, 1994). Research has shown that alcohol and other drug abuse is predicted by a number of risk factors in the individual and in the environment (Hawkins, Catalano, & Miller, 1992; Kandel, Simcha-Fagan, & Davies, 1986; Newcomb, 1995). Research has also identified protective factors that appear to mitigate the negative outcomes associated with exposure to risk (e.g., Garmezy, 1985; Werner, 1994). Moreover, the evidence indicates that the likelihood of alcohol and other drug abuse increases with exposure to more risk factors and that few children exposed to multiple risk factors also experience high levels of protection (Newcomb et al., 1987; Pollard, Hawkins, & Arthur, 1999). Finally, an increasing number of interventions that reduce risks and enhance protection have had positive results at preventing substance abuse in well-designed evaluation studies (Mrazek & Haggerty, 1994; Sloboda & David, 1997). These converging lines of evidence support the hypothesis that interventions that reduce multiple risk factors while promoting protective influences in family, school, peer, and community environments hold promise for alcohol and other drug abuse prevention.

Social Development Model

The social development model provides a theoretical basis for alcohol and other drug abuse risk-reduction efforts (Catalano & Hawkins, 1996; Farrington & Hawkins, 1991; Hawkins & Weis, 1985). The model builds on social control theory (Hirschi, 1969) and social learning theory (Akers, 1977; Bandura, 1977) and postulates that two key protective processes inhibit the development of antisocial behaviors. The first is bonding to pro-social units, such as family, school, community, and positive peers. Bonding consists of attachment and commitment to social groups and belief in their shared values. Bonding is viewed as an important protective factor against behavior that is outside of a group's norms. It is believed to provide motivation for the individual to live according to the norms of the group to which the individual is bonded. Clear norms against drug use are a second protective factor against alcohol and other drug abuse. Such norms provide the behavioral guidelines for those who are bonded to the social units promoting the norms.

The social development model hypothesizes that bonding is produced by processes involving three constructs: opportunities, skills, and reinforcements. As posited in the model, providing a young person with opportunities for active involvement, skills for successful participation, and consistent rewards for successful involvement and moderate and consistent punishment for misbehavior will lead to the development of a bond of attachment, commitment, and belief between that young person and the social unit in which he or she is participating. This is hypothesized to be true in all social groups, whether in a family, in a classroom, in a neighborhood, in a community, or in a group of friends.

The social development model provides a theoretical framework to guide risk-reduction efforts by specifying protective processes that are believed to operate in a similar manner across domains. According to the theory, risk factors in different domains can be reduced, mediated, or moderated by increasing the protective factors of pro-social bonding and clear norms in parallel fashion across different domains. The model directs risk-reduction programs to increase opportunities and rewards for active, positive involvement in families, communities, schools, and peer groups; to promote the development of skills needed to perform successfully in those social domains without violating acceptable standards for behavior; and to ensure that children's social environments provide consistent reinforcement for positive behavior and clear norms against alcohol and other drug use.

Community Mobilization

Despite the empirical and theoretical bases for risk-reduction interventions, they cannot succeed unless they are adequately implemented. In order to reduce the incidence and prevalence of adolescent problem behaviors in a community, research-based interventions that reduce multiple risk factors while enhancing protective factors must be implemented with enough scope and fidelity to effect the community as a whole. Studies of the diffusion of social innovations indicate that widespread implementation of innovative interventions is contingent on two basic conditions: community members must first recognize a problem or need; then they must put the new idea into a form that addresses the problem as they perceive it (Rogers, 1995). Local "ownership" is a vital component of successful community health promotion interventions (Bracht & Kingsbury, 1990). Community members who feel they can influence how their community's problems are defined and how these problems are addressed are likely to support such efforts.

Community planning boards have been used to mobilize communities in risk-reduction efforts, such as the Minnesota Heart Health Project and Project COMMIT (Bracht & Kingsbury, 1990), and in substance abuse prevention programs, such as the Center for Substance Abuse Prevention's Community Partnership Demonstration Program (Kaftarian & Hansen, 1994). From the perspective of the social development model, widespread involvement of community members in comprehensive risk-reduction efforts increases the impact of the intervention by promoting greater interaction and bonding among community members (Cottrell, 1976; Eng & Parker, 1990), thereby increasing the first key protective factor specified in the model. Moreover, the greater the number of community members who participate in the risk-reduction efforts, the greater the number of individuals who would be expected to express norms against alcohol and other drug abuse and promote the second key protective factor. Combining a theoretically grounded risk-reduction strategy with a vehicle for stimulating community participation and ownership of the risk-reduction efforts is hypothesized to increase the potential for successful risk reduction on a broad scale.

However, little is known about the processes that influence community coalitions to implement science-based prevention strategies (Butterfoss, Goodman, & Wandersman, 1993; Harachi Manger et al., 1992; Florin, Mitchell, & Stevenson, 1993). In fact, despite substantial investment in community coalitions to prevent substance use, there is a gap between the scientific base for effective prevention and the practice of prevention in communities (e.g., Altman, 1995; Morrissey et al., 1997). An emerging challenge for the field of prevention is to translate science-based knowledge about risk and protective factors, and about tested strategies for reducing risk and increasing protection, into widespread practice in communities (Biglan, 1995).

To understand the processes that influence the effectiveness of community-level interventions to reduce the prevalence of substance abuse, it is necessary to examine the extent of community mobilization and ownership of the prevention approach that the interventions produce. This chapter presents findings from process evaluations of two distinct community mobilization interventions. A key feature of the interventions is the active involvement of community members in the design and implementation of risk-reduction strategies for substance abuse prevention. Two independent statewide community mobilization efforts initiated in 1990 are examined—the Oregon TOGETHER! Project and the Washington State Community Youth Activity Program (CYAP). Community prevention planning boards in each project received training on risk and protective factors for alcohol and other drug abuse, how to assess and prioritize risk factors in their communities, and how to develop strategic action plans tailored to the prioritized risks. Evaluations of the two projects assessed the success of these boards at developing risk-reduction plans and programs.

TABLE 6.1. Comparison of Programs: Oregon TOGETHER! and Washington CYAP

Oregon TOGETHER!	Washington CYAP
Mobilization processes	
Mobilized communities in Oregon State.	Mobilized communities in Washington State.
Administered collaboratively by the University of Washington, Social Development Research Group and Oregon State's Office of Alcohol and Drug Abuse Programs.	Administered by Washington State's Division of Alcohol and Substance Abuse.
Mobilized new boards and a few preexisting groups.	Many participating groups were preexisting groups.
Funding	
Did not offer initial funding.	Offered $11,000 per community team at the outset.
Recruitment	
Emphasized recruitment and involvement of key leaders.	Emphasized recruitment and involvement of youth.
Orientation/training	
Training used Communities That Care model.	Training used Together We Can model.
1-day Key Leader Orientation session.	No orientation of community leaders.
Teams attended two 3-day workshops.	Team representatives attended one 2-day workshop.
The entire team attended training.	Two adult and two youth representatives attended training.
Training included explanation of empirical base for risk factors.	Training did not include an explanation of how risk factors were identified.
Expectations and requirements for participation clarified at key leader orientation and board trainings.	Expectations and requirements for participation were not explicit at the outset.
Processes	
Participants collected archival and/or survey data to identify priority risk factors.	Participants conducted key leader interviews, brainstormed and voted to identify priority risk factors.
Participants were provided with descriptions of strategies for reducing risk factors.	Training did not include strategies for reducing risk factors.

Overview of the Interventions

The Oregon TOGETHER! project and the Washington State CYAP project (Table 6.1) shared a common risk-reduction paradigm and theoretical basis, and both used a technology-transfer approach to promote science-based prevention (Backer, David, & Soucy, 1995). However, they used different strategies to mobilize, train, and support community teams through the risk- and protection-focused assessment, planning, and program implementation.

The Oregon TOGETHER! project, for example, explicitly involved key community leaders as well as grassroots community members during the community mobilization process. In contrast, the Washington State CYAP project focused its mobilization effort on grassroots community members and youths. The Oregon TOGETHER! project used a series of three training sessions, applying the Communities That Care model (Hawkins, Catalano, & Associates, 1992) to guide the community boards through the process. The Washington State CYAP project used a single training session and the Together We Can planning kit (Gibbs & Bennett, 1990). Initial participation in the Oregon TOGETHER! project did not include a promise of funding to community boards. The Washington State CYAP project announced at the outset that up to $11,000 would be made available to each participating community team to implement prevention activities.

This chapter examines the success of the two projects at mobilizing communities to develop community prevention boards, complete community risk assessments, complete comprehensive risk-reduction action plans, and implement strategic risk reduction activities. The results of these efforts provide important information about processes that influence the effectiveness of community mobilization efforts to implement science-based strategies to prevent alcohol and other drug abuse. Findings from the two projects are contrasted and discussed in terms of their implications for further research and intervention using community mobilization for risk reduction as a strategy for preventing alcohol and other drug abuse.

METHOD

A comparative analysis of process evaluation data from the two projects assessed the extent of (1) community mobilization and key leader and youth involvement; (2) adoption of the risk- and protective-factor prevention planning strategy, including completion of community risk and resource assessments and development of strategic action plans; and (3) implementation of risk- and protection-focused prevention strategies.

The process evaluation designs developed for the Oregon TOGETHER! and Washington State CYAP projects addressed three common questions (Harachi Manger et al., 1992; Hawkins et al., 1991):

1. Can communities be mobilized by training community members in risk and protective factors and encouraging them to organize a community prevention board or team?
2. To what extent do community boards or teams adopt the risk- and protective-factor prevention framework and follow a process to develop a comprehensive prevention plan?
3. To what extent do boards or teams develop and implement prevention activities that focus on reducing identified risk factors and enhancing protective factors?

Data Collection

To address these questions, the Oregon TOGETHER! project conducted telephone surveys of community board members during the Spring of 1992, approximately 1 year following the third and final training workshop provided to participating communities, to assess each board's progress in developing action plans and implementing activities to reduce risks for substance abuse. In addition, action plans submitted by the community boards were analyzed to assess the completeness of the plans and the potential effectiveness of planned strategies for reducing identified risk factors and enhancing protective factors.

The Washington State CYAP project collected information about the development and activities of each team through follow-up telephone interviews with team leaders and members in December 1991, 10 months following the CYAP leader training workshop. These interviews assessed team characteristics, members' understanding of the risk- and protective-factor model, and prevention activities carried out by the teams. In addition, the risk-reduction action plans were analyzed to assess completeness and the potential effectiveness of planned strategies.

Data Analysis

Data from the telephone interviews were used to create a profile of each team. The profiles indicated:

- whether the teams were active at the follow-up assessment,
- whether they had completed an assessment of risk factors among youth in their communities and what types of data were used in their assessment, and
- whether they had implemented any prevention activities during the past year and, if so, what types of activities they reported.

Action plans submitted by each team were also examined, and the following elements were added to each community's profile:

- whether the team had submitted an action plan,
- which of four specific components were included in the plan, and
- what types of activities were described in the plan.

The four plan components included (1) the indicators of community risk factors gathered during the risk assessment, (2) a clear indication of the priority risk factors selected by the planning board, (3) clearly defined positive outcomes for each priority risk factor, and (4) a clear description of the strategies selected to achieve the positive outcomes, with a detailed task timeline for implementing each strategy.

To assess the success of each project at transferring the prevention technology to the communities, a 4-point rating scale was developed by the authors to evaluate the activities proposed and implemented in terms of their potential effectiveness at reducing risk factors (0 = no activity; 1 = ineffective risk-reduction strategy; 2 = moderately effective risk-reduction strategy; 3 = effective risk-reduction strategy). Criteria used to rate effectiveness included the extent to which an activity clearly targeted an empirically established risk or protective factor, the intensity or strength of the proposed activity, and the duration of the activity. For example, an occasional drug-free activity was rated as ineffective due to a lack of intensity and duration. A regular schedule of drug-free activities or a drug-free teen center was rated as moderately effective because they lack intensity but are sustained over a long period of time. Strategies such as parent training workshops, social skills training curricula, and tutoring or mentoring were rated as clearly effective because they met each of the three criteria. Note that the ratings refer to the potential effectiveness of the strategy selected and not to the effectiveness of the actual activity as implemented. Many factors related to implementation influence an activity's effectiveness at reducing risk, and more extensive evaluation of the actual activities would be needed to judge their effectiveness.

The first two authors of this chapter made independent ratings of the activities planned and implemented by each prevention board or team, and each team was assigned two scores reflecting the highest rated activity they had planned and the highest rated activity they had implemented. Inter-rater agreement for the ratings of planned activities was 94% (Kappa = .78), while inter-rater agreement for the ratings of activities implemented was 90% (Kappa = .85).

RESULTS

Community Mobilization

While the goal of the Oregon TOGETHER! project was to recruit 25 communities for participation, the recruitment methods used in the project (see Harachi Manger et al. (1992) for a description of these methods) resulted in 40 Oregon communities sending teams of at least four key community leaders to the 1-day project orientation training. Some key leader groups represented counties, some represented single communities, some represented pairs of neighboring communities, and one represented several neighborhoods served by a single high school in a large metropolitan area. Thirty-seven (92.5%) of these key leader groups subsequently recruited community members to form 36 community prevention boards. A total of 306 prevention board members representing the 36 community boards (an average of 8.5 members per community) participated in the first community board training (CB-I) 3 months after the key leader orientation. This training focused on methods for assessing risk and protective factors in the community.

Five months later, following the community risk and resource assessment phase of the project, 35 community prevention boards (87.5%) had been successfully mobilized to initiate the community risk and resource assessment and action planning components of the Communities That Care strategy. These 35 community prevention boards sent 206 board members to participate in the second community board training (CB-II) that focused on action planning to reduce targeted risk factors while enhancing protective factors. These results are consistent with findings from a previous analysis (Harachi Manger et al., 1992) which concluded that the CTC approach is effective at recruiting key community leaders to mobilize their communities around the issue of alcohol and other drug abuse prevention. Twenty months after the initial key leader training and a year after the second community board training, 31 (77.5%) prevention boards were still active.

In contrast to the Oregon TOGETHER! project, the Washington State CYAP project relied on county prevention staff instead of community leaders to mobilize community teams and offered up to $11,000 in financial support to participating community teams. This approach was also successful at recruiting community teams. Each county initially mobilized at least one team or identified an existing community group to participate in the project, and 14 of the 26 targeted counties mobilized more than one team. The State Division of Alcohol and Substance Abuse (DASA) allocated funds for one to three teams per county, depending on the size of the population under age 18. Three counties mobilized more teams than the Washington State DASA had planned to fund, while only one county was unable to mobilize its allotted number of teams. This resulted in funding planned for 43 teams initially being divided among 48 teams.

Also in contrast to the Oregon TOGETHER! project, not all of the Washington State CYAP teams participated in the risk reduction training workshops. Approximately 150 team members representing 42 community teams attended 1 of the 4 training workshops offered in different regions of the state. Still, by the 10-month follow-up, 39 (81%) of the 48 original teams had been active for at least 4 months (long enough to plan some prevention activities) and 36 (75%) were still active. Of the 42 teams whose leaders attended the training workshops, 36 (86%) were active for at least 4 months and 30 (71%) were active at the 10-month follow up. Table 6.2 summarizes the results of the mobilization processes used in the Oregon TOGETHER! and Washington State CYAP projects.

Transfer of the Science-Based Prevention Technology

After mobilizing community planning teams, the second major objective of both the Oregon TOGETHER! and Washington State CYAP projects was to transfer knowledge about risk and protective factors for adolescent substance abuse and to provide a risk-reduction planning framework to the community teams. The Communities That Care (CTC) framework used by the Oregon TOGETHER! project and the Together We Can (TWC) framework used by the Washington State CYAP project were both designed to provide a method for teams to (1) assess risk factors in their

TABLE 6.2. Comparison of Community Mobilization Processes: Oregon TOGETHER! And Washington CYAP

Oregon TOGETHER!	
Number of communities at Key Leader Orientation	40
Number of communities mobilized	35 (88%)
Number of communities active at follow-up (11 months)[a]	31 (78%)
Washington CYAP	
Number of communities initially targeted	48
Number of communities mobilized	39 (81%)
Number of communities active at follow-up (10 months)[a]	36 (75%)

[a]Following training.

communities, (2) prioritize risk factors based on these assessments, (3) develop clear and specific plans of action to address the prioritized risk factors, and (4) implement prevention activities designed to reduce the prioritized risk factors and strengthen protective factors. The evaluations of the technology transfer process in both projects examined the extent to which the teams completed risk assessments, prioritized risk factors, and developed risk-focused action plans based on those assessments.

Completion of Community Risk Assessments

A large majority of the community boards in each project completed some form of community risk assessment as a basis for planning prevention activities. All of the 35 prevention boards mobilized for the Oregon TOGETHER! project assessed risk factors in their communities, and 31 of the 39 (79%) community teams mobilized for the Washington State CYAP project reported that they conducted a community risk assessment. A slightly greater proportion of Oregon TOGETHER! prevention boards (66%) than Washington State CYAP teams (56%) reported that they had assessed risk factors by asking local key informants about alcohol and other drug abuse issues in their community. More striking differences between the two projects were apparent in the proportions of boards or teams that used quantitative data in their risk assessments. All 35 of the Oregon TOGETHER! boards used existing archival data, such as school, police, or health department records, while only 20 of the 39 Washington State CYAP teams used archival data. Moreover, more than half (57%) of the Oregon TOGETHER! boards conducted surveys to assess risk factors, while only 21% percent of the Washington State CYAP teams conducted surveys. Of the 8 Washington State CYAP teams that did not complete risk assessments, 4 reported that they brainstormed ideas as a team, while 4 did not attempt to identify risk factors.

Completion of Risk-Reduction Action Plans

Once community risk and resource assessments were completed, the community prevention boards or teams in both projects were instructed to use the data they had collected to prioritize specific risk factors to target with new or expanded programs and to complete detailed action plans to guide implementation of the prevention activities. Although Oregon TOGETHER! boards initially were not required to submit their action plans for review, approximately 1 year after the CB-II training workshops the Oregon Office of Alcohol and Drug Abuse Programs announced the availability of

TABLE 6.3a. Completion of Action Plans: Oregon TOGETHER! and Washington State CYAP

	Oregon TOGETHER!	Washington CYAP
Number of teams mobilized	35	39
Submitted a complete action plan	28 (80%)	13 (33%)
Submitted an incomplete action plan	3 (9%)	7 (18%)
Did not submit an action plan	4 (11%)	19 (49%)

mini-grants of up to $5,000 to Oregon TOGETHER! boards that submitted clear, risk-focused action plans. These mini-grants were provided to support the risk reduction strategies described in these plans. In response to this offer, 31 (89%) of the 35 teams that had been mobilized submitted action plans. Twenty-eight boards (80%) submitted complete plans that included each of the following components: (1) the indicators of community risk factors gathered during the risk assessment, (2) a clear indication of the priority risk factors selected by the planning board, (3) clearly defined positive outcomes for each priority risk factor, and (4) a clear description of the strategies selected to achieve the positive outcomes with a detailed task timeline for implementing each strategy. Three other boards submitted incomplete action plans that did not include all four components (Table 6.3a). In the Washington State CYAP project, the teams were instructed to submit their action plans to the Washington State DASA as soon as they were completed, although CYAP funding was not contingent on completing a plan. Examination of the action plans submitted suggests that the TWC leader training workshops and kits were not as effective as the CTC training sessions in guiding teams through the risk-focused planning process. Only 13 of the 39 (33%) Washington State CYAP teams completed an action plan that included each of the four components. Seven other teams (18%) submitted action plans that were incomplete. Nineteen teams had not submitted action plans by the 10-month follow up.

As a further measure of the effectiveness of the two approaches at transferring the risk-reduction technology to the community prevention boards or teams, the ratings of prevention activities described in the community plans were compared (Table 6.3b). Based on these ratings, 26 (74%) of the Oregon TOGETHER! teams included effective risk-reduction strategies in their action plans. One team (3%) planned moderately effective activities, 4 teams (11%) planned activities rated as ineffective at reducing risk, and 4 teams (11%) did not submit an action plan. In contrast, only 12 (31%) of the 39 Washington State CYAP teams submitted action plans that were rated as including effective risk-reduction strategies. Five teams (13%) submitted plans that were rated as including moderately effective risk-reduction strategies, 3 teams (8%) submitted plans that were rated as including ineffective risk-reduction strategies, and 19 teams (49%)

TABLE 6.3b. Rating of Risk Reduction Strategies Proposed in Action Plans: Oregon TOGETHER! and Washington State CYAP[a]

	Oregon TOGETHER! (N = 35)	Washington CYAP (N = 39)
Effective risk-reduction strategy	26 (74%)	12 (31%)
Moderately effective risk-reduction strategy	1 (3%)	5 (13%)
Ineffective risk-reduction strategy	4 (11%)	3 (8%)
Did not submit an action plan	4 (11%)	19 (49%)

[a] $\chi^2 = 8.65$, $p < .01$.

TABLE 6.4. Rating of Prevention Activities Implemented: Oregon TOGETHER! and Washington CYAP[a]

	Oregon TOGETHER!	Washington CYAP
Active teams	35	39
Teams which implemented activities	31 (89%)	38 (97%)
Teams which implemented effective risk-reduction activities	21 (60%)	13 (33%)
Teams which implemented moderately effective risk-reduction activities	4 (11%)	6 (15%)
Teams which implemented ineffective risk-reduction activities	6 (17%)	19 (49%)

[a] $\chi^2 = 3.97$, $p < .05$.

did not submit a plan. Thus, a significantly higher proportion ($\chi^2 = 8.65$, $p < .01$) of Oregon TOGETHER! prevention boards than Washington State CYAP teams completed action plans that specified effective risk reduction activities.

Implementation of Risk-Reduction Activities

The final objective for the community boards in both projects was to implement risk- and protection-focused prevention strategies based on their action plans. Descriptions of the activities sponsored by each community prevention board in the two projects were rated according to the criteria described in the methods section. By the 1-year followup, before receiving any funding for implementing prevention activities, 21 (60%) of the 35 Oregon TOGETHER! boards had already implemented prevention activities that were clearly risk focused and based on their action plans (Table 6.4). Four boards (11%) had implemented activities rated as being moderately effective at reducing risk factors, while six boards (17%) had implemented activities rated as ineffective risk-reduction strategies. Four boards (11%) had not implemented activities. Thus, prior to receiving any outside funding, more than two-thirds (25 of 35) of the Oregon TOGETHER! teams had implemented risk- and protection-focused prevention activities within 1 year of the CTC training.

As expected, given the funding provided to Washington State CYAP teams, nearly all the Washington teams had implemented activities by the 10-month follow up. Thirty-eight (97%) of the 39 community teams mobilized for the Washington State CYAP project reported having implemented youth-oriented activities in their communities. However, only 13 teams (33%) reported implementation of activities rated as effective risk-reduction strategies. Six teams (15%) described activities rated as moderately effective at reducing risk, while 19 (49%) teams reported activities rated as ineffective risk-reduction strategies. In sum, although Washington State CYAP teams were slightly more likely than Oregon TOGETHER! teams to have implemented activities within 10 months following training, they were significantly ($\chi^2 = 3.97$, $p < .05$) less likely to have implemented risk-focused planning and action within their communities. See Table 6.5 for a listing of the types of prevention activities implemented in Oregon and Washington.

DISCUSSION

Findings from the process evaluations of these two community mobilization approaches to alcohol and other drug abuse prevention reveal similarities and differences which illustrate emerging issues regarding the mobilization of community coalitions to plan and implement science-based

TABLE 6.5. Activities Implemented: Oregon TOGETHER! and Washington CYAP

Oregon TOGETHER	
Effective risk-reduction activities	
Parent trainings	14 (40%)
Youth skills training	1 (3%)
Dropout prevention program or curriculum	9 (26%)
Early childhood education	3 (9%)
Mentoring program	4 (11%)
Moderately effective risk-reduction activities	
Regular program of drug-free activities	1 (3%)
Parent network or support group	1 (3%)
Policy change attempt	8 (23%)
Teen center	2 (6%)
Youth network or support group	5 (14%)
Media attempt	2 (6%)
Ineffective risk-reduction activities	
Occasional drug-free youth activities	12 (34%)
Single-shot media effort	11 (31%)
Sent youth to conference or camp	4 (11%)
Community awareness workshop or presentation	24 (69%)
Resource lists or libraries	8 (23%)
Washington CYAP	
Effective risk-reduction activities	
Parent trainings	7 (18%)
Youth skills training	4 (10%)
Dropout prevention program	3 (8%)
Community policy change	1 (3%)
Moderately effective risk-reduction activities	
Regular program of drug-free activities	3 (8%)
Parent network or support group	3 (8%)
Policy change attempt	4 (10%)
Teen center	1 (3%)
Youth network or support group	4 (10%)
Media attempt	4 (10%)
Ineffective risk-reduction activities	
Occasional drug-free youth activities	27 (69%)
Single-shot media effort	2 (5%)
Sent youth to conference or camp	19 (49%)
Community awareness workshop or presentation	15 (39%)
Resource lists or libraries	3 (8%)

prevention activities. Both approaches were successful at mobilizing community boards to plan and implement prevention activities. Both approaches were able to recruit and involve the types of community members they targeted on their planning boards. The Washington State CYAP project was successful at involving youth in planning youth-oriented activities. The Communities That Care process used in the Oregon TOGETHER! project was effective at involving key community leaders in organizing prevention boards in their communities.

However, the Oregon TOGETHER! project was more successful than the Washington State CYAP project at promoting planning and program activities aimed at specific, empirically based risk factors identified through a community risk assessment process. Even without funding, Oregon TOGETHER! prevention boards were more likely than the funded Washington CYAP community teams to collect empirical indicators of community risk and protective factors, develop action plans describing strategies to reduce prioritized risk factors, and implement programs aimed at reducing these risk factors. These findings have implications for risk-focused prevention programming and provide direction for further study of community coalitions and factors that may influence the adoption of emerging principles of prevention science (Coie et al., 1993).

Implications for Science-Based Prevention Programming

The success of both programs at mobilizing community prevention boards, many of which involved either youth or community leaders as well as other community members volunteering substantial amounts of time and energy, is important. Clearly, the prevention of alcohol and other drug abuse is an issue that many community members feel is worthy of their attention. Moreover, the results from the Oregon TOGETHER! project indicate that offering funding to local groups is not necessary to mobilize communities to plan and implement risk-reduction prevention activities. Community leaders and members can be engaged by offering a clear strategy for addressing an issue that is perceived as a major community concern. Offering communities a strategy that they believe will help them reduce a community concern can be an effective mobilization tool, even when outside funding is unavailable. This finding concurs with the work of Wandersman and his colleagues (Prestby et al., 1990; Wandersman et al., 1987), who found that members of voluntary block organizations were more likely to be active if they felt their organization was effective at addressing block problems.

The finding that the two programs differed in the degree to which participating communities adopted and implemented the risk-reduction prevention approach is also important. In times when funding for prevention programs is limited, the risk- and protective-factor prevention model offers an empirical basis for allocating funds to areas and programs where they may have the greatest impact. Periodic community risk and resource assessments also provide a means for tracking program effects on proximal outcome measures (such as local indicators of risk and protective factors) without requiring more complex and costly evaluation designs to assess impact on more distal outcomes, such as alcohol and other drug abuse.

Cottrell's (1976) concepts of the characteristics of a "competent" community and Wandersman's (1993) "open systems" model of community coalitions offer possible explanations for the observed differences between the programs. Among the "essential conditions" for a competent community hypothesized by Cottrell (1976) are commitment, role clarity, and articulateness. Each of these characteristics appear to distinguish the two projects. In the Oregon TOGETHER! Project, the commitment of participants to the risk-reduction approach and the clear definition and articulation of the approach's terms and goals were emphasized from the start. Key community leaders were oriented to the project in a 1-day session prior to mobilizing a community board. The steps in the project and requirements for key leaders and planning team members participating in the project were explained in detail. If they chose to participate, they were given detailed instructions about the steps for forming a community prevention board and were asked to make at least a 2-year commitment to the project and to their community prevention board.

In contrast, prior to the TWC leader training workshops, the county staff participants were not given clear and detailed information regarding the objectives of the project and the communities' requirements for participating, nor were community leaders oriented to the project. The project itself had two distinct objectives: to create opportunities for youth involvement in the planning of prevention programs, and to mobilize community teams to plan and implement risk-reduction prevention strategies. Although these objectives were not incompatible, the name of the project

(Community Youth Activity Project) emphasized the former objective and may have initially obscured the latter. Community groups were told it was necessary to send representatives to the training in order to receive funds from the state, but they were not given details about the content of the training or told what their responsibilities would be following the training. Moreover, they were not asked to make a commitment to the project or to their community team.

By the time the community prevention boards attended the CTC training sessions offered by the Oregon TOGETHER! project, they were committed to following the risk-focused planning process. In contrast, many of the participants in the TWC training offered by the Washington State CYAP project were present to satisfy a perceived requirement to get the funding offered by the project. Although most of the Washington State CYAP teams adopted at least part of the TWC process following the training, some of the training participants dropped out of the project soon after the workshops, and the information from the training was lost to their communities. Other participants simply refused to use the TWC process. Thus, some of the differences between the two projects in the extent of adoption of the risk- and protection-focused planning process may have resulted from differences in the clarity of program objectives and requirements and from differences in the involvement and commitment of community leaders who provided vision, status, and a sense of importance for the Oregon TOGETHER! community boards' work.

Another issue related to the clarity of program terms and objectives centers on the use of the terms "risk factor" and "risk indicator." The CTC approach used in the Oregon TOGETHER! Project limits its definition of risk factors to constructs that have consistently emerged from prospective, longitudinal studies as predicting greater risk for subsequent abuse of alcohol and other drugs (Hawkins, Catalano, & Miller, 1992). Similarly, CTC defines risk indicators as observable, empirical markers of a risk factor. For example, rates of retention in grade obtained from school records are an indicator of the risk factor "academic failure." In contrast, the TWC approach used in the Washington State CYAP project uses broader, conceptual definitions that are not based as directly on empirical data. The TWC materials define risk factors as influences that "increase the likelihood of alcohol and drug-abuse problems among youth" (Gibbs & Bennett, 1990, p. 7). The TWC materials present lists of risk factors in various social domains and at different developmental stages but do not give specific criteria for how these risk factors were selected, nor do they define risk indicators. The lack of specificity regarding the criteria for selecting risk factors and risk factor indicators may have been part of the reason why some CYAP teams identified things such as "bad kids," "boredom," "denial," and "the large migrant population" as risk factors.

Wandersman's "open systems" framework for analyzing community coalitions (Prestby & Wandersman, 1985; Wandersman, 1993) offers an additional interpretation for the observed differences between the two programs. The open systems framework identifies four components of organizational functioning: (1) resource acquisition, (2) organizational maintenance, (3) production, and (4) goal attainment. This framework suggests that factors such as external funding and community training, board organization and structure, leadership, technical assistance resources, and perceived efficacy are important considerations for community mobilization efforts to reduce risk and promote protective influences within the community. Differences between the two projects in the provision of external funding, key community leader involvement, and the structure of the training sessions offer potential explanations for the observed results.

The success of both projects at mobilizing and sustaining volunteer community prevention boards suggests that the external resources available were sufficient to maintain the boards. However, the resources used in the two projects differed, and this difference may account for some of the difference in community boards adopting the prevention science-based approach. The Oregon TOGETHER! project mobilized key community leaders to support their community prevention board's efforts, creating a sense of importance and legitimacy for the board's objectives and providing a mechanism for accessing local resources to support those objectives. The primary motivation that these key leaders had for allocating local resources to support the prevention board's objectives was the belief that the risk- and protection-focused approach would be more effective at preventing alcohol and other drug abuse than the community's existing system of prevention services. Thus, the Oregon TOGETHER! prevention boards were expected to adopt the risk reduction approach and were held accountable for doing so by their community leaders.

In contrast, the Washington CYAP community teams were provided an external resource (funding) that was not contingent on attending the training session or adopting the risk-reduction approach. Teams that did not attend training or submit risk-focused action plans were still able to use project funds to implement activities. Thus, Washington CYAP teams were given less motivation to adopt the risk-focused prevention approach than the Oregon TOGETHER! prevention boards.

Another difference between the projects in the external resources provided to communities lay in the timing and organization of the training workshops. The Communities that Care process used in the Oregon TOGETHER! project provided a series of three training workshops that divided the content of the risk-reduction approach into three components: community mobilization and board formation, community risk and resource assessment, and risk-factor prioritization and action planning. In contrast, the Together We Can process covered all three components in one training session and provided a kit that described seven steps to follow in completing the community assessment and risk-reduction action plan. While most CYAP teams reported that they liked the kits and followed some of the TWC steps, few teams reported that they followed the TWC process closely. Many of the CYAP team leaders who attended the training remarked that too much material was presented, though they also requested that the workshop be shortened from 2 1/2 days to 1 1/2 day. In contrast, the series of training workshops provided to Oregon TOGETHER! communities limited the breadth of information covered during a single training session and provided an opportunity for community members to refocus their efforts and discuss with the trainers any problems they encountered in translating the training material into action in their communities. The findings suggest that a series of content-specific training workshops are more effective than a single training session at transferring the prevention science-based technology to communities.

DIRECTIONS FOR FURTHER STUDY

Findings from the process evaluations of these two projects provide useful information regarding strategies for mobilizing communities to reduce risks for alcohol and other drug abuse. However, these findings are limited by the use of convenience samples of communities and a reliance on subjective reports of prevention board members and project staff for much of the data. Given the popularity of community coalitions for alcohol and other drug abuse prevention and many related health and community concerns, more systematic study of coalitions is needed (Butterfoss et al., 1993).

Future research should assess systematically the impact of community mobilization efforts to reduce risks and enhance protection against alcohol and other drug abuse. The findings reported here indicate that communities can be mobilized to assess and prioritize risk factors and to plan and implement risk reduction activities aimed at the prioritized risks. However, the impact of these activities on levels of risk and protective factors and the incidence and prevalence of alcohol and other drug abuse are unknown. Given the high costs associated with alcohol and other drug abuse in this country, the popularity of the community mobilization approach to prevention, and the empirical and theoretical basis for the use of a risk reduction/protective factor enhancement strategy in preventing substance abuse, it is important to study the effectiveness of this strategy.

REFERENCES

Akers, R. L. (1977). *Deviant behavior: A social learning approach* (2nd ed.). Belmont, CA: Wadsworth Press.

Altman, D. G. (1995). Sustaining interventions in community systems: On the relationship between researchers and communities. *Health Psychology, 14,* 526–536.

Backer, T. E., David, S. L., & Soucy, G. (Eds., 1995). *Reviewing the behavioral science knowledge base on technology transfer.* Washington, DC: National Institute on Drug Abuse.

Bandura, A. (1977). Self-efficacy: Toward a unifying theory of behavioral change. *Psychological Review, 84,* 191–215.

Biglan, A. (1995). Translating what we know about the context of antisocial behavior into a lower prevalence of such behavior. *Journal of Applied Behavior Analysis, 28,* 479–492.

Bracht, N., & Kingsbury, L. (1990). Community organization principles in health promotion: A five-stage model. In N. Bracht (Ed.), *Health promotion at the community level* (pp. 66–88). Beverly Hills, CA: Sage.

Butterfoss, F. D., Goodman, R. M., & Wandersman, A. (1993). Community coalitions for prevention and health promotion. *Health Education Research, 8,* 315–330.

Catalano, R. F., & Hawkins, J. D. (1996). The social development model: A theory of antisocial behavior. In J. D. Hawkins (Ed.), *Delinquency and crime: Current theories* (pp. 149–197). New York, NY: Cambridge University Press.

Coie, J. D., Watt, N. F., West, S. G., Hawkins, J. D., Asarnow, J. R., Markman, H. J., Ramey, S. L., Shure, M. B., & Long, B. (1993). The science of prevention: A conceptual framework and some directions for a national research program. *American Psychologist, 48,* 1013–1022.

Cottrell, L. S. (1976). The competent community. In B. H. Kaplan, R. Wislon, & A. H. Leighton (Eds.), *Further explorations in social psychiatry* (pp. 195–211). New York: Basic Books.

Dryfoos, J. G. (1990). *Adolescents at risk: Prevalence and prevention.* New York: Oxford University Press.

Eng, E., & Parker, E. (1990, October). *Community competence and health: Definitional, conceptual, and measurement issues.* Paper presented at the meeting of the American Public Health Association, New York, NY.

Farrington, D. P., & Hawkins, J. D. (1991) Predicting participation, early onset, and later persistence in officially recorded offending. *Criminal Behaviour and Mental Health, 1,* 1–33.

Florin, P., Mitchell, R., & Stevenson, J. (1993). Identifying training and technical assistance needs in community coalitions: A developmental approach. *Health Education Research, 8,* 417–432.

Garmezy, N. (1985). Stress-resistant children: The search for protective factors. In J. E. Stevenson (Ed.), Recent research in developmental psychopathology. New York: Pergaman Press. *Journal of Child Psychology and Psychiatry, 4,* (suppl.) 213–233.

Gibbs, J., & Bennett, S. (1990). *Together we can reduce the risks of alcohol and drug abuse among youth.* Seattle, WA: Comprehensive Health Education Foundation.

Harachi Manger, T., Hawkins, J. D., Haggerty, K. P., & Catalano, R. F. (1992). Mobilizing communities to reduce risks for drug abuse: Lessons on using research to guide prevention practice. *Journal of Primary Prevention, 13,* 3–22.

Hawkins, J. D., Arthur, M. W., & Catalano, R. F. (1995). Preventing substance abuse. In M. Tonry & D. Farrington (Eds.), *Crime and Justice: Vol. 19. Building a safer society: Strategic approaches to crime prevention* (pp. 343–427). Chicago: University of Chicago Press.

Hawkins, J. D., Catalano, R. F., & Associates. (1992). *Communities That Care: Action for drug abuse prevention.* San Francisco: Jossey-Bass.

Hawkins, J. D., Catalano, R. F., & Miller, J. Y. (1992). Risk and protective factors for alcohol and other drug problems in adolescence and early adulthood: Implications for substance abuse prevention. *Psychological Bulletin, 112,* 64–105.

Hawkins, J. D., Harachi Manger, T., Peterson, P. L., & Horn, M. (1991). *Evaluation of the Community Youth Activity Program grant.* Unpublished manuscript, University of Washington, Social Development Research Group, Seattle.

Hawkins, J. D., & Weis, J. G. (1985). The social development model: An integrated approach to delinquency prevention. *Journal of Primary Prevention, 6,* 73–97.

Hirschi, T. (1969). *Causes of delinquency.* Berkeley: University of California Press.

Johnston, L. D., O'Malley, P. M., & Bachman, J. G. (1998). *National survey results on drug use from the Monitoring the Future Study, 1975–1997. Volume 1: Secondary school students.* Rockville, MD: National Institute on Drug Abuse.

Kaftarian, S. J., & Hansen, W. B. (1994). Community Partnership Program. *Journal of Community Psychology,* CSAP Special Issue.

Kandel, D. B., Simcha-Fagan, O., Davies, M. (1986). Risk factors for delinquency and illicit drug use from adolescence to young adulthood. *Journal of Drug Issues, 16,* 67–90.

Morrissey, E., Wandersman, A., Seybolt, D., Nation, M, Crusto, C., & Davino, K. (1997). Toward a framework for bridging the gap between science and practice in prevention: A focus on evaluator and practitioner perspectives. *Evaluation and Program Planning, 20,* 367–377.

Mrazek, P. J., & Haggerty, R. J., (Eds., 1994) *Reducing risks for mental disorders: Frontiers for preventive intervention research.* Washington, DC: Institute of Medicine, National Academy Press.

National Institute on Drug Abuse and National Institute on Alcohol Abuse and Alcoholism. (1998). *The economic costs of alcohol and drug abuse in the United States 1992.* Rockville, MD: US Department of Health and Human Services.

Newcomb, M. D. (1995). Identifying high-risk youth: Prevalence and patterns of adolescent drug abuse. In E. Rahdert, D. Czechowicz, & I. Amsel (Eds.), *Adolescent drug abuse: Clinical assessment and therapeutic intervention* (pp. 7–38). Rockville, MD: National Institute on Drug Abuse.

Newcomb, M. D., Maddahian, E., Skager, R., & Bentler, P. M. (1987). Substance abuse and psychosocial risk factors among teenagers: Associations with sex, age, ethnicity and type of school. *American Journal of Drug and Alcohol Abuse, 13,* 413–433.

Office of National Drug Control Policy. (1999). *National Drug Control Strategy: 1999.* Washington, DC: Author.

Pollard, J. A., Hawkins, J. D., Arthur, M. W. (1999). Risk and protection: Are both necessary to understand diverse behavioral outcomes in adolescence? *Social Work Research, 23,* 145–158.

Prestby, J. E., & Wandersman, A. (1985). An empirical exploration of a framework of organizational viability: Maintaining block organizations. *Journal of Applied Behavioral Science, 21,* 287–305.

Prestby, J. E., Wandersman, A., Florin, P., Rich, R. C., & Chavis, D. (1990). Benefits, costs, incentive management and participation in voluntary organizations: A means to understanding and promoting empowerment. *American Journal of Community Psychology, 18,* 117–149.

Resnick, M. D., Bearman, P. S., Blum, R. W., Bauman, K. E., Harris, K. M., Jones, J., Tabor, J., Beuhring, T., Sieving, R. E., Shew, M., Ireland, M., Bearinger, L. H., and Udry, J. R. (1997). Protecting adolescents from harm: Findings from the National Longitudinal Study on Adolescent Health. *Journal of the American Medical Association, 278,* 823–832.

Rogers, E. (1995). *Diffusion of innovations* (4th ed.). New York: Free Press.

Sloboda, Z., & David, S. L. (1997). *Preventing drug use among children and adolescents: A research-based guide.* Rockville, MD: National Institute on Drug Abuse.

Wandersman, A. (1993). *Understanding coalitions and how they operate: An 'open systems' organizational perspective.* Unpublished manuscript, University of South Carolina, Department of Psychology.

Wandersman, A., Florin, P., Friedmann, R., & Meier, R. (1987). Who participates, who does not, and why? An analysis of voluntary neighborhood associations in the United States and Israel. *Sociological Forum, 2,* 534–555.

Werner, E. E. (1994). Overcoming the odds. *Journal of Developmental and Behavioral Pediatrics, 15,* 131–136.

CHAPTER 7

Community-Focused Drug Abuse Prevention

Barry M. Kibel
Harold D. Holder

INTRODUCTION

Incidents of problem use of alcohol and other drugs can be found in all types of communities—in urban, suburban, and rural America. A recently released report funded by the Centers for Disease Control and Prevention, the Youth Risk Behavior Surveillance (Kann, et al., 1997), based on a nationwide survey of 16,262 students ages 10 to 24, found that almost 80% of respondents reported having tried alcohol, with 33% having had five or more drinks in the past month. Nearly 50% said they used marijuana during the previous month; almost 10% had tried cocaine during the previous month, and one-third had ridden in the past month with someone who had been drinking.

Attempting to understand, anticipate, and prevent such alarming alcohol and drug use and the associated problems is a monumental undertaking because each such problem has complex causes. Additionally, many of the problem areas are interrelated: They influence and are influenced by the others. For example, alcohol and drug abuse can lead to violence, poor school work, and poor job performance. It can also be argued that these problems can, in turn, increase the probability of alcohol and drug abuse. Adding to the complexity, these problems operate in dynamic environments subject to powerful social, economic, media, political, cultural, racial, and other influences. As these environments change, so do the characteristics of the problems and the strategies that might best be applied to prevent them.

Barry M. Kibel • Pacific Institute for Research and Evaluation, Chapel Hill, North Carolina 27514
Harold D. Holder • Pacific Institute for Research and Evaluation, Berkeley, California 94704

A natural response to drug-related problems—from a prevention as well as a problem-solving standpoint—is to focus on individuals who are currently or potentially most at risk for such problems. After all, these are the persons most likely to create the problems—or so it might seem. And clearly, higher rates of alcohol- and drug-linked traffic accidents and fatalities, crime, violence, abuse, and other social ills can be linked to the more risky segments of the population. Still, many public health and social problems are best addressed from a community systems perspective (Holder, 1998). For example, there is little evidence that decisions of adolescents about criminal behavior and the pursuit of criminal careers are strictly the consequences of individual malfunctioning. Psychological, social, cultural, economic, and physical environmental factors can all contribute to producing young criminals. To date, efforts to reduce crime rates among adolescents through individually focused counseling and education or through law enforcement and the courts have not been successful (Whitehead & Lab, 1989).

Aspects of systems strategies have been used in community public health initiatives, including some disease- and cancer-prevention trials. Public health projects have succeeded in getting low-fat alternatives offered on restaurant menus, low-salt food products available and prominently displayed in grocery stores, warning labels on the hazards of smoking installed at points of sale for cigarettes, and the number of nonsmoking areas in public spaces and in the workplace increased.

A systems approach to alcohol and other drug abuse prevention is based on the following axioms (Holder, 1998):

1. Substance abuse problems are multicausal in nature, highly interrelated with other social and public health problems, and resistant to single, "magic bullet" cures.
2. Even the most promising prevention interventions delivered superbly, but in relative isolation from other efforts, such as those by law enforcement, schools, media, health agencies, and employers, will yield only small community effects that are unlikely to be sustained over time.
3. Effective responses to these problems require coordinated, multifaceted action at the local level, supported by regulatory action and resources from local, state, and federal bodies.

This chapter argues for types of planning, evaluation, and research that promote action-oriented and highly collaborative community responses in the development of effective alcohol and drug abuse prevention practices.

THE EMERGENCE OF COALITIONS

Community and organizational coalition activity has become a principal force for coordinating and mobilizing efforts to curtail the abuse of alcohol and other drugs. This push toward community-based initiatives was not grounded in research findings. Rather, it was spurred by a large influx of funding for such initiatives, common-sense positions which held that a whole-community response was needed for a whole-community problem, and widely felt frustration at the ineffectiveness of isolated approaches in making and sustaining an impact on large numbers of community members.

A 1992 study conducted by the Pacific Institute for Research and Evaluation for Join Together (a national project for communities fighting substance abuse, funded by The Robert Wood Johnson Foundation) found coalition-based prevention activities underway in every state and territory, all 25 of the nation's largest cities, and literally thousands of communities of every size (Join Together, 1992). Throughout the mid-1990s, Robert Wood Johnson and federal agencies, such as the Center for Substance Abuse Prevention, provided long-term (5 years or more) support and technical assistance activities for hundreds of U.S. communities to tackle local substance abuse issues. Following their lead, state agencies and other foundations provided resources and incentives to promote coalition-based problem solving.

The majority of these coalitions boasted representation and shared leadership by professionals, local organizations, lay people, activists, and government officials. For example, coalitions surveyed (Join Together, 1993) included representatives from schools (90%), local law enforcement (85%), prevention and treatment providers (over 70%), parents (72%), religious organizations (61%), health service agencies (56%), and volunteers (71%). Volunteers, in particular, provided a critical resource for sustaining the activities of these partnerships, which frequently promised more than they could deliver with the budgets and staff resources at hand.

The challenge of simply getting people from different professional, racial, economic, and institutional backgrounds to sit around the table and work together proved to be formidable. Joining together seemed to make sense; but figuring out how to work together to tackle complex social problems—often decades or more in the making—proved exceedingly difficult, at best. Granted, there were hundreds of local success stories in the form of new programs, stronger regulations, and transformed youths and adults. And lessons for effective community mobilization were learned from them. For example, chances for success increased proportionately to the ability of the coalition to (1) produce and maintain a heightened sense of community, (2) master the difficult art of community mobilization, and (3) orchestrate a multicycle action-planning process (Kibel & Stein-Seroussi, 1997). But definitive impact studies demonstrating that coalition efforts resulted in significant and sustained drops in local alcohol and drug use indicators have not yet emerged.

Coalitions did not find "magic bullets" with which to arm their communities in the fight against alcohol and drug abuse. They were—and continue to be—challenged to improvise strategies involving multiple, complementary, and result-reinforcing interventions. They are still learning how best to do this. Few coalitions have mastered the art of effective community systems planning. Few have made maximum use of evaluation feedback. Few have accessed the latest and best research and translated its findings into action alternatives (including avoiding activities and programs that researchers have determined do not work).

To gauge their success, as well as to justify their continued existence, coalitions need to know what interventions are working, both singly and particularly in combination with others. Local and national planners, evaluators, and researchers can help provide this essential information; but to be responsive to the call, professionals must recognize the need to become partners within the coalitions. In an arena of give-and-take and learning by doing, there simply is no appropriate place for a sideline observer. Action planning, collaborative evaluation, and community systems research are the emerging arsenal of tools needed to support successful community-based prevention efforts.

BEYOND SIMPLE SYSTEM SOLUTIONS

Why are new approaches and tools required for effective community-based prevention? A partial answer can be derived from two basic concepts from general systems theory. First, since the advent of this field in the mid-1960s (VonBertalanffy, 1968), systems theorists have used the concept of relative complexity to distinguish among different types of systems. Simple systems are easy to model and, where problems emerge within them, are fairly easy to fix. More complex systems (typically characterized by more interacting components) pose tricky modeling challenges and, should they become problematic, will often defy immediate and straightforward solutions. Exceedingly complex systems (invariably involving the interplay of free choice and other human factors) are very hard to model (note, for example, the struggles the U.S. Army Research Office

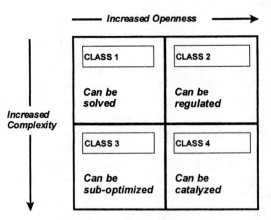

FIGURE 7.1. Classes of systems.

has faced over the past 2 decades in constructing artificial intelligence systems that mirror human thought processes); and, when problems emerge within them, those problems may defy solution. As Edward deBono (1990) noted:

> In many problems, we cannot find the cause. Or, we can find it but cannot remove it—for example, human greed. Or, there may be a multiplicity of causes. What do we do then? We analyze it further and analyze the analysis of others (so-called scholarship). [However,] more and more analysis is not going to help, because what is needed is design. We need to design a way out of the problem or a way of living with it.

Second, systems theorists have made wide use of the concept of the relative openness of a system (Levine & Fitzgerald, 1992). A closed system is a mechanical system that is totally self-contained and hence a rarity. As systems become more open, the numbers and types of interactions with their environment (and corresponding dependencies) increase. An exceedingly open system is one that exists in dynamic interplay with its environment and is shaped by, and in turn helps shape, that environment.

In Figure 7.1, four classes of systems are depicted. These are distinguishable by (1) their relative simplicity versus complexity and (2) their relative closure versus openness.

Mechanical systems (such as an electrical or heating system) are relatively simple and closed (Class 1). Their simplicity is reflected in the small number of components and operations that describe them. Their closure means that they are essentially self-contained and not influenced by factors or events beyond their boundaries during normal operations. (An exception would be an areawide power outage that would render an electrical system inoperative. Thus, the point where this relatively closed system is most vulnerable is where it is most open to the rest of the world.)

Communities, in contrast to mechanical systems, are highly complex, highly open systems (Class 4). Their complexity is apparent in the diversity and variability of the economic, sociocultural, and psychological interactions that continually engage their populations. Their openness is perhaps best expressed through their dependence on outside sources for sustenance (such as food) and stimulation (television).

Closed, simple systems (Class 1) are equilibrium-seeking. Undisturbed by outside factors, they tend to stabilize at some static point or dynamic operating condition. However, as their integrity is challenged (Class 2), they lose predictability and orderliness. At the extreme, when uncontrollable forces are continually intruding from outside, they become chaotic.

Problems in Class 2 systems cannot be solved unless the systems can be completely regulated, rendered relatively closed, and transformed to Class 1 systems. An example of a Class 2 system is the Mexico–U.S. border. Attempts to stop the entry into the United States by illegal immigrants have proved futile because the border is highly porous. Down the road from expensive, highly controlled border crossings, individuals crawl under barbed-wire fences to enter the country. A similar situation exists with regard to the only partially successful efforts to eliminate the flow of drugs into the United States. To the extent that relatively simple systems cannot be closed, problems within them cannot be solved. They can, at best, be regulated to approximate solutions.

As closed systems become increasingly complex, through the addition of new components and operations, they lose their equilibrium, and problems within them cease to be solvable through simple and routine adjustments. The components and operating rules of Class 3 systems (for example, a football game between two outstanding teams) may be completely known, yet no strategy can be formulated and followed to the letter to guarantee success. Class 3 systems can, at best, be suboptimized. This means that solutions can be found that work in some, but not in all, cases or that address problems in part of the system while not necessarily making the entire system ultimately better off.

There is no guarantee that the suboptimal solution to a problem in a Class 3 system will actually improve the system as a whole. There may be secondary interactions or chain reactions created by the interplay of the components that produce unanticipated and undesired consequences. In the prevention field, for example, some research has suggested that educational programs aimed at making youngsters more aware of the dangers of drugs piqued their curiosity and actually contributed to increased experimentation with drugs. This education strategy was based on the simple cause-and-effect logic that awareness leads to rational action. The rational processes of the youngsters turned out to be more complex than was assumed. As a second example, consider the effects of the Anti-Drug Abuse Act on the nation's court systems. This legislation increased funds available for drug enforcement leading to significant increases in the number of drug-related court cases. However, felony court systems began having great difficulty in handling their caseloads. By some measures, their capacity deteriorated (Milkman et al., 1993). Consequences of increased enforcement included increased average time from arrest to disposition and between conviction and sentencing, recidivism, overburdened court dockets, overworked felony court teams, and overcrowded jails and prisons.

Class 4 systems are highly complex and relatively open to outside influences that cannot be controlled from within the system. Hence, they cannot be solved, completely regulated, or even effectively suboptimized. In short, they are out of direct human control through manipulation. Society at large is an example of a Class 4 system. Despite the best intentions and best thinking of world leaders and scholars, war and violence pervade the planet. Hunger and poverty prevail. World economies are unstable. The ecological balance is threatened.

The standard problem-solving response to crises emerging within Class 4 systems is to pretend that they are not Class 4 systems. By pretending that they are Class 3 systems, they can be suboptimized (and perhaps the problem will go away without the problem solvers creating a bigger problem). By pretending that they are Class 2 systems, they can be regulated (and perhaps there will be no holes in the dike downriver). By pretending that they are Class 1 systems, they can be tinkered with to create the illusion of a solution—until the critics start pointing to the parts that have been ignored.

A more rational response (where rationality means applying our best thinking in light of the best available information rather than pretending that something is true when we know it is not) is to tackle problems in Class 4 systems on their own terms. This means developing responses that are themselves complex and open. Such "solutions" must be multifaceted, experimental, and prone to change as experience is gained. In short, these are solutions-in-process that must be constantly readapted to the complexity of the environments in which they are implemented.

To survive in dynamic, global economies, private-sector businesses are struggling to master Class 4 problem solving. Peters (1987) characterized healthy organizations as those engaged in constant improvement of services and products, endless experimentation, inspired leadership that promotes creativity, participatory management and widespread empowerment, and ubiquitous measurement systems that pinpoint and correct mistakes while highlighting successes. There are few guarantees that what worked yesterday or is working today will work tomorrow. In fact, what worked is likely not to work. The challenge is to keep inventing new solutions that are workable.

DRUG ABUSE PREVENTION: WHAT WORKS

As noted, most communities are Type 4 systems. They are exceedingly complex, and they are quite open to influences beyond their physical boundaries. Hence, communitywide problems, such as those linked to alcohol and drug use, will likely defy simple or even complex solutions. What is required is not problem solving. Instead, community leaders (both formal and informal) must take the risk of admitting out loud that community reinvention is what is demanded and, further, that the contributions of many are required for success to be realized.

For example, in 1993, the chief judge of the Rochester, New York, City Court, declared publicly that the community's approach to dealing with persons arrested for drug-related crimes was not working and could not be fixed by tinkering with the existing approaches (Schwartz & Schwartz, 1998). He had witnessed, on a daily basis, the revolving door of drug use, crime, jail, release, drug reuse, and crime. He saw tax dollars being wasted on jails to shelter and feed repeat offenders and an even greater cost in terms of the eroding sense of confidence in the criminal justice system. Building on a model that had shown some success in Miami, he mobilized needed community support and created the Rochester Drug Court, which is now serving more than 700 drug abusers through care-managed treatment rather than through incarceration or probation without treatment.

There are few single interventions (neither program, service, nor policy) that alone can produce a significant impact on a communitywide problem. A recently completed guide to effective programs, commissioned by the U.S. Department of Education, stated clearly:

> Because substance abuse and violence are complex human behaviors often related to other factors in the home or wider community and society, prevention is more likely to be successful when efforts directed at altering individual behavior are paired with those directed at altering the environment. (Scattergood et al., 1998)

The guide calls for programs to implement a combination of strategies that aim to involve families and communities, influence the larger social and legal context, create or enforce existing laws and regulations, and provide alternatives to substance abuse and violence through social and recreational activities and mentoring.

A dramatic example of an apparent exception was the federal pressure put on states in the mid-1980s to either raise the legal drinking age to 21 or lose highway funds. Significantly fewer crashes and deaths involving youths now occur on America's highways because of this intervention. But the intervention's effects were buttressed by increased enforcement of seatbelt laws and the 55-mile-per-hour maximum speed limit. Efforts of Mothers Against Drunk Driving, Students Against Destructive Decisions, and other groups to discourage drinking and driving contributed to the impact. General downward shifts in alcohol consumption, coupled with school-based education programs, contributed even further. And while morbidity and mortality rates linked to alcohol use have not risen to the pre-1980 levels, alcohol use and abuse among teens remains a national problem and an issue of continuing community concern, as the CDC report cited at the start of this chapter makes clear.

Two types of community efforts appear to be the most successful in reducing the problems of alcohol and drug abuse. The first, environmental strategies, involves creating and seriously enforcing policies that restrict or moderate use of alcohol and drugs. The entire community is blanketed with this single intervention. The second type involves the creation of what we term "oases of stability" within communities. In this case, there are multiple points of intervention, each offering somewhat unique responses to address the needs of the community.

Environmental Strategies

Holder (1993a) identifies five policy areas that researchers have demonstrated can lead to decreased alcohol availability and, thus, have the potential to reduce future alcohol-related problems. These are (1) minimum age for purchasing alcohol (now 21 in all states), (2) server intervention or responsible beverage service, (3) server or dram shop liability, (4) low- and nonalcoholic beverages, and (5) warning labels. None of these policies alone should be expected to "solve" the alcohol-related problems of a community; but if well executed and responsibly enforced these policies can contribute toward a reduction in alcohol abuse.

Perhaps the most striking example of effective prevention policy as applied to illicit drug use is random drug testing in the military. Declines in observed and reported drug use have been dramatic since urinalysis testing began in 1981 (Bray et al., 1990). Workplace drug testing has led to less dramatic but significant reductions (Kibel & Luckey, 1991), although in many cases drug testing is restricted to applicant and new-employee screening. However, widespread use of this policy has met with considerable resistance. Critics argue that (1) such testing tends to single out weekend marijuana users, while missing heavy drinkers and "hard drug" users; (2) decisions may be made by employers based on false positives from relatively inexpensive and correspondingly inaccurate screening tests; (3) poor protocols allow individuals to beat the system; and (4) urine testing represents an infringement of basic individual rights.

Oases of Stability

This is a term we coined to capture the range of interventions used to (1) buffer the target population from potentially negative outside influences while (2) providing consistent and positive support and encouragement. In a report prepared for the North Carolina legislature on dropout prevention, Kibel (1988) noted that successful prevention programs across the nation tended to incorporate these ABCs: academic alternatives; bonuses, benefits, and bribes; and caring and committed counselors. The alternative learning opportunities based on these ABCs and provided to students who had previously dropped out or were at risk of drop out were oases of stability for such youths.

African-American churches are a second example of this type of intervention. Since the first such church was founded in Philadelphia in 1787, Black churches have been the single most dominant institution controlled by African-Americans for their political and social advancement. In addition to serving the needs of its membership, church leaders have reached out to play important roles in the African-American community as a whole. In recent years, with government support for social programs shrinking, Black churches have had to feed and clothe the hungry, shelter the homeless, provide jobs, attempt to rein in young gang members, and respond to neighborhood violence. And the church is constantly challenged to do more. As expressed by one noted preacher, "The coming-to-church-for-personal-salvation days are over. Now we are looking not only for personal salvation, but for social salvation" (Murray, 1993). In short, the Black church is being challenged to reinvent itself to meet the challenges of the day.

The Friday Nite/Club Live programs in California offer a contrasting third example. With the assistance of state funding and technical support, student chapters have been formed in high schools and middle schools throughout the state with membership in excess of 1 million young-sters. These chapters are student organized and student run. Promoting drug-free lifestyles, the chapters sponsor social events and public projects (such as cleaning the local beaches of trash, followed by a beach party). Critics of the programs argue that the highest at-risk youths are not typically members of the chapters. But, in the spirit of Class 4 systems thinking, one should not demand that these programs "solve" all the state's problems. The oases of stability afford social structure for more than one million youths and, by social program standards, at relatively low cost.

To be successful, the designs for oases of stability must be both client and community fo-cused. For example, the University of Colorado's Center for the Study and Prevention of Violence (1998) recently completed a review of more than 400 delinquency, drug, and violence prevention programs. The center selected 10 programs as "Blueprints for Violence Prevention." The assess-ment criteria used in the selection included an experimental design, replication, and demonstrated effectiveness by at least one additional site and evidence that the deterrent effect was sustained for at least 1 year following the intervention. The programs selected shared at least some of these features: adult mentoring and peer-group support; communication and problem-solving skills training; life skills and social-resistance skills training; engagement of the family in prob-lem solving and relation building; mobilization and full use of community resources (including volunteers); and educational enrichment and related incentives, such as job opportunities.

Again, there are no "quick fixes" to the problems associated with alcohol and drug use. The hope for improvement lies in experimentation based on the best available research and thinking. This domain must extend beyond scholarly endeavors to include wider and wider segments of the community. In fact, the lead responsibility must be transferred from professionals to the community—hence, the importance of coalitions. In this regard, Lisbeth Schorr (1997) notes: "There is no simple model that can just be 'parachuted' in. Rather, successful programs are shaped to respond to the needs of local populations and to assure that local communities have a genuine sense of ownership. . . . Being community based means more than being located in the neighborhood. Increasingly, successful programs are not just in but of the community." This new arena for community problem tackling presents new challenges and opportunities for planners, evaluators, and researchers.

NEW CHALLENGES FOR
COMMUNITY-FOCUSED PLANNING

Planning processes are essential, but they frequently get bogged down for two reasons. First, communities believe (or are told by funding sources) that they must produce a complete, com-prehensive plan before they can act. Second, they believe (or are told) that any action taken must be anticipated in that plan. Enormous time, effort, and community goodwill are wasted perform-ing needs assessments, conducting endless rounds of meetings at which groups posture behind preestablished mindsets, debating issues with little hope of reconciliation, and producing formal plans that will never be fully implemented. Planning needs to be reality based and meaningful to local practitioners in order for the process to enhance implementation of science-based policies, practices, and program models.

It is particularly easy for a community to get pulled in competing directions when it comes to tackling alcohol and other drug abuse prevention. Should the focus be on youngsters before they begin experimenting with substances? Should the community focus exclusively on alcohol, which is a significant contributor to violence, crime, lost work hours, family instability, and teenage traffic deaths? Should the focus be on police enforcement and crackdowns on those who violate federal and local laws regarding illicit drug use? All these foci, and a dozen more that could be suggested, offer legitimate strategic options. The challenge for a community is not to limit its foci but to tackle each of these areas in a coherent, practical, and decisive manner.

The most sensible way to plan in an open, complex, dynamic system is through informed action and reaction. As Bunker and Alban (1997) note, participation is key: "When people have the important information about a system and are allowed to become collaboratively and fully engaged with others around these issues, they become highly motivated to take responsibility for change and improvement."

The approach needs to be commonsensical. For example, start anywhere a problem exists and where there are individuals willing to act to resolve the problem. Spend some time (3 to 4 hours) considering the logic of proposed courses of action and how these might link with other activities already under way or being planned in the community. If a logical, politically acceptable, mutually compatible, and locally feasible strategy emerges, then spend a bit more time (3 to 4 hours) developing a plan of action and an accompanying monitoring system. Then act, monitor, and adjust the action as needed. Encourage all parties in the process to ask hard questions and search together for responsible answers at any point in the process.

Meanwhile, start somewhere else and replicate the same process. The challenge for the community is to keep generating and sustaining informed action leading away from problems and toward desired community conditions. A spirit of experimentation should prevail, provided these experiments are small in scale, easily adjusted as they proceed, and lessons are learned. Planning, action, and assessment happen continuously as three aspects of a single process.

NEW CHALLENGES FOR
COMMUNITY-FOCUSED EVALUATION

Planning and evaluation are more closely akin than is generally recognized. Both functions are based on asking questions in a timely manner that contribute to creative thinking, realistic assessment, and informed action. Too frequently, however, planners pose questions about what will be (before the fact), evaluators pose questions about what was (after the fact), and the two functions are not merged. For maximum results, effective planning and evaluation must function in concert.

The evaluation function is typically subdivided between "process assessments" and "outcome measurements." In short, process evaluation focuses on the procedures and actions under way to produce results; outcome evaluation focuses on the results generated. Effective process evaluation for community-based initiatives involves constant monitoring of interventions as they are implemented and frequent readjustment to keep the interventions on track. In this regard, the evaluation is akin to quality assurance: (1) paying attention to detail at every step of the design and implementation process, (2) treating each step as if it were the step most critical to the success of the entire process, (3) soliciting feedback from everyone involved in the process, (4) being continually sensitive to the needs and expectations of the ultimate clients, and (5) continually striving to add quality at lower cost (Deming, 1982; Ishikawa, 1985).

Effective process evaluators must go beyond report writing; they should provide ongoing information on the design and execution of programs to the planners and program staff. This information may help in overcoming obstacles, avoiding pitfalls, forming alliances, and refining action plans while the action is in progress. Rather than standing apart as "objective" observers (Is anyone truly objective?), the evaluators must join forces and talents with the planners and program staff.

Action-oriented evaluation does not sacrifice rigor. A full range of community outcomes can be gauged and analyzed. However, the outcome evaluation must incorporate the right types and mix of measures. These include time-series social indicators that track progress in impacting the community through broad-scale policies and their enforcement. They also include results of diverse outcome studies under way in the community, particularly where the strategies being assessed are delivered to community members with fidelity and are of sufficient dosage to justify their link to outcomes. They also include systematic documentation and analysis of a community's prevention success stories to gain greater understanding of what works best, for whom, and most frequently in the community's oases of stability (Kibel, 1998).

NEW CHALLENGES FOR COMMUNITY-FOCUSED RESEARCH

Despite a flurry of program activity, research directed at comprehensive, community-based prevention programming remains a largely uncharted domain. Communities need to know what will work in their specific contexts. Too often, decisions are made about prevention strategies based on research or hearsay evidence of success in communities that may not be comparable. Furthermore, there is little available research on multicomponent intervention. Yet the essential question that communities ask is: Which mix of interventions will yield maximum reduction in alcohol- and drug-related problems in our community?

Community-focused researchers must pay attention to both the complexity of implementing multi-component strategies and the selection and implementation of these strategies through communitywide, participatory planning processes rather than through research hypotheses and controlled experiments. As Giesbrecht et al. (1991), at the Addiction Research Center, Toronto, Ontario, note:

1. Researchers and community members often have divergent priorities. The former are concerned with increasing the body of relevant knowledge. The latter are concerned with developing programs that match local conditions and address perceived needs.
2. Community members are prone to accept local "truths" and discard or distrust research propositions that conflict with these beliefs. Hence, they may not agree that a certain intervention does not work until they try it for themselves. And they may reject an intervention proposed by researchers because it does not sound like it has a chance of working locally.
3. Researchers may carry their own baggage into the community and consciously or otherwise embed these within their assumptions. For example, they may argue that the intervention has to be implemented in a specific way to permit comparisons across treatments. The communities, for their part, may insist on putting their own particular twist on the intervention to make it appear or actually be locally relevant.
4. Researchers may assume that community members possess the requisite knowledge and insights to grasp research that recommends a particular approach, and fail to take the time to explain the approach so that it is embraced locally. And rather than admit to confusion, community members may counter with expressions of impatience and discard potentially valuable research.

One solution to these challenges lies in increasing involvement of community members in the actual research effort. This is reinforced by Orlando (1992) in a monograph on culturally sensitive evaluation that calls for local research that respects local cultures and accommodates local realities when testing or evaluating new initiatives.

A methodological approach that holds promise with multicomponent prevention strategies is developing, testing, and experimenting with computer-based simulation models of local communities. These models are designed to first replicate the historical dynamics of target communities with regard to substance availability, use, and problems, and then simulate future outcomes and dynamics under alternative assumptions and prevention interventions. Amatetti (1987) and Holder and Blose (1983, 1987) have used such models to construct structural relationships that reflect alternative theories or explanations for important processes (such as the relationship between the availability of a drug and its subsequent consumption by one or more groups within the community). Community groups can use the models to explore the anticipated impacts of alternative mixes of interventions prior to finalizing their plans for actual implementation. These models permit the testing of changes in key economic and demographic parameters, national and local cultural norms, public pressures, and regulatory controls that moderate alcohol and drug use, misuse, and abuse. See Holder (1998) for a detailed discussion of how simulation can be applied to alcohol-problem prevention.

A second example of a form of research that recognizes communities as Class 4 systems is seen in work recently completed by the Prevention Research Center (Berkeley, CA). The Community Prevention Trials project attempted to reduce alcohol-involved injuries and death through a comprehensive 5-year program of community education and alcohol-related prevention activities. To achieve this goal, the project implemented and researched community-based activities in five prevention areas: community knowledge, values, and mobilization; responsible beverage service; underage drinking reduction; risk of drinking and driving reduction; and access to alcohol. Interventions were adjusted as they were implemented in response to learning that occurred within the community and discussions between researchers and community members based on this learning (see Holder, 1993b).

CONCLUSION

Challenged to react responsively to prevent alcohol and other drug problems, communities need to know what will work and how to achieve results quickly. However, the complexity of communities and their lack of closure make traditional planning, research, and evaluation methods inadequate for this task. Planning must address the problems as those of an open, complex community for which there are no simple solutions. The type of planning needed promotes actions that can be undertaken immediately, seeks to coordinate and implement as many actions as possible, and depends on meaningful levels of participation by the wider community.

In addition, addressing the problems of alcohol and drug abuse in a complex system calls for evaluation that is participatory and collaborative and is an active part of the entire planning, design, and implementation process. Its aim is to help the community achieve maximum possible results using a variety of quantitative and qualitative measures to track movement toward these results. And finally, research is needed that reflects the complex character of the communities in which it is to be applied and that will indicate to communities what multicomponent approaches will work best for them.

REFERENCES

Amatetti, S. L. (1987). The use of computer models to evaluate prevention strategies. *Alcohol Health and Research World, 1*, 18–21, 47.

Bray, R. M., Marsden, M. E., Rachal, J. V., & Peterson, M. R. (1990). Drugs in the military workplace: Results of the 1988 worldwide survey. *Drugs in the workplace: Research and evaluation data. Vol. II.* Rockville, MD: Research Monograph 100, National Institute on Drug Abuse.

Bunker, B. B., & Alban, B. T. (1997). *Large group interventions: Engaging the whole system for rapid change.* San Francisco: Jossey-Bass.

Center for the Study and Prevention of Violence (1998). *Ten Blueprints.* University of Colorado at Boulder, Boulder, CO: The Center for the Study and Prevention of Violence.

deBono, E. (1990). *I am right—You are wrong.* New York: Viking.

Deming, W. E. (1982). *Out of the crisis.* Cambridge, MA: Massachusetts Institute of Technology.

Giesbrecht, N., Hyndman, B. K., Bernardi, D. R., Coston, N., Douglas, R. R., Ferrecne, R. G., Gliksman, L., Goodstadt, M. S., Graham, D. G., & Loranger, P. D. (1991). Community action research projects: Integrating community interests and research agenda in multicomponent initiatives. Paper presented at 36th International Institute on the Prevention and Treatment of Alcoholism, Stockholm, Sweden, June 2–7.

Holder, H. D. (1993a). Changes in access to and availability of alcohol in the United States: Research and policy implications. *Addiction, 88,* 67S–74S.

Holder, H. D. (1993b). Prevention of alcohol-related accidents in the community. *Addiction, 88,* 1003–1012.

Holder, H. D. (1998). *Alcohol in the community: A systems approach to prevention.* Cambridge: Cambridge University Press.

Holder, H. D., & Blose, J. O. (1983). Prevention of alcohol-related traffic problems: Computer simulation of alternative strategies. *Journal of Safety Research, 14,* 115–129.

Holder, H. D., & Blose, J. O. (1987). The reduction of community alcohol problems: Computer simulation experiments in three counties. *Journal of Studies on Alcohol, 48,* 124–135.

Ishikawa, K. (1985). *What is total quality control? The Japanese way.* Englewood Cliffs, NJ: Prentice-Hall.

Join Together (1992). *Who really fights the war on drugs? A national study of community-based anti-drug and alcohol activity in America.* Boston: Boston University School of Public Health.

Join Together (1993). *Community leaders speak out against substance abuse.* Boston: Boston University School of Public Health.

Kann, L., Kinchen, S. A., Williams, B. I., Ross, J. G., Lowry, R., Hill, C. V., Grunbaum, J., Blumson, P. S., Collins, J. L., & Kolbe, L. J. (1997). *Youth risk behavior surveillance—United States 47*(SS-3) 1–89.

Kibel, B. (1988). *Study of school dropout factors in the secondary schools of North Carolina: Volume 1—Literature review* (Prepared for the Joint Legislative Commission on Governmental Operations of the North Carolina General Assembly.)

Kibel, B. (1998). *Success stories as hard data.* New York: Plenum Press.

Kibel, B., & Luckey, J. (1991). *Quarterly reports on employee drug testing results from commercial drug testing laboratories in the United States.* Prepared for the National Institute on Drug Abuse.

Kibel, B., & Stein-Seroussi, A. (1997). *Effective community mobilization: Lessons from experience.* Implementation Guide. Substance Abuse and Mental Health Services Administration.

Levine, R. L., & Fitzgerald, H. E. (1992). *Analysis of dynamic psychological systems.* New York: Plenum Press.

Milkman, R. H., Beaudin, B. D., Tarmann, K., & Landson, N. (1993). *Drug offenders and the courts.* The Lazar Institute, McLean, VA: Public Policy paper No. 921.

Murray, C. (1993). As quoted in: Lewis, Gregory. New role thrust on the black church. *San Francisco Examiner, February 28,* B-1, B-4.

Orlando, M. A. (Ed., 1992). *Cultural competence for evaluators* (pp. 1–22). OSAP Cultural Competence Series I. DHHS Pub. No. (ADM)92-1884. Washington, DC: Superintendent of Documents, U.S. Government Printing Office.

Peters, T. (1987). *Thriving in chaos: Handbook for a management revolution.* New York: Harper & Row.

Scattergood, P., Dash, K., Epstein, J., & Adler, M. (1998). *Applying effective strategies to prevent or reduce substance abuse, violence, and disruptive behavior among youth.* Washington, DC: U.S. Department of Education.

Schorr, L. B. (1997). *Common purpose: Strengthening families and neighborhoods to rebuild America.* New York: Anchor Books.

Schwartz, J. R., & Schwartz, L. P. (1998). The Drug Court: A New Strategy for Drug Use Prevention. *Obstetrics and Gynecology Clinics of North America, 25*(1), 255–268.

VonBertalanffy, L. (1968). *General systems theory.* New York: George Braziller.

Whitehead, J. T., & Lab, S. P. (1989). A meta-analysis of juvenile correctional treatment. *Journal of Research in Crime & Delinquency, 26,* 276–95.

CHAPTER 8

Drug Abuse Prevention in the Workplace

ROYER F. COOK

INTRODUCTION

Illicit drug use prevalence rates are highest in the unemployed and criminal populations, but the number of users in those groups is dwarfed by the number of users among the working population. In fact, most users of illicit drugs and heavy users of alcohol are employed adults, many of whom did not become regular drug users or problem drinkers until adulthood. Little wonder that in recent decades issues of substance abuse in the workplace have gained increasing attention from the public health community, employers, and drug abuse researchers and theorists. Not only is the afflicted population huge but also the associated problems have enormous health and economic consequences. For employers and their managed-care programs, there are several powerful reasons to address these problems—from improved productivity to the promise of reduced health-care costs. For public-health entities, the workplace offers tantalizing targets of opportunity for implementing innovative measures of prevention and control. Drug abuse researchers see all of these things and more in the workplace—a setting for prevalence studies, a set of sociocultural forces to be measured and (at least potentially) manipulated, and a test bed for trying new techniques of prevention and intervention for employees and their families.

This chapter provides a brief description of the scope of substance abuse problems among working adults, including prevalence studies and estimates of the impact of substance abuse on worker health and productivity. It also discusses major theoretical perspectives and models and provides recent data on the nature and effectiveness of the primary approaches to preventing substance abuse among workers and their families. The concept of prevention as addressed in this chapter is rather broadly cast, including a fairly wide range of approaches from primary prevention

---

ROYER F. COOK • The ISA Group, Alexandria, Virginia 22314

to interventions that lie just this side of medical treatment. However, the emphasis is on the more recent tests of preventive interventions, programs that attempt to promote healthful behavior and reduce the use of drugs (including nicotine), not only in the workplace but also among workers—a public health perspective that is being increasingly adopted throughout the field.

THE SCOPE OF THE PROBLEM: THE PREVALENCE AND IMPACT OF SUBSTANCE ABUSE IN THE WORK FORCE

Accurate estimates of the prevalence of substance abuse among working adults are notoriously difficult to obtain, but estimation methods and indices have improved in recent years. Much of this improvement is due to the inclusion of an expanded set of workplace-related items in the National Household Survey of Drug Abuse (NHSDA) and by methodological advances in drug use prevalence assessments. For example, a recent report from the Office of Applied Studies in the Substance Abuse and Mental Health Services Administration (SAMHSA) provides data on the nature and scope of alcohol and other drug use in the work force (Hoffman, Larrison, & Sanderson 1997). Using data from the 1994 NHSDA (the first time the survey included a special module designed to gather nationally representative data on drug use among U.S. workers and company drug use policies and programs), the report shows that adults employed full time constitute 69% of all current illicit drug users aged 18 to 49. Current drug use is defined as the use of any illicit drug in the past 30 days. However, although most drug users are employed adults, the large majority of employed adults are not drug users: Only 7.6% of full-time workers report current drug use. Marijuana is by far the most commonly used drug (83.3% of users) among these current users followed by psychotherapeutics (prescription-type psychoactive drugs used for nonmedical reasons) at 18.8% and cocaine at 12.7%. Similarly, 77% of all heavy alcohol users aged 18 to 49 (defined as those drinking 5 or more drinks on 5 or more occasions in the past 30 days) are full-time workers. Heavy alcohol users represent only 8.4% of all full-time workers. Although disturbing, these current rates for illicit drug use among workers represent a decline from 1985 and have remained virtually unchanged since 1991. Heavy alcohol use among workers has changed little over the past decade.

The NHSDA data on age of first use have significant implications for workplace-based prevention. These data have consistently shown that a substantial proportion of drug users do not begin drug use until after they enter the work force. Although the mean age of first use of marijuana has been in the 16- to 18-year-old range for the past decade, the mean age of first use of cocaine has been in the range of 19 to 23 years of age, and first use of heroin in the range of 19 to 25 years of age (SAMHSA, 1996).

The SAMHSA report also provides a revealing picture of the correlates of the drug-using worker. Higher rates of drug use tend to occur among white males in smaller organizations (1 to 24 employees) where there are less likely to be employee assistance programs (EAPs) and written policies on drug abuse. The drug-using worker is also more likely to have an unstable recent work history. Rates of drug use vary considerably by occupation, with the highest rates found in the blue-collar trades of construction, machine operators, handlers and helpers, and workers in bars and restaurants.

Because the NHSDA estimates are based on self-reports and therefore susceptible to the suppressive effects of reactive bias, it is possible (some would say likely) that actual use rates are considerably higher. Indeed, recent workplace research by Cook and his associates comparing self-reports and bioassays indicated that sole reliance on self-reports can produce prevalence rates that are approximately two-thirds of those produced by self-reports combined with bioassays (Cook, Bernstein, & Andrews. 1997).

The many injurious effects of substance abuse, from productivity losses to negative health consequences, are well documented. Illicit drug use has been linked to increased absenteeism (Lehman et al., 1990; Normand, Salyards, & Mahoney, 1990; Rosenbaum et al., 1992), higher accident rates (Alleyne, Stuart, & Copes, 1991; CONSAD, 1989; Moody et al., 1990), more costly use of benefits (Winkler & Sheridan, 1989), and job withdrawal (Lehman & Simpson, 1992).

Although illicit drug and alcohol use rates are high among workers, illicit drug use is not highly prevalent in the actual workplace (Cornell/Smithers, 1992; MacDonald, Wells, & Fry, 1993; Normand, Lempert, & O'Brien, 1994). Most surveys reviewed by Normand et al. (1994) found that fewer than 10% of workers reported alcohol or other drug use on the job during the past 12 months. While most current workplace programs are aimed at on-the-job substance use/impairment, it is increasingly recognized that there are many workers who, though they may never use drugs at work, may experiment with drugs or drink heavily and come to the workplace "ragged and frayed" from their off-the-job drug- and alcohol-using behaviors (Shain, Suurvali, & Boutilier, 1986). From the perspective of primary prevention, as Ames has suggested, substance abuse problems in the workplace should be viewed as any alcohol or other drug use that has negative consequences for the employee or the employer. Drug use and drinking practices in the work force that put workers at risk for a variety of health and social problems, from family disruption to premature death (Ames, 1993; Lewis, 1990), are public-health problems that require attention. In this respect, the field seems to be moving from a concern with substance abuse in the workplace to substance abuse in the work force. Moreover, based on the data on age of first use, it seems that primary prevention efforts—which are currently targeted almost exclusively at children and adolescents—need to be applied to younger adult workers as well.

THEORETICAL PERSPECTIVES

The roots of workplace substance abuse theory are imbedded in, and still heavily influenced by, the occupational alcoholism literature of the past 40 years (Sonnenstuhl & Trice, 1987; Trice & Roman, 1972). This perspective was shaped largely by the disease model of alcoholism and by sociological traditions that emphasize sociocultural influences and view the work group and its norms as central determinants of substance use practices (Ames & Janes, 1987; Delaney & Ames, 1993; Sonnenstuhl, 1996). More recently, theorists of this school have broadened their conceptualizations to include a more diverse range of influences on worker substance abuse; but their research still focuses largely on alcohol as opposed to other drugs.

Sonnenstuhl and Trice (1987) identified five factors that can contribute to substance abuse problems in the workplace: workplace culture, social control, alienation, occupational stress, and the availability of drugs. Reduction of those work-related risks is seen as the most effective means of preventing substance abuse in the work force.

Ames (1993) focuses on the identification and management of environmental risk factors that lead to unhealthy work-related drinking patterns. She and her associates recently stated that "striking differences in alcohol consumption rates by job category indicate that the work environment may affect drinking norms and drinking patterns" and cited nine studies conducted in a variety of occupations and work environments that document the link between work environment and drinking patterns (Ames, Grube, & Moore, 2000, p. 203). Their latest study found significant differences in work-related drinking practices between two work environments with contrasting alcohol policies and the extent to which they were enforced. The results of analyses support their conceptual model—that social controls (enforced policies) influence drinking norms, which in turn influence work-related drinking. Interestingly, there were almost no differences between work sites in overall drinking, coming to work with a hangover, and heavy drinking.

Similarly, Mangione and his associates (Howland et al., 1996; Mangione et al., 1999) have been researching the effects of work-site variation on worker drinking. Based on data from 16 work sites and 6,540 workers, a recent study found that self-reported work performance problems (such as missed work, did less work, did poor-quality work) varied as a function of employee drinking practices, with moderate-to-heavy and heavy drinkers reporting more work performance problems than employees who drank less. In addition to the drinking measures, both self-reported use of marijuana and use of prescription drugs for anxiety and depression were independently and positively associated with work performance problems. Based on these findings Mangione and his associates recommend that, along with clear policy statements, organizations promote educational interventions for alcohol and drugs similar to those targeted to wellness topics, such as exercise and nutrition (Mangione et al., 1999).

The broadly inclusive "integrative" model of Walsh and her associates (1993) combines three groups of theories designed to guide research on problem drinking in the workplace. The theory groups include cultural theories, which hold that some workers become involved with problem-drinking subcultures because the workplace supports drinking on or off the job; job-design theories that emphasize ways in which dehumanizing or stressful jobs create or exacerbate problem drinking; and psychosocial theories, which assume that individuals predisposed to alcohol abuse select jobs in which their drinking goes undetected.

In contrast to models that emphasize the role of the social environment, Shain et al. (1986), Cook and Youngblood (1990), and Snow (1996) take a more health-oriented view, developing models rooted in psychological theories of individual behavior change (Abrams et al., 1986; Fishbein, 1983; Lazarus & Folkman, 1984). The effects of stress and specific interventions aimed at reducing stress occupy a particularly prominent role in these models. Although these researchers clearly place special emphasis on the role of individual psychology in the development of substance abuse problems in adult workers, their theoretical stance appears to be shaped, at least in part, by their desire to develop and test interventions that focus more specifically on individual behavior change.

The substance abuse prevention/health-behavior model developed by Cook and Youngblood (1990) draws on existing social–cognitive and health-behavior theories, including Shain's research, the work of Rosenstock, Strecher, and Becker (1988) on self-efficacy, the research of Abrams et al. (1986) on the role of social support in health-behavior change, and Cook's (1985) model of healthful alternatives to substance abuse. The model emphasizes (1) raising awareness of the risks of substance abuse and the benefits of healthful behaviors, (2) increasing motivation for avoiding substance abuse and embracing healthful practices (by boosting self-efficacy—social supports, for example), and (3) transmitting skills, such as drink refusal, that are crucial to successfully moving toward healthful practices and away from substance abuse.

Recently, Cook and his associates revised and expanded their model of workplace substance abuse prevention to reflect the findings from field tests of their workplace programs (Cook, Back, & Trudeau, 1996a,b) as well as other, broader theoretical perspectives from the literature (e.g., Ames, 1993; Vicary, 1994). The revised model (shown in Figure 8.1) retains most of the chief elements of the original Cook and Youngblood model: the social–cognitive framework, the focus on raising awareness, motivation, and skills with respect to health and substance use; and the view that avoidance of substance abuse occurs as healthful practices provide rewards and as the social environment (workplace and community) provides support for such behavior. It continues to include primary prevention efforts and to accommodate the mainstream of workers,

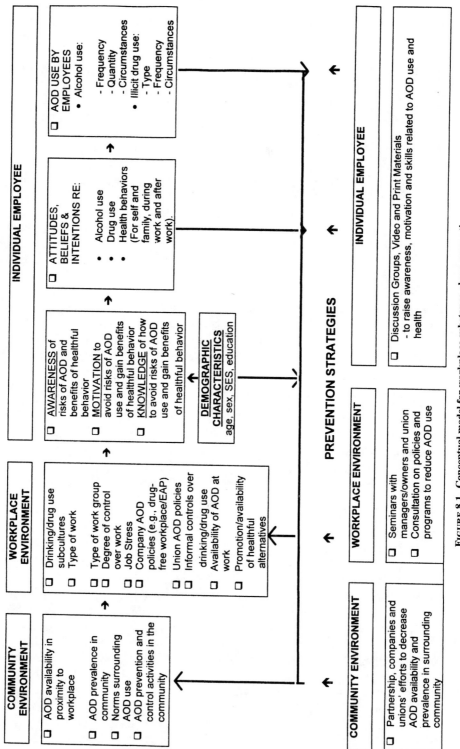

FIGURE 8.1. Conceptual model for workplace substance abuse prevention.

not just those with advanced substance abuse problems. However, in the revised model, the role of the social environment in fostering substance abuse or healthful behavior is expanded and more explicitly identified. The current model recognizes that the use of alcohol and other drugs is substantially shaped by powerful forces in the community and by the characteristics of the workplace, especially the presence of drinking and drug use subcultures, as documented by Ames (1993) and Sonnenstuhl (1996). Similarly, the existence of a variety of prevention and deterrence strategies in the community and the workplace, from media campaigns to drug testing, can potentially have a significant impact on the alcohol and other drug practices of working adults (Center for Substance Abuse Prevention; 1994; Cook et al., 1996a; Roman & Blum, 1996). The prevention strategies shown in the lower portion of the framework are examples of the types of interventions that research has indicated as promising for reducing substance abuse in the workforce (e.g., Cook et al., 1996b; Sonnenstuhl, 1996). The evidence supporting the efficacy of these strategies is, however, uneven (see following), and their presence in the model is designed mainly to encourage further research rather than serve as an endorsement of their effectiveness. In its current form, the model also reflects the view that individuals typically do not abruptly engage in major changes in substance use or health practices but instead proceed through stages and cycles of change, as indicated by the research of Prochaska, DiClemente, and Norcross (1992). From this perspective, changes in motivations and intentions can be important precursors of reductions in drinking and drug use; programs that move individuals toward contemplating specific substance use or health practices are seen as accomplishing important achievements, especially in the short term. Another significant addition to the model is the feedback loop. Although the main causal flow is from left to right (from community to workplace to individual), the reverse can also occur. As individual workers begin changing their attitudes and practices, they will begin to change the norms and practices of their community and their workplace.

PROGRAMS, PRACTICES, AND DATA

To date, the primary vehicles for addressing substance abuse in the work force have been EAPs and drug testing. Very few organizations currently engage in explicit prevention education programs aimed at the mainstream of workers, and such interventions have only recently gained the attention of researchers.

Employee Assistance Programs

EAPs began appearing in organizations in increasing numbers in the 1970s; and by the mid-1980s they had become commonplace throughout industry. By 1991, Blum estimated that 45% of the entire U.S. work force was covered by EAPs. These programs offer identification, assessment, referral, and follow-up procedures to employees who have drug or alcohol problems, as well as to those with a variety of other problems. They can serve an important prevention function by addressing problems in their early stages before they progress to full-blown chemical dependency (Roman, 1990). However, the focus of EAPs remains on the tertiary end of the prevention continuum, seeking to ensure that employees with serious alcohol problems receive the treatment they need. Only in the "megabrush" concept of Erfurt, Foote, and Heirich (1992), in which EAPs are explicitly integrated with wellness functions—a rarity in practice—do EAPs embrace prevention as a central activity.

Sonnenstuhl (1996) reports that EAPs have been "relatively successful" at helping alcoholic employees gain sobriety, with recovery rates of 70% or better. However, he also notes that EAPs have had "limited" success at deterring harmful drinking practices (such as on-the-job drinking) in some occupations.

Roman and Blum (1996) conducted a review of the impact of work-site interventions (mostly EAPS and the like) on health and behavioral outcomes. After reviewing 24 studies from the peer review literature, they concluded that there was evidence to support the general efficacy of interventions that are fashioned after the EAP model in "rehabilitating employees with alcohol problems," but that beyond this generalization, the research literature offered very little insight into "what works." Moreover, the authors described the methodological quality of these collective studies as "weak," characterized by problems of self-selection and lack of randomized designs. Interestingly, nearly all of the studies reviewed focused on the effectiveness with which programs identified and treated employees with alcohol problems; only two of the interventions were aimed at preventing alcohol problems in the general work force.

There is little doubt that EAPS provide a useful function, particularly with respect to the identification and referral of alcohol- and drug-dependent employees. It is also likely that they operate as a generalized, diffuse force for the prevention of substance abuse, raising awareness, and nudging norms toward more responsible drinking. However, it is the rare EAP that actively pursues genuine prevention strategies with the mainstream of workers—strategies designed to alter drinking practices before they become harmful, halt experimentation with illicit drugs before dependence develops, or help employees keep their children off drugs. Such primary and secondary prevention targets seem to be off the radar screen of virtually all EAPS.

Drug Testing Programs

There are three types of workplace drug testing programs: (1) pre-employment testing of job applicants (by far the most prevalent type), (2) for-cause testing of employees (such as after an accident), and (3) random testing of employees (Normand et al., 1994). Although concerns continue about the accuracy of drug testing, the standard urinalysis technique of screening urine specimens with relatively inexpensive radioimmunoassays and confirming positives with the more expensive and highly accurate gas chromatography/mass spectrometry is generally considered highly reliable, particularly when conducted by certified laboratories in the context of proper chain-of-custody procedures. During the past decade, these types of drug testing programs have become increasingly commonplace in both government and industry. A 1995 survey conducted by the American Management Association (AMA) revealed that nearly 80% of surveyed firms test employees for drugs (AMA, 1995). Walsh (1995) estimated that approximately 30 million American workers will be tested annually for illicit drug use. There are numerous reasons for the explosive growth in workplace drug testing, including its presumed impact on safety, productivity, and employer costs. However, perhaps the main impetus for the widespread adoption of drug testing was the passage in 1988 of the federal Drug-Free Workplace Act and the subsequent promotion by the federal government of drug testing in the workplace.

Although a variety of studies have attempted to assess the impact of drug testing on the work force, evidence of its preventive effects are less clear cut than generally assumed. Indeed, when Normand and his associates reviewed the research on the topic, they concluded that "Despite beliefs to the contrary, the preventive effects of drug testing programs have never been adequately demonstrated" (Normand et al., 1994). The authors admit that there are "some suggestive data that allude to the deterrent effect of pre-employment testing," but they found no "conclusive scientific evidence" of such effects. A close examination of these studies (e.g., Parish, 1989; Blank & Fenton, 1989) and those from the military (e.g., Bray et al., 1991) clearly support their conclusion: While the evidence for the impact of drug testing is consistent and often seemingly dramatic, properly controlled studies have yet to be conducted.

In a recent review of drug testing, Trice and Steele (1995) attributed the popularity of drug testing to a combination of promotion by the federal government, media hype of the "drug epidemic" (at a time when drug abuse was clearly declining), and "corporate imitation and ritual." These authors join Normand in concluding that the evidence supporting the deterrent effects of drug testing is scientifically weak. As an example, they describe the U.S. Navy experience with drug testing, often cited as a dramatic demonstration of drug testing's deterrence effectiveness. When the drug testing program began in the Navy in 1981, nearly half of the enlisted personnel were found positive; by 1984, the positive rate was below 5%. The inference that the sharp decrease was caused by drug testing alone is, however, scientifically insupportable since the Navy program included a wide variety of anti-drug actions in addition to drug testing. Although lamenting the rather sweeping and uncritical acceptance of drug testing, Trice and Steele acknowledge that drug testing can support the mission of EAPs by (1) sensitizing organizations to the drug abuse issue, (2) providing objective corroboration of a supervisor's suspicion of drug use, and (3) promoting referrals to the EAP.

The evidence in support of the deterrent effects of drug testing, though not scientific, is not without its persuasive power. For example, Walsh (1995) points out that data from the NHSDA show that as drug testing became prevalent in the workplace (along with many other drug-free workplace programs) between 1985 and 1990, the number of full-time workers who were current users of illegal drugs was reduced by one-half. Walsh also cites the example of the 28% decrease in accidents in the railroad industry from 1987, when the drug testing requirements went into effect, to 1993. More significantly, in 1987, twenty-one percent of railroad accidents involved workers who tested positive for drug use; by 1993 that number had dropped to 5% (Walsh, 1995). Obviously, there are myriad factors besides drug testing to which the reductions may be attributed, from altered management policies to secular trends in drug use. That is why there is a great need for rigorously conducted studies. (Indeed, the central thrust of Walsh's paper is the need for research on the issue.) But there seems little question that the preventive power of drug testing is, at the very least, a hypothesis in urgent need of testing. Walsh and his associates are currently conducting a research project that will involve the systematic manipulation of drug testing frequency, offering the appealing possibility that some hard evidence of drug testing's deterrence power will be in hand in the near future (personal communication).

Health Promotion Approaches

Health promotion has been defined as "the science and art of helping people change their lifestyle to move toward a state of optimal health" (O'Donnell & Harris, 1994). Health promotion programs are designed to raise awareness and change behavior in a variety of lifestyle areas—such as improving diet, reducing stress, and increasing exercise. With the exception of smoking cessation activities, substance abuse topics have been virtually nonexistent in most workplace health promotion programs. In the following section, we will describe very briefly the status of workplace smoking-cessation activities, then discuss health-promotion-based approaches to the prevention of alcohol and illicit drug abuse.

Workplace smoking control programs typically have three major elements: smoking policies and restrictions, smoking-cessation programs, and incentives (Sofian et al., 1994). The Community Intervention Trial for Smoking Cessation found a substantial need to increase the level of work-site smoking-cessation activities (Glasgow et al., 1996). Effective smoking-cessation programs recognize that smokers move in distinct stages in their efforts to stop smoking (DiClemente et al.,

1991). Group-based classroom programs typify company smoking-cessation offerings (Sofian et al., 1994). These group-based approaches are generally not consonant with the need to tailor messages to stage-of-change; they are expensive and dependent upon the leadership of the group. Self-administered programs are considered a promising means of delivering smoking cessation because of their ability to reach a broad audience at relatively low cost (Glynn, Boyd, & Gruman, 1990). The Working Well Trial involving 111 work sites and a sophisticated theoretical framework (including social learning theory and stage-of-change theory) sought to improve a variety of behaviors associated with reducing cancer risk—including tobacco use. Sorensen and her colleagues found only a 1% reduction in smoking prevalence; and Jeffrey and his associates, in a study of a work-site health promotion program, found a 4% reduction in smoking prevalence after 2 years (Jeffery et al., 1993). Later studies, however, focusing exclusively on smoking interventions in the workplace, found a 12% reduction in smoking rates after 6 months (Sorensen, Lando, & Pechacek, 1993).

Over the years several researchers have suggested that health promotion programs could be effective in preventing and reducing substance abuse, either indirectly, through the adoption of more healthful practices that would tend to supplant substance abuse, or directly, by including substance-abuse prevention components explicitly in such programs—or both. Among the first researchers of record to test this approach in the workplace were Shain and his associates (Shain et al., 1986), who found that after workers attended a 15-hour course in stress management, moderate drinkers showed significant decreases in alcohol consumption (although heavy drinkers maintained their consumption levels). No such decreases were found in the comparison group. In a related study, Shehadeh and Shain (1990) surveyed transportation workers in Ontario and found that 15 to 20% of drinking workers were concerned about their alcohol consumption and interested in a variety of health topics; such as exercise, nutrition, stress management, and weight loss. The "concerned heavy drinker" that emerged from this survey was a male, blue-collar smoker who was overweight—precisely the person most in need of health improvement. These data seemed to suggest that health promotion programs may be able to address substance abuse issues in the context of general health promotion topics.

In another survey-based study of the relationship between wellness and substance use, Bennett and Lehman (1997) administered an organizational wellness scale designed to assess employee perceptions of the "health" of their work environment, along with a comprehensive measure of personal substance use, to 780 employees from a municipal organization. Workers with high scores on the organizational wellness scale reported less personal use of alcohol and drugs (legal and illicit) than those with low scores. Although the causal dynamics are unclear, these findings suggest that organizational dysfunction is associated with worker substance use.

Erfurt and his associates tested the effectiveness of four program models in reducing obesity, smoking, and high blood pressure over a 3-year period (Erfurt et al., 1992). One model was a fitness center; the other three models were various combinations of health education, outreach, and counseling. At sites with personal outreach and counseling, there was considerable impact in all three areas. Without such components there was virtually no impact.

Similar findings on the positive impact of follow-up contact and support have been reported in other studies (e.g., Gomel et al., 1993), and a recent review of studies of multicomponent work-site health promotion programs concluded that providing opportunities for individual risk reduction counseling for high-risk employees within a comprehensive program may be the critical component of such programs (Heaney & Goetzel, 1997). The Heaney and Goetzel review included 36 studies, only 5 of which included alcohol use as a targeted outcome (none included illicit drug use). Interestingly, all 5 studies reported some impact on alcohol use, typically on average weekly consumption.

Heirich and Sieck recently tested the effectiveness of a cardiovascular wellness program as a route to preventing alcohol abuse in the work force (Heirich & Sieck, 2000). Based on a social-learning model, their approach emphasizes raising the salience of alcohol abuse as a potential health risk, developing one's confidence to make successful behavior changes, providing social support for making the changes, and providing information on alternative health behaviors. They assessed the effectiveness of a cardiovascular risk reduction education program that included unsafe drinking as a cardiovascular risk, comparing a classroom-based approach with indivi-dualized proactive follow-up counseling. In a work site of 4,000 employees, 2,000 employees were recruited for initial screening, then randomly assigned to the proactive counseling or health education classes. One-half of this sample were followed up for rescreening. At rescreening, 43% of the employees who had been identified as at-risk drinkers were either not drinking or had reduced their consumption to safe levels. In addition, overall health risks improved among all study groups. The proactive counseling intervention was more effective than health education classes in reducing the proportion of heavy drinkers (and smokers) from initial screening to rescreening. The authors attribute much of the success of the counseling approach to the highly visible, proactive outreach of the program, as well as to the individualized nature of the counseling. The authors also point out that this type of intervention is labor intensive and costly, although they believe it to be more cost effective (as well as more effective) than health education classes.

For the past several years, Snow and Kline have been testing the effects of preventive inter-ventions in the workplace on a variety of psychiatric outcomes, focusing mainly on abilities to cope with stress, psychological outcomes (anxiety, depression, and somatic complaints), as well as alcohol and tobacco use (Kline & Snow, 1994; Snow & Kline, 1995). Their approach is based on stress and coping theories (e.g., Lazarus & Folkman, 1984; Pearlin & Schooler, 1978) and has typically taken the form of 10 to 15 hour-long training sessions designed to teach workers a wide range of adaptive strategies for coping with stress. Although the sessions have covered a wide range of stress coping topics and strategies, they have rarely explicitly addressed substance abuse issues. Until recently their subject samples have been mainly female workers. Their research has been marked by methodological strengths, including careful conceptualization and measurement, randomized designs, attrition analysis, and long-term follow-ups (6 months and 22 months). Re-sults have generally been positive, showing an impact on some stress coping skills, psychological symptoms, and tobacco and alcohol use (Kline & Snow, 1994; Snow & Kline, 1995). Snow re-cently tested his coping skills intervention approach on a sample of 468 male and female workers from three company sites, randomly assigned to a coping skills intervention condition or a control group and assessed at four points in time (although only pretest, post-test, and 6-month results are currently available). Effects were largely concentrated in the coping measures, although the intervention impact on alcohol (number of drinks per month) was significant at post-test and, for a subsample of higher alcohol users only, at 6 months. This program of research has shown rather consistently that interventions that teach workers skills for coping with stress can have an impact on alcohol and tobacco use.

Kishuk and her associates (1994) conducted one of the rare tests of a workplace intervention aimed specifically at promoting "healthy alcohol consumption." A sample of mostly male, blue-collar workers ($n = 268$) were randomly assigned to the alcohol prevention sessions, nutrition ses-sions, or a control condition. The alcohol prevention program was based on cognitive–behavioral approaches, adapted for "normal drinkers." Topics included controlled consumption techniques, drink refusal skills, and stress management. Among the eight measures of alcohol knowledge, attitudes, and consumption gathered at pretest and post-test, two measures were significantly dif-ferent between the alcohol program group and the other two groups: The alcohol group showed more socially responsible attitudes and lower number of drinks per week.

During the past decade, Cook and his associates conducted a series of studies testing approaches to substance abuse prevention in the workplace. The approaches were based on the health-promotion-oriented conceptual model developed by Cook and Youngblood (1990; described previously) and typically involved multimedia presentations (video, print, and lecture–discussion) to small groups of workers. Specially developed videos were central to this approach, offering unique capabilities for behavioral modeling, boosting self-efficacy, and transmitting specific skills. For example, opportunities for behavioral modeling are provided through the use of carefully scripted, engaging dramatic vignettes that show people successfully addressing the challenges of reducing their alcohol consumption; viewer self-efficacy is boosted by video segments that present individuals ("real people") describing how they made improvements in their lifestyle. In this approach, the film and video arts—including casting, music, graphics, and script development—are harnessed to bring about behavior change. In addition to being ideally suited to the implementation of social–cognitive learning techniques, film and video can be attractive and engaging, helping make health promotion and substance abuse prevention a positive, interesting experience for the participant.

In the first field test of this model, 371 employees of a manufacturing facility in the northeast United States were randomly assigned to a health promotion/substance abuse prevention program (HP/SAP) or to a control condition (Cook et al., 1996a). The HP/SAP program consisted of three 1-hour sessions delivered by a trainer using video and print materials interweaving health promotion concepts and strategies (such as techniques and rewards of a healthy lifestyle and effective approaches to behavior change) with techniques for examining and controlling alcohol consumption and avoiding illicit drug use. Significant differences were found between the HP/SAP and the control groups on three of the four measures of health: health and work control, measures of internal control, and health self-efficacy. The HP/SAP group showed a significant increase in "desire to reduce drinking" (a single item), but there were no effects on alcohol consumption. Only 4% of the sample reported any drug use in the past 30 days at pretest, so these data were not further analyzed. These results indicated that when substance abuse prevention materials are integrated with health promotion materials, desired effects on health attitudes and beliefs can be achieved. However, there seemed to be virtually no impact on alcohol and other drug use.

In a second field test of their workplace substance abuse prevention approach, Cook and associates (1996b) presented an alcohol prevention program in a health promotion framework; but this time greater emphasis was placed on the hazards of alcohol abuse and strategies for reducing alcohol use. Somewhat less emphasis was placed on health promotion strategies per se. In a quasiexperimental pretest/post-test design, employees from two sites of a medium-sized printing company were invited to participate in an alcohol prevention program. Initial questionnaires were administered to 200 employees, but only 108 (38 program participants and 70 comparison-group subjects) completed the post-test questionnaire. Program effects were demonstrated on alcohol consumption (number of drinking days in past month and number of days having five or more drinks), motivation to reduce consumption, and problem consequences of drinking. No effects were found on health beliefs or self-efficacy to reduce drinking. The findings were qualified by self-selection, but nonetheless suggested that alcohol consumption can be reduced among workers who participate in this kind of program. It seems clear, however, that any workplace program identifiable as "alcohol prevention" was likely to be sparsely attended.

In their most recent field test, Cook and his associates tested a "third way" to integrate health promotion and substance abuse prevention (Cook et al., in press). In this approach, substance abuse prevention messages and materials are inserted into popular health promotion offerings. Workers at a property casualty insurance company in the southeast United States were invited to participate in one of two health promotion programs—a stress-management program or a nutrition-/weight-management program (called "Healthy Eating"). In each program, participants ($n = 416$) were randomly assigned to a health-promotion-only condition or a condition in which they received substance abuse prevention materials and messages along with the health promotion program. The substance abuse prevention materials (videos and print materials) were specially developed for relevance to either stress management or healthy eating. Both programs were delivered in three group sessions of approximately 45 minutes.

Participants were assessed on a self-administered questionnaire during private interviews at three points in time (pretest, initial post-test, and 8 months later). The questionnaire administered to all subjects contained measures of alcohol and other drug use, drinking and drug use intentions, connections between health and substance use, health and job control, and risks of alcohol and drug use. For participants in the stress management program, the questionnaire also contained five measures of stress: work pressures, personal pressures, symptoms of distress and stress, and stress-relief strategies (a scale that measured the extent to which the respondent used nondrug means to gain relief from stress). For participants in the healthy-eating program, the questionnaire also included five other measures: eating practices, attitudes toward healthy eating, nutritional facts, exercise practices, and exercise self-efficacy.

Two major hypotheses were central to the research: (1) participants will display positive changes in measures of stress and healthy eating, regardless of the presence or absence of the substance abuse prevention component; and (2) participants in the condition that included the substance abuse prevention component will exhibit positive changes in substance abuse measures, but participants in the condition without the substance abuse prevention component will not exhibit such changes. Preliminary results indicate that hypothesis No. 1 has been resoundingly confirmed, while hypothesis No. 2 was only partly confirmed.

On all five measures of stress and all five measures of healthy eating, significant positive changes occurred for all participants (experimental and control subjects) from pretest to post-test, including use of nondrug means to relieve stress. All the changes in the stress measures held up through the second post-test, while changes on healthy-eating measures were maintained on three of the five measures. As hypothesized, there were virtually no differences between experimental and control groups on the stress and healthy-eating measures. Participants showed similar, significant improvement regardless of the presence of the substance abuse prevention material.

On measures of substance abuse, the stress management participants showed significant improvement at initial post-test on the three attitude/perceptions measures, regardless of whether they were in the experimental or the control group. Similarly, both experimental and control groups in the stress management program showed significant decreases in alcohol and other drug use from pretest to post-test. Among participants who were drinkers, significantly more reduced the number of drinking days and the number of drinks in the past 30 days than increased or stayed the same. Moreover, among the 16 stress-management participants who reported using illicit drugs at pretest, 11 reported no use at the first post-test, a significant decrease (McNemar test significant at .02). In some contrast, the healthy-eating participants in the experimental group showed improvement on two of the three attitude/perceptions measures, improvements that held through second post-test; the control group showed no such improvements. Neither experimental nor control participants in the healthy-eating program exhibited significant reductions in their consumption of alcohol or other drugs. These findings indicate that workers will change important attitudes, perceptions, and practices regarding substance abuse if they are exposed to stress management sessions—regardless of whether explicit substance-abuse prevention materials are presented to them. Participants in healthy-eating sessions (and perhaps other health promotion offerings) will also change substance abuse attitudes and perceptions, but only if they receive the substance-abuse prevention materials.

Improvements in substance use attitudes and behavior seemed to occur as a result of learning healthful stress management practices as much as—perhaps more than—exposure to explicit substance-abuse prevention materials, findings that are congruent with those of Snow and his associates (described previously).

Two current studies by Cook and his associates are exploring further the effects of health-oriented interventions. In one study four groups of construction workers—an occupational group that typically displays high levels of substance abuse—were randomly assigned either to a stress management program with substance abuse prevention materials or to one without, after having been assessed through a self-administered questionnaire and bioassays (hair and urine tests). This study should shed further light on the impact of stress management and explicit substance abuse prevention materials on the drinking and drug use practices of a high-prevalence occupational group.

The second study currently being conducted by the author and his associates is part of a larger program sponsored by the Center for Substance Abuse Prevention, involving eight other grantees in an exploration of the broad impact of substance abuse prevention interventions in the context of workplace managed care. How can substance abuse prevention and other behavioral health strategies be efficiently implemented in the workplace, and what are their effects on worker health and medical claims? These and related questions are being addressed in the course of this multiyear study.

CONCLUSION

Data on the prevalence of substance abuse in the work force indicate that although the use of illicit drugs has declined since 1985, it has not changed significantly in the past several years; and both illicit drug use and heavy drinking by members of the American work force remain disturbingly high, particularly among young males in blue-collar occupations. Moreover, recent methodological studies of prevalence assessment indicate that estimates based solely on self-reports (as are most current estimates) may substantially underestimate the level of drug use in the work force and that more accurate (and higher) estimates may be obtained by combining self-reports with bioassays, particularly urinalysis. In addition, data on the mean age of first use of alcohol and illicit drugs indicate that the initial use of some illicit drugs does not occur for many workers until after they have joined the work force.

An examination of the major theoretical perspectives on substance abuse in the workplace shows that the theories tend to cluster into two types: sociocultural theories that emphasize the influence of the work group and work environment on drug use and more psychological frameworks that place greater emphasis on individual variables. The former theories have been associated with research that sought mainly to identify correlates of alcohol abuse in the work force; the latter have been used to guide research on preventive interventions in the workplace. Cook's recent conceptual model, although more closely identified with the psychological view, is an example of a theoretical framework designed to accommodate both perspectives.

A review of current interventions and programs designed to prevent substance abuse points to three types of preventive approaches: drug testing, EAPs, and health-oriented preventive interventions. Drug testing appears to offer considerable promise as a preventive/deterrent technique; but rigorous, well-designed evaluations of drug testing have yet to be conducted.

The findings from a recent review of the impact of EAPs indicated that although the evidence supports EAPs as having beneficial effects, the research has been marked by weak designs and other methodological flaws. Moreover, it seems clear that EAPs seldom engage in primary prevention activities aimed at the broad mainstream of workers. However, this focus may be entirely appropriate. Perhaps EAPs should continue to concentrate on identifying and assisting seriously troubled employees, but it appears that a potentially useful force for prevention is being underutilized.

Some of the more promising prevention approaches are the health-oriented preventive interventions that Snow, Kishuk, Cook, Heirich, and others have been testing in the workplace. Based on social–cognitive learning theories, these interventions are being tested and shaped in a series of rigorous field experiments (randomized designs are typical) in a variety of worksites. Findings to date indicate that such interventions can alter drinking and (perhaps) drug use practices, as well as important mediator variables, such as perceived risk of alcohol and drug use. These studies represent a refreshing change from the decades of survey-based research on the correlates of alcohol and drug use. Although survey-based studies have been—and will continue to be—necessary and illuminating forms of investigation, rigorous field tests of preventive interventions aimed at the mainstream of workers offer the promise of enhancing both the science and the practice of workplace drug abuse prevention.

REFERENCES

Abrams, D. B., Elder, J. P., Carleton, R. A., Lasater, T. M., & Artz, L. M. (1986). Social learning principles for organizational health promotion: An integrated approach. In M. F. Cataldo & T. J. Coates (Eds.), *Health and industry: A behavioral medicine perspective.* New York: Wiley.

Alleyne, B. C., Stuart, P., & Copes, R. (1991). Alcohol and other drug use in occupational facilities. *Journal of Occupational Medicine, 3,* 496–500.

American Management Association (1995). *The 1995 AMA Survey: Workplace drug testing and drug abuse policies.* New York: AMA.

Ames, G. M. (1993). Research and strategies for the primary prevention of workplace alcohol problems. *Alcohol, Health and Research World 17*(1), 19–27.

Ames, G., Grube, J. W., & Moore, R. S. (2000). Social control and workplace drinking norms: A comparison of two organizational studies. *Journal of Studies on Alcohol, 61,* 203–219.

Ames, G. M., & Janes, C. R., (1987). Heavy and problem drinking in an American blue-collar population. *Social Sciences and Medicine, 25,* 949–960.

Bennett, J. B., & Lehman, W. E. (1997). Employee views of organizational wellness and the EAP: Influence on substance use, drinking climates, and policy attitudes. *Employee Assistance Quarterly, 13*(1), 55–71.

Blank, D. L., and Fenton, J. W., (1989). Early employment testing for marijuana: demo-graphic and employees retention patterns. In S. W. Gust, & J. M., Walsh (Eds.), *Drugs in the workplace: Research and evaluation data.* Rockville, MD: NIDA Research Monograph No. 91, National Institute on Drug Abuse.

Bray, R. M., Kroutil, L. A., Luckey, J. W., Wheeless, S. C., Iannacchoine, V. G., Anderson, D. W., Marsden, M. E., & Dunteman, G. H. (1991). *Worldwide survey of substance abuse and health behaviors among military personnel.* Research Triangle Park, NC: Research Triangle Institute, Research Triangle Institute.

Center for Substance Abuse Prevention (1994). National evaluation of the Community Partnership Demonstration Program: Third annual report, 1993. Washington, DC: U.S. Department of Health and Human Services, Public Health Service.

CONSAD Corporation (1989). Analysis of occupational substance use and workplace safety: Final report. Pittsburgh, PA: CONSAD Research Corporation.

Cook, R. F. (1985). The alternatives approach revisited: A bio-psychological model and guidelines for application. *International Journal of the Addictions, 20*(a), 1399–1419.

Cook, R. F., & Back, A. (Executive Producers) (1993). *Working people: Decisions about drinking.* Washington, DC: ISA Associates, Inc.

Cook, R. F., Back, A. S., & Trudeau, J. (1996a). Substance abuse prevention in the workplace: Recent findings and an expanded conceptual model. *The Journal of Primary Prevention, 16*(3), 319–338.

Cook, R. F., Back, A. S., & Trudeau, J. (1996b). Preventing alcohol use problems among blue-collar workers: A field test of the Working People program. *Substance Use & Misuse, 31*(3), 255–275.

Cook, R. F., Back, A. S., Trudeau, J. V., & McPherson, T. (in press). Integrating substance abuse prevention into health promotion programs in the workplace. In J. Bennett & W. Lehman (Eds.), *Beyond drug testing: Innovative approaches to dealing with employee substance abuse.* Washington: APA Books.

Cook, R. F., Bernstein, A. D., & Andrews, C. M. (1997). Assessing drug use in the workplace: A comparison of self-report, urinalysis and hair analysis. In L. Harrison & A. Hughes (Eds.), *The validity of self-reported drug use: Improving the accuracy of survey estimates.* Washington, DC: NIDA Research Monograph 167, NIH Pub. No. 96-4147.

Cook, R. F., & Youngblood, A. (1990). Preventing substance abuse as an integral part of worksite health promotion. *Occupational Medicine: State of the Art Reviews, 5*(4), 725–738.

Cornell/Smithers (1992). *Report on workplace substance abuse policy.* Ithaca, NY: Smithers Institute, Cornell University.

Delaney, W., & Ames, G. (1993). Shop steward handling on alcohol-related problems. *Addiction, 88,* 1205–1214.

DiClemente, C. C., Prochaska, J. O., Fairhurst, S. K., Velicer, W. F., Velasquez, M. M., & Rossi, J. S. (1991). The process of smoking cessation: An analysis of precontemplation, contemplation, and preparation stages of change. *Journal of Consulting Clinical Psychology, 59,* 295–304.

Erfurt, J. C., Foote, A., & Heirich, M. A. (1992). Integrating employee assistance and wellness: Current and future core technologies of a megabrush program. *Journal of Employee Assistance Research, 1*(1), 1–31.

Fishbein, M. (1983). Factors influencing health behaviors: An analysis based on a theory of reasoned action. In R. Landry (Ed.), *Health risk estimation, risk reduction and health promotion.* Papers presented at the 18th Annual Meeting of the Society of Prospective Medicine, Quebec City, Oct. 20–23, 1982. Ottawa: Canadian Public Health Association.

Glasgow, R. E., Sorensen, G., Giffen, C., Shipley, R. H., Corbett, K., & Lynn, W. (1996). Promoting worksite smoking control policies and actions: The Community Intervention Trial for Smoking Cessation (COMMIT) experience. *Preventive Medicine, 25,* 186–194.

Glynn, T., Boyd, G., & Gruman, J. (1990). Essential elements of self-help/minimal intervention strategies for smoking cessation. *Health Education Quarterly, 17,* 329–345.

Gomel, M., Oldenburg, B., Simpson, J., & Owen, N. (1993). Worksite cardiovascular risk reduction: A randomized trial of health risk assessment, education, counseling, and incentives. *American Journal of Public Health, 87*(9), 1231–1238.

Heaney, C., & Goetzel, R. (1997). A review of health-related outcomes of multi-component worksite health promotion programs. *American Journal of Health Promotion, 11*(4), 290–307.

Heather, N. (1989). Brief intervention strategies. In R. Hester & W. Miller (Eds.), *Handbook of alcoholism treatment approaches: Effective alternatives* (pp. 93–116). New York: Pergamon Press.

Heirich, M., & Seick, C. J. (2000). Worksite cardiovascular wellness programs as a route to substance abuse prevention. *Journal of Occupational and Environmental Medicine, 42,* 47–56.

Hoffman, J. P., Larrison, C., & Sanderson, A. (1997). *An analysis of worker drug use and workplace policies and programs.* Rockville, MD: SAMHSA, Office of Applied Studies.

Howland, J., Mangione, T., Kuhlthan, K., Bell, N., Heeren, T., Lee, M., & Levine, S. (1996). Worksite variation in managerial drinking. *Addiction, 91*(7), 1007–1017.

Jeffery, R. W., Forster, J. L., French, S., Kelder, S. A., Lando, H., McGovern, P., Jacobs. D., & Baxter, J. (1993). Healthy Worker Project: A work site intervention for weight control and smoking cessation. *American Journal of Public Health, 83,* 395–401.

Kishuk, N., Peters, C., Towers, A., Sylvester, M., Bourgault, C., & Richard, L. (1994). Formative and effectiveness evaluation of a worksite program promoting healthy alcohol consumption. *American Journal of Health Promotion, 8*(5), 353–362.

Kline, M., & Snow, D. (1994). Effects of a worksite coping skills intervention on the stress, social support and health outcomes of working mothers. *Journal of Primary Prevention, 15*(2), 105–121.

Lehman, W. E. K., Holcom, M. L., & Simpson, D. D. (1990). *Employee health and performance in the workplace: A survey of municipal employees of a large southwest city.* Unpublished manuscript, Institute of Behavioral Research, Texas Christian University, Fort Worth.

Lehman, W., & Simpson, D. (1992). Employee substance use and on-the-job behaviors. *Journal of Applied Psychology, 77,* 309–321.

Lazarus, R. S., & Folkman, S. (1984). *Stress, appraisal, and coping.* New York: Springer.

Lewis, R. J. (1990). Day-night patterns in workplace accidental deaths: Role of alcohol abuse as a contributing factor. In *Chronobiology: Its Role in Clinical Medicine, General Biology and Agriculture. Part B. Progress in Clinical and Biological Research* (pp. 327–335). New York: Liss.

MacDonald, S., Wells, S., & Fry, R. (1993). The limitations of drug screening in the workplace. *International Labor Review 132*(1), 95–113.

Mangione, T. W., Howland, J., Amick, B., Cote, J., Lee, M., Bell, N., & Levine, S. (1999). Employee drinking practices and work performance. *Journal of Studies on Alcohol, 60,* 261–270.

Moody, D. E., Crouch, D. J., Andrenyak, D. M., Smith, R. P., Wilkins, D. G., Hoffman, A. M., & Rollins, D. E. (1990). Mandatory post accident drug and alcohol testing for the Federal Railroad Administration (FRA). In S. W. Gust & J. M. Walsh (Eds.), *Drugs in the workplace: Research and evaluation Data Vol. II* (NIDA Research Monograph No. 100, pp. 79–96). Rockville, MD: National Institute on Drug Abuse.

Normand, J., Lempert, R. O., & O'Brien, C. P. (Eds., 1994). *Under the influence? Drugs and the American work force.* National Research Council/Institute of Medicine. Washington, DC: National Academy Press.

Normand, J., Salyards, S., & Mahoney, J. J. (1990). An evaluation of pre-employment drug testing. *Journal of Applied Psychology, 75,* 629–639.

O'Donnell, M. P., & Harris, J. S. (1994). *Health promotion in the workplace.* Albany, NY: Delmore Publishers.

Parish, D. C. (1989). Relation of the pre-employment drug testing result to employment status: A one-year follow-up, *J. Gen. Med., 4,* 44.

Pearlin, L. I., & Schooler, C. (1978). The structure of coping. *Journal of Health and Social Behavior, 19,* 2–21.

Prochaska, J. O., DiClemente, C. C., & Norcross, J. C. (1992). In search of how people change: Applications to addictive behaviors. *American Psychologist, 47*(9), 1102–1114.

Rice, D. P., Kelman, S., Miller, L. S., & Dunmeyer, S. (1990). *The economic costs of alcohol and drug abuse and mental illness: 1985.* San Francisco: University of California, Institute for Health and Aging.

Roman, P. M. (1990). The salience of alcohol problems in the work setting: Introduction and overview. In P. M. Roman, *Alcohol problem intervention in the workplace: Employee assistance programs and strategic alternatives* (pp. 1–16). New York: Quorum Books.

Roman, P., & Blum, T. (1996). Alcohol: A review of the impact of worksite interventions on health and behavioral outcomes. *American Journal of Health Promotion, 11*(2), 136–149.

Rosenbaum, A. L., Lehman, W. E. K., Olson, K. E., & Holcom, M. L. (1992). *Prevalence of substance use and its association with performance among municipal workers in a southwestern city.* Unpublished manuscript. Institute of Behavioral Research. Texas Christian University, Fort Worth.

Rosenstock, I. M., Strecher, V. J., & Becker, M. H. (Summer, 1988). Social learning theory and the health belief model. *Health Education Quarterly, 15*(2).

SAMHSA (1996). Preliminary estimates from the 1995 national household survey on drug abuse. Washington, DC: U.S. Public Health Service.

Shain, M., Suurvali, H., & Boutilier, M. (1986). *Healthier workers: Health promotion and employee assistance programs.* Lexington, MA: Lexington Books, D.C. Heath.

Shehadeh, V., & Shain, M. (1990). *Influences on wellness in the workplace: A multivariate approach.* Toronto: Addiction Research Foundation.

Snow, D. (1996). *A workplace intervention to address work and family stressors: Effects on coping and alcohol use.* Paper presented at Conference on Research on Alcohol Problems in the Worksite: Moving toward Prevention Research. Washington, DC, April.

Snow, D., & Kline, M. (1995). Preventive interventions in the workplace to reduce negative psychiatric consequences of work and family stress. In C. M. Mazure (Ed.), *Does stress cause psychiatric illness?* (pp. 220–270). Washington, DC: American Psychiatric Press.

Sofian, N. S., McAfee, T., Doctor, J., & Carson, D. (1994). Tobacco control and cessation. In M. P. O'Donnell M. P. & J. S. Harris (Eds.), *Health promotion in the workplace* (pp. 343–366). Albany, NY: Delmar.

Sonnenstuhl, W. (1996). *Working sober: The transformation of an occupational drinking culture.* Ithaca, NY: Cornell University Press.

Sonnenstuhl, W., & Trice, H. (1987). The social construction of alcohol problems in a union's peer counseling program. *Journal of Drug Issues, 17*(3), 223–254.

Sorensen, G., Lando, H., & Pechacek, T. (1993). Promoting smoking cessation in the workplace: Results of a randomized controlled intervention study. *Journal of Medicine, 35,* 121–126.

Trice, H. M., & Roman, P. M. (1972). *Spirits and demons at work.* Ithaca, NY: ILR Press.

Trice, H. M., & Steele, P. D. (1995). Impairment testing: Issues and conversion with employee assistance programs. *Journal of Drug Issues, 25*(2), 471–503.

Vicary, J. R. (1994). Primary prevention and the workplace. Presentation: Alcohol, Tobacco, and Other Drug Problems in the Workplace: Incentives for Prevention. San Diego, CA, May 12–14, 1994.

Walsh, J. M. (1995). Is workplace drug-testing effective: Let's see the data! Guest editorial in *MRO Update,* October.

Walsh, D. C., Rudd, R., Biener, L., & Mangione, T. (1993). Researching and preventing alcohol problems at work: Toward an integrative model. *American Journal of Health Promotion 7*(4), 289–295.

Winkler, H., & Sheridan, J. (1989). An examination of behavior related to drug use at Georgia Power Company. Presentation: National Institute on Drug Abuse Conference on Drugs in the Workplace: Research and Evaluation Data. Bethesda, MD.

CHAPTER 9

Prevention Approaches in Methadone Treatment Settings: Children of Drug Abuse Treatment Clients

RICHARD F. CATALANO

KEVIN P. HAGGERTY

RANDY R. GAINEY

INTRODUCTION

Children from families in which parents are substance abusers are at elevated risk for developing problem behaviors (Deren, 1986, Goodwin, 1985; Kumpfer, 1987; Kolar et al., 1994; Sloboda & David, 1996). Evidence also suggests that the behavior, attitudes, and interaction patterns of family members play a significant role in either preventing or encouraging children's involvement in adolescent problem behaviors, including drug abuse, delinquency, and other forms of antisocial behavior (Chassin et al., 1993; Gainey et al., 1997; Hawkins, Catalano, & Miller, 1992; Kumpfer 1999). Although a number of selective prevention programs have been developed to reduce children's risk of drug abuse when one or both parents have a substance abuse problem (Falco, 1992; Gross & McCaul, 1992; Haskett et al., 1992; Russell & Free, 1991; Springer et al.,

RICHARD F. CATALANO AND KEVIN P. HAGGERTY • Social Development Research Group, University of Washington, Seattle, Washington 98115
RANDY R. GAINEY • Department of Sociology and Criminal Justice, Old Dominion University, Norfolk, Virginia 23529

1992), few rigorous experimental evaluations of these programs have been published (Catalano et al., 1997; DeMarsh & Kumpfer, 1985; Friedman, 1989).

The Institute of Medicine (Mrazek & Haggerty, 1994) developed a framework for delivering prevention interventions and defined three types of prevention programs: universal, selected, and indicated. Universal prevention approaches serve the entire population without regard to who may be at risk. Selected approaches serve those who may be at risk for problem behaviors but who have not yet manifested the behavior to be prevented. Indicated approaches serve those who have initiated the problem behavior but have not yet developed a serious chronic behavior problem.

The effects of universally applied prevention approaches for substance abuse and other problems are well documented (Hansen, Tobler, & Graham, 1990; Hawkins, Catalano, & Miller, 1992), but less attention has been given to the effects of selected or indicated prevention approaches, particularly those for children whose parents are drug addicts. This chapter describes evidence that establishes the importance of selective interventions to prevent intergenerational drug addiction among families whose parents are in drug treatment. The chapter also describes a specific selective prevention intervention, Focus on Families (FOF), a program to prevent substance abuse among children whose parents are in methadone treatment.

Traditionally, the focus in drug abuse treatment has been on addict behavior, which often extends to the role of the family in influencing addiction (Stanton & Todd, 1982; Surgeon General, 1988). However, little attention has been given to the role of recovering addicts serving as drug abuse prevention agents for their own children. Few addicts wish their children to grow up to be addicts. In fact, most parents in drug abuse treatment express concern for their children and the impact their drug use has had on them. Yet, these children are often at high risk for substance abuse because of parental modeling, favorable parental attitudes toward drug use, and poor parenting practices. In addition to placing the children at high risk for drug abuse, these conditions also place them at risk for other problem behaviors, including school dropout, delinquency, and teenage pregnancy (Brewer et al., 1995; Dryfoos, 1990; Mrazek & Haggerty, 1994).

The premise of this chapter is that to prevent dysfunction it is essential to eliminate, reduce, or mitigate the factors that put people at risk for dysfunction (Hawkins et al., 1992). A risk- and protective-focused approach to prevention of substance abuse seeks to prevent drug abuse by eliminating, reducing, or moderating risk factors for substance abuse while enhancing protective factors. Although research has not yet definitively established risk factors as causes, enough research exists to demonstrate longitudinal relationships between risk factors and substance abuse. Undoubtedly, some risk factors will eventually turn out to be "markers" rather than causes of the development of problem behavior, but risk and protective factors offer an empirical foundation to begin preventive efforts.

RISK FACTORS FOR TEENAGE DRUG ABUSE

Just as public health researchers have identified certain factors that increase the likelihood of heart and lung disease, research has identified risk factors that predict teenage drug abuse (Hawkins, Arthur, & Catalano, 1995; Mrazek & Haggerty, 1994; Newcomb et al., 1987; Simcha-Fagan, Gersten, & Langner, 1986). Risk factors have been identified in individuals as well as in the environments within which they develop. Contextual community factors include economic and social deprivation, low neighborhood attachment and community disorganization, community laws and norms favorable to drug abuse, and the availability of drugs. Family risk factors include family history of addiction; family management problems including conflict, inadequate monitoring, inconsistent or harsh discipline, and lack of clear rules and expectations; family conflict; parental drug use; and positive parent and sibling attitudes toward use. School risk factors include low commitment to school, academic failure, and early antisocial behavior in kindergarten through third grade. Peer and individual risk factors include biologic and genetic predispositions, alienation or rebelliousness, early antisocial behavior, friends who use drugs, favorable attitudes toward drug use, and early first drug use.

The lives of families whose parents are in methadone treatment are characterized by many of these risk factors. Children living in these families face social isolation and entrapment of parents in extreme poverty, poor living conditions, and low-status occupations (Kumpfer & DeMarsh, 1986). Biological factors, such as genetic susceptibility or a child's early temperamental and behavioral difficulty resulting from a mother's drug use during pregnancy may place children at especially high risk for developing later problem behaviors, including substance abuse (Azuma & Chasnoff, 1993; Berstein et al., 1984). Difficult life circumstances, such as trouble with the law, frequent moves, frequent arguments, illness, drug and alcohol use by household members, and abusive relationships, make parenting more challenging (Kolar et al., 1994; Mercer, 1990; Spieker & Booth, 1988; Tableman & Katzenmeyer, 1985). These circumstances produce families that are generally disorganized, have few home management skills, low family cohesion, high stress, and financial troubles (Kumpfer, 1987; Kumpfer & DeMarsh, 1986). Life for children in these families is often chaotic and unpredictable. The following account of one family in our study of parents in methadone treatment offers a glimpse into the world in which drug addicts, even those abstaining from use, are rearing their children.

> My first trip to the client's house was in the evening so that I could have a chance to meet her two sons, aged 14 and 11. When I arrived, I saw a woman sitting in a wheelchair about two feet from a large color television screen. It was the client's mother, and it was evident that the client was responsible for taking care of this woman who was nearly blind and confined to the house. The house was dimly lit and cluttered, with things piled on every surface.

> The older son, already involved with the juvenile justice system for assaulting his mother and younger brother, had again assaulted his younger brother and had another referral, this time for wrapping a bathrobe belt around his brother's neck and causing a burn serious enough to warrant reports to Children's Protective Services by the school and psychiatrist. The younger son was developmentally disabled.

> The client's ex-husband was unemployed and hung around the house a lot. He injured his shoulder and was having surgery soon. The client warned me that her ex was an alcoholic but said, "I don't let him drink at our house any more"—although during one meeting after he'd disappeared for awhile, it was clear that he'd been drinking.

This case illustrates the chaotic lives of many of these families and the elevated risk faced by many children of addicts.

Opiate-addicted parents experience serious problems in many areas of their lives, spend fewer hours with their children each week, and usually have poor parenting practices (Kolar et al., 1994; Sowder & Burt, 1980). In addition, family-management problems are likely to be elevated because of parental drug use and the children's increased likelihood of behavioral problems. Our sample of methadone-treated parents provided the following verbatim answers when asked for the best parental response to specific situations:

A 4-year-old wants more cereal, but there isn't any in the house. She begins to bang on her bowl with her spoon and says, "I hate you, I hate you," to her parent. In this situation what should the parent do?

Responses:

"Give her a candy bar instead. I always keep a box around."

"Restrain her. Take the spoon away and bowl away from her. Take her down from the chair and put her in her bed."

"Put the child to bed. Explain that there is no cereal. Find something else to eat."

A 13-year-old girl cusses and swears at her parents when they ask her to clean her room. In this situation, what should a parent do?

"Lock her in her room till it's clean. If it's not, then—slam her to the floor. Someone better be in charge."

"She should punish her, wash her mouth out with soap. Then put her on restriction."

"I'd slap her first for disrespecting, then send her downstairs. Tell her not to ever disrespect family members again or anybody else."

"Don't accept it. Nine out of ten I'd whip her ass when I feel she is way out of control with herself."

Some parents gave skillful responses in these situations, but most responses were of this nature.

Numerous studies have found that parental conflict characterizes the homes of substance abusers (Brewer, Fleming, et al., 1998; Kumpfer & DeMarsh, 1986; McCord, 1979; Moos et al., 1979; Robins, 1980). Simcha-Fagan et al. (1986) found that the use of heroin and other illicit drugs is strongly associated with marital discord. Fiks, Johnson, and Rosen (1985) found that among methadone mothers living with male partners during pregnancy, 45.7% reported ambivalent or negative relationships, compared to 25.9% in the non-drug-abusing control group.

Family environments influence risk for substance abuse through their effects on other factors that increase risks. Early variety and frequency of antisocial behavior in the primary grades is a risk factor for later drug abuse (Hawkins et al., 1987; Patterson, 1982) that can arise through poor family-management practices (Loeber & Stouthamer-Loeber, 1986), which are more likely in families with parents who are substance abusers (Kolar et al., 1994). The predictive power of early antisocial behavior for teenage drug use has been demonstrated from as early as 5 years of age (Gittleman et al., 1985; Lerner & Vicary, 1984; Lewis, Robins, & Rice, 1985). Furthermore, in studies focused on adolescent conduct disorders, troublesome childhood behavior—including acting out, impulsivity, defiance, aggressiveness, and other maladaptive behavior—as early as age 4 has been found to be predictive of a range of adolescent problem behaviors 5 to 9 years later (Loeber & Dishion, 1983; Shedler & Block, 1990).

School failure, regardless of its direct cause, has been shown to be associated with adolescent substance abuse (Newcomb et al., 2002; Weng, Newcomb, & Bentler, 1988); and many children's habits and predilections toward school are formed in the home (Epstein, 1994). Evidence suggests that academic failure may be a stable predictor of delinquency and drug use between late elementary school and early junior high school (Brophy & Good, 1986). Likewise, low commitment to education and low attachment to school are risk factors with etiological ties to the family environment (Johnston, O'Malley, & Bachman, 1985; Kandel, 1982).

Peer factors, including association with drug-using peers and perceived use of substances by others, are strongly associated with adolescent substance abuse (Hawkins et al., 1997); and such friendship patterns can be influenced by family-management and supervision techniques (Patterson & Dishion, 1985). Attitudes and beliefs conducive to drug use and deviance, including parent and sibling attitudes favorable to drug use, have been shown to increase the risk of children's later substance abuse (Hawkins et al., 1997).

In sum, children of addicted parents are generally exposed to multiple risk factors within their families. Evidence suggests that exposure to the number of risk factors is frequently more consequential than the type of individual factor (Felix-Ortiz & Newcomb, 1999) and that risk increases exponentially with exposure to multiple factors (Newcomb et al., 1987; Rutter, 1980). The evidence also suggests the importance of the family in the etiology of adolescent drug abuse. If one accepts the premise that effective prevention entails intervening to eliminate or buffer

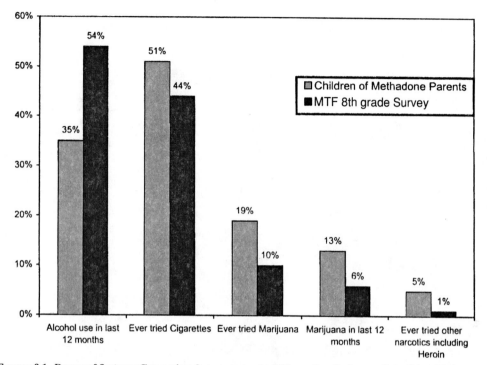

FIGURE 9.1. Degree of first use: Comparison between sample children of methadone patients (11 to 14-year-olds) and Monitoring the Future 1991 survey of 8th grade students. (Source: Monitoring the Future, Institute for Social Research, The University of Michigan.

factors implicated in the causal processes, there is reason to expect that interventions targeting the family can effectively reduce drug abuse among children of substance abusers. Risk factors provide a framework for identifying targets of intervention for parents in drug abuse treatment.

In addition to targeting risk factors, it is important to identify at what age children are exposed to risk. Baseline data from focus on families (FOF), our study of children of methadone-treated parents, shows that 48.4% of 11- to 14-year-olds had seen adults use drugs in the prior year, 65.1% had seen an adult drunk in the prior 3 months, and nearly 16% of 6- to 10-year-olds had used alcohol. When compared with respondents in the Monitoring the Future Survey (MTF) of Secondary School Students (Johnston et al., 1992), it is clear that children of drug addicts have higher rates of initiation, especially with illegal drugs, such as marijuana and heroin. Figure 9.1 illustrates the prevalence of early first use by 11- to 14-year-old children of heroin addicts in methadone treatment, compared to the MTF study at eighth grade (age equivalent 13 to 14). Each measure of use is higher among the children of methadone clients than among eighth-grade students in the MTF study, with the exception of alcohol use in the prior 12 months, which is curiously lower. The lower rate of alcohol use may be due in part to the slight differences in items (our item explicitly excludes sips of alcohol, which the MTF study does not exclude) and to the younger age of some participants in our sample compared with the MTF study.

In addition to early initiation, children of addicts appear to experience higher levels of risk at earlier ages in other areas. Figure 9.2 compares initiation of early problem behaviors by 12- to 14-year-old children of drug addicts and a public school population of eighth-grade students in the same urban area (Seattle, WA). Children in the methadone sample are significantly more likely to initiate cigarette and marijuana use. Their rate of being picked up by the police is more

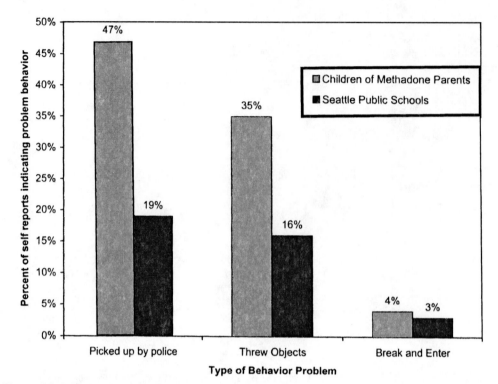

FIGURE 9.2. Initiation of early problem behaviors: comparison between sample of children of methadone patients (11–14 years old) and Seattle eighth-grade students. (Source: Seattle Social Development Project. P.I.: J. David Hawkins Reprinted with permission. Note: SSDP sample size range from 474 to 490. FOF sample sizes 63.)

than double that of the public school student population. It is important to note that the higher rates of initiation of problem behavior by the FOF sample, despite their younger age, suggest that early intervention may be particularly important for this population.

PREVENTION IN A TREATMENT CONTEXT

Parental drug use may be one of the single most important risk factors for children. Parental addiction is not only likely to add biological or genetic aspects to their children's risk but also likely to affect other factors, such as family conflict, family management (including abuse and neglect), parent modeling of and favorable attitudes toward use, friends who use, and early first use. In addition, parents who are addicted are not as likely to provide consistent economic support for their families. Keeping parents drug free has significant preventive value for their children (Fleming et al., 1997).

Although treatment programs of various modalities have demonstrated effectiveness in reducing use during treatment, post-treatment use is common across all treatment modalities (Brewer, Catalano, et al., 1998; Surgeon General, 1988). About two-thirds of treated substance abusers experience at least one relapse in the year after treatment (Surgeon General, 1988).

In addition to identifying risk factors for the development of substance abuse, research has also identified environmental and situational predictors of post-treatment relapse. (See Surgeon General (1988), for an in-depth review of relapse factors for alcohol, opiate, and tobacco use.)

Treatment adjuncts to reduce these factors during and after treatment are likely to enhance the effectiveness of treatment, reduce relapse, and help prevent substance abuse among children of parents in treatment. Relapse factors for adults include family conflict, lack of family support, drug use among other family members, lack of involvement in nondrug leisure activities, association with substance-abusing peers, skill deficits, high life stress, and lack of needed services. All of these factors have been shown to increase the likelihood that adults will relapse following treatment (Surgeon General, 1988).

Such relapse factors often characterize the lives of drug-treatment patients. Many of these individuals traditionally lack adequate coping or problem-solving skills with which to address their often serious, longstanding problems (Hawkins, Catalano, & Wells, 1986). Their lives are often characterized by lack of social support and lack of support for abstinence in particular (Hawkins & Fraser, 1983). Stark (1989, p. 172) notes that methadone clients are frequently without adequate social support. Often, their family and community of origin have been negative influences or are completely lost to them; and their current associates are likely to be involved in drug use and criminal behavior.

Negative emotional states, such as depression, also contribute to the risk of post-treatment relapse. In our study of methadone-treated patients, 73% of respondents ($n = 165$) show signs of significant depression. Other studies confirm high rates of psychopathology, especially depression, among methadone clients (Stark, 1989). With little social support, low tolerance for stress and frustration, and a high degree of impulsiveness, many methadone clients relapse or continue to use drugs and alcohol while in treatment (Catalano et al., 1997). Reducing parental drug use during treatment is a necessary tool for preventing substance abuse among their children.

The evidence is clear. Children of parents in methadone treatment are exposed to multiple risk factors for substance abuse, and their parents' lives are characterized by continued drug use or high risk for relapse. Given the importance of parental drug use as a risk factor for these children, it is essential that we reach parents during treatment with prevention interventions. As shown in Table 9.1, a number of relapse and risk factors can be influenced by the family. In fact, a synergy may be achieved by addressing these factors because they are likely to be related to, and interact with, one another. For example, successfully setting clear expectations for children's behavior

TABLE 9.1. Focus on Families: Family-Influenced Risk Factors

Teenage drug abuse	Post-treatment relapse
Family history of drug abuse	Drug use in the family
Parental drug use and positive attitudes toward use	Family and peer drug use
Family conflict	Family conflict
Family management problems	Little family support for abstinence
Early antisocial behavior	
Friends who use	Friends who use
Extreme economic deprivation	High life stress
Transitions and mobility	Unemployment
	Residential instability
Alienation and rebelliousness	Low family bonding
	Lack of nondrug leisure activities
	Isolation
Low commitment to school	
Academic failure	
(Hawkins, Catalano, & Miller, 1992)	(Surgeon General, 1988)

could effectively reduce life stress and family conflict. Furthermore, if a clear family policy is established against drug use, family support for abstinence could be strengthened.

PROTECTIVE FACTORS

There is evidence that the effects of exposure to risk can be mitigated by a variety of individual and social characteristics. Three broad categories of protective factors against stress in children have been identified: (1) individual characteristics, including resilient temperament, positive social orientation, and intelligence (Radke-Yarrow & Sherman, 1990); (2) family or external social supports that are characterized by warm, supportive relationships or bonding (Catalano & Hawkins, 1996; Resnick et al., 1997); and (3) healthy beliefs and clear standards that promote prosocial behavior (Brook et al., 1990; Resnick et al., 1997; Werner, 1989). Critical for children of substance-abusing parents is the interaction between parent drug use, bonding, and child's drug use. Parental bonding plays a protective role when parents have stopped using drugs but increases risk when parents are unable to abstain (Fleming et al., 1997). Distinct from risk factors, protective factors are hypothesized to operate indirectly through interaction with risk factors, mediating or moderating the risk exposure (Hawkins, Catalano, & Miller, 1992; Rutter, 1985).

In addition to being exposed to multiple risk factors, children of addicted parents are likely to have few protective factors in their lives. To illustrate, comparing our samples of 11- to 14-year-old children of heroin addicts in methadone treatment with children in high-risk urban public schools in the same city, children of substance abusers are significantly less attached to both their mothers and fathers and indicate significantly greater attachment and loyalty to their best friend than do those in the public school sample (Hoppe et al., 1998). In addition, as previously discussed, children of heroin addicts are likely to be in conflict with their parents, may have a difficult temperament due to being affected *in utero* and be in a family environment that is not characterized by healthy beliefs and clear standards.

PRINCIPLES FOR TREATMENT PROGRAMS
FOR CHILDREN

The evidence on risk and protective factors led us to develop the following five principles for creating prevention programs for children whose parents are in treatment for drug abuse:

1. Programs must focus on reducing known risk factors for relapse and on youthful drug abuse that can be affected by family action. Family factors that are important predictors of relapse and adolescent substance abuse include family history of addiction, family-management problems, parental drug use and positive attitudes toward use, family conflict, and family drug use. In addition to these family factors, several factors are under the influence of family, such as early antisocial behavior, academic failure, low commitment to school, friends who use drugs and early first use, little family support for abstinence, high life stress, and lack of involvement in non-drug-use leisure activities. These factors are likely to be important in the development of children's problem behaviors and should be addressed in prevention intervention strategies aimed at interrupting the causal process.
2. Programs working with recovering parents should seek to enhance protective factors while reducing risks. Enhancing protection while reducing risk provides double protection. Factors associated with risks should be reduced in ways that strengthen relationships and at the same time promote prosocial beliefs and standards. It is especially necessary

among substance-abusing parents to combine the promotion of strong relationships with risk reduction and the creation of strong pro-social beliefs and standards. Without clear abstinence policies and beliefs that drug use is unhealthy, promoting strong bonding between parent and child may increase risk for both parent and child. In situations where parents are still using drugs and ignoring the health consequences of use, strong bonds between parent and child are likely to promote rather than deter use (Fleming et al., 1997; Foshee & Bauman, 1992).

3. Programs must address risk factors at the appropriate developmental stage. Effective prevention efforts are targeted at the appropriate developmental stage of the child. Different risk factors for substance abuse become salient at different ages. Programs should develop different activities and foci for parents of children of different ages, based on the prominent risk factors for these children.

4. Prevention interventions in treatment programs should have strong links with treatment. Treatment efforts first need to focus on the client's recovery (Surgeon General, 1988), and parents must be committed to their own recovery. Ideally, parents will have been involved with a treatment program for a minimum of 90 days before focusing on parenting issues. After progress toward cessation has been accomplished, a prevention focus in treatment settings helps shift the focus of recovery away from the individual and toward the broader context of family issues. Creating linkages between treatment and prevention programs is critical.

5. Effective programs include intensive and comprehensive program elements (family, peers, school, and community). Because parents in treatment have multiple problems and their children are exposed to multiple risks, intensive, sustained interventions are needed. It is likely that access to a wide array of comprehensive services is critical to reduce the risk of relapse and children's substance abuse. Such an array may include family services (such as family-involvement training, family-management training, and conflict reduction); economic services (housing, medical, financial, employment); social services (mental health, abstinence supports, network development, leisure activities, stress coping and social skills strategy, and relapse prevention); and school services (educational support for children and self).

FOCUS ON FAMILIES

FOF was an 8-year field experiment funded by the National Institute on Drug Abuse that incorporated the previously cited five principles. The goals of the project were (1) to reduce the risk of post-treatment relapse among methadone-treated parents, (2) to reduce the risk of drug abuse by children of methadone-treated parents, and (3) to increase protective factors against drug abuse among children of methadone-treated parents. The program sought to create conditions for bonding within the family and with others outside the family by enhancing opportunities, skills, and recognition for social involvement, and encouraging families to set clear family policies on drug use (Catalano & Hawkins, 1996).

FOF served parents enrolled in two methadone programs in Seattle, Washington, who had children between the ages of 3 and 14. Parents had to meet the following eligibility criteria: (1) voluntarily agree to participate and be randomly assigned to experimental conditions, (2) have a child living with them at least 50% of the time, and (3) have completed at least 90 days of treatment before assignment to one of the experimental conditions (parent training and case management plus standard methadone treatment or a methadone-treatment-only control group). Parents and their children received a pretreatment baseline interview; parents only received a post-test interview after the parent-training sessions; and parents and children were interviewed at 6 months, 12 months, and 24 months following post-test. Parents in the program came from a three-county area and lived in both urban and rural settings. One hundred thirty families were randomly assigned to receive either the treatment-enhanced FOF intervention ($n = 75$) or a non-treatment-enhanced control condition ($n = 55$). Of the 144 parents who enrolled in the project, 94% were interviewed immediately after completion of the intervention, 94% were interviewed 6 months later, 92% completed a 12-month follow-up interview, and 92% completed the 24-month follow-up interview.

The average age of participating parents was 35 years; 75% were female. Seventy-seven percent of the parents were European-American, 18% were African-American, and 5% were of other ethnic backgrounds. Sixty-six percent of the parents had two or more children between the ages of 3 and 14. The average age of first heroin use by parents was 19.14 years. Although participants were receiving methadone treatment at baseline, 54% had engaged in illicit drug use in the prior month.

The 130 families in the project included 178 children, 97 experimental and 81 control. Children were interviewed if they were age 6 or older. Mean age of child participants was 10.5 ($SD = 2.4$).

The project had two components: parent and child skill training and home-based case management. Systematic training was provided in relapse prevention and coping, appropriate developmental expectations, communication, anger control, family involvement, and skills to set limits, monitor, praise, and provide appropriate consequences for children's behavior. Parents also learned how to support their children's academic progress and how to teach them refusal and problem-solving skills. Case managers worked with families in their homes to help them maintain the skills they learned and to generalize these skills to their natural environment. Case managers also worked with children to encourage their involvement in prosocial opportunities outside the family and helped parents access other needed services. The rationale and description for each component are described in the following, and an overview is provided in Figure 9.3.

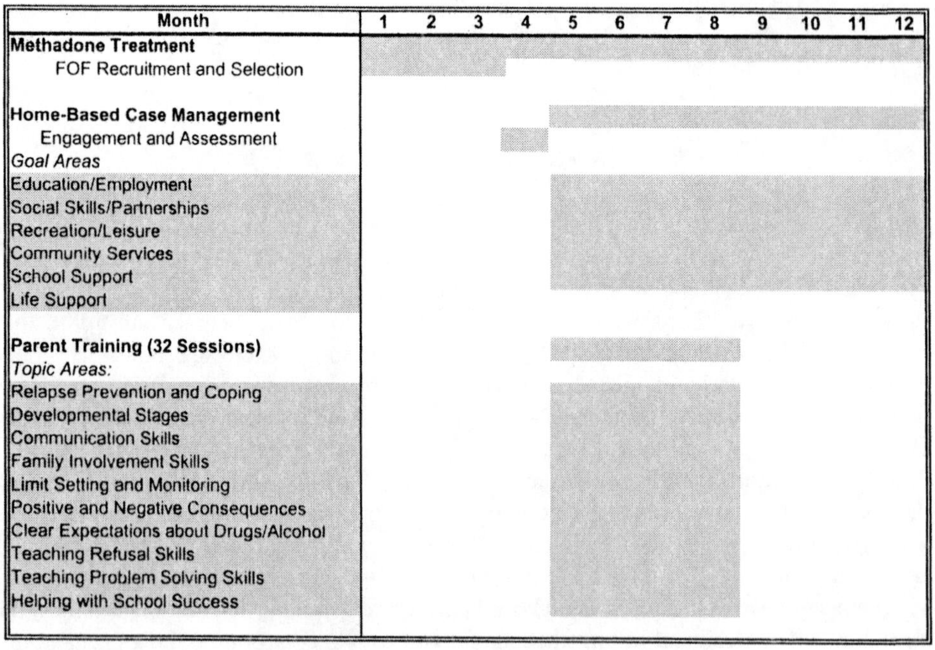

FIGURE 9.3. Focus on families timeline overview.

The FOF program addressed the following risk factors for teen drug abuse through parent training and case management: family-management problems (lack of clear expectations, lack of monitoring and supervision, severe or inconsistent discipline, and family conflict); parental drug use and positive attitudes toward use; family history of addiction; early antisocial behavior; early first use; academic failure; low commitment to school; and friends who use drugs. In addition, FOF addressed the following risk factors for relapse by parents: drug use in the family, peer drug use, family conflict, lack of involvement in non-drug-use leisure activities, and little family support for abstinence and isolation.

Parent Training

Parent-training approaches are supported by evidence from controlled studies showing that family-management problems and antisocial behavior can be reduced through parenting training (Dishion & Andrews, 1995; Dumas, 1989; Serketich & Dumas, 1996). Parent training that teaches skills in family-management practices and in clarifying and creating consistency in rewards and punishments has produced short-term improvements in family interactions and in reducing delinquency and other problem behaviors (Bry & Krinsley, 1992; Fraser, Hawkins, & Howard, 1988; Yoshikawa, 1994). Parenting skills training combined with social skills training for disruptive kindergarten boys reduced school adjustment problems and delayed the onset of delinquent behavior (Tremblay et al., 1992). Randomized experimental tests of parenting skills training have shown significant reductions in preadolescent problem behaviors (Patterson, Chamberlain, & Reid, 1982) and in reducing other maladaptive adolescent behaviors (Briar & Conte, 1978; Forehand, Griest, & Wells, 1979; Loeber & Stouthamer-Loeber, 1986). Parent training has also demonstrated effectiveness in improving family-management practices (Catalano et al., 1999; Spoth et al., 1995) and in improving school achievement (Fraser et al., 1988). Promising outcomes have been observed for children from socioeconomically disadvantaged families and for children who have experienced conduct disorders (Hawkins, Catalano, Morrison et al., 1992). Parent training has also demonstrated increases in protective factors and processes, including increases in communication and decision-making skills (Grady, Gersick, & Boratynski, 1986) and increases in parent–child bonding (Rose, Battjes, & Leukefeld, 1984). DeMarsh and Kumpfer (1986) found significant improvements in parent–child interactions and in parents' ratings of their own and their children's behaviors after involvement in the Strengthening Families program. DeMarsh and Kumpfer (1985) reported that parents were successfully trained to develop more effective discipline methods, that their children had fewer behavior problems after treatment, and that the children had decreased intentions to smoke and use alcohol.

Three major challenges in working with parents exposed to multiple risk factors have been noted in tests of parent-training interventions. First, it is difficult to recruit these parents (Grady et al., 1986; Hawkins et al., 1987). Second, it is clear that short-term programs (8 to 10 sessions) are unlikely to succeed because of the multiplicity of problems (Patterson & Reid, 1973). Clinical reports suggest that these parents may require twice as many hours of training as parents from the general population to achieve the same level of change in their own and in their children's behavior (Patterson, 1974; Patterson & Fleishman, 1979). Third, parent training alone may not be potent enough to produce substantial, lasting changes in families exposed to multiple risk factors (Reid, 1993; Tremblay et al., 1992; Serketich & Dumas, 1996). The FOF intervention attempted to address each of these issues.

Parents in methadone treatment are good candidates for such a program, because they have already made a commitment to examine their drug use and have begun to work on making changes in their lives. Their regular attendance at the clinic provides ready availability for parent-training sessions. The program is of long duration, pays particular attention to recruitment and retention mechanisms, and offers other supportive services. The FOF intervention lasted 9 months (4 months of parent-training groups, 9 months of home-based services). The program was also linked with other treatment services, such as housing, child welfare, and employment, when appropriate.

The FOF parent-training curriculum consists of a 5-hour family retreat and thirty-two $1^1/_2$–hour parent-training sessions. The curriculum was developed after a number of parent-training and skill-based curricula were reviewed (see Appendix). Sessions are conducted twice a week over a 16-week period. Children attend 12 of the sessions to practice developmentally appropriate skills with their parents. Parent-only sessions are held in the morning; the sessions children attend are generally conducted in the evening when the children are not in school. Session topics are targeted at specific developmental risk and protective factors and include the following:

1. Family goal setting. The 5-hour kick-off retreat focuses on goal setting and bringing families together to share a common, trust-building experience. This session empowers families to work together to develop goals for their participation in the family sessions. Case managers later work with individual families to identify the small steps they need to take in order to reach their identified goals.
2. Relapse prevention. These four sessions cover material including identification of relapse signals or triggers, anger and stress control, and creating and practicing a plan to follow in case a relapse occurs. The impact of relapse on the client's children is emphasized, and skills are taught to prevent and cope with relapse and relapse-inducing situations. Parents learn that they are responsible for their behavior and its consequences. They are taught to identify the cognitive, behavioral, and situational antecedents (signals) of relapse and to use self-talk to anticipate the consequences of their drug-using behavior (Hawkins et al., 1986). In addition to self-talk, parents are taught to use "urge surfing" and distractions as preventive measures against relapse (Marlatt & Gordon, 1985).
3. Family communication skills. The skills of paraphrasing, open questions, and "I" messages are taught during these sessions. Families practice using the skills during two practice sessions. All subsequent groups reinforce the use of the communication skills taught in these early sessions. Families then use these skills to develop family expectations, to conduct regular family meetings, and to make family play and fun time successful.
4. Family-management skills. Parents learn and practice setting clear and specific expectations, monitoring expected behavior, rewarding, and providing appropriate consequences for negative behaviors. Parents practice implementing "the law of least intervention," using the smallest intervention to get the desired behavior from their child. A variety of discipline skills learned and practiced by parents include praise, ignoring, expressing feelings, using "if-then" messages, time-outs, and privilege restrictions. The pros and cons of using spanking as a discipline technique are discussed, and parents review tips for reducing spanking. In addition, parents target one behavior to work on with each of their children. Parents chart both their own behavior (for consistency) and their children's behavior to aid in recognizing and reinforcing the desired behaviors. Parents are referred to outside resources for children's behavioral problems if needed.
5. Creating family expectations about drugs and alcohol. Families work together to define and clarify expectations about drugs and alcohol in their families. Parents are taught how to involve their children in creating clear and specific expectations, how to monitor, and how to provide appropriate consequences for violations of the expectations. Families work together to establish written policies for tobacco, alcohol, and other drug use.

They apply previously learned skills of family involvement, communication, and family management to develop and implement the policy.

6. Teaching children skills. Parents learn how to teach their children two important types of skills—refusal skills and problem-solving skills—using a five-step process: (1) "Sell/ Tell"—sell the skill to your children and tell them the steps; (2) "Show"—model the skill steps for your child; (3) "Do"—provide guided practice steps for the child; (4) provide "Feedback" accentuating the strengths; and (5) plan for "Application" to real-life situations. Parents teach and practice the skills with their children during sessions so trainers can guide parent-teaching practices.

7. Helping children succeed in school. Parents build on the previously learned skills to create, monitor, and provide appropriate consequences in a home-learning routine for their children. Parents identify time, place, and consequences for homework completion. Strategies to assist children with homework are taught and practiced. Parents review communication skills and practice using the skills to communicate with school personnel.

Parent sessions are conducted with groups of six to eight families. Given the severity of these parents' dysfunction (Kolar et al., 1994), it is necessary to provide practice opportunities as well as skill components that address specific recurring problem behaviors. The parent-training format combines a peer-support and skill training model. The training curriculum teaches skills using "guided participant modeling" (Rosenthal & Bandura, 1978). Skills are modeled by trainers and other group members and then discussed by participants. Skill steps are reviewed and then practiced by parents. Videotape is frequently used in modeling the skills or to give feedback after skill practice. To maximize effectiveness, the training focuses on affective and cognitive as well as behavioral aspects of performance (W. T. Grant Consortium on the School-Based Promotion of Social Competence, 1992).

The FOF curriculum allows participants to practice in situations they currently face with their own children. Parents complete home extension exercises after each session to generalize the skills from the training setting to the home setting (Goldstein & Kanfer, 1979). After parents learn and practice skills, parents and children practice using their new skills together in family sessions.

Following their graduation from the parent-training group, families are invited to a monthly potluck. The potluck acts as a booster session for families and helps them maintain behavior changes learned in parent-training sessions. At each potluck, families review their progress toward their goals, go over skill steps, and discuss their use of skills at home.

Home-Based Case Management

The complex nature of many families in treatment and the multiple risks facing the children of these families make it necessary to combine the resources of community, school, a positive peer network, and positive extended family to achieve a level of support adequate to ensure recovery, reduce risks, and increase protective factors. Increasingly, case management is used as an intervention strategy for those who present multiple problems, including children with emotional disturbances and delinquency (Haggerty et al., 1989) and drug abusers (Grant et al., 1996; Rapp, Siegal, & Fisher, 1992). Historically, case management has been defined as having five functions: assessment, planning, advocacy, linkage, and monitoring—acting as a "brokerage" of services to clients (Kaplan, 1990). More recently, however, case management models have generally been expanded to include interventions that emphasize relationship development, intense involvement with clients, and outreach (Chamberlin & Rapp, 1991; Dunst & Trivette, 1988).

Some research suggests that home visiting has brought improvements in the birth weight of babies of high-risk pregnancies and reductions in child abuse and neglect when visits are continued postpartum (Olds & Kitzman, 1990). Other results include better school performance at follow-up than control students (Gordon & Guinagh, 1978), higher cognitive development during preschool (Gray & Ruttle, 1980), and reduced need for out-of-home placements for children of families in crisis (Fraser & Haapala, 1987/1988). These programs involve tailoring services to the specific needs of each family.

Despite the research documenting the success of home-based interventions with families that include infants and preschool children (Mrazek & Haggerty, 1994), few studies evaluating the effectiveness of home-based case management among drug-abusing families with school-age children have been conducted; and few service delivery models exist (Olds & Kitzman, 1990). However, the use of home-based case management services with addicted populations appears to hold promise for engaging reluctant families in the process of reducing family risks and enhancing family protective factors.

Fraser and Haapala (1987/1988) identified two important characteristics of home-based services that may lead to successful interventions. First, interventions conducted in the home are filled with opportunities to demonstrate *in vivo* the family-management and problem-solving skills being addressed in parent-training sessions. Second, when home-based services meet tangible, hard service needs of families, such as housing, education, financial, and medical services, the families appear to have superior outcomes.

The FOF case management definition focuses on habilitation: the process of developing an empowering relationship with families to reduce risk and at the same time enhance family strengths, integrate skills into the family, strengthen family bonds, and create and reinforce clear norms opposed to drug use. Case managers facilitate participation in parenting groups by contacting clients before each session to make sure they are planning to attend and by reducing barriers to participation, such as transportation or child care. When clients miss a group session, case managers conduct home visits and provide families with the content materials and workbooks and provide opportunities for practicing the skills before the next group session.

The goal of home-based case management is to empower families and facilitate their ability to identify the changes they want to make. Case managers work with families to define specific goals they want to work on, both individually and as a family, and to identify the steps they need to take to meet those goals. Case managers play a key role in encouraging families to participate in the parent-training sessions and in helping them generalize skills to "real-life" situations outside the group. They show families how participation in parent training helps them make the necessary changes to meet the goals they defined. Case managers help families recognize that they are in control of their recovery and have the power to change patterns of behavior. Initially, case managers assist families in solving their problems, then gradually teach them a process for their own problem solving. Eventually, case managers provide opportunities for families to demonstrate parenting and problem-solving competencies. Case managers also facilitate access to needed services and provide linkages to other agencies, such as school and leisure activities. Finally, case managers provide support to help keep families focused on their goals during crises.

The FOF case management system uses a six-step model:

STEP 1: JOINING AND ENGAGING WITH FAMILIES. This is perhaps the most critical aspect of case management. Case managers seek to build a trusting relationship not only with the addicted parent but with all family members. Although the addicted parent is the client initially, after the first meeting the case manager shifts the focus from the client as addict to the client as parent, and then from the addict-parent as client to the family as client.

FOF case managers use several strategies to engage families. Frequent visits are used to build trust. Clients are initially met at the clinic, often informally, and an invitation is extended to go for a cup of coffee. This provides a neutral setting to conduct an informal assessment of the family, meet the parent, and develop a plan to meet the rest of the family. Soon afterward, case managers visit the home where they meet the rest of the family and begin the assessment process. Case managers engage in fun, non-threatening activities with the children, such as games, sports, or walks, in order to establish themselves as caring and competent adults who can help the family. The main goal of this relationship-building period is to create a strong enough bond with the family so that members will want to attend the parent-training sessions.

Case managers develop their relationships with families in concrete ways. They establish themselves immediately as family advocates by assisting in solving critical problems, such as housing, child care, and treatment issues, and by providing concrete services, such as assistance with power bills, diapers, or transportation.

STEP 2: RISK AND RELAPSE ASSESSMENT. FOF case managers use an assessment form to identify family strengths, weaknesses, and risk potential. Assessments are organized into seven sections:

1. Parenting Skills assesses parents' norms and rules against the use of drugs and alcohol, general family rule structure, family-management style, monitoring behavior, discipline practices, family interactions, and fun time spent with the child or children.
2. Social Skills/Relationships assesses relationships with other family members, spouse, and peers; degree of isolation; degree of family conflict; family-related stress; respite from child care; and children's relationships with parent or parent figures and children's friends.
3. Community Services assesses current services being utilized and the client's degree of comfort in using services.
4. Employment/Education assesses current employment status, job history, job satisfaction, and career goals.
5. Recreation/Leisure assesses parents' and children's leisure activities outside the home.
6. School Support assesses children's academic success, commitment to school, home learning routine, opportunities for learning, and parent involvement in school.
7. Life Support assesses negative life events and stress in the areas of housing, legal, and financial stress, and medical and dental problems. The case manager conducts this assessment informally with the family and uses it to develop a service plan.

STEP 3: SERVICE PLAN AGREEMENT. Case managers work with families to identify potential risk areas and jointly develop goals for the priority areas identified in the assessment. Families are encouraged to create and develop the goals they want for their family, and these goals become the center of the case management service plan. In the treatment service agreement, case managers identify the target behaviors to be changed, graduated outcomes, and strategies to reach the outcomes. In some instances, case managers may identify specific goals for the family based on their assessment, which the family has not identified.

STEP 4: SERVICE PLAN IMPLEMENTATION. Given the broad areas of assessment and client goals, case managers need to have the knowledge and ability to apply a variety of therapeutic interventions. These may include couples therapy, strategic family therapy, skills training, problem solving, and crisis intervention. Effective home visits require that case managers respect their clients and use some fundamental helping skills, such as active listening and open-ended questions (see Wasik, Bryant, & Lyons, 1990) and skills to motivate and encourage steps toward recovery (see Miller & Rollnick, 1991). Case managers empower families by providing opportunities for practicing and using the skills they learned in parent training and by implementing the service plan in ways that are consistent with the family's goals.

Case management with drug-affected families requires that individual family members be confronted with the reality of their behaviors, so case managers also need supportive confrontation skills. For example, a parent who wants his or her 5-year-old to stop swearing yet swears continually him- or herself needs to be confronted directly on this behavior. Likewise, a parent who is concerned about his or her daughter's use of alcohol and yet is smoking marijuana in front of the children needs to be confronted directly on this behavior. FOF works under the assumption that no parent intends or wants his or her child to grow up to be a drug addict. Consequently, behaviors that increase the risk of the child's drug abuse are pointed out to parents clearly and specifically, focusing on the behavior rather than on the person.

A discretionary fund was available for families to provide financial support when needed for leisure activities, crisis intervention, and services. For example, one client established a goal of controlling her anger, and funds were made available to pay for her intake interview at an anger-management program. In other cases, funds were used to pay fees for critically needed services or to pay for part of a family leisure activity, such as summer camp, or for memberships in organizations such as Boys' and Girls' Clubs.

STEP 5: MONITORING, EVALUATING, AND REVISING SERVICE PLANS. Case managers are responsible for monitoring the outcomes of their clients' progress toward goals. Monitoring service plans keeps both case managers and clients accountable for the family's goals. Each month case managers review progress toward goals with their clients. Regular monitoring of the service plan serves two purposes: It helps clients know where they are and where they are headed with regard to their goals, and it provides focus and accountability for services from case managers. Service plans are revised if planned goal steps are too big. New goals are added if clients have achieved targeted goals.

STEP 6: TERMINATING WITH CLIENTS. FOF case management services are provided for nine months. This means that case managers must work with their clients proactively to terminate services. Termination includes providing clients with alternate resources they can access on their own; assisting them in developing at least one strong, healthy pro-social relationship; and modeling ending a relationship in a healthy, nonaggressive manner. Case managers evaluate minimum outcomes expected with each family. These include:

1. Parents refrain from using illegal drugs in front of their children.
2. There is no physical abuse in the family.
3. The family has carried out one successful family meeting without case managers present.
4. The family has a written family drug policy.
5. All school-age youth regularly attend school.
6. Families have an established home learning routine.
7. Families use communication skills of "I" messages, paraphrasing, and open questions.
8. Each family has one new resource in their network.
9. Each family will attend at least two follow-up groups.

Outcomes on family-defined goals were rated by the case manager at termination. Sixty-three percent of families were rated as having attained a significant change or preferred outcome on their first goal; 51% were rated as having made at least a significant change or preferred outcome on their second goal; and 62% were rated as having made at least a significant change or preferred outcome on their third goal.

PROGRAM IMPLEMENTATION ISSUES

FOF emphasizes intervention fidelity. Manuals guide all interventions. Weekly clinical meetings review case management practices and highlight the week's action plans for each family receiving services. The clinical director supervises all case managers and group leaders weekly. In addition, parent-training sessions are observed through two full sessions to ensure the training's fidelity to the manual.

Recruiting and retaining high-risk parents for training events is critical. The literature suggests that attrition rates are commonly 40 to 60% (DeMarsh & Kumpfer, 1986; Firestone & Witt, 1982; Fraser et al., 1988; Spoth & Redmond, 1994). Considerable effort on the part of project staff resulted in high rates of attendance at parent-training sessions. Preliminary data show that 54% of all those assigned to the experimental treatment condition completed at least 16 sessions. Of those who actually initiated parent training, that is, attended at least 1 session, 63% completed at least 16 sessions. This compares favorably with other parenting programs, especially given the intensity of FOF training, the number of sessions offered (33), and the multiple problems and barriers faced by these families.

Two important factors contributed to high attendance rates in the project. First, case managers encouraged participation. The trusting relationship developed between family members and their case manager gives them an incentive to attend the groups. Second, certain barriers to attendance were removed. Transportation, child care, money for parking, and group scheduling were made available to provide maximum opportunity for involvement. We also offered a small incentive for attending each session ($3) and for completing home practice ($2). Parents attending at least half of the sessions completed an average of 61% of the homework assignments.

OUTCOME SUMMARY

Overall, research results suggest that the FOF intervention improved treatment outcomes (see Catalano et al., 1997, 1999, in press). Parents in the experimental groups used significantly less heroin at the end of parent training and at 12-month follow-up and less cocaine at the 12-month follow-up, than did parents in the control group. Experimental- and control-group parents displayed similar levels of marijuana use during the evaluation period. Biochemical measures to assess veracity of self-reports of drug use were used with a random sample of participants at each time period, and no experimental–control differences in veracity were discovered.

Although no statistically significant differences between experimental- and control-group children were found in the areas of drug use or delinquency at 6- and 12-month follow-up, the direction of differences favored the experimental group in all but one of the comparisons made in these two areas. Secondary analysis of individual items in the delinquency scale revealed that children in the experimental group were less likely than control group children to have reported stealing in the 6 months prior to the 6-month interview (26% vs. 10%, odds ratio = 0.31, $p < .10$, $n = 77$). At the 24-month follow-up, children under the experimental condition continued to display lower rates of substance use and other problem behavior, although again these experimental versus control differences were not significantly different.

BENEFITS AND COSTS

A blueprint for a benefit-cost analysis of the FOF program was developed (Plotnick, 1994) to measure the effects of the program at the 6-month follow-up time point (Plotnick et al., 1998). Few statistically significant differences were found between treatment and control families. Although parents in the experimental condition showed significant improvement in relapse prevention and coping skills, as well as reduced frequency of opiate use, no significant evidence of positive monetary benefit was found at the 6-month follow-up time point, suggesting that improvements in risk and protective factors may not translate rapidly into differences in employment, health, or criminal involvement.

CONCLUSION

Working with parents, many of whom are ambivalent about progressing toward recovery, can be difficult and emotionally challenging, but several lessons we learned may help with future implementation of prevention programs in treatment settings. First, parents must have at least some degree of commitment to recovery. Parents who are preoccupied with continuing their drug use cannot focus on effective parenting strategies, and creating stronger bonds between such parents and their children may actually have a deleterious effect on the children. Second, family members should be screened and assessed for any biological or neurological disorders, including fetal alcohol syndrome and mental health problems. Such screenings should take into account other prescription drugs being used by methadone clients so that the impact of multiple drug use on the family can be explored. Positive assessments of these problems would not exclude families from participation in the program but might indicate the need for a broader array of services. The assessment can also help case managers identify limitations they may face in helping certain families. Third, and perhaps most important, specialists working with this population must consider not only the addicted parent but also the entire family as the client. It is often easy, given the crisis-prone nature of these families, to focus on treatment issues for the parents and overlook the risk potential for the children. A clear and ever-present focus must be on the children as well as on the parents.

Finally, this intensive and coordinated program requires a high level of commitment on the part of the parent trainers, case managers, and treatment professionals. For too long, the fields of treatment and prevention have been viewed as separate and distinct. The FOF staff depended on developing strong bonds with treatment providers. Quarterly coordinating meetings assisted in this effort. FOF staff members attended monthly all-staff meetings at the treatment agency and were considered adjunct staff members. The development of clear lines of communication between treatment and prevention strengthened the trusting relationship. This strong link with the treatment agency provided the foundation a reason for continuing this selective prevention intervention after the study was completed.

Breaking the cycle of intergenerational addiction can be approached while parents are in treatment by targeting both parents' and their children's risk for future drug abuse. Successful interventions seek to reduce factors that place youth at risk for drug abuse and factors that place parents at risk for relapse while enhancing factors that mitigate or protect against drug abuse. FOF is a program designed to use these principles to prevent drug abuse by children of drug addicts. Training parents during their own treatment to act as prevention agents for their children holds promise for intervening and breaking the cycle of addiction.

APPENDIX: CURRICULA REVIEWED IN FOCUS
ON FAMILIES DEVELOPMENT

Addict Aftercare: A Manual for Self-Help
Training (1985)
Fred Zackon & William Mcaullife, Ch'ien,
J.M.N.
Department of Behavorial Sciences,
Harvard School of Public Health,
Boston, MA

Catch 'Em Being Good (1983)
Susan P. McCarthy & Edward O. Brown
National Institute for Juvenile Justice
and Delinquency Prevention,
Office of Juvenile Justice and
Delinquency Prevention, Washington, DC

Developing Capable People (1991)
H. Stephen Glenn with Jane Nelson
Sunset Books, Tapes, & Videos, Provo, UT

Effective Black Parenting (1990)
Kirby Alvy, Ph.D., & Marilyn K. Marigana,
M.S.W.
Center for the Improvement of Child Caring,
Studio City, CA

Growing Up Again: Parenting Ourselves,
Parenting our Children (1989)
Jean Illsley Clarke & Connie Dawson
Hazelden Books, HarperCollins,
New York, NY

Los Niños Bien Educados
Kirby Alvy, Ph.D., & Lupita Montoya
Tannatt, M.Ed.
Center for the Improvement of Child Caring,
Studio City, CA

Nurturing Program for Families and Parents
(1985)
Stephen Bavolek, Ph.D., & Christine
Comstock
Family Development Resources, Inc., Eau
Claire, WI

The Parents & Children Videotape Series
(1989)
Carolyn Webster-Stratton
University of Washington, School of Nursing,
Seattle, WA

Parenting As Prevention: Weaving
Together Tradition, Knowledge and Hope
(1990)
Bostain & Associates
Washington State Division of Alcohol and
Substance Abuse, Olympia, Washington

Preparing for the Drug Free Years (1989)
J. D. Hawkins & R. F. Catalano
Developmental Research and Programs,
Seattle, WA

Project ADAPT: A Program For Successful
Reintegration of Institutionalized
Youth (1987)
Kathleen Burgoyne et al.
University of Washington,
Social Development Research Group,
Seattle, WA

Project AFTER: Alternatives for Teens
Through Education and Resources (1988)
Distributed by Seattle/King County Dept. of
Public Health
Kevin P. Haggerty et al.
University of Washington, School of Social
Work, Seattle, WA

Project Skills (1985)
Richard F. Catalano et al.
University of Washington, Seattle, WA

Strengthening Families Program (1989)
Karol L. Kumpfer, Joseph DeMarsh, &
Wendy Child
University of Utah, Salt Lake City, UT

REFERENCES

Azuma, S. D., & Chasnoff, I. J. (1993). Outcome of children prenatally exposed to cocaine and other drugs: A path analysis of three-year data. *Pediatrics, 92,* 396–402.

Berstein, V., Jeremy, R. J., Hans, S. L., & Marcus, J. (1984). A longitudinal study of offspring born to methadone-maintained women: II. Dyadic interaction and infant behavior at 4 months. *American Journal of Drug and Alcohol Abuse, 10,* 161–193.

Brewer, D. D., Catalano, R. F., Haggerty, K. P., Gainey, R. R., & Fleming, C. B. (1998). A meta-analysis predictors of continued drug use during and after treatment for opiate addiction. *Addiction, 93,* 73–92.

Brewer, D. D., Fleming, C. B., Haggerty, K. P., & Catalano, R. F. (1998). Drug use predictors of partner violence in opiate-dependent women. *Violence and Victims, 13,* 107–115.

Brewer, D. D., Hawkins, J. D., Catalano, R. F., & Neckerman, H. J. (1995). Preventing serious, violent, and chronic juvenile offending: A review of selected strategies in childhood, adolescence, and the community. In J. C. Howell, B. Krisberg, J. D. Hawkins, & J. J. Wilson (Eds.), *A sourcebook: Serious, violent, and chronic juvenile offenders* (pp. 61–141). Thousand Oaks, CA: Sage.

Briar, S., & Conte, J. R. (1978). Families. In H. S. Mass (Ed.), *Social service research: Reviews of studies* (pp. 9–38). Washington, DC: National Association of Social Workers.

Brook, J. S., Brook, D. W., Gordon, A. S., Whiteman, M., & Cohen, P. (1990). The psychosocial etiology of adolescent drug use: A family interactional approach. *Genetic, Social, and General Psychology Monographs, 116* (Whole No. 2).

Brophy, J., & Good, T. L. (1986). Teacher behavior and student achievement. In M. C. Wittrock (Ed.), *Handbook of research on training* (3rd ed.) (pp. 328–375). New York: Macmillan.

Bry, B. H., & Krinsley, K. E. (1992). Booster sessions and long-term effects of behavioral family therapy on adolescent substance use and school performance. *Journal of Behavior Therapy and Experimental Psychiatry, 23,* 183–189.

Catalano, R. F., Gainey, R. R., Fleming, C. B., Haggerty, K. P., & Johnson, N. O. (1999). An experimental intervention with families of substance abusers: One-year follow-up of the Focus on Families project. *Addiction, 94,* 241–254.

Catalano, R. F., Haggerty, K. P., Fleming, C. B., Brewer, D. D., & Gainey, R. R. (2002). Children of substance-abusing parents: Current findings from the Focus on Families project. In R. J. McMahon & R. D. Peters (Eds.), *The Effects of Parental Dysfunction on Children* (pp. 179–204). New York: Kluwer Academic/Plenum Publishers.

Catalano, R. F., Haggerty, K. P., Gainey, R. R., & Hoppe, M. J. (1997). Reducing parental risk factors for children's substance misuse: Preliminary outcomes with opiate-addicted parents. *Substance Use and Misuse, 32,* 699–721.

Catalano, R. F., & Hawkins, J. D. (1996). The social development model: A theory of antisocial behavior. In J. D. Hawkins (Ed.), *Delinquency and crime: Current theories* (pp. 149–197). New York: Cambridge University Press.

Chamberlin, R., & Rapp, C. A. (1991). A decade of case management: A methodological review of outcome research. *Community Mental Health Journal, 27,* 171–187.

Chassin, L., Pillow, D. R., Curran, P. J., Molina, B. S. G., & Barrera, M., Jr. (1993). Relation of parental alcoholism to early adolescent substance use: A test of three mediating mechanisms. *Journal of Abnormal Psychology, 102,* 3–19.

DeMarsh, J., & Kumpfer, K. L. (1985). Family-oriented interventions for the prevention of chemical dependency in children and adolescents. In S. Griswold-Ezekoye, K. L. Kumpfer, & W. J. Bukoski (Eds.), *Childhood and chemical abuse: Prevention and intervention* (pp. 117–151). New York: Haworth.

Deren, S. (1986). Children of substance abusers: A review of the literature. *Journal of Substance Abuse Treatment, 3,* 77–94.

Dishion, T. J., & Andrews, D. W. (1995). Preventing escalation in problem behaviors with high-risk young adolescents: Immediate and 1-year outcomes. Special Section: Prediction and prevention of child and adolescent antisocial behavior. *Journal of Consulting and Clinical Psychology, 63,* 538–548.

Dryfoos, J. G. (1990). *Adolescents at risk: Prevalence and prevention.* New York: Oxford University Press.

Dumas, J. E. (1989). Treating antisocial behavior in children: Child and family approaches. *Clinical Psychology Review, 9,* 197–222.

Dunst, C. J., & Trivette, C. M. (1988). An enablement and empowerment perspective of case management. *Topics in Early Childhood Special Education, 8,* 87–102.

Epstein, J. L. (1994, October–November). *Perspectives and previews on research policy for school, family, and community partnerships.* Paper presented at national symposium, Family-school links: How do they affect educational outcomes? Penn State University.

Falco, M. (1992). *The making of a drug-free America: Programs that work.* New York: Times Books.

Felix-Ortiz, M., & Newcomb, M. D. (1999). Vulnerability for drug use among Latino adolescents. *Journal of Community Psychology, 27,* 257–280.

Fiks, K. B., Johnson, H. L., & Rosen, T. S. (1985). Methadone maintained mothers: Three-year follow-up of parental functioning. *International Journal of the Addictions, 20,* 651–660.

Firestone, P., & Witt, J. E. (1982). Characteristics of families completing and prematurely discontinuing a behavioral parent-training program. *Journal of Pediatric Psychology, 7,* 209–222.

Fleming, C. B., Brewer, D. D., Gainey, R. R., Haggerty, K. P., & Catalano, R. F. (1997). Parent drug use and bonding to parents as predictors of substance use in children of substance abusers. *Journal of Child and Adolescent Substance Abuse, 6,* 75–86.

Forehand, R. L., Griest, D., & Wells, K. C. (1979). Parent behavior training: An analysis of the relationship among multiple outcome measures. *Journal of Abnormal Child Psychology, 7,* 229–242.

Foshee, V., & Bauman, K. E. (1992). Parental and peer characteristics as modifiers of the bond-behavior relationship: An elaboration of control theory. *The Journal of Health and Social Behavior, 33,* 66–76.

Fraser, M., & Haapala, D. (1987/1988). Home-based family treatment: A quantitative-qualitative assessment. *The Journal of Applied Social Sciences, 12,* 1–22.

Fraser, M. W., Hawkins, J. D., & Howard, M. O. (1988). Parent training for delinquency prevention. *Family Perspectives in Child and Youth Services, 11,* 93–125.

Friedman, A. S. (1989). Family therapy vs. parent groups: Effects on adolescent drug abusers. *The American Journal of Family Therapy, 17,* 335–347.

Gainey, R. R., Catalano, R. F., Haggerty, K. P., & Hoppe, M. J. (1997). Deviance among the children of heroin addicts in treatment: Impact of parents and peers. *Deviant Behavior, 18,* 143–159.

Gittleman, R. S., Mannuzza, R. S., Shenker, R., & Bonagura, N. (1985). Hyperactive boys almost grown up: I. Psychiatric status. *Archives of General Psychiatry, 42,* 937–947.

Goldstein, A. P., & Kanfer, F. H. (1979). *Maximizing treatment gains: Transfer enhancement in psychotherapy.* New York: Academic Press.

Goodwin, D. W. (1985). Alcoholism and genetics: The sins of the fathers. *Archives of General Psychiatry, 42,* 171–174.

Gordon, I. J., & Guinagh, B. J. (1978). A home learning center approach to early stimulation. *JSAS Catalog of Selected Documents in Psychology, 8,* 6 (MS No. 1624).

Grady, K., Gersick, K., & Boratynski, M. (1986). Preparing parents for teenagers: A step in the prevention of substance abuse. *Journal of Drug Education, 16,* 203–220.

Grant, W. T. (1992). Consortium on the School-Based Promotion of Social Competence Drug and alcohol prevention curricula. In J. D. Hawkins, R. F. Catalano, & Associates, *Communities that care: Action for drug abuse prevention.* San Francisco: Jossey-Bass.

Grant, T. M., Ernst, C. C., Streissguth, A. P., Phibbs, P., & Gendler, B. (1996). When case management isn't enough: A model of paraprofessional advocacy for drug and alcohol abusing mothers. *The Journal of Case Management, 5*(1), 3–11.

Gray, S. W., & Ruttle, K. (1980). The Family-Oriented Home Visiting Program: A longitudinal study. *Genetic Psychology Monographs, 102,* 299–316.

Gross, J., & McCaul, M. E. (1992). An evaluation of a psychoeducational and substance abuse risk reduction intervention for children of substance abusers. *Journal of Community Psychology, OSAP Special Issue,* 75–87.

Haggerty, K. P., Wells, E. A., Jenson, J., Catalano, R. F., & Hawkins, J. D. (1989). Delinquents and drug use: A model program for community reintegration. *Adolescence, 24,* 439–456.

Hansen, W. B., Tobler, N. S., & Graham, J. W. (1990). Attrition in substance abuse prevention research: A meta-analysis of 85 longitudinally followed cohorts. *Evaluation Review, 14,* 677–685.

Haskett, M. E., Miller, J. W., Whitworth, J. M., & Huffman, J. M. (1992). Intervention with cocaine-abusing mothers. *Families in Society, 73,* 451–461.

Hawkins, J. D., Arthur, M. W., & Catalano, R. F. (1995). Preventing substance abuse. In M. Tonry & D. Farrington (Eds.), *Crime and Justice, Vol. 19, Building a safer society: Strategic approaches to crime prevention,* (pp. 343–427). Chicago: University of Chicago Press.

Hawkins, J. D., Catalano, R. F., Jones, G., & Fine, D. (1987). Delinquency prevention through parent training: Results and issues from work in progress. In J. Q. Wilson & G. C. Loury (Eds.), *From children to citizens: Vol. III. Families, schools, and delinquency prevention* (pp. 186–204). New York: Springer-Verlag.

Hawkins, J. D., Catalano, R. F., & Miller, J. Y. (1992). Risk and protective factors for alcohol and other drug problems in adolescence and early adulthood: Implications for substance abuse prevention. *Psychological Bulletin, 112,* 64–105.

Hawkins, J. D., Catalano, R. F., Morrison, D. M., O'Donnell, J., Abbott, R. D., & Day, L. E. (1992). The Seattle Social Development Project: Effects of the first four years on protective factors and problem behaviors. In J. McCord & R. E. Tremblay (Eds.), *Preventing antisocial behavior: Interventions from birth through adolescence* (pp. 139–161). New York: Guilford Press.

Hawkins, J. D., Catalano, R. F., & Wells, E. A. (1986). Measuring effects of a skills training intervention for drug abusers. *Journal of Consulting and Clinical Psychology, 54,* 661–664.

Hawkins, J. D., & Fraser, M. W. (1983). Social support networks in treating drug abuse. In J. K. Whittaker, J. Garbarino, & Associates (Eds.), *Social support networks: Informal helping in the human services* (pp. 355–380). New York: Aldine.

Hawkins, J. D., Graham, J. W., Maguin, E., Abbott, R. D., Hill, K. G., & Catalano, R. F. (1997). Exploring the effects of age of alcohol use initiation and psychosocial risk factors on subsequent alcohol misuse. *Journal of Studies on Alcohol, 58,* 280–290.

Hoppe, M. J., Wells, E. A., Haggerty, K. P., Simpson, E. E., Gainey, R. R., & Catalano, R. F. (1998). Bonding in a high-risk and a general sample of children: Comparison of measures of attachment and their relationship to smoking and drinking. *Journal of Youth and Adolescence, 27,* 59–82.

Johnston, L. D., O'Malley, P. M., & Bachman, J. G. (1985). *Use of licit and illicit drugs by America's high school students, 1975–1984.* Rockville, MD: National Institute on Drug Abuse.

Johnston, L. D., O'Malley, P. M., & Bachman, J. G. (1992). *Smoking, drinking, and illicit drug use among secondary school students, college students, and young adults: Vol. 1. Secondary school students.* Washington, DC: U.S. Department of Health and Human Services.

Kandel, D. B. (1982). Epidemiological and psychosocial perspectives on adolescent drug use. *Journal of the American Academy of Clinical Psychiatry, 21,* 328–347.

Kaplan, K. O. (1990). Recent trends in case management. In L. Ginsberg & K. Shanti (Eds.), *Encyclopedia of social work* (18th ed.) (pp. 60–77). Silver Spring, MD: National Association of Social Workers.

Kolar, A. F., Brown, B. S., Haertzen, C. A., & Michaelson, M. A. (1994). Children of substance abusers: The life experiences of children of opiate addicts in methadone maintenance. *American Journal of Drug and Alcohol Abuse, 20,* 159–171.

Kumpfer, K. L. (1987). Special populations: Etiology and prevention of vulnerability to chemical dependency in children of substance abusers. In B. S. Brown & A. R. Mills (Eds.), *Youth at high risk for substance abuse* (pp. 1–72). Washington, DC: U.S. Government Printing Office.

Kumpfer, K. L. (1999). Factors and processes contributing to resilience: The resilience framework. In M. D. Glantz, & J. L. Johnson (Eds.), *Resilience and development: Positive life adaptations. Longitudinal research in the social and behavioral sciences* (pp. 179–224). New York: Kluwer Academic.

Kumpfer, K. L., & DeMarsh, J. P. (1986). Family environmental and genetic influences on children's future chemical dependency. In S. Ezekoye, K. Kumpfer, & W. Bukoski (Eds.), *Childhood and chemical abuse: Prevention and intervention* (pp. 49–91). New York: Haworth.

Lerner, J. V., & Vicary, J. R. (1984). Difficult temperament and drug use: Analyses from the New York longitudinal study. *Journal of Drug Education, 14,* 1–8.

Lewis, C. E., Robins, L. N., & Rice, J. (1985). Association of alcoholism with antisocial personality in urban men. *Journal of Nervous and Mental Disease, 173,* 166–174.

Loeber, R., & Dishion, T. (1983). Early predictors of male delinquency: A review. *Psychological Bulletin, 93,* 68–99.

Loeber, R., & Stouthamer-Loeber, M. S. (1986). Family factors as correlates and predictors of juvenile conduct problems and delinquency. In M. Tonry & N. Morris (Eds.), *Crime and justice: An annual review of research* (Vol. 7, pp. 29–149). Chicago: University of Chicago Press.

Marlatt, G. A., & Gordon, J. R. (1985). *Relapse prevention: Maintenance strategies in the treatment of addictive behaviors.* New York: Guilford.

McCord, J. (1979). Some child-rearing antecedents of criminal behavior in adult men. *Journal of Personality and Social Psychology, 37,* 1477–1486.

Mercer, R. T. (1990). *Parents at risk.* New York: Springer.

Miller, W. R., & Rollnick, S. (1991). *Motivational interviewing: Preparing people to change addictive behavior.* New York: Guilford.

Moos, R. H., Bromet, E., Tsu, V., & Moos, B. (1979). Family characteristics and the outcome of treatment for alcoholism. *Journal of Studies on Alcohol, 40,* 78–88.

Mrazek, P. J., & Haggerty, R. J., Eds.; Committee on Prevention of Mental Disorders, Institute of Medicine. (1994). *Reducing risks for mental disorders: Frontiers for prevention intervention research.* Washington, D. C.: National Academy Press.

Newcomb, M. D., Abbott, R. D., Catalano, R. F., Hawkins, J. D., & Battin, S. R. (2002). *Mediational and deviance theories of high school failure: Process roles of structural strains, academic competence, and general versus specific problem behaviors. Journal of Counseling Psychology, 49,* 172–186.

Newcomb, M. D., Maddahian, E., Skager, R., & Bentler, P. M. (1987). Substance abuse and psychosocial risk factors among teenagers: Associations with sex, age, ethnicity, and type of school. *American Journal of Drug and Alcohol Abuse, 13,* 413–433.

Olds, D. L., & Kitzman, H. J. (1990). Can home visitation improve the health of women and children at environmental risk? *Pediatrics, 86,* 108–116.

Patterson, G. R. (1974). Interventions for boys with conduct problems: Multiple settings, treatments, and criteria. *Journal of Consulting and Clinical Psychology, 42,* 471–481.

Patterson, G. R. (1982). The management of disruption in families. In G. R. Patterson (Ed.), A social learning approach: Vol. 3. *Coercive family process* (pp. 215–236). Eugene, OR: Castalia.

Patterson, G. R., Chamberlain, P., & Reid, J. B. (1982). A comparative evaluation of a parent training program. *Behavior Therapy, 13,* 638–650.

Patterson, G. R., & Dishion, T. J. (1985). Contributions of families and peers to delinquency. *Criminology, 23,* 63–79.

Patterson, G. R., & Fleishman, M. J. (1979). Maintenance of treatment effects: Some considerations concerning family systems and follow-up data. *Behavior Therapy, 10,* 168–185.

Patterson, G. R., & Reid, J. B. (1973). Intervention for families of aggressive boys: A replication study. *Behavior Research Therapy, 11,* 383–394.

Plotnick, R. D. (1994). Applying benefit-cost analysis to substance use prevention programs. *International Journal of the Addictions, 29,* 339–359.

Plotnick, R. D., Young, D. S., Catalano, R. F., & Haggerty, K. P. (1998). Benefits and costs of a family-focused methadone treatment and drug abuse prevention program: Preliminary findings. In W. J. Bukoski & R. I. Evans (Eds.), NIDA Research Monograph: Vol. 176 *Cost benefit/cost effectiveness research of drug abuse prevention: Implications for programming and policy* (pp. 161–183). Rockville, MD: National Institute on Drug Abuse.

Radke-Yarrow, M., & Sherman, T. (1990). Children born at medical risk: Factors affecting vulnerability and resilience. In J. Rolf, A. S. Masten, D. Cicchetti, K. H. Nuechterlein, & S. Weintraub (Eds.), *Risk and protective factors in the development of psychopathology* (pp. 97–119). Cambridge, England: Cambridge University Press.

Rapp, R. C., Siegal, H. A., & Fisher, J. H. (1992). A strengths-based model of case management/advocacy: Adapting a mental health model to practice work with persons who have substance abuse problems. In R. S. Ashety (Ed.), NIDA Research Monograph: Vol. 127. *Progress and issues in case management* (pp. 79–91). Rockville, MD: National Institute on Drug Abuse.

Reid, J. B. (1993). Prevention of conduct disorder before and after school entry: Relating interventions to developmental findings. *Development and Psychopathology, 5,* 243–262.

Resnick, M. D., Bearman, P. S., Blum, R. W., Bauman, K. E., Harris, K. M., Jones, J., Tabor, J., Beuhring, T., Sieving, R. E., Shew, M., Ireland, M., Bearinger, L. H., & Udry, J. R. (1997). Protecting adolescents from harm: Findings from the National Longitudinal Study on Adolescent Health. *JAMA, 278,* 823–832.

Robins, L. N. (1980). The natural history of drug abuse. *Acta Psychiatrica Scandinavica, 62*(Suppl. 284), 7–20.

Rose, M., Battjes, R., & Leukefeld, C. (1984). *Family life skills training for drug abuse prevention* (NIDA Publication). Washington, DC: US Government Printing Office.

Rosenthal, T., & Bandura, A. (1978). Psychological modeling: Theory and practice. In S. Garfield, & A. E. Bergin (Eds.), *Handbook of psychotherapy and behavior change: An empirical analysis.* New York: Wiley.

Russell, F. F., & Free, T. A. (1991). Early intervention for infants and toddlers with prenatal drug exposure. *Infants and Young Children, 3,* 78–132.

Rutter, M. (1980). *Changing youth in a changing society.* Cambridge, MA: Harvard University Press.

Rutter, M. (1985). Resilience in the face of adversity: Protective factors and resistance to psychiatric disturbance. *British Journal of Psychiatry, 147,* 598–611.

Serketich, W. J., & Dumas, J. E. (1996). The effectiveness of behavioral parent training to modify antisocial behavior in children: A meta-analysis. *Behavior Therapy, 27,* 171–186.

Shedler, J., & Block, J. (1990). Adolescent drug use and psychological health: A longitudinal inquiry. *American Psychologist, 45,* 612–630.

Simcha-Fagan, O., Gersten, J. C., & Langner, T. (1986). Early precursors and concurrent correlates of illicit drug use in adolescents. *Journal of Drug Issues, 16,* 7–28.

Sloboda, Z., & David, S. L. (1996). *Preventing drug use among children and adolescents: A research-based guide.* Rockville, MD: National Institute on Drug Abuse.

Sowder, B. J., & Burt, M. R. (1980). *Children of heroin addicts: An assessment of health, learning behavioral, and adjustment problems.* New York: Praeger.

Spieker, S. J., & Booth, C. L. (1988). Maternal antecedents of attachment quality. In J. Belsky & T. Nezworski (Eds.), *Clinical implications of attachment* (pp. 95–134). Hillsdale, NJ: Erlbaum.

Spoth, R., & Redmond, C. (1994). Effective recruitment of parents into family-focused prevention research: A comparison of two strategies. *Psychology and Health, 9,* 353–370.

Spoth, R., Redmond, C., Haggerty, K., & Ward, T. (1995, May). A controlled parenting skills outcome study examining individual difference and attendance effects. *Journal of Marriage and the Family, 57,* 449–464.

Springer, F., Phillips, J., Phillips, L., Cannady, L. P., & Derst-Harris, E. (1992). CODA: A creative therapy program for children in families affected by abuse of alcohol or other drugs. *Journal of Community Psychology, OSAP Special Issue,* 55–74.

Stanton, M. D., & Todd, T. C. (1982). *The family therapy of drug abuse and addiction.* New York: Guilford.

Stark, M. J. (1989). A psychoeducational approach to methadone treatment. *Journal of Substance Abuse Treatment, 6,* 169–181.

Surgeon General (1988). *The health consequences of smoking: Nicotine addiction.* A report of the Surgeon General. Rockville, MD: U.S. Department of Health and Human Services.

Tableman, B., & Katzenmeyer, M. (1985). *Infant mental health services: A newborn screener.* Lansing, MI: Michigan Department of Mental Health.

Tremblay, R. E., Vitaro, F., Bertrand, L., LeBlanc, M., Beauchesne, H., Boileau, H., & David, L. (1992). Parent and child training to prevent early onset of delinquency: The Montreal Longitudinal-Experimental Study. In J. McCord & R. Tremblay (Eds.), *Preventing antisocial behavior: Interventions from birth through adolescence* (pp. 117–138). New York: Guilford.

Wasik, B. H., Bryant, D. M., & Lyons, C. M. (1990). *Home visiting: Procedures for helping families.* Newbury Park, CA: Sage.

Weng, L., Newcomb, M. D., & Bentler, P. M. (1988). Factors influencing noncompletion of high schools: A comparison of methodologies. *Educational Research Quarterly, 12,* 8–22.

Werner, E. E. (1989). High-risk children in young adulthood: A longitudinal study from birth to 32 years. *American Journal of Community Psychology, 9,* 411–423.

W. T. Grant Consortium on the School-Based Promotion of Social Competence. (1992). Drug and alcohol prevention curricula. In J. D. Hawkins, R. F. Catalano, Jr., & Associates (Eds.), *Communities That Care. Action for drug abuse prevention* (pp. 129–148). San Francisco: Jossey-Bass.

Yoshikawa, H. (1994). Prevention as cumulative protection: Effects of early family support and education on chronic delinquency and its risks. *Psychological Bulletin, 115,* 28–54.

PART III

PREVENTION AS SOCIAL CONTROL

CHAPTER 10

Drug Tests in Prevention Research

ROBERT L. DUPONT
KEITH E. SAYLOR

INTRODUCTION

If you know that you might be tested for drugs and that testing positive means that you could lose your job, or your scholarship, or face other unpleasant consequences, you might decide not to use drugs. This seems logical and suggests that drug testing could be a useful tool in preventing drug abuse in some settings. However, the role of drug testing in prevention research has not been widely studied. Most prevention outcome studies continue to rely on self-reports of drug use even though it is well known that many drug users, from occasional users to hard-core addicts, under-report their drug use (Wish, Hoffman, & Nemes, 1997). For example, less than half of the alcohol consumed in the United States can be explained through population studies based on self-reports (DuPont, 1997a). The same is true for tobacco consumption. Unlike illicit drugs, for which consumption must be estimated, good data exist on the actual amount of both alcohol and tobacco consumed annually. When it comes to illicit substance use, especially now when illicit drug use is more highly stigmatized than in previous years, the probability of accurate responses to questions about recent use is lower than that for licit substance use, even in anonymous settings (Wish, 1998).

The need to overcome potential under-reporting of recent drug use is the reason drug treatment programs and the criminal justice system have used drug testing for more than 2 decades. For the same reason, drug testing has become widespread in the American workplace in the past decade (Office of National Drug Control Policy, 1998).

There are many reasons why most research on drug use has not used drug testing more widely (General Accounting Office, 1993). Drug tests provide evidence of recent use of specific drugs

ROBERT L. DUPONT • Institute for Behavior and Health, Inc.; Bensinger, DuPont & Associates, Rockville, Maryland 20852
KEITH E. SAYLOR • NeuroScience, Inc., Bethesda, Maryland 20814

but do not reveal patterns of use over time, the amount of drugs used, or information about drug dependence and other consequences of drug use. There is also concern about the accuracy and reliability of drug tests, about the intrusiveness of sample collection, about racial bias, about the possibility that passive exposure could lead to positive drug test results, and finally, about the costs of drug tests. And there are other limitations. Drug tests typically identify a far narrower range of drugs than do self-reports. Drug tests may be negative even when a subject has recently used a specific drug. Drug tests provide no information about the route of administration, the costs of drug use, or the subject's reasons for using drugs. When the self-report is positive and the drug test is negative, the self-report is likely to be correct. When a self-report is negative for recent drug use and the drug test is positive (a more common occurrence), it means either that the subject did not know that he or she was taking a particular drug (not a rare occurrence for illicit drugs) or that the subject chose not to report the use. Despite these concerns and limitations, drug testing can provide valuable information that supplements the information found in self-reports. Drug tests are not a way of validating (or impeaching) self-reports but of providing different and important data on a subject's drug use in the days or months prior to the test, information that can be useful in prevention research.

This chapter reviews these and related issues, the literature on drug testing, psychological mechanisms associated with drug testing in prevention, and the biology of drug tests.

LITERATURE REVIEW

Although the literature on drug testing is voluminous, we are aware of no studies that specifically address the role of drug testing in prevention research. There is evidence, however, that drug testing reduces drug use when used in settings in which drug use is relatively *common* or at least considered normative. In these situations, drug testing is considered a deterrent to further use for those who already use and a prevention tool for those who do not use yet but may be considering it. In either case, drug use as a whole is reduced by the possibility of testing.

What is missing in the prevention literature is a true test of the role of drug testing in prevention. Such research would assess the impact of drug testing on drug use in a cohort at risk for drug use but in which drug use at the start of the study is relatively *uncommon*. Subjects assigned randomly to drug testing or no testing would be compared over time to see the prevalence of nonmedical drug use in each group. Although it is widely believed that the rate of new drug use and the overall prevalence of drug use would be far lower for the group subject to drug testing, no study can yet make this claim.

Given the existing literature about drug testing and the prevalence of drug use, it could be argued that such randomized studies are unnecessary. Drug testing could be assumed to have proved its value in a variety of circumstances and that any attempt to use it in prevention is justified. The cost and policy implications of drug testing, coupled with the heated philosophical arguments for and against the use of drug tests, give credibility to both the ardent empiricists and those who say they argue from a more practical perspective. Instead of attempting to decide these arguments, this chapter describes the current state of drug testing and its associated pros and cons.

Because of the enormous emotional and financial costs associated with drug use and addiction, there is clearly a need for effective methods to reduce drug use. The *Monitoring the Future* surveys of college and secondary-school students show a reversal beginning in 1992 in the long-term downward trend of drug use by youth (Johnston, 1996, 1997; Johnston, O'Malley, & Bachman, 1996). Approximately 12.8 million Americans aged 12 and older use illegal drugs on a past-month basis (Office of National Drug Control Policy, 1998). Seventy-one percent of illicit drug users aged 18 and older are employed either full time (5.4 million workers) or part time (1.9 million workers) (Substance Abuse and Mental Health Services Administration (SAMHSA), 1996).

The effects of illicit drug use on the job include increased absenteeism (Normand, Salyards, & Mahoney, 1990; Winkler & Sheridan, 1989), higher accident rates (Crouch et al., 1989) and increased use of medical benefits (Winkler & Sheridan, 1989). A study by the U.S. Postal Service showed that absenteeism is 66% higher among drug users, use of health benefits is 84% greater in dollar terms, disciplinary actions are 90% higher, and there is significantly higher employee turnover (National Institute on Drug Abuse (NIDA), 1990). Drug-using employees are more likely to have had three or more employers in the past year than are those who do not use drugs (32.1 vs. 17.9%); to have taken an unexcused absence from work in the past month (12.1 vs. 6.1%); to have voluntarily quit work in the past year (25.8 vs. 13.6%); and/or to have been fired in the past year (4.6 vs. 1.4%) (de Bernardo, 1998; SAMHSA, 1997). In 1991, the reported cost of drug abuse to the business community was $75 billion annually, or approximately $640 per employed person, based on 117 million U.S. workers (Tasco, 1991).

In response to the problem of illicit drug use and its associated costs, many employers have established drug-testing programs. Some adopted drug testing only after failed attempts at other approaches (such as employee assistance or addiction treatment). In 1997 more than 40 million workplace drug tests were conducted in the United States, a 1,000% increase in the past 10 years (Lappe, 1998). Purposes for drug testing in the workplace include pre-employment detection of illicit drug use, determination of fitness to work, maintenance of workplace safety, and confirmation of suspected illicit drug or alcohol use. Drug tests can also serve as a prevention tool, as a referral mechanism to addiction treatment programs, or as a complement to other policies regarding substance use in the workplace (Moreland & McPhaul, 1988).

Those who adopt drug-screening programs must weigh the benefits against the costs. Benefits include increased attendance, higher productivity, and fewer accidents (Cohen (1984) cited in Crant & Bateman (1989)). Costs include technical, ethical, and legal concerns (e.g., Crown & Rosse, 1988; Dogoloff & Angarola, 1985), such as questions about the efficacy and fairness of drug-testing programs (Crant & Bateman, 1989), the reliability of drug tests, and issues surrounding privacy and confidentiality (Bible & McWhirter, 1990). These concerns are addressed later in this chapter (DuPont, 1997b), but it is important to point out that effective drug-testing programs are achieved through diligent attention to quality control, documentation, chain of custody, technical expertise, and ability to produce data that are secure from false positives (Hawks, 1986). Laboratories that perform drug-detection services must comply with established procedures and guidelines, such as the Mandatory Guidelines for Federal Workplace Drug Testing Programs (1994).

Drug Testing in the Workplace

FEDERAL AND PRIVATE SECTORS. In government agencies workplace drug testing has become more common since federal guidelines were established through the Drug-Free Workplace Act in 1988 (Willette, 1986). The federal government tests about 345,00 employees in sensitive positions (including agency heads, presidential appointees, law enforcement officers, and employees with access to classified information or in positions involving national security) in 42 executive branch agencies (U.S. Department of Justice, 1992). The Department of Transportation tests another 30,000 workers, including air traffic controllers (U.S. Department of Justice, 1992). The four U.S. military services test all applicants and most service personnel on active duty. The federal government also requires drug testing in many regulated industries, such as defense contracting and nuclear energy.

Less is known about the extent of private-sector efforts, since most information has been drawn from small segments of private industry with samples that do not represent employers as a whole (Hayghe, 1990). Generally, larger companies (those with more than 1,000 employees) are more likely than small businesses (those with fewer than 50 employees) to have drug-testing programs and employee assistance programs (EAPs). For example, 43% of large businesses had drug-testing programs compared to only 2% of small firms (U.S. Department of Labor, 1989). Similarly, 76 versus 9% had EAPs. Relatively few employees are tested for drugs, even when a workplace drug-testing program exists (Hayghe, 1990). Most workplace drug-testing programs (85%) target job applicants rather than employees. Programs that test current employees focus primarily on those who are suspected of substance abuse or are in safety-sensitive jobs.

The consequences for testing positive for illicit drugs vary from company to company. Drug-positive employees may be terminated immediately or may be required to enroll in an EAP or seek treatment or counseling. Those who do not complete treatment successfully or who test positive for drugs a second time may be fired (Willette, 1986). In a sample of 1,090 companies, 8% fired employees for the first positive drug tests, and the remainder either suspended employees or gave warnings along with EAP referrals (Masi, 1987). Other surveys found that 22% of companies immediately fired drug-positive employees, 21% either suspended employees or put them on probation, and 70% issued referrals for treatment or counseling (Greenberg, 1988, 1989, 1990). Although little research has been conducted on sanctions for drug use in the workplace, other studies on the effect of sanctions on illicit behaviors found that outcome expectations play a significant role in behavior (Bandura, 1986; Harris & Heft, 1992). If the anticipated outcome of drug use at work is job loss, employees would be less likely to use drugs. It follows that companies that terminate drug-positive employees will have less drug use than companies that use progressive discipline (Blum et al., 1992).

Programs in both the federal and private sectors have reduced the number of workers who test positive. In large and midsize companies, the rate of drug-positive test results decreased from 4.2% in 1990 to 2.7% in 1991 (Drug Testing Soars, 1992). Federal Aviation Administration data show a drop from 0.95% in 1992 to 0.82% in 1993 (Peat, 1995). Drug use in the U.S. military services has dropped dramatically as a result of a random drug-testing program based on standardized testing procedures, rehabilitation, and strict disciplinary action (Peat, 1995; Willette, 1986). Six worldwide surveys report nearly a 90% decrease in drug use by military personnel since 1980 (Substance Abuse in the Military, 1996).

For many businesses, urine drug testing has resulted in significant economic benefits, especially from decreased absenteeism and employee turnover. For industry, major direct costs linked to drug abuse include accidents, health and welfare services, worker's compensation, insurance claims, and property damages. Although both direct and indirect costs are large, there is no consensus on how large (Lehman & Simpson, 1990). However, a longitudinal study conducted by the U.S. Postal Service reported savings of more than $100 million on one annual set of new employees over a 10-year period, or about $19,000 savings for each drug-positive applicant not hired (Peat, 1995).

Much of the available literature on drug-testing programs focuses on the workplace because of the severity of the problem and its associated costs, as well as the enormous potential for positive change. Other areas, however, also are receiving increased attention, including the criminal justice system, athletic programs, and high schools and colleges. The U.S. Supreme Court recently concluded 6 to 3 that mandatory random testing is constitutionally acceptable in public school athletes (*Vernonia School District 47J v. Wayne Acton*, 1995).

Drug Testing in the Criminal Justice System

The criminal justice system uses drug testing to detect illicit drug use in arrestees, probationers, parolees, and inmates. The purposes of this drug testing are to deter drug use, to reduce criminal behavior, to ensure public safety, to reduce prison overcrowding by referring drug users to treatment programs, and to track trends in drug use (U.S. Department of Justice, 1992; Wish, 1988a,b). The results of drug tests are used to make decisions about bail, personal recognizance, compliance with parole or probation conditions, and violations of prison drug use rules (Collins, 1990).

Reliable drug-testing programs in the criminal justice system help ensure that offenders are held accountable for their drug use. Random drug testing with escalating sanctions for repeat positive tests deters drug use (Bureau of Justice Assistance, 1991). Typically, offenders are informed in writing about the consequences (such as revocation of parole or other administrative sanctions) of either a positive test or a refusal to be tested (Bureau of Justice Assistance, 1991). Criminal justice officials report that urinalysis programs have had a deterrent effect on drug use (Collins, 1990). Drug-court programs in which frequent, random drug testing (ranging from once a week to five times a week) and continuous supervision are key components have been especially successful in preventing drug use. Participants in drug-court programs reduce drug use substantially while in the program; and 50 to 65% eliminate use completely (Drug Court Clearinghouse and Technical Assistance Project (DCCTAP), 1997). Furthermore, recidivism for drug-court participants ranges between 5 and 28% and is lower than 4% for graduates, compared with a 45% recidivism rate for nonparticipating defendants (DCCTAP, 1997).

Drug Testing in Athletic Programs

In response to heightened awareness of drug use among athletes, the National Collegiate Athletic Association and many of its affiliated universities have implemented mandatory drug-testing programs for student athletes. These programs protect the health and safety of all competitors, provide assistance for those found to engage in substance abuse, and prevent an unfair competitive edge by those who abuse certain performance-enhancing substances (University Policy Statement, 1987). The same applies to drug testing of professional and Olympic athletes (Skolnick, 1996). Drug-positive athletes may be suspended immediately from participation or may be referred for counseling and then re-tested randomly.

Tested athletes show significantly less marijuana, LSD, and barbiturate use than do nontested athletes (Coombs & Ryan, 1990). Nearly two-thirds of athletes (62.4%) believe that drug testing is effective in preventing drug use, and 76% think that mandatory testing deters some athletes from using drugs (Coombs & Ryan, 1990). Many athletes are motivated to stay drug free in order to maintain athletic scholarships or their standing on the team. More than half (52.8%) said that drug testing gave them a socially acceptable excuse for refusing drugs (Coombs & Ryan, 1990). Despite drug testing, however, some athletes continue to use drugs, their rationale being that drug testing is not foolproof and that the consequences rarely are severe—often only a warning for first offences (Coombs & Ryan, 1990). However, drug testing is expected to increase in athletics despite the limitations these programs have (Jacobs & Samuels, 1995).

Drug Testing of Youth

The incidence of drug use among youth has grown since 1991. For example, lifetime illicit drug use among eighth-graders is up 57% from 18.7 to 29.4% over the past 6 years (Johnston, 1997). In 1995, 10.9% of all youngsters 12 to 17 years of age had used illicit drugs in the past month, compared with 8.2% in 1994, 5.7% in 1993, and 5.3% in 1992 (SAMHSA, 1996). The 1997 *Monitoring the Future* study reported that more than half (54.3%) of all high school students have used illicit drugs by the time they graduate (Johnston, 1997). Because adolescents typically do not refer themselves for assessments of illicit drug use, mandatory drug-testing programs may serve to detect current users or to prevent drug use altogether. Use of random drug-testing programs is growing in high schools and colleges, although this practice is far from widespread (Fudala et al., 1994).

Home-drug-testing kits using either urine or hair samples are also available. Like athletes, adolescents who are subject to drug testing at home or at school may use the tests as a socially acceptable excuse not to use drugs. Or the expectation of being drug tested may prevent them from initiating illicit drug use or continuing occasional use.

PSYCHOLOGICAL MECHANISMS OF DRUG TESTING: A SOCIAL COGNITIVE PERSPECTIVE

How do a person's beliefs, observations, attitudes, and behaviors shape perceptions about the power and persuasiveness of drug testing and its associated consequences? Because there are no empirical reports about these psychological mechanisms of action, this discussion relies primarily on the tenets of social cognitive theory to explain how the specter of drug testing might result in successful regulation of behavior through cognitive mediation.

Social cognitive theory proposes that behavior is shaped through interaction among behavioral, cognitive, and environmental factors (Bandura, 1986). Within the social cognitive framework, individuals are not passive actors but rather take part actively in creating their environment. Two distinguishing features of social cognitive theory especially germane to this discussion are outcome expectations and perceived self-efficacy, both of which are crucial to successful behavioral management and change.

Outcome Expectations

One's behavior is regulated largely by the anticipated or experienced outcomes (Bandura, 1986). For someone who is contemplating whether to use drugs, an *outcome expectation* is a judgment about the likely consequences of engaging, or not, in drug use. If a person knows that he or she might be tested for drugs and that unpleasant consequences are attached to a positive test result, the outcome expectancy may be sufficient to inhibit drug use. The outcome expectation would be further enhanced if the individual believed that the test was precise and fair and had seen people similar to himself or herself experience adverse consequences related to drug use. The judgments attached to the decision not to use drugs would compete against the outcome expectancies in favor of use, such as peer approval, feelings of affiliation, and the good feelings expected from use of the drug. For workers committed to keeping their jobs, for athletes who want to remain in competition, or for persons in the military who wish to avoid discipline or discharge, the drug test may serve as a prevention tool in that the outcome expectations for nonuse override the anticipated outcomes for use.

Perceived Self-Efficacy

Motivation and behavior are influenced not only by expected outcomes but also by an individual's judgment about the level of performance that he or she can achieve. *Perceived self-efficacy* is a judgment about one's capability to act in a way that brings about a desired outcome (Bandura, 1986). Self-efficacy differs across areas or domains in a person's life. For example, a person may have a high level of confidence about his or her athletic performance but low levels of confidence about maintaining good eating habits. Within domains (such as exercise or diet), a person's self-efficacy varies depending on the specifics of different situations. Beliefs about athletic performance on one's home turf, for example, may be higher than percepts about performance when playing out of town. A sense of personal efficacy enables control over events. Self-doubt may intrude on an individual's efforts to change, but a strong sense of self-efficacy can bolster efforts even in the face of uncertain outcomes.

Self-efficacy can be increased through various feedback sources, such as verbal persuasion, behavioral rehearsal, and actual accomplishment. A sense of personal competency is enhanced by experiences of progressive mastery or goal attainments. Actions associated with positive internal and external experiences usually are repeated, whereas those associated with negative internal and external experiences are discontinued (Bandura, 1986). Individuals who know that a drug test is forthcoming may act in a way to ensure that they won't get caught. For example, to avoid a positive drug test at work or school, a person may refuse drugs offered in a social setting. Or an occasional user may use drugs at a party, get caught through a drug test at work, and decide to forgo future use to avoid getting caught again and possibly losing his or her job. The drug test thus serves as an inducement to practice stricter behavioral management, which would increase and generalize self-percepts of coping efficacy.

WHY USE DRUG TESTS IN RESEARCH?

It is reasonable to question why prevention researchers should consider measuring drug use with a biological assay. Biological specimens may be messy and uncomfortable to obtain, and the adoption of testing requires that the researcher learn about a new and perhaps intimidating domain of information and costly techniques. If research participants could be relied upon to provide accurate histories of their drug use, drug testing might not be necessary. There are a number of reasons, however, that can make people unable or unwilling to report their drug use accurately. First and foremost, possession and sale of many drugs of abuse are illegal acts, involving severe criminal sanctions. Second, the admission of illicit drug use may place a person at risk for school suspension, job loss, or political reprisal. Third, substance abuse is often marked by extreme denial of the existence of a problem or even denial of drug use. Finally, even if a person is willing to report drug use, the uncontrolled nature of the illicit drug marketplace makes it impossible for the purchaser to know exactly what substance is obtained. Given these barriers to accurate reporting, it is not surprising that researchers using biological measures of drug use have frequently found that their subjects substantially underreport their use of drugs.

The measurement of drug use by structured research interviews has been an established technique in the social sciences. Numerous studies conducted in the 1970s and early 1980s concluded that respondents provide valid information about their illicit drug use when the interviews are conducted by trained interviewers in a nonthreatening setting and when the respondents feel reasonably secure that their disclosures will not result in adverse consequences (Harrell, 1985; Hubbard et al., 1989). Indeed, the federal government spends millions of dollars on surveys of household members and student populations that rely solely on respondents' willingness to report their illicit drug use accurately (General Accounting Office, 1993).

Now, researchers have begun to question the early assumptions about the validity of self-reports of drug use. Most of the validity studies were based primarily on indirect measures of validity, usually assessments of internal consistency or the construct validity of responses. If a respondent's reports of drug use were internally consistent or correlated with other variables in theoretically expected ways (construct validity), the findings were interpreted as supporting the validity of the drug use self-reports. However, an important limitation of such indirect estimates of validity is that a respondent who lied consistently during the interview would have been judged to be providing valid responses. Thus, a person who underreported both his or her drug use and other deviant behaviors would have exhibited the expected correlation between low drug use and low deviance. (See Magura et al., (1987) for an example of such a spurious relationship.) The same spurious association would be found if respondents were prone to over-reporting deviance and drug use.

Even attempts to validate self-reported drug use by comparisons with official record information may lead to what at first glance appears to be evidence of the validity of self-reported drug use information. For example, Wish (1988a,b) found the expected relationship between self-reported drug dependence and the number of prior drug arrests in respondents' criminal justice records in an arrestee cohort in which there was considerable under-reporting of recent drug use in comparison to the urine-test results.

The substantial technological advances that have been made in the sensitivity of biological measures of recent drug use have provided researchers with new tools to measure recent drug use directly and to estimate validity more accurately. However, while urine-test results have been used by researchers for almost 25 years to validate self-reports of drug use, the technology has improved so much that the new findings cast doubt on the findings of the early validity studies (Mieczkowski, 1990).

The first urine drug tests used a process called thin-layer chromatography (TLC), a time-consuming and subjective laboratory test. As drug tests were perfected and became more sensitive and easier to interpret, it became clear that TLC had greatly underdetected the recent use of drugs, especially cocaine and opiates (Wish et al., 1993). Because TLC underdetected the use of these drugs, the concordance between self-reported use and the urine tests was inflated in persons who were concealing their drug use. Drug users who reported that they had not used a drug appeared to be telling the truth because the TLC failed to detect the drug in their urine samples. The early urinalysis-based validity studies conducted before the advent of the more sensitive immunoassay screening tests were likely to overestimate the validity of the self-reports of drug use.

The social changes that have occurred with regard to attitudes toward illicit drug use may also have lessened the applicability of the findings from the early validity studies. Since the beginning of the cocaine and crack epidemic and related street violence in the mid-1980s, and the emerging AIDS epidemic among injection drug users (IDUs), the public has become more intolerant of drug use (Musto, 1991). The earlier studies of the validity of self-reports of drug use were conducted at times when individuals may have been more likely than now to reveal their drug use in a research interview.

Researchers have begun to reassess the limitations and determinants of self-report measures of drug use using the more sensitive urinalysis and hair analysis (Magura & Kang, 1995). The weight of the evidence suggests that the relationship between a respondent's self-reports of drug use and actual drug use behavior is more complex and variable than had been understood. For example, the evidence is overwhelming that persons under the supervision of the criminal justice system greatly underreport their recent use of illicit drugs even when they are interviewed by researchers under conditions of anonymity and confidentiality (Dembo et al., 1990; Mieczkowski et al., 1991; Wish and Gropper, 1990). Even arrested youths interviewed by experienced research interviewers under conditions of confidentiality 6 months after their release have been found to conceal much of their recent drug use (Magura et al., 1995). Moreover, an experiment that tried to enhance reporting among arrestees by obtaining a urine specimen prior to an anonymous research interview and telling respondents that the test results would be compared to their interview responses found that less than one-half of the arrestees who tested positive for cocaine reported using the drug in the 72 hours prior to the interview (Wish, Gray, & Sushinsky, 1998).

It may be expected that persons who are interviewed while they are under the supervision of the criminal justice system or after release may never feel secure enough to disclose their illicit drug use in research interviews. However, studies of noncriminal populations have also found under-reporting of recent drug use. Of the patients seeking treatment in a medical clinic who tested positive for cocaine by urinalysis, only 28% reported recent use of the drug in the nurse-administered medical intake interview (McNagy & Parker, 1992). Marques, Tippetts, and Branch (1993) studied a sample of infants and their postpartum mothers using interviews and urine and hair analyses. They found that while the cocaine levels in infant hair were correlated with analyses of maternal urine ($r = .28$) and hair ($r = .43$), the maternal self-reports of cocaine use did not correlate ($r = .06$) with the infant-hair results. The authors concluded that self-reported drug use information routinely collected by interviewers should be interpreted cautiously.

Cook et al. (1995, 1997) found that fewer than one-half of the employees of a steel manufacturing plant who tested positive by urine or hair analysis reported their drug use in anonymous research interviews or group-administered questionnaires. The largest amount of under-reporting was found for cocaine/crack use. And a telephone interview study of occupants of shelters and residents of single-occupancy hotels in New York City and state found that only one-third of those who tested positive for cocaine by hair analysis reported ever using the drug, even though all had been informed that they would be tested (Appel, 1995). Under-reporting of recent drug use in comparison to urinalysis results was also reported by another study of the homeless in New York City (New York City Commission on the Homeless, 1992).

While the evidence suggests that traditional interview studies in which a researcher conducts a one-time interview or periodic interviews with a research subject may be open to underreporting, it has been suggested that more sustained, ethnographic, community-based interview procedures may obtain more valid self-reports of drug use. Weatherby et al. (1994) found that when community outreach workers recruited admitted drug injectors to participate in an AIDS risk-assessment study, the urine-test results confirmed their self-reported drug use. However, Wish and Mieczkowski (1994) pointed out that because the study's findings came from persons recruited and interviewed because they had previously reported their drug use to the recruiter and had been informed of the impending urine test, the likelihood that the urine tests would detect underreporting in the research interview was diminished. Moreover, Falck et al. (1992) reported considerable underreporting of cocaine and opiate use in their study of a similar sample of not-in-treatment, nonincarcerated IDUs who were not given advance notice of the urine test.

It could be argued that persons in contact with the criminal justice system, the homeless, and employees may have significant reasons for underreporting their drug use, even in confidential research interviews. One might expect, however, that drug abuse treatment clients would find little reason to conceal their drug use, especially at admission to treatment. Assessment and diagnostic tools generally rely on the person's accurate reporting of recent drug use and associated problems. Moreover, treatment evaluation studies often depend on self-report measures of drug use at intake and at follow-up to assess treatment outcomes. Systematic under-reporting of drug use would greatly bias the results of such studies.

The evidence suggests, however, that drug abuse treatment clients may systematically under-report their drug use. Magura et al. (1987) found that only 35% of the persons receiving treatment at methadone programs who tested positive for opiates by urinalysis testing reported using the drug in the prior 30 days. Reporting was higher for cocaine (85%) and benzodiazepines (61%). But these results underestimated the level of potential under-reporting because individuals were classified as having used a drug if they reported current use or use in the past 30 days, rather than use in the past 2 or 3 days, the period to which the urine tests were sensitive.

A comparison of the urinalysis results and self-reported drug use for clients in the Treatment Outcome Prospective Study 24 months after treatment found that only 33% of those positive for opiates reported using heroin in the prior 3 days (Research Triangle Institute, 1994). That study also found that only 40% of the cocaine-positive clients reported using the drug in the prior 3 days.

More recently, the *Early Retrospective Study of Cocaine Treatment Outcomes,* a study of clients receiving treatment for cocaine at a subset of Drug Abuse Treatment Outcome Study (DATOS) programs found that only 26% of the 109 clients who tested positive for cocaine by urinalysis at follow-up 12 months after treatment reported using the drug in the prior 72 hours. Fewer than one-half (43%) of the cocaine-positive clients admitted using the drug in the prior 2 weeks. Even when the researchers expanded their measure to compare the concordance between any drug-positive urine test and a self-report of the use of any drug in the prior 72 hours, they reported, "but still two-thirds of those who tested positive for any drug did not report use of any drug in the past 72 hours" (Research Triangle Institute, 1994; pp. 4–10).

Magura et al. (Magura et al., 1992) obtained interview, urine, and hair test information to investigate the validity of hair analysis among clients receiving methadone treatment. They found that 81% of clients positive for cocaine by urinalysis and 73% positive by hair analysis reported using the drug in the confidential research interview. The numbers were smaller for heroin—57 and 64%, respectively.

Hinden et al. (1994) found that most of the persons who tested positive by hair analysis for heroin (96%) or cocaine (89%) at the inception of residential treatment had reported their use of these drugs during the admission interview. However, at the post-treatment interview, only 67% of those positive for heroin and 51% of those positive for cocaine reported using the drugs. The authors speculated that people may be less likely to report drug use after treatment or when not in the protected treatment environment. Similar concerns have been raised by Magura and Kang (1995) and Wish et al. (1997).

Overall, the recent research literature raises important questions about the validity of self-report measures of drug use in a variety of contexts. It can no longer be assumed that research subjects will accurately report on their illicit drug use when queried during confidential research interviews. The accuracy of the information obtained varies depending upon the research context, the type of respondents, and even the type of drug use being measured. Prevention researchers would be well served to use biological assays along with interviews when attempting to identify recent drug use among persons at risk for substance abuse.

DRUG TESTS AND HOW THEY WORK

Biology of Drug Use

Drug users take drugs because they like the feelings that the drugs produce. This is because the drugs stimulate specific reward centers in the brain, particularly the nucleus accumbens and the ventral tegmental area, the pleasure centers mediated by the neurotransmitter dopamine (DuPont & Gold, 1995). Drug users consume drugs in a variety of ways, including smoking, swallowing, injecting, and snorting. Once in the body, the drugs are rapidly disseminated to every part of the body. Because the target organ of abused drugs is the brain, abused drugs are all lipid soluble so they can easily pass the blood brain barrier. The concentration of abused drugs in the blood falls within several hours after use, although drug use can sometimes be detected for 12 to 36 hours in blood samples.

Drugs are primarily metabolized to more water-soluble chemicals (metabolites) in the liver and excreted by the kidney. Therefore, drug substances are often concentrated in the urine, and urine tests can be positive for 1 to 3 days after a single drug-using episode. While drugs are present in the blood, they are also found in the sweat and saliva (which are in equilibrium with the blood). Drug chemicals and metabolites are also laid down in the hair as it is produced in the hair follicle and in fingernails and toenails. Because head hair grows at about 1½-inch a month, a 1½-inch sample of head hair contains a record of drug use in the prior 90 days.

See Table 10.1 for a description of various commonly used samples to detect drug use.

Drug-Testing Technology

The standard drug test today is an immunoassay test based on antibodies produced by cloned bacteria. The three primary immunoassays differ primarily in the ways the antibody–antigen reaction is measured, either by a visual density scale, a radioactive marker, or by a fluorescent marker. Antibodies have been developed that are highly specific for the drug or drug metabolite being identified so that cross-reactivity (a positive reaction to drugs other than that being tested for), which was a minor problem with the early immunoassays, has been all but eliminated. This is especially true for the marijuana, cocaine, and PCP assays. Opiate and amphetamine/methamphetamine antibodies are exceptions because they identify closely related families of substances, such as some stimulant cold preparations that can mimic amphetamines. In addition, codeine can be confused with morphine or heroin on an immunoassay screening test.

In workplace drug testing, where an employee's job can be placed in jeopardy with a single positive test, the standard test has become an immunoassay followed by a gas chromatography/mass spectrometry (GC/MS) test. When the immunoassay screening test is positive, the sample is re-tested using an entirely different laboratory technology. Only when the second, confirming test, is positive is the sample declared positive. The GC/MS test is the "gold standard" of drug identification. With the GC/MS test, there is no cross-reactivity, and the drug identified is unmistakably the single drug (or metabolite) identified on the GC/MS result.

Research testing can use the workplace standard; but it can also use the unconfirmed result since there are few samples that do not confirm, and there is no danger to a subject's livelihood or other risk to be considered. If testing is limited to the immunoassay test, that limitation can be noted. This avoids the substantial cost of the confirming test.

Workplace testing has generally been limited to just five drugs or groups of drugs: marijuana, cocaine, PCP, amphetamine/methamphetamine, and codeine/morphine. Many other abused drugs can be identified, but they are not tested for in most workplace drug testing. These drugs include LSD, MDMA (Ecstasy), barbiturates, benzodiazepines, methaqualone, and a variety of synthetic narcotics such as methadone, Demerol, Dilaudid, and others.

Other Methods

There are a variety of alternatives to the standard immunoassay screen with GC/MS confirmation, including the old TLC and a number of newer high-tech techniques. None is likely to replace the currently used standard approaches, but the drug-testing technology is evolving rapidly.

Samples Tested

The most commonly used sample is urine, which, in the criminal justice system and in drug abuse treatment, is collected under direct observation to reduce the risk of adulteration or sample

TABLE 10.1. Blood, Urine, Hair, and Sweat Patch Testing for Drugs of Abuse

	Blood	Urine	Hair	Sweat Patch
Immunoassay screen	Yes	Yes	Yes	Yes
GC/MS confirmation option	Yes	Yes	Yes	Yes
Chain-of-custody option	Yes	Yes	Yes	Yes
Retained positives for re-test option	Yes	Yes	Yes	Yes
Medical review officer option	Yes	Yes	Yes	Yes
Surveillance window	3–12 hours	1–3 days	7–90 days	1–21 days
Intrusiveness of collection	Severe	Moderate	None	Slight
Re-test of same sample	Yes	Yes	Yes	Yes
Re-test of new sample if original test disputed	No	No	Yes	No
Number of drugs screened (NIDA-5)	Unlimited[a]	Unlimited	5[b]	3[c]
Cost/sample (NIDA-5)	About $200	About $15–$30	About $20, $40–$65	
Permits distinction between light, moderate and heavy use	Yes, acutely no	Yes,	Yes, chronically	Chronically
Resistance to cheating	High	Low	High	High
Best applications	Post-accident and overdose testing for alcohol and other drugs; Alcohol BAC level	Reasonable cause and random testing; Frequent testing of high-risk groups such as post-treatment follow-up and CJS	Pre-employment testing treatment; Random and periodic testing	Post-testing; Maintaining abstinence
Best applications		Testing to determine severity of drug use for poppy seed referral to treatment; Testing subjects suspected of seeking to evade urine test detection	Opiate addicts claiming "false-positive"	
Best applications		Opiate addicts claiming poppy seed "false-positive"		

[a] Blood testing for alcohol is routine, costing about $25 per sample, but blood testing for drugs is done by only a few laboratories in the country. Blood testing for drugs is relatively expensive, costing about $60 for each drug detected.

[b] Currently hair testing is available only for NIDA-5 (cocaine, opiates, marijuana, amphetamines, and PCP).

[c] Morphine/codeine, cocaine, marijuana, amphetamine/methamphetamine, and PCP (HHS-5). Additional sweat-patch tests will become available for alcohol.

substitution, common problems with drug addicts. In workplace testing a variety of strategies have been developed to avoid the need to directly observe urine collection, including checking the sample temperature to be sure it is freshly voided.

Hair samples are collected by snipping about 40 to 50 strands of hair, about the amount of hair that equals the diameter of a pencil lead, close to the scalp. The 1½ inches of hair closest to the scalp is tested, revealing drug use during the prior 90 days, minus the approximately 1 week it takes hair to grow out of the follicle long enough to be easily cut.

Sweat patches can be placed on the arm or body and then removed at the time of testing, up to about 2 or 3 weeks. Patches cannot be worn for a longer time because the skin sloughs over time, and the patches fall off after about 4 or 5 weeks.

Saliva samples can also be used for drug tests; and, like blood tests, they are positive usually for only up to about 12 hours after the most recent drug use.

Issues

FALSE NEGATIVES.   Subjects can use drugs and still produce negative drug-test results. Small amounts of drug use are often insufficient to trigger a positive urine drug-test result, especially when a relatively long time has elapsed since the use and when the subject has drunk a lot of water in the hour or two before the test. Tests are all conducted using cutoff levels that eliminate the risk of giving positive results after passive exposure to low levels of drug substances. For this reason, even though testing technology is getting more and more sensitive, there are limits to the ability of tests to identify low levels of drug use. For marijuana, the most commonly used illicit drug, a single joint or two will produce a positive test at the 100-nanogram cutoff level for up to 3 days and at the 20-nanogram cutoff level for up to 5 days. However, as many as 50% of people who smoke a joint or two will be negative even the day after smoking at these cutoff levels. Virtually all people who have used a drug more than a few days prior to the sample collection will be negative on urine testing. Hair testing will identify drug use for up to 90 days, but subjects who use small amounts of drugs in the 90 days prior to testing will test negative on hair tests.

Thus, many people who use drugs, unless they use them frequently and at high levels, test negative on all drug tests. However, hair testing has a longer surveillance window than does urine testing. When hair samples are compared to urine samples, there are more positives on hair testing than on urine testing largely because of this longer surveillance window (Wish et al., 1997).

FALSE POSITIVES.   The greatest concern in workplace drug tests has been that a positive test will falsely identify a subject as a drug user. Great care has been used to insure that this does not happen. The modern drug-testing system, including chain-of-custody, immunoassay screen and GC/MS confirmation, the services of a medical review officer, and the retained positive sample, help ensure that there are no false-positive results (DuPont, 1990).

Particular attention has been given to the problem of passive exposure, which can occur when a person goes to a concert or is in a room with a person who is smoking marijuana. Urine tests have been used in a variety of settings, all showing that no real-life situation has produced a sample measuring higher than 7 nanograms per milliliter, substantially below the lowest cutoff level used, 20 nanograms. Hair testing and urine testing involve cutoff levels designed to prevent this problem. For hair testing, samples are extensively washed prior to testing to ensure that external drug exposure is washed off the hair (DuPont & Baumgartner, 1995).

Practical Questions

HOW TO COLLECT SAMPLES. Urine samples can be collected using temperature-measuring devices built into the collection cup that give good reliability in terms of sample substitution. Most sources of adulteration can be easily identified at the lab and require that the subject be prepared well before collection to falsify the sample. Hair testing is resistant to falsification, since a hair sample is collected under direct observation. No manipulation of the hair, including perming, dying, or washing, is effective at removing the drugs and drug metabolites embedded in the protein matrix of the hair. Sweat patches also resist tampering since they cannot be peeled off and then reattached to the skin. If they are still in place, you can be sure they have not been removed.

HOW MUCH DOES IT COST? Unconfirmed immunoassay screens can be conducted for about $5 to $15 a sample, depending on which drugs are tested for. With confirmation the testing can cost from $25 to $50 a sample. Hair testing costs about $40 a sample with GC/MS confirmation. Sweat patches cost about the same as hair tests.

CONCLUSION

Firm, clear, and consistent consequences, such as termination from employment or suspension from athletic participation, enhance the preventive effects of drug tests, since outcome expectations and perceived self-efficacy influence people's actions and behaviors. The drug-testing programs of the U.S. military services illustrate the dramatic effects that can be achieved by use of random drug testing based on standardized testing procedures and backed by strict disciplinary consequences. These findings from two decades of experience are ripe for study in prevention research. While drug-testing programs have also reduced illicit drug use in many arenas, including the workplace, the criminal justice system, and athletic competitions, broader and more consistent efforts are needed in prevention research. Based on these results, it appears that model drug-testing programs in prevention research need to be developed to advance the use of reliable and cost-effective drug-testing programs. More study is also needed on the preventive effects of drug testing on adolescents and young adults. Random drug testing has been implemented in several U.S. school districts, including Dade County, Florida, but the practice is uncommon, and outcome data are unavailable. Research is needed on the results of these pioneering programs. Overall, drug testing provides valuable information to researchers on preventing drug use and extends the information provided by self-reported data on drug use.

REFERENCES

Appel, P. W. (1995). *Substance abuse among adults in transient housing in New York State: Validation of self-report by use of hair analysis.* New York State Office of Alcoholism and Substance Abuse Services and Research Institute on Addictions.

Bandura, A. B. (1986). *Social foundations of thought and action: A social cognitive theory.* Englewood Cliffs, NJ: Prentice-Hall.

Bible, J. D., & McWhirter, D. A. (1990). *Privacy in the workplace: A guide for human resource managers.* New York: Quorum Books.

Blum, T. C., Fields, D. L., Milne, S. H., & Spell, C. S. (1992). Workplace drug testing programs: A review of research and a survey of worksites. *Journal of Employee Assistance Research, 1,* 315–349.

Bureau of Justice Assistance (1991, July). *American Probation and Parole Association's drug testing guidelines and practices for adult probation and parole agencies* (Monograph). Washington, DC: Bureau of Justice Assistance.

Collins, W. C. (1990). *Drugs of abuse testing in the criminal justice system.* San Jose, CA: Syva Company.

Cook, R. F., Bernstein, A. D., Arrington, T. L., & Andrews, C. M. (1997). Methods for assessing drug use prevalence in the workplace: A comparison of self-report, urinalysis and hair analysis. In L. Harrison & A. Hughes (Eds.), *The validity of self-reported drug use: Improving the accuracy of survey estimates* (pp. 247–272). Rockville: NIDA Research Monograph 167, NIH Publication No. 97-4147.

Cook, R. F., Bernstein, A. D., Arrington, T. L., Andrews, C. M., & Marshall, G. A. (1995). Methods for assessing drug use prevalence in the workplace: A comparison of self-report, urinalysis and hair analysis. *International Journal of the Addictions, 30,* 403–426.

Coombs, R. H., & Ryan, F. J. (1990). Drug testing effectiveness in identifying and preventing drug use. *American Journal of Drug and Alcohol Abuse, 16,* 173–184.

Crant, J. M., & Bateman, T. S. (1989). A model of employee responses to drug-testing programs. *Employee Responsibilities and Rights Journal, 2,* 173–190.

Crouch, D. J., Webb, D. O., Peterson, L. V., Buller, P. F., & Rollins, D. W. (1989). A critical evaluation of the Utah Power and Light Company's substance abuse management program: Absenteeism, accidents, and costs. In S. W. Gust & J. M. Walsh (Eds.), *Drugs in the workplace: Research and evaluation data.* NIDA Research Monograph 91 (pp. 169–193). Rockville, MD: National Institute on Drug Abuse.

Crown, D. F., & Rosse, J. G. (1988). A critical review of the assumptions underlying drug testing. *Journal of Business and Psychology, 3,* 22–41.

de Bernardo, M. A. (1998, June 5). Statement on employer drug-testing and drug-abuse prevention programs and in support of H.R. 3853—The Drug-Free Workplace Act of 1998, The Private-Sector Drug-Free Workplace Act, and The Public and Employe Safety Assurance Act. Testimony before the Government Reform and Oversight's Subcommittee on National Security, International Affairs, and Criminal Justice. Hearing transcript (in press).

Dembo, R., Williams, L., Wish, E. D., & Schmeidler, J. (1990). *Urine testing of detained juveniles to identify high-risk youth.* National Institute of Justice Research in Brief. Washington, DC: National Institute of Justice.

Dogoloff, L. I., & Angarola, R. T. (1985). In S. C. Price (Ed.), *Urine testing in the workplace* (pp. 5–31). Rockville, MD: American Council for Drug Education.

Drug Court Clearinghouse and Technical Assistance Project (DCCTAP) (1997). *Summary assessment of the drug court experience.* Washington, DC: American University.

Drug Testing Soars among Big and Midsize Businesses (1992, March). *Small Business Employee Assistance,* p. 1.

DuPont, R. L. (1990). Medicines and drug testing in the workplace. *Journal of Psychoactive Drugs, 22,* 451–459.

DuPont, R. L. (1997a). *The selfish brain: Learning from addiction.* Washington, DC: American Psychiatric Press, Inc.

DuPont, R. L. (1997b). Drug testing. In N. S. Miller, M. S. Gold, & D. E. Smith (Eds.), *Manual of therapeutics for addictions* (pp. 86–94). New York: Wiley-Liss, Inc.

DuPont, R. L., & Baumgartner, W. A. (1995). Drug testing by urine and hair analysis: Complementary features and scientific issues. *Forensic Science International, 70,* 63–76.

DuPont, R. L., & Gold, M. S. (1995). Withdrawal and reward: Implications for detoxification and relapse prevention. *Psychiatric Annals, 25,* 663–668.

Falck, R., Siegel, H. A., Forney, M. A., Wang, J., & Carlson, R. G. (1992). The validity of injection drug users' self-reported use of opiates and cocaine. *Journal of Drug Issues, 22,* 823–832.

Fudala, P. J., Fields, L., Kreiter, N. A., & Lange, W. R. (1994, May). An examination of current and proposed drug-testing policies at U.S. colleges and universities. *Journal of Adolescent and Child Health, 42,* 267–270.

General Accounting Office (1993). *Drug use measurement.* Washington, DC: General Accounting Office.

Greenberg, E. R. (1988). Workplace testing: Results of a new AMA survey. *Personnel, 65,* 36.

Greenberg, E. R. (1989). Workplace testing: Who's testing whom? *Personnel, 66,* 39.

Greenberg, E. R. (1990). Workplace testing: The 1990 AMA survey, Part 2. *Personnel, 67,* 26.

Harrell, A. V. (1985). Validation of self-report: The research record. In B. A. Rouse, N. J. Kozel, & L. G. Richards (Eds.), *Self-report methods of estimating drug use: Meeting current challenges to validity* (pp. 12–21). National Institute on Drug Abuse Research Monograph 57, DHHS Pub. No. (ADM) 85–1402. Washington, DC: Superintendent of Documents, U.S. Government Printing Office.

Harris, M. S., & Heft, L. L. (1992). Alcohol and drug use in the workplace: Issues, controversies, and directions for future research. *Journal of Management, 18,* 239–266.

Hawks, R. L. (1986). Establishing a urinalysis program—Prior considerations. In R. L. Hawks & C. N. Chiang (Eds.), *Urine testing for drugs of abuse* (pp. 1–4). Research Monograph Series 73. Rockville, MD: National Institute on Drug Abuse.

Hayghe, H. (1990). Survey of employer anti-drug programs. In S. W. Gust, J. M. Walsh, L. B. Thomas, & D. J. Crouch (Eds.), *Drugs in the workplace: Research and evaluation data* (Vol. II). Research Monograph 100. Rockville, MD: National Institute on Drug Abuse.

Hinden, R., McCusker, J., Vickers-Lahti, M., Bigelow, C., Garfield, F., & Lewis, B. (1994). Radioimmunoassay of hair for determination of cocaine, heroin and marijuana exposure: Comparison with self-report. *International Journal of the Addictions, 29,* 771–789.

Hubbard, R., Marsden, M. E., Rachal, J. V., Harwood, H. J., Cavanaugh, E. R., & Ginzburg, H. M. (1989). *Drug abuse treatment: A national study of effectiveness.* Chapel Hill, NC: University of North Carolina Press.

Jacobs, J. B., & Samuels, B. (1995). The drug testing project in international sports: Dilemmas in an expanding regulatory regime. *Hastings International and Comparative Law Review, 18,* 557–589.

Johnston, L. D. (principal investigator) (1996, December 19). The rise in drug use among American teens continues in 1996. News release, *Monitoring the future study.* Ann Arbor, MI: University of Michigan, Institute for Social Research.

Johnston, L. D. (principal investigator) (1997, December 18). Drug use among American teens shows some signs of leveling after a long rise. News Release, *Monitoring the future study.* Ann Arbor, MI: University of Michigan, Institute for Social Research.

Johnston, L. D., O'Malley, P. M., & Bachman, J. G. (1996). *National survey results on drug use from The Monitoring the Future Study, 1975–1995–Volume I—Secondary school students.* U.S. Department of Health and Human Services, Public Health Service, National Institutes of Health, National Institute on Drug Abuse. NIH Publication No. 96-4139. Washington, DC: Superintendent of Documents, U.S. Government Printing Office.

Lappe, M. I. (1998, June 5). Components of superior workplace substance-abuse testing programs. Testimony before the Government Reform and Oversight's Subcommittee on National Security, International Affairs, and Criminal Justice. Hearing transcript (in press).

Lehman, W. E., & Simpson, D. C. (1990). Patterns of drug use in a large metropolitan workforce. In S.W. Gust, J. M. Walsh, L. B. Thomas, & D. J. Crouch (Eds.), *Drugs in the workplace: Research and evaluation data* (Vol. II), Research Monograph 100. Rockville, MD: National Institute on Drug Abuse.

Magura, S., Freeman, R., Siddiqi, Q., & Lipton, D. S. (1992). The validity of hair analysis for detecting cocaine and heroin use among addicts. *International Journal of the Addictions, 27,* 54–69.

Magura, S., Goldsmith, D., Casriel, C., Goldstein, P. J., & Lipton, D. S. (1987). The validity of methadone clients' self-reported drug use. *International Journal of the Addictions, 22,* 727–749.

Magura, S., & Kang, S. W. (1995). *Validity of self-reported drug use in high risk populations: A meta-analytic review.* New York: National Development and Research Institute, Inc.

Magura, S., Kang, S. W., & Shapiro, J. L. (1995). Measuring cocaine use by hair analysis among criminally-involved youth. *Journal of Drug Issues, 25,* 683–701.

Mandatory Guidelines for Federal Workplace Testing Programs (1994). *Federal Register, 59,* 29,908–29,931.

Marques, P. R., Tippetts, A. S., & Branch, D. G. (1993). Cocaine in the hair of mother-infant pairs: Quantitative analysis and correlations with urine measures and self-report. *American Journal of Drug and Alcohol Abuse, 19,* 159–175.

Masi, D. (1987). Company responses to drug abuse from AMA's nationwide survey. *Personnel, 64,* 40.

McNagy, S. E., & Parker, R. M. (1992). High prevalence of recent cocaine use and the unreliability of patient self-report in an inner-city walk-in clinic. *Journal of the American Medical Association, 267,* 1106–1108.

Mieczkowski, T. (1990). The accuracy of self-reported drug use: An evaluation and analysis of new data. In R. Weisheit (Ed.), *Drugs, crime and the criminal justice system* (pp. 275–302). Cincinnati, OH: Anderson Publishing.

Mieczkowski, T., Barzelay, D., Gropper, B., & Wish, E. D. (1991). Concordance of three measures of cocaine use in an arrestee population: Hair, urine and self-report. *Journal of Psychoactive Drugs, 23,* 241–246.

Moreland, R. F., & McPhaul, K. M. (1988, March). Drug testing: A preventive approach. *AOHN Journal, 36,* 119–122.

Musto, D. (1991, July). Opium, cocaine and marijuana in American history. *Scientific American,* 40–47.

National Institute on Drug Abuse. (1990). *Research on drugs and the workplace: NIDA Capsule 24.* Rockville, MD: U.S. Department of Health and Human Services.

New York City Commission on the Homeless (1992). *The way home, a new direction in social policy.* New York: New York City Commission on the Homeless.

Normand, J., Salyards, S., & Mahoney, J. J. (1990). An evaluation of pre-employment drug testing. *Journal of Applied Psychology, 75,* 629.

Office of National Drug Control Policy (1998). *The national drug control strategy, 1998—A ten year plan—1998–2007.* Washington, DC: Executive Office of the President.

Peat, M. A. (1995). Financial viability of screening for drugs of abuse. *Clinical Chemistry Forum, 41,* 805–808.

Research Triangle Institute (1994). *Early retrospective study of cocaine treatment outcomes, overview and findings.* Draft technical report Number 1, Volume I, submitted to the National Institute on Drug Abuse. Research Triangle Park, NC: Research Triangle Institute.

Skolnick, A. A. (1996). Tougher drug tests for Centennial Olympic games. *Journal of the American Medical Association, 275,* 348–349.

Substance Abuse and Mental Health Services Administration (1996). *Preliminary estimates from the 1995 National Household Survey on Drug Abuse.* Rockville, MD: Substance Abuse and Mental Health Services Administration, Office of Applied Studies, U.S. Department of Health and Human Services.

Substance Abuse and Mental Health Services Administration (SAMHSA) (1997). *An analysis of worker drug use and workplace policies and programs.* Rockville, MD: Substance Abuse and Mental Health Services Administration, Office of Applied Studies, U.S. Department of Health and Human Services.

Substance Abuse in the Military Shows Significant Decrease (1996, August 19). *Alcoholism and Drug Abuse Weekly,* 6–7.

Tasco, F. T. (1991, November 15). Address to President Bush and the President's Drug Advisory Council by the Chairman of the President's Drug Advisory Council. (Unpublished paper).

University Policy Statement on Drug Education and Testing Program for Student Athletes (1987). National Collegiate Athletic Association.

U.S. Department of Justice (1992). *Drugs, crime, and the justice system: A national report.* Washington, DC: U.S. Department of Justice.

U.S. Department of Labor, Bureau of Labor Statistics (1989). *Survey of employer anti-drug programs.* Washington, DC: U.S. Department of Labor.

Vernonia School District 47J v. Wayne Acton, et ux., Guardians Ad Litem for Acton, 115 S.Ct. 2386, 515 U.S. 646 (1995).

Weatherby, N. L., Needle, R., Cesari, H., Booth, R., McCoy, C. B., Watters, J. K., Williams, M., & Chitwood, D. D. (1994). Validity of self-reported drug use among injection drug users and crack cocaine users recruited through street outreach. *Evaluation and Program Planning, 17,* 347–355.

Willette, R. E. (1986). Drug testing programs. In R. L. Hawks & C. N. Chiang (Eds.), *Urine testing for drugs of abuse. Research Monograph Series 73* (pp. 5–12). Rockville, MD: National Institute on Drug Abuse.

Winkler, H., & Sheridan, J. (1989). *An examination of behavior related to drug use at Georgia Power Company.* Paper presented at the NIDA Conference on Drugs in the Workplace, Bethesda, MD.

Wish, E. D. (1988a). Identifying drug-abusing criminals. In C. G. Leukefeld, & F. M. Tims (Eds.), *Compulsory treatment of drug abuse: Research and clinical practice* (pp. 139–159). National Institute on Drug Abuse Research Monograph 86, DHHS Publication No. (ADM) 88-1578. Washington, DC: Superintendent of Documents, U.S. Government Printing Office.

Wish, E. D. (1988b). In *National Institute of Justice Crime File Study Guide.* Washington, DC: U.S. Department of Justice.

Wish, E. D. (1998, July 22). On the validity of self-reported illicit drug use. Testimony before the Government Reform and Oversight's Subcommittee on National Security, International Affairs, and Criminal Justice. Hearing transcript (in press).

Wish, E. D., Gray, T., & Sushinsky, J. (1998). An experiment to enhance the reporting of drug use by arrestees. College Park, MD: Center for Substance Abuse Research. (Unpublished final report).

Wish, E. D., & Gropper, B. A. (1990). Drug testing by the criminal justice system: Method, research and applications. In J.Q. Wilson & M. Tonry (Eds.), *Drugs and crime* (pp. 321–339). Chicago: University of Chicago Press.

Wish, E. D., Hoffman, J. A., & Nemes, S. (1997). The validity of self-reports of drug use at treatment admission and followup: Comparisons with urinalysis and hair assays. In L. Harrison & A. Hughes (Eds.), *The validity of self-reported drug use: Improving the accuracy of survey estimates* (pp. 200–226). NIDA Research Monograph 167, NIH Publication No. 97-4147. Rockville, MD: National Institute on Drug Abuse.

Wish, E. D., Johnson, B., Strug, D., Chedekel, M., & Lipton, D. S. (1993). *Are urine tests good indicators of the validity of self-reports of drug use? It depends on the test.* New York: Narcotic and Drug Research, Inc.

Wish, E. D., & Mieczkowski, T. (1994). Comment on Weatherby et al., Validity of self-reported drug use among injection drug users and crack cocaine users recruited through street outreach. *Evaluation and Program Planning, 17,* 356–357.

CHAPTER 11

Anti-Drug-Abuse Policies as Prevention Strategies

Mary Ann Pentz

INTRODUCTION

Drug use in the United States, particularly tobacco and marijuana use among 8th- and 10th-grade students, increased between 1991 and 1996, following several years of decline or level use (Johnston, O'Malley, & Bachman, 1996). Then, in 1997, there appears to have been some leveling off or slight decrease in use, primarily among 8th-grade students (Johnston, Bachman, & O'Malley, 1997). This cyclic pattern suggests that the national drug abuse problem may ebb and flow with attention to the problem and implementation of prevention programs. The decrease in drug use among adolescents, for example, appears to be related to the their perceived risk of harm from using drugs, national media attention to the drug abuse problem, and participation in drug abuse prevention programs (Pentz, 1998, 1999). Fortunately, the limited reductions in drug use that have been achieved from carefully evaluated social influences-based prevention programs with adolescents suggest that such programs have the potential to overcome cyclical changes if they are disseminated widely and implemented and over long periods (Pentz et al., 1990). If drug abuse is a cyclical problem in the United States, drug abuse prevention efforts may have to be population-based, continuous, and systems (rather than person) oriented in order to bring about larger and longer declines than would be predicted from historical trends (Musto, 1995; Pentz, 1998).

Unfortunately, several factors limit the capacity of prevention programs to affect whole populations for long periods. These limitations include inadequate technologies for transferring knowledge of effective prevention programs from researchers to lay communities (Pentz, 1986), limited community, and school resources to support and monitor the quality of program implementation

MARY ANN PENTZ • Department of Preventive Medicine, University of Southern California, Alhambra, California 91803

(Pentz et al., 1990); lack of sufficient precedent for institutionalizing drug prevention programs in communities (Goodstadt, 1989); and a relative lack of research on systems approaches to preventing drug use (Moscowitz, 1989). Specific limitations include the individual behavior-change focus of most programs in which skills training, education, or intervention is delivered to small groups of individuals. This face-to-face method yields stronger immediate effects than do mass media or broad-based community education efforts (Farquhar et al., 1990) but is too labor and time intensive to be used on a community wide basis. In addition, the small-group method of program delivery typically reaches only those who agree to participate. School dropouts, for example, will not be affected by in-school programs. Finally, recent research suggests that the primary mechanism by which the more effective social influences programs change behavior is by building the perception that drug use is not acceptable to peers, parents, and the public (Hansen, 1992; MacKinnon et al., 1991). But a person's perceived change in social norms may be short-lived if it is not reinforced by evidence of an actual change, such as a change in a community's policy about liquor outlets or monitoring of drug-free zones around schools. Bringing about such obvious changes in social norms is beyond the scope of most small prevention programs.

A logical complement to current drug prevention programs is comprehensive policies for drug abuse prevention. Such policies would be less subject to community limitations and constraints and would reach more individuals, including high-risk populations. Policies for drug abuse prevention are designed to affect all individuals in a specified area (state, county, or community) regardless of whether they choose to participate in a drug abuse prevention program. For example, school dropouts no longer affected by a school-based drug abuse prevention program will still be subject to work-site policies about tobacco, alcohol, or drug use if they work and to community policies about use, sales, taxation of use, removal of promotional materials regarding drug use, and drunk driving laws regardless of whether they work, return to school, or participate in any prevention program. In addition to reaching larger and more segments of the population than do most prevention programs, local prevention policies would also be less expensive to implement. Most such policies can be disseminated through inexpensive local print media.

WHAT IS PREVENTION POLICY?

Public policy is generally designed to reflect societal values by specifying actions to be taken for social improvement. In the field of drug abuse control, policy consists of both formal laws, regulations, requirements, and court orders, as well as informal guidelines and directions for action (Lynch & Bonnie, 1994; Pentz, Bonnie, & Shopland, 1996). For purposes of this chapter, prevention policy refers to both formal and informal regulations intended to reduce drug supply and demand among youth who have not yet tried drugs, as opposed to those who are regular users in need of treatment or have violated a formal regulation or law.

Formal Regulations and Informal Directives

There are four types of formal legal regulations (Pentz et al., 1996). One establishes the conditions under which a potentially harmful substance is available by either prohibiting its production or distribution for nonmedical uses or by regulating its price, and the conditions under which it is accessible. These are supply-side strategies. A second type of formal regulation controls the flow of information regarding the use of a particular substance through mandatory warnings or certain types of messages. These are demand-side strategies. A third is direct regulation of consumption, either by prescribing and imposing sanctions for use or by withholding benefits to which an individual would otherwise be entitled if not a user. These sanctions include total bans on possession and consumption of controlled substances, bans on consumption of alcohol by persons under the minimum age, and situational or partial bans against using alcohol or smoking in public areas. A fourth type of formal regulation is a declaration of illegality that may serve an educational role. Specification of a minimum drinking age, warning labels on alcoholic beverages and cigarette packages, and sanctions for possession of illicit drugs may all generate symbolic or declarative effects directed at users (demand-side) or distributors (supply-side).

Supply and Demand Reduction

The national drug abuse control strategy consists of both supply and demand reduction goals and actions (Office of National Drug Control Policy, 1997). Supply reduction consists of any programs, interventions, or policies that are aimed at controlling or reducing access to and use of drugs (Pentz et al., 1996). The primary method used to control access to illicit drugs has been interdiction, including policies that dictate procedures, budget, and consequences to judiciary and law enforcement agencies (Goldstein & Kalant, 1990). Direct interdiction policies that could be considered preventive in their focus on youth include drug testing at schools, athletic events, and workplaces; road-side alcohol testing by law enforcement officials; higher minimum drinking age laws; lower minimum blood alcohol content (BAC) laws; drug and alcohol possession checks at schools and public events; identification checks where tobacco and alcohol are sold; and confiscation of tobacco, as is now required by California Penal Code 308. Among these policies, road-side checks and testing, lower BAC and higher age, and identification checks have been evaluated and found to have resulted in decreased alcohol-related accidents and tobacco purchases by youth, with effects lasting from several months up to 3 years (Forster et al., 1997; Hingson et al., 1996; Holder, 1993).

Indirect interdiction policies that are preventive are those that focus on the vendor as a means of controlling access to and availability of substances. Removal of cigarette vending machines, sting operations conducted where tobacco and alcohol are sold, threat of tobacco or alcohol license revocation, and alcohol server training policies have all been found to have significant effects on decreasing the access of youths to tobacco and alcohol (Altman et al., 1991; Forster et al., 1997; Perry et al., 1996). The effects of designated driver educational directives on youth are less clear (cf. Holder, 1993).

Research on supply reduction policies, such as raising the drinking age and limiting access to tobacco and alcohol in public bars, restaurants, and stores, has shown such policies to be associated with reductions in tobacco and alcohol consumption and sales, DUI arrests, and alcohol and drug-related accidents for periods of up to 3 years (e.g., Altman et al., 1991; Forster et al., 1997; Hingson et al., 1996; Lynch & Bonnie, 1994; Moscowitz, 1989).

In recent years, public health experts have begun to focus heavily on the use of supply-side interventions for legal drugs, especially tobacco. The two main strategies are increasing the excise tax (to reduce tobacco use by youths, who are especially price sensitive) and tightening enforcement of access restrictions (Chaloupka, 1996; Grossman & Coate, 1988; Lynch & Bonnie, 1994). For alcohol, raising the drinking age to 21 and increasing the level of enforcement have had a significant effect on the intensity of youthful alcohol consumption.

Local community supply reduction strategies have included restricting and monitoring merchant licensing, server training, removal or monitoring of vending machines, and local campaigns to support voluntary restricted access (Altman et al., 1991; Casswell & Gilmore, 1989; Forster et al., 1997; Hingson et al., 1996; Holder, 1993; Lynch & Bonnie, 1994; Pentz, Mihalic, & Grotpeter, 1997). Most of these strategies have shown significant short-term effects on lowering tobacco and alcohol use. Although sources of data and types of drug use measures vary considerably across studies of supply reduction and differ considerably from studies of demand reduction, the magnitude of the effect of local tobacco and alcohol policy interventions is considered to be at least comparable to the short term (6 months to 3 years) net reductions of 20 to 40% in use of these substances reported from school-based demand reduction programs (c.f., Goodstadt, 1989; Hansen, 1992; Holder, 1993; Moscowitz, 1989; Pentz, 1993).

Demand reduction consists of programs, interventions, or policies aimed at increasing an individual's ability to resist drugs (Pentz et al., 1996). While most demand reduction strategies consist of educational programs, several policies also focus on demand reduction, either directly or indirectly. For example, alcohol and tobacco warning label legislation represent declarative policies aimed directly at reducing demand by increasing the perceived harmfulness or risk of use. Alcohol warning labels have had a small effect on changing the beliefs of youths about the harmfulness of alcohol use but have had no significant effect on alcohol use (e.g., MacKinnon, Pentz, & Stacy, 1993). School policies of suspension for use of alcohol or drugs are also aimed directly at demand reduction by increasing the perceived risk of the consequences of use (Moscowitz & Jones, 1988). Similarly, alcohol and tobacco taxation has significantly reduced purchases by youths by rendering tobacco and alcohol too expensive for many (Chaloupka, 1996; Grossman & Coate, 1988). Road-side checks and blood alcohol testing are indirect efforts at demand reduction that threaten loss of driving privileges and punitive legal consequences (Hingson et al., 1996; Holder, 1993). Although these policies have had an effect on decreasing drunk driving accidents, it is not clear whether the effect is either direct or mediated by increased perceived risk.

Levels of Prevention Policy: Federal, State, and Local

Federal policy consists of the overall national drug control strategy and legislation that applies to all states. The national drug control strategy, developed by the Office of National Drug Control Policy (ONDCP), consists of 5 goals and 30 measurable objectives (ONDCP, 1997). The first goal—to educate and enable youth to reject drugs—has the most relevance to prevention policy at the national, state, and local levels, with 8 of the 10 objectives translatable to policy. These objectives include informal guidelines to provide funding and education for caregivers to support prevention practices, informal guidelines and declarative regulations (such as banning tobacco and alcohol ads or developing and broadcasting counter-advertising) for the mass media to warn about the risks of use, formal zero tolerance policies in schools, workplaces, and the community, formal and informal policies for setting aside funds and resources in schools for effective drug prevention programming, informal directives for establishing mandated programs, informal guidelines to assist in the development of community coalitions and media/sports partnerships for prevention, and declarative regulations for disseminating research on the consequences of legalizing drugs. Formal and informal prevention policies under the framework of the national drug control strategy are administered through funds provided by the Safe and Drug-Free Schools Act (Bukoski, 1990). Specific funding levels are mandated for prevention and disbursed first to states, and through states, to local communities and schools for implementation of policies at the local level. A recent amendment to this act under consideration would require that communities and schools implement only research-based prevention programs in order to receive prevention funds (Sloboda & David, 1997).

Recent federal legislation aimed at youth includes the alcohol warning label legislation and the Synar Amendment (Hingson, Donnay, & Zakocs, unpublished manuscript). The warning label is required on all alcohol beverage containers. As noted earlier, this legislation has had a small effect on attitudes and beliefs about risk but no effects on use (e.g., MacKinnon et al., 1993). The Synar Amendment is a federal tobacco access policy that requires communities to refuse and monitor tobacco sales to youth or risk loss of federal prevention funds (Hingson et al., unpublished manuscript). There is no research yet available on the efficacy of this legislation.

Examples of state laws relevant to prevention with youth include the State Block Grant program, which mandates 20% set-aside funds for prevention, minimum age drinking laws, BAC level regulations, tobacco and alcohol tax legislation (e.g., California's Proposition 99, Massachusetts and Minnesota taxation and prevention planning), and penalties for possession of tobacco (such as California's Penal Code 308, which requires that youths provide community service if caught in possession of tobacco and/or submit to a tobacco cessation program). Of these, minimum age and BAC regulations have had a significant impact on accidents. Taxation has decreased purchases by youths, and overall taxation linked to prevention planning in one case (California) has decreased adult but not youth smoking (Farkas et al., 1996; Grossman & Coate, 1988; Join Together, 1997a, b). The set-aside funds, prevention program planning, and penalties for possession, while legislated at the state level, are implemented at the community level. The effects of state legislation, as a whole, have been evaluated in at least two studies. Both have shown no effects on tobacco use by youths (Farkas et al., 1996; Murray et al., 1992). However, whether effects of specific components of state legislation, such as mandated tobacco education, have been effective cannot be evaluated independently of other components.

Examples of formal local ordinances or policies relevant to prevention of drug use by youths include no-smoking ordinances, removing cigarette vending machines, establishing and monitoring drug-free zones in schools and neighborhoods, vendor training and license revocation for tobacco and alcohol sales to minors, mandating cessation programs for youths caught in possession of tobacco, drug testing and no-smoking policies in work sites that employ youths, and mandated educational programs in youth-service agencies or student-assistance programs in schools (Normand, Salyards, & Mahoney, 1990; Swisher et al., 1993). Of these, no-smoking ordinances, removing vending machines, and vendor training and licensing have had significant effects on decreasing tobacco and alcohol use and purchases, although the effects thus far appear to be short term, lasting only a few months (e.g., Altman et al., 1991; Forster et al., 1997; Jason et al., 1991; Perry et al., 1996). The effectiveness of these policies depends on the level of implementation and enforcement by relevant policy officials (e.g., Pentz, Brannon et al., 1989), as well as on assistance from law enforcement officials. For example, policing of drug-free zones around schools may be assisted by DARE officers or other police trained in community-watch methods (Clayton, 1990). Drug-free zones and mandated programming as part of school policy have yet to be systematically evaluated, but some research suggests that prevention-orientation and mandated prevention education policies in schools have more of an effect on decreasing adolescent smoking than does restrictiveness (Pentz, Brannon, Charlin, et al., 1989). Mandated programs have shown no significant effects on drug use, but voluntary enrollment of adolescent smokers in smoking cessation or student-assistance programs focused on coping skills have had some marginal effect on increasing readiness to quit and decreasing use (cf., Pentz, 1997; Swisher et al., 1993).

Other community policies are informal, particularly those that attempt to operationalize the objectives of the first goal of the national drug control strategy: education for caregivers, guidelines or training for mass communications, developing set-aside funds and resources for prevention programming and selecting and institutionalizing evidence-based programming, and developing community coalitions and media/sports partnerships. Federal legislation has provided funds for technical assistance and dissemination of guides to communities to carry out these objectives through federal research agencies, such as the Center for Substance Abuse Prevention

Community Partnerships Program (Yin et al., 1997), the Office of Juvenile Justice and Drug Prevention, Blueprints publications (Pentz et al., 1997), and the National Institute on Drug Abuse Prevention Works publication (Sloboda & David, 1997). In addition, private foundations have developed public policy panels and guides for communities, such as the community action guides published by Join Together, a Robert Wood Johnson Foundation program that refers communities to successful community action projects and to policymakers (Join Together, 1997a, b).

How Local Policy Change Fits the Federal Agenda

Local policy change, that is, change at the city or community level, fits the federal agenda for drug abuse prevention in three ways. First and foremost, local policy change provides accountability to the federal government that communities have complied with mandates of the U.S. Anti-Drug Abuse Acts by developing drug free zones, limiting access to and availability of drugs, and institutionalizing prevention education through set-aside funds for teacher training program implementation and materials (Bukoski, 1990; Inciardi, 1990; Library of Congress, 1989; Schuster, 1989). This accountability, while currently voluntary, is the primary means by which the U.S. Congress receives feedback about expenditures of Drug-Free Schools and Communities monies. Second, local policy change ostensibly represents a formal statement by a community that it supports a non-drug-use social norm (Pentz et al., 1997). Developing an anti-drug abuse or no-tolerance climate was and is the intention of the Anti-Drug Abuse Acts and the Office of National Drug Control Policy. Third, policy, particularly formal, written policy that is regularly enforced, has the potential to diffuse effective prevention programs more rapidly through whole communities than is possible by other means (Goodstadt, 1989; Pentz, Brannon, Charlin, et al., 1989; Wallack & Corbett, 1987). Currently, "other means" of diffusion include a single school's, work-site's, or community's individual choice to adopt a particular program, limited implementation of experimental programs as part of a research study, haphazard word-of-mouth among potential program users from the same occupation or system, and media-dependent diffusion in response to an immediate crisis, such as a community's rapid adoption of a drunk-driving campaign in response to a drunk-driving death that receives media attention (Hingson et al., 1996). None of these "other means" is predictable or systematic enough to evaluate and replicate.

THEORETICAL SUPPORT FOR LOCAL POLICY CHANGE

In order to develop an overall approach to considering the effects of local policy on drug prevention, several theories can be integrated. First are attributional, behavior-change, and learning theories related to motivation, participation in, and reactance to policy adoption (Ajzen & Fishbein, 1990; Bandura, 1977; Rotter, 1954). These theories require that a sequence of change occur within the individuals of a community before a local policy change can be considered, adopted, implemented, complied with, and maintained. This sequence includes (1) awareness of the need for policy change and policy options, (2) knowledge of the policy's content and potential consequences, (3) a positive attitude toward the policy and a belief that it can change drug use behavior, (4) a personal weighting of the relative value of policy change versus other options for prevention, (5) expectations that the policy change will result in positive outcomes for the community and positive personal consequences, (6) self-efficacy or self-confidence in supporting and complying with the policy under consideration, (7) initial personal behaviors that demonstrate support for and compliance with policy change, and (8) mastery of these behaviors through repeated practice. For example, basic learning and social learning theories posit that adequate population awareness and knowledge of a policy is required before behavior change in the form of policy revision or new policy adoption can occur (Bandura, 1977; Rotter, 1954). Adoption will occur to the extent that policymakers have the self-efficacy to reach consensus about the change or the group self-efficacy or empowerment to carry the change forward to the implementation stage. Implementation, or enforcement, of a policy change will be consistent to the extent that implementors (such as law enforcement personnel) perceive their local policymakers (community or local government leaders) as models of the policy message (such as not smoking). Expectancy-value theories posit that the selection of policy options and subsequent change in policy will depend on the policymakers' assessment of benefit over risk of changing policy, including beneficial consequences for individuals and the community (such as a change in smoking rates) (Ajzen & Fishbein, 1990; Rotter, 1954). Perceived social normative expectations about the extent of the drug use problem (thus, the need for policy change) and perceived community disapproval of use should also predict policy change and help bring about changes in behavior (e.g., MacKinnon et al., 1991).

Second are social support and consensus theories related to inclusion of environmental interventions designed to support policy change (Barrera, 1986; Butterfoss, Goodman, & Wandersman, 1996). For example, whether initial trial behaviors that demonstrate a social group's support of a policy change are repeated will depend on that group's reinforcing communication with and feedback from others in the community. Based on previous research, compliance of policy implementors with enforcement and compliance of the community with policy regulations will depend on how much the community supports the policy (e.g., Glasgow et al., 1996). Group social support (such as workers in support of a no-smoking policy and in support of assisting co-workers to quit) should, in turn, increase policy implementation (Pentz, Brannon, Charlin, et al., 1989; Galaif, Sussman, & Bundek, 1996).

Third are communications theories related to settings or channels for policy delivery and methods of policy dissemination (e.g., Rogers, 1987). Diffusion of innovation theory suggests that the idea of a policy change must be embraced first by credible, highly visible innovators in the community and then "passed on" for first trial implementation to credible early adopters who have high levels of self-efficacy, behavioral skills, population access, and who can communicate implementation across multiple channels of policy delivery (Rogers, 1987). While this sequence of diffusion has not been evaluated experimentally, nonexperimental studies of policy adoption in the prevention field support this theory, most notably, the national diffusion of DARE across police departments in the United States and from police departments to communities (Rogers, 1993). In most communities there are several systems that provide important day-to-day communication and social functions and have the potential for implementing prevention programs and policies. These systems are ideal channels for policy delivery and dissemination. Schools, for example, provide major communication, social, and educational functions on a regular basis, and most schools have some precedent for drug abuse prevention education and/or a drug free zone policy. Thus, local policy change implemented throughout a community's school system might have a higher likelihood of diffusing rapidly throughout a community than would a policy change attempted in systems that do not meet these communication and diffusion criteria.

Organizational development and community action models are relevant to implementation and support of policy change (Bracht, 1990; Butterfoss, Goodman, & Wandersman, 1996). These models, based on learning, group process, and systems theories, posit that certain fundamental conditions must be met by policymakers before policy adoption and implementation can occur (Bracht, 1990; Klitzner, 1993; Pentz, 1995). Evaluation and research trials involving community organization for drug abuse prevention suggest that several factors are associated with more rapid adoption of prevention mandates. These include centralized versus decentralized distribution of tasks, developing of a climate of cooperation prior to formal community organization, and a trial period of prevention programming prior to adoption of prevention policy and institutionalizing of programs (Bracht, 1990; Butterfoss et al., 1996; Giesbrecht, Consley, & Denniston, 1990; Goodman & Streckler, 1990; Mansergh et al., 1996; Pentz & Montgomery, unpublished manuscript; Rothman, 1979; Saxe et al., 1997; Wagenaar et al., 1994; Yin et al., 1997). Interim results of the CSAP Community Partnership Programs and the RWJ Fighting Back Communities indicate that some communities more than others demonstrate effective organization, timely implementation of local policy and prevention initiatives, and longevity (beyond 3 years). These are communities that aligned themselves with stronger, credible organizations at the outset of planning; maintained centralized regular communication among organization members, with prevention messages disseminated through the community; focused on prevention rather than on personal issues; established short timelines for task completion (months versus years); used a centralized system or hierarchy for task distribution, such as through subcommittees; and had or could acquire adequate resources for implementation (Mansergh et al., 1996; Saxe et al., 1997; Yin et al., 1997).

Other research on community tobacco, alcohol, and drug abuse prevention trials suggests that the complementarity of prevention program messages and timing of program delivery with policy contributes to support for a policy and its implementation (e.g., Forster et al., 1997; Pentz & Sussman, 1997; Pentz, 1997; Perry et al., 1996). However, research has not determined whether top-down (leader-initiated) versus bottom-up (citizen-initiated), authoritarian versus democratic, or lateral versus hierarchical organizational models are more or less effective in mobilizing a community for prevention policy change.

These theories, collectively, represent reciprocal interactions between person, social situational (group), and environmental factors that can be expected to affect drug use in a community (Pentz, 1999). Hypothesized causal relationships between these factors and policy change and the effects of policy change on drug use behavior are shown in Figure 11.1.

RESEARCH SUPPORT FOR LOCAL POLICY CHANGE

Studies of the effects of policy change on cigarette smoking and alcohol use are more prevalent than are studies of other types of drug use among adolescents. The predominance of cigarette and alcohol studies may reflect a wider public recognition of the negative health consequences of these substances, compared with other drugs, and a relatively longer history of prevention research evaluating gateway drugs (cigarettes, alcohol, marijuana), compared with other substances. A summary of the results of policy research suggests the following. At national, state, and county levels, studies have used forecasting and time series analyses to evaluate the effects of changes in drunk driving penalties, the use of roadblocks as checkpoints, BAC levels, legal driving age, price, and monitoring of liquor outlets on associated changes in adult, and to a lesser extent, late adolescent drinking patterns (e.g., see Casswell & Gilmore, 1989; Giesbrecht et al., 1990; Grossman & Coate, 1988; Hingson et al., 1996; Holder, 1993; Join Together, 1997a; Moskowitz, 1989). Studies indicate that these policies, overall, have yielded moderate, statistically significant declines in heavy drinking for periods of six months to three years after policy change. At the community level, studies have used trend and regression analyses as well as simple analysis of variance to evaluate differences between communities involved or not involved in restricting access by youth to alcohol and tobacco (e.g., see Altman et al., 1991; Forster et al., 1997; Perry et al., 1996). These studies suggest that policy change is associated with short-term declines in the

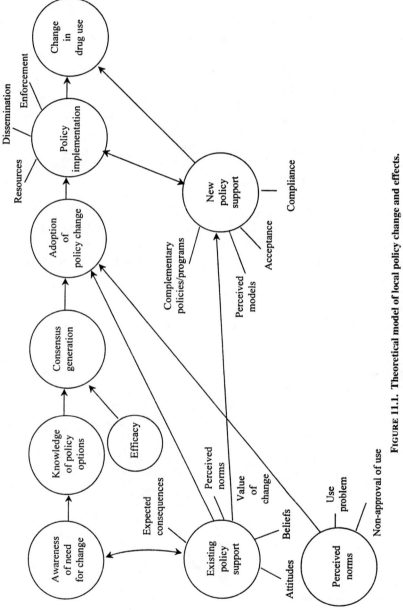

FIGURE 11.1. Theoretical model of local policy change and effects.

amount and prevalence rates of adolescent smoking; effects on adolescent drinking are less clear. Studies at the workplace level have used pre–post change analyses and simple tests for group differences to evaluate the effects of smoking restrictions and smoking bans on adult employee smoking (e.g., Glasgow et al., 1996). Most of these studies have shown changes in amount and patterns of smoking associated with policy change but not in prevalence rates of smoking. Studies have also been conducted on the effects of drug testing in the workplace. Results of one large study suggest that drug testing is associated with lower rates of absenteeism and drug use among new hires (Normand et al., 1990). At the school level, studies using regression analyses and analysis of variance suggest that lower adolescent smoking and other drug use are associated with policies that are regularly enforced and prevention oriented, as opposed to punishment oriented (see Moskowitz & Jones, 1988; Pentz, Dwyer, MacKinnon, et al., 1989). Notably absent are studies of the effects of policy change on drug use at the neighborhood or service agency level within communities.

Interestingly, in recent years, populationwide support of drug policy change has been greater than might have been expected, given public arguments that have heretofore hindered the consideration of policy change as a viable drug use prevention strategy for communities (e.g., Forster et al., 1997; Perry et al., 1996; Wagenaar et al., 1994). Most arguments have focused on the violation of individual rights, such as invasion of privacy through drunk driving and drug use tests and on the interpretation of what constitutes punishable abuse versus acceptable, or tolerated, use levels (Jeffrey et al., 1990; Library of Congress, 1989; MMWR, 1987; Moskowitz, 1989). For example, smokers have been shown to be more accepting and supportive of no-smoking policies in the workplace and restricted smoking in public settings than has been previously assumed (Galaif et al., 1996; Glasgow et al., 1996). The generally high levels of support for such policies in recent years may reflect a general trend toward acceptance of policy as a drug prevention intervention strategy in the United States.

Overall, the results of policy research suggest that local policy changes can have an effect on youth and adult drug use, implementation of other preventive interventions not withstanding. With one exception (Forster et al., 1997), policy effects on cigarette smoking by youth have been limited to the number of cigarettes smoked among current smokers, rather than on decreasing prevalence rates of smoking. Thus, for cigarette smoking, local policy change alone may not be as effective as smoking prevention and cessation programs that have shown significant reductions in prevalence rates. The effects of policy on alcohol use, particularly of policies aimed at pricing and limiting availability, appear to be stronger than current alcohol prevention and treatment programs, which have reported weak, short-lived effects, or effects limited to delaying onset of drinking rather than preventing drunk driving (c.f., Grossman & Coate, 1988; Moskowitz, 1989; Pentz, 1993). The effectiveness of local policy change regarding other drug use is not yet known.

MAJOR PREVENTION POLICY
RESEARCH ISSUES

Theory and previous research suggest several conceptual directions for studies of local prevention policy change. Before mounting quasiexperimental and experimental studies that have the capacity to determine the effects of such change, appropriate research methods need to be developed to address three major issues. These issues include (1) quantifying policy (according to prevention orientation, restrictiveness, enforcement, dissemination, population awareness, and population support criteria), (2) modeling longitudinal effects (hypothesizing linear, quadratic, or sudden drop effects of policy change), and (3) evaluating causal effects (differentiating the effects of policy from those of ongoing prevention programs and prevention-related events in a community and determining whether policy effects are uni- or bidirectional.)

Quantifying policy is an issue, because previous research has treated policy simply as a dichotomous independent variable for its effects on drug use (for example, a state initiates a higher minimum age drinking law, yes or no, or before or after implementation of that law) (Holder, 1993) with little regard for the contribution of implementation and support factors that have already been shown to influence compliance (e.g., Glasgow et al., 1996). Modeling longitudinal effects according to different assumptions about how policy influences behavior is also important, since previous research has tended to assume a "drop-off" effect. That is, as soon as a policy is initiated, use will drop (e.g., Jason et al., 1991). Alternative possibilities should also be explored, such as a gradual linear decline in drug use as policy knowledge is disseminated throughout a community, or a u-shaped function that shows an initial dramatic drop off followed by a gradual increase in use again as the novelty effect of a new policy wears off. Finally, most evaluations of policy effects do not control for the effects of other interventions that are occurring either simultaneously with policy implementation or have been affected by policy, such as the effects of the timing of new prevention programs in schools. Figure 11.2 partially illustrates the complexity of modeling the causal effects of local policy and policy change within a community vis-à-vis existing local government structures and functions, community organization efforts applied to the problem of drug abuse prevention, and prevention program effects (Pentz, 1995).

PROPOSED RESEARCH METHODS

Formative Evaluation Research

The evaluation of local prevention policies may require developing at least two relatively new components of formative evaluation: systemic epidemiology and content and process of policy change. Both of these can be defined and elaborated on in a series of formative evaluation studies of several months up to 3 years duration, the length of time previous research suggests may be required for a community to mobilize to the point of adopting a policy (e.g., see Altman et al., 1991; Bracht, 1990; Butterfoss et al., 1996; Giesbrecht et al., 1990; Goodman & Streckler, 1990; Pentz & Montgomery, unpublished manuscript; Rothman, 1979; Saxe et al., 1997; Yin et al., 1997).

Systemic Epidemiology

The first component of formative evaluation research on local policy change can be referred to as "systemic epidemiology" studies, research on factors that work their way through the systems, organizations, and community leader networks and either contribute to or inhibit the spread of local policy change (Butterfoss et al., 1996; Goodman & Streckler, 1990; Klitzner, 1993). Systemic epidemiology is different from behavioral epidemiology studies of drug abuse, which focus on intrapersonal (person) and interpersonal (situational) factors that contribute to drug use or prevention. Systemic epidemiology studies would focus on environmental factors that affect the functioning of a community, such as the negative effects of political corruption on community leader empowerment and subsequently on poor school achievement, defaced neighborhoods, and failure to enforce drug-free zone policies (cf. Sampson, Raudenbush, & Earls, 1997). Based on

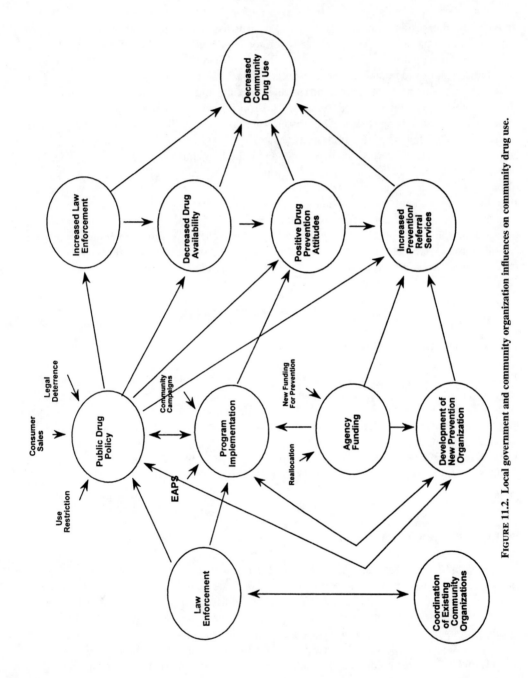

FIGURE 11.2. Local government and community organization influences on community drug use.

community organization, social action, and community psychology studies, likely factors include empowerment of community leaders, the centrality and density of community leader and community agency networks, the level of consensus building among community leaders and agencies on other health initiatives, previous positive policy change and/or prevention programming, access to local funds, the clarity and rapidity of vertical and lateral communications among local government and community agencies, and positive local mass media support for policy change (see Bracht, 1990; Butterfoss et al., 1996; Giesbrecht et al., 1990; Pentz & Montgomery, unpublished manuscript; Rothman, 1979).

Content and Process of Policy Change

The second new component of formative evaluation would be developing and piloting a local policy as a preventive intervention. In the case of prevention programs, formative evaluation typically consists of needs assessment and reactions to theory-based material by the target consumer or intervention receiver group; discussion, feedback, and revision of initial drafts of program materials by researchers; reactions to and feedback by the consumer group; revision; piloting in a limited setting, with process and immediate post-test evaluation; subsequent revision; and field application (Butterfoss et al., 1996). In this case, the role of the researcher is that of primary developer and, usually, implementor of the program (Mittlemark, 1990; Pentz, 1995). The researcher could follow the same procedures for developing policy as for an intervention. However, since researchers are not policymakers, the role of the researcher, on an active–passive continuum, changes to co-developer, advisor, or consultant to local government or community leaders who will eventually implement the policy (Mittlemark, 1990; Pentz, 1995). Regardless of the specific level of activity, the researcher's primary role is to inform the decision-making process that is ultimately decided and acted upon by others.

An important part of developing policy as an intervention is elucidating and validating hypothesized policy mediators, the mechanisms thought to move the process along in a positive and expedited fashion. Based on previous research, at least some of these mediators can be operationalized as a set of process and early interim outcome variables during the pilot phase of formative evaluation. These include consumer awareness and support of policy change, previous personal positive experience with a similar policy or a similar intervention, perceived positive consequences of policy adoption and compliance, and adequate time for community leaders to develop a climate of cooperation among policymakers (e.g., see Goodman & Streckler, 1990; Giesbrecht et al., 1990). To the extent that the content and process of the policy change intervention can induce and change these variables, they are considered policy change mediators.

Because of the short timelines for evaluation, and often, pressure from communities to initiate policy change, the utility of formative evaluation research is limited to developing measures and policy intervention strategies. Formative evaluation studies do not address the question of whether policy change is an antecedent, consequent, or mediator of other preventive intervention effects in a community, a causality question more suitable for study in research trials lasting several years.

Developing Prevention Policy Typology

Local drug prevention policies can differ on several parameters, including whether a drug is legal or illegal (Warner et al., 1990). Based on variation of policies shown in previous research, several parameters lend themselves to future study as independent or mediating variables of their effects on drug behavior:

- setting for local policy change (school, worksite, community);
- type of policy (passive, such as adherence to a no-smoking ordinance, or active, as in participation in drug-testing);
- direction of policy initiation (administration or "top-down," or grassroots/population or "bottom-up");
- extent of population involvement in policy change (high if a representative sample or the total population was involved in policy decision making, low if a selected sample was involved, none if decision making is limited to administration only);
- reason for policy initiation (reactive if in response to an immediate drug problem or complaint, or proactive if not in response to an immediate problem or complaint);
- evidence of support for policy (yes or no by target population and community leaders, and successful implementation of environmental change interventions designed to support the policy, such as modification of worksite employee assistance programs (EAPs) to provide intervention for employees testing positive from a drug testing policy);
- extent of policy dissemination through interpersonal and mass media (high if interpersonal and mass media are used, low if interpersonal or mass media are not used).

Based on previous policy reviews (Join Together, 1997a; President's Commission, 1992; Wallack & Corbett, 1987; Warner et al., 1990), a typology of prevention policy can be developed to guide formative evaluation studies of policy; construct appropriate research designs for later trials of policy change; and identify appropriate measures, variables, and analyses for evaluation of policy effects. To reflect the current status of drug abuse control strategies, the typology should include the following categories: source of policy (formal law or regulation or informal guideline), organization of policy (top-down, bottom-up, mixed), target (user, supplier, service provider), type of drug control approach (supply or demand reduction), and unit or boundary of policy (school, neighborhood, etc.).

One parameter is whether the policy is a formal, legal regulation or an informal guideline or a directive for action. Included in informal guidelines could be declarative regulations, since they serve an educational role and do not require enforcement. In some studies where local community support is assumed to contribute substantially to the success or failure of a policy, it might be hypothesized that an informal policy would be more effective than a formal policy because it invites community participation in policy planning and carries no punitive consequences. An example of an informal source is parents who agree to assist school and law enforcement personnel in monitoring school grounds for drug use. The policy is informal in its source (parents) and informal to the extent that it is not a written mandate provided by the school.

How a policy is formulated and adopted—top-down, bottom-up, or mixed—may determine its effectiveness in a community. Top-down refers to policies that are initiated, formulated, and adopted by a few administrators or community leaders with little input from community residents. Bottom-up is the reverse, whereby policies are initiated, formulated, and adopted by community residents (grass roots effort), and policymakers are pressured to adopt the policy. Mixed refers to policies that are initiated either top-down or bottom-up, but both residents and policymakers provide early and continuing input to policy formulation, adoption, and implementation. For example, a proposed policy change might be categorized as top-down if community leaders initiate consideration of the policy change, if leaders have been previously educated in policy options, and if limited dissemination of policy awareness and knowledge is required for policy adoption. A policy change would be bottom-up if it is initiated by community pressure or referendum, if new educational preparation of the population is required, and if rapid dissemination is required for adoption. A mixed model involving reciprocal communications, feedback, and decision making between community and government leaders; the general population is the third category, which has been used in several recent community-based trials for heart disease and drug abuse prevention (see Mittlemark, 1990; Pentz & Montgomery, unpublished manuscript).

Another parameter to include in the typology is the approach to drug abuse control: supply reduction versus demand reduction (see Bukoski, 1990; Inciardi, 1990; Nahas et al., 1986; Pentz et al., 1996; Schuster, 1989). As noted earlier, supply reduction policies include, but are not limited to, age restrictions, setting restrictions, and sales and use disruption through deterrence, interdiction, or retribution. Demand reduction policies include, but are not limited to, institutionalization of prevention education, price increase or taxation, reinforcement of nonuse practice through community recognition, and dissemination of nonuse messages through mass media (Join Together, 1997a). These apparently disparate policies can be organized further into four categories: (1) regulation (statutes and rules), (2) economic incentives, (3) information/education, and (4) assistance/support (cf. Lynch & Bonnie, 1994; Warner et al., 1990). They represent a continuum from most to least coercive to a population (cf. Warner et al., 1990).

An additional parameter is the focus or target of policy change: the user, supplier, or service provider (cf. Warner et al., 1990). A user focus is directed at changing user drug use; the other two are indirect or mediator targets that have the same eventual end point—changing user behavior. Most studies on youth have evaluated associations between policy change and behavior (e.g., Biglan et al., 1996; Forster et al., 1997; Jason et al., 1991; Pentz & Sussman, 1997), but a few have attempted to evaluate changes in supplier behavior by examining sales to youths (see Chaloupka, 1996; Grossman & Coate, 1988).

Finally, prevention policy can be categorized by its unit of influence or boundary. For example, a school tobacco policy covers the school but not the neighborhood surrounding the school. Some units of policy may be nested within others, such as school tobacco policy within neighborhood vendor policies on tobacco sales within community no-smoking ordinances. Conceptualizing units of policy influence can be useful in randomized and quasiexperimental trials, with assignment of appropriate units of policy influence to policy change or control conditions (such as neighborhoods to a neighborhood watch or control condition). Such units are also helpful in analyzing data with nested effects of each unit of policy in a community, for example, analyzing successive effects of school, neighborhood, and community policy on individual youth, using PROC.MIXED or hierarchical linear modeling (Chou, Bentler, & Pentz, 1998; Wagenaar et al., 1994).

Based on these parameters, a policy could be categorized according to the cells shown in Figure 11.3, which enables the researcher to develop appropriate policy content, identify the target consumer, and prioritize appropriate independent, dependent, and mediating variables for later evaluations. In its entirety, progressing from more general to more specific categories, the typology is a 3 (top, bottom, mixed organization) × 5 (community, neighborhood, worksite, service agency, school unit) × 8 (supply versus demand reduction × regulation, economic, education, assistance strategy) × 3 (user, supplier, service provider target) × 2 (informal, formal source) matrix.

Developing Measures and Variables

As others have noted, the length of time and complexity involved in producing policy change subjects almost all policy evaluation studies to potential confounds of intervening historical events and interventions, maturation and history effects, and possibly measurement decay (Boruch & Gomez, 1977; Cook & Campbell; 1979; Musto, 1995). One of the primary methods to interpret policy effects in the face of these potential confounds is the use of multiple measures from multiple data sources within a community, including self- and other-report, archival records, observations,

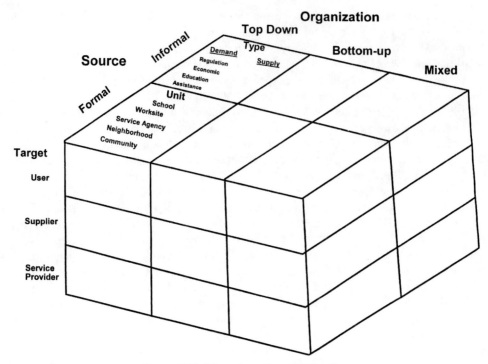

FIGURE 11.3. Dimensions of prevention policy.

and interviews from independent samples of users, suppliers, and service providers, regardless of which is the actual target of the policy intervention. Another is *a priori* specification of variables that are expected to behave as antecedent, consequent (interim or long-term outcome), or mediating (process or interim outcome) variables in the course of local policy change. Measures and variables also should provide data on potential confounds to interpretation of policy effects that can be included and adjusted for longitudinal analyses. Based on recent prevention intervention research, these include, but are not limited to, measures and variables that assess school and community demographic shifts; national and community secular trends for drug use; tobacco and alcohol sales tax revenues; and prevention and treatment service delivery rates and content, process, and implementation of other prevention programs, policies, and interventions in the community (e.g., Chaloupka, 1996; Grossman & Coate, 1988; Musto, 1995; Pentz, Dwyer, MacKinnon, et al., 1989, 1990).

The specification of variables should be time dependent (cf. Pentz et al., 1996). For example, in a 5-year longitudinal study, it might be hypothesized that initial implementation of a prevention education program in a community during the first 2 years is a catalyst for school district adoption of a policy in year 3 that guarantees set-aside funds, time, and teacher training for program implementation in later years. If this course of action is hypothesized *a priori,* then program implementation acts as an antecedent (independent) variable in years 1 and 2 to policy change in year 3, and policy change in year 3 is an antecedent to continued, and perhaps, improved, program implementation as a consequent (dependent) variable in years 4 and 5.

Based on research described thus far, Table 11.1 shows proposed measures and variables for the evaluation of local policy change, by phase of study (formative, process, summative), course of policy change hypothesized in Figure 11.1, and by illustrative types of policy drawn from Figure 11.3.

TABLE 11.1. Proposed Variables and Measures for Evaluation of Local Policy Change by Sample Types of Policy

Type	Source	Unit	Target	Phase of study	Variables[a]	Measures
Demand-education	Formal/mixed	School	User	Formative	IVs[a] = Program adoption, existing policy MVs[a] = Program implemention, use prevalence change DVs = Policy revision, implementation, dissemination	Archival policy, use infractions, youth, & staff surveys, meeting records
Demand-regulation	Informal/bottom-up	Neighborhood	User + supplier	Process	IVs = Precipitating event, resident dissatisfaction & fear, sales & use MVs = Resident support, communication DVs = Adoption, implementation, dissemination of monitoring system	Observations, interviews, meeting records
Supply-economic	Formal/top-down	Community	User + supplier	Summative	IVs = Existing revenue MVs = Tax DVs = Sales & use	Sales/revenue records, observations
Demand + supply-assistance	Informal/mixed	Service agency	Service provider	Process	IVs = Provider dissatisfaction with service implementation MVs = Change in service delivery procedures, client participation DVs = Client use prevalence	Survey, observation, agency records

[a]IVs, Independent/antecedent variables; MVs, mediating or interim dependent variables; DVs, endpoint dependent variables.

Taking the first row of Table 11.1 as an example, a formative evaluation study of a demand reduction policy that focuses on institutionalizing prevention programming in a school could be designed as follows. The target of such a policy would be students. The independent variables would consist of existing policy (level of enforcement and severity of consequences for policy violation) and policy support (attitudes toward policy, perceived use norms, and policy compliance) and whether the demand reduction prevention program had been adopted. Mediating variables would consist of the level or quality of prevention program implementation before policy mandates the program and interim program effects on drug use prevalence as an indication to school administrators and parents that the program is worth institutionalizing in a policy change. Dependent variables would then consist of evidence of policy revision to include institutionalization of the prevention program (set-aside funds, standardized teacher training, curriculum fit, specification of teacher and student program materials) and subsequent evaluation of implementation and dissemination of the policy change.

Research and Measurement Designs

Because of the opportunistic nature of most policy studies to date (a researcher finds out about a policy change that is about to or has just occurred and decides to evaluate it), few if any studies have been under researcher control (Chaloupka, 1996; Holder, 1993). Most studies, therefore, have used pre-experimental or quasiexperimental designs to evaluate policy change, with the relatively more methodologically advanced quasiexperimental research designs including multiple contrasted groups and/or randomized planned variations within policy cells, and measurement designs that include extended baseline or time series measurement (Biglan et al., 1996). If assigning units of policy implementation randomly to policy or control group conditions is not an option, regression discontinuity and nested randomized variations within policy conditions may be superior to other quasiexperimental designs for controlling biases associated with history, maturation, or regression (Pentz, 1994).

With few exceptions (e.g., Forster et al., 1997; Perry et al., 1996; Wagenaar et al., 1994) local policies have not been manipulated experimentally in randomized designs with large numbers of sites. Rather, previous studies have been based on sites that were ready for or needed the policy change. Several researchers have discussed the ecological validity of research designs that are based on need, merit, readiness or additional factors other than randomization (Boruch & Gomez, 1977; Butterfoss et al., 1996; Pentz, 1994; Saxe et al., 1997). While these alternative designs may improve the ecological validity of a study, they are not readily accepted by the scientific community. Since it is difficult to randomly assign and control policies in communities, the external validity of studies using alternative non- or quasiexperimental designs may depend on multiple replications of effect.

One possible design alternative to randomization is developing a pool of communities ready and with the requisite resources to implement policy change, matching the communities on demographic and population behavior variables predictive of drug use and support for prevention, and assigning matched communities to alternative theory-driven types of policies, such as policies that are primarily deterrent or punitive in focus versus policies that are support and education focused. At least one study has already shown that prevention-oriented policies focused on institutionalizing smoking prevention programs in schools are more effective in reducing the number of cigarettes smoked by adolescents than are cessation- or punishment-oriented policies (Pentz, Brannon, Charlin, et al., 1989).

Development and Refinement of Analysis Methods

Several analytic strategies have been developed for use either in longitudinal prevention intervention research or in studies of policy effects at levels larger than the community. Conceivably, these strategies could be integrated into longitudinal studies of local prevention policy effects. These strategies include methods to statistically model the complexity of the environmental units in which policy change occurs in order to aid experimental assignment and adjustment for antecedent and confounding variables. They also include methods for adjusting other confounds discussed earlier in this chapter, and—perhaps particularly relevant to drug prevention policy research—methods for modeling linear, quadratic, reciprocal, drop off, and recidivistic drug use trends in a community.

These strategies include:

- using multiattribute utility measurement (MAUM) strategies to match and assign communities and community subunits to experimental conditions (Graham et al., 1984);
- using analysis methods that model the nested effects of multiple policies on individuals in communities, such as hierarchichal linear modeling (Chou et al., 1998);
- modeling fixed environmental effects and comparing these to collective community demographic effects (Dwyer et al., 1989; Pentz, 1994);
- pooling environmental units for analysis to minimize missing data due to temporary rather than permanent attrition (Dwyer et al., 1989; Graham et al., 1984);
- adjusting for attrition and target subject movement through multiple attrition analysis methods, including forward missing values imputation (Chou et al., 1998);
- covariate adjustment of process, implementation, and secular trend data (Pentz et al., 1990);
- using proportional hazards and Markov models to estimate movement of a community population from one behavioral state to another as a result of policy change (Norton et al., 1996);
- incorporating cost-effectiveness analyses into evaluation of prevention policy effects on drug use behavior (Kim et al., 1995).

AN IDEAL PREVENTION POLICY

An ideal prevention policy, implemented at the community level, should incorporate three features: (1) a plan for linking and cross-referring compatible polices across segments or subsets of the community; (2) simultaneous implementation of policies that complement or enhance the effects of each other; and (3) strategic use of prevention programs to increase support for policy, policy change, and its effects on drug use.

Linking Compatible Policies

A plan for policy change in one community setting could include provisions for linking the change with compatible policies in other settings, or for promoting compatible policies in other settings if policies do not already exist. For example, a smoking, alcohol, and drug prevention policy in one worksite might be shared as a model for other worksites through a local Chamber of Commerce or Rotary Club. For parents of school-age children, a work-site policy that includes drug prevention education and family intervention as part of an EAP could be linked to drug prevention education and policy changes occurring in local schools. Company directors could link directly with local school superintendents to share information about their policies that affect the same families or neighborhoods. Quasiexperimental research methods will be required to determine the relative efficacy of comprehensive, multichannel policies before this recommendation can be made. For example, between-community designs could be used to evaluate the effects of public ordinances concerning no-smoking or monitoring of liquor sales to minors, with or without integration of school policies concerning the development and monitoring of smoking- and alcohol-free zones around schools. Within-community designs could evaluate the effects of individual school policies for staff and student smoking, with and without involvement of local convenience stores in limiting the availability of tobacco products.

Support for a local policy change should be solicited from representatives of the target population as well as from community leaders. Plans for and subsequent implementation of environmental change interventions that support the policy should also be included. For example, a school policy change to institutionalize drug prevention education as part of the regular school curriculum could also include community plans to collect, monitor, and revise curriculum materials on a regular basis, as was done as part of a community prevention program in both Kansas City and Indianapolis (Pentz, Dwyer, MacKinnon, et al., 1989; Newman, unpublished manuscript). The efficacy of environmental support could be evaluated using designs with large numbers of communities assigned to various support–no-support conditions, or in single replicated community designs using time series analysis of preintroduction, introduction, and postintroduction of environmental support interventions.

Local dissemination of information about a policy change within the setting affected by the policy is probably required to produce immediate compliance from the target population. However, broader, positive mass media coverage of the policy change could improve long-term compliance and promote chain reactions of compatible policy changes in other community settings. For example, a change in city government worker policy to include prevention education for families of workers referred to an EAP for drug treatment could be communicated to all employees through city government departmental memos, newsletters, and office posters. If the policy change were also positively communicated to the general public, the interest generated among community residents could be expected to both reinforce employees and increase their public commitment to comply with the policy. These principles of behavior change are routinely applied in preventive interventions with youth (Pentz, 1986, 1993, 1998; Tobler, 1997). Furthermore, community interest could put pressure on other worksites to appear as civic leaders and innovators by quickly adopting either similar or even expanded policies (Pentz, 1995). The relative effectiveness of "small" media (within-setting) versus mass media (communitywide) dissemination of a policy could be evaluated in research designs that randomly assign matched worksites, schools, or other local organizations, by community, to dissemination conditions. Alternatively, dissemination effectiveness might be evaluated in a modified ABAB1 applied behavioral analysis design in which a single worksite is followed from baseline (A), to small media dissemination (B), to removal of small media dissemination (A), to reinstatement of small media and addition of mass media dissemination (B1) (see Biglan et al., 1996).

Implementation of Mutually Enhancing Policies

Implementing mutually enhancing policies refers to the use of different policies that contribute to the effectiveness or efficiency of each other within the same population. For example, in the case of tobacco and alcohol use, local policy interventions aimed at youth might include a two-pronged effort. The first would focus on controlling access at stores and other points of legal purchase for adults through (1) limiting and reviewing license applications to merchants, (2) monitoring merchant compliance in checking identification and refusing sales to minors, (3) revoking licenses if necessary, and (4) conducting sting operations with community support. The second effort would integrate local store access strategies with other policy interventions, including (1) ordinances to limit the number and types of tobacco and alcohol outlets in communities; (2) standardizing identification checking for alcohol purchases at 21 and tobacco purchases at 18; (3) raising the purchase price by at least $1.00 for a pack of cigarettes; and (4) mandating education of local merchants for legal server responsibility, procedures for checking identification, and criteria for license application and maintenance.

Use of Prevention Programs To Enhance Policy

Using program intervention first, followed by policy intervention, may have the strongest impact on preventing drug abuse by youths (Pentz et al., 1996). Resistance skills, anti-use norms, and compliance are directly affected early by the program intervention and subsequently contribute to access and resistance. Awareness and support for population or communitywide policy change can be built in by implementing a successful program intervention first. Successful program intervention then contributes to community recognition of the need for policy change that includes institutionalizing the successful program.

Integrating supply and demand reduction strategies may require policies that include funding and institutionalizing demand reduction programs, education for lobby groups to support prevention and prevention-oriented drug policies, and maintenance of healthy community partnerships that bring together policymakers and educators. An interdependent relationship between policymakers and educators can affect both supply and demand reduction, and produce a greater reduction in community drug use than could be achieved by either alone, perhaps doubling the effects found from either program or policy interventions.

SUMMARY

This chapter has examined the potential of local policy to change drug use behavior. As more research is conducted in this area and more attention is drawn to the potential of using policy as a preventive intervention in and of itself, more systematic and representative evaluations of the effects of policy on drug use behavior will become available. This is an area of research that has been lacking in the drug prevention field as well as in the health and social sciences in general. Without more systematic research, recommendations for the most effective policy a community might implement, or for efficacy trials of policies, are premature. However, several community action researchers have attempted to outline components of community preventive interventions, including local policy changes that could be expected to maximize effects on health behavior based on principles of behavior change, public health, and social marketing (Bracht, 1990; Butterfoss et al., 1996; Pentz et al., 1996; Saxe et al., 1997). Based on these principles, an ideal prevention policy would:

- be implemented in settings that are convenient to reach, appropriate for drug prevention messages, and least disruptive to normal functioning;
- address multiple stages of drug use behavior change and intervention needs, from prevention of onset through relapse prevention;

- focus on small, realistically achievable behavior goals;
- specify substances, settings, and mechanisms for change;
- vary environmental support interventions for policy and messages to disseminate policy;
- be comprehensive by including multiple settings within a community;
- utilize existing or reorganized social networks and media to disseminate policy;
- involve the target population in developing or choosing the policy;
- provide positive socializing experiences or other reinforcements for policy compliance;
- provide for systematic training for policy disseminators and administrators and educate for the target population in the skills needed to implement and participate in policy objectives; and
- include guidelines and/or funds to encourage independent activities that maintain interest and support of the policy change over the long term.

REFERENCES

Ajzen, I., & Fishbein, M. (1990). *Understanding attitudes and predicting social behavior.* Englewood Cliffs, NJ: Prentice-Hall.

Altman, D. G., Rasenick-Douss L., Foster, V., & Tye, J. B. (1991). Sustained effects of an educational program to reduce sales of cigarettes to minors. *American Journal of Public Health, 81,* 891–893.

Bandura, A. (1977). *Social learning theory.* Englewood Cliffs, NJ: Prentice Hall.

Barrera, M., Jr. (1986). Distinctions between social support concepts, social support inventory. Measure and models. *American Journal of Community Psychology, 14*(4), 413–445.

Biglan, A., Ary, D., Yudelson, H., Duncan, T. E., Hood, D., James, L., Koehn, V., Wright, Z., Black, C., Levings, D., Smith, S., and Gaiser, E. (1996). Experimental evaluation of a modular approach to mobilizing anti-tobacco influences of peers and parents. *American Journal of Community Psychology, 24*(3), 311–39.

Boruch, R. F., & Gomez, H. (1977). Sensitivity, bias, and theory in impact evaluations, *Professional Psychologist, 8,* 411–434.

Bracht, N. F. (Ed., 1990). *Health promotion at the community level.* Newbury Park, CA: Sage.

Bukoski, W. J. (1990). The federal approach to primary drug abuse prevention and education. In J. A., Inciardi, (Ed.), *Handbook of drug control.* Westport, CT: Greenwood Publishing Group, Inc.

Butterfoss, F. D., Goodman, R. M., & Wandersman, A. (1996). Community coalitions for prevention and health promotion: Factors predicting satisfaction, participation and planning. *Health Education Quarterly, 23*(1), 65–79.

Casswell, S., & Gilmore, S. (1989). An evaluated community action project on alcohol. *Journal of Studies on Alcohol, 50*(4), 339–346.

Chaloupka, F. (1996). *Price, tobacco control policies, and youth smoking.* Cambridge, MA: National Bureau of Economic Research.

Chou, C-P., Bentler, P. M., & Pentz, M. A. (1998). Comparisons of two statistical approaches to study growth curve: The hierarchical linear model and the latent curve model. *Structural Equation Modeling.* (51) pp. 247–266.

Clayton, R. R. (1990). The National Institute on Drug Abuse (NIDA) Longitudinal DARE Evaluation. Presented at the Alcohol, Tobacco, and Other Drugs Conference in San Diego, CA, October 1990.

Cook, T. D., & D. T. Campbell. (1979) *Quasi-experimentation: design and analysis issues for field settings.* Rand McNally: Chicago.

Dwyer, J. H, MacKinnon, D. P., Pentz, M. A., et al. (1989). Estimating intervention effects in longitudinal studies. *Am J Epidemiol., 130,* 781–795.

Farkas, A. J., Pierce, J. P., Zhu, S. H., Rosbrook, B., Gilpin, E. A., Berry, C., & Kaplan, R. M. (1996). Addiction versus stages of change models in predicting smoking cessation. *Addiction, 91*(9), 1271–1280.

Farquhar, J. W., Fortmann, S. P., Flora, J. A., Taylor, C. B., Haskell, W. L., Williams, P. T., Maccoby, N., Wood, P. D. (1990). Effects of communitywide education on cardiovascular disease risk factors: the Stanford Five-City Project. *JAMA, 264,* 359–365.

Forster, J. L., Wolfson, M., Murray, D. M., Wagenaar, A. C., & Claxton, A. J. (1997). Perceived and measured availability of tobacco to youths in 14 Minnesota communities: the TPOP Study. Tobacco Policy Options for Prevention. *American Journal of Preventive Medicine, 13*(3), 167–174.

Galaif, E. R., Sussman, S., & Bundek, N. (1996). The relations of school staff smokers attitudes about modeling smoking behavior in students and the receptivity to no-smoking policy. *Journal of Drug Education, 26*(4). 313–322.

Giesbrecht, N., Consley, P., & Denniston, R. W. (Eds., 1990). *Research, action, and the community: experiences in the prevention of alcohol and other problems, OSAP Prevention Monograph 4.* U.S. Department of Health and Human Services.

Glasgow, R. E., Soreson, G., Giffen, C., Shipley, R. H., Corbett, K., & Lynn, W. (1996). Promoting worksite smoking control policies and actions: the Community Intervention Trial for Smoking Cessation (COMMIT) experience. The COMMIT Research Group. *Preventive Medicine, 25*(2), 186–195.

Goldstein, A., & Kalant, H. (1990). Drug policy: Striking the right balance. *Science, 29*(4976), 1513–1521.

Goodman, R. M., & Streckler, A. (1990). A model for the institutionalization of health promotion programs. *Family and Community Health, 11,* 63–78.

Goodstadt, M. S. (1989). Substance abuse curricula vs. school drug policies. *Journal of School Health, 59*(6), 246–250.

Graham, J. W., Flay, B. R., Johnson, C. A., Hansen, W. B., & Collins, L. M. (1984). Group comparability: A multi-attribute utility measurement approach to the use of random assignment with small numbers of aggregated units. *Evaluation Review 8,* 247–260.

Grossman, M., & D. Coate. (1988). Effects of alcoholic beverage prices and legal drinking ages on youth. *National Bureau of Economic Research, Inc., 31*(1012), 145–171.

Hansen, W. B. (1992). School-based substance abuse prevention: a review of the state-of-the-art in curriculum, 1980–1990. *Health Education Research, 7*(3), 403–430.

Hingson, R., Donnay, G., & Zakocs, R. (unpublished manuscript). *Current state laws and programs regarding the access of minors to tobacco and plans for implementation of the Synar amendment.* Boston University School of Public Health, 1–30.

Hingson, R., McGovern, T., Howland, J., Heeren, T., Winter, M., & Zakocs, R. (1996). Reducing alcohol-impaired driving in Massachusetts: the Saving Lives program. *American Journal of Public Health, 86*(6), 791–797.

Holder, H. D. (1993). Prevention of alcohol-related accidents in the community. *Addiction, 88*(7), 1003–1012.

Inciardi, J. A. (1990). *Handbook of drug control.* Westport, CT: Greenwood Publishing Group, Inc.

Jason, L. A., Li, P. Y., Anes, M. D., & Birkhead, S. H. (1991). Active enforcement of cigarette control laws in the prevention of cigarette sales to minors. *Journal of the American Medical Association, 266*(22), 3159–3161.

Jeffrey, R. W., Forster, J. L., Schmid, T. L., McBride, C. M., Rooney, B. L., & Pirie, P. L. (1990). Community attitudes toward public policies to control alcohol, tobacco, and high-fat food consumption. *American Journal of Preventive Medicine, 6*(1), 12–19.

Johnston, L., Bachman, J. G., & O'Malley, P. M. (1997). *Drug use among teens shows some signs of leveling after a long rise.* The University of Michigan News and Information Services, Press Release, December 18 (24).

Johnston, L. D., O'Malley, P. M., & Bachman, J. G. (1996). *National survey results on drug use from the Monitoring the Future study, 1975–1995. Vol. 1, secondary school students.* Rockville, MD, U.S. Department of Health and Human Services (NIH Publication No. 94-3809).

Join Together (1997a). *Alcohol and drug abuse in America: Policies for prevention.* Join Together, Boston, MA.

Join Together (1997b). *Community action guide to policies for prevention: The Recommendations of the Join Together Policy Panel on Preventing Substance Abuse.* Join Together, Boston, MA.

Kim, S., Coletti, S. D., Crutchfield, C. C., Williams, C., & Hepler, N. (1995). Benefit-cost analysis of drug prevention programs: A macroscopic approach. *Journal of Drug Education, 25*(2), 111–127.

Klitzner, M. (1993). A public health/dynamic systems approach to community-wide alcohol and other drug initiatives. In R. Davis, R. C. Davis, A. J. Lurigio, D. P. Rosenbaum (Eds.), *Drugs and Community.* Springfield, IL: Charles C Thomas.

Library of Congress (1989). *Anti-drug abuse act of 1988: Summary of major provisions (Publication CRS 89-288).* Washington, DC: Congressional Research Service.

Lynch B. S., & Bonnie, R. J. (Eds., 1994). *Growing up tobacco-free: Preventing nicotine addiction in children and youths.* Committee on Preventing Nicotine Addiction in Institute of Medicine Report, Washington DC: National Academy Press.

Mansergh, G., Rohrbach, L., Montgomery, S. B., Pentz, M. A., & Johnson, C. A. (1996). Process evaluation of community coalitions for alcohol and other drug prevention: Comparison of two models. *Journal of Community Psychology, 24,* 118–135.

MacKinnon, D. P., Johnson, C. A., Pentz, M. A., Dwyer, J. H., Hansen, W. B., Flay, B. R., & Wang, W. E. (1991). Mediating mechanisms in a school-based drug prevention program: One year effects of the Midwestern Prevention Project. *Health Psychology, 10*(3), 164–172.

MacKinnon, D. P., Pentz, M. A., & Stacy, A. W. (1993). First year effects of the alcohol warning label. *American Journal of Public Health. 83*(4), 585–587.

Mittlemark, M. (1990). Balancing the requirements of research and the needs of communities. In N. Bracht, (Ed.), *Health promotion at the community level.* Newberry Park, CA: Sage.

MMWR (1987). Survey of worksite smoking policies—New York City. *Morbidity and Mortality Weekly Report, 36*(12), 177–179.

Moskowitz, J. M. (1989). The primary prevention of alcohol problems: A critical review of the research literature. *Journal of Studies on Alcohol, 50,* 54–88.

Moskowitz, J. M., & Jones, R. (1988). Alcohol and drug problems in the schools: Results of a national survey of school administrators. *Journal of Studies on Alcohol 49*(4), 299–305.

Murray, D. M., Perry, C. L., Griffin, G., Harty, K. C., Jacobs, D. R., Jr., Schmid, L., Daly, K., & Pallonen, U. (1992). Results from a statewide approach to adolescent tobacco use prevention. *Preventive Medicine, 21*(4), 449–472.

Musto, D. (1995). Perception and regulation of drug use: The rise and fall of the tide. *Annals of Internal Medicine, 123*(6), 468–469.

Nahas, G. G., Frick, H. C., Gleaton, T., Schuchard, K., & Moulton, O. (1986). A drug policy for our times. *Bulletin on Narcotics, 38*(1–2), 3–14.

Newman, T. L. (Unpublished manuscript). *The relationship betweeen high school anti-smoking policies and adolescent cigarette use.*

Normand, J., Salyards, S., & Mahoney, J. J. (1990). An evaluation of preemployment drug testing. *Journal of Applied Psychology, 75*(6), 629–639.

Norton, E. C., Bieler, G. S., Ennett, S. T., & Zarkin, G. A. (1996). Analysis of prevention program effectiveness with clustered data using generalized estimating equations. *Journal of Consulting and Clinical Psychology, 64*(5), 919–926.

Office of National Drug Control Policy (1997). *The National Drug Control Strategy,* Washington, DC.

Pentz, M. A. (1986). Community organization and school liaisons: How to get programs started. *Journal of School Health, 56,* 382–388.

Pentz, M. A. (1993). Primary prevention of adolescent drug abuse. In C. B. Fisher & R. M. Lerner (Eds.), *Applied developmental psychology.* New York: McGraw-Hill.

Pentz, M. A. (1994). Adaptive evaluation strategies for estimating effects of community-based drug abuse prevention programs. *J Community Psych, CSAP Special Issue,* 26–51.

Pentz, M. A. (1995). A comprehensive strategy to prevent the abuse of alcohol and other drugs: Theory and methods. In R. Coombs & D. Ziedonis (Eds.), *Handbook on drug abuse prevention* (pp. 69–92). Boston, MA: Allyn & Bacon.

Pentz, M. A. (1997). *High school smoking cessation clinics: results of a pilot.* San Francisco, CA: Society for Behavioral Medicine's 18th Annual Scientific Sessions, April 16–19.

Pentz, M. A. (1995). Alternative models of community prevention research in ethnically and culturally diverse communities. In P. Langton, L. G. Epstein, & M. A. Orlandi (Eds.), *Challenge of participatory research: Preventing alcohol-related problems in ethnic communities* (pp. 69–104). CSAP Cultural Competence Series 3, Rockville, MD: Center for Substance Abuse Prevention.

Pentz, M. A. (1999). Prevention aimed at individuals: An integrative transactional perspective In B. S. McCrady & E. E. Epstein (Eds.), *Addictions: A comprehensive guidebook for practitioners.* Oxford University Press: New York. pp. 555–1572.

Pentz, M. A. (1998). In Z. Sloboda & W. B. Hansen (Eds.), *Preventing drug abuse through the community: Multi-component programs make the difference.* NIDA Research Monograph. 98, pp. 73–86.

Pentz, M. A., Bonnie, R. J., Shopland, D. S. (1996). Integrating supply and demand reduction strategies for drug abuse prevention. *American Behavioral Scientist, 39*(7), 897–910.

Pentz, M. A., Brannon, B. R., Charlin, V. L., Barrett, E. J., MacKinnon, D. P., & Flay, B. R. (1989). The power of policy: The relationship of smoking policy to adolescent smoking. *American Journal of Public Health, 79*(7), 857–862.

Pentz, M. A., Dwyer, J. H., MacKinnon, D. P., Hansen, W. B., Wang, E. Y. I., & Johnson, C. A. (1989). A multi-community trial for primary prevention of adolescent drug abuse: Effects on drug use prevalence. *Journal of the American Medical Association, 261*(22), 3259–3266.

Pentz, M. A., Mihalic, S. F., & Grotpeter, J. K. (1997) The Midwestern Prevention Project. In D. S. Elliot (Ed.), *Blueprints for violence prevention.* Boulder, CO: Center for the Study and Prevention of Violence, Institute of Behavioral Science, University of Colorado.

Pentz, M. A., & S. B. Montgomery (unpublished manuscript). Research-based community coalitions for drug abuse prevention: Guidelines for replication. *Health Education Research.*

Pentz, M. A., Trebow, E. A., Hansen, W. B., MacKinnon, W. B., Dwyer, J. H., Flay, B. R., Daniels, S., Cormack, C., & Johnson, C. A. (1990). Effects of program implementation on adolescent drug use behavior: The Midwestern Prevention Project (MPP). *Evaluation Review, 14*(3), 264–289.

Pentz, M. A., Sussman, S., & Newman, T. (1997). The conflict between least harm and no-use tobacco policy for youth: Ethical and policy implications. *Addiction, 92*(9), 1165–1173.

Perry, C. L., Williams, C. L., Veblen-Mortenson, S., Toomey, T. L., Komro, K. A., Anstine, P. S., McGovern, P. G., Finnegan, J. R., Forster, J. L., Wagenaar, A. C., & Wolfson, M. (1996). Project Northland: Outcomes of a community-wide alcohol use prevention program during early adolescence. *American Journal of Public Health, 86*(7), 956–965.

President's Commission on Model State Drug Laws (1992). Final report: Five volume report, including Drug-Free Families, Schools, and Workplaces.

Rogers, E. M. (1987). The diffusion of innovations perspective. In N. D. Weinstein, (Ed.), *Taking care: Understanding and encouraging self-protective behavior* (pp. 79–94). New York: Cambridge University Press.

Rogers, E. M. (1993). Diffusion and re-invention of Project DARE. In T. E. Backer, & E. M. Rogers (Eds.), *Organizational aspects of health communication campaigns: What works?* Newbury Park, CA: Sage.

Rothman, J. (1979). Three models of community organization practice, their mixing and phasing. In F. M. Cox, J. L. Ehrlich, J. Rothman, J. E. Tripman, (Eds.), *Strategies of community organization* (3rd ed.). Itaska, IL: F. E. Peacock Publishers.

Rotter, J. B. (1954). *Social learning and clinical psychology.* New York: Prentice-Hall.

Sampson, R. J., Raudenbush, S. W., & Earls, F. (1997). Neighborhoods and violent crime: A multilevel study of collective efficacy. *Science, 277*(5328), 918–924.

Saxe, L., Reber, E., Hallfors, D., Kadushin, C., Jones, D., Rindskopf, D., & Beveridge, A. (1997). *Think global, act local: Assessing the impact of community-based substance abuse prevention.* Evaluation and Program Planning. 20(3) 357–366.

Schuster, C. R. (1989). Implications for research of the 1988 Anti-Drug Abuse Act. *NIDA Research Monograph Series, 95,* 16–22.

Sloboda, Z., & David, S. L. (1997). *Preventing drug abuse among children and adolescents: A research-based guide.* Washington, DC: NIDA/NIH Publication #97-4212.

Sussman, S. (1991). Curriculum development in school-based prevention research. *Health Education Research, 6*(3), 339–351.

Swisher, J. D., Baker, S. B., Barnes, D., Gebler, M. K., Hadleman, D. E., & Kophaz, K. M. (1993). An evaluation of student assistance programs in Pennsylvania. *Journal of Drug and Alcohol Education, 39*(1), 1–18.

Tobler, N. S. (1997). Meta-analyses of adolescent drug prevention programs: Results of the 1993 meta-analysis. *NIDA Research Monograph, 170,* 5–68.

Wagenaar, A. C., Murray, D. M., Wolfson, M. Forster, J. L., & Finnegan, J. R. (1994). Communities mobilizing for change on alcohol: Design of a randomized community trial. *Journal of Comparative Psychology, 22,* 79–101. OSAP Special Issue.

Wallack, L., & Corbett, K. (1987). Alcohol, tobacco and marijuana use among youth: An overview of epidemiological, program and policy trends. *Health Education Quarterly, 14*(2), 223–249.

Warner, K. E., Citrin, T., Pickett, G., Rabe, B. G., Wagenaar, A., & Stryker, J. (1990). Licit and illicit drug policies: A typology. *British Journal of Addiction, 85,* 255–262.

Yin, R. K., Kaftarian, S. J., Yu, P., & Jansen, M. A. (1997). Outcomes from CSAP's Community Partnerships Program: Findings from the National Cross-Site Evaluation. *Evaluation & Program Planning, 20*(3), 345–356.

PART IV

THEORETICAL AND EMPIRICAL FOUNDATIONS OF PREVENTION

CHAPTER 12

Forging a Relationship between Drug Abuse Epidemiology and Drug Abuse Prevention

ZILI SLOBODA

INTRODUCTION

The marriage of epidemiology and prevention has long been recognized and encouraged in public health. This marriage took place in the 18th and 19th centuries with observations such as those of Bernoulli, who determined the long-term effects of smallpox inoculation; Snow, who associated the outbreak of cholera in London with the use of a particular water pump; Louis, whose studies on bloodletting altered medical practice; and Simmelweis, who pointed out the relationship between puerperal fever and the fact that medical staff did not wash their hands with soap or disinfectant between performing autopsies and delivering babies (Lilienfeld & Lilienfeld, 1980).

The marriage of epidemiology and prevention of drug abuse had also been proposed but was never fully consummated until the 1970s with the funding of general-population surveys and longitudinal studies that followed youngsters through their high risk-years into early adulthood. Such studies led to the development of causal hypotheses and theories about the etiology of drug-abusing behaviors to guide prevention programming and research, but large gaps remain in our knowledge of drug-abuse epidemiology and drug abuse prevention.

The goal of this chapter is to establish a link between drug abuse epidemiology and drug abuse prevention and show what contributions epidemiology has made to the field of prevention research and practice. It provides examples from past and current research and offers recommendations for further research. The emphasis is on research, however, and how this research can be translated for, and to, prevention practitioners.

ZILI SLOBODA • Department of Sociology, The University of Akron, Akron, Ohio 44325

THE ROLES OF EPIDEMIOLOGY
AND PREVENTION

Epidemiology

Epidemiology is an approach to organizing information on a health condition in order to identify its cause and ways to reduce or eliminate its impact. Epidemiologists accept that a certain percentage of the population will experience some negative health conditions (i.e., many health problems remain at endemic levels). For instance, some children will not be inoculated for measles or some children will be diagnosed with diabetes. However, when rates of a disease increase or if affected groups show differing characteristics, epidemiologists become concerned. They analyze existing data and generate hypotheses to explain the increases or changing characteristics. These hypotheses form the core of epidemiologic research, and findings from studies designed to address the hypotheses become the basis for prevention interventions and research.

For many in the field of drug abuse, epidemiology is synonymous with reports from school or household surveys on the percentages of people who are estimated to have used one or more illicit drugs during their lifetime, the year prior to the survey, or the month prior to the survey. Policymakers compare sequential years to determine whether the rates of drug use have gone up, down, or remained the same. These up-and-down movements are then used to rate the policies of the administration that implemented them. Drug abuse prevention researchers also cite them when discussing their research and its importance. Rarely are these movements or even longer time trends seen as suggestive of other societal changes that are taking place in this country or elsewhere.

Prevention

Prevention is the heart and soul of public health. It is clear that preventing the spread of some infectious diseases, such as small pox, yellow fever, and HIV, is more important than treating them in attempting to control their impact. By attacking the vectors of these infectious diseases—the virus or bacteria—one can impede their spread. For example, spraying areas in which there was mosquito infestation prevented the spread of yellow fever. Prevention of infectious diseases also includes attempts to change behaviors in the host that increase the risk of becoming infected. HIV prevention programs address behaviors that make transmission of the virus easier, such as unprotected sexual relations or sharing of injection equipment between an infected person and his or her uninfected partner. Along with the host or affected group and the vector or source of a health condition, the third "leg" on the epidemiology prevention stool is the environment. Prevention programs include such activities as improving sanitation, eliminating crowded housing conditions, and improving the water supply. Which aspect is emphasized depends on what stage of the condition is being addressed, whether it is preventing exposure, early morbidity, or later long-term impairment and mortality.

DEFINING DRUG ABUSE

Drug abuse, by its very nature, challenges the approaches traditional epidemiologists use to study a health problem. Indeed, there is even debate over whether drug addiction/dependence is a medical problem that can be diagnosed—at least with currently available tools. What is known is that drugs change the biochemistry of the brain, and with the use of imaging technology there has been an ever-increasing understanding of the impact of drugs on the brain and, therefore, on both emotions and behaviors. It is currently recognized that drugs are used initially, voluntarily for pleasure (DuPont, 1998). Whether that initial pleasurable sensation is retained over time or whether more biological processes take over is still unclear. At what point in the drug-using process do these biological processes occur has not been well documented although there is growing recognition that these processes may vary by drug type (Koob et al., 1998; Lyvers, 1998; O'Brien et al., 1998; Shaffer, 1997; Tiffany & Carter, 1998; Volkow & Fowler, 2000).

Two aspects of drug-using behaviors are of concern (1) habituation and (2) health effects. Habituation, addiction, and dependence have a physiological basis that is becoming better understood as our tools for brain imaging improve. Volkow and her colleagues (1991) and others (Altman, 1996; Childress et al., 1995) using new brain-imaging technologies, such as MRI, PET, and SPECT scans, have actually viewed the living human brain to learn about the basic mechanisms involved in drug abuse and addiction and to map the specific areas in the brain where these effects occur. Changes in those sections of the brain associated with emotions, cognition, and even movement have been observed. These researchers also have shown that the effects of drugs remain even after use of the drugs has stopped. Drugs alter the chemistry of the brain and the way it the produces natural biochemicals. This observation explains both short- and long-term effects of drugs on cognition, memory, and movement (Block & Ghoneim, 1993; Kouri et al., 1999; Pope & Yurgelun-Todd, 1996).

Studies on the impact of drugs on the health status of users have been few, but those that have been published show increased negative health effects among drug users (Andreasson & Allebeck, 1990; Cherubin & Sapira, 1993; Ghodse, Oyefeso, & Kilpatrick, 1998; Gore, 1999; Hulse et al., 1999; Neumark, Van Etten, & Anthony, 2000; Polen et al., 1993; Richards et al., 1999; Single et al., 2000; Solowij, 1995; Thomas, 1996) and that the effects can be passed *intra-utero* to the fetuses of drug-using women. One of the best longitudinal studies of the negative effects associated with prenatal exposure to drugs, mostly tobacco and marijuana, is being conducted by Peter Fried and his colleagues (e.g., Fried, 1995; Fried & Watkinson, 2000).

Even without additional studies on the health problems related to drug use, prevention researchers and practitioners want to focus on drug use before it becomes a problem. However, defining the various stages of drug use—from use to abuse to dependence—has been a challenge. Use of illicit drugs is easy to define. It includes the use of any illicit drug. Defining abuse and dependence is more difficult. Original definitions of abuse and dependence included behavioral markers for physiological problems and for drugs such as opiates. These markers of tolerance and withdrawal were useful. According to Jaffe, Knapp, and Ciraulo (1997; p. 161), "Physical dependence is usually defined as an altered state of biology induced by a drug, such that when the drug is withdrawn (or displaced from its receptors by an antagonist), a complex set of biologic events (withdrawal or abstinence phenomena) ensue that are typical for that drug (or class of drugs) and that are distinct from a simple return to normal function. . . . Physical dependence can be observed with a number of classes of pharmacological agents that have psychoactive effects, including opioids, CNS depressants, caffeine, and nicotine, to name but a few, as well as with drugs that are not ordinarily thought of as psychoactive agents."

Physical withdrawal symptoms were used in diagnosing drug dependence when opioids were the primary drug of choice. During the 1960s and 1970s, heroin was highly diluted with a variety of substances, and, therefore, withdrawal was often experienced without many of the more severe symptoms noted previously. Furthermore, other drugs were becoming available that did not meet the tolerance and withdrawal criteria. But users were having problems with them, showing up in emergency rooms with health problems and in treatment. Without any biological or diagnostic tests available, drug abuse professionals had to focus on the behavioral dimensions of abuse and dependence.

TABLE 12.1. Criteria for Drug Abuse and Dependence—DSM IV AND ICD-10

Diagnostic and Statistical Manual of Mental Disorders (4th edition)	Tenth Revision of the International Classification of Diseases
Three or more of	
(1) Tolerance	(i) A strong desire or sense of compulsion to take the substance
(2) Withdrawal	(ii) Difficulties in controlling substance-taking behavior in terms of its onset, termination or levels of use
(3) The substance is often taken in large amounts or over a longer period that was intended	(iii) Withdrawal
(4) Any unsuccessful effort or a persistent desire to cut down or control substance use	(iv) Tolerance
(5) A great deal of time is spent in activities necessary to obtain substance or recover from its effects	(v) Increased amounts of time necessary to obtain or take the substance or recover from its effects; progressive neglect of the alternative pleasures or interests.
(6) Important social, occupational, or recreational activities given up or reduced because of substance use	(vi) Persisting with substance use despite evidence of overly harmful problem consequences
(7) Continued substance use despite knowledge of having had a persistent or recurrent physical or psychological problems that are likely to be caused or exacerbated by the substance	
Dependence with physiological features of tolerance or withdrawal or without physiological features if three or more of items 3 through 7 are experienced.	
DSM-VI: Abuse	ICD-10: Harmful Use
One of more of the following occurring over the same 12-month period:	Clear evidence that the substance use was responsible for (or substantially contributed to) physical or psychological harm, including impaired judgment or dysfunctional behavior
(1) Recurrent substance use resulting in a failure to fulfill major role obligations at work, school, or home	
(2) Recurrent substance use in situations in which it is physically hazardous	
(3) Recurrent substance-related legal problems	
(4) Continued substance use despite having persistent or recurrent social or interpersonal problems caused or exacerbated by the effects of the substance	
Never met criteria for dependence	

Psychiatrists in the United States have developed The Diagnostic and Statistical Manual (DSM) to address mental illness, and the most recent versions, DSM-III, DSM-IIIR and DSM-IV, include drug abuse and dependence. The criteria from DSM-IV are shown in Table 12.1. In addition, an international classification of diseases was developed by the World Health Organization (for an excellent discussion see the chapter by Woody and Cacciola (1997)). There is comparability between DSM-IV and the 10th edition of the International Classification of Diseases (ICM-10) on many of the criteria for dependence (Table 12.1). Furthermore, a number of studies have been conducted comparing these criteria with each other, clinical judgement, and other instruments, such as the Addiction Severity Inventory (Feingold & Rounsaville, 1995; Kosten et al., 1987; Rounsaville et al., 1993; Ustun et al., 1997; Woody, Cottler, & Cacciola, 1993). There seems to be high concordance on dependence but less so on abuse or harmful use.

As mentioned previously there is wide consensus in the United States that use and abuse and dependence are endpoints of the continuum of drug-using behaviors. And there is agreement that one does not become an abuser of drugs or dependent on drugs unless one has begun using them. Epidemiologic evidence from both cross-sectional and longitudinal surveys, however, indicate that the percentage of those who initiate drug use and go on to abuse or become dependent on drugs varies by drug type, frequency of use, and the age at which drug use began (Anthony & Petronis, 1995; Coffey et al., 2000; DeWitt et al., 2000; Fergusson & Horwood, 2000; Grant & Pickering, 1998; Kandel & Chen, 2000; Kandel & Raveis, 1989; Perkonigg et al., 1999). For instance, for the Monitoring the Future study, the researchers from the University of Michigan developed noncontinuation rates calculated by subtracting the number of students who reported no past year use from those who reported lifetime use. Figure 12.1 shows that the drugs that have the highest noncontinuation rates are inhalants while the drug that has the lowest noncontinuation rate is marijuana.

Dependence measures, adapted from DSM-IV have been included on the National Household Survey on Drug Abuse. In the most recently available survey, 1999, the past year rate of dependence for any illicit drug was 1.6%. The rates varied by age with the oldest and youngest age groups having the lowest rates (0.2 through 0.7%), while those aged 18–25 had the highest dependence rate of 6.8%. These rates are similar to those found by Warner et al. (1995) from the National Comorbidity Survey.

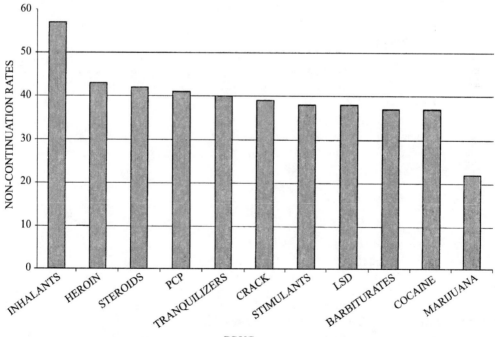

FIGURE 12.1. Noncontinuation rates for 8th-, 10th-, and 12th-graders by drug: Monitoring the Future Study, 1997.

Kandel and her colleagues, in their analyses of data from the National Household Survey on Drug Abuse (1991–1993), found that for marijuana, dependence rates were higher among adolescents than among adults. They found that both the frequency and quantity of use were related to the probability of dependence. These probabilities varied by age, with adolescents becoming dependent at lower levels of use than do adults (Chen, Kandel, & Davies, 1997; Kandel, 1994).

Despite the availability of this information from longitudinal studies, few published works discuss rates of dependence, continued use, or even cessation of use of illicit drugs. In 1989, Kandel and Raveis examined predictors of cessation of marijuana and cocaine use in a longitudinal study of a cohort of 1,222 young people. They found that the strongest predictor of cessation was degree of prior involvement with drugs for marijuana and friends' use for cocaine. In summary, they found that those who used drugs for social reasons were more likely to stop use than those who used them for psychological reasons. Chen and Kandel (1998) conducted subsequent event history analyses of data from 706 marijuana users from the above sample, who were followed into their 30s. Their findings continue to support the finding that those who use marijuana for social reasons are more likely to stop use than are those who use it for mood alteration.

DRUG USE AND ABUSE IN THE
UNITED STATES

In the United States, the major sources of information on the nature and extent of drug use are the National Household Survey on Drug Abuse (NHSDA) and the Monitoring the Future Study (MTF). The NHSDA, originally established by the National Institute on Drug Abuse (NIDA), has been conducted since 1975. Until 1991, when it became an annual survey, it was conducted every 2 or 3 years. The survey includes a sample of households in the United States and, within these households, selects individuals aged 12 and older for interview. Since 1992, the survey has been supported by the Substance Abuse and Mental Health Services Administration (SAMHSA). In 1999, close to 67,000 respondents had completed the survey. The latest information from the NHSDA can be seen at http://www.samhsa.gov/oas/oasftp.htm.

The Monitoring the Future Study, conducted by the University of Michigan under a grant from NIDA, has surveyed seniors each year from representative samples of public and private high schools since 1975. In 1991, the study was expanded to include 8th- and 10th-graders from representative samples of middle and high schools. In the 1999 survey, more than 50,000 eighth-, 10th-, and 12th-graders completed self-administered surveys in their classrooms. Information on the most recent information for the Monitoring the Future Study can be seen on http://www.nida.nih.gov.

In general, findings from these surveys report drug use not as stage of use, i.e., dependence or abuse, but rather as period of use:

- lifetime use—ever used (specific drug) at least once;
- annual use—used (specific drug) at least once in the 12 months prior to the survey; and
- current use—used (specific drug) at least once in the 30 days prior to the survey.

Information regarding frequency of use or "times" used is also available. In addition, the NHSDA has developed measures of problems associated with the use of specific drugs. There has been an effort to make these items comparable to DSM-III, -IIIR and -IV. Table 12.2 shows the questions as they appear in the 1999 survey form. The following sections summarize key findings from these two surveys.

TABLE 12.2. Dependence Questions from the National Household Survey on Drug Abuse[a]

For each drug type:

In the past 12 months, indicate

(1) If you wanted or tried to stop or cut down on your use of that drug but found that you couldn't;

(2) Whether you had built up a tolerance for the drug so that the same amount had less effect than before;

(3) Whether you had a period of 1 month or more when you spent a great deal of time getting or using the drug or getting over its effects;

(4) Whether you have used that kind of drug much more often or in larger amounts than you intended;

(5) Whether your use of the drug often kept you from working, going to school, taking care of children, or engaging in recreational activities;

(6) Whether your use of the drug caused you to have any emotional or psychological problems—such as feeling uninterested in things, feeling depressed, feeling suspicious of people, feeling paranoid, or having strange ideas;

(7) Whether your use of the drug caused you any health problems—such as liver disease, stomach disease, pancreatitis, feet tingling, numbness, memory problems, an accidental overdose, a persistent cough, a seizure or fit, hepatitis, or abscesses.

[a]Source: Office of Applied Studies, SAMHSA, National Household Survey on Drug Abuse, 1998.

Prevalence (Existing Cases) of Drug Use

Since the NHSDA began, the United States has experienced both up and down trends in illicit drug use. The peak year for use was in 1979, when it was estimated that 14.1% or 25 million people used an illicit drug in the month prior to interview. At that time and subsequently, use of marijuana was the major illicit drug used, with approximately 80% of the drug-using population reporting use of this drug. Over the next several years, the estimated rates of illicit drug use decreased until 1992. In 1992, past-month use was at its lowest point, 5.8%, involving approximately 12 million people. Since 1992, rates of illicit drug use have increased until 1997 when they began to level off (Substance Abuse and Mental Health Services Administration, 1995). In the 1999 Household Survey (Substance Abuse and Mental Health Services Administration, 2001), it was estimated that 6.7% of the population used an illicit drug at least once in the month prior to interview.

When rates of illicit drugs used during the year period prior to the 1999 survey are ranked, marijuana is the most prevalent illicit drug used. Marijuana use is followed by use of analgesics, hallucinogens, powder cocaine, inhalants, tranquilizers, and stimulants. It is estimated that 1 million people used crack-cocaine at least once in that time period while an estimated 400,000 used heroin.

In the United States, drug abuse is clearly a problem of young people. In Figure 12.2, it can be seen that the highest rates of past-month illicit drug use are for those aged 18 to 25, followed most recently by those aged 12 to 17. This pattern is maintained when specific drug categories are examined including marijuana, cocaine, and hallucinogens.

Although the 1-to-25 age group generally has the highest rates of drug use, it is the youngest age group, those 12 to 17, that has shown increased rates of marijuana and cocaine use since 1992. In general, the MTF study of 8th-, 10th-, and 12th-graders supports these trends. However, there appear to be large differences in the reported rates of drug use between these two surveys, with those from the MTF being higher (Table 12.3).

The drug use portions of both surveys are self-administered, but data collection for the MTF is done in the classroom while data for the NHSDA are collected in the home. The lower reported rates of use are thought to be related to the presence of parents, even if the parents are in another room. Researchers, such as Turner and Miller (1997) and Lessler and O'Reilly (1997), suggest that the

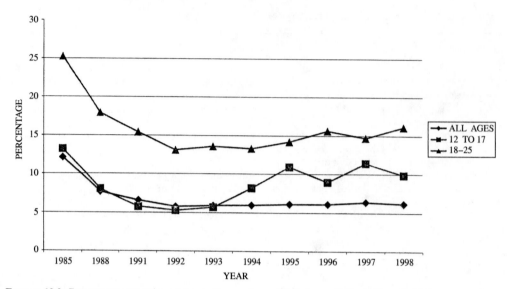

FIGURE 12.2. Percentages reporting past-month use of any illicit drug: National Household Survey on Drug Abuse—1985–1998.

use of audio computer-assisted self-interviewing approaches will help improve the reliability of self-reported use of drugs. This approach is currently being tested for the NHSDA.

What is not so clear are the reasons for different trends between these two surveys for marijuana, alcohol, and cigarette use. For instance, for marijuana the trends are similar for those 12 to 13 (8th-graders) and 14 to 15 (10th-graders) until 1995; thereafter they are quite different. The trends for the oldest adolescent group (ages 16 and 17, or 12th-graders) are comparable across time. Similar results are found when examining past-month rates of use for alcohol and cigarettes. Whether these differences are due to changes in the administration of the NHSDA, to other internal study features or to external, environmental factors needs to be assessed.

Incidence (New Cases) of Drug Use

From the NHSDA, it has been possible to develop mean ages at which persons initiate the use of illicit and licit substances. The estimated mean ages for initiating the use of marijuana, cocaine, inhalants, hallucinogens heroin, alcohol, and cigarettes have changed over time since the survey

TABLE 12.3. Comparison of Rates of Past-Month Use of Marijuana from the National Household Survey and the Monitoring the Future Study—1991–1997

Year	8th Grade	Age 12–13	10th Grade	Age 14–15	12th Grade	Age 16–17
1991	3.2	0.4	8.7	3.7	13.8	8.9
1992	3.7	0.9	8.1	3.8	11.9	7.8
1993	5.1	0.8	10.9	3.9	15.5	10.5
1994	7.8	1.9	15.8	5.0	19.0	11.8
1995	9.1	2.2	17.2	9.7	21.2	13.0
1996	11.3	1.2	20.4	6.7	21.9	13.1
1997	10.2	2.5	23.7	9.2	23.7	16.3

began, with all but cigarettes showing lower mean ages. The mean ages for the onset of daily cigarette use has remained level (SAMHSA, 1999; pp. 105–112).

Another important epidemiologic measure is age-specific rates of first use (i.e., rates per 1,000 person-years of exposure). These rates indicate that since the survey began in 1975 the highest rates for use of marijuana, inhalants, hallucinogens, heroin, alcohol, and cigarettes occurred in the period between 1996 and 1998 among those aged 12 to 17 (SAMHSA, 1999; pp. 105–112). Van Etten and Anthony (1999) and Van Etten, Neumark, and Anthony (1997) used the data from 1979 through 1994 to examine the relationship between opportunity to use marijuana, cocaine, hallucinogens, and heroin and transitions to first use. They report that the transition to use occurs within 1 year of the first opportunity to use. They calculated the probabilities of transition for all drugs and found that these have been increasing in recent years, particularly for hallucinogens.

Changing Trends in the Prevalence of Drug Use

This information raises several questions that have not been well addressed in the literature. The most important one is, why are more young people trying drugs? Analyses of data from both the NHSDA and the MTF attribute the up-and-down trends in drug use, particularly use of marijuana and cocaine, to changing perceptions of the harmful effects of the use of these drugs and of the level of social disapproval of the use of these drugs (Bachman et al., 1988, 1990, 1998; Office of Applied Studies, 1999). Although there seems to be a strong statistical association between these measures, it is not clear what characteristics define the groups that account for the increases and decreases in the prevalence trends. Brown et al. (2001) attempted to determine whether the characteristics of substance users have changed over time by examining the MTF data for 22 consecutive cohorts of high school seniors. They found a consistency in the factors that predicted use of most substances. These predictors were religious commitment, political beliefs, grade-point average, truancy, and evenings out. Some differences were found between substances. Many more studies of this nature are needed to understand differential trends in substance use over time, particularly those periods when rates go up and down.

Examination of changing trends in perceived harmfulness of drug use also sheds some light on what is happening. Looking specifically at perceptions of the risk of harm from the occasional use of marijuana by age groups from the NHSDA over time we find interesting changes in this variable for those aged 12 to 17 (Figure 12.3).

Between 1990 and 1993, this group perceived the risks associated with the occasional use of marijuana to be high, close to perceptions held by the oldest age group (aged 35 and older), which would include their parents. However, since 1994, perceptions of risk held by the youngest group have become more like those aged 18 to 25, the group that, as we have seen earlier, has had the highest rates of drug abuse since the survey began. In the past 5 years there has been a growing recognition that parents have a great deal of influence on their children's drug using behaviors, even during adolescence. The information presented suggests that parents are not talking to their children about their own perceptions about the harmfulness of drug use. This is an important area for research and has implications for prevention. Helping parents discuss drugs and the potential harm from their use, particularly for adolescents who are still developing physically, emotionally, and intellectually, needs to be emphasized in prevention programming. Most parents today grew up during the mid-1970s when drug use rates were at their highest levels. Parents may feel uncomfortable talking about the use of drugs or may not recognize how harmful they can be for their children. The challenge for prevention practitioners is to reach parents and provide them with the information they need on the effects of drugs on the brain and on the health of their children (Crowley et al., 1998).

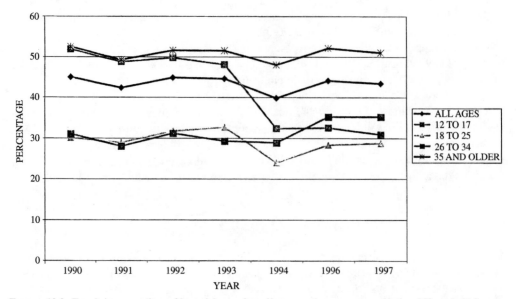

FIGURE 12.3. Trends in perceptions of harmfulness of marijuana use by age groups: National Household Survey on Drug Abuse—1990–1997.

Other changes that have been noted in these surveys over time include increased use of drugs by girls and by African-Americans. Boys and men have always had higher rates of drug use than did girls and women. In general, as with other deviant and antisocial behaviors, males tend to have higher rates of illicit drug use than do females and also different patterns of use. These differences, however, are changing. For instance, the rates of past-month use of illicit drugs were 19.2 and 9.4% for males and females, respectively, in the 1979 NHSDA. By 1988, these rates narrowed to 9.4 and 6%; and by 1997 to 8.5 and 4.5% (Office of Applied Studies, 1997, 1998). Yet examination of these gender differences by age and by type of drug show that the gap between males and females is smaller at younger ages and that there is some variation across drug types. This trend began to change over time particularly for adolescents and specifically for the use of marijuana and cocaine. Looking at the prevalence of both marijuana and cocaine by gender from NHSDA, changes are noted over time for those aged 12 to 17. Although males continue to have higher rates of use of past month use than females, the male to female ratio has decreased over time so that in 1997 it is 1.2:1. With cocaine, for the same age group, past month rates of use were similar for males and females in 1997 (1.1 and 0.9%, respectively).

More detailed analyses of the drug use patterns of the 12th-graders who used illicit drugs from the 1997 MTF study show that boys reported different patterns of drug use than did girls (National Institute on Drug Abuse, 1998). For instance, more boys report past year use of marijuana than do girls (41% of boys compared to 36% of girls). Meanwhile, annual rates of use of heroin, other opiates, cocaine, crack-cocaine, inhalants, and LSD for boys are one to two and one-half times higher than they are for girls. Also, in many cases, as with marijuana, boys tend to use drugs more frequently than do girls. Nonetheless, 12th-grade boys and girls have equivalent annual rates of use for stimulants. For younger adolescents, those in the 8th and 10th grades, the 1997 rates of use of stimulants, inhalants, and tranquilizers is higher for girls than it is for boys. This suggests avenues of research that have not been fully explored concerning the differences between boys and girls in drug use. As drug use rates have been higher for boys than for girls, the emphasis in the research has been either to focus on cohorts of boys or to combine genders in analyses of determinants of initiation of drug use. In response to the growing concern about the use of drugs by girls and women in the past few years there has been an effort on the part of researchers to explore these gender differences, and several epidemiologic studies have been funded to examine it. Reports of studies of differential origins of drug abusing behaviors are sparse but suggest that social factors are more influential for females initiating drug use and intrapersonal factors are more influential for males (Brady & Randall, 1999; Hoffman & Su, 1998; James & Moore, 1999; Jessor, Jessor, & Finney, 1973; Kaplan & Johnson, 1992; Lifrak et al., 1997; Rohrbach & Milam, 2002; Sanders-Phillips, 1999). If this is the case, then are girls today experiencing more social pressures to use drugs than prior cohorts? Are they experiencing more negative life events? These differences require more intensive research attention, particularly since they have implications for prevention.

When we examine past-month rates of illicit drug use for the general population, we find that African-Americans and Whites have higher rates of use than do Hispanics. This is not the case when we look at the rates of use in those years when drug use is initiated. For those aged 12 to 17, Whites tend to have higher initiation rates of drug use than do either Hispanics or African-Americans (Office of Applied Studies, 1998). In addition, historically, these racial/ethnic groups have differed by patterns of use. Prior to 1993, whites had the highest rates of past-month use of marijuana, but by 1993 rates of use for Whites, African-Americans, and Hispanics converged and increased. This pattern is different for cocaine use. For this age group, African-Americans had the lowest rates of past-month use of cocaine in 1997 with Whites and Hispanics having similar rates. In general, however, this picture changes among older age groups with African-Americans reporting higher rates of use.

Data from the MTF support what has been observed among the 12- to 17-year olds in the NHSDA. Overall, African-American students tend to report lower rates of use of most of the illicit and licit substances than do white or Hispanic students. By the 12th grade, Whites report higher lifetime and annual rates of use of inhalants, hallucinogens, opiates other than heroin, stimulants, barbiturates, tranquilizers, alcohol, cigarettes, and smokeless tobacco. Hispanic seniors report the highest lifetime and annual rates of use of cocaine, crack, and steroids. Examination of changes in rates of use over time indicate, again, that there are ethnic differences. African-American adolescents have increased their use of marijuana while decreasing their use of cocaine.

Information about the use of drugs by Asian and Native-American populations is based on local area studies. Estimates from the NHSDA indicate that Asians have lower rates of illicit drug use while Native-American groups have higher use rates of certain substances. (See chapters in this book by Chen and by Beauvais and Trimble for more detailed information regarding the prevalence of illicit and licit substance abuse in these populations.)

It is not clear whether the response to prevention programming differs across racial/ethnic groups. However, a number of studies suggest there may be a differential response. (Chapters by Chen, Beauvais and Trimble, Turner and Hinch, and Martinez et al., address special aspects of these groups that need to be incorporated in any prevention programming.)

Emerging Drug Abuse Patterns

Another source of information about drug-abuse patterns in the United States is the Community Epidemiology Work Group (CEWG), which grew out of a methodology developed in public health to estimate the extent and nature of an emerging public-health problem. Initially applied by the National Treatment Administration in Washington, DC, to estimate the need for the treatment of heroin, the technique was easily transferred to other geographic areas and other drugs (Sloboda &

Kozel, 1999). The Work Group consists of locally-based experts in drug abuse who collect existing data from treatment providers, law enforcement agencies, emergency rooms, coroners' or medical examiners' offices, school surveys, poison control centers, and local health departments. In contrast to the surveys that provide estimates of the incidence and prevalence of drug use, the CEWG researchers look for new characteristics of users, new drugs of abuse, and new ways of using drugs. They meet twice a year with support from NIDA to discuss their findings. The CEWG was instrumental in pointing out the emergence of crack cocaine in the 1970s, Rohypnol (the date-rape drug) in the 1990s, the increased use of marijuana among youth, the intranasal use of heroin that presaged the current growing heroin problem, and, most recently, the use of oxycotin. Twenty-one cities participate in the CEWG, representing the diversity of the U.S. population. The emergence of methamphetamine and "club" drugs such as MDMA, GHB, and GLB and the movement to synthetic or "laboratory" created drugs that are currently being watched by CEWG members are the most recent challenges to drug abuse experts. These changing patterns in drug use in an environment that is becoming more tolerant of the use of drugs is reminiscent of the 1970s. However, unlike the past, the decreasing age of initiation of drug use presents a greater risk since the effects of early exposure on the developing brain and body are not well-known and if drug use is not prevented, it could potentially become a major public-health problem in future decades. The latest findings from the CEWG are posted at: http://www.nida.nih.gov/CEWG/pubs.html#cewg or http://www.cdmgroup.com/cewg/pubs.htm.

Origins and Pathways to Drug Use and Abuse

Since the mid-1970s, several longitudinal, prospective studies as well as cross-sectional studies have been funded to determine the origins and pathways to drug use. It has only been since the 1990s that there has been a focus on the progression from use to abuse of drugs. Many researchers have made an effort to organize the findings from these studies so they could generate hypotheses about the origins of drug use and design prevention strategies (Hawkins, Catalano, & Miller, 1992; Pandina, 1998). These findings focus primarily on risk and, recently, on protective factors. The risk perspective covers a range of factors, from biological (i.e., having a parent or other close relative who is a substance user) to sociological (i.e., being alienated from prosocial groups) (Weinberg et al., 1998)

Several researchers found that although many adolescents are exposed to risks for drug use many do not abuse drugs. These researchers feel that protective factors temper the risks. They found that factors such as family bonding and bonding to prosocial groups, behaviors, and institutions are important (Brook et al., 1997). Currently, there is a growing focus on less well-articulated factors, such as resilience and positive assets (Benson, Galbraith, & Espeland, 1998; Glantz & Sloboda, 2000). All of these approaches to the same issue of onset lack specificity for drug abuse. Indeed, Jessor and his colleagues (Donovan, Jessor, & Costa, 1998; Jessor & Jessor, 1977) have developed a theory of problem behaviors that indicates common roots associated with a number of deviant behaviors. Recent work by Brook and her associates (1997, 1998) attempts to address specificity by comparing risk and protective factors that discriminate between adolescent boys who use drugs only and those who commit delinquent acts only. They found that 88% of the risks they included (covering the domains of personality, family, peer relationships, ecology, and acculturation) are statistically significant for both behaviors, which supports Jessor's theory.

Another area that has received a great deal of attention among drug abuse epidemiologists and prevention researchers is the sequence of the use of substances, particularly among adolescents, which was first discussed by Denise Kandel in the late 1970s and replicated in other longitudinal studies. There appears to be a sequencing of use from alcohol and/or tobacco and marijuana to other drugs of abuse (Kandel, 1975). We do not fully understand this sequencing and there has been a continuing debate as to whether the underlying mechanism for this sequencing of drug use has a biological or a social learning basis. The sequencing does not imply inevitability that everyone who smokes or drinks alcohol or even uses marijuana will move on to the next substance but that one who smokes or drinks alcohol or uses marijuana is tremendously more at risk to go on to the next substance than are those who did not use tobacco or alcohol or marijuana. In fact, the staff of the Division of Epidemiology, Services and Prevention Research of the National Institute on Drug Abuse (1996), calculated that someone who smokes cigarettes is 65 times more likely to use marijuana than is someone who does not smoke and that someone who uses marijuana is more than 100 times more likely to use cocaine than is someone who does not use marijuana.

Kandel has continued her research on the sequencing issue and has found that the sequencing model applies in late adolescence and young adulthood (Kandel, Yamaguchi, & Chen, 1992). Those who smoke or drink are more likely to use illicit drugs even after high school. Furthermore, those who smoked or drank more frequently are most at risk (Chen et al., 1997). Patterson and his associates (1988) also find confirmation of Kandel's sequencing hypothesis. As a result of these consistent findings across studies, tobacco and alcohol have been called "gateway" substances and are the target of many of the drug abuse prevention programs delivered to children in the United States.

The failure to refine our diagnosis of drug use and abuse is probably the core reason for our failure to specify risk. There is a need for drug abuse molecular and clinical epidemiologic studies to begin work in this area. Why these two areas have not evolved is not clear, yet there has been little dialogue among drug abuse epidemiologists, drug abuse treatment specialists and neuroscientists. Surely, these are conversations that need to be held in order to develop the needed cross-disciplinary research.

Dependence

Most of the studies on origins and pathways for drug use have used initiation of use as an endpoint. In order to examine the issue of progression to abuse/dependence, Glantz and Pickens, held a meeting at NIDA and requested that researchers with longitudinal data bases analyze their data to determine factors related to maintenance of drug use over time (or abuse of drugs). These analyses were extremely important to the field. They showed that the process of initiating drug use was driven primarily by social factors. The process leading to drug abuse is more biological. In fact, in the introduction to the book that included the presented papers, Glantz and Pickens state: "In general, drug use appears to be more a function of social and peer factors, whereas abuse appears to be more a function of biological and psychological processes" (Glantz & Pickens, 1992; p. 9). Risk factors found to be associated with use include: "bad" friends, friends using drugs, peer influences on use, drug availability, bad conduct, unconventionality, low involvement with traditional value-oriented institutions (i.e., family, religious institutions, school), poor academic achievement, poor-quality relations with (and attachment to) parents, and having parents with problems. The more risk factors experienced, the more likely that drug abuse will occur (Bry, McKeon, & Pandina, 1982). It is clear that abuse must follow from use, however, two use characteristics were found to be associated with abuse: early age at onset of use and high frequency of the use of drugs. Other factors found to be associated with abuse include the functioning of the family and, possibly, genetic influences (parental substance abuse and antisocial behavior, a family history of psychopathology, and family disruption); neurobiologic dysfunctions, and psychopathologies, such as antisocial personality, conduct disorder, criminal behavior, acting out, aggressiveness, and a risk-factor cluster that includes emotional/behavioral arousal, self-regulation difficulties, impulsivity and hyperactivity/attention deficit disorder. These findings are supported by the results of other studies (Kandel et al., 1999; Kendler & Prescott, 1998; Yamaguchi & Kandel, 1984).

TRANSLATING EPIDEMIOLOGY FOR PREVENTION

Over the past 100 years, efforts to address the societal impact of drugs have focused on halting the production and distribution of drugs both here and in other countries. These supply-reduction activities include interdiction at the point of entry into the country and destruction of opium, coca, and marijuana crops and the laboratories where they are transformed into heroin and crack-cocaine and where other types of drugs, such as MDMA, PCP, or methamphetamines, are created. It also includes reducing the diversion of prescription drugs from medical to nonmedical use. Although these efforts can be considered preventive from a public-health perspective, drug abuse prevention professionals tend to focus on demand-reduction activities, which include efforts to impact drug users. Tension exists between these two approaches because of funding discrepancies, with supply-reduction groups receiving up to 70% of available resources, and because demand-reduction groups must demonstrate through systematic studies that their programs and activities are effective in reducing demand while supply-reduction efforts are rarely held to these same requirements. Indeed, reports of the impact of supply reduction are usually in terms of amounts of drugs seized, illicit laboratories dismantled, and hectares of crops destroyed without any knowledge of exactly how much of which drugs are produced, how many illicit laboratories exist, or how many hectares are planted with poppies, coca, or marijuana.

Tensions also exist because professionals involved in supply and demand reduction have different types of training. Those in supply reduction detect, attack, and destroy and tend to be trained mostly in law enforcement or military strategies. Demand-reduction professionals focus on protecting populations vulnerable to drug abuse and are mostly educators or social and behavioral scientists. Despite these tensions, however, the two groups are both in the business of prevention; their jobs would be all that more difficult without each other. Almost all epidemiologic studies are geared to demand reduction. They tend to focus on consumers of drugs, not necessarily on consumption, which would provide useful information to those in supply reduction prevention efforts.

Prevention researchers have become skillful in taking advantage of available epidemiologic information to design their prevention strategies and measures to evaluate these strategies. The key epidemiologic findings that have influenced prevention researchers have been:

- age of initiation: 13 to 16-interventions are targeted at children either prior to the age of initiation or in the early teen years
- types and sequencing of drugs used: adolescents who use tobacco and alcohol are at greater risk to use marijuana–interventions target tobacco and alcohol as well as inhalants and marijuana
- sources of influence on drug use: adolescents are introduced to drugs by drug-using peers and by pressures in the media to use alcohol and tobacco–interventions establish anti-drug norms, confront misconceptions about how many youngsters use drugs, and address media manipulation strategies
- harmful effects of drug use: surveys have found that there is an inverse relationship between perceptions of the harmful effects of drugs, such as marijuana and cocaine, and the reported

use of these drugs—interventions incorporate findings from neurological studies on how the brain and body are affected by drugs and from epidemiologic findings on increased negative short- and long-term compromised behavioral, cognitive, emotional, and health statuses

- comorbidity: surveys and epidemiologic studies indicate that other problem behaviors are associated with drug use–interventions address drug use and these problem behaviors
- risk and protective factors: interventions emphasize one or more factors including prosocial bonding, improved academic performance, and improved parental monitoring.

Our understanding of risk and protective factors has been important for classifying prevention programs. Until the late 1980s, both drug abuse and mental-health prevention experts relied on the public-health classification of interventions. This classification was based on the stage of disease—whether it was prior to onset (primary prevention), at the time that an individual showed signs of disease (secondary prevention), or a progressive stage of disease (tertiary prevention). However, because this system was not found to be relevant or appropriate to mental illness or drug abuse, drug-abuse and mental-illness prevention experts drafted a new model for prevention focused on the risk status of the host (Mzarek & Haggerty, 1997). This model has proved to be quite helpful to the field. It defines three categories of prevention: universal, selective, and indicated. Universal prevention programs target both those who are and are not at risk for drug abuse. Selective programs target groups at risk or particular subsets of the general population, such as children of drug abusers. Indicated programs are designed for groups who are already using drugs or who exhibit other risk-related behaviors.

Based on this model, drug abuse prevention programs address particular aspects of risk status believed to lead to the initiation of drug use or to the progression from use to abuse and dependency. Many universal drug abuse prevention programs are school-based, either as part of the curriculum or as efforts to change the school environment. Curriculum-based programs are usually delivered in middle school and have booster sessions in high school. They emphasize communication, decision making, and resistance skills. They also focus on altering belief systems by focusing on short- and long-term negative effects of drug use on the brain and behavior and by correcting misconceptions regarding norms about drug use. Life Skills Training and Project STAR (Botvin et al., 1995; Pentz et al., 1989) are two of the many universal programs that have demonstrated long-term success in more than one population.

Programs designed to alter the school environment tend to address factors and processes that have been found to protect children against using drugs. Common features of these programs include initiation in the early grades in an attempt to make children successful in the school environment. They train teachers in skills that serve to improve learning and classroom behaviors. Examples of these types of programs include the Seattle Social Development Project (Hawkins et al., 1999) and the Baltimore Mastery Program and Good Behavior Games (Kellam & Anthony, 1998). Many prevention programs target the use of tobacco, alcohol, and illicit drugs as well as other problem behaviors, such as poor academic performance and delinquency.

Fewer selective programs have demonstrated effectiveness. The shared feature of these programs is that they include components that address parent–child relationships, teaching parents parenting skills, and helping children define their role in the family.

There are even fewer indicated programs with demonstrated effectiveness. Such programs are designed to teach children skills to deal with school, family, and peers and to moderate the early signs of drug use. An excellent example of one such program is the Reconnecting Youth Program (Thompson et al., 1997), which was designed for adolescents in grades 9 through 12 who are not doing well in school or who are frequently absent from school.

Most programs that address the environment focus on tobacco and alcohol use and have not been well assessed relative to drug abuse (Holder et al., 2000; MacKinnon et al., 2000). In the drug abuse field, the impact of school policies on drug abuse within the school has only recently been addressed (Pentz et al., 1989). The impact of law enforcement on trafficking and distribution of drugs within a community has not been well investigated nor have other environmental programs. Ennett and her colleagues (1997) and Bobashev and Anthony (1998) examined patterns in marijuana use by school and neighborhoods and found clustering. However, the reasons for these differences have not been fully explored. Such findings underscore the need for communities to assess their own patterns of drug use and to select preventive interventions that are most appropriate.

CONCLUSION

The marriage of epidemiology and drug abuse prevention has been a productive one but its continued success will require close communication between the partners. In the past, the field of drug abuse prevention drew heavily on epidemiology, but this appears to have been a one-way exchange. Now it is time for epidemiology to take note of the advances being made in drug abuse prevention research. With the increasing successes of prevention strategies, theories of prevention are evolving. The constructs from these theories need to be incorporated into epidemiologic studies to further our understanding of the pathways to drug use. Perhaps as prevention researchers conduct more mediational analyses and publish their results, epidemiologists will include these variables in their research.

On the other hand, prevention researchers may have to recommit themselves to epidemiology. The history of success in the area of drug abuse prevention is tied very closely to the evolution and growth of an epidemiologic knowledge base. Some of the exchange between prevention and epidemiologic researchers was due to the involvement of the early epidemiologic researchers with prevention, such as J. David Hawkins and Sheppard Kellam. But the influence of epidemiologic findings on prevention has leveled off in recent years, and changing and emerging trends observed in epidemiologic data bases have not been fully addressed by prevention researchers. Among these trends are (1) the declining age at which children begin to use drugs, (2) newer types of drugs, (3) declining ratio of male to female use among young people, and (4) declining differential in rates of use by ethnicity. There are important questions related to the appeal of drug experimentation to preadolescents and to those groups, such as girls, who were thought to be "protected." Are the increases we are seeing among these groups associated with increased risk or decreased protection? Are girls facing different pressures today than they faced 20 years ago? What will the next several decades present for young people? We need further analyses of the existing survey data but we also need to have hypothesis-generated research that can help answer such questions.

We are better prepared to address these new challenges than were our predecessors in many respects. We have a better understanding of dependence and addiction. We have better ways to reach young people with effective prevention strategies. Now we need to build on this knowledge base in order to be more responsive to dramatic changes in drug abuse and the problems they pose for the future.

REFERENCES

Altman, J. (1996). A biological view of drug abuse. *Molecular Medicine Today,* June.
Andreasson, S., & Allebeck, P. (1990). Cannabis and mortality among young men: a longitudinal study of Swedish conscripts. *Scandinavian Journal of Social Medicine, 18*(1), 9–15.

Anthony, J. C., & Petronis, K. R. (1995). Early-onset drug use and risk of later drug problems. *Drug and Alcohol Dependence, 49*(1), 9–15.

Bachman, J. G., Johnston, L. D., & O'Malley, P. M. (1990). Explaining the recent decline in cocaine use among young adults: Further evidence that perceived risks and disapproval lead to reduced drug use. *Journal of Health and Social Behavior, 31*(2), 173–184.

Bachman, J. G., Johnston, L. D., & O'Malley, P. M. (1998). Explaining recent increases in student's marijuana use: Impacts of perceived risks and disapproval: 1976–1996. *American Journal of Public Health. 88*(6), 887–892.

Bachman, J. G., Johnston, L. D., O'Malley, P. M., & Humphrey, R. H. (1988). Explaining recent decline in marijuana use, differentiating the effects of perceived risks, disapproval, and general lifestyle factors. *Journal of Health and Social Behavior, 29,* 92–112.

Benson, P. L., Galbraith, J., & Espeland, P. (1998). *What kids need to succeed: Proven practical ways to raise good kids.* Minneapolis: Free Spirit Publishing, Inc.

Block, R. I., & Ghoneim, M. M. (1993). Effects of chronic marijuana use on human cognition. *Psychopharmacology 110,* 219–228.

Bobashev, G. V., & Anthony, J. C. (1998). Clusters of marijuana use in the United States. *American Journal of Epidemiology, 148*(12), 1168–1174.

Botvin, G. J., Baker, E., Dusenbury, L., Botvin, E. M., & Diaz, T. (1995). Long-term followup results of a randomized drug abuse prevention trial in a white middle-class population. *Journal of the American Medical Association 273*(14), 1106–1112.

Brady, K. T., & Randall, C. L. (1999). Gender differences in substance use disorders. *Psychiatric Clinics of North America 22*(2), 241–252.

Brook, J. S., Balka, E. B., Gursen, M. D., Brook, D. W., Shapiro, J., & Cohen, P. (1997). Young adult's drug use: a 17-year longitudinal inquiry of antecedents. *Psychological Reports, 80*(3 Pt. 2), 1235–1251.

Brook, J. S., Whiteman, M., Balka, E. B., & Cohen, P. (1997). Drug use and delinquency: shared and unshared risk factors in African American and Puerto Rican adolescents. *Journal of Genetic Psychology, 158*(1), 25–39.

Brook, J. S., Whiteman, M., Balka, E. B., Win, P. T., & Gursen, M. D. (1998). Similar and different precursors to drug use and delinquency among African American and Puerto Ricans. *Journal of Genetic Psychology, 159*(1), 13–29.

Brown, T. N., Schulenberg, J., Bachman, J. G., O'Malley, P. M., & Johnston, L. D. (2001). Are risks and protective factors for substance use consistent across historical time?: National data from the high school classes of 1976 through 1997. *Prevention Science, 2*(1), 29–43.

Bry, B. H., McKeon, P., & Pandina, R. J. (1982). Extent of drug use as a function of number of risk factors. *Journal of Abnormal Psychology, 91*(4), 273–279.

Chen, K., & Kandel, D. B. (1998). Predictors of cessation of marijuana use: An event history analysis. *Drug and Alcohol Dependence, 50*(2), 109–121.

Chen, K., Kandel, D. B., & Davies, M. (1997). Relationship between frequency and quantity of marijuana use and last year proxy dependence among adolescents and adults in the United States. *Drug and Alcohol Dependence, 46*(1–2), 53–67.

Cherubin, C. E., & Sapira, J. D. (1993). The medical complications of drug addiction and the medical assessment of the intravenous drug user: 25 years later. *Annals of Internal Medicine, 119*(10), 1017–1028.

Childress, A. R., Mozley, D., Fitzgerald, J., Reivich, M., Jaggi, J., & O'Brien, C. P. (1995). Limbic activation during cue-induced cocaine craving. *Society for Neuroscience Abstracts, 21*(3), 1956.

Coffey, C., Lynskey, M., Wolfe, R., & Patton, G. C. (2000). Initiation and progression of cannabis use in a population-based Australian adolescent longitudinal study. *Addiction, 95*(11), 1679–1690.

Crowley, T. J., Macdonald, M. J., Whitmore, E. A., & Mikulich, S. K. (1998). Cannabis dependence, withdrawal, and reinforcing effects among adolescents with conduct symptoms and substance use disorders. *Drug and Alcohol Dependence, 50*(1), 27–37.

DeWit, D. J., Hance, J., Offord, D. R., & Ogborne, A. (2000). The influence of early and frequent use of marijuana on the risk of desistance and of progression to marijuana-related harm. *Preventive Medicine, 31*(5), 455–464.

Donovan, J. E., Jessor, R., & Costa, F. M. (1998). Syndrome of problem behavior in adolescence: A replication. *Journal of Consulting and Clinical Psychology, 56*(5), 762–765.

DuPont, R. L. (1998). Addiction: A new paradigm. *Bulletin of the Menninger Clinic, 62*(6), 231–242.

Ennett, S. T., Flewelling, R. L., Lindroth, R. C., & Norton, E. C. (1997). School and neighborhood characteristics associated with school rates of alcohol, cigarettes, and marijuana use. *Journal of Health and Social Behavior, 38*(1), 55–71.

Feingold, A., & Rounsaville, B. (1995). Construct validity of the abuse-dependence distinction as measured by DSM-IV criteria for different psychotic substances. *Drug and Alcohol Dependence, 39*(2), 99–109.

Fergusson, D. M., & Horwood, L. J. (2000). Cannabis use and dependence in a New Zealand birth cohort. *New Zealand Medical Journal, 113*(1109), 156–158.

Fried, P. A. (1995). Prenatal exposure to marihuana and tobacco during infancy, early and middle childhood: effects and an attempt at synthesis. *Archives of Toxicology, Supplement, 17,* 233–260.

Fried, P. A., & Watkinson, B. (2000). Visuoperceptual functioning differs in 9- to 12-year olds prenatally exposed to cigarettes and marihuana. *Neurotoxicology and Teratology, 22*(1), 11–20.

Ghodse, H., Oyefeso, A., & Kilpatrick, B. (1998). Mortality of drug addicts in the United Kingdom 1967–1993. *International Journal of Epidemiology, 27*(3), 473–478.

Gore, S. M. (1999). Fatal uncertainty: death-rate from use of ecstasy or heroin. *Lancet, 354*(186), 1265–1266.

Glantz, M. D., & Pickens, R. W. (1992). Vulnerability to drug abuse: Introduction and overview. In: Glantz, M.D. & Pickens, R.W. (Eds.). *Vulnerability to Drug Abuse* (pp. 1–14). Washington, D.C.: American Psychological Association.

Glantz, M. D., & Sloboda, Z. (1999). Analysis and reconceptualization of resiliency. In M. D. Glantz & J. Johnson (Eds.), *Resilience and development: Positive life adaptations.* New York: Kluwer Academic/Plenum Press.

Grant, B. R., & Pickering, R. (1998). The relationship between cannabis use and DSM-IV cannabis abuse and dependence: results from the National Longitudinal Alcohol Epidemiologic Survey. *Journal of Substance Abuse, 10*(3), 255–264.

Hawkins, J. D., Catalano, R. F., Kosterman, R., Abbott, R., & Hill, K.G. (1999). Preventing adolescent health-risk behaviors by strengthening protection during childhood. *Archives of Pediatric and Adolescent Medicine, 153*(3), 226–234.

Hawkins, J. D., Catalano, R. F., & Miller, J. Y. (1992). Risk and protective factors for alcohol and other drug problems in adolescence and early adulthood: Implications for substance abuse prevention. *Psychological Bulletin. 112*(1), 64–105.

Hoffman, J. P., & Su, S. S. (1998). Stressful life events and adolescent substance use and depression: Conditional and gender differentiated effects. *Substance Use and Misuse, 53*(11), 2219–2262.

Holder, H. D., Gruenwald, P. J., Ponicki, W. B., Treno, A. J., Grube, J. W., Saltz, R. F., Voas, R. B., Reynolds, R., Davis, J., Sanchez, L., Gaumont, G., & Roeper, P. (2000). Effect of community-based interventions on high-risk drinking and alcohol-related injuries. *Journal of the American Medical Association, 284*(18), 2341–2347.

Hulse, G. K., English, D. R., Milne, E., & Holman, C. D. (1999). The quantification of mortality resulting from the regular use of illicit opiates. *Addiction, 94*(2), 221–229.

Jaffe, J. H., Knapp, C. M., & Ciraulo, D. A. (1997). Opiates: Clinical aspects. In J. H. Lowinson, P. Ruiz, R. B. Millman, & J. G. Langrod (Eds.), *Substance abuse: A comprehensive textbook.* Baltimore: Williams & Wilkins.

James, W. H., & Moore, D. D. (1999). Examining the relationship between gender and drug-using behaviors in adolescents: The use of diagnostic assessments and biochemical analyses of urine samples. *Journal of Drug Education, 29*(3), 235–249.

Jessor, R., & Jessor, S. L. (1977). *Problem behavior and psychosocial development: A longitudinal study of youth.* New York: Academic Press.

Jessor, R., Jessor, S. L., & Finney, J. (1973). A social psychology of marijuana use: Longitudinal studies of high school and college youth. *Journal of Personality and Social Psychology, 26*(1), 1–15.

Kandel, D. (1975). Stages of adolescent involvement in drug use. *Science, 190,* 912–914.

Kandel, D. B., & Chen, K. (2000). Types of marijuana users by longitudinal course. *Journal of Studies on Alcohol, 61*(3), 367–378.

Kandel, D. B., Johnson, J. G., Bird, H. R., Weissman, M. M., Goodman, S. H., Lahey, B. B., Regier, D. A. & Schwab-Stone, M. E. (1999). Psychiatric comorbidity among adolescents with substance use disorders: findings from the MECA Study. *Journal of the American Academy of Child and Adolescent Psychiatry, 38*(6), 693–699.

Kandel, D. B., & Raveis, V. H. (1989). Cessation of illicit drug use in young adulthood. *Archives of General Psychiatry, 46*(2), 109–116.

Kandel, D. B., Wu, P., & Davies, M. (1994). Maternal smoking during pregnancy and smoking by adolescent daughters. *American Journal of Public Health, 84*(9), 1407–1413.

Kandel, D. B., Yamaguchi, K., & Chen, K. (1992). Stages of progression in drug involvement from adolescence to adulthood: Further evidence for the gateway theory. *Journal of Studies of Alcohol, 53,* 447–457.

Kaplan, H. B., & Johnson, R. J. (1992). Relationships between circumstances surrounding initial illicit drug use and escalation of drug use: Moderating effects of gender and early adolescent experiences. In M. Glantz & R. Pickens (Eds.), *Vulnerability to drug abuse* (pp. 299–358). Washington, DC: American Psychological Association.

Kellam, S. G., & Anthony, J. C. (1998). Targeting early antecedents to prevent tobacco smoking: findings from an epidemiologically based randomized field trial. *American Journal of Public Health, 88*(10), 1490–1495.

Kendler, K. S., & Prescott, C. A. (1998). Cannabis use, abuse, and dependence in a population-based sample of female twins. *American Journal of Psychiatry, 155*(8), 1016–1022.

Koob, G. F., Rocio, M., Carrera, A., Gold, L. H., Heyser, C. J., Maldonado-Irizarry, C., Markou, A., Parsons, L. H., Roberts, A. J., Schulteis, G., Stinus, L., Walker, J. R., Weissenborn, R., & Weiss, F. (1998). Substance dependence as a compulsive behavior. *Journal of Psychopharmacology, 12*(1), 39–48.

Kosten, T. R., Rounsaville, B. J., Babor, T. F., Spitzer, R. L., & Willams, J. B. (1987). Substance-use disorders in DSM-IIIR. Evidence for the dependence syndrome across different psychoactive substances. *British Journal of Psychiatry, 151,* 834–843.

Kouri, E. M., Pope, H. G., & Lukas, S. E. (1999). Changes in aggressive behavior during withdrawal from long-term marijuana use. *Psychopharmacology, 143,* 302–308.

Lessler, J. T., & O'Reilly, J. M. (1997). Mode of interview and reporting of sensitive issues: Design and implementation of audio computer-assisted self-interviewing. *National Institute on Drug Abuse Research Monograph, 167,* 366–382.

Lifrak, P. D., Mckay, J. R., Rostain, A., Alterman, A. I., & O'Brien, C. P. (1997). Relationship of perceived competencies, perceived social support and gender to substance abuse in young adolescents. *Journal of the American Academy of Child and Adolescent Psychiatry, 36*(7), 933–940.

Lilienfeld, A. M., & Lilienfeld, D. E. (1980). *Foundations of epidemiology.* New York: Oxford University Press.

Lyvers, M. (1998). Drug addiction as a physical disease: The role of physical dependence and other chronic drug-induced neurophysiological changes in compulsive drug self-administration. *Experimental and clinical psychopharmacology, 6*(1), 107–125.

MacKinnon, D. P., Nohre, L., Pentz, M. A., & Stacy, A. W. (2000). The alcohol warning and adolescents: 5-year effects. *American Journal of Public Health, 90*(10), 1589–1594.

Mrazek, P. J., & Haggerty, R. J. (Eds., 1994). *Reducing risks for mental disorders: Frontiers for prevention intervention research.* Washington, DC: National Academy Press.

National Institute on Drug Abuse (1996). Calculations derived from the 1994 National Household Survey on Drug Abuse by staff of the Division of Epidemiology. Services and Prevention Research, National Institute on Drug Abuse, National Institutes of Health.

National Institute on Drug Abuse (1998). *National survey results on drug use from the monitoring the future study, 1975–1997. Volume 1: Secondary School Students.* NIH Publication No. 98-4345.

Neumark, V. D., Van Etten, M. L., & Anthony, J. C. (2000). 'Drug dependence' and death: Survival analysis of the Baltimore ECA sample from 1981 to 1995. *Substance Use and Misuse, 35*(3), 313–327.

O'Brien, C. P., Childress, A. R., Ehrman, R., & Robbins, S. J. (1998). Conditioning factors in drug abuse: can they explain compulsion? *Journal of Psychopharmacology, 12*(1), 15–22.

Office of Applied Studies, Substance Abuse and Mental Health Services Administration (1997). *National household survey on drug abuse main findings 1998.* Washington, DC: U.S. Department of Health and Human Services.

Office of Applied Studies, Substance Abuse and Mental Health Services Administration (1998). *National household survey on drug abuse main findings 1996.* Washington, DC: U.S. Department of Health and Human Services.

Office of Applied Studies, Substance Abuse and Mental Health Services Administration (1999). *National household survey on drug abuse 1998.* http://www.samhsa.gov/statistics/statistics.html.

Pandina, R. J. (1998). Risk and protective factor models in adolescent drug use: Putting them to work for prevention. *National conference on drug abuse prevention research: Presentations, papers, and recommendations* (pp. 17–26). NIH Publication No. 98-4293.

Patterson, E. W., Myers, G., & Gallant, D. M. (1988). Patterns of substance use on a college campus: A 14-year comparison study. *American Journal of Drug and Alcohol Abuse, 14*(2), 237–246.

Pentz, M. A., Brannon, B. R., Charlin, V. L., Barrett, E. J., MacKinnon, D. P., & Flay, B. R. (1989). The power of policy: the relationship of smoking policy to adolescent smoking. *American Journal of Public Health, 79*(7), 857–862.

Pentz, M. A., Dwyer, J. H., MacKinnon, D. P., Flay, B. R., Hansen, W. B., Wang, E. Y., & Johnson, C. A. (1989). A multi-community trial for primary prevention of adolescent drug abuse: Effects of drug use prevalence. *Journal of the American Medical Association, 261,* 3259–3266.

Perkonigg, A., Lieb, R., Hofler, M., Schuster, P., Sonntag, H., & Wittchen, H. U. (1999). Patterns of cannabis use, abuse and dependence over time: incidence, progression and stability in a sample of 1228 adolescents. *Addiction, 94*(11), 1663–1678.

Polen, M. R., Sidney, S., Tekawa, I. S., Sadler, M., & Friedman, G. D. (1993). Health care use by frequent marijuana smokers who do not smoke tobacco. *The Western Journal of Medicine, 158*(6), 596–601.

Pope, H. G., Jr., & Yurgelun-Todd, D. (1996). The residual cognitive effects of heavy marijuana use in college students. *JAMA 275*(7), 521–527.

Richards, J. R., Johnson, E. B., Stark, R. W., & Derlet, R. W. (1999). Methamphetamine abuse and rhabdomyolsis in the ED: a 5-year study. *American Journal of Emergency Medicine, 17*(7), 681–685.

Rohrbach, L. A., & Milam, J. (2002). Gender issues in substance abuse prevention. In Z. Sloboda and W. J. Bukoski (Ed.), Handbook of drug abuse prevention (351–359). Kluwer Academic/Plenum Publishers.

Rounsaville, B. J., Bryant, K., Babor, T., Kranzler, H., & Kadden, R. (1993). Cross system agreement for substance use disorders: DSM-IIIR, DSM-IV and ICD-10. *Addiction, 88*(3), 337–348.

Sanders-Phillips, K. (1999). Ethnic minority women, health behaviors, and drug abuse: A continuum of psychosocial risks. In M. D. Glantz & C. R. Hartel (Eds.), *Drug abuse origins and interventions* (pp. 191–222). Washington, DC: American Psychological Association.

Shaffer, H. J. (1997). The most important unresolved issue in the addictions: Conceptual chaos. *Substance Use and Misuse, 32*(11), 1573–1580.

Single, E., Rehm, J., Robson, L., & Truong, M. V. (2000). The relative risks and etiologic fractions of different causes of death and disease attributable to alcohol, tobacco and illicit drug use in Canada. *Canadian Medical Association Journal, 162*(12), 1669–1675.

Sloboda, Z., & Kozel, N. J. (1999). Frontline surveillance: The Community Epidemiology Work Group on Drug Abuse. In M. D. Glantz & C. R. Hartel, (Eds.), *Drug abuse origins and Interventions* (pp. 47–62). Washington, DC: American Psychological Association.

Solowij, N. (1995). Do cognitive impairments recover following cessation of cannabis use? *Life Sciences, 56* (23–24), 2119–2126.

Substance Abuse & Mental Health Services Administration (1995). *National Household Survey on Drug Abuse: Main Findings 1992.* DHHS Publication No. (SMA) 94-3012.

Substance Abuse & Mental Health Services Administration (1999). *Summary of findings from the 1998 National Household Survey on Drug Abuse.* DHHS Publication No. (SMA) 99-3328.

Substance Abuse & Mental Health Services Administration (2001). *National Household Survey on Drug Abuse.* http://www.samhsa.gov/statistics/statistics.html.

Thomas, H. (1996). A community survey of adverse effects of cannabis use. *Drug and Alcohol Dependence, 42*(3), 201–207.

Thompson, E. A., Horn, M., Herting, J. R., & Eggert, L. L. (1997). Enhancing outcomes in an indicated drug prevention program for high-risk youth. *Journal of Drug Education, 27*(1), 19–41.

Tiffany, S. T., & Carter, B. L. (1998). Is craving the source of compulsive drug use? *Journal of Psychopharmacology, 12*(1), 23–30.

Turner, C. F., & Miller, H. G. (1997). Monitoring trends in drug use: strategies for the 21st century. *Substance Use and Misuse, 32*(14), 2093–2103.

Ustun, B., Compton, W., Mager, D., Babor, T., Baiyewu, O., Chatterji, S., Cottler, L., Gogus, A., Mavreas, V., Peters, L., Pull, C., Saunders, J., Smeets, R., Stipec, M. R., Vrasti, R., Hasin, D., Room, R., Van den Brink, W., Regier, D., Blaine, J., Grant, B. R., & Sartourius, N. (1997). WHO Study on the reliability and validity of the alcohol and drug use disorder instruments: overview of methods and results. *Drug and Alcohol Dependence, 47*(3), 161–169.

Van Etten, M. L., & Anthony, J. C. (1999). Comparative epidemiology of initial drug opportunities and transitions to first use: marijuana, cocaine, hallucinogens and heroin. *Drug and Alcohol Dependence, 54*(2), 117–125.

Van Etten, M. L., Neumark, Y. D., & Anthony, J. C. (1997). Initial opportunity to use marijuana and the transition to first use: United States, 1979–1994. *Drug and Alcohol Dependence, 49*(1), 1–7.

Volkow, N. D., & Fowler, J. S. (2000). Addiction, a disease of compulsion and drive: involvement of the orbitofrontal cortex. *Cerebral Cortex, 10*(3), 318–325.

Volkow, N. D., Fowler, J. S., Wolf, A. P., Hitzemann, R., Dewey, S., Bendriem, B., Alpert, R., & Hoff, A. (1991). Changes in brain glucose metabolism in cocaine dependence and withdrawal. *American Journal of Psychology, 148*, 621–626.

Warner, L. A., Kessler, R. C., Hughes, M., Anthony, J. C., & Nelson, C. B. (1995). Prevalence and correlates of drug use and dependence in the United States. Results from the National Comorbidity Survey. *Archives of General Psychiatry, 52*(3), 219–229.

Weinberg, N. Z., Rahdert, E., Colliver, J. D., & Glantz, M. D. (1998). Adolescent substance abuse: A review of the past 10 years. *Journal of the American Academy of Child and Adolescent Psychiatry, 37*(3), 252–261.

Woody, G. E., & Cacciola, J. (1997). Diagnosis and classification: DSM-IV and ICD-10. In Lowinson, J. H., Ruiz, P., Millman, R. B., & Langrod, J. G. (Eds.), *Substance abuse: A comprehensive textbook,* Baltimore: Williams & Wilkins.

Woody, G. E., Cottler, L. B., & Cacciola, J. (1993). Severity of dependence: data from the DSM-IV field trials. *Addiction, 88*(11), 1573–1579.

Yamaguchi, K., & Kandel, D. B. (1984). Patterns of drug use from adolescence to young adulthood: III. Predictors of progression. *American Journal of Public Health, 74*(7), 673–681.

CHAPTER 13

Risk and Protective Factors of Adolescent Drug Use: Implications for Prevention Programs

JUDITH S. BROOK
DAVID W. BROOK
LINDA RICHTER
MARTIN WHITEMAN

INTRODUCTION

Drug use and abuse are costly problems that affect the health and well-being of individuals and families. Despite a decline in drug use during the early 1990s, there has been an increase in use in recent years (Bachman et al., 1997). Many youngsters use drugs, and the personal, social, medical, and legal costs are considerable (Newcomb & Bentler, 1988). Furthermore, there is the risk of dependence and deviance, particularly among young users of drugs (Kaplan, 1995).

This chapter presents an integration of findings from several cross-sectional and longitudinal studies conducted over the past 2 decades on the psychosocial etiology of the risk and protective factors for drug use. Risk factors precede and increase the probability of drug use. Protective factors "ameliorate" the effect of risk factors on drug use or "enhance" *the beneficial effects of* other protective factors and lead to less drug use. Numerous studies conducted since the 1970s have

JUDITH S. BROOK, DAVID W. BROOK, AND MARTIN WHITEMAN • Department of Community and Preventive Medicine, Mount Sinai School of Medicine, New York, New York 10029
LINDA RICHTER • The National Center on Addiction and Substance Abuse, Columbia University, New York, New York 10027

contributed to our understanding of the etiology of drug use (Brook et al., 1990; Hawkins, Catalano, & Miller, 1992; Kumpfer, 1989; Oetting & Donnermeyer, 1998; Pandina & Johnson, 1999; Petraitis, Flay, & Miller, 1995; Szapocznik & Coatsworth, 1999) and have important implications for prevention and policy decisions. In this chapter, we use our research as a base from which to discuss the major empirical and theoretical issues related to the causes of adolescent drug use and identify effective prevention programs that address psychosocial risk factors for drug use and abuse.

A DEVELOPMENTAL MODEL

The main goal of our research has been to understand the underlying causes of adolescent drug use and to test hypothetical relationships among developmental, familial, personality, peer, and contextual factors. The data from these studies appear in a number of publications (Brook, Balka et al., 1997; Brook, Brook, & Whiteman, 2000; Brook et al., 1990; Brook, Brook et al., 1997; Brook, Cohen, & Brook, 1998; Brook, Tseng, & Whiteman, 1998; Brook, Richter, & Whiteman, 2000; Brook, Whiteman et al., 1997; Brook, Whiteman et al., 1998; Brook et al., 1995, 2000) and are generally consistent with the findings of others in the field.

Family interactions provide a framework for the developmental model that is the basis of our research on adolescent drug use. This model, based on family interactional theory, has been tested and supported in cross-sectional and longitudinal studies (Brook et al., 1990, Brook et al., 1993). Figure 13.1 outlines the model and the basic pathways that lead to nonuse of marijuana. They are

1. Internalization of societal values by the parent leads to a warm, conflict-free parent–child attachment, which is linked with the youngster's identifying with the parent.
2. A consequence of this attachment and the child's close identification with the parent is the child's incorporation of the parent's personality traits, attitudes, and behaviors, which then manifest themselves in the adolescent's own personality, attitudes, and behaviors.
3. These adolescent characteristics (such as conventionality and control of emotions) are then expressed in affiliations with peers who do not use drugs, which in turn leads to the adolescent's nonuse of marijuana.

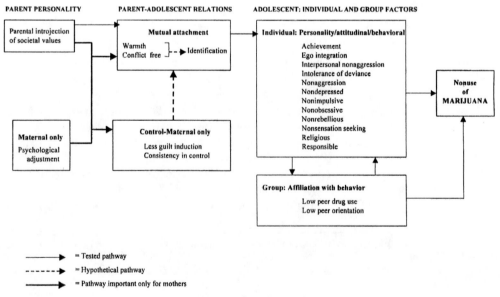

FIGURE 13.1. The developmental model.

Our studies have focused on various developmental domains believed to be relevant to adolescent drug use. Figure 13.2 depicts the domains that have direct effects on drug use as solid arrows between boxes A, B, and C and adolescent drug use. Dashed arrows between the boxes indicate mediated effects on drug use. Parental personality, for example, does not have a direct effect on adolescent drug use but does have an effect on parent–adolescent relations, which do effect drug use.

The Influence of Each Domain

THE MARITAL RELATIONSHIP.   Because the family consists of husband-wife relations in addition to parent–child relations, the marital context needs to be considered in attempts to understand childhood development (e.g., Gable, Belsky, & Crnic, 1992). Marital conflict is likely to interfere with the development of mutual attachment between parents and child, reducing the opportunity for the parent to influence the child and have the child internalize adaptive norms and conventional rules. Marital conflict may, therefore, ultimately result in an increased risk of drug use. Researchers have also found that family conflict and having parents who are not emotionally supportive are associated with a higher risk for delinquency and drug use (Johnson & Pandina, 1991; Simcha-Fagen, Gersten, & Langner, 1986). Indeed, parental conflict may be a greater risk factor for adolescent drug use than is parental absence (Farrington, 1991).

PARENTAL DRUG USE AND PERSONALITY.   Parental drug use has been found by many investigators to be related to a child's drug use (Brook, Whiteman, Gordon, & Brook, 1983; Hops et al., 1990; McDermott, 1984; Peterson et al., 1995). The transmission from parent to child may be based on genetic factors and/or be a result of parental drug modeling. Moreover, when both parents use drugs, there is a synergistic effect. That is, the effect of two parents using drugs is greater than the effect of the sum of both parents using drugs. The effects of parental drug use on the adolescent's use of drugs is indirect (Hansen et al., 1987) in that parental drug use is associated with youngsters selecting friends who use drugs, which in turn is related to the adolescent's drug use. Not only is parental drug use important, parental attitudes toward drug use also play a role in the adolescent's use of drugs. Parents who are tolerant of drug use are more likely to have children who use drugs (Brook, Gordon, Whiteman, & Cohen, 1986; Oetting et al., in press).

Parent personality factors also play a significant role in an adolescent's use of drugs (Brook, Gordon, & Brook, 1987; Brook, Whiteman, Gordon, & Brook, 1986, Brook et al., 1990). As noted earlier, children who have close relationships with their parents often adopt their parents' personality traits. In the case of mothers, but not fathers, psychological adjustment is also important in the child's drug use, perhaps because mothers traditionally spend more time with their youngsters than do fathers.

THE PARENT–ADOLESCENT RELATIONSHIP

Mutual Attachment.   The parent–child attachment relationship is very important both directly and indirectly in terms of its effect on adolescent drug use (Bailey & Hubbard, 1990; Hundleby & Mercer, 1987; Selnow, 1987; Wills, Mariani, & Filer, 1996). Parents of nonusers, in comparison with parents of users, tend to report greater warmth (more child centeredness, affection, and communication) and a less conflicted relationship. Jessor and Jessor (1977) found that marijuana users reported significantly less parental warmth than did nonusers. Furthermore, in a study

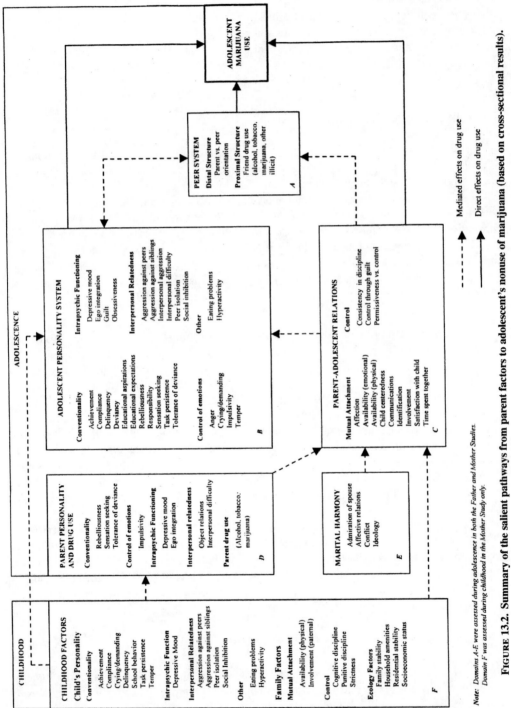

FIGURE 13.2. Summary of the salient pathways from parent factors to adolescent's nonuse of marijuana (based on cross-sectional results).

Note: Domains A-E were assessed during adolescence in both the Father and Mother Studies.
Domain F was assessed during childhood in the Mother Study only.

of almost 3,000 men (ages 20 to 30), O'Donnell and Clayton (1979) found that the family influences that predicted less marijuana use included closeness to mothers, closeness to fathers, and communication with parents. Other similar and promising findings highlight the crucial role of attachment and demonstrate the importance of this variable in adolescent drug use (e.g., Barnes, Farrell, & Banerjee, 1995; Hirschi, 1969; Newcomb & Felix-Ortiz, 1992).

These findings suggest that an affectionate and nonconflicted parent–adolescent attachment relationship helps shape a youngster's behavior in ways that lead to less drug use. This can be explained by the following factors: (1) parental warmth, which makes the parent important to the child and obviates the need for severe forms of discipline; (2) parental models of controlled behavior; (3) a conflict-free relationship, which results in less frustration, aggression, and need to rebel; and (4) a youngster's greater identification with the parent, which results in the incorporation of parental values and behavior.

Hawkins, Catalano, & Miller (1992) have suggested that the parent–adolescent attachment may inhibit drug use in much the same way that parental bonding inhibits delinquency. In our own research we have found common family bonding variables that inhibit both drug use and delinquency (Brook & Cohen, 1992). When risk factors, such as negative peer influences, are controlled for, adolescents who have good communications with their parents are less likely to use drugs.

Control Variables.   Another way parents help shape the behavior of their children is through control, referring to both physical discipline and psychological methods of control. O'Donnell and Clayton (1979) reported that family control can be used to predict drug use. Brook, Whiteman, and Gordon (1983) found that disciplinary structure serves as a barrier to adolescent drug use (see also Kandel & Andrews, 1987). Appropriate parental monitoring has also been found to be effective in reducing delinquency and substance abuse (Fletcher, Darling, & Steinberg, 1995; Patterson, Reid, & Dishion, 1992). On the other hand, several investigators have found little association between parental permissiveness and marijuana use (see Penning & Barnes, 1982). In general, structure and consistency appear to be beneficial, power assertive techniques may be detrimental, and permissiveness appears to have no effect (Brook et al., 1990).

To our knowledge, there are no drug studies comparing the differential impacts of maternal and paternal control. However, maternal techniques of control appear to be far more important than paternal techniques in explaining adolescent marijuana use. For example, maternal control patterns that involve setting clear requirements for mature and responsible behavior result in less marijuana use. Maternal control through guilt, which appears to make use of as well as threaten the love relationship, is correlated with greater drug use. Perhaps maternal control is more effective than paternal control because it is more often accompanied by a higher degree of involvement (Brook et al., 1990).

Siblings.   Siblings, like parents, can have an effect on drug use. Some relevant research includes a study by Conger, Reuter, and Conger (1994), who found that the substance use by older siblings increases the chances of substance use by younger ones. Duncan, Duncan, and Hops (1996) conducted a longitudinal study demonstrating that siblings are a continuing source of influence on the adolescent's drug use patterns and that these influences extend into adulthood. Our research examined the role of older brothers in a younger brother's drug use (Brook et al., 1991) and identified two mechanisms by which an older brother can influence a younger brother's drug use. The first is a personality influence mechanism through which the older brother's personality influences the younger brother's personality through identification and modeling. This identification is likely to lead to common values, attitudes, and behavioral orientation. An older brother's deviance and attitude to deviance were associated with deviant orientations and behavior in the younger brother. On the other hand, similarities between brothers could also be a result of genetic factors or similar upbringing (Rowe, Rodgers, & Meseck-Bushey, 1992).

The second mechanism involves the relationship between brothers. A difficult sibling relationship marked by jealousy and low degrees of nurturing, admiration, satisfaction, and sibling identification may lead to increased psychological distress that can be manifested as a lack of responsibility or other signs of unconventional behavior in the younger brother, *including drug use*. The sibling relationship can also interact with parental factors. For instance, if an adolescent has a conflicted relationship with the parents, a close relation with a sibling can buffer these negative influences.

CHILDHOOD ATTRIBUTES.   Individual personality traits strongly affect adolescent drug-using behavior. A child who is irritable, easily distractible, has temper tantrums, fights often with siblings, and shows early signs of delinquent behavior is more likely to use drugs in adolescence and young adulthood (Brook, Whiteman, Gordon, & Cohen, 1986; Brook et al., 1996). This is because certain personality dispositions related to later drug use, such as antisocial behavior and aggression, appear to be moderately stable from childhood through adolescence (Cohen & Brook, 1987; Kagan & Moss, 1962; Moffitt, 1993). Early childhood signs of social inhibition, anger, and low aspirations are related to similar characteristics years later. Some of these stable characteristics are part of a general category of unconventionality, which is closely related to drug use. For example, the adolescent's attitude toward deviance may have evolved to some extent from childhood characteristics, such as problem behavior (Brook & Newcomb, 1995).

Childhood Psychopathology.   Childhood psychopathology is often a risk factor for problem behaviors later in life. For example, early antisocial behavior and deviance are risk factors for both drug use and drug abuse (Robins & McEvoy, 1990). Two psychopathologies that have been identified as *being among the most common* risk factors for substance abuse are depression and antisocial personality disorder (Grove et al., 1990). Studies of clinical and epidemiological samples also suggest that drug abuse and psychopathology are often linked (Kessler et al., 1996). Surveys reveal that psychiatric disorders related to increased risk of alcoholism and drug abuse include conduct and oppositional disorder, attention deficit disorder, and anxiety disorders, particularly phobic disorders and depression (Fergusson, Horwood, & Lynskey, 1994; Kessler et al., 1996; Riggs et al., 1995). In contrast to drug abuse, psychopathology does not play a major role in drug use.

PEERS.   *Peer influences* contribute greatly to drug use. In fact, the percentage of variance in drug use contributed by the peer *domain* is more than that of any other intrapersonal or interpersonal domain. In general, the findings regarding the importance of the peer group are consistent in a variety of studies (Donovan, 1996; Oetting & Beauvais, 1987a,b; Oetting & Beauvais, 1990; Oetting & Donnermeyer, 1998). Newcomb and Bentler (1986) found that peers had a greater effect than parents on a youngster's drug use for several *ethnic* groups, including White, African, Asian, and Hispanic-Americans. Oetting and his colleagues have developed an in-depth understanding of the mechanisms involved in peer influence on drug use (see Chapter 5). According to their Peer Cluster Theory (Oetting & Beauvais, 1987a,b), adolescent drug use takes place within the context of peer clusters, which consist of best friends or very close friends. The theory describes the dynamics of peer groups and notes that peers are effective in establishing the attitudes, beliefs, and group norms for drug behavior. Oetting and his colleagues also describe the linkages between peer clusters and specific psychosocial clusters. Their empirical data are consistent with their developmental model, which suggests that families and schools influence the formation of peer clusters, which in turn affect drug use. The connection between personality and peers may also be a function of general peer factors such as warmth, conventionality, values, and academic achievement, as well as the more specific drug-related factors of peer pressure, imitation, and identification (Kandel, 1996; Oetting, Donnermeyer, & Deffenbacher, 1998).

Finally, there is the possibility of reciprocal causality and the likelihood that "feedback loops" are operating between peer drug use and self drug use. If an adolescent is using drugs, he or she is more likely to associate with drug-using peers. This, in turn, increases the chance of the adolescent's maintaining or increasing his or her drug involvement. In other words, drug-prone adolescents tend to select deviant peers who share characteristics similar to their own personality attributes. *This is known as assortative pairing* (Brook & Cohen, 1992; Kaplan, 1995). The deviant peers in turn influence deviant attitudes and behavior via role modeling (Kaplan, 1995), which further increases the probability of adolescent drug use.

ADOLESCENT PERSONALITY. Adolescent personality characteristics have a very strong impact on a youngster's use of drugs (Bachman et al., 1997; Brook et al., 1990; Kaplan, 1996; Pandina, Labouvie, & White, 1984; Petraitis et al., 1995). There are four distinct aspects to the adolescent personality domain: (1) conventionality versus unconventionality, (2) emotional control, (3) intrapsychic functioning, and (4) interpersonal relatedness. Of these, the most powerful predictors of more frequent drug use are the unconventionality variables, namely, sensation seeking, risk-taking, rebelliousness, tolerance of deviance, and low school achievement.

Adolescents with an orientation toward sensation seeking probably require greater stimulation from outside sources and may use drugs as external or new stimulation. Adolescents who are rebellious, having fewer internalized personal controls and rules, may seek out that which is forbidden (marijuana or other illegal substances or acts). Adolescents who have not incorporated socially acceptable attitudes and ethics, as reflected in the tolerance of deviance measures, may lack the requisite conviction to avoid illegal and socially unacceptable drugs.

Less important in terms of drug use than the conventionality dimension are the remaining three dimensions—emotional control, intrapsychic functioning, and interpersonal relatedness, although aspects of each are significantly related to drug use. Donovan (1996) found that tolerance of deviance, deviant behavior, low achievement, and a critical attitude toward society were all associated with marijuana use. Johnston, O'Malley, and Bachman (1985) found that adolescents who expect to attend college are less likely to use hallucinogens, cocaine, heroin, stimulants, or other illicit drugs. In our research (e.g., Brook, Balka et al., 1997), dimensions of unconventionality affected drug use independently of family or peers. That is, despite benign family and peer conditions, drug-prone personality traits contributed to involvement in drug use.

BIOLOGY. During the past 2 decades, a great deal of progress has been made in understanding the biological and genetic risk factors for drug use and drug abuse. Family studies have been undertaken to identify genetic vulnerability for drug abuse; for example, one line of research suggests that sons and daughters of alcoholics have a three- to fourfold risk for developing alcoholism (Institute of Medicine, 1996). While family studies report genetic vulnerability, they cannot definitively determine the effects of genes versus the environment on the development of alcoholism or drug abuse.

Another approach to the study of genetic vulnerability is twin studies, which have been used to identify the role of genetic factors in the etiology of substance abuse in twins. Overall, the results of these studies indicate that genetic factors do explain a proportion of the variance in the development of drug abuse. Furthermore, a proportion of the heritability of drug abuse in adulthood may be attributed to the same genetic factors as those that underlie the development of behavior problems in childhood (Grove et al., 1990). In addition to twin studies, adoption studies have been used to examine the respective roles of genetic and environmental factors in problem behavior, alcoholism, and drug abuse (Braungart-Rieker et al., 1995). Children of alcoholics who are raised by nonalcoholic parents have been shown to have a three- to fourfold increased risk for alcohol abuse compared to adoptees whose biological parents were not alcoholics (Cloninger, Bohman, & Sigvardsson, 1981).

Physiological vulnerability has also been suggested as a possible source for exacerbating the individual's vulnerability to drug and alcohol abuse. Such physiological influences include neurochemical impairment and metabolic variations in susceptibility to drugs (Cloninger, 1987). Indeed, there are large interindividual and interethnic variations in the physiological suscepti- bility to drugs and alcohol. For example, in contrast to Caucasians, some Asian populations are believed to be biologically protected from becoming alcoholics because of the effects of genetic polymorphism of two liver enzymes: aldehyde dehydrogenase and alcohol dehydrogenase-. The inability to metabolize a drug may be a protective factor in preventing continued exposure. In contrast, efficient metabolism may permit higher levels of exposure, which is more conducive to the development of abuse and dependence. Finally, there are certain biochemical markers for drug and alcohol abuse, such as monoamine oxidase, that have decreased activity levels among alcohol abusers (Tabakoff et al., 1988).

CONTEXT. In the context domain, environmental factors, such as drug availability, ad- verse economic conditions, a high crime rate, and neighborhood disorganization have all been found to be related to drug use (Robins, 1984; Sampson, 1985). Aspects of the larger sociocultural environment, including media advertising and social and legal policies, have important effects on drug use as well. As shown in Figure 13.3, the influence of cultural and ecological factors on drug use is mediated by their effects on family relations, personality, and peer factors.

CULTURE. A related area of great importance that has received relatively little attention is the influence of cultural factors on drug use (Brook, Whiteman, Balka, Win et al., 1998; Felix- Ortiz, & Newcomb, 1992). Our research (Brook, Brook et al., 1998) has found that in Colombia, South America, a country in which drug availability and violence exceeds that of the United States, several cultural characteristics serve as protective factors to counter the numerous psychosocial

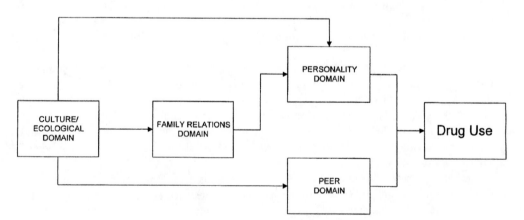

FIGURE 13.3. The role of cultural/ecological factors in the pathway to drug use.

and environmental risk factors that exist there. For example, religion, familism (a system of values that places the needs and rights of the family and community over individual needs and rights), and a respect for one's elders and authority all serve as protective or mitigating factors for drug use. The study demonstrated that, similar to other cultures and groups we have studied, a family interactional framework can best explain the pathways to adolescent marijuana use among Colombian youth.

While some researchers have found a number of commonalities in the risk factors for drug use among different ethnic and cultural groups (e.g., Brook, Whiteman, Balka, Win, & Gursen, 1997; Warheit et al., 1995), others have found differences. For example, among Mexican-Americans, several risk factors such as low socioeconomic status, higher school dropout rates, and living in barrios in large cities have been found to exacerbate drug use (Carter & Wilson, 1991). On the other hand, family influence among Mexican-Americans may have a stronger and more direct positive or protective effect than is the case among White youngsters. This may be particularly true for females and seems to be related to the family's identification with traditional Hispanic culture (Swaim et al., 1989).

Similarly, the cultural and ecological factors unique to Colombian youth provide an added dimension to the more commonly observed risk and protective factors involved in adolescent drug use. Some notable differences in specific risk factors for marijuana use found in our study included the finding that interpersonal distress (depression, anxiety, interpersonal difficulty, and obsessiveness), peer drug use, violence, and drug availability all had a greater impact on drug use in Colombia than in the United States. Furthermore, two important cultural factors, religion and familism, were more likely to protect the youngsters from drug use in Colombia than in the United States.

INTERACTIONS OF PERSONALITY, PARENTAL, AND PEER FACTORS

Certainly, one goal of prevention programs should be the reduction of risk factors related to drug use. Another goal should be the enhancement of factors that protect against risk or enhance the effects of other protective factors (Jessor et al., 1995; Werner, 1989). Our research (Brook et al., 1990) has focused on two mechanisms involved in the interaction of personality, parent, and peer factors. In the first (risk/protective), risk factors are attenuated by protective factors in the adolescent's personality. The second (protective/protective) is a synergistic interaction in which one protective factor potentiates another protective factor so that the combined effect is greater than the sum of the two protective factors.

These two mechanisms are illustrated in Figures 13.4 and 13.5. Figure 13.4 depicts a maternal risk variable ameliorated by an adolescent protective variable. As shown by the solid, sloping line, low adolescent rebelliousness offsets the potential risk of the mother's high interpersonal difficulty, leading to a low level of marijuana use. Figure 13.5 shows a paternal protective variable enhanced by an adolescent protective variable. When the father has high ego integration, the adolescent is less likely to use marijuana if he or she is intolerant of deviance than if he or she is tolerant of deviance.

Risk/Protective Interactions

Certain factors buffer, or protect, individuals from the potentially negative influences of risk factors. Evidence has shown, for example, that even in the most damaging environment many adolescents survive relatively unscathed. A greater comprehension of why certain adolescents

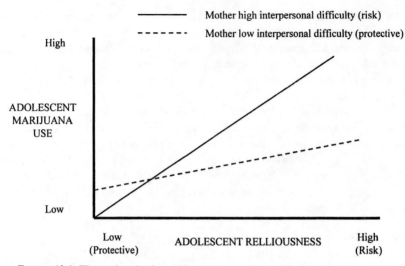

FIGURE 13.4. Illustrative plot for a risk variable ameliorated by a protective variable.

are not irreversibly affected by risk factors would certainly provide a strong foundation for the development of optimally effective drug prevention and treatment programs. Our studies have identified a number of leads that should prove useful for these purposes. They include the following: (1) the importance of adolescent conventionality as a buffer against risks that lead to drug use; (2) factors that buffer against peer risks leading to drug use; and (3) the extent to which one parent can offset risk factors posed by the other parent.

ADOLESCENT CONVENTIONALITY AS A BUFFER. Adolescent conventionality, particularly for girls, can offset risks leading to drug use from a variety of sources, including the parental personalities, the parent-adolescent relationship, and the peer group. From a preventive or

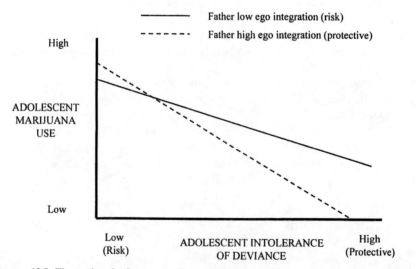

FIGURE 13.5. Illustrative plot for a protective variable enhanced by another protective variable.

treatment perspective, these findings clearly suggest that strengthening aspects of the adolescent's conventionality would be of great assistance in offsetting risks from parents or peers that lead to drug use. The crucial ways that aspects of conventionality serve as buffers include low-sensation seeking, internalization of traditional societal values, the development of internal controls, and, above all, putting a high value on achievement (Rutter, 1980).

INTERPERSONAL FACTORS AS BUFFERS FOR PEER RISKS.   As previously mentioned, involvement in drug-using peer groups is one of the greatest potential risks in terms of a youngster's own drug use, making it essential to identify protective factors that can offset the risk of having friends who use drugs. A number of interpersonal protective factors have been identified that serve as buffers against peer drug risks, including parental conventionality and a strong parent–adolescent attachment.

What is it about these various protective factors that allows them to act as buffers against peer risk factors? One might speculate that parental models of low drug use, conventionality, and adjustment counteract to some degree the drug-using models presented by the peer group. A strong mutual attachment between parent and child may offset such peer risk factors because parental attachment, in which the adolescent identifies with the parent, may provide for adolescents a feeling of being loved, a sense of predictability in their life situation, a recognition of their self-worth, and a general expectation of support, all of which would help to mitigate peer drug influences. In accord with social learning theory, it is likely that close relationships and identification with parents decrease the need for adolescents to depend on peers for approval, which in turn reduces adolescent vulnerability to peer pressure for conformity to peer norms.

These findings suggest that prevention and treatment efforts aimed at enhancing the adolescent's conventionality or the attachment with the parents could go a long way toward reducing one of the prime risks implicated in adolescent drug use–that of a drug-using peer group.

PARENTAL FACTORS AS BUFFERS FOR OTHER PARENT RISKS.   To our knowledge there has been no systematic study of the differential impact of the influence of one parent on risk factors compared with the influence of the other parent. However, risks stemming from conflicted paternal-child relationships and paternal use of drugs can be offset by the mother's conventionality and psychological adjustment and by a close mother-child attachment (Brook et al., 1990). For the prevention and treatment of adolescent drug use, to offset the influence of paternal risk factors, one should work toward strengthening the mother's psychological adjustment, her conventionality, and the mother–child attachment.

Protective/Protective Interactions

As a result of our research into the extent to which protective factors are further enhanced by other protective factors in reducing the likelihood of adolescent drug use, the most outstanding finding is the crucial role of the father in protective/protective interactions. Protective father characteristics (i.e., his general emotional stability, a strong father–adolescent bond) enhanced other protective aspects, such as adolescent conventionality, positive maternal characteristics (nonuse of drugs, positive child-rearing practices), and marital harmony. Thus, by including the father in prevention and treatment efforts, one adds to the adolescent's ability to resist drug use.

In sum, our findings suggest that in designing intervention programs, it is necessary to reduce risk factors and enhance protective factors. Programs that reduce risks at the same time that they enhance protective factors from many domains will be most effective.

IMPLICATIONS FOR PREVENTION
AND TREATMENT

Prevention Implications of Individual Domain Findings

In regard to personality attributes and behavioral domains, every effort should be made to enhance the development of the attributes of conventionality, such as nonrebelliousness and intolerance of deviance. The childhood component of an intervention program should attempt to increase conventional behavior and problem-solving behavior and focus on treating any existing early conduct disorder. Because intrapsychic stress has also been found to be related to drug use, adolescents must learn how to reduce levels of intrapsychic stress without turning to the use of drugs. For adolescents at risk, special access to psychiatric treatment or special classes that emphasize human growth and development or handling stress may be helpful. Teachers can be taught to recognize adolescents at risk for drug use and can provide help through classes and school programs as well as make appropriate referrals for timely intervention by school authorities. Prevention programs should train teachers in the use of proactive classroom management and cooperative learning techniques. The use of these techniques strengthens a youngster's attachment to school. A closer attachment to school should lead to an increase in conventionality and academic success and, ultimately, to a decrease in drug use.

In regard to the parent–child relationship, drug use is ameliorated by an affectionate mutual attachment between parents and children. In such families, parents spend more time with their children, interact more with their children, and set more reasonable limits for them than do parents in families in which drug use is more likely to occur. Stronger earlier attachment bonds between parents and children leads to increased identification of the child with the parent and a stronger attachment bond in adolescence. Parents must be emotionally available and responsive to children, spend adequate time with them, and communicate some of their beliefs to them, ideally in a manner that is tactful and considerate and does not induce guilt or parent–child conflict.

Within the family domain, parental encouragement of conventional behavior should help to prevent drug use, as should discouragement of unconventional behavior, drug use, and associations with drug-using peers. Of course, this is easier for parents to do if they themselves are conventional and do not use drugs. Treatment of parental emotional disturbance or helping parents avoid drug use ought to be useful in preventing their children's drug use. Teaching parents, especially mothers, to set appropriate limits while avoiding an authoritarian attitude would probably be helpful since appropriate maternal control is especially important. Education for parenting should help parents learn how to disagree with their children while still showing consideration of their feelings. Interventions focused on improving parenting practices may lower the risk for adolescent drug use.

As noted earlier, since parental drug abuse is a risk factor for drug abuse by offspring (Merikangas, Rounsaville, & Prusoff, 1992), parents should avoid drug use of any kind unless medically indicated. Parents who use recreational drugs or drink alcohol encourage children to do the same through modeling. While some people believe that it is better for children and adolescents to smoke, drink, or use drugs at home with parental knowledge rather than away from home without parental knowledge or supervision, the data support the social influence model, which indicates that adolescents imitate the drug-using behavior of significant others in their environment, especially parents.

In regard to the peer domain, the influence of friends has consistently been found to play a critical role in adolescent drug use. Nevertheless, it is important to note that the effects of peers may have been somewhat overestimated in some studies (Kandel, 1996; Krohn et al., 1996; Labouvie, 1996). Indeed, *many* social influence programs are based on the assumption that pressure from peers is the main influence on an adolescent's use (or nonuse) of drugs. The use of prosocial peer groups to enhance the development of desirable personality attributes and to decrease the likelihood of drug use should be encouraged and supported by the community and the school. At the same time, methods to decrease adolescent involvement in deviant peer groups should be utilized.

Several programs have targeted peer risk factors identified in etiologic studies. Programs that train children in social influence resistance skills to avoid drugs have had some success. Some of these programs also incorporate training in social competence. Evaluation of these programs has shown a decrease in cigarette smoking (Botvin, 1986; Botvin 1995; Bukoski, 1986) and a later onset of alcohol or marijuana use (Botvin, 1986; Pentz et al., 1989b).

As noted by Oetting and Lynch (in press), drug use is more likely to change if peer clusters and their shared behaviors change. Thus, prevention needs to be aimed not only at the norms developed by peer clusters, but also at attributes that can alter peer clusters. They argue that prevention programs need to establish general social norms against substance use. These alterations will diminish the chances that peer clusters will get involved with drugs. The media and the schools are likely candidates for creating a climate in which drug use is frowned upon. In the past several years, a number of advertising firms and the media have joined together to provide anti-drug advertising. Research suggests that there has been some change in social norms as a result of such campaigns (Black, 1989). Indeed, Johnston, Bachman, and O'Malley (1981) reported an increase in perceived risk associated with marijuana use.

Finally, in terms of the implications of the findings relating to the context or ecological domain, our research indicates that a positive learning environment and decreased school conflict are associated with less drug use (Brook, Nomura, & Cohen, 1989). Certainly, prevention programs should take into account these important school factors. Religious and other social institutions can also provide structure and organization and set healthier peer norms and goals. Several community interventions have had some success (Perry et al., 1992; Smith & Davis, 1993). Broader social issues, such as neighborhood environmental factors (including the quality of housing, sanitation, access to playgrounds, and outdoor facilities), adequate nourishment, and access to general health care, should also be considered in the development of prevention and treatment programs. In economic terms, the more we know about etiology, prevention, and treatment, the less expensive it is to take effective action. In addition, using an empirical approach has a heuristic value and enables us to enhance our understanding and to target our interventions more accurately.

Implications of Domain Linkage Findings

As depicted in Figures 13.1 and 13.2, parental traditionality is associated with an affectionate and nonconflicted parent–adolescent relationship, which leads to increased identification of the child with the parents. This, in turn is associated with increased conventionality in the adolescent, which is related to friendships with peers who do not use drugs, ultimately leading to nonuse of drugs. In our research, we have also found that some aspects of the adolescent personality led directly to drug use and some of the peer influences leading to drug use were mediated by adolescent personality traits.

These findings suggest at least four possible targets for therapeutic or preventive intervention during adolescence: the parent alone, the parent and the adolescent, the adolescent alone, and the peer group. If one wished to intervene earlier in the causal chain of events, intervention should take place at the parent/child level. Intervention intended to alter parental personalities in the direction of greater conventionality and psychological adjustment ought to lead to a more enduring and affectionate parent–child bond. A slightly later point of intervention involves working with both the parent and the child, although not necessarily together, on *any* disturbances in their attachment relationship. If parent and adolescent are not both available, separate work with either one could develop a stronger and more affectionate parent-child bond.

Changes in the attachment relationship ought to lead to changes in an adolescent's personality characteristics. As we have theorized, mutual attachment and a strong parent–child bond can lead to strong internalization of parental values, behavior, and attitudes. A strong parent–child attachment relationship may also provide children with the feeling that they can control what happens to them and that they can and will acquire the problem-solving skills needed to do so. It may also result in increased maturity and self-esteem, which would further enable adolescents to develop in an optimal manner.

Intervention at a later point might be directed at altering an adolescent's personality toward greater conventionality (e.g., achievement), which should lead to affiliations with drug-resistant peer groups (as well as to less drug use). Our data identified a number of specific predictors of conventionality associated with friendships with peers who did not use drugs. These include responsibility, intolerance of deviance, and a lack of rebelliousness and sensation seeking.

Finally, one might intervene at the peer-group level. Placing at-risk individuals in pro-social peer groups ought to decrease the risk of drug use. Overall, the implication of these personality and peer connections is that one can break into the causal chain leading to drug use at the level of the adolescent's personality or at the link connecting it with the peer group's influence.

The points at which to intervene in the causal pathway (parent, adolescent, personality, or peer) can be determined by a number of factors. For example, if parents are not available and their ways of relating to their children are extremely disturbed and ingrained, one might attempt to alter personality or peer factors. Similarly, if one cannot effect changes in the adolescent, one might focus on parents or peers. For clinicians working with adolescents, knowledge concerning all these areas of the adolescent's life should enable them to determine which have the most potential for successful intervention.

Implications of the Interactive Findings

The foremost implication of the interactive findings from our research on risk and protective factors in adolescent drug use is that when a particular area of the youngster's life is strengthened (i.e., personality, family), a double benefit accrues. First, these strengths (which we have deemed protective characteristics) may offset risks in other areas, such as having drug-using peers. Second, protective characteristics enhance one another synergistically. In both cases, the likelihood of adolescent drug use is considerably reduced. For example, non-drug-use by both parents leads to the greatest resistance of the child to use drugs.

To the degree that treatment and prevention efforts can be carried out with the adolescents themselves, we would highlight the importance of building up the adolescent's *attribute of* conventionality (especially achievement) to offset interpersonal (parental and peer) risks and enhance positive interpersonal factors. We have found this particularly effective for girls.

We also found that the parental factors are crucial. Prevention and treatment programs ought to include work with parents. The results from our studies highlighted the interactive importance of parental conventionality, parental adjustment (mainly for the mother) and, most pointedly, a strong mutual attachment between parent and child in offsetting risk factors in adolescence, such as friends who use drugs. In addition, interactive effects between parental factors are important in different ways. While the mother serves as a powerful buffer to paternal risk, the father is more effective as an enhancer of maternal protective factors.

Finally, some very important implications for prevention and treatment can be derived from the interactive findings related to peer drug use, generally considered to be the most potent factor in the etiology of adolescent self drug use. The most exciting finding is that peer drug risks can be offset by a number of protective factors, including adolescent and parental conventionality, maternal adjustment, and a strong parent–child *mutual* attachment *relationship*. This means that prevention and treatment efforts aimed at strengthening these nonpeer factors can help reduce the greatest risk implicated in adolescent drug use.

EFFECTIVE PREVENTION AND TREATMENT PROGRAMS

The following review of prevention programs cites programs that have been evaluated for effectiveness. It is organized according to three main themes: (1) those programs that focus on the developmental timing of the programs; (2) those that focus specifically on the family as the main target of intervention; and (3) those that take a multidimensional or broad-based approach to prevention and treatment.

Developmental Timing of the Intervention

Prevention and treatment tend to be more successful if begun at an early age. It is usually assumed that it is better, easier, and more effective in promoting health to prevent unhealthy behavior or disease than to change the unhealthy behavior or cure the disease once it has occurred. In a review of the predelinquency interventions, Zigler, Taussig, and Black (1992) concluded that the effects are more powerful if begun prior to the emergence of delinquency rather than afterwards. This conclusion is supported by research demonstrating that problem behavior in childhood is associated with later drug use and delinquency (Brook, Whiteman, Gordon, & Cohen, 1986; Loeber, 1991; Loeber & Dishion, 1983, 1987).

Clinical experience suggests that it is easier to work therapeutically with children than adolescents. Children's personalities are less formed, more flexible, and easier to modify. Symptoms are often less fixed and more amenable to change. Childhood drug-prone personality traits and adverse childhood experiences seem to determine to some extent both drug-prone personality traits in the adolescent and a weak bond between parent and child. Because the indirect effects of adverse childhood personality traits and experiences are long lasting, logic dictates that one try to break the chain of noxious influences early in the child's development. Since poor achievement, poor control of behavior, and early signs of delinquency are frequently present in children at risk for drug use, it should be possible to identify children who would benefit from treatment by studying their school records and by using some of the childhood predictors identified earlier. However, this must be done in a way that will not infringe on the privacy of either the child or the family.

Children who experience positive intervention programs in early childhood are better prepared to start school, which results in better relations with teachers and other adults (Berrueta-Clement et al., 1984). One might hypothesize that positive relations with adults, such as teachers, help enhance cognitive functioning in children, which may increase the likelihood of later academic achievement. Because poor academic achievement and deviant behavior are related, enhancing the factors that contribute to higher levels of academic achievement may help diminish the chances that the child would later engage in deviant behaviors, such as drug use. Findings from several longitudinal studies suggest that prevention programs begun in childhood may decrease some of the risk factors that are associated with drug use, delinquency, and other anti-social behaviors.

A number of such programs have made strides in combating adolescent problem behavior by intervening early in the child's life. Among these is the Perry Preschool Project, which provided young children with high-quality, cognitively oriented schooling. Parents participated in the program and were encouraged to take part in the education of their children. Data collected from the children some 15 years later indicated that the children in the experimental group were more socially competent and achievement oriented than the children in the control group (Berrueta-Clement et al., 1984).

Another promising program is the Seattle Social Development Program developed by Hawkins and Catalano. The program, which begins at an early age, focuses on the socializing agents of family, school, peers, and community influences. Data suggest that youngsters who took part in the program scored lower on alcohol initiation and on the risk factors for drug use compared to a control group (Hawkins et al., 1992). Other programs that have been shown to reduce deviant behavior are the Syracuse University Family Development Research Project and the Yale Child Welfare Research Program.

Positive programs, such as the ones described previously, are not likely to have long-term effects unless followed by appropriate interventions at later developmental periods in the youngster's life. Unless such early programs are followed by continuous interventions, the benefits are likely to decrease or fade with time (Zigler et al., 1992).

As children grow older, the influence of the family on their behaviors declines as the influence of their peer group increases. Therefore, family interventions are generally more effective earlier in childhood, whereas interventions involving peers are generally more effective in adolescence. Nevertheless, it is never too late to effect some beneficial change, and the timing and nature of the interventions are important in determining their success. Particularly helpful in deterring drug use are prevention and treatment measures that foster responsible behavior in adolescents, enhance their ability to cope with intrapsychic conflict and strong emotions, and assist them in learning to postpone immediate gratification and use internal controls.

Family Interventions

There are several main approaches to family interventions. For the past 2 decades, Patterson (e.g., Patterson, Chamberlain, & Reid, 1982) has focused on behavioral parent training to decrease negative parenting. More recently, he and his colleagues have expanded their approach to study how "coercive" parenting promotes susceptibility to negative influences in other domains (Dishion et al., 1991). They maintain that modifying family functioning is a necessary, but not sufficient prerequisite to reducing risk, in part, because it mediates other influences.

Another approach is exemplified by Szapocznik and colleagues in their work with adolescent drug abusers. In addition to its attention to poor disciplinary practices, this approach focuses on changing emotional disengagement, ineffective family problem solving, and unsatisfying interactions in the family. In addition, their program addresses the values and beliefs of the specific cultural groups that the interventions target and has been quite effective in reducing later drug use in at-risk youth (Szapocznik & Kurtines, 1989).

Kumpfer and DeMarsh's Strengthening Families Program (DeMarsh & Kumpfer, 1986) focuses on enhancing parent-child communication and monitoring the child's behavior. The program is consistent with current empirical research and has had considerable success.

Finally, Liddle and colleagues argue that one of the most promising approaches for dealing with adolescent drug abuse is family therapy, in which the multidimensional nature of the disorder is highlighted along with the concomitant need to operate within a broad-based, developmental, and contextual therapeutic framework (Liddle & Dakof, 1995a,b; Liddle et al., 1992). Liddle emphasizes the need for in-depth knowledge of the issues faced by adolescents, family risk factors for adolescent drug abuse, and the typical transitions and transformations that occur in the parent-adolescent relationship. These issues are integrated into his Multidimensional Family Therapy (MDFT) approach to intervention.

Multidimensional, Broad-Based Interventions

Several of the effective intervention programs have taken a multidomain approach to delinquency and drug use, rather than focusing on a particular domain, such as the effects of the peer group. Such programs have included health care and parenting programs, school, community, and media programs, as well as social support and services to children (Rohrbach et al., 1995). Since intrapersonal, interpersonal, and contextual factors all influence drug use, a multidisciplinary approach to drug use prevention is essential (Brook, Balka et al., 1997; Donovan, 1996; Kaplan, 1996). Similarly, since multiple direct and indirect paths lead to drug use, there is a great need to develop multiple interventions. Because the risk factors related to drug use derive from different domains, comprehensive prevention approaches that target the whole child, as compared with narrow approaches, are more likely to be effective. Prevention programs that foster healthy families and children and pay attention to the child's other social settings would go a long way in dealing with the prevalent problem of drug use. Another advantage of broad-based programs that support the child's interaction with multiple systems is that they are likely to affect the child's behavior in multiple domains. Certainly, programs that assist the child in relating to others, in achieving success in school, and in using community supports are more likely to produce children who avoid drug use.

The success of the broad-based multidomain approach in reducing delinquency and drug use in children and in increasing their competence is evident in several programs. In addition to the Perry Preschool Project (Berrueta-Clement et al., 1984) described earlier, one such program is the Midwestern Prevention Project (MPP). The basic component of this program is a 10-session, school-based peer-resistance and social skills curriculum (Pentz et al., 1989a; Pentz, MacKinnon et al., 1989). Students in this program work with the parents on a number of homework assignments. The program is supplemented by media campaigns and community leader involvement. The children in the experimental program were less likely to use tobacco, alcohol, marijuana, and cocaine. Other broad-based programs that have been successful include the Seattle Social Development Program (Hawkins, Catalano, Morrison et al., 1992), the program of Patterson et al. (1982), and the program of Tremblay et al. (1990). Another promising program (Conduct Problems Prevention Research Group, 1992) encompasses universal components (the school curriculum) and selective interventions (family and social skills modules). The program is targeted at children who display disruptive behavior in kindergarten. Despite the success of these programs, comprehensive intervention programs are difficult to evaluate because it is not always clear which aspects of the program significantly reduce drug use.

Only a few programs have been cited here; others are presented in other chapters in this book. Overall, those prevention programs that have incorporated findings from etiological studies that emphasize the importance of the parent-child mutual attachment relationship, the significance of improving parent-child communication, and the importance of appropriate and consistent control techniques have achieved the goals of reducing drug use, delinquency, and increasing the child's social competence.

Selective or Targeted Intervention Programs

Many of the prevention programs described above are universal and based on the fact that all young people are potentially at risk for experimenting with drug use (IOM, 1996). Recent research has indicated, however, that some youngsters are at greater risk for drug use than others (Glantz & Pickens, 1992). Consequently, it is important to develop: (1) selective preventive interventions targeted at those assumed to be most "at risk;" and (2) specific therapeutic interventions targeted at those who exhibit some clinically demonstrable abnormality (IOM, 1996).

CONCLUSION

In conclusion, the current interest in the study of adolescent drug use is likely to broaden inquiry and yield a sounder base of evidence, both of which augur well for future investigations, for further comprehension of the etiology of drug use, and for prevention programs. Should the effect of prevention programs that address the childhood and adolescent risk factors identified in etiologic studies result in reduced drug use and abuse in future evaluations, empirical data will then be available that may yield further knowledge about the benefits of prevention programs.

REFERENCES

Bachman, J. G., Wadsworth, K. N., O'Malley, P. M., Johnston, L. D., & Schulenberg, J. E. (1997). *Smoking, drinking, and drug use in young adulthood. The impacts of new freedoms and new responsibilities.* NJ: Erlbaum.

Bailey, S. L., & Hubbard, R. L. (1990). Developmental variation in the context of marijuana initiation among adolescents. *Journal of Health and Social Behavior, 31,* 587–593.

Bandura (1997). *Self-efficacy: The exercise of control.* New York: Freeman.

Barnes, G. M., Farrell, M. P., & Banerjee, S. (1995). Family influences on alcohol abuse and other problem behaviors among black and white adolescents in a general population sample. In G. M. Boyd, J. Howard, & R. A. Zucker (Eds.), *Alcohol problems among adolescents: Current directions in prevention research* (pp. 13–31). Hillsdale, NJ: Erlbaum.

Berrueta-Clement, J. R., Schweinhart, L. J., Barnett, W. S., Epstein, A. S., & Weikart, D. P. (1984). *Changed lives: The effects of the Perry Preschool Program on youths that are through age 19.* Ypsilanti, MI: High/Scope Press.

Black, G. S. (1989). *The attitudinal basis of drug use—1987 and changing attitudes toward drug use—1988: Reports from the Media Advertising partnership for a Drug-Free America, Inc.* Rochester, NY: Gordon S. Black.

Botvin, G. J. (1986). Substance abuse prevention research: Recent developments and future directions. *Journal of School Health, 56,* 369–374.

Botvin, G. J., Baker, E., Dusenbury, L., Botvin, E. M., & Diaz, T. (1995). Long-term follow-up results of a randomized drug abuse prevention trial in a white middle-class population. *Journal of the American Medical Association, 273,* 1106–1112.

Braungart-Rieker, J., Rende, R. D., Plomin, R., DeFries, J. C., & Fulker, D. W. (1995). Genetic mediation of longitudinal associations between family environment and childhood behavior problems. *Development and Psychopathology, 7,* 233–245.

Brook, D. W., Brook, J. S., Whiteman, M., Win, P. T., Gordon-Maloul, C., Roberto, J., Masci, J. R., Amundsen, F., & de Catalogne, J. (1997). Psychosocial risk factors for HIV transmission in female drug abusers. *American Journal on Addictions, 6*(2), 124–134.

Brook, J. S., Balka, E. B., Gursen, M., Brook, D. W., Shapiro, J., & Cohen, P. (1997). Young adults' drug use: A 17-year longitudinal inquiry of antecedents. *Psychological Reports, 80,* 1235–1251.

Brook, J. S., Brook, D. W., De La Rosa, M., Duque, L. F., Rodriguez, E., Montoya, I. D., Min, D., & Whiteman, M. (1998). Pathways to marijuana use among adolescents: Cultural/ecological family, peer, and personality influences. *Journal of the American Academy of Child and Adolescent Psychiatry, 37*(7), 759–766.

Brook, J. S., Brook, D. W., & Whiteman, M. (2000). The influence of maternal smoking during pregnancy on the toddler's negativity. *Archives of Pediatrics and Adolescent Medicine, 154,* 381–385.

Brook, J. S., Brook, D. W., Whiteman, M., Gordon, A. S., & Cohen, P. (1990). The psychosocial etiology of adolescent drug use and abuse. *Genetic, Social and General Psychology Monographs, 116*(2).

Brook, J. S., & Cohen, P. (1992). A developmental perspective on drug use and delinquency. In J. McCord (Ed.), *Advances in criminological theory: Vol. 3: Crime facts, fictions, and theory* (pp. 231–251). New Brunswick, NJ: Transactions Publishers.

Brook, J. S., Cohen, P., & Brook, D. W. (1998). Longitudinal study of co-occurring psychiatric disorders and substance use. *Journal of the American Academy of Child and Adolescent Psychiatry, 37,* 322–330.

Brook J. S., Gordon, A. S., & Brook, D. W. (1987). Fathers and daughters: Their relationship and personality characteristics associated with the daughter's smoking behavior. *Journal of Genetic Psychology, 148*(1), 31–44.

Brook, J. S., Gordon, A. S., Whiteman, M., & Cohen, P. (1986). Some models and mechanisms for explaining the impact of maternal and adolescent characteristics on adolescent stage of drug use. *Developmental Psychology, 22,* 460–467.

Brook, J. S., & Newcomb, M. D. (1995). Childhood aggression and unconventionality: Impact on later academic achievement, drug use, and workforce involvement. *Journal of Genetic Psychology, 4,* 393–410.

Brook, J. S., Nomura, C., & Cohen, P. (1989). Prenatal, perinatal, and early childhood risk factors and drug involvement in adolescence. *Genetic, Social and General Psychology Monographs, 115*(2), 221–241.

Brook, J. S., Richter, L., & Whiteman, M. (2000). Effects of parent personality, upbringing, and drug use on the parent-child attachment relationship. *Journal of the American Academy of Child and Adolescent Psychiatry, 39*(2), 240–248.

Brook, J. S., Tseng, L. J., & Whiteman, M. (1998). Three-generation study: Intergenerational continuities and discontinuities and their impact on the toddler's anger. *Genetic, Social, and General Psychology Monographs, 124*(3), 335–353.

Brook, J. S., Whiteman, M., Balka, E. B., Win, P. T., & Gursen, M. D. (1997). African-American and Puerto Rican drug use: A longitudinal study. *Journal of the American Academy of Child and Adolescent Psychiatry, 36*(9), 1260–1268.

Brook, J. S., Whiteman, M., Balka, E. B., Win, P. T., & Gursen, M. D. (1998). Similar and different precursors to drug use and delinquency among African-Americans and Puerto Ricans. *Journal of Genetic Psychology, 159*(1), 13–29.

Brook, J. S., Whiteman, M., Brook, D. W., & Gordon, A. S. (1991). Sibling influences on adolescent drug use: Older brothers on younger brothers. *Journal of the American Academy of Child and Adolescent Psychiatry, 30*(6), 958–966.

Brook, J. S., Whiteman, M., & Finch, S. (1993). The role of mutual attachment in adolescent drug use: A longitudinal study. *Journal of the American Academy of Child and Adolescent Psychiatry, 32*(5), 982–989.

Brook, J. S., Whiteman, M., Finch, S., & Cohen, P. (1995). Aggression, intrapsychic distress, and drug use: Antecedents and intervening processes. *Journal of the American Academy of Child and Adolescent Psychiatry, 34*(8), 1076–1084.

Brook, J. S., Whiteman, M., Finch, S., & Cohen, P. (1996). Young adult drug use and delinquency: Childhood antecedents and adolescent mediators. *Journal of the American Academy of Child and Adolescent Psychiatry, 35*(12), 1584–1592.

Brook, J. S. Whiteman, M., Finch, S., & Cohen, P. (2000). Longitudinally foretelling drug use in the late twenties: Adolescent personality and social environmental antecedents. *Journal of Genetic Psychology, 161*(1), 37–51.

Brook, J. S., Whiteman, M., & Gordon, A. S. (1983). Stages of drug use in adolescence: Personality, peer, and family correlates. *Developmental Psychology, 19,* 269–277.

Brook, J. S., Whiteman, M., Gordon, A. S., & Brook, D. W. (1986). Father-daughter identification and its impact on her personality and drug use. *Developmental Psychology, 22,* 743–748.

Brook, J. S., Whiteman, M., Gordon, A. S., & Brook, D. W. (1983). Paternal correlates of adolescent marijuana use in the context of the mother-son and parental dyads. *Genetic Psychology Monographs, 108,* 197–213.

Brook, J. S., Whiteman, M., Gordon, A. S., & Cohen, P. (1986). Dynamics of childhood and adolescent personality traits and adolescent drug use. *Developmental Psychology, 22,* 403–414.

Bukoski, W. J. (1986). School based substance abuse prevention: A review of research. In S. Griswold-Ezekoye, K. L. Kumpfer, & W. J. Bukoski (Eds.), *Childhood and chemical abuse* (pp. 95–115). New York: Haworth.

Carter, D. J., & Wilson, R. (1991). *Ninth annual status report: Minorities in higher education.* Washington, DC: American Council on Education.

Cloninger, C. R. (1987). Neurogenetic adaptive mechanisms in alcoholism. *Science, 236,* 410–416.

Cloninger, C. R., Bohman, N., & Sigvardsson, S. (1981). Inheritance of alcohol abuse: Cross-fostering analysis of adopted men. *Archives of General Psychiatry, 36,* 861–868.

Cohen, P., & Brook, J. S. (1987). Family factors related to the persistence of psychopathology in childhood and adolescence. *Psychiatry, 50,* 332–345.

Conduct Problems Prevention Research Group (1992). A developmental and clinical model for the prevention of conduct disorders: The FAST Track program. *Development and Psychopathology, 4,* 509–527.

Conger, R. D., Reuter, M. R., & Conger, K. J. (1994). The family context of adolescent vulnerability and resilience to alcohol use and abuse. *Sociological Studies of Children, 6,* 55–86.

DeMarsh, J., & Kumpfer, K. L. (1986). Family-oriented interventions for the prevention of chemical dependency in children and adolescents. In A. Griswold-Ezekoye, K. L. Kumpfer, & W. J. Bukoski (Eds). *Childhood and chemical abuse: Prevention and intervention* (pp. 117–151). New York: Haworth.

Dishion, T. J., Patterson, G. R., Stoolmiller, M., & Skinner, M. L. (1991). Family, school, and behavioral antecedents to early adolescent involvement with antisocial peers. *Developmental Psychology, 27*(1), 172–180.

Donovan, J. E. (1996). Problem-behavior theory and the explanation of adolescent marijuana use. *Journal of Drug Issues, 26*(3), 379–404.

Duncan, T. E., Duncan, S. C., & Hops, H. (1996). The role of parents and older siblings in predicting adolescent substance use: Modeling development via structural equation latent growth methodology. *Journal of Family Psychology, 10,* 158–172.

Farrington, D. P. (1991). Childhood aggression and adult violence: Early precursors and later life outcomes. In D. J. Pepler and K. H. Rubin (Eds.). *The development and treatment of childhood aggression* (pp. 5–29). Hillsdale, NJ: Lawrence Erlbaum.

Felix-Ortiz, M., & Newcomb, M. D. (1992). Risk and protective factors for drug use among Latino and White adolescents. *Hispanic Journal of Behavioral Science, 14,* 291–309.

Fergusson, D. M., Horwood, L. J., & Lynskey, M. (1994). The childhood of multiple problem adolescents: A 15-year longitudinal study. *Journal of Child Psychology and Psychiatry, 35,* 1123–1140.

Fletcher, A. C., Darling, N. E., & Steinberg, L. (1995). Parental monitoring and peer influences on adolescent substance use. In J. McCord (Ed.), *Coercion and punishment in long-term perspectives* (pp. 259–271). New York: Cambridge University Press.

Gable, S., Belsky, J., & Crnic, K. (1992). Marriage, parenting, and child development: Progress and prospects. Special Issue: Diversity in contemporary family psychology. *Journal of Family Psychology, 5,* 276–294.

Glantz, M., & Pickens, R. (1992). *Vulnerability to drug abuse.* Washington, DC: American Psychological Association.

Grove, W., Eckert, E., Heston, L., Bouchard, T., Segal, N., & Lykken, D. (1990). Heritability of substance abuse and antisocial behavior: A study of monozygotic twins reared apart. *Biological Psychiatry, 27,* 1293–1304.

Hansen, W. B., Graham, J. W., Sobel, J. L., Shelton, D. R., Flay, B. R., & Johnson, C. A. (1987). The consistency of peer and parent influences on tobacco, alcohol, and marijuana use among young adolescents. *Journal of Behavioral Medicine, 10,* 559–579.

Hawkins, J. D., Catalano, R. F., & Miller, J. Y. (1992). Risk and protective factors for alcohol and other drug problems in adolescence and early adulthood: Implications for substance abuse prevention, *Psychological Bulletin, 112*(1), 64–105.

Hawkins, J. D., Catalano, R. F., Morrison, D. M., O'Donnell, J., Abbott, R. D., & Day, L. E. (1992). The Seattle Social Development Project: Effects of the first four years on protective factors and problem behaviors. In J. McCord & R. Tremblay (Eds.), *The prevention of antisocial behavior in children.* New York: Guilford Press.

Hirschi, T. (1969). *Causes of delinquency.* Berkeley: University of California Press.

Hops, H., Tildesley, E., Lichtenstein, E., Ary, D., & Sherman, L. (1990). Parent-adolescent problem-solving interactions and drug use. *American Journal of Drug and Alcohol Abuse, 16,* 239–258.

Hundleby, J. D., & Mercer, G. W. (1987). Family and friends as social environments and their relationship to young adolescents' use of alcohol, tobacco, and marijuana. *Journal of Clinical Psychology, 44,* 125–134.

Institute of Medicine (IOM) (1996). *Pathways of addiction: Opportunities in drug abuse research.* Washington, DC: National Academy Press.

Jessor, R., & Jessor, S. L. (1977). *Problem behavior and psychosocial development: A longitudinal study of youth.* San Diego, CA: Academic Press.

Jessor, R., Van Den Bos, J., Vanderryn, J., Costa, F. M., & Turbin, M. S. (1995). Protective factors in adolescent problem behavior: Moderator effects and developmental change. *Developmental Psychology, 31*(6), 923–933.

Johnson, V., & Pandina, R. J. (1991). Effects of the family on adolescent substance use, delinquency, and coping styles. *American Journal of Drug and Alcohol Abuse, 17,* 71–88.

Johnston, L. D., Bachman, J. G., & O'Malley, P. M. (1981). *Student drug use in America 1975–1981* (DHHS Publication No. ADM 82-1208). Washington DC: U.S. Government Printing Office.

Johnston, L. D., O'Malley, P. M., & Bachman, J. G. (1985). *Use of licit and illicit drugs by American high school students: 1975–1984.* Rockville, MD: National Institute of Drug Abuse.

Kagan, J. & Moss, H. A. (1962). *Birth to maturity: A study in psychological development.* New York: Wiley.

Kandel, D. B. (1996). The parental and peer contexts of adolescent deviance: An algebra of interpersonal influences. *Journal of Drug Issues, 26*(2), 289–315.

Kandel, D. B., & Andrews, K. (1987). Processes of adolescent socialization by parents and peers. *International Journal of Addictions, 22,* 319–342.

Kaplan, H. B. (1995). Drugs, crime, and other deviant adaptations. In H. B. Kaplan (Ed.), *Drugs, crime, and other deviant adaptations* (pp. 3–46). New York: Plenum.

Kaplan, H. B. (1996). Empirical validation of the applicability of an integrative theory of deviant behavior to the study of drug use. *Journal of Drug Issues, 26*(2), 345–377.

Kessler, R. C., Nelson, C. B., McGonagle, K. A., Edlund, M. J., Frank, R. G., & Leaf, P. J. (1996). The epidemiology of co-occurring addictive and mental disorders: Implications for prevention and service utilization. *American Journal of Orthopsychiatry, 66,* 17–30.

Krohn, M. D., Lizotte, A. J., Thornberry, T. P., Smith, C., & McDowall, D. (1996). Reciprocal causal relationships among drug use, peers, and beliefs: A five-wave panel model. *Journal of Drug Issues, 26*(2), 405–428.

Kumpfer, K. L. (1989). Prevention of alcohol and drug abuse: A critical review of risk factors and prevention strategies. In D. Shaffer, I. Philips, & N. B. Enzer (Eds.), *Prevention of mental disorders, alcohol, and other drug use in children and adolescents.* OSAP Prevention Monograph No. 2. Rockville, MD: Office of Substance Abuse Prevention.

Labouvie, E. (1996). Maturing out of substance use: Selection and self-correction. *Journal of Drug Issues, 26*(2), 457–476.

Liddle, H. A., & Dakof, G. A. (1995a). Family-based treatments for adolescent drug use: State of the science. In E. Rahdert & D. Czechowicz (Eds.), *Adolescent drug abuse: Clinical assessment and therapeutic interventions* (pp. 218–254). NIDA Research Monograph No. 156, NIH Publication No. 95-3908. Rockville, MD: National Institute on Drug Abuse.

Liddle, H. A., & Dakof, G. A. (1995b). Efficacy of family therapy for drug abuse: Promising but not definitive. *Journal of Marital and Family Therapy, 21,* 511–544.

Liddle, H. A., Dakoff, G., Diamond, G. Holt, M., Arroyo, J., & Watson, M. (1992). The adolescent module in multidimensional family therapy. In J. W. Lawson & A. W. Lawson (Eds.) Adolescent Substance Abuse, etiology, treatment, and prevention. (pp. 165–186). Rockville, MD: Aspen.

Loeber, R. (1991). Antisocial behavior: More enduring than changeable? *Journal of the American Academy of Child and Adolescent Psychiatry, 30,* 393–397.

Loeber, R., & Dishion, T. J. (1983). Early predictors of male delinquency: A review. *Psychological Bulletin, 94,* 68–99.

Loeber, R., & Dishion, T. J. (1987). Antisocial and delinquent youths: Methods for early identification. In J. D. Burchard & S. N. Burchard (Eds.), *Primary prevention of psychopathology: Vol. 10. Prevention of delinquent behavior* (pp. 75–89). Newbury Park, CA: Sage.

McDermott, D. (1984). The relationship of parental drug use and parent's attitude concerning adolescent drug use. *Adolescence, 19,* 89–97.

Merikangas, K. R., Rounsaville, B. J., & Prusoff, B. A. (1992). Familial factors in vulnerability to substance abuse. In M. D. Glantz & R. W. Pickins, (Eds.), *Vulnerability to drug abuse* (pp. 75–98). Washington, DC: American Psychological Association Press.

Moffitt, T. E. (1993). Adolescence-limited and life-course persistent antisocial behavior: A developmental taxonomy. *Psychological Review, 100,* 674–701.

Newcomb, M. D., & Bentler, P. M. (1986). Substance use and ethnicity: Differential impact of peer and adult models. *Journal of Psychology, 120,* 83–95.

Newcomb, M. D., & Bentler, P. M. (1988). *Consequences of adolescent drug use: Impact on the lives of young adults.* Newbury Park, CA: Sage.

Newcomb, M. D., & Felix-Ortiz, M. (1992). Multiple protective and risk factors for drug use and abuse: Cross-sectional and prospective findings. *Journal of Personality and Social Psychology, 63,* 280–296.

O'Donnell, J. A., & Clayton, R. R. (1979). *Determinants of early marijuana use.* In G. M. Beschner & A. S. Friedman (Eds.), *Youth drug abuse: Problems, issues, and treatment* (pp. 63–110). Lexington, MA: Lexington Books.

Oetting, E. R., & Beauvais, F. (1987a). Common elements in youth drug abuse: Peer clusters and other psychosocial factors. *Journal of Drug Issues, 17*(1&2), 133–151.

Oetting, E. R., & Beauvais, F. (1987b). Peer cluster theory, socialization characteristics and adolescent drug use: A path analysis. *Journal of Counseling Psychology, 34*(2), 205–213.

Oetting, E. R., & Beauvais, F. (1990). Adolescent drug use: Findings of national and local surveys. *Journal of Consulting and Clinical Psychology, 58*(4), 385–394.

Oetting, E. R., & Donnermeyer, J. F. (1998). Primary socialization theory: The etiology of drug use and deviance. Part I. *Substance Use and Misuse, 33*(4), 995–1026.

Oetting, E. R., Donnermeyer, J. F., Deffenbacher, J. L. (1998). Primary socialization theory: The influence of the community on drug use and deviance. III. *Substance Use and Misuse, 33,* 1629–1665.

Oetting, E. R., Edwards, R. W., Kelly, K., & Beauvais, F. (1997). Risk and protective factors for drug use among rural American youth. In Z. Sloboda, G. Boyd, E. Robertson, & L. Beatty (Eds.), *Rural substance abuse: State of knowledge and issues* (NIDA Research Monograph). Rockville, MD: National Institute on Drug Abuse.

Oetting, E. R., & Lynch, R. S. (in press). Peers and the prevention of adolescent drug use. In W. J. Bukoski & Z. Sloboda (Eds.), *Handbook for drug abuse prevention: Theory, science, and practice.* New York: Plenum Press.

Pandina, R. J., & Johnson, V. L. (1999). Why people use, abuse, and become dependent on drugs: Progress toward a heuristic model. In M. D. Glantz & C. R. Hartel (Eds.). *Drug abuse: Origins and interventions. Washington, DC: American Psychological Association.*

Pandina, R., Labouvie, E., & White, H. (1984). Potential contribution of the life span developmental approach to the study of adolescent alcohol and drug use: The Rutgers Health and Human Development Project, a working model. *Journal of Drug Issues, 14,* 253–268.

Patterson, G., Chamberlain, P., & Reid, J. (1982). The comparative evaluation of a parent training program. *Behavior Therapy, 13,* 638–650.

Patterson, G., Reid, J., & Dishion, T. (1992). *Antisocial boys.* Eugene, OR: Castalia.

Penning, M., & Barnes, G. E. (1982). Adolescent marijuana use: A review. *International Journal of Addictions, 17,* 749–791.

Pentz, M. A., Dwyer, J., MacKinnon, D., Flay, B. R., Hansen, W. B., Wang, E. Y., & Johnson, C. A. (1989a). A multicommunity trial for primary prevention of adolescent drug abuse. *Journal of the American Medical Association, 261,* 3259–3266.

Pentz, M. A., Dwyer, J. H., MacKinnon, D. P., Flay, B. R., Hansen, W. B., Wang, E. Y. I., & Johnson, C. A. (1989b). The power of policy: Relationship of smoking policy to adolescent smoking. *American Journal of Public Health, 79,* 857–862.

Pentz, M. A., MacKinnon, D. P., Flay, B. R., Hansen, W. B., Johnson, C. A., & Dwyer, J. H. (1989). Primary prevention of chronic diseases in adolescence: Effects of the Midwestern Prevention project on tobacco use. *American Journal of Epidemiology, 130,* 713–724.

Perry, C. L., Kelder, S. H., Murray, D. M., & Kepp, K.-I. (1992). Community-wide smoking prevention: Long-term outcomes of the Minnesota Heart Health Program and the Class of 1989 Study. *American Journal of Public Health, 82,* 1210–1216.

Peterson, P. L., Hawkins, J. D., Abbott, R. D., & Catalano, R. F. (1995). Disentangling the effects of parental drinking, family management, and parental alcohol norms on current drinking by black and white adolescents. In G. M. Boyd, J. Howard, & R. A. Zucker (Eds.), *Alcohol problems among adolescents; Current directions in prevention research* (pp. 35–59). Hillsdale, NJ: Erlbaum.

Petraitis, J., Flay, B. R., & Miller, T. Q. (1995). Reviewing theories of adolescent substance use: Organizing pieces in the puzzle. *Psychological Bulletin, 117,* 67–86.

Riggs, P. D., Baker, S., Mikulich, S. K., Young, S. E., & Crowley, T. J. (1995). Depression in substance-dependent delinquents. *Journal of the American Academy of Child and Adolescent Psychiatry, 34*(6), 764–771.

Robins, L. N. (1984). The natural history of adolescent drug use. *American Journal of Public Health, 74,* 656–657.

Robins, L. N., & McEvoy, L. (1990). Conduct problems as predictors of substance abuse. In L. Robins & M. Rutter (Eds.), *Straight and devious pathways from childhood to adulthood* (pp. 242–258).Cambridge, England: Cambridge University Press.

Rohrbach, L. A., Hodgson, C. S., Broder, B. I., Flay, B. R., Hansen, W. B., & Pentz, M. A. (1995). Parental participation in drug abuse prevention: Results from the Midwestern Prevention Project. In G. M. Boyd, J. Howard, & R. A. Zucker (Eds), *Alcohol problems among adolescents: Current directions in prevention research* (pp. 173–194). Hillsdale, NJ: Erlbaum.

Rowe, D. C., Rodgers, J. L., & Meseck-Bushey, S. (1992). Sibling delinquency and the family environment: Shared and unshared influences. *Child Development, 63,* 59–67.

Rutter, M. (1980). *Changing youth in a changing society.* Cambridge, MA: Harvard University Press.

Sampson, R. J. (1985). Neighborhood and crime: The structural determinants of personal victimization. *Journal of Research on Crime and Delinquency, 22,* 7–40.

Selnow, G. W. (1987). Parent-child relationships and single and two parent families: Implications for substance usage. *Journal of Drug Education, 17,* 315–326.

Simcha-Fagen, O., Gersten, J. C., & Langner, T. (1986). Early precursors and concurrent correlates of illicit drug use in adolescents. *Journal of Drug Issues, 16,* 7–28.

Smith, B. E., & Davis, R. C. (1993). Successful community anti-crime programs: What makes them work? In: R. C. Davis, A. J. Lurgio, & D. P. Rosenbaum (Eds.), *Drugs and the community: Involving community residents in combating the sale of illegal drugs* (pp. 123–137). Springfield, IL: Charles C. Thomas.

Swaim, R. C., Oetting, E. R., Edwards, R. W., & Beauvais, F. (1989). The links from emotional distress to adolescent drug use: A path model. *Journal of Cross Cultural Psychology, 15*(2), 153–172.

Szapocznik. J., & Coatsworth, J. D. (1999). An ecodevelopmental framework for organizing the influences on drug abuse: A developmental model of risk and protection. In M. D. Glantz & C. R. Hartel (Eds.) *Drug abuse: Origins & interventions.* Washington, DC: American Psychological Association.

Szapocznik, J., & Kurtines, W. M. (1989). *Break-through in family therapy with drug abusing and problem youth.* New York: Springer.

Tabakoff, B., Hoffman, P. L., Lee, J. M., Saito, T., Willard, B., & De Leon-Jones, F. (1988). Differences in platelet enzyme activity between alcoholics and nonalcoholics. *New England Journal of Medicine, 318,* 134–139.

Tremblay, R. E., McCord, J., Boileau, H., Leblanc, M., Gagnon, C., Charlebois, P., & Larivee, S. (1990, November). *The Montreal prevention experiment: School adjustment and self-reported delinquency after three years of follow-up.* Paper presented at the 42nd Annual Meeting of the American Society of Criminology, Baltimore, MD.

Warheit, G. J., Biafora, F. A., Zimmerman, R. S., Gil, A. G., Vega, W. A., & Apospori, E. (1995). Self-rejection/derogation, peer factors, and alcohol, drug, and cigarette use among a sample of Hispanic, African-American, and white non-Hispanic adolescents. *International Journal of the Addictions, 30,* 97–116.

Werner, E. E. (1989). High-risk children in young adulthood: A longitudinal study from birth to 32 years. *American Journal of Orthopsychiatry, 59,* 72–81.

Wills, T. A., Mariani, J., & Filer, M. (1996). The role of family and peer relationships in adolescent substance use: In G. R. Pierce, B. R. Sarason, & I. G. Sarason (Eds.), *Handbook of social support and the family* (pp. 521–549). New York: Plenum.

Zigler, E., Taussig, C., & Black, K. (1992). Early childhood intervention: A promising preventative for juvenile delinquency. *American Psychologist, 47,* 997–1006.

CHAPTER 14

Bridging the Gap between Substance Use Prevention Theory and Practice

BRIAN R. FLAY
JOHN PETRAITIS

INTRODUCTION

In theory, there is nothing so practical as a good theory. When it comes to substance use (SU) there is no shortage of theories (Flay, Petraitis, & Miller, 1995). In fact, Lettieri, Sayers, and Pearson (1980) reviewed 43 different theories of SU 20 years ago, and the list has grown measurably since then. Unfortunately, there is a gap between SU theories and SU prevention. Years of work developing and refining theories has rarely resulted in practical changes in how prevention programs are planned, implemented, or evaluated. This chapter examines different forms of SU, different causes of SU, and different approaches to SU prevention. It offers one theory of SU prevention as an example of the practical applications of theory and goes on to discuss how theory has gained prominence historically and how theory can become even more important in SU prevention.

DIFFERENCES IN SU AND SU PREVENTION

To have its greatest influence on the design, implementation, and evaluation of SU prevention programs, prevention specialists and SU theorists must be explicit about what they mean by SU. It is not simply a black-and-white, dichotomous construct that has the same meaning for all theorists and prevention planners; it is, of course, a continuous variable that has degrees or varying

BRIAN R. FLAY • Preventive Research Center, University of Illinois at Chicago, Chicago, Illinois 60607
JOHN PETRAITIS • Department of Psychology, University of Alaska, Anchorage, Anchorage, Alaska 99508

shades of gray and an assortment of meanings. Some of the gray comes from the fact that for any particular substance there are at least four levels of use. It is widely recognized that the use of a substance, such as alcohol, progresses from no use through trial and experimental use, regular use, and, for some people, abuse and dependence (Clayton, 1992; Flay et al., 1983; Leventhal & Cleary, 1980; Mayhew, Flay, & Mott, 2000). It is also widely recognized that with a variety of substances available, there are at least four different patterns of SU. As Kandel (1989; Kandel & Yamaguchi, 1993) and others (e.g., Graham et al., 1991) note, people typically experiment with alcohol and/or tobacco first, progress to alcohol intoxication, move to marijuana use (if at all), and only advance to other substances, such as cocaine, after gaining experiences with tobacco, alcohol, and marijuana. If the different levels of use are crossed with the different patterns, the term "substance use" potentially has at least 16 different meanings, ranging at the lowest end of trial or experimental use of alcohol or tobacco to the high end of dependence on illicit drugs. Acknowledging the various definitions of su is important because some theories, such as the social development model of Hawkins and Weis (1985), have more obvious implications for the prevention of lower levels and earlier patterns of SU. Other theories, such as Sher's (1991) model of vulnerability, have more implications for the prevention of advanced levels and patterns of SU. Accordingly, a theory is only capable of improving the design, implementation, and evaluation of a prevention program when the theory and the program focus on the same range of SU.

Similarly, before theory can contribute to prevention practices, theorists and prevention specialists must be clear about what they mean by "prevention"—a term that has different meanings depending on the type of program used to alter behaviors or prevent certain conditions. The Institute of Medicine (IOM, 1994) suggests that programs aimed at reducing the risk of psychological disorders fall into three general categories. *Universal prevention* uses relatively non-intrusive interventions, delivers the interventions through people who are not necessarily experts in prevention, and aims at either the general public or large subpopulations who, as a group, have "not been identified on the basis of individual risk" (IOM, p. 24). *Selective prevention,* by contrast, tailors more intensive programs for smaller subpopulations that have above-average risk for developing a particular disorder. It is not assumed that the effects of selective programs will generalize to a broader cross-section of the public. Finally, *indicated prevention* uses experts to deliver more intensive interventions to individuals (as opposed to subpopulations) who, through individual screening, are found to have a strong pattern of risk factors or who exhibit early symptoms that foreshadow the full development of clinical disorder.

At the heart of the IOM typology is the recognition that programs that aim to prevent psychological disorders differ in their breadth (from those that try to affect millions of people at once to those that aim at a few people at a time) and depth (from those that are fairly brief or non-intrusive to those that are longer or more intensive). The same is true of programs that aim to prevent SU. The Television, School, and Family Project (TVSFP) was an example of a broad-based program (Flay et al., 1988). The goal of the TVSFP was to reduce or prevent tobacco use in a broad cross-section of adolescents by providing standardized school- and media-based messages that were integrated into usual activities at school, at home, and with parents. Although the project was designed for breadth and involved adolescents in numerous activities for several weeks, it was not designed to provide the depth of other programs, such as the Strengthening the Families Program (SFP, Kumpfer, Molgaard, & Spoth, 1996). The SFP tries to prevent adolescent SU with fairly intensive training of parents (through discussion of reinforcement principles, family communication, problem solving, and limit setting), children (through discussion of emotions, social skills, and resistance to peer pressure, among many other things), and entire families (through family therapy and role playing among family members). Although SFP was designed with more depth than TVSFP, it has less breadth because it was designed specifically for children whose parents were substance abusers (see Chapter 4).

It follows from the above discussion that prevention programs can differ in (1) the levels and patterns of SU they try to prevent, (2) the degree to which they target the general public or more high-risk individuals, and (3) the intensity of their effort. Considering each of these factors can help prevention planners identify the goals of their programs. However, considering these factors does not identify the means of achieving those goals. That is, the above considerations tell prevention planners where they want to go but not how to get there. Knowing, for example, that they want to prevent alcohol onset with a broad program tells prevention planners nothing about how to design a program that actually reduces alcohol onset in the most efficient manner. For that, prevention planners need a basic understanding of the causes of SU.

MAJOR INFLUENCES ON SU

There have been several reviews of the correlates and predictors of SU, including reviews of research on cigarette smoking (see Conrad, Flay, & Hill, 1992; Mayhew et al., 2000), illicit substance use (see Petraitis et al., 1998) and both licit and illicit substance use (see Hawkins et al., 1992). The following are some of the major influences on SU.

Substance-Specific Cognitions

Expectations—although not always accurate—abound about the immediate physiological effects of, the social reactions to, the likely legal consequences of, and the less immediate health consequences of SU (Stacy et al., 1996). For example, preteens might expect that smoking their first cigarette will make them feel instantly nauseous, will eventually help them look mature, and probably will not give them lung cancer in the long-term future. Numerous longitudinal studies of cigarette smoking and illicit SU suggest that substance-related beliefs play an important role in SU (for reviews, see Conrad et al., 1992; Petraitis et al., 1998). For instance, Kandel, Kessler, and Margulies (1978) found that 16-year-olds were more likely to use marijuana if, as 15-year-olds, they did not consider its use to be personally harmful, and if they did not fear any negative consequences of its use. Similarly, Jessor, Donovan, and Costa (1991) concluded that adolescents who thought the benefits of marijuana use exceeded its costs were more likely to use marijuana as young adults.

Prior Experience with SU

Beliefs about SU do not arise from thin air. They can grow from prior experiences with SU, and it is widely assumed that one of the best predictors of future behavior is past behavior. This holds true with SU (see Petraitis et al., 1998). Several studies have found that past levels of use of a given substance, such as tobacco, can predict future levels of use of that substance. Furthermore, prior use of one substance, such as alcohol, can predict use of other substances, such as marijuana. For instance, we found 14 longitudinal studies in which prior levels of alcohol use significantly predicted subsequent levels of marijuana use, and we found no studies in which alcohol use was not a significant predictor of marijuana use (Petraitis et al., 1998).

Substance-Related Attitudes and Behaviors of Other People

Beliefs about SU no doubt also arise when people listen to others—especially peers, parents, and other family members—as they voice their endorsement of or opposition to SU, and when people watch as others either use or abstain from substances. Although the relationship is less robust than often assumed, studies have shown that adolescent SU is more common in families in which the parents have favorable attitudes toward SU and engage in some SU themselves (see Petraitis et al., 1998). The relationship between peer SU and an adolescent's own SU is, by contrast, very robust: study after study has fairly consistently found that the substance-related attitudes and behaviors of peers predict an adolescent's use of cigarettes (see Conrad et al., 1992) and illicit substances (see Petraitis et al., 1998). Thus, having friends who have positive attitudes toward SU and who use substances might put people at risk for SU. We say "might" because there is mounting evidence that the link between peer SU and an adolescent's own might arise, in large part, because adolescents who are inclined toward SU select friends who also use or are inclined to use substances (Bauman & Ennett, 1996).

Family Environment

In our review of longitudinal studies of illicit SU (Petraitis et al., 1998) we found that the childhood home environments of people who are more heavily involved in SU are different from the home environments of people who are less involved in SU. For instance, longitudinal studies generally (although not consistently) suggest that the people who are at greater risk for SU are those who come from homes with (1) higher socioeconomic status; (2) divorced or separated parents; (3) parents who were abusive, negligent, or offered little emotional support; and (4) a discrepancy between the quality of parent–child relations that the children wanted and the quality that they obtained. There is also some evidence that children are at risk for SU later in life if they come from homes where a parent has a history of a psychiatric disorder or the parents were permissive with the child (see Petraitis et al., 1998).

Deviant Behaviors and Unconventional Values

For some people, SU is not the result of difficult home environments or the substance-related attitudes of other people. Rather, it is the result of a rejection of conventional values and an attraction to unconventional behaviors. Our review of longitudinal studies (Petraitis et al., 1998) found that adolescents were at risk for SU if they either (1) rejected traditional values, (2) were critical of mainstream society, (3) were tolerant of deviance, (4) were politically detached or alienated, (5) were not religious, or (6) were not committed to education. Moreover, several studies found that adolescents were at risk for SU if they had a history of disobedience or deviant behavior, such as vandalism.

Personality Traits and Affective States

For other people, SU might be driven either by basic and stable personality characteristics or by more transient affective states. In line with this, several studies have shown that SU is more common among people who characteristically (1) lack persistence or the will to achieve long-term goals, (2) lack emotional stability or emotional control, (3) are disinhibited and seek thrills, (4) are rebellious, (5) are assertive, or (6) are aggressive or hostile toward others (see Petraitis et al., 1998). Furthermore, there is some evidence that SU is more common after periods of anxiety, low self-esteem, and depressed mood. However, the evidence concerning anxiety, self-esteem, and depression generally shows that these affective states are not consistently or strongly related to SU (see Petraitis et al., 1998).

Biological Influences

Not only does SU tend to run in families (see Sher, 1991) it is also linked to a variety of biological factors (see Cloninger, 1987; Phil, Peterson, & Finn, 1990; Tarter, Alterman, & Edwards, 1985). For instance, studies have shown that cigarette use among girls (but not boys) is positively related to testosterone levels (Bauman, Foshee, & Haley, 1992); the early onset of puberty predicts the onset of cigarette use (Wilson et al., 1994); and levels of serotonin and dopamine influence cocaine consumption among rats (White, 1997).

There are two likely mechanisms by which biological influences contribute to SU. First, biological factors, such as genetic differences or interuterine exposure to substances, might affect SU indirectly through more direct effects on personality characteristics that increase the risk of SU. For example, genetics might contribute to risk-taking characteristics, which in turn might contribute to SU. In line with this type of indirect effect, research suggests that substance abuse among adolescents is more common among those with difficult temperaments (particularly high activity levels) than among adolescents with less difficult temperaments (Tarter et al., 1990). Second, biological factors might affect SU more directly by making some people either more susceptible to the reinforcing physiological effects, such as relaxation, of various substances or have stronger physiological cravings for specific substances. Certainly, some people are genetically more sensitive to the physiological effects of substances. As examples: dopamine metabolism in adults might be affected by *in utero* exposure to substances (Middaugh & Zemp, 1985); similarly, maternal smoking during pregnancy seems to increase the risk that children will smoke during adolescence (Kandel, Wu, & Davies, 1994); and Asians who have inherited a genetic mutation of mitochondrial aldehyde dehydrogenase or human alcohol dehydrogenase metabolize alcohol more slowly, have stronger alcohol-flush reactions, and are less susceptible to alcoholism than Asians who do not have these genetic variants (Thomasson et al., 1993). In the case of cigarette use, some research suggests that the strength of physiological reactions—be they pleasing or aversive—to substances is a risk factor for SU. In particular, Pomerleau et al. (1993) demonstrated that people who have the strongest physiological reactions (either positive or negative) to nicotine are at greatest risk to escalate from experimental smoking to regular smoking.

Comorbidity

A startling number of people who have problems with substance abuse or dependence also have other psychological disorders (Mueser, Bennett, & Kushner, 1995). For instance, having a major depressive episode triples the odds that a person will also have an abuse or dependence problem within a year, and having bipolar disorder increases the odds by more than 600% (Kessler et al., 1996; see also Johnson, Posner, & Rolf, 1995.) Moreover, when people have histories of psychological disorders and SU problems, the chances are extremely high that the psychological disorder came first. Specifically, Kessler et al. (1996) found that when people had a history of both a psychological disorder and a SU problem, only 12.8% reported that the SU problem clearly preceded the psychological disorder, whereas 83.5% reported that the psychological problem predated the SU problem, suggesting that psychological problems might cause SU problems.

Self-Medication

Some researchers (e.g., Khantzian, 1985) have suggested that SU arises when people try to cope with difficult emotional challenges, such as divorce, or, as indicated earlier, when people try to control the symptoms of psychological problems. In line with this, Bibb and Chambless (1986) found that 43% of nonalcoholic patients with agoraphobia reported using alcohol to medicate their anxiety, and 90% of agoraphobics with alcoholism turned to alcohol to reduce their anxiety. Although there is compelling evidence that people with psychological problems have high levels of SU, in general, there is far less evidence that people selectively seek out specific substances that effectively counteract the symptoms of their disorders. For instance, people with depression do not seem to seek out stimulants to combat lethargy, and people with anxiety do not seem to seek out the calming influences of marijuana any more than people who do not suffer from anxiety. In fact, Mueser et al. (1995) concluded that clinical diagnoses are not a major determinant of which substance people use and that people with clinical diagnoses are at risk for abusing whichever substances are most available to them.

THE THEORY OF TRIADIC INFLUENCE

Understanding SU is a bit like cooking. Preparing a dish requires two things: a list of ingredients and a recipe that tells how those ingredients get combined. Similarly, understanding SU requires a list of factors that contribute to SU and an understanding of how those factors work together to influence SU. That is, before we can understand SU we need to understand what factors are involved, what causal processes link one factor to another, which factors affect SU directly and which factors affect SU more indirectly, which factors mediate the effects of other factors, and which ones moderate the effects of others. For this, we need theories. This section describes a theory that identifies many of the factors involved in SU and examines how those factors might mediate or moderate each other. Specifically, it describes the theory of triadic influence (TTI) and shows how it, as just one example of SU theory, can be used to advance SU prevention.

Three Streams and Multiple Levels of Influence

The TTI argues that three basic types or streams of influences contribute to SU and its prevention (Flay & Petraitis, 1994). First, there are cultural factors that might contribute primarily to attitudes toward SU. An unfavorable (or favorable) media depiction of SU is just one example of a cultural/attitudinal influence, and beliefs or expectations about SU would be another. Second, there are social or interpersonal factors that might contribute primarily to the social pressures people experience that lead them to believe that SU is either acceptable or not. Growing up in a home where alcohol is not (or is) consumed is an example of such an influence. Having negligent parents or bonding with substance-using peers are two more examples of situational or microenvironmental factors that might contribute to social pressures to use substances. Third, there are intrapersonal factors that might affect one's motivation to use or abstain

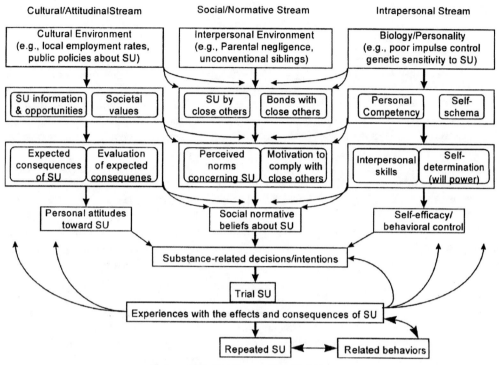

FIGURE 14.1. The theory of triadic influence.

from substances or might affect one's ability to resist pressures to use substances. Weak impulse control, genetic sensitivity to substances, and self medication are examples of intrapersonal influences.

The TTI also argues that within each stream of influence there are several levels or tiers of influence. As shown in Figure 14.1, variables at the top of each stream are the furthest removed from SU (e.g., rigid parenting style, neighborhood unemployment rate, and sociability). As such, the effects of such "ultimate" influences are the most distal, the most mediated, and often the most difficult for anyone or any program to change. Below the ultimate-level influences are distal influences (e.g., bonding to deviant role models and rebelliousness). When compared to ultimate-level influences, distal-level influences are less numerous, less far removed from SU, have effects on SU that are less mediated, and are usually less difficult to change. Then, near the bottom of Figure 14.1, there is a smaller set of proximal influences (e.g., substance-related attitudes, normative beliefs, resistance skills) that probably have direct effects on intentions to use substances and actual SU and might be the easiest for individuals or programs to alter (at least in the short run).

Within-Stream Mediating Processes

Mediation lies at the core of TTI. The theory does more than just provide a list of variables that contribute to SU; it offers suggestions about the numerous mediating processes that link each variable to other variables and SU. In another paper (Flay & Petraitis, 1994), we describe in detail the mediating processes by which the effects of ultimate-level influences in the attitudinal stream begin to filter down through distal- and proximal-level influences. Some of that filtering process is depicted in the left side of Figure 14.1. For example, in the cultural/attitudinal stream, we suggest a process by which ultimate-level attitudinal influences, such as media depictions of SU, might contribute to SU by contributing to distal-level attitudinal influences, such as subjective beliefs about the general consequences of SU. These distal-level attitudinal influences, in turn, probably contribute to the proximal-level and attitudes towards SU. Although we are not aware of any studies that assessed the mediating processes involving ultimate-level attitudinal influences, several studies support the mediating processes between distal and proximal attitudinal influences. Stacy, Newcomb, and Bentler (1991) found that adolescents who lack conventional values (a distal variable) have more positive expectations for alcohol use (a proximal variable) and are at greater risk for SU. Webb et al. (1993) found that an adolescent's tolerance for deviance contributes to positive expectations for alcohol use which, in turn, contributes to SU.

A similar filtering process (from ultimate, through distal, to proximal) is probably at work with social influences as well. As depicted in the center of Figure 14.1, inadequate schools, poor home environments, and negative parenting styles might contribute to SU by weakening conventional bonds and increasing exposure to role models who use substances. Weakened bonds and exposure to SU by role models might, in turn, affect the amount of social pressure people feel to use or avoid substances. In line with the mediating processes among TTI's social influences, Rodriquez, Adrados, and De La Rosa (1993) found that weak involvement of parents in the lives of their adolescents (an ultimate-level social influence) is replaced by increased involvement with deviant peers (a distal influence); involvement with deviant peers, in turn, contributes to SU among the adolescents. Also in line with TTI, Flay et al. (1994) found that smoking by parents and friends (distal influences) contributes to beliefs that smoking is widespread and socially acceptable (proximal influences); and these beliefs, in turn, influence intentions to smoke and subsequent smoking.

In addition, the previously cited filtering process probably exists with the intrapersonal influences. Therefore, as depicted on the right side of Figure 14.1, genetic traits and basic personality characteristics (such as behavioral control and emotional control) might contribute to SU indirectly by contributing to a person's self-concept and competence in various social roles. Self-concept and competencies then contribute to the strength of someone's determination to use or avoid substances and to his or her skills in situations where SU is being considered. Unfortunately, empirical support for the mediating processes among TTI's intrapersonal influences is weak because few studies have assessed the links among the different levels of intrapersonal influences. However, Dielman et al. (1989) found that having an external health locus of control (an ultimate-level influence) contributes to low self-esteem (a more distal influence) which, in turn, contributes to alcohol use among adolescents. Similarly, Newcomb and Harlow (1986) found that an external locus of control contributes to a sense of meaningless and lack of direction in life which, in turn, contributes to SU.

Between-Stream Influences

Although mediation within streams lies at the core of TTI, some mediating processes flow between streams in Figure 14.1. For instance, Ellickson and Hays (1992) found that weak bonds to school (a distal variable) contribute to positive expectations for SU (a proximal variable) which, in turn, contribute to SU. Another example is that poor behavioral control (an ultimate-level intrapersonal influence) might contribute to SU through its contribution to involvement with substance-using peers (a distal-level social influence). In fact, Wills et al. (1994) found just such an effect. Similarly, social influences might be mediated by attitudinal influences. For instance, Ellickson and Hays found that weak bonds to school (a distal-level social influence) contribute to positive expectations for SU (a proximal-level attitudinal influence) which, in turn, contribute to SU.

In addition to mediating influences between streams, there are moderating processes, or interactions, between streams. For example, we do not believe that poor behavioral control (an ultimate-level intrapersonal influence) increases or decreases parental SU (a distal-level social influence). However, it might alter the effects of parental SU so that parental SU has a stronger effect on adolescents who lack behavioral control but might have no effect on adolescents who have strong behavioral control. In a similar manner, exposure to a program (an ultimate-level attitudinal influence) that teaches refusal skills might have no effect on adolescents who already have strong social skills (a distal-level intrapersonal influence) but might have its strongest effect on adolescents who have the weakest social skills.

Developmental Influences

Experimentation with SU is largely a phenomenon of adolescence and young adulthood. Although TTI has no developmental stream, it recognizes that three milestones of adolescent development might contribute to the three streams of TTI. First, attitudinal processes might be affected by the development of formal operational thought and the ability to think hypothetically, consider various alternatives, envision possible outcomes, and plan ahead. Until these complex mental skills are fully developed, young adolescents have limited capacities to understand or foresee the long-term consequences of their behavior (Orr & Ingersoll, 1991). This, paired with generally good health (Brindis & Lee, 1991), might contribute to an adolescent's cavalier attitudes about health (Levenson, Morrow, & Pfefferbaum, 1984) and tendency to underestimate personal risks from health-compromising behaviors (Millstein, 1991), such as SU. Second, intrapersonal processes might be affected by an adolescent's search for self-identity or sense of self—a search that might lead to experimentation with different ideas, values, and lifestyles. The search is not easy, and during it adolescents are psychologically vulnerable (Konopka, 1991), self-conscious, concerned about social appearances (Elkind & Bowen, 1979), and highly self-critical (Lowenthal, Thurner, & Chiriboga, 1975; Rosenberg, 1985), possibly because for the first time they can envision discrepancies between who they are and who they want to be or ought to be (Damon, 1991; Higgins, 1987). SU might serve as a coping mechanism as adolescents search for an identity and feel vulnerable and self-conscious during this stage of intrapersonal flux (Flammer, 1991). Finally, social processes might be influenced by the independence adolescents seek from parents. Usually beginning at puberty, positive interactions between adolescents and parents diminish (Steinberg, 1991), and adolescents begin seeking independence from their parents (Montemayor & Flannery, 1991). Their independence from parents is replaced by greater dependence on peers, and relations with peers "become more pervasive, more intense, and carry greater psychological importance" (Foster-Clark & Blyth, 1991; p. 786) during adolescence. Not too surprisingly, adolescents are more susceptible to and compliant with social pressures than are children or adults (Berndt, 1979; Landsbaum & Willis, 1971). This is especially true of pressures to engage in deviant acts (Brown, Clasen, & Eicher, 1986), like SU.

THE ROLE OF THEORY IN SU PREVENTION

Careful attention to theories about the onset of and prevention of SU is necessary for the proper development, implementation, and evaluation of SU prevention. Following are six specific ways in which theory functions in the advancement of prevention (see also Flay & Petraitis, 1991).

1. Theories can identify risk and protective factors. All prevention programs must provide some intervention (such as information about SU or access to adult supervision after school) designed to decrease or delay SU. However, program developers need to know what to provide. And, this is the first function of theory: theory guides the development of interventions by helping identify protective factors (knowledge about the dangers of SU) and risk factors (lack of adult supervision after school) for SU. It is no coincidence that SU prevention programs only started teaching refusal skills after Bandura's (1977) theoretical work on self-efficacy. In this and countless other cases, theories have suggested the basic content that has gone into developing new and more effective approaches to prevention.

2. Theories can expand the list of risk and protective factors. Not only must interventions provide something, they probably must provide many things. Like TTI, most theories of SU suggest that a great many risk and protective factors influence SU. Therefore, theories can remind us that the most effective interventions are probably those that target a wide range of risk and protective factors. Accordingly, theories help us design more effective approaches to prevention. For instance, one glance at Figure 14.1 reminds prevention planners that SU has its roots in numerous cultural/attitudinal, social/normative, and intrapersonal influence and reminds planners that simple interventions are likely to have modest effects. Moreover, Figure 14.1 reminds planners that among the three streams of influences, only a few factors probably affect SU fairly directly (such as attitudes toward SU) and that most factors probably have indirect effects (genetically inherited traits).

3. Theories can point toward intervening variables and modifiable risk and protective factors. Having a thorough list of risk and protective factors is not enough. Program developers also need to focus their intervention on risk and protective factors that are modifiable (such as self-esteem) rather than permanent (such as gender), inflexible, or difficult to modify (poverty). Knowing, for example, that rural males are at high risk for dependence on smokeless tobacco is of little use in developing effective prevention programs for them. Their gender, after all, is not something program providers can change. However, if program developers understand the causal processes and intervening variables that link gender and smokeless tobacco use they are in a better position to develop an effective program. Theories, in conjunction with empirical support, explicitly articulate the intervening causal process that link unmodifiable variables with SU. Consequently, theories give program developers more than a list of risk and protective factors: theories also give developers a list of protective factors (knowing that smokeless tobacco can cause cancer) that can be modified and enhanced by a program and a list of risk factors (poor refusal skills) that can be modified and reduced by the program.

4. Theories can point toward the appropriate audience. In addition to telling us what to provide, theories also tell us for whom to provide it. That is, theories can tell us for whom an intervention is likely to be most effective. Not all people have the same level of risk, and, consequently, not all people ought to be targeted for equal levels of SU prevention. Furthermore, not all people will have the same reaction to a program. For instance, a program that emphasizes the dangers of SU might reduce the SU of low risk-takers but might promote SU among high risk-takers. Thus, theories—especially theories that articulate moderating or interaction effects—can suggest populations for which programs ought to be delivered, populations for which the program should not be delivered, and

variables that might moderate a program's effect. Consequently, theories can suggest whether prevention efforts should be universal, selective, or indicated.

5. Theories can help anticipate program power. Theories can also lead to consensus regarding the potential magnitude of program effects. Because theories often include a variety of causes, they can alert us to the fact that prevention programs that target one or two causes of su might have only modest effects because they do not address the other factors that contribute to su. Judging the potential impact of a program against TTI, for example, might help program planners more realistically anticipate the size of their program's impact. No doubt well-intended su prevention efforts have been conducted around the country under the assumption that simply teaching kids about the dangers of su will, by itself, have a meaningful impact on their audience. However, if program providers realized that information about substances and su is only one variable in a more complex web of variables, they would come to expect more modest effects from their programs. In short, theories help us anticipate whether prevention programs will have small, medium, or large effects.

6. Theories point toward likely program effects. Finally, theories can help locate the various effects of an intervention. All programs are probably designed to have an immediate effect on some variables that are expected to have subsequent effects on su. For instance, prevention programs might try to increase knowledge about the negative consequences of su in the hope that such knowledge will change attitudes toward su and, eventually, reduce su. By spelling out the intervening variables, theories allow us to measure the appropriate variables and help us locate the immediate, intermediate, and long-term effects of a program. Theories, like TTI, suggest exactly which variables are most likely to be affected by a program.

Efforts To Incorporate Theory in su Prevention

Although a good theory has these and other practical benefits, the use of theories in su prevention has varied over the past decades. Beginning in the 1960s, the use of theory in su prevention progressed through five generations, relying on increasingly complex theories of su.

KNOWLEDGE-BASED TRAINING. The first generation of prevention efforts—popular during the 1960s—followed a universal approach to prevention and attempted to deter su by presenting information about its harmful consequences. This knowledge-based approach relied on the assumption that adolescents would stay away from su if they knew about the risks involved in su, especially the long-term risks to personal health.

Although such efforts appealed to common sense, their attention to theory was fairly limited, and the programs were usually unsuccessful for several reasons. First, the novel information they provided about drugs sometimes increased su (Goodstadt, 1978). Second, their effects were limited by an emphasis on the long-term consequences of su—consequences that are of little importance or value to youth (Evans, 1976). Third, they focused on only one aspect of su (the consequences of su) while not focusing on other determinants. As noted previously, altering only one determinant of a behavior will not be of much use if the unaltered determinants are important. Fourth, although these programs might have provided information about the negative consequences of su, they only provided one source of information about su, while competing sources of information (such as peers and the media) might have overpowered the effects of knowledge provided by the programs. Fifth, these programs adopted a strategy of universal prevention, providing a relatively modest intervention across the board. As such, they provided unnecessary information to people who were never at risk for SU, and they provided too little intervention for those who were at greatest risk for SU.

VALUES-BASED TRAINING. The first generation of prevention attempted to deter SU by educating adolescents about the consequences of SU. The second generation tried to deter SU by changing adolescents' values with regard to SU and by teaching students how to make decisions using their knowledge and evaluations of consequences. These affective approaches—popular during the 1970s—relied on the assumption that adolescents need to know more than the risks involved in SU; they need to have negative values about SU and its consequences and positive values about nonuse and its consequences. For example, student athletes might be deterred from SU if they were taught to think about their values and realize that SU might interfere with athletic performance.

However, like knowledge-based efforts, values-based efforts did not rely heavily on theory and had limited success in part because they generally focused on only one cause of SU (evaluations of the consequences of SU), tried to alter values with only one source of information (such as a health educator) that might have been overwhelmed by other sources (peers and the media), and provided universal prevention when more selective or indicated prevention was warranted. The success of values-based efforts hinges on the ability of relatively short-lived and superficial presentations to change relatively long-standing and central values of adolescents—something that now seems unrealistic. As a result, values-based efforts might have taught adolescents about values but might not have permanently changed those values or had a lasting effect on SU.

RESISTANCE SKILLS TRAINING. The first two generations were characterized by getting adolescents to recognize and appreciate the risks involved in SU. The third generation focused on teaching adolescents to recognize and say "no" to social pressures to use drugs. During the 1980s, prevention researchers focused on the role of social influences (particularly from peers and the media) as determinants of SU and developed approaches to making youth aware of the extent to which their behavior is influenced by peers and the mass media, raising their awareness of the misperceptions of their peers' behavior, and teaching them skills to resist social pressures.

Like earlier prevention efforts, resistance skills efforts tended to adopt a strategy of universal prevention, providing the program, for example, to all youth in school without knowing their individual risks for SU or whether they came from a subpopulation with elevated risk. These approaches had more success than the previous approaches, but their effects were still small, fragile (Flay, 1985), and short term (Flay, Koepke, et al., 1989; Murray et al., 1989), perhaps because (1) most of them still focused on only some of the major determinants of SU and generally did not consider other determinants (such as knowledge and values); (2) the interventions tended to be of short duration; (3) the social influences in adolescents' social environments were not changed by the interventions; and (4) the interventions tended to be more universal than selective or indicated, thereby delivering more program than was necessary for some individuals but far less than was necessary for individuals at greatest risk for SU. Interventions developed and tested by Botvin (1996; Botvin et al., 1990) at Cornell University were the exception in that they tended to be more like, and foreshadowed, the fourth-generation approaches.

COMPREHENSIVE INTERVENTIONS. Since the mid-1980s, researchers like Botvin (1996), Pentz et al. (1989), Biglan et al. (1995, 1996), and Dishion et al. (1996) have emphasized more comprehensive approaches to prevention. First, they focused simultaneously on several major determinants of SU. For example, Botvin's Life Skills Training program tried to prevent SU by teaching adolescents (1) better decision-making and problem-solving skills, (2) skills for controlling anxiety and anger, (3) techniques for self reinforcement, (4) social skills and ways to overcome shyness, and (5) about SU and pressures toward SU (such as direct peer pressure and media influences). Second, they were comprehensive and tried to curb more than just SU. For instance, Botvin's program tried to enhance social skills, improve personal decision-making skills, and promote self-control skills. Third, their programs used multiple agents to deliver the intervention. These included health professionals, teachers, older peers, parents, the mass media, schools, and other community organizations (such as the American Lung Association). Such programs not only involved these agents in the educational or change process but also aimed to change the schools and communities in which youth grow up. And finally, the interventions were of longer duration. It is clear that short-term programs will have short-term effects because most of the influences that contribute to SU will continue to exist long after a short program has ended. As such, more recent programs have included booster sessions that occur months or years after the initial intervention ended.

INTENSIVE SELECTIVE INTERVENTIONS. Despite the improved effects of comprehensive universal interventions, it is clear from the TTI model that for programs to have larger effects that persist over time, they must change the social context or the broader cultural environment in which youth spend most of their time. Accordingly, another trend among more recent programs has been a move toward more selective and/or indicated interventions. For example, both Dishion et al. (1996) and Kumpfer et al. (1996) have developed interventions that not only have strong theoretical foundations but rely on theory to screen for individuals who are at greatest risk for SU. These programs are not universally provided to everyone in a geographic area or school. Rather, they are only provided to those individuals who show a strong pattern of risk factors. For example, Dishion et al.'s Adolescent Transitions Program focuses on adolescents who have four or more risk factors.

COMPREHENSIVE MULTILEVEL INTERVENTIONS. The emerging generation of preventive interventions will (1) involve universal, selective, and indicated levels of prevention activities; (2) target multiple levels of influence, from ultimate to proximal; and (3) address multiple behaviors or problems in a single, integrated program. The FAST Track project by the Conduct Problems Prevention Research Group (CPPRG: Bierman, Greenberg, & CPPRG, 1996; CPPRG, 1992; McMahon, Slough, & CPPRG, 1996) already provides one example of this approach. In education, some Comprehensive School Reform models also exemplify such a strategy. (Flay, 2002, Flay, Allred, & Ordway, 2001.)

CONCLUSION

Reducing SU has been an elusive goal, and SU prevention programs for the past 30 years have had, at best, only modest success. Although programs have relied increasingly on theory and increasingly more comprehensive theory, they still have a long way to go to make full use of SU theories. Therefore, it is our belief that SU could be reduced further if program planners relied more on theory when designing their programs. A heavy reliance on theory could build programs upon a foundation of (1) less than obvious risk and protective factors, (2) multiple risk and protective factors that are modifiable within the context of the intervention, (3) careful consideration of how audience characteristics might moderate or interact with program effects, and (4) realistic considerations of the magnitude and immediacy of program effects. Without a heavy reliance on comprehensive theory, su prevention might only continue its 30-year trend of modest success.

REFERENCES

Bandura, A. (1977). Self-efficacy: Toward a unifying theory of behavior change. *Psychological Bulletin, 84,* 58–70.

Bauman, K. E., & Ennett, S. T. (1996). On the importance of peer influence for adolescent drug use: Commonly neglected considerations. *Addiction, 91,* 185–198.

Bauman, K. E., Foshee, V. A., & Haley, N. J. (1992). The interaction of sociological and biological factors in adolescent cigarette smoking. *Addictive Behaviors 17,* 459–467.

Berndt, T. J. (1979). Developmental changes in conformity to peer and parents. *Developmental Psychology, 15,* 608–616.

Bibb, J. L., & Chambless, D. L. (1986). Alcohol use and abuse among diagnosed agoraphobics. *Behavior Research Therapy, 24,* 49–58.

Bierman, K. L., Greenberg, M. T., & the Conduct Problems Prevention Research Group. (1996). Social skills training in the Fast Track Program. In R. DeV. Peters & R. J. McMahon (Eds.), *Preventing childhood disorders, substance abuse, and delinquency* (pp. 65–89). Thousand Oaks, CA: Sage.

Biglan, A., Henderson, J., Humphreys, D., Yasui, M., Whisman, R., Black, C., & James, L. (1995). Mobilizing positive reinforcement to reduce youth access to tobacco. *Tobacco Control, 4,* 42–48.

Biglan, A., Ary, D. V., Koehn, V., Levings, D., Smith, S., Wright, Z., James, L., & Henderson, J. (1996.) Mobilizing positive reinforcement in communities to reduce youth access to tobacco. *American Journal of Community Psychology, 24*(5), 625–638.

Botvin, G. J. (1996). Substance abuse prevention through life skills training. In R. DeV. Peters & R. J. McMahon (Eds.), *Preventing childhood disorders, substance abuse, and delinquency.* Thousand Oaks, CA: Sage.

Botvin, G. J., Baker, E., Dusenbury, L., Tortu, S., & Botvin, E. M. (1990). Preventing adolescent drug abuse through a multimodal cognitive-behavioral approach: Results of a 3-year study. *Journal of Consulting and Clinical Psychology, 58,* 437–446.

Brindis, C. D., & Lee, P. R. (1991). Adolescents conceptualization of illness. In R. M. Learner, A. C. Petersen & J. Brooks-Gunn (Eds.), *Encyclopedia of adolescence* (pp. 534–540). New York: Garland Publishing.

Brown, B. B., Clasen, D. R., & Eicher, S. A. (1986). Perceptions of peer pressure, peer conformity dispositions, and self-reported behavior among adolescents. *Developmental Psychology, 22,* 521–530.

Clayton, R. R. (1992). Transitions in drug use: Risk and protective factors. In M. Glantz & R. Pickens (Eds.), *Vulnerability to drug abuse* (pp. 15–51). Washington, DC: American Psychological Association.

Cloninger, C. R. (1987, April 24). Neurogenetic adaptive mechanisms in alcoholism. *Science, 236,* 410–416.

Conduct Problems Prevention Research Group (1992). A developmental and clinical model for the prevention of conduct disorders: The FAST Track Program. *Development and Psychopathology, 4,* 509–527.

Conrad, K. M., Flay, B. R., & Hill, D. (1992). Why children start smoking cigarettes: Predictors of onset. *British Journal of Addiction, 87,* 1711–1724.

Damon, W. (1991). Adolescent self-concept. In R. M. Learner, A. C. Petersen & J. Brooks-Gunn (Eds.), *Encyclopedia of adolescence* (pp. 987–991). New York: Garland Publishing.

Dielman, T. E., Shope, J. T., Butchart, A. T., Campaneilli, P. C., & Caspar, R. A. (1989). A covariance structure model test of antecedents of adolescent alcohol misuse and a prevention effort. *Journal of Drug Education, 19*(4), 337–361.

Dishion, T. J., Andrews, D. W., Kavanagh, K., & Soberman, L. H. (1996). Preventive intervention for high-risk youth: The adolescent transitions program. In R. DeV. Peters & R. J. McMahon (Eds.), *Preventing childhood disorders, substance abuse, and delinquency.* Thousand Oaks, CA: Sage.

Elkind, D., & Bowen, R. (1979). Imaginary audience behavior in children and adolescents. *Developmental Psychology, 15,* 33–44.

Ellickson, P. L., & Hays, R. D. (1992). On becoming involved with drugs: Modeling adolescent drug use over time. *Health Psychology, 11,* 377–385.

Evans, R. I. (1976). Smoking in children: Developing a social psychological strategy of deterence. *Preventive Medicine, 4,* 449–488.

Flammer, A. (1991). Self-regulation. In R. M. Learner, A. C. Petersen & J. Brooks-Gunn (Eds.), *Encyclopedia of adolescence* (pp. 1001–1003). New York: Garland Publishing.

Flay, B. R. (1985). Psychosocial approaches to smoking prevention: A review of findings. *Health Psychology, 4,* 449–488.

Flay, B. R. (2002) Positive youth development requires comprehensive health promotion programs. *American Journal of Health Behavior, 26*(6), 407–424.

Flay, B. R., Allred, C. G., & Ordway, N. (2002) Effects of the positive action program on achievement and discipline: Two matched-control comparisons. *Prevention Science, 2*(2), 71–90.

Flay, B. R., Brannon, B. R., Johnson, C. A., Hansen, W. B., Ulene, A., Whitney-Saltiel, D. A., Gleason, L. R., Sussman, S., Gavin, M. D., Glowacz, K. M., Sobol, D. F., & Spielgel, D. C. (1988). The television, school, and family smoking prevention/cessation project: I. Theoretical basis and television program development. *Preventive Medicine, 17,* 585–607.

Flay, B. R., d'Avernas, J. R., Best, J. A., Kersell, M. W., & Ryan, K. B. (1983). Cigarette smoking: Why young people do it and ways of preventing it. *Mass communication for public health.* Newberry Park, CA: Sage.

Flay, B. R., Hu, F. B., Siddiqui, O., Day, E. L., Hedeker, D., Petraitis, J., Richardson, J., & Sussman, S. (1994). Differential influences of parental and friends' smoking on adolescent initiation and escalation of smoking. *Journal of Social and Health Behavior, 35,* 248–265.

Flay, B. R., Koepke, D., Thomson, S. J., Santi, S., Best, J. A., & Brown, K. S. (1989). Six-year follow-up of the first Waterloo smoking prevention trial. *American Journal of Public Health, 79,* 1371–1376.

Flay, B. R., & Petraitis, J. (1991). Methodological issues in drug abuse prevention research: Theoretical foundations. In C. Leukfeld & W. Bukoski (Eds.) *Drug abuse and prevention research: Methodological issues.* Washington, DC: National Institute of Drug Abuse Research Monographs.

Flay, B. R., & Petraitis, J. (1994). The theory of triadic influence: A new theory of health behavior with implications for preventive interventions. In G. Albrecht (Ed.), *Advances in Medical Sociology (Vol. 4)* (pp. 19–44). Greenwich, CT: JAI Press.

Foster-Clark, F. S., & Blyth, D. A. (1991). Peer relations and influences. In R. M. Learner, A. C. Petersen & J. Brooks-Gunn (Eds.), *Encyclopedia of adolescence* (pp. 767–771). New York: Garland Publishing.

Goodstadt, M. S. (1978) Alcohol and drug education: Models and outcomes. *Health Education Monographs, 6*(3), 263–279.

Graham, J. W., Collins, L. M., Wugalter, S. E., Chung, N. K., & Hansen, W. B. (1991). Modeling transitions in latent stage-sequential processes: A substance use prevention example. *Journal of Consulting and Clinical Psychology, 59,* 48–57.

Hawkins, J. D., Catalano, R. F., & Miller, J. Y. (1992). Risk and protective factors for alcohol and other drug problems in adolescence and early adulthood: Implications for substance abuse prevention. *Psychological Bulletin, 112,* 64–105.

Hawkins, J. D., & Weis, J. G. (1985). The social development model: An integrated approach to delinquency prevention. *Journal of Primary Prevention, 6,* 73–97.

Higgins, E. T. (1987). Self-discrepancy: A theory relating self and affect. *Psychological Review, 94,* 319–340.

Institute of Medicine (1994). *Reducing risks for mental disorders: Frontiers for preventive intervention research.* Washington, DC: National Academy Press.

Jessor, R., Donovan, J. E., & Costa, F. M. (1991). *Beyond adolescence: Problem behavior and young adult development.* New York: Cambridge University Press.

Johnson, V. (1988). Adolescent alcohol and marijuana use: A longitudinal assessment of a social learning perspective. *American Journal of Drug and Alcohol Abuse, 14,* 419–439.

Johnson, J. L., Posner, N. E., & Rolf, J. E. (1995). The comorbidity of substance use and mental illness among adolescents. In A. F. Lehman & L. B. Dixon (Eds.), *Double jeopardy: Chronic mental illness and substance use disorders.* Chur, Switzerland: Harwood Academic Press.

Kandel, D. B. (1989). Issues of sequencing of adolescent drug use and other problem behaviors. *Drugs and Society, 3,* 55–76.

Kandel, D. B., Kessler, R. C., & Margulies, R. Z. (1978). Antecedents of adolescent initiation into stages of drug use: A developmental analysis. In D. B. Kandel (Ed.), *Longitudinal research on drug use: empirical findings and methodological issues* (pp. 73–99). Washington, DC: Hemisphere.

Kandel, D. B., Wu, P., & Davies, M. (1994). Maternal smoking during pregnancy and smoking by adolescent daughters. *American Journal of Public Health, 84,* 1407–1413.

Kandel, D. B., & Yamaguchi, K. (1993). From beer to crack: Developmental patterns of drug involvement. *American Journal of Public Health, 83,* 851–855.

Kessler, R. C., Nelson, C. B., McGonale, K. A., Edlund, M. J., Frank, R. G., & Leaf, P. J. (1996). The epidemiology of co-occurring addictive and mental disorders: Implications for prevention and service utilization. *American Journal of Orthopsychiatry, 66,* 17–31.

Khantzian, E. J. (1985). The self-medication hypothesis of addictive disorders: Focus on heroin and cocaine dependence. *American Journal of Psychiatry, 142,* 1259–1264.

Konopka, G. (1991). Adolescence, concept of, and requirements for a healthy development. In R. M. Learner, A. C. Petersen & J. Brooks-Gunn (Eds.), *Encyclopedia of adolescence* (pp. 10–13). New York: Garland Publishing.

Kumpfer, K. L., Molgaard, V. L., & Spoth, R. (1996). The Strengthening Families Program for the prevention of delinquency and drug use. In R. DeV. Peters & R. J. McMahon (Eds.), *Preventing childhood disorders, substance abuse, and delinquency.* Thousand Oaks, CA: Sage.

Landsbaum, J., & Willis, R. (1971). Conformity in early and late adolescence. *Developmental Psychology, 4,* 334–337.

Lettieri, D. J., Sayers, M., & Pearson, H. W. (Eds, 1980). *Theories on drug abuse: Selected contemporary perspectives.* (Research Monograph 30). Rockville, MD: National Institute on Drug Abuse.

Levenson, P. M., Morrow, J. R., & Pfefferbaum, B. J. (1984). Attitudes toward health and illness: A comparison of adolescent, physician, teacher, and school nurse views. *Journal of Adolescent Health Care, 5,* 254–262.

Leventhal, H., & Cleary, P. D. (1980). The smoking problem: A review of the research and theory in behavioral risk modification. *Psychological Bulletin, 88,* 370–405.

Lowenthal, M., Thurner, M., & Chiriboga, D. (1975). *Four stages of life.* San Francisco: Jossey-Bass.

Mayhew, K., Flay, B. R., and Mott, J. (2000). Stages in the development of adolescent smoking. *Drug and Alcohol Dependence, 59* Suppl. 1(2), 61–81.

McMahon, R. J., Slough, N. M., & the Conduct Problems Prevention Research Group. (1996). Family-based intervention in the Fast Track Program. In R. DeV. Peters & R. J. McMahon (Eds.), *Preventing childhood disorders, substance abuse, and delinquency* (pp. 90–110). Thousand Oaks, CA: Sage.

Middaugh, L. D., & Zemp, J. W. (1985). Dopaminergic mediation of long-term behavioral effects of in utero drug exposure. *Nueurobehavioral Toxicology and Teratology, 7,* 685–689.

Millstein, S. G. (1991). Health beliefs. In R. M. Learner, A. C. Petersen & J. Brooks-Gunn (Eds.), *Encyclopedia of adolescence* (pp. 445–448). New York: Garland Publishing.

Montemayor, R., & Flannery, D. J. (1991). Parent-adolescent relations in middle and late adolescence. In R. M. Learner, A. C. Petersen & J. Brooks-Gunn (Eds.), *Encyclopedia of adolescence* (pp. 729–734) New York: Garland Publishing.

Mueser, K. T., Bennett, M., & Kushner, M. G. (1995). Epidemiology of substance use disorders among persons with chronic mental illnesses. In A. F. Lehman & L. B. Dixon (Eds.), *Double jeopardy: Chronic mental illness and substance use disorders.* Chur, Switzerland: Harwood Academic Press.

Murray, D. M., Pirie, P., Luepker, R. V., Pallonen, U. (1989). Five and six-year followup results from four seventh-grade smoking prevention strategies. *Journal of Behavioral Medicine, 12,* 207–218.

Newcomb, M. D., & Harlow, L. L. (1986). Life events and substance use among adolescents: Mediating effects of perceived loss of control and meaninglessness in life. *Journal of Personality and Social Psychology, 51,* 564–577.

Orr, D. P., & Ingersoll, G. (1991). Cognition and health. In R. M. Learner, A. C. Petersen & J. Brooks-Gunn (Eds.), *Encyclopedia of adolescence* (pp. 130–132). New York: Garland Publishing.

Pomerleau, O. F., Collins, A. C., Shiffman, S., & Pomerleau, O. F. (1993). Why some people smoke and others do not: New perspectives. *Journal of Consulting and Clinical Psychology, 61,* 723–731.

Pentz, M. A., Dwyer, J. H., MacKinnon, D. P., Flay, B. R., Hansen, W. B., Wang, E. Y. I., & Johnson, C. A. (1989). A multi-community trial for primary prevention of adolescent drug abuse: Effects on drug use prevalence. *Journal of the American Medical Association, 261*(22), 3259–3266.

Petraitis, J., Flay, B. R., & Miller, T. Q. (1995) Reviewing theories of adolescent substance abuse: Organizing pieces of the puzzle. *Psychological Bulletin, 117*(1), 67–86.

Petraitis, J., Flay, B. R., Miller, T. Q., Torpy, E. J., & Greiner, B. (1998). Illicit substance use among adolescents: A matrix of prospective predictors. *Substance Use & Misuse, 33,* 2561–2604.

Phil, R. O., Peterson, J., & Finn, P. (1990). An heuristic model of the inherited predisposition to alcoholism. *Psychology of Addictive Behaviors, 4,* 12–25.

Rodriguez, O., Adrados, J. R., & De La Rosa M. R. (1993). Integrating mainstream and subcultural explanations of drug use among Puerto Rican Youth, In M., De La Rosa & J. R. Adrados, (Eds.), *Drug abuse among minority youth: Methodological issues and recent research advances. NIDA Research Monograph 130.* NIH Publication No. 93-3479.

Rosenberg, M. (1985). Self-concept and psychological well-being in adolescence. In R. Leahy (Ed.), *The development of the self* (pp. 205–242). New York: Academic Press.

Sher, K. J. (1991). *Children of alcoholics.* Chicago: University of Chicago Press.

Stacy, A. W., Galaif, E. R., Sussman, S., & Dent, C. W. (1996). Self-generated drug outcomes in high-risk adolescents. *Psychology of Addictive Behaviors, 10,* 18–27.

Stacy, A. W., Newcomb, M. D., & Bentler, P. M. (1991). Personality, problem drinking, and drunk driving: Mediating, moderating, and direct-effect models. *Journal of Personality and Social Psychology, 5,* 795–811.

Steinberg, L. (1991). Parent-adolescent relations. In R. M. Learner, A. C. Petersen & J. Brooks-Gunn (Eds.), *Encyclopedia of adolescence* (pp. 724–728) New York: Garland Publishing.

Tarter, R. E., Alterman, A. O., & Edwards, K. L. (1985). Vulnerability to alcoholism in men: A behavioral-genetic perspective. *Journal of Studies on Alcoholism, 46,* 329–356.

Tarter, R. E., & Blackson, T. C. (1991, October). *An integrative approach to drug abuse etiology and prevention.* Paper presented at the first International Drug Abuse Prevention Symposium, Lexington, KY.

Tarter, R. E., Laird, S. B., Kabene, M., Bukstein, O., & Kaminer, Y. (1990). Drug abuse severity in adolescents is associated with magnitude of deviation in temperament traits. *British Journal of Addiction, 85,* 1501–1504.

Thomasson, H. R., Crabbe, D. W., Edenberg, H. J., & Li, T. (1993). Alcohol and aldehyde dehydrogenase polymorphism and alcoholism. *Behavior Genetics, 23,* 131–136.

Webb, J. A., Baer, P. E., Francis, D. J., & Caid, C. D. (1993). Relationship among social and intrapersonal risk, alcohol expectancies, and alcohol usage among early adolescents. *Addictive Behaviors, 18,* 127–134.

White, F. J. (1997). Cocaine and the serotonin sage. *Nature, 393,* 118–119.

Wills, T. A., Schreibman, D., Benson, G., & Vaccaro, D. (1994). Impact of parental substance use on adolescents: A test of a mediating model. *Journal of Pediatric Psychology, 19,* 537–556.

Wilson, D. M., Killen, J. D., Hayward, C., Robinson, T. N., Hammer, L. D., Kraemer, H. C., Vardy, A., & Taylor, C. B. (1994). Timing and rate of sexual maturation and the onset of cigarette and alcohol use among teenage girls. *Archives of Pediatric and Adolescent Medicine, 14,* 789–795.

CHAPTER 15

Preventive Intervention Targeting Precursors

JOHN E. LOCHMAN

INTRODUCTION

Childhood aggression, lack of social competence in children, and certain parenting practices can be precursors to adolescent substance abuse. This chapter reviews research on these precursors, or risk factors for substance abuse, and describes successful preventive interventions that target them.

CHILDHOOD AGGRESSION

Aggressive behavior, a stable trait in some children, is now known to be a precursor of, or risk factor for, substance abuse and other negative outcomes during adolescence and adulthood (Lynskey & Fergusson, 1995; Wills & Filer, 1996). For example, one type of adult alcoholism identified by Cloninger (Cloninger, Sigvardsson, & Bohman, 1988) is associated with high levels of impulsive-aggressive behavior and early onset of alcohol use and alcohol problems in adolescence (Hawkins, Catalano, & Miller, 1992). Longitudinal research has also found that childhood rebelliousness and low self-esteem are associated with adolescent marijuana and drug use (Kandel, 1982) and that childhood anger predicts substance use in adolescence (Swaim et al., 1989). Most importantly, a high level of aggression in elementary school has been linked to adolescent (Kellam & Brown, 1982; Kellam, Ensminger, & Simon, 1980; Lochman, 1992) and adult drug and alcohol use (Lewis, Robbins, & Rice, 1985). Children with conduct disorders have also been found to begin using drugs earlier and are more likely to abuse multiple substances, compared to children without

JOHN E. LOCHMAN • Department of Psychology, University of Alabama, Tuscaloosa, Alabama 35487

conduct disorders (Lynskey & Fergusson, 1995). This developmental pattern can lead to a chronic pattern of substance abuse (Anthenelli et al., 1994; Frick, 1998).

Much of the research on childhood aggression has focussed on boys (Crick & Grotpeter, 1995), but relational aggression has been found to be as prevalent among girls as overt aggression is among boys (Cairns et al., 1989; Crick & Grotpeter, 1995). Relational aggression can involve harming and controlling others by threatening to withdraw acceptance and using social exclusion and rumor spreading as forms of retaliation. Relationally aggressive children have been found to have significant difficulties with both externalizing and internalizing behavior problems, and they display social–cognitive distortions that parallel those of more overtly aggressive children (Crick, 1997).

Although boys appear to have problems with overt aggressive behavior at about twice the rate of girls (Lochman & Conduct Problems Prevention Research Group, 1995), there are relatively few differences in the behavioral symptoms of boys and girls who have early-onset conduct problems (Webster-Stratton, 1996). Unfortunately, overtly aggressive girls experience a larger disparity between their behavior and that of their same-sex peers, and this can lead to greater social difficulties for them (Webster-Stratton, 1996). Research indicates that overtly aggressive girls and relationally aggressive boys are significantly more maladjusted than are children who engaged in more gender-appropriate forms of aggression (Crick, 1997). For example, girls with conduct disorder and co-morbid anxiety disorder have more severe and chronic forms of conduct disorder (Frick, 1998; Zoccolillo, 1992), which enhances their risk for substance abuse.

There is growing evidence that these serious adolescent outcomes for aggressive children are even more prevalent among children who are in ethnic minorities (Lochman & Lenhart, 1993). Economic deprivation and family instability contribute to the higher level of aggression found in ethnic minorities, and aggression may serve a survival function at times in lower socioeconomic status (SES) environments which may be characterized by higher levels of violence (Graham, Hudley, & Williams, 1992). However, despite these larger environmental effects on the aggressive behavior of minority children, and indications that certain parenting practices may have different types of impact on children's aggressive behavior in minority families (Deater-Deckard et al., 1996; Florsheim, Tolan, & Gorman-Smith, 1996; Forehand & Kotchick, 1996), minority children's aggressive behavior appears to be influenced by the same general types of causal factors, such as social–cognitive difficulties (Graham et al., 1998), as would be the case for Caucasian children. Future research will need to further explore these findings of socioeconomic status, minority status, and gender on children's aggressive behavior.

Co-occurrence of Predictors

To further explore the role of conduct problems as predictors of escalating substance use, Miller-Johnson et al. (1998) examined the co-occurrence of conduct and depressive problems and later substance use in 340 young boys and girls when they were in grades 6, 8, and 10. In sixth grade they were grouped according to (1) co-occurring conduct and depressive problems, (2) conduct problems only, (3) depressive problems only, or (4) neither conduct nor depressive problems. Overall, the boys with conduct problems displayed the highest levels of substance use, although those in the co-occurring group had an earlier onset of substance use and displayed significantly higher levels of use by the eighth grade. Subjects with only depressive problems displayed levels of substance use equivalent to subjects in the no-problem group. These findings highlight the importance of examining co-occurring symptoms as well as possible synergistic effects between conduct and depressive problems (Capaldi, 1992; Loeber & Keenan, 1994; Lewinsohn et al., 1993). In addition, the combined presence of depressive disorders and conduct disorders in children and adolescents leads to increased risk for suicidal thinking and makes the possibility of suicide a serious clinical concern (Frick, 1998). Capaldi (1992) found that 31% of children with both conduct disorder and a depressive disorder, in comparison to 7% of children with conduct disorder only, reported suicidal ideation.

Another important co-occurring condition for children with aggressive behavior problems is attention-deficit hyperactivity disorder (ADHD). ADHD is the most common co-morbid diagnosis in children with conduct disorder, and children with both ADHD and conduct problems have more severe degrees of psychopathology, including earlier onset of severe conduct problems, more violent offending, and earlier and greater substance abuse (August et al., 1996; Frick, 1998; Thompson et al., 1996). Children with ADHD have a basic problem with self-control, are often impulsive, intrusive, and act without apparent regard for the needs of others (Gold, 1998; Barkeley, 1997). These behavioral difficulties are hypothesized to be due to deficits in children's executive cognitive functioning, which are the result of mild dysfunctions in the prefrontal cortex. Lesions in this area of the brain have been found to lead to impulsivity, cognitive rigidity, and disorganized, uninhibited, and aggressive behavior (Giancola et al., 1996).

Executive cognitive functioning involves self-regulation of goal-directed-behavior and encompasses higher-order cognitive abilities, such as attention control, cognitive flexibility, planning, and self-monitoring (Giancola et al., 1996). Executive cognitive functioning deficits, assessed with neuropsychological tests, have been found to predict reactive aggressive behavior 2 years later in boys whose fathers had a history of substance abuse (Giancola, Moss, et al., 1996). These boys were initially assessed between 10 and 12 years of age. The reactive aggressive behavior assessed in early adolescence involved impulsive hostile reactions committed with little forethought. This relationship between executive cognitive functioning deficits and aggressive behavior has been found in girls as well (Giancola, Mezzich, & Tarter, 1998) and occurs even when children's intellectual functioning and socioeconomic status are controlled for (Giancola, Martin, et al., 1996). Most importantly, low executive cognitive functioning has been found to be associated with more severe drinking among adults (Giancola, Zeichner et al., 1996) and to be a better predictor than overactive behavior of adolescent tobacco, marijuana, and drug use and of severity of drug involvement (Aytaclar et al., 1998).

Co-morbidity of Outcomes

A particular concern for developmental psychopathology and for prevention is that substance use tends to co-occur with a variety of adolescent problem behaviors, including violence, school failure and dropout, depression, teen parenthood, and risky sexual practices. These problems increase sharply from early to middle adolescence. Delinquent behavior approximately doubles between the ages of 9 and 15 before and begins to decline at around the age of 17 (Achenbach, 1991). Similarly, alcohol and drug use increases rapidly from the sixth to the ninth grade and then increases only gradually throughout the late high school years in both rural and urban children (Oetting & Beauvais, 1990). Initial substance use typically occurs in seventh or eighth grade (Wills et al., 1996). Between ages 10 and 15, youths also have a threefold increase in depressed mood and a dramatic increase in affective disorder (Compas, Ey, & Grant, 1993; Kazdin, 1989). In addition, their sexual activity and pregnancy rates increase during this period. The surge in rates of these problem behaviors occurs as delinquency (Gillmore et al., 1991). Problem youth typically do not differ from their peers on just one dimension, such as aggressiveness, but vary on multiple behavioral dimensions related to poor self control, which leads to the high correlation among delinquency, substance abuse, and depression (Wills & Filer, 1996). These empirical findings are consistent with the predictions made by Problem Behavior Theory (Jessor & Jessor, 1977) that deviance proneness would involve associations among a variety of adolescent problem behaviors, including heavy drinking, marijuana use, delinquency, and precocious sexual intercourse. As individuals accumulate increasing numbers of risky problem behaviors, their odds for violent behavior increase. By age 14, risk taking, drug selling, gang membership, violence, and peer delinquency all combine to become the strongest predictors of later violence (Herrenkohl et al., 1998).

It is also apparent that youth who display antisocial behavior early rather than late (Moffitt, 1993; Patterson, Capaldi, & Bank, 1991) are at greatest risk for surges in problem behavior. Coie et al. (1997) found that children who were highly aggressive and rejected by their peers in early elementary school had the sharpest increases in juvenile offending between the ages of 11 and 16. Similarly, when adolescents are classified as either non-users of drugs, minimal experimenters, late starters, or escalators (who have a steady increase in substance use from 12 to 18 years of age), the escalators will have had family and peer problems that are typical for early-starting antisocial youth (Wills et al., 1996). While these results indicate that preadolescent aggression does predate adolescent substance use, it is not clear if aggression merely serves as a risk predictor or if aggressive behavior is part of the actual causal chain leading to substance use (Windle, 1990). Accordingly, preventive approaches are needed that intervene directly on aggressive behavior, using powerful intervention models, and then observe the effects on drug use. These results also suggest that the optimal timing for preventive interventions would be in the childhood and preadolescent years, before surges in serious problem behaviors begin to occur and begin to become increasingly co-morbid.

SOCIAL COMPETENCE

While risk status may extend back to innate characteristics such as temperament (i.e., Hawkins et al, 1992; Tarter, Alterman, & Edwards, 1985), the focus in this chapter is on malleable, formative factors in a child's social and psychological development that are related to childhood aggression and later substance abuse. One correlate of childhood aggression is poor social competence (as marked by rejection by peers and participation in deviant peer groups), which may be among the direct causes of substance use and of other adolescent conduct problems (Dishion & Patterson, in press; Ledingham, 1990). Children who are rejected by their peers are often highly aggressive (Coie et al, 1992), display characteristic social competence difficulties (Crick & Dodge, 1994; Dodge, 1986), and are at risk for early-onset drug use and other, often associated, negative adolescent outcomes, such as school failure and criminality (Brook et al, 1986; Coie, 1990; Hawkins, Catalano, & Miller, 1992; Kellam et al., 1980).

One reason aggressive-rejected children have difficulties in social competence is that they have distortions in the initial appraisal stages of information processing. At the encoding stage, aggressive-rejected children attend to and remember hostile cues (such as words, tone of voice, or facial expression) more than nonhostile social cues (Dodge et al., 1986; Milich & Dodge, 1984). Aggressive preadolescent and adolescent boys, for example, have less accurate recall of social cues from videotaped vignettes (Lochman & Dodge, 1994). At the interpretation stage, aggressive-rejected children attribute more hostile intentions to peers than do nonaggressive children (Dodge et al., 1990; Lochman & Dodge, 1994) and they perceive themselves to be less aggressive than observers rate them to be (Lochman, 1987; Lochman & Dodge, in press). These distorted appraisal processes are more apparent in reactive-aggressive youth than in proactive-aggressive youth (Dodge et al., 1997) and could be influenced by deficits in executive cognitive functioning (Giancola, Moss, et al, 1996).

Socially incompetent children may also have deficiencies in social problem-solving skills. Preadolescent aggressive children think of more direct action solutions and fewer verbal assertion solutions and tend to think of more physically aggressive solutions than do nonaggressive children (Asarnow & Callan, 1985, Dodge et al., 1986; Lochman & Lampron, 1986; Richard & Dodge, 1982). Aggressive adolescents generate fewer bargaining and compromise solutions and are less able to accurately perceive others' motives in order to create solutions that integrate the needs of both themselves and others (Lochman, Wayland, & White, 1993). At the response decision stage, aggressive children choose aggressive responses because they believe such behavior will stop aversive behavior by others (Lochman & Dodge, 1994, Perry, Perry, & Rasmussen, 1986). Violent, highly aggressive youth have more of these social–cognitive deficiencies than do moderately aggressive youth (Dunn, Lochman, & Colder, 1997; Lochman & Dodge, 1994).

Because of the lack of acceptance by most of their peer group, socially incompetent children become susceptible to the influence of deviant peer groups in adolescence (Coie et al., 1995), and substance use by peers is among the strongest predictors of substance use (Elliott et al., 1985; Kandel & Andrews, 1987). Aggressive youth also tend to value social goals such as dominance and revenge and tend not to value social goals such as affiliation (Lochman, Wayland & White, 1993). This dominance-oriented social goal pattern contributes to their maladaptive problem-solving style, consisting of limited capacity for negotiation and bargaining and excessive reliance on physically and verbally aggressive strategies.

Physiological Arousal

Recent research has begun to explore how other factors are linked to the distorted and deficient social–cognitive processes of aggressive children. Williams, Lochman, Phillips, & Barry (under review), for example, evaluated the relationship between attributional processes and physiological and emotional arousal as they relate to aggression. The physiological arousal (heart rate), emotional experience (moment-to-moment self report ratings of emotional state, and retrospective self-reports of emotional experience), and social cognitions (attributions of intent as measured by hypothetical peer provocation situations) of 51 fifth- and sixth-grade boys at three levels of aggression were examined. Subjects were assessed at baseline, and changes were observed following an experimental manipulation in which they were led to believe that an unknown peer, who was waiting in another room, was agitated and threatening to initiate a conflict with them. Data were analyzed to evaluate differences between high (HA), moderate (MA), and low aggressive (LA) boys' physiological and emotional reactions and attributional style in response to learning that a challenge to fight may be imminent. At baseline, HA boys had the lowest resting heart rates, while LA boys had the highest. After hearing about a possible threat, HA boys had the largest increase in heart rate and had relatively more hostile attributional biases on a hypothetical vignette measure. This study is the first to indicate a clear relationship ($r = .41$) between increases in heart rate and increased hostility of attribution. The results suggest the need for interventions to address aggressive children's abilities to regulate their physiological arousal; as their arousal dissipates, they may become less impulsive and less likely to over infer hostility in others.

Prior Expectations

In a recent study, we explored how the distorted perceptions of aggressive boys are maintained over time. Lochman and Dodge (1998) examined distorted self and peer perceptions in 48 aggressive and 48 nonaggressive boys at preadolescent and early adolescent age levels. Subjects completed semantic differential ratings of themselves and of their peer partners following two brief competitive discussion tasks and following a cooperative game-playing task. Subjects also rated their expectations for self and peer behavior prior to the first competitive interaction. Research assistants later rated videotapes of the interactions. Aggressive boys overestimated aggression in their partners and underestimated their own aggressiveness. These distorted perceptions of aggression carried over for aggressive boys into a cooperative task, indicating that aggressive boys have difficulty modulating their perceptions even when the overt threat of conflict is no longer present. Regression analyses results also indicated that aggressive boys' perceptions of their own behavior after the first interaction task are substantially affected by their prior expectations. Nonaggressive boys base their perceptions of themselves more on what they were observed to do than on what they expected to do. Aggressive boys' schemas for interpersonal behavior are rigid and relatively impermeable; they perceive what they expect to perceive, and this often involves distorted views of the threats coming from others.

Dominance Behaviors

Dominance-oriented social goals and resulting dominance behaviors are also likely to contribute to children's aggressiveness. Levy, Lochman, & Wells (1998) used a microanalytic behavioral coding system to examine the partner-oriented dominance (POD) and task-oriented-dominance (TOD) behavior of aggressive and non-aggressive boys engaged in a brief competitive verbal discussion. Coders viewing videotapes of these interactions attained adequate inter-rater reliability on eight specific behaviors related to POD and TOD. Aggressive boys did not have higher overall rates of POD, but they did respond with significantly higher levels of POD following a partner's TOD behaviors on the task. This indicates that the controlling, bossy behaviors (POD) of aggressive boys occur largely in response to assertive but competent (TOD) behaviors of their peers. High levels of POD behaviors were also seen in boys whose parents provided high levels of punishment and low levels of facilitation responses on hypothetical vignettes of parent–child difficulties. More authoritarian parenting styles, which involve high levels of parental control in the absence of parental warmth and support, appear to be related to boys' internalization of dominance goals and reactive dominance behaviors. These findings reinforce the need to help aggressive boys coping with lower-level assertion and dominance behaviors by peers and to intervene with parents to promote more authoritative parenting styles that provide both control and warmth. Cognitive–behavioral prevention programs, working with high-risk children and parents in structured groups, would be an effective way to address these maladaptive dominance reactions of children and parents (Lochman & Wells, 1996).

Stress and Coping

Wills and Filer (1996) reviewed the results of a series of research studies and propose a stress-coping model for understanding adolescent substance abuse. In this model, the strongest precursor of adolescent substance use is a complex of poor coping abilities, which reflect the adolescent's perception that he or she is unable to cope with problems. Certain temperament factors, such as high activity level and dysregulated moods, have been found to lead to poor behavioral coping, poor self-control, more negative life events, and more anger and helplessness. Unregulated anger and frustration (Swaim et al., 1989) and low levels of emotional restraint (Farrell & Danish, 1993) have been found to have direct effects on adolescent drug use, independent of the equally malignant effects of associating with drug-using peers. When faced with stressful situations, an adolescent's use of active behavioral coping (characterized by direct verbal and nonverbal behaviors that resolve perceived problems) and low use of avoidant coping (characterized by withdrawal, helplessness, and anger) have been found to be related to avoidance of substance use (Wills & Filer, 1996). Because active coping moderates, or reduces, the negative impact of avoidant coping, intervention should attempt to enhance active coping efforts. Unfortunately, substance use can have a coping function itself. Adolescents tend to use drugs as a coping mechanism when they have limited and ineffective active coping resources (Wills & Filer, 1996). Smoking and heavy drinking have been found to be motivated by efforts to regulate emotion by calming down, by cheering up, or by relieving boredom (Wills & Filer, 1996). Therefore, a task of preventive intervention should be to use cognitive–behavioral programs to help adolescents develop active coping skills, emotional regulation abilities, and positive problem-solving abilities in order to forestall later substance use (Lochman & Wells, 1996).

Deviant Peer-Group Associations

As a result of poor social competence and active social rejection by peers (often because of highly aggressive, noxious behavior directed toward peers), children and adolescents may gravitate to a deviant peer group in early adolescence (Coie, 1990). These socially rejected and disliked youth still typically have social goals that place a substantial value on affiliating with peers (Lochman, Wayland, & White, 1993) and begin to spend time with the only type of peer group that will usually accept them, namely, peers who are similarly socially rejected and antisocial (Cairns et al, 1988; Coie et al., 1992; Coie et al., 1995). As youth begin to spend increasing amounts of time in a deviant peer group they are exposed to frequent negative referent models, reinforcement of negative attitudes and behaviors, and peer pressure to engage in increasingly antisocial behavior. Highly antisocial dyads have been found to reinforce each others' delinquent talk more than low antisocial dyads (Dishion, Patterson, & Griesler, 1994). They often increase their rates of school truancy and dropout, placing themselves in even more contact with each other, which leads directly to increased rates of delinquency (e.g., Coie et al., 1995, 1997). Exposure to high levels of peer substance abuse within the deviant peer groups is also associated with high levels of concurrent drug use by adolescents (Dishion et al., 1988; Kandel, 1982) and with escalating use of drugs over time (Wills et al., 1996). The steepest growth of substance use occurs among adolescents with drug-using peers (Chassin et al., 1996). Preventive intervention should, thus, increase children's social competence so they can more successfully become involved with average and pro-social peer groups and decrease their involvement with deviant peer groups. The latter goal *of decreasing children's involvement with deviant peers* can also be accomplished through intervention with parents, especially by increasing *parents'* monitoring skills, as discussed in the following.

PARENTING PRACTICES

Family and parenting factors exert a direct effect on adolescent substance abuse (Bry et al., in press; Chassin et al., 1996)) as well as indirect effects through their association with childhood aggression and antisocial behaviors, poor social competence, and academic failure (Santisteban, Szapocznik, & Kurtines, 1994). Aggressive childhood behavior can be the result of early experiences with parents who provide harsh discipline, poor problem-solving models, vague commands, and poor monitoring of children's behavior (Patterson, 1986; Patterson & Bank, 1989). Poor parenting is exacerbated in a reciprocal manner by the child's aggressive, oppositional behavior. Parental child-rearing styles are also accompanied, and maintained, by the parents' own dysregulated anger and hostile attributional biases (Dix & Lochman, 1990).

Recent research suggests that harsh parenting, poor monitoring, and lack of parental warmth are mediating factors often related to children's conduct problems and to adolescent substance use in complex ways. This set of mediating factors should be a focus for preventive parent intervention research programs. Recent research has also begun to examine how children's traits moderate the relationship between parenting practices and children's behavior and how parental social cognition appears to provide the socializing framework for children's social cognition (Colder, Lochman, & Wells, 1997; Lochman, Wells, & Colder, 1997).

Harsh Parenting

Substantial research over the past 30 years has indicated that harsh parenting practices can contribute to the development of children's oppositional and aggressive behavior, which in turn can be a risk marker for subsequent substance use (e.g., Lochman & Wayland, 1994). Evidence for the link between harsh parenting and childhood conduct problems comes from research involving direct observation of parent–child interactions in naturalistic and laboratory settings (e.g., Patterson, 1982, 1986; Patterson & Banks, 1989; Wahler & Graves, 1983) and from parental self-reports of their behavior toward their children, often using measures such as the Conflict Tactics Scale (Dodge, Bates, & Pettit, 1990). Some research indicates that marital disharmony may predict negative outcomes (Jenkins & Smith, 1991). However, Jouriles, Barling, and O'Leary (1987) found that even among families experiencing severe marital violence, direct parent-to-child aggression often predicts childhood conduct problems. In these studies, harsh parenting typically involves the relatively frequent use of physical and verbal aggression toward children and may include actual physical abuse (e.g. Dodge et al., 1990).

Once harsh parenting has contributed to an escalating cycle of aggressive behavior in a child, the child's later movement toward more severe conduct problems and substance abuse may be more the result of continuity in the behavior itself, rather than ongoing harsh parenting. For example, Farrington and Hawkins (1991) found that harsh and erratic punishment is associated with the early onset of delinquency but minimally related to later persistence in crime. In a similar finding, but at a much earlier age, Bates, Pettit, and Dodge (1995) found that self-reported coercive discipline practices are associated with aggressiveness in kindergarten (using teachers and peer ratings), but that only kindergarten aggression predicted first grade aggression. In these two studies, harsh parental discipline seemed to have its primary effect early in the developmental sequence, and highly aggressive behavior, once activated, tended to be self-maintaining and demonstrated continuity.

In a recent study, Maughan, Pickles, and Quinton (1995) further explored whether harsh parenting has its negative effects primarily because the aggressive behavior is self-maintaining or because there are later effects of early harsh parenting. Based on a high-risk sample of parents receiving psychiatric services and a general population sample from London, boys and girls were found to receive equivalent amount of harsh parenting, according to both prospective and retrospective measures. For males in particular, the effects of harsh parenting were clearly mediated through the development of childhood conduct disorder, which led to difficulties in functioning in adult life. Prospective measures indicated that harsh parenting is related to the development of conduct disorder in childhood and has less effect on the persistence of problems or on the onset of new problems in adulthood. However, the potentially more biased retrospective measures did suggest some additional latent effects for early harsh parenting on adult adjustment, with women being more vulnerable to hostile relations with their fathers.

Part of the reason for the stability and continuity of aggressive behavior is the effect of harsh parenting on the development of social–cognitive distortions and deficiencies that then mediate the relationship between harsh parenting and subsequent self-sustaining childhood aggressive behavior. Harsh and restrictive physical punishment has been found to contribute to children's maladaptive information processing in terms of poor cue encoding, hostile attributional bias, action-oriented solution generation, and positive expectations for the effects of aggressive behavior (Pettit et al., 1991; Weiss et al., 1992).

This research on harsh parenting suggests the importance of intervening with parents early (in the preschool and very early elementary years) to prevent the stabilization of an aggressive behavioral pattern and the child's associated social-cognitive difficulties. It also suggests that later intervention will probably need to be provided within a package of other interventions directed at the child's social–cognitive and academic difficulties in order to interrupt the stabilized behavior pattern evident among children with early-onset conduct disorder.

Poor Monitoring

One of the strongest links between parenting practices and substance abuse involves poor parental monitoring. Monitoring involves adequate awareness and supervision of children's behavior, even when the children are not physically in the presence of the parent. High levels of parental monitoring can insulate children from drug and alcohol use and a broad range of other antisocial behaviors (Snyder, Dishion, & Patterson, 1986; Steinberg, 1987). According to the Oregon Social Learning Center model (e.g., Dishion, Reid, & Patterson, 1988), ineffective parental monitoring and parenting skills lead to poor social skills and aversive behavior among children, which in turn leads to association with deviant peer groups and to drug and alcohol use.

Fletcher, Darling, and Steinberg (1995) examined the joint influence of parental monitoring and peer drug use on substance use. High school students provided self-report information about parental monitoring, substance use, and their closest friends at two annual assessments. Cross-sectional analyses indicated that parental monitoring was negatively associated with levels of substance use for boys and girls. Longitudinal analyses indicated that high levels of parental monitoring (1) discouraged boys and girls from beginning to use drugs, (2) encouraged boys to lessen their involvement with drugs when they were already heavily involved, and (3) encouraged girls to move from experimentation to nonuse. However, parent monitoring did not affect boys' movement from experimentation to heavier use or nonuse over time; instead boys moved toward the levels of substance use reported by their immediate friends. Thus, for transitions from the experimenting stage, both parent monitoring and peer groups influenced changes for girls. For boys, the peer group was critical.

The implications for prevention are that promoting parental monitoring is an appropriate strategy for deterrence and prevention of initial experimentation with drugs and that monitoring can assist girls in reversing their initial experimentation with drugs. For boys who are already experimenting with drugs, monitoring may be useful in potentially disrupting their association with deviant peers. Fletcher et al. (1995) note that parental monitoring can help to deter children's substance use and their association with drug-using peers, making children "double-protected."

Parental Warmth

Authoritative, as opposed to authoritarian, parents have adolescents who tend to be less engaged in substance use (Baumrind, 1991; Lamborn et al., 1991). Authoritative parents are both responsive and demanding. They provide firm and consistent limit setting but also relate to their adolescents in a respectful, warm manner. The combination of parents in two-parent families can produce a form of authoritative parenting in which maternal affection and paternal nonpermissiveness are related to lower rates of adolescent substance use (Brook, Whiteman, & Gordon (1983). Firm limit setting is not the same as rigid parental control or directiveness. Parents who display high levels of rigid control have boys who display higher expectations that aggressive behavior will work to meet their needs (Lochman, Cohen, & Wayland, 1991). This suggests that a parent's rigid directiveness may increase children's aggressiveness and thus increase their risk for substance use.

Recent research on positive parenting behaviors supports the bidirectional nature of parenting and children's behavior (Kandel & Wu, 1995). In a longitudinal study of 208 mothers and children, who were interviewed twice over a 6-year interval, parental reports of positive (closeness to children, close supervision) and negative parenting (punitive discipline) and of children's behavior (aggression, control problems, positive relations with parent, well-adjusted) were collected. Negative parenting was found to reinforce negative behavior in children more than positive parenting was able to reduce children's negative behavior. Most importantly, negative behavior in children was found to evoke significant decreases in positive reinforcing behaviors by parents as well as small increases in negative parenting. In this regard, negative childhood behavior was found to have more effects on parental behavior than did positive childhood behavior.

These results again suggest the need for early preventive intervention to avoid deterioration in the level of positive, supportive parental behavior, which may have been present at the early elementary school age. For later indicated prevention efforts with parents of aggressive early-adolescent children, a primary goal may be to reengage levels of positive parental behaviors that may have been present when the child was younger.

Parenting and Childhood Temperament

A study by Colder, Lochman, and Wells, (1997) assessed the moderating effects of children's activity level and fear on relations between parenting practices and childhood aggression and depressive symptoms in 64 fourth- and fifth-grade boys. Findings from multiple regression analyses showed that poorly monitored active boys and fearful boys who were exposed to harsh discipline exhibited high levels of aggression. However, less active and less fearful boys were less affected by negative parenting behavior. In addition, boys characterized by high fear who were exposed to harsh discipline or whose parents were extremely over involved showed elevated levels of depressive symptoms. These findings suggest that integrating children's individual differences with parenting models enhances our understanding of the etiology of childhood disorders. Specifically, the results indicate that certain deficient parenting practices are likely to be associated with children's behavioral problems, primarily when the children have certain temperamental features involving high activity and high fear. In a similar pattern of findings, ineffective parenting has been found to lead to conduct problems primarily in children with callous, unemotional traits (Wootton et al., 1997). Accordingly, intervention should more heavily emphasize altering these parenting practices (harsh discipline, poor monitoring) when children rate high on activity and fear.

Parental and Childhood Social-Cognitive Processes

Sayed, Lochman, and Wells (1998) examined relationships between parental thoughts about their child-rearing practices and children's solutions to social problems in 147 high-risk children and their parents using two hypothetical vignettes. Problem-solving strategies on the Problem-Solving Measure for Conflict (Lochman & Lampron, 1986) were aggregated into five clusters: aggressive solutions, negative verbal solutions, action-oriented/indirect verbal solutions, direct verbal solutions, and irrelevant solutions. Child-rearing strategies on the Structured Child-Rearing Style Inventory (Lochman, Cohen, & Wayland, 1991) were also consolidated into four clusters: punishment, directive, facilitative, and nonconfrontational. Facilitative parenting was related to children's use of more direct verbal solutions and fewer irrelevant solutions, while punishment was related to more action-oriented/indirect verbal solutions and more irrelevant solutions. Lochman, Wells, and Colder, (June, 1997) extended this line of research by examining the relationship between children's and parent's social–cognitive processes and children's social goals and aggressive behavior. The sample consisted of preadolescent boys and their primary caretakers: three-quarters of the sample were part of an aggressive high-risk group. Data collected during individual assessments consisted of responses to hypothetical vignettes, audiotaped stimuli, and questionnaires. Children's aggressive behaviors were assessed with teacher ratings. Multiple regression findings indicated that distinct patterns of social–cognitive processes were associated with dominance and affiliation goals. Boys with high dominance goals reported little sadness in response to situations that typically evoke sadness. Boys with high affiliation goals had competent attribution and problem-solving skills, low levels of trait anger, and parents who used noncontrolling parenting strategies. Aggressive behavior in boys was predicted by high levels of dominance and low levels of affiliation as well as by poor accuracy in affect labeling, external locus of control, and low levels of an authoritative parenting style. Both children's and parental social–cognitive processes were useful in predicting children's aggressive behavior, and they did so in relatively direct and additive ways rather than being mediated through each other. These results have implications for the etiology of children's social cognitions and indicate that cognitive–behavioral interventions could be usefully directed at both children and parents due to the additive nature of these effects on children's behavior. These interventions could address children's social problem-solving skills in children's groups and parental methods of disciplining their children and facilitating their children's development of competent problem-solving skills.

PREVENTIVE INTERVENTION

Since childhood aggression has been demonstrated to be a relatively stable behavior pattern and a significant risk factor for subsequent substance use difficulties, indicated prevention effects should be directed at elementary school children identified as aggressive and disruptive (Gelfand et al., 1986). Indicated prevention involves early identification of children who are just beginning to manifest adjustment difficulties and provision of an intervention to reduce their risk status, if possible, and prevent further, more severe maladjustment (Institute of Medicine, 1994). Earlier intervention can ameliorate problems completely and with less intensive effort, since the problems are less well developed and ingrained (Allen et al., 1976). However, conceptual models for the development of adjustment disorder are crucial for universal and indicated preventive interventions (Conduct Problems Prevention Research Group, 1992).

In our conceptual model, the principal formative factors that influence the development of adolescent substance abuse include parenting practices and children's social competence. Parenting practices are in turn affected by background factors, such as parental psychopathology, parental insularity, and marital discord. Preventive interventions with aggressive children who are at risk for substance abuse, therefore, should target malleable mediator processes, such as parenting practices and children's social competence.

Cognitive–Behavioral Intervention

Our Coping Power Program used two types of intervention: a behavioral intervention with parents that focuses on reducing poor parenting practices and a cognitive behavior intervention with children that focuses on changing distorted or deficient social cognitive processes and enhancing social competence and self regulation. Controlled studies have shown that cognitive behavior intervention with aggressive preadolescent children can produce reductions in disruptive and aggressive behavior in both school and home settings (Kazdin et al., 1989, 1987a,b, 1991; Lochman et al, 1984, 1989; Lochman & Curry, 1986). Follow-ups during the first year after intervention indicate that these behavioral gains are maintened (Kazdin et al., 1987a,b; Lochman & Lampron, 1988). A 3-year follow up (Lochman, 1992) found that aggressive boys who had received school-based cognitive–behavioral intervention in elementary school had lower levels of marijuana, drug, and alcohol involvement than did untreated aggressive children. The treated boys were functioning in a range typical for nonaggressive, low-risk children. They maintained their gains in social problem-solving skills and self-esteem. However, the reduction in off-task and classroom behavior were only maintained in a subset of boys who received a second-year booster program. These results illustrate the potential buffering effect of social problem-solving skills and perceived competence on preventing subsequent drug use among high-risk aggressive children (Hawkins et al., 1992). Similar effects (reduced alcohol use) were found for a classroom-based universal prevention program focusing on social problem-solving skills, assertiveness skills, and development of pro-social networks (Caplan et al., 1992).

Social competence promotion programs have also been successfully used to focus directly on drug use reduction (Schinke, Botvin, & Orlandi, 1991). These programs combine social influence resistance approaches with training in problem solving and decision making. Such programs have yielded reductions in the prevalence and onset of cigarette smoking, alcohol use, and marijuana use (e.g., Botvin, 1986; Hansen et al., 1988; Pentz et al., 1989). Prevention effects were still evident one to 8 years later in some studies (Botvin et al., 1990).

Multicomponent Prevention Programs for Parents and Children

Research indicates that parent-directed interventions designed to prevent substance use can be effective (Bry, 1993). For example, De Marsh and Kumpfer (1986) found that drug-abusing parents can be successfully trained in more effective parenting styles, which results in reduced rates of behavioral problems in their children and in children's decreased self-report of intentions to smoke and use alcohol.

Hawkins et al. (1992) suggest that a promising line for prevention research lies in testing interventions that target multiple early risk factors for drug abuse. In one series of studies, Kazdin and his colleagues (Kazdin et al., 1987; Kazdin, Siegel, & Bass, 1992) combined behavioral parent training with cognitive problem-solving skills training for preadolescents to reduce antisocial behavior in children. The combined intervention was more effective than either parent training or problem-solving skills training alone in placing a greater proportion of children within the range of normal functioning. These results were maintained at a 1-year follow up.

Multicomponent prevention trials have also been directed at substance abuse in youth. Pentz and colleagues (Johnson et al., 1990; Pentz et al., 1989) developed a multicomponent program including a 10-session school program emphasizing drug use resistance skills for children in grade 6 or 7. It included homework sessions with children and parents, training of parents in positive parent–child communication skills, training of community leaders, and mass-media coverage. Randomly assigned control schools received only the latter two components. Three years after their involvement, children in the program had reduced prevalence rates of monthly cigarette smoking and marijuana use. These results were obtained for both high-risk and low-risk children.

Although the results of these multicomponent studies are encouraging, a study by Dishion and Andrews (1995) raises troubling concerns about possible iatrogenic effects of child-focused group interventions. Children in sixth through eighth grades and their parents were randomly assigned to parent-focus-only, teen-focus-only, combined parent and teen focus, and a control condition for self-directed change. These four groups were also compared to a quasiexperimental control group that was not randomly assigned. Interventions involved 12 weekly 90-minute sessions. Both the children's and the parent's interventions produced reductions in coercive behavior by children and parents during observed parent–child interactions. However, the parent-only intervention produced short-term behavioral improvements at school (which faded at the 1-year follow-up) while the teen-only intervention produced higher levels of tobacco use and higher teacher-rated behavior problems by the one-year follow-up. The teen-only intervention appeared to produce this iatrogenic effect through peer reinforcement of deviant talk during group sessions.

Because of these marked differences in findings, future research should explore whether, and under which conditions, childhood interventions can augment parental intervention. Ongoing multicomponent studies, such as the Coping Power Program (Lochman & Wells, 1996) and the Fast Track Program (Conduct Problems Prevention Research Groups, 1992), which are discussed in the following, may be useful in generating hypotheses about how the composition, timing, and content of childhood intervention programs may affect outcomes. For example, in preliminary analyses of the Coping Power Program, immediate postintervention effects with two cohorts of children and with 1-year follow-up effects of the first cohort in the Coping Power Program, we find indications of the importance of additive effects of intervention as well as for timing of intervention at important developmental transition points. In the two cohorts, 183 boys identified as being at risk for substance abuse because of high levels of teacher-rated aggression in 4th or 5th grades were randomly assigned to three conditions. The first two conditions were a school-based children's component and combined children and parents component. The third was a no-treatment condition. The children's component focused on the social–cognitive difficulties of aggressive children and was based on an anger coping program (Lochman, 1992). This component was provided in a group format in boys' elementary and middle schools and lasted for 33 sessions over 1 1/4 years. The parent's component was provided in a group format in community and school settings. It consisted of 16 sessions over the same 1 1/4-year intervention period. The parental intervention addressed alternate, less harsh methods of discipline, increased monitoring, and stress management for the parents.

The initial outcome analyses indicate that the Coping Power intervention has had broad effects at postintervention and at follow-up on the boys' social competence, social information processing, locus of control, temperament and on parenting behavior, parental social cognition, the marital relationship, and children's behavior (Lochman & Wells, in press a, in press b). Not all variables were influenced by the intervention at each time point and some effects were qualified by grade level and level of aggression. However, the Coping Power intervention produced substantial change on a range of factors that would be expected to reduce these boys' future risk for substance use and substance abuse. Perhaps most importantly, the effects appear to be generally maintaining at the 1-year follow-up for Cohort 1. Most intervention effects, especially for children's social competence, social information processing, and school behavior were apparent in both intervention groups; but certain effects, such as parental sense of efficacy and satisfaction with their parenting and aspects of their marital relationship, were affected only by the Coping Power Program condition and appear to be a result specifically of the parental intervention.

The results indicate that the age and aggression levels are important moderator variables for this intervention. Positive intervention effects were more apparent on social information-processing, perceived competence, and school behavior variables for boys who received interventions in the fourth and fifth grades than in fifth and sixth grades. This is likely due to the relatively greater ease in delivering school-based groups in elementary school than in middle school and to changes in the relative openness to intervention of elementary-school versus middle-school boys. Pragmatic difficulties in delivering the group intervention in middle school included a reduced time for group sessions due to more rigid class schedules, school counselors who had less time and interest in serving as co-leaders, and teachers who knew each child's behavior less intensively because students changed classes during the day. In contrast, certain parent-rated effects (home aggression and externalizing behavior at post-test intervention and marital satisfaction and marital aggression at follow up) were most evident for fifth- and sixth-grade intervention boys, perhaps because parental motivation to participate in the intervention was increased due to the parental concerns about their children's transition to middle school and its attendant behavior, social, and academic changes. When initial aggression level served as a moderator for the intervention effects, it primarily indicated that the intervention was more successful with highly aggressive boys (e.g., Lochman & Dodge, 1994).

The Fast Track Program (Conduct Problems Prevention Research Group, 1992) is an extensive, comprehensive, long-lasting prevention program that is specifically targeted at high-risk children who are displaying early-onset disruptive behaviors in kindergarten. Following the kindergarten screening by teachers, the high-risk children who had been randomly assigned to the intervention began receiving social skills training, tutoring, peer-pairing activities with non-risk peers, and teacher-administrated, classroom-wide social competence training in first grade. The latter program served to provide universal prevention as well as to reinforce positive concepts and skills with the high-risk children in the classroom. The parents of the high-risk children participated in parent groups, in parent–child activities, and in home visits. These developmentally guided interventions continued with the high-risk children through the elementary school grades. Adolescent-phase interventions will continue with high-risk children through the 10th grade to prevent an array of adolescent problem behaviors, including substance abuse, conduct disorder, and delinquency. Initial analyses indicate that the intervention children, in comparison to control children, have begun showing significant improvements in social cognition skills, reading achievement, social acceptance by peers, and reductions in problem behaviors in the early elementary school years (Conduct Problems Prevention Research Group, 1999, 2002).

These results suggest that preventive intervention that focuses directly on established, mutable precursors of substance use can have immediate and sustained effects. Social competence, parenting practices, and children's aggressive behavior can be effectively targeted by preventive interventions delivered at key developmental transition points. Future longitudinal research should continue to explore whether intervention-produced changes in these precursors to substance abuse produce clear preventive effects on adolescent substance use and abuse.

REFERENCES

Achenbach, T. M. (1991). *Integrative guide for the 1991 CBCL/4–18, YSR and TRF Profiles.* Burlington: University of Vermont.

Allen G., Chinsky, J., Larcen, S., Lochman, J., & Selinger, H. (1976). *Community psychology and the schools: A behaviorally oriented multilevel preventive approach.* New York: Wiley.

Anthenelli, R. M., Smith, T. L., Irwin, M. R., & Schuckit, M. A. (1994). A comparative study of criteria for subgrouping alcoholics: The primary/secondary diagnostic scheme versus variations of the type 1/type 2 criteria. *American Journal of Psychiatry, 151,* 1468–1474.

Asarnow, J. R., & Callan, J. W. (1985). Boys with peer adjustment problems: Social cognitive processes. *Journal of Consulting and Clinical Psychology, 53,* 80–87.

August, G. J., Realmuto, G. M., MacDonald, A. W., III, Nugent, S. M., & Crosby, R. (1996). Prevalence of ADHD and comorbid disorders among elementary school children screened for disruptive behavior. *Journal of Abnormal Child Psychology, 34,* 571–595.

Aytaclar, S., Tarter, R. E., Kirisci, L., & Lu, S. L. (1998). *Association between hyperactivity and executive cognitive functioning in childhood and substance use in early adolescence.* Unpublished Manuscript, University of Pittsburgh.

Barkley, R. A. (1997). *ADHD and the nature of self control.* New York: Guilford.

Bates, J. E., Pettit, G. S., & Dodge, K. A. (1995). Family and child factors in stability and change in children's aggressiveness in elementary school. In: J. McCord (Ed.) *Coercion and punishment in long-term perspectives* (pp. 124–138). Cambridge University Press, Cambridge England.

Baumrind, D. (1991). The influence of parenting style of adolescent competence and substance use. *Journal of Early Adolescence, 11,* 56–95.

Baumrind, D. (1983, October). *Why adolescents take chances-And why they don't.* Paper presented at the National Institute of Child Health and Human Development, Bethesda, MD.

Botvin, G. (1986). Substance abuse prevention efforts: Recent developments and future directions. *Journal of School Health, 56,* 369–374.

Botvin, G., Baker, E., Dusenbury, L., Torfu, S., & Botvin, E. M. (1990). Preventing adolescent drug abuse through a multi-modal cognitive-behavioral approach: Results of a 3-year study. *Journal of Consulting and Clincial Psychology, 58,* 437–446.

Brook, J. S., Gordon, A. S., Whiteman, M., & Cohen, P. (1986). Some models and mechanisms for explaining the impact of maternal and adolescent characteristics on adolescent stage of drug use. *Developmental Psychology, 22,* 460–467.

Brook, J. S., Whiteman, M., & Gordon, A. S. (1983). Stages of drug use in adolescence: Personality, peer and family correlates. *Developmental Psychology, 19,* 269–277.

Bry, B. H. (1993). Research on family setting's role in substance abuse. *NTIS No. PB94-175692,* Piscataway, NJ, Rutgers—The State University of New Jersey.

Bry, B. H., Catalano, R. F., Kumpfer, K., Lochman, J. E., & Szapocznik, J. (1999). Scientific findings from family prevention intervention research. In R. Ashery (Ed.), *Family-based prevention interventions.* Rockville, MD: National Institute of Drug Abuse (pp. 103–129).

Cairns, R. B., Cairns, B. D., Neckerman, H. J., Ferguson, L. L., & Gariepy, J. L. (1989). Growth and aggression: 1. Childhood to early adolescence. *Developmental Psychology, 25,* 320–330.

Cairns, R. B., Cairns, B. D., Neckerman, H. J., Gest, S. D., & Gariepy, J. L. (1988). Social networks and aggressive behavior: Peer support or peer rejection? *Developmental Psychology, 24,* 815–823.

Capaldi, D. M. (1992). Co-occurrence of conduct problems and depressive symptoms in early adolescent boys: II. A 2-year follow-up at Grade 8. *Development and Psychopathology, 4,* 125–144.

Caplan, M., Weisberg, R. P., Grober, J. S., Sivo, P. J., Grady, K., & Jacoby, C. (1992). Social competence promotion with inner-city and suburban young adolescents: Effects on social adjustment and alcohol use. *Journal of Consulting and Clinical Psychology, 60,* 56–63.

Chassin, L., Curran, P. J., Hussong, A. M., & Colder, C. R. (1996). The relation of parent alcoholism to adolescent substance use: A longitudinal follow-up study. *Journal of Abnormal Psychology, 105,* 70–80.

Cloninger, C. R., Sigvardsson, S., & Bohman, M. (1988). Childhood personality predicts alcohol abuse in young adults. *Alcoholism, 12,* 494–503.

Coie, J. D. (1990). Toward a theory of peer rejection. In S. R. Asher & J. D. Coie (Eds.), *Peer rejection in childhood* (pp. 365–402). New York: Cambridge University Press.

Coie, J. D., Lochman, J. E., Terry, R., & Hyman, C. (1992). Predicting early adolescent disorders from childhood aggression and peer rejection. *Journal of Consulting and Clinical Psychology, 60,* 783–792.

Coie, J. D. Miller-Johnson, S., Terry, R., Maumary-Gremaud, A., Lochman, J. E., & Hyman, C. (1997). *The influence of peer rejection, aggression, and deviant peer associations on juvenile offending among African-American Adolescents.* Unpublished manuscript, Duke University.

Coie, J. D., Terry, R., Lenox K., Lochman, J., & Hyman, C. (1995). Childhood peer rejection and aggression as predictors of stable patterns of adolescent disorders. *Development and Psychology, 7,* 697–713.

Coie, J. D., Terry, R., Zakriski, A., & Lochman, J. E. (1995). Early adolescent social influences on delinquent behavior. In J. McCord (Ed.), *Coercion and punishment in long-term perspectives* (pp. 229–244). New York: Cambridge University Press.

Colder, C. R., Lochman, J. E., & Wells, K. C. (1997). The moderating effects of children's fear and activity level on relations between parenting practices and childhood symptomatology. *Journal of Abnormal Child Psychology, 25,* 251–263.

Compas, B. E., Ey, S., & Grant, K. E. (1993). Taxonomy, assessment and diagnosis of depression during adolescence. *Psychology Bulletin, 114,* 323–344.

Conduct Problems Prevention Research Group (in alphabetical order: K. Bierman, J. Coie, K. Dodge, M. Greenberg, J. Lochman, & R. McMahon) (1992). A developmental and clinical model for the prevention of conduct disorders: The FAST Track Program. *Development and Psychopathology, 4,* 505–527.

Conduct Problems Prevention Research Group (1999). Initial impact of the Fast Track prevention trial for conduct problems: I. The high-risk sample. *Journal of Consulting and Clinical Psychology, 67,* 631–647.

Conduct Problems Prevention Research Group (2002). Evaluation of the first three years of the Fast Track prevention trial with children at high risk of adolescent conduct problems. *Journal of Abnormal Child Psychology, 30,* 19–35.

Crick, N. R. (1997). Engagement in gender normative versus nonnormative forms of aggression: Links to social-psychological adjustment. *Developmental Psychology, 33,* 610–617.

Crick, N. R., & Dodge, K. A. (1994). A review and reformulation of social information-processing mechanisms in children's social adjustment. *Psychology Bulletin, 115,* 74–101.

Crick, N. R., & Grotpeter, J. K. (1995). Relational aggression, gender, and social-psychological adjustment. *Child Development, 66,* 710–722.

Deater-Deckard, K., Dodge, K. A., Bates, J. E., & Pettit, G. S. (1996). Physical discipline among African American and European American mothers: Links to children's externalizing behaviors. *Developmental Psychology, 32,* 1065–1072.

DeMarsh, J., & Kumpfer, K. (1986). Family-oriented interventions for the prevention of chemical dependency in children and adolescents. In. S. Griswold-Ezekoye, K., Kumpfer, & W. J. Bukoski (Eds), *Childhood and chemical abuse: Prevention and intervention* (pp. 117–151). New York: Haworth.

Dishion, T. J., & Andrews, D. W. (1995). Preventive escalation in problem behavior with high-risk young adolescents: Immediate and 1-Year Outcomes. *Journal of Consulting and Clinical Psychology, 63,* 538–548.

Dishion, T. J., & Patterson, G. R. (1993). Childhood screening for early adolescent problem behavior: A multiple gating stratefy. In M. Singer & L. Singer (Eds.), *Handbook for screening adolescents at psychosocial risk.* Lexington, MA: Lexington Books (pp. 375–399).

Dishion, T. J., Patterson, G. R., & Griesler, P. C. (1994). Peer adaptations in the development of antisocial behavior: A confluence model. In L. R. Huesmann (Eds.), *Aggressive behavior: Current perspectives* (pp. 61–95). New York: Plenum Press.

Dishion, T. J., Reid, J. B., & Patterson, G. R. (1988). Empirical guidelines for a family intervention for adolescent drug use. *Journal of Chemical Dependency Treatment, 2,* 181–216.

Dix, T., & Lochman, J. E. (1990). Social cognition and negative reactions to children: A comparison of mothers of aggressive and nonaggressive boys. *Journal of Social and Clinical Psychology, 9,* 418–438.

Dodge, K. A. (1986). A social information processing model of social competence in children. In M. Perlmutter (Eds.), *Cognitive perspectives on children's social and behavioral Development* (pp. 77–125). Hillsdale, NJ: Earlbaum.

Dodge, K. A., Bates, J. E., & Pettit, G. S. (1990). Mechanisms in the cycle of violence. *Science, 250,* 1678–1683.

Dodge, K. A., Lochman, J. E., Harnish, J. D., Bates, J. E., & Pettit, G. S. (1997). Reactive and proactive aggression in school children and psychiatrically-impaired chronically-assaultive youth. *Journal of Abnormal Psychology, 106,* 37–51.

Dodge, K. A., Pettit, G. S., & Bates, J. E. (1997). *Adolescent stories.* Unpublished manuscript. Vanderbilt University, Nashville, TN.

Dodge, K. A., Pettit, G. S., McClaskey, C. L., & Brown, M. M. (1986). Social competence in children. *Monographs of the Society for Research in Child Development, 51* (2 Serial No. 213).

Dodge, K. A., Price, J. M., Bachorowski, J., & Newman, J. P. (1990). Hostile attributional biases in severely aggressive adolescents. *Journal of Abnormal Psychology, 99,* 385–392.

Dunn, S. E., Lochman, J. E., & Colder, C. (1997). Social problem-solving skills in boys with conduct and oppositional defiant disorders. *Aggressive Behavior, 23,* 457–469.

Elliott, D. S., Huizinga, D., & Ageton, S. S. (1985). *Explaining delinquency and drug use.* Beverly Hills, CA: Sage.

Farrell, A. D., & Danish, S. J. (1993). Peer drug associations and emotional restraint: Causes or consequences of adolescents' drug use? *Journal of Consulting and Clinical Psychology, 61,* 327–334.

Farrington, D. P., & Hawkins, J. D. (1991). Predicting participation, early onset and later persistence in officially recorded offending. *Criminal Behavior and Mental Health, 1,* 1–33.

Fletcher, A. C., Darling, N. E., & Steinberg, L. (1995). Parental monitoring and peer influences on adolescent substance use. In J. McCord (Ed.), *Coercion and punishment in long-term perspectives* (pp. 259–271). New York: Cambridge University Press.

Florsheim, P., Tolan, P. H., & Gorman-Smith, D. (1996). Family processes and risks for externalizing behavior problems among African American and Hispanic boys. *Journal of Consulting and Clinical Psychology, 64,* 1222–1230.

Forehand, R., & Kotchick, B. A. (1996). Cultural diversity: A wake-up call for parent training. *Behavior Therapy, 27,* 187–206.

Frick, P. J. (1998). *Conduct disorders and severe antisocial behavior.* New York: Plenum.

Gelfand, D. M., Ficula, T., & Zarbatany, L. (1986). Prevention of childhood behavior disorders. In B. A. Edelstein & L. Michelson (Eds.), *Handbook of prevention.* New York: Plenum.

Giancola, P. R., Martin, C. S., Tarter, R. E., Pehlam, W. E., & Moss, H. B. (1996). Executive cognitive functioning and aggressive behavior in preadolescent boys at high risk for substance abuse/dependence. *Journal of Studies on Alcohol, 57,* 352–359.

Giancola, P. R., Mezzich, A. C., & Tarter, R. E. (1998). Executive cognitive functioning, temperament and antisocial behavior in conduct-disordered adolescent females. *Journal of Abnormal Psychology, 107,* 629–641.

Giancola, P. R., Moss, H. B., Martin, C. S., Kirisci, L., & Tarter, R. E. (1996). Executive cognitive functioning predicts reactive aggression in boys at high risk for substance abuse: A prospective study. *Alcoholism: Clinical and Experimental Research, 20,* 740–744.

Giancola, P. R., Zeichner, A., Yarnell, J. E., & Dickson, K. E. (1996). Relation between executive cognitive functioning and the adverse consequences of alcohol use in social drinkers. *Alcoholism: Clinical and Experimental Research, 20,* 1094–1098.

Gillmore, M. R., Hawkins, J. D., Catalano, R. F., Jr., Day, L. E., Moore, M. & Abbot, R. (1991) Structure of problem behaviors in preadolescence. *Journal of Consulting and Clinical Psychology, 59,* 499–506.

Gold, P. W. (1998). Lack of attention from loss of time. *Science, 281,* 1149–1150.

Graham, S., Hudley, C., & Williams, E. (1992). Attributional and emotional determinants of aggression among African American and Latino young adolescents. *Developmental Psychology, 28,* 731–740.

Hansen, W. B., Graham, J. W., Wolkenstein, B., & Lundy, B. Z. (1988). Differential impact of three alcohol prevention curricula on hypothesized mediating variable *Journal of Drug Education, 18,* 143–153.

Hawkins, J. D., Catalano, R. F., & Miller, J. Y. (1992). Risk and protective factors for alcohol and other drug problems in adolescence and early adulthood: Implications for substance abuse prevention. *Psychological Bulletin, 112,* 64–105.

Herrenkohl, I. T., Maguin, E., Hill, K. G., Hawkins, J. D., Abbott, R. D., & Catalano, R. F. (1998). *Developmental predictors of violence in late adolescence.* Unpublished manuscript, University of Washington.

Hundleby, J. D., & Mercer, G. W. (1987). Family and friends as social environments and their relationship to young adolescents' use of alcohol, tobacco, and marijuana. *Journal of Clinical Psychology, 44,* 125–134.

Institute of Medicine (1994). *Reducing risks for mental disorders: Frontiers for preventive intervention research.* Washington, DC: National Academy Press.

Jenkins, J. M., & Smith, M. A. (1991). Marital disharmony and children's behavior problems: Aspects of a poor marriage that affect children adversely. *Journal of Child Psychology and Psychiatry, 32,* 793–810.

Jessor, R., & Jessor, S. L. (1977). *Problem behavior and psychosocial development: A longitudinal study of youth.* New York: Academic Press.

Johnson, C. A., Pentz, M. A., Weber, M. D., et al. (1990). Relative effectiveness of comprehensive community programs for drug abuse prevention with high risk and low-risk adolescents. *Journal of Consulting and Clinical Psychology, 58,* 447–456.

Jouriles, E. N., Barling, J., & O'Leary, K. D. (1987). Predicting child behavior problems in maritally violent families. *Journal of Abnormal Child Psychology, 15,* 165–173.

Kandel, D. B. (1982). Epidemiological and psychosocial perspective on adolescent drug use. *Journal of American Academic Clinical Psychiatry, 21,* 328–347.

Kandel, D. B., & Andrews, K. (1987). Processes of adolescent socialization by parents and peers. *International Journal of the Addictions, 22,* 319–342.

Kandel, D. B., & Wu, P. (1995) Disentangling mother-child effects in the development of antisocial behavior. In J. McCord (Ed.), *Coercion and punishment in long-term perspectives* (pp. 106–123). New York: Cambridge University Press.

Kazdin, A. E. (1989). Developmental difficulties in depression. *Advances in clinical child psychology, 12* (pp. 193–219). New York: Plenum Press.

Kazdin, A. E., Bass, D., Siegel, T., & Thomas, C. (1989). Cognitive-behavioral therapy and relationship therapy in the treatment of children referred for antisocial behavior. *Journal of Consulting and Clinical Psychology, 57,* 522–535.

Kazdin, A. E., Esveldt-Dawson, K., French, N. H., & Unis, A. S. (1987a). Effects of parent management training and problem-solving skills training combined in the treatment of antisocial child behavior. *Journal of the American Academy of Child and Adolescent Psyciatry, 26,* 416–424.

Kazdin, A. E., Esveldt-Dawson, K., French, N. H., & Unis, A. S. (1987b). Problem-solving skills training and relationship therapy in the treatment of antisocial child behavior. *Journal of Consulting and Clinical Psychology, 55,* 76–85.

Kazdin, A. E., Siegel, T., & Bass, D. (1992). Cognitive problem-solving skills training and parent management training in the treatment of antisocial behavior in children. *Journal of Consulting and Clinical Psychology, 60,* 733–747.

Kellam, S. G., and Brown, H. (1982). *Social adaptational and psychological antecedents of adolescent pyschopathology ten years later.* Baltimore: Johns Hopkins University.

Kellam, S. G., Ensimger, M. E., & Simon, M. B. (1980). Mental health in first grade and teenage drug, alcohol, and cigarette use. *Drug and Alcohol Dependence, 5,* 273–304.

Kendall, P. C., Ronan, K. R., & Epps, J. (1991). Aggression in children/adolescents: Cognitive-behavioral treatment perspectives. In D. Pepler & K. Ruebin (Eds.), *Development and treatment of childhood aggression.* Toronto: Erlbaum.

Lamborn, S. D., Mounts, N. S., Steinberg, L., & Dornbusch, S. M. (1983). Patterns of competence and adjustment among adolescents from authoritative, authoriarian, indulgent and neglectful families. *Child Development, 62,* 1049–1065.

Ledingham, J. E. (1990). Recent developments in high risk research. In B. B. Lahey and A. E. Kazdin (Eds.), *Advances in clinical child psychology: Volume 13* (pp. 91–137). New York: Plenum.

Levy, D., Lochman, J. E., & Wells, K. C. (1998). *Children's frequencies of dominance attempts related to aggression status and parent disciplinary style.* Unpublished manuscript, Duke University.

Lewinsohn, P. M., Hops, H., Roberts, R. E., Seeley, J. R., & Andrews, J. A. (1993). Adolescent psychopathology I. *Journal of Abnormal Psychology, 102,* 133–144.

Lewis, C. E., Robins, L. N., & Rice, J. (1985). Association of alcoholism with antisocial personality in urban men. *Journal of Nervous and Mental Disease, 173,* 166–174.

Lochman, J. E. (1985). Effects of different treatment lengths in cognitive behavioral interventions with aggressive boys. *Child Psychiatry and Human Development, 16,* 45–56.

Lochman, J. E. (1987). Self and peer perceptions and attributional biases of aggressive and nonaggressive boys in dyadic interactions. *Journal of Consulting and Clinical Psychology, 55,* 404–410.

Lochman, J. E. (1992). Cognitive-behavioral intervention with aggressive boys: Three Year Follow-up and preventive effects. *Journal of Consulting and Clinical Psychology, 60,* 426–432.

Lochman, J. E., Burch, P. R., Curry, J. F., & Lampron, L. B. (1984). Treatment and generalization effects of cognitive behavioral and goal setting interventions with aggressive boys. *Journal of Consulting and Clinical Psychology, 52,* 915–916.

Lochman, J. E., Cohen, C., & Wayland, K. (April, 1991). *Outcome expectations for aggressive boys' developmental effects and parent-child rearing styles.* Paper presented at the Biennial Convention of the Society for Research in Child Development. Seattle, WA.

Lochman, J. E., & the Conduct Problems Research Group (1995). Screening of child behavior problems for prevention programs at school entry. *Journal of Consulting and Clinical Psychology, 63,* 549–559.

Lochman, J. E., & Curry, J. F. (1986). Effects of social problem-solving training and of self instruction training with aggressive boys. *Journal of Clinical Child Psychology, 15,* 159–164.

Lochman, J. E., & Dodge, K. A. (1998). Distorted perception in dyadic interactions of aggressive and nonaggressive boys: Effects of prior expectations, context, and boys' age. *Development and Psychopathology, 10,* 495–512.

Lochman, J. E., & Dodge, K. A. (1994). Social-cognitive processes of severely violent, moderately aggressive and nonaggressive boys. *Journal of Consulting and Clinical Psychology, 62,* 366–374.

Lochman, J. E., & Lampron, L. B. (1986). Situational social problem-solving skills and self-esteem of aggressive and nonaggressive boys. *Journal of Abnormal Child Psychology, 14,* 605–617.

Lochman, J. E., & Lampron. L. B. (1988). Cognitive behavioral interventions for aggressive boys: Seven months follow-up effects. *Journal of Child and Adolescent Psychotherapy, 5,* 15–23.

Lochman, J. E., Lampron, L. B., Gemmer, T. C., Harris, R., & Wyckoff, G. M., 1989). Teacher consultation and cognitive-behavior interventions with aggressive boys. *Psychology in the Schools, 26,* 179–188.

Lochman, J. E., & Lenhart, L. A. (1993). Anger coping intervention for aggressive children: Conceptual models and outcome effects. *Clinical Psychology Review, 13,* 785–805.

Lochman, J. E., & Wayland, K. K. (1994). Aggression, social acceptance and race as predictors of negative adolescent outcomes. *Journal of the American Academy of Child and Adolescent Psychiatry, 33,* 1026–1035.

Lochman, J. E., Wayland, K. K., & White, K. J. (1993). Social goals: Relationship to adolescent adjustment and to social problem solving. *Journal of Abnormal Child Psychology, 21,* 135–151.

Lochman, J. E., & Wells, K. (1996). A social-cognitive intervention with aggressive children: Prevention effects and contextual implementation issues. In R. D. Peters & R. J. McMahon (Eds.), *Prevention and early intervention: Childhood disorders, substance use, and delinquency* (pp. 111–143). Newbury Park, CA: Sage.

Lochman, J. E., & Wells, K. C., (in press-a). The Coping Power Program at the middle school transition: Universal and indicated prevention effects. *Psychology of Addictive Behaviors.*

Lochman, J. E., & Wells, K. C., (in press-b). Contextual social-cognitive mediators and child outcome: A test of the theoretical model in the Coping Power Program. *Development and Psychopathology.*

Lochman, J. E., Wells, K. C., & Colder, C. (June, 1997). *Parent and child social cognitive processes among aggressive and nonaggressive boys and their parents.* Paper presented at the meeting of the International Society for Research in Child and Adolescent Psychopathology, Paris, France.

Loeber, R. (1990). Development and risk factors of juvenile antisocial behavior and delinquency. *Clinical Psychology Review, 10,* 1–42.

Loeber, R., & Keenan, K. (1994). Interaction between conduct disorder and its comorbid conditions: Effects of age and gender. *Clinical Psychology Review, 14,* 497–523.

Lynskey, M. T., & Fergusson, D. M. (1995). Childhood conduct problems attention deficit behaviors, and adolescent alcohol, tobacco, and illicit drug use. *Journal of Abnormal Child Psychology, 23,* 281–302.

Maughan, B., Pickles, A., & Quinton, D. (1995). Parental hostility, childhood behavior, and adult social functioning. In J. McCord (Ed.) *Coercion and punishment in long-term perspectives* (pp. 34–58). Cambridge, England: Cambridge University Press.

Milich, R., & Dodge, K. A. (1984). Social information processing in child psychiatric populations. *Journal of Abnormal Child Psychology, 12,* 471–490.

Miller-Johnson, S., Lochman, J. E., Coie, J. D., Terry, R., & Hyman, C. (1998). Co-occurrence of conduct and depressive problems at sixth grade: Substance use outcomes across adolescence. *Journal of Abnormal Child Psychology, 26,* 221–232.

Moffitt, T. E. (1993). Adolescence-limited and life-course-persistent antisocial behavior: A development taxonomy. *Psychology Review, 100,* 674–701.

Muthén, B. O. (1991). Analysis of longitudinal data using latent models with varying parameters. In L. M. Collins & J. L. Horn (Eds.), *Best methods for the analysis of change: recent advances, unanswered questions, future directions.* APA: Washington DC.

Norem-Hebeisen, A., Johnson, D. W., Anderson, D., & Johnson, R. (1984). Predictors and concomitants of changes in drug use patterns among teenagers. *The Journal of Social Psychology, 124,* 43–50.

Oetting, E. R., & Beauvais, F. (1990). Adolescent drug use: Findings of national and local surveys. *Journal of Consulting and Clinical Psychology, 58,* 385–394.

Ollendick, T. H., Weist, M. D., Borden, M. D., & Greene, R. W. (1992). Sociometric status and academic, behavioral, and psychological adjustment: A five year longitudinal study. *Journal of Consulting and Clinical Psychology, 60,* 80–87.

Patterson, G. R. (1982). *Coercive family process.* Eugene, OR: Castalia.

Patterson, G. R. (1986). Performance models for antisocial boys: *American Psychologist, 41,* 432–444.

Patterson, G. R., & Bank, C. L. (1989). Some amplifying mechanisms for pathological processes in families. In M. R. Gunnary & E. Thelen (Eds.), *Systems and development: the minnesota symposia on child psychology, 22,* (pp. 167–209). Hillsdale, NJ: Erlbaum.

Patterson, G. R., Capaldi, D. M., & Bank, C. L. (1991). An early-starter model for predicting delinquency. In D. J. Pepler & K. H. Rubin (Eds.), *The development and treatment of childhood aggression* (pp. 139–168). Hillsdale, NJ: Lawrence Erlbaum.

Pentz, M. A., Dwyer, J. H., MacKinnon, D. P., Flay, B. R., Hansen, W. B., Wang, E. Y. I., & Johnson, C. A. (1989). A multicommunity trial for primary prevention of adolescent drug abuse: Effects on drug use prevalence. *Journal of the American Medical Association, 261,* 3259–3266.

Perry, D. G., Perry, L. C., & Rasmussen, P. (1986). Cognitive social learning mediators of aggression. *Child Development, 57,* 700–711.

Pettit, G. S., Harris, A. W., Bates, J. E., & Dodge, K. A. (1991). Family interaction, social cognition, and children's subsequent relations with peers at kindergarten. *Journal of Social and Personal Relationships, 8,* 383–401.

Richard, B. A., & Dodge, K. A. (1982). Social maladjustment and problem-solving and school-aged children. *Journal of Consulting and Clinical Psychology, 50,* 226–233.

Robins, L. N. (1979). Follow-up studies. In H. C. Quay & J. S. Werry, (Eds.), *Psychopathological disorders of childhood, second edition.* New York: Wiley.

Santisteban, D. A., Szapocznik, J., & Kurtines, M. W. (1994). Behavioral problems among Hispanic youth: The family as moderator of adjustment. In J. Szapocznik (Ed.), *A Hispanic/Latino family approach to substance abuse prevention* (pp. 19–39). Rockville, MD: Center for Substance Abuse Prevention.

Sayed, J. C., Lochman, J. E., Wells, K. C. (1998). *Children's social problem-solving strategies: Relationships to parental child-rearing practices.* Unpublished manuscript, Duke University.

Schinke, S. P., Botvin, G. J., & Orlandi, M. A. (1991). *Substance abuse in children and adolescents: Evaluation and intervention.* Newbury Park, CA: Sage.

Simcha-Fagan, O., Gersten, J. C., & Langer, T. (1986). Early precursors and concurrent correlates of illicit drug use in adolescents. *Journal of Drug Issues, 16,* 7–28.

Snyder, J., Dishion, T. J., & Patterson, G. R. (1986). Determinants and consequences of associating with deviant peers during preadolescence and adolescence. *Journal of Early Adolescence, 6,* 29–43.

Steinberg, L. (1987). Single parents, stepparents, and the susceptibility of adolescents to antisocial peer pressure, *Child Development, 58,* 269–275.

Swaim, R. C., Oetting, E. R., Edwards, R. W., & Beauvais, F. (1989). Links from emotional distress to adolescent drug use: A path model. *Journal of Consulting and Clinical Psychology, 57,* 227–231.

Tarter, R. E., Alterman, A. I., & Edwards, K. L. (1985). Vulnerability of alcoholism in men: A behavior genetic perspective. *Journal of Studies on Alcohol, 46,* 329–356.

Thompson, L. L., Riggs, P. D., Mikulich, S. E., & Crowley, T. J. (1996). Contributions of ADHD symtpoms to substance problems and delinquency in conduct-disordered adolescents. *Journal of Abnormal Child Psychology, 24,* 325–348.

Wahler, R. G., & Graves, M. G. (1983). Setting events in social networks: Ally or enemy in child behavior therapy, *Behavior Therapy, 14,* 19–36.

Webster-Stratton, C. (1996). Early-onset conduct problems: Does gender make a difference? *Journal of Consulting and Clinical Psychology, 64,* 540–551.

Weiss, B., Dodge, K., Bates, J. F., & Pettit, G. S. (1992) Some consequences of early harsh discipline: Child aggression and a maladaptive social information processing style. *Child Development, 63,* 1321–1335.

Williams, S. C., Lochman, J. E., Phillips, N. C., & Barry, T. D. Aggressive and non-agressive boys' physiological and cognitive processes in response to peer provocations. Unpublished manuscript, University of Alabama (submitted for publication).

Wills, T. A., & Filer, M. (1996). Stress-coping model of adolescent substance use. In T. H. Ollendick & R. J. Prinz (Eds.), *Advances in clinical child psychology, volume 18* (pp. 91–132). New York: Plenum.

Wills, T. A., McNamara, G., Vaccaro, D., & Hirkey, A. E. (1996). Escalated substance use: A longitudinal grouping analysis from early to middle adolescence. *Journal of Abnormal Child Psychology, 105,* 166–180.

Windle, M. (1990). A longitudinal study of antisocial behavior in early adolescence as predictors of late adolescent substance use: Gender and ethnic group differences. *Journal of Abnormal Psychology, 99,* 86–91.

Wooten, J. M., Frick, P. J., Shelton, K. K., & Silverthorn, P. (1997). Ineffective parenting and childhood conduct problems. The moderating role of callous-unemotional traits. *Journal of Consulting and Clinical Psychology, 65,* 301–308.

Zoccolillo, M. (1993). Gender and the development of conduct disorder. *Development and Psychopathology, 5,* 65–78.

CHAPTER 16

Designing Prevention Programs: The Developmental Perspective

Marvin W. Berkowitz
Audrey L. Begun

INTRODUCTION

To prevent a problem, one needs to understand how it emerges and develops. In other words, etiology is at the heart of prevention (Hawkins et al., 1986). And prevention research is at its best when it involves discovery of developmentally important antecedents and conditions and targets those antecedents for preventive intervention (Kellam, 1994; p. 38). Therefore, because certain conditions relevant to later substance abuse exist even during prenatal development, the field of substance abuse prevention must adopt a developmental perspective and incorporate the sciences of human development and behavioral genetics to maximize its efficacy (Kellam & VanHorn, 1997; Tarter & Vanyukov, 1994). In order to design effective prevention programs for children and adolescents, with elements appropriate for specific developmental levels (Dryfoos, 1990), it is necessary to understand the unique developmental capacities, limitations, and needs of children and adolescents at different developmental levels.

This chapter explores the role of developmental knowledge in the design of drug and alcohol abuse prevention efforts. It focuses on childhood and early adolescence because that is when a great deal of drug and alcohol related behavior begins. However, it takes a life-span perspective and addresses relevant developmental issues from earlier and later periods in life. It discusses specific stages in the life span and identifies developmental issues relevant to the design of substance abuse prevention programs.

Marvin W. Berkowitz • College of Education, University of Missouri at St. Louis, St. Louis, Missouri 63121
Audrey L. Begun • University of Wisconsin-Milwaukee, Milwaukee, Wisconsin 53211

A DEVELOPMENTAL PERSPECTIVE

A true developmental perspective does more than simply characterize or describe the nature of a particular age group, such as adolescents (e.g., Baumrind & Moselle, 1985; Howard, Boyd, & Zucker, 1995) or young adults (e.g., Bachman et al., 1997). Such an approach ignores the processes of human development and limits our understanding of the individuals involved. A true developmental perspective attempts to understand human development as a continuously changing interplay of biological, intrapsychic, social, and cultural forces. Any particular aspect of development is embedded in a flow of prior interactions and later developments and is the result of both intrinsic and extrinsic forces. Therefore, the onset (or absence of onset) of substance use is one point in a continuous flow of interacting forces and the result of an interplay of intrinsic "vulnerability and resilience" factors, such as genetics, neuropsychology, disability, constitution, temperament and personality, with extrinsic "risk and safety" factors, such as behavioral models (peers, siblings, elders, and media representatives), accessibility of substances, stressors present in the environment, reinforcement, and punishment. This interplay, in turn, is mediated by a host of factors that include the person's cognitions, morality, past learning, information processing style, attitudes, and social skills.

There is also an element of chance, since many developmental phenomena depend on a convergence of specific experiences and developmental timing; both means and opportunity must coincide in order for change to occur. For example, fetal exposure to the rubella virus can result in serious birth defects if it occurs during the specific prenatal period when vulnerable organ systems are emerging; earlier and later exposure have little or no long-term impact. Such windows of opportunity, or "periods of peak sensitivity," are times during development when an individual is most sensitive to certain inputs. For example, children's babbling will mimic the sounds and intonations of their native language if they hear that language during the first 6 months of life. If they do not hear it until much later in life, they may develop language capacities, but the language and intonations will have different qualities.

The developmental perspective also considers reciprocal determinism, or *circularity of influence*. This means that there is an interactive pattern of influence between an individual and the environment, with the environment having the power to shape aspects of an individual's development and the individual having the power to shape the environment and to respond in different ways to environmental factors (Coie et al., 1993). In short, an individual is neither entirely passive nor totally directive in the process of development. For example, a sixth-grader's social development is influenced by interactions with a peer group, but that child also has an impact on the peer group. Association with deviant peers can lead a child to try illicit drugs, but the personality of the child may encourage peers to entice the child to join their deviant behavior.

The developmental perspective also presumes an element of continuity in the course of development. For example, the influence of peers on adolescent drug use is not a phenomenon segregated in time (Petersen, 1982). Susceptibility to peer influences is a product, in part, of what has transpired in the child's development during the preceding decade and has implications for how the individual will function during later adolescence and adulthood. The choices made during adolescence, or any period of the life span, are born in prior development and lay the foundations for later development.

Proximal versus Distal Causes

For any behavior, including substance abuse, there will be a host of proximal influences that occur just prior to the behavior as well as distal influences that occurred long before the behavior.

Prevention efforts that focus on proximal causes of substance abuse (or any other developmental outcome) tend to be most popular, but the developmental perspective emphasizes the importance of distal causal factors (e.g., Block, Block, & Keyes, 1988; Brook et al., 1990). One reason prevention efforts tend to focus on the more temporally proximal factors is salience. When looking at a current problem, such as substance abuse, those factors that immediately precede it are more salient to the observer (and more obviously related to the behavior) than are distally related factors. A second reason is cost-effectiveness. Short-term studies are much easier to execute (and easier to fund) than are long-term studies. A third reason is simplicity. The links between proximal phenomena and their developmental consequences are usually more direct and less complex than those between distal phenomena and the same developmental consequences.

Despite the temptation to focus on proximal causes, the developmental perspective argues for consideration of distal as well as proximal factors in attempts to understand how change occurs over time. This is because early influences can be as, or even more, important than later influences. Psychoanalytic theory, for example, argues that the earliest stages of personality development are the foundation upon which later personality is built. Therefore, disruptions in the earliest stages are most traumatic and produce the most serious and intractable pathology. In other words, distortions of one's life course that occur during early, formative periods will have more pervasive and more serious effects and become more resistant to intervention than disruptions that occur at nonformative periods in one's developmental history (Erikson, 1963). This is, in part, because subsequent experiences are processed through whichever filters of adaptation or dysfunction are developed through earlier experiences. Therefore, prevention efforts are likely to have the most impact if they are introduced either early in the developmental process (Coie et al., 1993) or at "nodal" points in the life span. Nodal points are those periods in development when individuals are at their peak of sensitivity for certain types of experiences that can affect the subsequent course of development. Substance abuse prevention strategies often focus on periods immediately prior to onset, but the developmental perspective argues for prevention strategies targeted at earlier age periods and at more distal causes. In fact, what is often considered primary prevention (e.g., addressing proximal factors, such as treating the anti-personality disorder, teaching social skills to an asocial child, reducing impulsivity) may indeed be only secondary prevention because each of the symptoms may be the result of early disruptions in parenting (the distal factor).

Early influences are especially influential, in part, because they tend to be associated with general, or global, development. During periods of rapid developmental change, such as infancy, toddlerhood, or early adolescence, the individual is changing in multiple domains simultaneously. As a result, a single significant event has the potential to intrude on several developmental processes at once. Furthermore, the effects are often more dramatic because a younger individual may have relatively few mechanisms for coping or may be less resilient. (A notable exception to this is the relative plasticity or functional malleability of the infant's and young child's neurobiology in comparison to that of older children, adolescents, and adults.) In addition, both behaviorally and biologically, as an organism develops, it becomes more differentiated (Werner, 1948). Hence, earlier impacts tend to have more diffuse and pervasive impacts than do later influences.

Distal causes are also important because much in development depends on multiple exposures and cumulative experiences, rather than on single events. This is particularly true of complex developmental phenomena, such as language, social cognition, moral reasoning, gender roles, and ethnic identity. These complex elements of development generally require multiple exposures in multiple contexts over time in order for the individual to develop a clear understanding of the entire concept or phenomenon. For example, young children require many experiences paired with consistent consequences before learning that eating is "good" only when edibles are consumed; eating is "bad" when dirt, hair, pet food, or rocks are consumed. And, this categorization concept is relatively simple compared to some of the complex ideas that an individual is able to acquire over time.

Developmental Tasks

Each stage of human development is associated with a unique constellation of developmental capacities and requirements. Robert Havighurst (1974) coined the phrase "developmental tasks" to describe a set of tasks that are endemic to and significant for each stage in the life span. Developmental tasks are the psychological "work" that must be done at a particular stage in one's development. For example, in the process of developing their personal identities and autonomy (a developmental task of adolescence), adolescents examine (through challenges, debates, and experimentation) the beliefs, values, attitudes, and rules which are imposed by members of the social context—peers, parents, social institutions, media heroes, and others. In doing so, the adolescent is sorting out the elements for a good versus poor fit for the emerging persona, and negativism and autonomy become developmental necessities. Adolescents *need* to discover their own answers in order to become competent, confident individuals. Accordingly, it is not surprising to see a marked increase in substance use and in other risky behaviors during the adolescent years. For example, delinquency peaks in adolescence, and in most cases is a short-lived lifestyle that begins and ends in adolescence. The need to be autonomous may even explain in part the finding that adolescents who experiment with drugs have healthier psychological profiles than adolescents who abuse or abstain entirely from the use of substances (Baumrind & Moselle, 1985; Shedler & Block, 1990). The "work" of forming an identity, however, is strongly influenced by earlier experiences and developmental tasks that have affected self-confidence and a sense of self-efficacy, as well as by the current context. In summary, each stage in the life span continues the work of prior developmental stages and prepares the way for later developmental tasks.

DEVELOPMENTAL STAGES AND PREVENTION

Each stage of human development has significant characteristics that are relevant to substance abuse prevention. Childhood and adolescence are perhaps the most important. However, because of the necessity of planning prevention efforts that address distal causal factors, this section takes a life-span developmental approach to prevention, beginning before birth.

Prenatal Development

Prenatal exposure to harmful substances, including substances of abuse, such as alcohol, nicotine, and cocaine, can damage the developing fetus and have long-term effects. Preventive efforts at this stage of development should attempt to prevent exposure to harmful substances and provide a safe environment in which the fetus can develop. Four factors determine the result of exposure to a substance: (1) dosage and duration of exposure, (2) nature of the substance, (3) timing of exposure, and (4) the constitution of the individual exposed.

DOSAGE. The impact of a specific drug on the developing fetus may not be related directly to the mother's dosage or a drug's impact on her system. The mother's more mature organ systems (i.e., liver and kidneys) may process and eliminate the drug with far greater efficiency than do those of the fetus; in fact, the placental tissue and amniotic fluid can trap some of the drug (or its byproducts) and actually increase exposure of the fetus to the drug (Freeman, 1992). The relative dosage to the fetus may be many times higher and last for many more hours (or days) than is experienced by the mother (Gandelman, 1992). It is difficult to identify dosage and exposure curves of maternal–fetal exposure in human models because many uncontrolled variables affect circulating doses of a drug, including the quality of the drug and whether it is taken orally, intravenously, intramuscularly, or inhaled. In many studies, however, it seems that higher doses correlate with greater harm to the fetus when other variables are constant or controlled.

NATURE OF THE SUBSTANCE.   The next important set of variables are those related to the actual type of drugs or substances used. It is not surprising that different substances have different impacts on the developing fetus because each has a unique chemical composition and set of effects on the adult. For example, prenatal exposure to alcohol has been labeled the single greatest cause of mental retardation in the United States (Abel & Sokol, 1987). Alcohol use can have a deleterious impact on the developing facial features, on growth rate and birth weight, and on the central nervous system of an exposed fetus. Alcohol consumption during pregnancy can result in full-blown fetal alcohol syndrome or a host of fetal alcohol effects that include a wide range of mild to severe cognitive, behavioral, and growth delays (Mattson et al., 1998). Fetal alcohol syndrome occurs in about 1 of 750 births in the United States. Many thousands more are born with fetal alcohol effects.

Drugs other than alcohol can also have significant negative effects on fetal development. It is not clear that fetal exposure to marijuana has lasting effects on child development, but early childhood deficits in cognitive abilities have been noted, though these deficits appear to diminish by school age (Chandler et al., 1996). Fried and his colleagues (Fried & Watkinson, 2000; Fried, Watkinson, & Gray, 1998; Fried, Watkinson, & Siegal, 1997) have demonstrated both long-term deficits (until adolescence) of prenatal marijuana exposure and different cognitive and visual–perceptual effects than caused by prenatal exposure to the products of maternal cigarette smoking. Cocaine is known to have a deleterious effect on placental blood flow (resulting in oxygen deprivation or fetal death), high rates of premature delivery (resulting in a range of respiratory and central nervous system complications), and low birth weight (associated with growth and central nervous system complications) (DeCrisofaro & LaGamma, 1995; Madden, Payne, & Miller, 1986). Cocaine has also been found in fetal brain tissue (Gandelman, 1992). Newborns who are known to have been exposed to cocaine prenatally are likely to have temperament difficulties, including irritability, state lability, disturbed sleep patterns, and transient EEG shifts (Gandelman, 1992), as well as inadequate control over behavioral state, depressed social interactions, poorly organized responses to stimuli from the environment, tremors, abnormally sensitive startle responses, irritability, poor feeding, and abnormal sleep patterns. The developmental impacts of prenatal exposure to cocaine range from the extreme and fatal to the subtle, and some appear to persist into early childhood (Waller, 1993). These outcomes, in turn, can be responsible for disruptions in bonding and attachment relationships. This, and the lack of many life skills in some abusing mothers, can result in such infants being be abused, neglected, and/or placed in foster care (Regan, Ehrlich, & Finnegan, 1987). Mothers who use cocaine during pregnancy tend to also use other drugs and accurate use histories are difficult to obtain. Therefore, conclusions about the impact of prenatal cocaine exposures must be tentative.

TIMING.   The timing of exposure to a substance is another important variable in predicting its effect. The substance to which a fetus is exposed might have a specific action that either coincides with or misses a period of peak sensitivity. For example, fetal exposure to alcohol, even at relatively low doses, has its greatest impact on development if it occurs early in the first trimester or at any time during the third trimester (Gandelman, 1992). This is because the developing fetus has different periods of peak sensitivity to alcohol. For this reason, among others, chronic substance use throughout the course of pregnancy is likely to have a harmful effect because it increases the probability that the actions of a specific drug will be present during a critical developmental point. Poly-drug-use also increases the probability that a specific action will interact with a particular developmental point. Prevention efforts, in addition to encouraging abstinence throughout pregnancy, might be directed towards short-term goals of abstinence during periods of peak sensitivity.

HEALTH.   If a pregnant woman is well nourished, free of disease, and relatively unstressed, her fetus may be able to fight off the effects of small exposures to harmful substances. However, alcohol and cocaine users are frequently malnourished (Gandelman, 1992). Mothers who abuse substances are often exposed to diseases and stress and may have less healthy reproductive systems than their nonusing counterparts. In short, their constitutions and the constitutions of their developing fetuses may be compromised and relatively nonresilient. Primary prevention would obviously include efforts to stop the mothers from using substances; secondary and tertiary prevention would address exposure to disease, stress reduction, nutrition, and other aspects of health.

In addition to obvious biological effects, prenatal drug exposure to alcohol is correlated with difficulties in learning and forming social ties and attachments as well as with difficulties in temperament, hyperactivity, and self-soothing. This may be the result of alcohol interfering with the transfer of nutrients through the placenta, oxygen deprivation during metabolism of alcohol, interference with hormonal pathways, and/or suppression of fetal activity during exposure (Hoyseth & Jones, 1989). The effects of such exposure can be indirect. For example, in the case of fetal alcohol exposure, there may be subtle central nervous system problems that result in IQ decrements, learning difficulties, and poor psychomotor performance (Gandelman, 1992; Streissguth, Sampson, & Barr, 1989). These decrements may, in turn, can result in academic (or other activity) performance difficulties or parent–infant bonding difficulties. The experience of repeated failure is recognized as a cause, or at least a correlate of, poor self-esteem and poor social relations. Thus, the fetal exposure is a distal factor in the child's later development in these domains.

Children who experience fetal exposure to harmful substances may grow up to have difficulties with substance abuse, themselves. It may be that their central nervous systems have been sensitized to these substances as a result of exposure during critical periods of intrauterine development, which alters their susceptibility in a direct manner. It is also likely that genetic factors can predispose children of substance abusers to difficulties with substance use. There is also evidence of a more indirect pathway of influence: these children have relatively high incidence rates of attention-deficit problems, and adolescents with attention-deficits have higher rates of substance abuse (Kumpfer, 1987). Furthermore, animal models suggest that individuals exposed to alcohol prenatally have decrements in response inhibition and require more trials in learning to avoid punishment than do nonexposed individuals (Gandelman, 1992). These impaired capacities may translate into greater difficulty in discovering the negative consequences of substance use and in inhibiting substance use, despite being aware of its consequences.

In summary, whether the causal pathways are direct or indirect, fetal exposure to drugs has long-range, far-reaching implications for the prevention of substance abuse and other social problems. Clearly, fetal drug exposure has an important distal influence on later substance use, and primary prevention strategies should address the issues of prenatal exposure.

Infant and Toddler Development

Infancy and toddlerhood are marked by the emergence of sociability, language, sophisticated cognition, psychomotor skills, and many other essential skills. But perhaps the singlemost psychologically significant event during this stage of development is the formation of what Bowlby (1969) calls the attachment bond with primary caregivers. The attachment bond is the foundation for the development of personality and the template for all future relationships. Erikson (1963) argues that basic trust or mistrust is born in an infant's relationship to his or her parents. Nurturing, consistent, and responsive parenting produces trusting, secure children; neglectful, inconsistent, or abusive parenting produces insecure or conflicted children. The failure to form secure attachments during infancy predicts the development of serious social and emotional difficulties later in life; this has been observed in work with both humans (Bowlby, 1969; Jacobson & Wille, 1986) and other primates (Harlow & Harlow, 1962; Suomi, Mineka, & DeLizio, 1983).

Unfortunately, the relationship between attachment formation and later substance use is not entirely clear, perhaps because of the tendency to neglect distal causes of substance use. A general picture can be sketched, however. The formation of secure attachments within the family during infancy serves as a template for the formation of later life social bonds. Youth who have experienced disrupted or anxious early attachments may not have the requisite skills or confidence to form positive peer relationships or appropriate relationships with adults later in their lives. The finding that drug-using youth are more likely than nonusing youth to have difficulties in peer relationships (e.g., Baumrind, 1991; Elliott, Huizinga, & Ageton, 1985) is consistent with findings from the attachment literature, which show that difficulties in peer relations result from poor early attachments (e.g., Erickson, Sroufe, & Egeland, 1985; Matas, Arend, & Sroufe, 1978; Rutter, 1979). Similarly, research demonstrating poor school achievement and school orientation among drug-using youth (e.g., Brook et al., 1986) corresponds to findings for individuals lacking a healthy early attachment history (Bowlby, 1973). Conscienceless youth crime (Magid & McKelvey, 1987) and antisocial behavior (Ewing, 1990) may also be related to the distal factor of unhealthy attachment relationships in infancy. Clearly, substance abuse use is heavily implicated as a proximal factor in these behaviors (Kusserow, 1992). Furthermore, it has been argued that:

> If there are problems in the parent-child bond, then children may also be deprived of a number of mechanisms typically learned in infancy through receiving 'good enough' mothering that could later help them deal with stress and other unpleasant feelings. One such mechanism has been termed 'self-soothing.' Children who are adequately comforted by a parent when upset eventually learn to comfort or soothe themselves when they feel frustrated or afraid.... Recovering individuals with developmental deficits originating in infancy may face issues of concern in recovery that are analogous to those of the period of 'trust vs. mistrust.' These include intense fears of abandonment, the inability to tolerate anxiety or to engage in 'self-soothing' behaviors, and difficulties with intimate relationships. Alcohol or drugs may have been used to cope with these inadequacies. (Wallen, 1993; p. 18)

Based on attachment theory, interventions during infancy and toddlerhood should be geared toward reinforcing the development of trust and attachments. Such interventions could provide cement for the foundation of the individual's emerging sense of efficacy, self-esteem, social competency, and self-preservation—each of which is an important resilience factor related to substance use. Research on attachment also demonstrates that the attachment formed in infancy continues to affect one's development throughout life (Kaplan, 1995). There is evidence that the nature of the attachment bond in adolescence affects the likelihood of substance abuse (Brook et al., 1990). It is clear that a healthy attachment bond can improve the trajectory of development and may even counteract the effects of prenatal drug exposure (Johnson, Glassman, et al., 1990).

In addition to these issues of infant social development, it is important to remember that the brain and central nervous system continue to develop at a rapid rate during the first years of life (Tanner, 1970) and that infants and toddlers, like fetuses, are susceptible to negative developmental consequences as a result of exposure to drugs and alcohol. Unfortunately, some parents or caregivers use alcohol and paregoric (an opium/alcohol elixir) to calm babies with colic or to help them sleep through the night. Little is known of the potential long-term effects of these practices, but most pediatricians are likely to discourage them. Another unfortunate way in which infants and toddlers are exposed to alcohol and other drugs is through accidental ingestion of a family member's substances. Prevention interventions should address the fact that infants and toddlers learn about the world through oral explorations that can result in their exposure to harmful substances that are too easily accessible. Prevention efforts should also focus on creating a safe environment for vulnerable infants, toddlers, and children.

Preschool Development

Self-concept emerges during the preschool years (roughly ages 2 to 6 years). Interactions with the environment shape the preschooler's developing ego (Erikson, 1963), the sense of self as competent, effective, and independent, and the child's sense of purpose and goal directedness. Preschool-aged children become increasingly aware of and integrated into the social world, both within and outside of the family. Their understanding of the social world (social cognitions) derives largely from observing and imitating others and from experiencing the results of the many experiments they conduct each day. This is also the time when the basis of the moral sense emerges (beginning at around 18 months of age) (Lamb & Feeny, 1995). Conscience has its roots in this part of the life span, according to both psychoanalytic (Emde, Johnson, & Easterbrooks, 1987) and social-personality perspectives (Kochanska, 1993).

Preschoolers develop many of their categorizations and understanding of the world through social referencing, the process by which they use the emotional expressions and responses of others as cues for interpreting confusing, ambiguous events. In other words, if the child does not understand a situation, the reactions of others to that situation will be used in the child's assessments. Preschool-aged children are very sensitive to, and keenly aware of, the behavior of others (peers and adults), and they are quite adept at remembering another's behavior. However, their ability to understand social phenomena remains quite immature; they have a poor understanding of the covert experiences of others—thoughts and motivations. They have a propensity to imitate adults but cannot understand the reasons behind what they imitate. They are also much more susceptible to an adult's overt, observable behaviors than they are to verbal dictates (i.e., they are more likely to do what an adult does than to do what an adult says to do).

Children at this stage can also develop attitudes about drug and alcohol use through observation of significant people in their lives. The desire to imitate is powerful: parents who drink alcohol, smoke cigarettes, or use other substances are strong role models. Some parents of preschool-aged children even share their drinks and drugs with their children because they enjoy satisfying the child's desire to be like them or think of the imitation as "cute" or funny. Furthermore, among some nonabusing, substance-using adults there is a belief that "experimental" amounts of these substances will not harm the child and, in fact, may teach the child responsible use. However, this adult-centered logic is ill suited to the child's cognitive capacities at this age. The child does not distinguish between a "good amount" and a "bad amount," only between some and none, and thinks that it is "good" because someone they admire is giving it to them.

During the preschool years children also take major steps toward mastering self-control. Russian psychologists such as Vygotsky and Luria, as well as western psychologists such as Mischel, have clearly demonstrated the marked gains in self-control between 3 and 6 years of age (for a full review of this research, see Berkowitz (1982)). Such self-control is necessary for the later ability to resist temptations to engage in substance use (Block, Block, & Keyes, 1988). Likewise, the ability to tolerate frustration and delay gratification is critical to resistance (Shedler & Block, 1990). Clearly, before children develop the ability to resist temptation and control their impulses, it is necessary to create an environment in which controls are more external to the child. This is precisely why most parents put prescription drugs out of reach of small children and why they put child-proof latches on cabinets that hold dangerous substances (such as cleaning supplies). Once children develop better internal controls, the external controls can be eased.

Prevention in the preschool years is typically distal primary prevention. It should therefore focus on building the protective factors that are most developmentally appropriate to this period in the life span, such as those just reviewed: conscience, self-control, social perspective-taking, and attitudes toward substance use. Berkowitz and Grych (1998) have reviewed the parenting research and identified five parenting behaviors (induction, modeling, demandingness, nurturance, democratic family processes) that promote the development of central psychological strengths in early childhood. They have also applied those findings to guidelines for early childhood educators (Berkowitz & Grych, 2000).

Elementary School Development

The elementary school years (approximately 7 to 11 years of age) are often described as a time of skill building and eagerness to learn. This is seen in numerous ways: from the obvious acquisition of the "three R's" in formal schooling, to the ego dominance of the psychoanalytic latency stage, to the beginning mastery of logical thinking in the Piagetian stage of concrete operational reasoning (Piaget, 1970).

Erikson (1963) considers the key developmental task of this period to be resolving the tension between a sense of industry ("I can do things well") and a sense of inferiority. A sense of inadequacy is the result of children experiencing repeated failures, few successes, and negative, discouraging criticisms of their work. A sense of industry, or the belief that one can be an effective worker and producer, is fostered by an encouraging, rewarding environment. Curiosity and achievement are also suppressed in children who are exposed to inappropriate challenges—either too many that are too easily conquered (so that there is no pride to be gained despite succeeding) or too many that are too difficult. Many of these experiences occur in school, and a host of school- and achievement-related factors, including school failure, low-achievement orientation, and alienation, appear to be related to later substance use (Anhalt & Klein, 1976; Robins, 1980; Kumpfer & DeMarsh, 1986). According to Wallen (1993, p. 29):

> A number of individuals who become attracted to drugs and alcohol during junior high or high school years have learning disabilities that make school achievement difficult and unrewarding. They learn to rely on alcohol and drugs or substance-abusing peers for their sense of well-being and fail to develop motivation and work patterns that support success in an educational or work setting.

Elementary school is also a time when peer influences expand beyond their earlier modeling and social experimentation roles. Peers affect development in many spheres of a child's life but particularly as authorities on peer culture and peer relational issues. Until this time, "good friends" are those who serve an instrumental function (e.g., they share their toys with you, or play interesting games, or have a pet that you enjoy). In the elementary school years, even though the instrumental perspective on friendship continues to be significant, friendship also becomes understood and valued for its relational and emotional character. "Good friends" are now people who care for you, offer companionship, and like you (Selman, 1980).

Status in the peer network is clearly related to social skills and competencies (Asher, 1978). The preferred peer is one who makes people feel good about themselves. The socially skilled peer delivers many positive remarks, is appealing and interesting, and is someone who others choose to emulate. Once again, the quality of parenting and family atmosphere play a key role. Negative, sarcastic, verbally abusive, or discouraging family messages result in children who treat their peers poorly. These children are not desirable companions and often end up as "loners" and are socially rejected. Studies have shown that such children are at risk for developing substance abuse problems (Kellam, Brown, & Fleming, 1982; McCord, 1988a,b). Despite such studies and Sullivan's (1953) identification of the intimate friendships of this period as therapeutic and developmentally critical, little research has focused on preadolescent peer associations as possible predictors of subsequent drug initiation or abuse or the potential for peer-focused interventions prior to the junior high school years (Hawkins et al., 1986, p. 28)

One of the cognitive hallmarks of the elementary school years is the child's propensity and newly developed capacity for ordering the world. Piaget (Piaget & Inhelder, 1969) calls this the stage of concrete operations, which is highlighted by development of the ability for logical categorization. Unlike preschool children, elementary school children can create logical categories and distinctions between categories and can embed them in logical hierarchies. They also seem highly disposed to applying this skill robustly. They have a strong tendency to sort their experiences, often into rather rigid and stark, mutually exclusive categories. Phenomena tend to be either good or bad, large or small.

This characteristic offers a prime opportunity to influence the child's categorization of substance use and related phenomena. Children at this stage (and the preceding stage) are likely to have difficulty understanding how "good" people could use "bad" drugs. The 1990's "Hang Tough Milwaukee" media campaign relied on simple peer-delivered messages about the undesirability of substance use. From an adult perspective, these messages were too simplistic, but the targeted group (10- to 12-year-olds) tended to absorb such messages in an age-appropriate dualistic way (i.e., drugs are bad). Problems arise when children of this age receive conflicting messages about the acceptability of a particular behavior, such as when they receive anti-drug messages in school but see their parents using drugs at home.

Children at the end of this stage also tend to begin to use logical reasoning but make the mistake of assuming that the product of their deductive thought is equivalent to the truth. Hence, they are often logically confrontational and seem to be quite arrogant and stubborn. Elkind (1974) calls this developmental complexity "cognitive conceit." It can make arguing with children about drugs a difficult task if they have concluded that you are wrong.

Moral reasoning at this age tends to be markedly instrumental. In other words, the moral correctness of a behavior is determined by the likely consequences to the person. School-aged children begin to take into consideration the covert intentions of the person, not just overt, observable actions, when judging whether the person acted rightly or wrongly. Therefore, at this age, it may appear to be morally acceptable to use drugs if nothing bad happens to you but morally wrong if the risk of negative consequences is calculated to be high. Preventive efforts at this stage could focus on the concrete negative personal consequences of substance use. Research clearly indicates the strong association between the perceived harmfulness of a substance and the prevalence of its use (Johnson, O'Malley, & Bachman, 1996). Interestingly, this strategy is not developmentally indicated for adolescents.

A primary factor in the attraction toward or avoidance of the use of substances in the elementary school years is the nature of the school experience. The Center for Substance Abuse Prevention (CSAP) has identified the Child Development Project (CDP), a comprehensive character and academic school reform model, as one of the most effective elementary school drug prevention programs. This is despite the fact that the CDP was never intended to be a prevention model and never explicitly addresses substance use. Nonetheless, their focus on developing pro-social attitudes and behaviors in a caring school community significantly reduces such use (Battistich et al., 2000). Comprehensive, high-quality character education is an important prevention element in the elementary school years (Berkowitz, 2000).

Middle School and Early Adolescent Development

The middle school years (approximately 12 to 14 years of age), or early adolescence, are also a time of rapid developmental change. One of the most significant developments of this period is puberty, a complex set of physiological changes that coincide with dramatic shifts in social expectations and demands and changes in psychological and cognitive functioning—all of which have implications for substance abuse prevention.

The process begins gradually, long before the most visible "growth spurts" and changes in sexual characteristics. Many hormonal changes precede the visible appearance of pubertal changes. There exists tremendous heterogeneity among individuals as to the rate, age, and timing of pubertal processes (Katchadourian, 1977).

Puberty has powerful social and psychological implications well beyond the obvious physical changes and evolving interest in sexually oriented social relations. Research suggests, for example, that parents treat their children differently before and after puberty becomes apparent (Steinberg, 1981). Parents become much more permissive and allow increased autonomy in their adolescent offspring once they show signs of pubertal maturation. Early versus late maturation during this period has also been associated with significant differences in how individuals feel about themselves (self-esteem) and how the social world relates to them. The longevity of this impact is uncertain (Eichorn, 1963; Simmons & Blyth, 1987) and seems to differ markedly for males and females. However, rate of maturation does appear to have a significant impact on development during the adolescent period. Furthermore, there is evidence for the relation of pubertal timing (early vs. late) on problem behaviors including substance use (Magnusson, Stattin, & Allen, 1986), although it is unclear if this is an increase in deviance or an attempt to "catch up" to older peers who are at the same pubertal level (Silbereisen et al., 1989).

Not much is known about how the physiological changes of puberty interact with drug use, but pharmacologists often use the chronological age of 12 as the beginning point for adult doses of medications. For obvious ethical reasons, however, controlled research has not tested the differential effects of illicit drugs or alcohol on children versus adolescents. Nonetheless, it seems quite likely that there may be important differences in drug effects, sensitivities, and usage for pre- and postpubertal youth. This hypothesis is based on observations of the vast physiological differences between pre- and postpubertal children in response to prescription drugs.

Pre- and postpubertal differences in thinking also have implications for prevention. At about the age of 12, "the age of reason," young adolescents acquire the ability to use formal logic (Inhelder & Piaget, 1958; Muuss, 1988). This allows them to engage in hypothetico-deductive scientific problem solving; to reason about reason; to reason about abstractions, propositions, and hypothetical situations; and to engage in self-reflection. Because of these abilities, prevention specialists need to refine their interventions. It is no longer sufficient to rely on the relatively simplistic, dualistic thinking and the simple categorical labeling of younger children. Fallible logic will be exposed quickly by these more sophisticated thinkers who also have a larger pool of general knowledge on which to draw when reasoning about the world. For example, they are no longer satisfied with categorizing drug use as "bad" because it has bad effects on a person; they now recognize that drug use occurs because it also has some desirable effects or is pleasurable. It is critical that prevention interventions develop reactions to this aspect of substance use.

An intriguing and elusive aspect of development in these years is the advent of what David Elkind (1974) calls "adolescent egocentrism." Elkind describes a two-part phenomenon that peaks during the middle school years and slowly decreases throughout adolescence. The first part involves an "imaginary audience" phenomenon in which adolescents confuse their own self-preoccupations with being the object of their peers' thoughts (i.e., they assume that others are always monitoring them as they are monitoring themselves). Hence, they tend to "perform" for their peers—despite the fact that their peers may not be paying attention and may not even be physically present. Much adolescent behavior, including substance abuse, may be in response to the presumed regard and sanctioning of peers.

The second part of adolescent egocentrism is called the "personal fable," in which the adolescent labors under a myth of exaggerated personal uniqueness. One's experiences and life are presumed to be unique and extraordinary: one's own emotions are more extreme than those of others, relationships are deeper, disappointments harsher, successes more magnificent. This kind of thinking has two implications. The first has to do with one's own unique invulnerability. When asked why they got into potentially avoidable trouble, such as getting caught shoplifting or vandalizing property, middle-school-aged children are likely to say: "I never thought it could happen to me." Children of this age may not really believe that the reputed risks of substance use can happen to them. This heightened sense of invulnerability in adolescence is a controversial issue (Quadrel, Fischoff, & Davis, 1993), but there is empirical evidence that this form of egocentrism is related to greater substance use in adolescence (Arnett, 1990; Gross & Billingham, 1990).

Second, children operating from the personal fable perspective do not believe that the experiences of others are relevant to their unique situations. Parents and other adults often weaken their communication attempts by relaying their own personal experiences during adolescence in an attempt to convey the message that "I know what you are going through." Adolescents engulfed by personal fable thinking will reject such messages and are not likely to receive the important aspects of the prevention messages that are attached. With this age group, prevention efforts need to be responsive to the individual adolescent and may be most effective if individuals are encouraged to develop their own personal views with guidance from others rather than adopting the "ready made" answers created by others. It is also important to note that the relation of the personal fable to substance use is clearer for males than for females (Colwell, Billingham, & Gross, 1995; Gross & Billingham, 1990) and that no research has investigated this relation with early or middle adolescents, when adolescent egocentrism is understood to be most prevalent.

One adolescent characteristic that has been integrated into the substance use prevention field is peer conformity. Many recent prevention programs rely on attempts to train adolescents in how to resist negative peer pressure and about manipulations of assumptions about peer norms concerning substance use (Schinke, Botvin, & Orlandi, 1991). Indeed, adolescents tend to be highly oriented to peers and to be highly conformist, particularly during early adolescence. It has been reported that friends' use of substances is the strongest correlate of adolescent use, and that peer influence is stronger for substance abusing adolescents than for other adolescents (Coombs, Paulson, & Richardson, 1991). Furthermore, this shift may occur fairly early in regards to substance use. Webb et al. (1995) report that intentions to use alcohol are most strongly predicted by family factors for fifth-graders but by peer factors for sixth graders. Understanding this dynamic may be helpful in prevention efforts. However, there are differences between males and females regarding the importance of peer orientation. The impact of peer orientation also differs for the use of different substances and depending on relationships with parents (Kandel & Davies, 1992). Furthermore, peers can serve as a protective factor if the peer group norm is anti-substance use (Hawkins, Catalano, & Miller, 1992).

High School and Middle to Late Adolescent Development

The adolescent high school years (approximately 15 to 18 years of age) are a time of exploring options, waiting in limbo, and tolerating contradictions. The characterization of adolescence as a time of psychological turbulence (Hall, 1904) is no longer widely held and certainly not empirically supported (Bandura, 1964; Offer, 1969; Powers, Hauser, & Kilner, 1989).

During puberty, adolescents find themselves thrust into uncharted territory. Their bodies have undergone rapid transformations. Adult perceptions and expectations of their maturity have changed and they are treated differently than before—but inconsistently ("Stop acting like a child!" coincides with "You are still my child and will follow my rules!"). Adolescents become more independent but continue to display a great degree of dependency (Gould, 1978; Pipp et al., 1985). They are often unsure of themselves, as seen in an increase in self-consciousness during early adolescence, which decreases minimally into the high school years (Simmons, Rosenberg, & Rosenberg, 1973). And being unsure, they turn to others, usually peers, for help in charting the new territory. If those peers use substances, they are likely to begin using substances. One powerful predictor of adolescent substance use is the substance use behavior and related attitudes of their friends (Kandel, 1985). Affiliation with peers who use substances is an important factor in leading adolescents to become users themselves (Wills, DuHamel, & Vaccaro, 1995).

One reason adolescents follow the lead of their peers is that peers offer the best source of expertise and guidance regarding peer culture and experience. Adolescents also use peer relationships to practice social skills and to define right and wrong. Kohlberg (1984) defines adolescent morality as typically a morality of dyadic relationships. Right is what maintains relationships and what those one has relationships with say is right. Right is what will be lauded by significant others. Hence, the adolescent zeitgeist is not only for peers to be valued for their social influence and expertise but actually to be perceived as the criterion for moral rightness. More mature moral reasoners in adolescence tend to use less drugs (Berkowitz et al., 1991; Berkowitz, Zweben, & Begun, 1992).

There are two additional intrapsychic reasons for the powerful influence of peers. First, Erikson (1968) suggests that the core developmental task of adolescence is the formation of a personal identity (i.e., answering the questions of "Who am I?" and "Where do I fit in?") This is accomplished, in part, through introspection but also through social comparison and considering the reactions of others to oneself. Peers serve as social mirrors for the adolescent. Second, Kegan's cognitive–structural theory (1982) of ego development suggests that social relationships are central to the adolescent's developing ego; in adolescence, one does not *have* relationships, one *is* the relationships. Both of these models underscore the centrality of identity formation to adolescent development and, therefore, its importance to prevention efforts.

Adolescents who are frequent substance users (compared to experimenters) appear to be unable to derive meaning from their personal relationships (Shedler & Block, 1990), and heavy substance users often lack empathy for the feelings of others. The same is true for antisocial youth who show heavy patterns of substance use (Gibbs, Potter, & Goldstein, 1995; IOM, 1994). Such individuals are alienated from their peers—a characteristic that can be identified during the early school years and may have its roots in individual temperament and early relationship experiences with caregivers.

It has been argued that the role of peers in the lives of adolescents has been overemphasized, while that of parenting has been underplayed. According to Brook et al. (1990; p. 114),

> The relative influence of the family has been somewhat muted. [However,] the developmental analyses that have been made of adolescent drug-use data point to both the direct and indirect effect of parental factors.

These "indirect" effects may be the result of the distal causes highlighted earlier in this chapter. The overemphasis on peer factors may be due to their more proximal nature. There is, however, evidence of a relationship between parenting style (i.e., the parents' particular manner of interacting with and, particularly, controlling the behavior of their children) and substance use later in childhood and adolescence (Baumrind, 1985; Dornbusch & Ritter, 1991). In reviewing the relevant literature, Glynn and Haenlein (1988) conclude that "the near unanimous conclusion is that a positive relationship between the child and his or her parents can serve as a deterrent to the use of drugs" (p. 44). Families in which poor parenting skills are evidenced are disproportionately represented among those whose children use substances (Kumpfer, 1987). On the other hand, parental supportiveness is a protective factor against adolescent substance use (Wills et al., 1995). It is not entirely clear whether this is the result of proximal or distal effects of parenting style. However, in light of the findings on substance abuser's peer difficulties (Shedler & Block, 1990) and the relation of attachment disruption to later social deficits, it seems quite plausible that both proximal and distal parenting factors interact in producing substance use.

A process central to the adolescent task of identity formation is what Erikson calls the psychosocial moratorium, a "time-out" for experimentation and exploration (Erikson, 1968). Our culture appears to tolerate adolescent fickleness and erratic behavior and to understand that such behavior is an appropriate aspect of adolescent development. The degree of this tolerance varies by social class, by culture and family ethnicity, by historical period, and possibly by gender. Unfortunately, the only empirical reports on the relation of identity formation to adolescent substance use are two case studies (Bron, 1975; Osorio, 1993). Nonetheless, reports of greater psychological health for adolescents who merely experiment with drugs relative to abstaining or abusing adolescents suggest support for this relation (Baumrind & Moselle, 1985; Shedler & Block, 1990).

The complexity of logical and sociomoral reasoning increases as individuals proceed through adolescence. They become increasingly adept at applying formal logic to arguments and analyses. They become more philosophical and are better equipped to comprehend arguments about abstract concepts, such as justice. They also begin to attach affective responses to such abstract concepts. Indeed, they have a tendency to become quite idealistic, largely due to their new discovery of the infinite possibilities that exist in the world of the logically possible (Cowan, 1978; Inhelder & Piaget, 1958). Adolescents become increasingly able to engage in sophisticated social reasoning, including the ability to adopt multiple perspectives and the perspectives of social systems (Selman, 1980). Hence, they may be able to understand the societal implications of drug use that extend beyond the implications for an individual. For example, arguments about the effects of the drug trade on the welfare of the community are likely to have greater meaning than at earlier developmental stages. Interestingly, adolescents tend not to focus on effects on others and predominantly focus on effects (e.g., harm) for oneself (Giese & Berkowitz, 1997; Nucci, Guerra, & Lee, 1991).

Adult Development

The transition to adulthood from adolescence is a high-risk period for the development of binge drinking problems (Schulenberg, Wadsworth, & O'Malley, 1996) and perhaps for the use of other substances. There appears to be a circular pattern of influence in operation: adolescents who drink heavily or frequently engage in binge drinking appear to have more difficulty in negotiating the transition to adulthood (Schulenberg, O'Malley, & Bachman, 1996) while difficulty in negotiating the transition to adulthood may result in greater difficulties with substance abuse.

Adult substance abuse may be a response to normative stressors, paranormative events, or a combination of the two. Normative stressors are those that relate to specific developmental transitions, such as leaving home, job challenges, and building intimate relationships. Paranormative events are those that are generally seen as "atypical," either because of their timing, such as becoming a parent as a teenager or being widowed or "orphaned" during early adulthood, or because of they are unusual at any time of the life span, such as being raped, being injured in an airplane disaster, divorce, having a child with disabilities, giving birth to triplets, or certain military experiences. Normative and paranormative developmental transitions require tremendous expenditures of adaptation and adjustment energies, regardless of type, and therefore represent developmentally significant (nodal) periods in the developmental life course. Developmental transitions are especially risky periods for substance abuse.

Levinson (1978) identified a number of adulthood transitions that are highly stressful: the transition into early adulthood (17 to 22 years of age), the age-30 transition (28 to 33 years of age), and the midlife transition (40 to 45 years of age). Each transition is associated with specific stressors. The first involves accepting the status of being a novice in an unfamiliar adult world. The next concerns confrontations with success and failure in the spheres of adult achievement and the resulting self-assessments of progress in those domains. The third involves issues of mortality and the loss of youth as one faces middle age, along with a final assessment of the young adult project of "moving up the ladders" of adult achievement. Other normative life events that may produce stress are marriage, parenthood, the launching of one's own children, and retirement.

Both normative and nonnormative crises must be understood from the life-span perspective; they occur in the context of one's developmental history. How one reacts to these events, and sometimes the nature of the event itself, are products of what transpired before. Indeed, individuals often refer to their solutions to past stressful events in coping with current events (Aldwin, Sutton, & Lachman, 1996). Research suggests that how one responds to life crises is largely a product of one's lifelong coping style. Whether or not one marries, marries on time or off time, or marries successfully are partly derived from one's developmental history. The adult developmental transitions then help to construct the probabilities of one's future development. Furthermore, the contexts in which the transition occurs seem to have relevance to the outcome: persistent drug use is associated with making the transition to adulthood under conditions of extraordinary deprivation. Adults with risky coping styles should be targeted for prevention efforts, especially preceding or during those transitions and stages that present the greatest stress.

IMPLICATIONS FOR PREVENTION

Three general issues must be considered when designing substance abuse prevention interventions: the source and focus of the prevention message, phenomenology of receiving prevention messages, and developmental appropriateness of the intervention.

Source and Focus of the Prevention Message

Substance abuse deterrence messages vary on a number of dimensions, including the source of the message (whether it be a representative of a peer group, the law, or remorseful substance abusers) and the focus of the message. From a developmental perspective, it is clear that particular sources and foci will vary in effectiveness at different developmental levels. Young children are relatively responsive to messages from adults but are most responsive to messages from appealing figures, such as a sports hero or a beloved cartoon character. However, more research is needed to fully understand the relative impact of different message sources and models in childhood. For example, recent research has demonstrated the ineffectiveness of the Drug Abuse Resistance Education (DARE) program, which is delivered to children by police officers (Ennett et al., 1994).

As children grow into adolescence, there are significant shifts in the categories of people to whom they will be most responsive. Young and Ferguson (1979) found that adolescents in grades 5, 7, 9, and 12 favored parents and unrelated adults over peers for advice on moral issues. They also favored both categories of adults for advice on factual issues, but with clear age trends: parents were favored by fifth-graders, but respect for parental factual expertise systematically diminished with increasing age. Unrelated adults came in a distant second at fifth grade and increased steadily in importance thereafter, being the preferred factual source from seventh grade on. Peers remained a nonpreferred source at all ages. A markedly different pattern emerged for advice on social issues. Peers remained the preferred source at all ages but gained markedly in influence from fifth grade (when the three sources had largely equivalent influence) to ninth grade (when peers were preferred at least 4 to 1 over parents). Parents lost influence slightly during the same period. Adults outside the family dropped markedly in influence from fifth to seventh grade. Of course, these data merely address whom the adolescents consider to be more influential, not who actually is most influential. They may be the same or they may be different. Further research will make this clear. However, research suggests that peer influence on substance use increases in adolescence (Webb, Baer, & McKelvey, 1995) and is strongest for substance abusing adolescents (Coomb et al., 1991).

These data suggest that the design of a prevention program needs to consider the complex interaction of the age of the target audience, the source of the message, and the focus or content of the message. It would be a mistake for factual messages to be given to high school students primarily by parents or other adults, but it would be quite appropriate for them to be the primary factual source for elementary school children. Parents, teachers, and peers are roughly interchangeable sources of social information for fifth graders, but peers are much more influential at later ages. The "Hang Tough Milwaukee" drug and alcohol prevention media campaign addressed this issue when it was designed. It was aimed at preteens and presented entirely by peers. It includes an emphasis on what a "real friend" is and whether a "real friend" would pressure you to use substances.

Phenomenology of Receiving Prevention Messages

The complex interplay of message variables suggests another important point about developmental perspectives in designing prevention programs. The qualitative shifts in developmental status point out a flaw in assuming that the message sent is the message actually received. It is generally important to consider how individuals perceive risky behaviors differently (Severson, Slovic, & Hampson, 1993), but this is even more central when taking a life-span perspective. Individuals at different developmental stages will interpret messages differently (Glynn, Leventhal, & Hirschman, 1990). As noted previously, Young and Ferguson (1979) asked children and adolescents to recommend sources of advice concerning three advice domains (factual, moral, social). It is less clear, however, how subjects assign phenomena to one or another of those three domains. For example, would substance use be a moral or social issue (Berkowitz, Guerra, & Nucci, 1991)? Cognitive–developmental psychology (e.g., Piaget, 1970) emphasizes that individuals tend to construct meaning out of their experiences, and the nature of their constructions is determined in large part by the developmental level of their thinking. A lunar eclipse may connote a juxtaposition of heavenly bodies to an adolescent or an adult, but a preschooler may construe it as the moon playing "peek-a-boo." To an adult, the "Golden Rule" may mean logical reciprocity (do unto others what would be acceptable for them do unto you), but to an elementary-school child the focus is on instrumental exchange (do unto others so that they will do unto you, or do unto others what they did unto you).

In an attempt to explore this phenomenological aspect of substance use, we established Project Decide, a National Institute on Drug Abuse project that explores the role of moral reasoning in adolescents' decisions to use or not use drugs and alcohol. Relying on the theoretical and empirical work of Elliot Turiel (1983) and his colleagues, we have been asking adolescents and their parents whether they consider a broad range of substance use behaviors to be moral issues, social conventional issues, or personal lifestyle issues. We found that most substance use behaviors are considered to be moral issues (with notable exceptions, such as cigarette smoking and occasional alcohol consumption), although with a primary focus on harm to oneself (Berkowitz et al., 1992). We also found that mothers tend to be more moralistic than their adolescent sons and daughters. We also noted that one's categorization of substance use behavior is significantly related to one's self-reported use of the same substance. Those who consider use to be a moral issue report significantly less use than those who consider it to be a matter of personal lifestyle choice. Furthermore, analyses (Giese & Berkowitz, 1997) suggest that how adolescents make meaning of the personal relevance of use is critical to whether or not they use substances, how much they use, and even activates other protective factors. In a parallel study of adolescent reasoning about drugs, Killen, Leviton, and Cahill (1991) concluded "that educational programs about drugs and their usage should be sensitive to the aspects that individuals consider important when evaluating drug use" (p. 355).

Developmental Appropriateness

The developmental perspective suggests that intervention approaches need to be adapted to the developmental status of the target population. This may seem obvious, but it is actually a significant problem. For example, efforts to prevent substance use initiation during early adolescence have been somewhat successfully directed toward the modification of parenting skills, altering school teacher practices, and expansion of individual social skills during late childhood and/or early adolescence (O'Donnell, Hawkins, & Catalano, 1995). These are the domains of influence with greatest impact during the preinitiation period of development.

For younger children, it may be more effective to design prevention programs around general developmental strengths and not focus on substance use per se. With the current proliferation of character education programs at the elementary school level, there is an opportunity to focus on broader developmental issues (Benson, 1997) that represent some of the distal factors related to substance abuse. Although character education programs are rarely evaluated well and even less frequently include substance use as an outcome variable (Berkowitz, 2000), the best implemented and evaluated character education project, The Child Development Project, has demonstrated the prevention effectiveness of its intervention (Battistich et al., 2000).

Certainly a focus on developmental level also implies a return to the consideration of distal and proximal factors. Prevention researchers often begin with the assumption that interventions should be optimally targeted to the immediate preuse era, typically late elementary or middle school. However, if one considers the relative power of distal factors, such as infant abuse or the failure to develop adequate social skills in the early elementary school years, then later prevention efforts are handicapped by the failure to intervene when those risk factors were first developing. To complicate matters, and perhaps explain the emphasis on proximal factors, is the tendency of distal factors to have their effects through more proximal factors. For example, Brook et al. (1986) report that elementary school personality predicts adolescent substance use only as mediated through adolescent personality; child personality affects adolescent personality, which affects drug use. One could statistically conclude that the strongest predictor of adolescent drug use in this study is adolescent personality. But how does one most effectively intervene with personality development in adolescence? Most likely by addressing formative personality factors in infancy and early childhood.

Another problem is that so many intervention models are designed for school-age children and typically are delivered in school settings. A more effective approach might be to design broad, community-based efforts (Johnson, Pentz, et al., 1990; Pentz et al., 1989) with a focus on early parenting competencies (such as the *Birth to Three Program* and *Strengthening America's Families*).

CONCLUSION

The field of substance abuse prevention, indeed any prevention endeavor, is inextricably related to developmental science (Coie et al., 1993). In order to prevent a phenomenon, an understanding of its etiology and influential factors is essential. This chapter has considered the usefulness of developmental knowledge in designing substance use prevention programs by highlighting significant conceptual and methodological developmental issues and by describing central developmental phenomena at various points in the life span.

Prevention efforts should pay particular attention to the developmental needs, capabilities, and tasks of the relevant periods in the life span and incorporate a developmental perspective when considering both the population being addressed and the phenomena being prevented. This includes recognizing the dialectical nature of development, the qualitative distinctiveness of developmental periods, and the interdependency of the stages in the life span. It also includes the need to examine more temporally distal causal factors in the prevention recipe. The developmental perspective also entails a phenomenological core and points to the need for considering developmental differences both in how the prevention message is received and in which messengers are most likely to be positively received.

The substance use prevention field has embraced the science of development to a significant degree, but it may need to go even further if we are to avoid what Schinke et al. (1991) describe as approaches to substance abuse prevention that may alter attitudes or knowledge but fail to alter behavior.

REFERENCES

Abel, E. L., & Sokol, R. J. (1987). Incidence of fetal alcohol syndrome and economic impact of FAS-related anomalies. *Drug & Alcohol Dependence, 19,* 51–70.

Aldwin, C. M., Sutton, K. J., & Lachman, M. (1996). The development of coping resources in adulthood. *Journal of Personality, 64,* 837–871.

Anhalt, H. S., & Klein, M. (1976). Drug abuse in junior high school populations. *American Journal of Drug & Alcohol Abuse, 3,* 589–603.

Arnett, J. (1990). Drunk driving, sensation seeking, and egocentrism among adolescents. *Personality and Individual Differences, 11,* 541–546.

Asher, S. R. (1978) Children's peer relations. In M. E. Lamb (Ed.), *Social and personality development* (pp. 91–113). New York: Holt, Rinehart & Winston.

Bachman, J. G., Wadsworth, K. N., O'Malley, P. M., Johnston, L. D., & Schulenberg, J. E. (1997). *Smoking, drinking, and drug use in young adulthood.* Mahwah, NJ: L. Erlbaum.

Bandura, A. (1964). The stormy decade: Fact or fiction? *Psychology in the schools, 1,* 224–231.

Battistich, V., Schaps, E., Watson, M., Solomon, D., & Lewis, C. (2000). Effects of the Child Development Project on students' drug use and other problem behaviors. *Journal of Primary Prevention, 21,* 75–99.

Baumrind, D. (1985). Familial antecedents of adolescent drug use: A developmental perspective. In C. L. Jones & R. J. Battjes (Eds.), *Etiology of drug abuse: Implications for prevention* (NIDA Research Monograph No. 56, pp. 13–44). Rockville, MD: National Institute on Drug Abuse.

Baumrind, D. (1991). The influence of parenting style on adolescent competence and substance abuse. *Journal of Early Adolescence, 11,* 56–94.

Baumrind, D., & Moselle, K. A. (1985). A developmental perspective on adolescent drug abuse. In J. S. Brook, D. J. Lettieri, & D. W. Brook (Eds.), *Alcohol and substance abuse in adolescence* (pp. 41–68). New York: The Haworth Press.

Benson, P. L. (1997). *All kids are our kids: What communities must do to raise caring and responsible children and adolescents.* San Francisco: Jossey-Bass.

Berkowitz, M. W. (1982). Self-control development and relation to prosocial behavior: A response to Peterson. *Merrill-Palmer Quarterly, 28,* 223–236.

Berkowitz, M. W. (2000). Character education as prevention. In W. B. Hansen, S. M. Giles, & M. D. Fearnow-Kenney (Eds.), *Improving prevention effectiveness.* Greensboro, NC: Tanglewood Research, 37–45.

Berkowitz, M. W., Gimenez, J., Begun, A., & Zweben, A. (July, 1991). *Moral thinking and drug and alcohol use.* Paper presented at the biennial conference of the International Society for the Study of Behavioral Development, Minneapolis.

Berkowitz, M. W., & Grych, J. H. (1998). Fostering goodness: Teaching parents to facilitate children's moral development. *Journal of Moral Education, 27,* 371–391.

Berkowitz, M. W., & Grych, J. H. (2000). Early character development and education. *Early Education and Development, 11,* 55–72.

Berkowitz, M. W., Guerra, N., & Nucci, L. (1991). Sociomoral development and drug and alcohol abuse. In W. M. Kurtines & J. L. Gewirtz (Eds.), *Handbook of moral behavior and development (Volume 3)* (pp. 35–53). Hillsdale, NJ: L. Erlbaum.

Berkowitz, M. W., Zweben, A., & Begun, A. (1992). *Adolescent moral thinking and drug use.* Paper presented at the annual conference of the American Educational Research Association, San Francisco.

Block, J., Block, J. H., & Keyes, S. (1988). Longitudinally foretelling drug usage in adolescence: Early childhood personality and environmental precursors. *Child Development, 59,* 336–355.

Bowlby, J. (1969). *Attachment.* New York: Basic Books.

Bowlby, J. (1973). *Separation: Anxiety and anger.* New York: Basic Books.

Bron, B. (1975). Crisis of identity and drug abuse in juveniles. *Zeitschrift fuer Psychosomatische Medizin und Psychoanalyse, 21,* 129–150.

Brook, J. S., Brook, D. W., Gordon, A. S., Whiteman, M., & Cohen, P. (1990). The psychosocial etiology of adolescent drug use: A family interactional approach. *Genetic, Social, and General Psychology Monographs, 116,* 111–267.

Brook, J. S., Whiteman, M., Gordon, A. S., & Cohen, P. (1986). Dynamics of childhood and adolescent personality traits and adolescent drug use. *Developmental Psychology, 22,* 403–414.

Chandler, L. S., Richardson, G. A., Gallagher, J. D., & Day, N. L. (1996). Prenatal exposure to alcohol and marijuana: Effects on motor development of preschool children. *Alcoholism, Clinical & Experimental Research, 20,* 455–461.

Coie, J. D, Watt, N. F., West, S. G., Hawkins, J. D., Asarnow, J. R., Markman, H. J., Ramey, S. L., Shure, M. B., & Long, B. (1993). The science of prevention: A conceptual framework and some directions for a national research program. *American Psychologist, 48,* 1013–1022.

Colwell, B., Billingham, R., & Gross, W. (1995). Reasons for drinking, cognitive processes and alcohol consumption. *Health Values, 19,* 30–38.

Coombs, R. H., Paulson, M. J., & Richardson, M. A. (1991). Peer vs. parental influence in substance use among Hispanic and Anglo children and adolescents. *Journal of Youth and Adolescence, 20,* 73–88.

Cowan, P. A. (1978). *Piaget with feeling: Cognitive, social and emotional dimensions.* New York: Holt, Rinehart, & Winston.

DeCristofaro, J. D., & LaGamma, E. F. (1995). Prenatal exposure to opiates. *Mental Retardation and Developmental Disabilities Research Reviews, 1,* 177–182.

Dornbusch, S. M., & Ritter, P. L. (1991). *Family decision-making and authoritative parenting.* Paper presented at the biennial conference of the Society for Research in Child Development, Seattle.

Dryfoos, J. G. (1990). *Adolescents at risk: Prevention and prevalence.* New York: Oxford University Press.

Eichorn, D. (1963). Biological correlates of behavior. In H. W. Stevenson (Ed.), *Child psychology.* Chicago: University of Chicago Press.

Elkind, D. (1974). *Children and adolescents: Interpretive essays on Jean Piaget (2nd ed.).* New York: Oxford University Press.

Elliott, D. S., Huizinga, D., & Ageton, S. S. (1985). *Explaining delinquency and drug use.* Beverly Hills, CA: Sage.

Emde, R. N., Johnson, W. F., & Easterbrooks, A. (1987). The do's and don'ts of early moral development: Psychoanalytic tradition and current research. In J. Kagan & S. Lamb (Eds.), *The emergence of morality in young children* (pp. 245–276). Chicago: University of Chicago Press.

Ennett, S. T., Tobler, N. S., Ringwalt, C. L., & Flewelling, R. L. (1994). How effective is drug abuse resistance education? A meta-analysis of Project DARE outcome evaluations. *American Journal of Public Health, 84,* 1394–1401.

Erikson, E. H. (1963). *Childhood and society (2nd ed.).* New York: W. W. Norton.

Erikson, E. H. (1968). *Identity: Youth and crisis.* New York: W. W. Norton.

Erickson, M. F., Sroufe, L. A., & Egeland, B. (1985). The relationship between quality of attachment and behavior problems in preschool in a high-risk sample. In I. Bretherton & E. Waters (Eds.) *Growing points of attachment theory and research (Monographs of the Society for Research in Child Development), 209* (pp. 147–166).

Ewing, C. P. (1990). *When children kill: The dynamics of juvenile homicide.* Lexington, MA: Lexington Books.

Freeman, E. M. (1992). Addicted mothers—Addicted infants andchildren: Social work strategies for building support networks. In E. M. Freeman (Ed.), *The addiction process: Effective social work approaches* (pp. 108–122). New York: Longman.

Fried, P. A., & Watkinson, B. (2000). Visuoperceptual functioning differs in 9- to 12-year olds prenatally exposed to cigarettes and marijuana. *Neurotoxicology & Teratology, 22*(1) Jan.–Feb., 11–20.

Fried, P. A., Watkinson, B., & Gray, R. (1998). Differential effects on cognitive functioning in 9- to 12-year olds prenatally exposed to cigarettes and marijuana. *Neurotoxicology & Teratology, 20*(3) May–June, 293–306.

Fried, P. A., Watkinson, B., & Siegel, L. S. (1997). Reading and language in 9- to 12-year olds prenatally exposed to cigarettes and marijuana. *Neurotoxicology & Teratology, 19*(3) May–June, 171–183.

Gandelman, R. (1992). *Psychobiology of behavioral development.* New York: Oxford University Press.

Gibbs, J. C., Potter, G. B., & Goldstein, A. P. (1995). *The EQUIP program: Teaching youth to think and act responsibly through a peer-helping approach.* Champaign, IL: Research Press.

Giese, J. K., & Berkowitz, M. W. (1997, May). *Understanding the personal meaning of adolescent alcohol use.* Poster presented at the annual meeting of the Midwestern Psychological Association, Chicago.

Glynn, T. J., & Haenlein, M. (1988). Family theory and research on adolescent drug use: A review. In R. H. Coombs (Ed.) *The family context of adolescent drug use* (pp. 39–58). New York: The Haworth Press.

Glynn, K., Leventhal, H., & Hirschman, R. (1990). A cognitive developmental approach to smoking prevention. In C. S. Bell & R. Battjes (Eds.), *Prevention research: Deterring drug abuse among children and adolescents* (NIDA Research Monograph No. 63, pp. 130–152). Rockville, MD: National Institute on Drug Abuse.

Gould, R. L. (1978). *Transformations: Growth and change in adult life.* New York: Simon and Schuster.

Gross, W. C., & Billingham, R. E. (1990). Relationship between egocentrism, alcohol consumption and reasons given for drinking. *Psychological Reports, 67,* 459–464.

Hall, G. S. (1904). *Adolescence.* New York: Appleton.

Harlow, H., & Harlow, M. K. (1962). Social deprivation in monkeys. *Scientific American, 207,* 136–144.

Havighurst, R. J. (1974). *Developmental tasks and education* (3rd ed.). New York: D. McKay Co.

Hawkins, J. D., Catalano, R. F., & Miller, J. Y. (1992). Risk and protective factors for alcohol and other drug problems in adolescence and early adulthood: Implications for substance abuse prevention. *Psychological Bulletin, 112*(1), 64–105.

Hawkins, J. D., Lishner, D. M., Catalano, R. F., & Howard, M. O. (1986). Childhood predictors of adolescent substance abuse: Toward an empirically grounded theory. In S. Grizwold-Ezekoye, K. L. Kumpfer, & W. J. Bukoski (Eds.), *Childhood and chemical abuse: Prevention and intervention* (pp. 11–48). New York: The Haworth Press.

Howard, J., Boyd, G. M., & Zucker, R. A. (1995). An overview of issues. In G. M. Boyd, J. Howard, & R. A. Zucker (Eds.), *Alcohol problems among adolescents: Current directions in prevention research* (pp. 1–12). Hillsdale, NJ: L. Erlbaum.

Hoyseth, K. S., & Jones, P. J. (1989). Ethanol induced teratogenesis: Characterization, mechanisms and diagnostic approaches. *Life Sciences, 44,* 643–649.

Inhelder, B., & Piaget, J. (1958). *The growth of logical thinking from childhood to adolescence.* New York: Basic Books.

Institute of Medicine (1994). *Reducing risk for mental disorders: Frontiers for preventive intervention research.* Washington, DC: National Academy Press.

Jacobson, J. L., & Wille, D. E. (1986). The influence of attachment pattern on developmental changes in peer interaction from the toddler to the preschool period. *Child Development, 57,* 338–347.

Johnson, H. L., Glassman, M. B., Fiks, K. B., & Rosen, T. S. (1990). Resilient children: Individual differences in developmental outcome of children born to drug abusers. *The Journal of Genetic Psychology, 151,* 523–539.

Johnson, L. D., O'Malley, P. M., & Bachman, J. G. (1996). *National survey results on drug use from the Monitoring the Future study, 1975–1995 (Volume 1: Secondary school students).* Rockville, MD: National Institute on Drug Abuse.

Johnson, C. A., Pentz, M. A., Weber, M. D., Dwyer, J. H., Baer, N., MacKinnon, D. P., & Hansen, W. B. (1990). Relative effectiveness of comprehensive community programming for drug abuse prevention with high-risk and low-risk adolescents. *Journal of Consulting and Clinical Psychology, 58,* 447–456.

Kandel, D. B. (1985). On processes of peer influences in adolescent drug use: A developmental perspective. In J. Brook, D. Lettieri, & D.W. Brook (Eds.), *Alcohol and substance abuse in adolescence* (pp. 139–164). New York: The Haworth Press.

Kandel, D. B., & Davies, M. (1992). Progression to regular marijuana involvement: Phenomenology and risk factors for near-daily use. In M. Glantz & R. Pickens (Eds.), *Vulnerability to drug abuse* (pp. 211–254). Washington, DC: American Psychological Association.

Kaplan, L. J. (1995). *No voice is every wholly lost: An exploration of the everlasting attachment between parent and child.* New York: Touchstone.

Katchadourian, H. (1977). *The biology of adolescence.* San Francisco: W. H. Freeman.

Kegan, R. G. (1982). *The evolving self: Problems and process in human development.* Cambridge, MA: Harvard University Press.

Kellam, S. G. (1994). Testing theory through developmental epidemiologically based prevention research. In A. Ca'zares & L. A. Beatty (Eds.), *Scientific methods for prevention intervention research* (NIDA Research Monograph 139 pp. 37–57). Rockville, MD: National Institute on Drug Abuse.

Kellam, S. G., Brown, C. H., & Fleming, J. P. (1982). Social adaptation to first grade and teenage drug, alcohol and cigarette use. Journal of School Health, *52,* 301–306.

Kellam, S. G., & VanHorn, Y. V. (1997). Life course development, community epidemiology, and preventive trials: A scientific structure for prevention research. *American Journal of Community Psychology, 25,* 177–188.

Killen, M., Leviton, M., & Cahill, J. (1991). Adolescent reasoning about drug use. *Journal of Adolescent Research, 6,* 336–356.

Kohlberg, L. (1984). *Essays on Moral Development. Volume 2: The psychology of moral development.* San Francisco: Harper & Row.

Kochanska, G. (1993). Toward a synthesis of parental socialization and child temperament in early development of conscience. *Child Development, 64,* 325–347.

Kumpfer, K. L. (1987) Special populations: Etiology and prevention of vulnerability to chemical dependency in children of substance abusers. In B. S. Brown & A. R. Mills (Eds.), *Youth at high risk for substance abuse* (pp. 1–71). Rockville, MD: NIDA.

Kumpfer, K. L., & DeMarsh, J. (1985). Family environmental and genetic influences on children's future chemical dependency. *Journal of Children in a Contemporary Society, 18,* 49–91.

Kusserow, R. P. (1992). *Youth and alcohol: Dangerous and deadly consequences.* U.S. Department of Health and Human Services: Office of the Inspector General.

Lamb, S., & Feeny, N. C. (1995). Early moral sense and socialization. In W. M. Kurtines & J. L. Gewirtz (Eds.), *Moral development: An introduction* (pp. 497–510). Boston: Allyn & Bacon.

Levinson, D. J. (1978). *The seasons of a man's life.* New York: Knopf.

Madden, J. D., Payne, T. F., & Miller, S. (1986). Maternal cocaine abuse and effect on the newborn. *Pediatrics, 77,* 209–211.

Magid, K., & McKelvey, C. A. (1987). *High risk: Children without conscience.* New York: Bantam Books.

Magnusson, D., Stattin, H., & Allen, V. L. (1986). Differential maturation among girls and its's relevance to social adjustment: A longitudinal perspective. In D. L. Featherman & R. M. Lerner (Eds.), *Life-span development and behavior, vol. 7* (pp. 135–172). New York: Academic Press.

Matas, L., Arend, R., & Sroufe, L. A. (1978). Continuity of adaptation in the second year: The relationship between quality of attachment and later competence. *Child Development, 49,* 547–556.

Mattson, S. N., Riley, E. P., Gramling, L., Delis, D. C., & Jones, K. L. (1998). Neuropsychologicalcomparison of alcohol-exposed children with or without physical features of fetal alcohol syndrome. *Neuropsychology, 12,* 146–153.

McCord, J. (1988a). Alcoholism: toward understanding genetic and social factors. *Psychiatry, 51,* 131–141.

McCord, J. (1988b). Identifying developmental paradigms leading to alcoholism. *Journal of Studies on Alcohol, 49,* 357–362.

Muuss, R. E. (1988). *Theories of adolescence (5th ed.).* New York: Random House.

Neuspiel, D. R., Hamel, S. C., Hochberg, E., Greene, J., & Campbell, D. (1991) Maternal cocaine use and infant behavior. *Neurotoxicology and Teratology, 13,* 229–233.

Nucci, L., Guerra, N., & Lee, J. (1991). Adolescent judgments of the personal, prudential, and normative aspects of drug usage. *Developmental Psychology, 27,* 841–848.

O'Donnell, J., Hawkins, J. D., & Catalano, R. F. (1995). Preventing school failure, drug use, and delinquency among low-income children: Long-term intervention in elementary schools. *American Journal of Orthopsychiatry, 65,* 87–100.

Offer, D. (1969). *The psychological world of the teen-ager: A study of normal adolescent boys.* New York: Basic Books.

Osorio, L. C. (1993). The delinquential syndrome: A study of adolescent psychopathology. *International Journal of Adolescent Medicine and Health, 6,* 59–68.

Pentz, M. A., Dwyer, J. H., MacKinnon, D., Flay, B. R., Hansen, W. B., Wang, E. Y. I., & Johnson, C. A. (1989). A multi-community trial for primary prevention of adolescent drug abuse: Effects on drug use prevalence. *Journal of the American Medical Association, 261,* 3259–3266.

Petersen, A. C. (1982). Developmental issues in adolescent health. In T. J. Coates, A. C. Petersen, & C. Perry (Eds.), *Promoting adolescent health: A dialog on research and practice* (pp. 61–71). New York: Academic Press.

Petraitis, J., Flay, B. R., & Miller, T. Q. (1995). Reviewing theories of adolescent substance use: Organizing pieces in the puzzle. *Psychological Bulletin, 117,* 67–86.

Piaget, J. (1970). Piaget's theory. In P. M. Mussen (Ed.) *Carmichael's manual of child psychology (3rd ed.)* (pp. 703–732). New York: Wiley.

Piaget, J., & Inhelder, B. (1969). *The psychology of the child.* New York: Basic Books.

Pipp, S., Shaver, P., Jennings, S., Lamborn, S., & Fischer, K. W. (1985). Adolescents' theories about their development of their relationships with parents. *Journal of Personality and Social Psychology, 48,* 991–1001.

Powers, S. I., Hauser, S. T., & Kilner, L. A. (1989). Adolescent mental health. *American Psychologist, 44,* 200–208.

Quadrel, M. J., Fischoff, B., & Davis, W. (1993). Adolescent (In)vulnerability. *American Psychologist, 48,* 102–116.

Regan, D. O., Ehrlich, S. M., & Finnegan, L. P. (1987). Infants of drug addicts: At risk for child abuse, neglect, and placement in foster care. *Neurotoxicology & Teratology, 9,* 315–319.

Robins, L. N. (1980). The natural history of drug abuse. *Acta Psychiatrica Scandinavica. 62,* 7–20.

Rousseau, J. J. (1962). In W. Boyd (Ed.), *The Emile of Jean Jacques Rousseau.* New York: Columbia Teachers College (Original publication, 1762).

Rutter, M. (1979). Maternal deprivation 1972–1978: New findings, new concepts, new approaches. *Child Development, 50,* 283–305.

Schinke, S. P., Botvin, G. J., & Orlandi, M. A. (1991). *Substance abuse in children and adolescents: Evaluation and intervention.* Newbury Park, CA: Sage.

Schulenberg, J. E., O'Malley, P. M., & Bachman, J. G. (1996). Getting drunk and growing up: Trajectories of frequent binge drinking during the transition to young adulthood. *Journal of Studies on Alcohol, 57*(xx), 289–304.

Schulenberg, J. E., Wadsworth, K., & O'Malley, P. M. (1996). Adoescent risk factors for binge drinking during the transition to young adulthood: Variable- and pattern-centered approaches to change. *Developmental Psychology, 32*(3), 659–74.

Selman, R. (1980). *The development of interpersonal understanding.* New York: Academic Press.

Severson, H. H., Slovic, P., & Hampson, S. (1993). Adolescents perception of risk: Understanding and preventing high risk behavior. *Advances in Consumer Research, 20,* 1–6.

Shedler, J., & Block, J. (1990). Adolescent drug use and psychological health: A longitudinal inquiry. *American Psychologist, 45*(5), 612–630.

Silbereisen, R. K., Petersen, A. C., Albrecht, H. T., & Kracke, B. (1989). Maturational timing and the development of problem behavior: Longitudinal studies in adolescence. *Journal of Early Adolescence, 9,* 247–268.

Simeonsson, R. J. (Ed) (1994). *Risk, resilience & prevention: Promoting the well-being of all children.* Baltimore: Paul H. Brookes Publishing Co.

Simmons, R. G., & Blyth, D. A. (1987). *Moving into adolescence.* Hawthorne, NY: Aldine.

Simmons, R., Rosenberg, F., & Rosenberg, M. (1973). Disturbance in the self-image at adolescence. *American Sociological Review, 38,* 553–568.

Steinberg, L. (1981). Transformations in family relations at puberty. *Developmental Psychology, 17,* 833–840.

Streissguth, A. P., Sampson, P. D., & Barr, H. M. (1989). Neurobehavioral dose-response effects of prenatal alcohol exposure in humans from infancy to adulthood. *Annals of the New York Academy of Sciences, 562,* 145–158.

Sullivan, H. S. (1953). *The interpersonal theory of psychiatry.* New York: W. W. Norton.

Suomi, S. J., Mineka, S., & DeLizio, R. D. (1983). Short- and long-term effects of repetitive mother-infant separations on social development in Rhesus monkeys. *Developmental Psychology, 19,* 770–786.

Tanner, J. M. (1970). Physical growth. In P. Mussen (Ed.) *Carmichael's manual of child psychology* (Vol. 1, pp. 77–156). New York: Wiley.

Tarter, R. E., & Vanyukov, M. (1994). Alcoholism: A developmental disorder. *Journal of Consulting & Clinical Psychology,* 1096–1107.

Turiel, E. (1983). *The development of social knowledge: Morality and convention.* New York: Cambridge University Press.

Wallen, J. (1993). *Addiction in human development: Developmental perspectives on addiction and recovery.* New York: Haworth Press.

Waller, M. B. (1993). *Crack-affected children: A teacher's guide.* Newbury Park, CA: Corwin Press.

Webb, J. A., Baer, P. E., & McKelvey, R. S. (1995). Development of a risk profile for intentions to use alcohol among fifth and sixth graders. *Journal of the American Academy of Child and Adolescent Psychiatry, 34,* 772–778.

Werner, H. (1948). *Comparative psychology of mental health.* New York: International Universities Press.

Wills, T. A., DuHamel, K., & Vaccaro, D. (1995). Activity and mood temperament as predictors of adolescent substance use: Test of a self-regulation mediational model. *Journal of Personality and Social Psychology, 68,* 901–916.

Young, H., & Ferguson, L. (1979). Developmental changes through adolescence in the spontaneous nomination of reference groups as a function of decision context. *Journal of Youth and Adolescence, 8,* 239–252.

PART V

SPECIAL POPULATIONS

CHAPTER 17

Gender Issues in Substance Abuse Prevention

LOUISE ANN ROHRBACH

JOEL MILAM

INTRODUCTION

The costs to our nation of alcohol, tobacco, and other drug use in terms of mortality, morbidity, and lost productivity are very high (U.S. Department of Health & Human Services, 1990; U.S. General Accounting Office, 1996). Much of the problem of adult substance use takes root during adolescence, with early onset of drug use being a risk factor for later substance abuse and other problems (Kandel, 1980; Kandel et al., 1986). After several years of decline from a peak in the late 1970s, rates of substance use resumed a sharp upward trend in the 1990s (Johnston, O'Malley, & Bachman, 1996; Substance Abuse and Mental Health Services Administration, 1996). Recent trends in substance use among youth show increasing rates of illicit drug use, in particular, marijuana use. In addition, rates of cigarette smoking among adolescents have increased, and levels of drunkenness and problematic alcohol use among high school and college students remain unacceptably high (Johnston et al., 1996).

Our nation has generally thought of alcohol and other drug abuse as a problem of men (Blumenthal, 1998). Because of this belief and the fact that past studies often used only male subjects, the extent and effects of drug abuse on women are not fully understood. However, the estimated number of women who use or abuse drugs is of considerable concern. Although drug use is more common among younger men than younger women, by the time people reach adulthood,

LOUISE ANN ROHRBACH • Institute for Health Promotion and Disease Prevention Research, University of Southern California, Alhambra, California 91803

JOEL MILAM • Institute for Health Promotion and Disease Prevention Research, University of Southern California, Los Angeles, California 90089

the use of alcohol, tobacco, and other drugs and the improper use of prescription medications takes a serious toll on the health and well-being of both men and women.

Recent research suggests that there are differences between the sexes in the etiology of drug abuse. It is important that practitioners understand these differences and consider the implications they have for prevention of drug abuse. This chapter reviews research findings on gender differences in the patterns and etiology of substance use, discusses gender-specific approaches to treatment and prevention, and explores the implications of these findings for prevention research and practice.

GENDER DIFFERENCES IN THE PREVALENCE
OF DRUG USE

For most substances, there is a greater prevalence of use among males than females. Data from the National Household Survey on Drug Abuse in 1992 showed that the proportion of those who had ever used an illicit drug was lower among women (32%) than men (41%) (Substance Abuse and Mental Health Administration, 1992). Surveys show that women are less likely to drink and less likely to report drinking-related problems than are men (Johnson, 1991). Differences between the sexes generally increase with age, and within age groups the gap between the sexes tends to increase at higher levels of drug use.

Among younger adolescents, sex differences in the lifetime prevalence of substance use are small. In fact, for some drugs, including inhalants, stimulants, tranquilizers, and cocaine, eighth-grade females have slightly higher rates of use than do males (Johnston et al., 1996). The one substance that is used almost exclusively by males is smokeless tobacco, with a 30-day prevalence of 2.2% among eighth-grade males and 0.3% among eighth-grade females in 1995 (Johnston et al., 1996).

Sex differences seem to emerge over the course of middle to late adolescence, with males more likely to use more types of substances, to use them in greater amounts, and to use them with greater frequency by the 12th grade. For instance, the annual prevalence of marijuana use among high school seniors in 1995 was 38% for males and 31% for females, and daily use of marijuana was even more concentrated among males (7% for males versus 2% for females). Senior males were also more likely to report daily use of alcohol (6% for males versus 2% for females) and drunkenness in the past 30 days (38% for males versus 29% for females). Since 1992, rates of 30-day and daily smoking have been higher among males than females, although smoking rates were higher among females in the late 1980s. During the past decade, the annual prevalence rates in the senior year of high school have tended to be one and one-half to two and one-half times higher among males than among females for heroin, other opiates, cocaine, crack cocaine, inhalants, and LSD. In addition, males accounted for an even greater share of the frequent or heavy users of these various classes of drugs. The only exception to the rule that males are more frequent users of illicit drugs than are females occurs for stimulant use in high school, where females are usually at the same level or slightly higher (Johnston et al., 1996).

GENDER DIFFERENCES IN ONSET AND STAGES
OF DRUG USE

Male and female adolescents differ in the time of onset and pattern of progression of drug use, with males being at higher risk for early onset of drug use than females (Kandel & Logan, 1984; Kandel & Yamaguchi, 1993). Kandel and her colleagues (1984, 1993) have shown that there are well-delineated stages and sequences of involvement in the use of drugs during adolescence. The use of alcohol and/or cigarettes marks the first stage, followed by the use of marijuana in the second stage, and the use of illicit drugs other than marijuana in the third stage. The sequence is somewhat different for females, in that cigarette smoking plays a more important role for women in the initiation of illicit drugs. A subgroup of females will not progress to illicit drug use unless they have already smoked cigarettes, but males progress to illicit drugs when they have used alcohol, whether or not they have smoked cigarettes (Kandel, Warner, & Kessler, 1998).

For the most part, the risk of developing dependence, once having used an illicit drug, is greater for men than for women. For instance, the rate of lifetime dependence on marijuana is twice as high among men (12%) as among women (6%). For alcohol as well, men are more than twice as likely to develop dependence (21%) than are women (9%). However, for nonmedical use of psychotropic drugs (such as sedatives), women (12%) are significantly more likely than men (7%) to develop dependence. There are only slight sex differences in the risk of developing dependence on tobacco (33% for men versus 31% for women), cocaine (18% for men versus 15% for women), and heroin (22% for men versus 25% for women) (Anthony, Warner, & Kessler, 1994).

Biological Factors

One of the explanations for sex differences in the prevalence and patterns of drug use is that men's and women's bodies respond differently to at least some substances. For instance, it has been shown that after consuming comparable amounts of ethanol, even with allowances for differences in size, women have higher blood alcohol concentrations than do men and thus more quickly feel the effects of alcohol or become drunk (Frezza et al., 1990; Jones & Jones, 1976). Women who abuse alcohol are also more susceptible to cirrhosis of the liver, circulatory disorders, and anemia than are male abusers (Hill, 1984; Saunders, Davis, & Williams, 1981). Women show considerable variation in day-to-day peak blood alcohol levels, which appear to be related to the phases of the menstrual cycle. Thus, women in general may be less able to accurately predict the effect of a given amount of alcohol on their bodies than are men.

Other research shows that women may metabolize cocaine at different rates than do males (Lukas et al., 1996). In addition, women may be more sensitive to nicotine, the primary pharmacological agent of addiction in tobacco, than are men (Battig, Buzzi, & Nil, 1982). Because of this, women may be more resistant to behavioral and pharmacological treatment strategies for smoking cessation than are men (U.S. Department of Health and Human Services, 1989).

RISK AND PROTECTIVE FACTORS FOR SUBSTANCE ABUSE

Risk factors can be used to explain the onset of drug use, transitions from experimental to regular use, and adverse consequences from drug use. This approach asserts that exposure to various risk and protective factors, together with variations in vulnerability to the impact of these factors, explains adolescent drug use and abuse (Hawkins, Catalano, & Miller, 1992). However, there has been relatively little research on gender differences in risk factors and differential pathways between those factors and the development of drug abuse. Most current knowledge about gender differences in risk factors comes from research on alcohol and tobacco use rather than on illicit drug use, and many of the studies have been cross-sectional, limiting the extent to which conclusions about causality can be drawn.

Reviews of the literature find that many risk factors are the same for males and females; however, in some cases different risk factors appear to exist for one sex and not for the other, and in other cases males and females are affected differentially by the same risk factors. Overall, the evidence provides support for the conclusion that there are differences in the processes by which risk factors affect substance use among males and females (Bodinger de Uriarte & Austin, 1991; Clayton, 1991). These will be discussed by category of risk factor.

Early Precursors of Substance Abuse

Several studies indicate that sex differences in factors known to be precursors of substance abuse, such as shyness and childhood aggression, appear as early as first grade. Kellam and colleagues found that shyness among first-grade males, but not females, inhibited substance use in adolescence (Kellam et al., 1983). Early aggressiveness appears to be an even more important predictor of substance use and other deviant behaviors in adolescence and early adulthood. Aggressiveness is far more common among first-grade males than females, and it is a strong predictor of increased substance use by males in adolescence, but not by females. However, other researchers have not found sex differences in the developmental path between childhood aggression and later drug use (Brook, Whiteman, & Finch, 1992).

Social Environment Factors

For both male and female adolescents, strong bonds to family are associated with lower use of some substances (Bodinger de Uriarte & Austin, 1991). However, several studies have found gender differences in the strength of association between family bonds and substance use. Although males generally have stronger family bonds than do females (Ensminger, Brown, & Kellam, 1982), low attachment to parents is more strongly correlated with cigarette smoking (Krohn et al., 1986), alcohol use (Johnson & Marcos, 1988), and marijuana use (Ensminger et al., 1982) among females than males. Furthermore, low parental monitoring (Krohn et al., 1986), low parental concern (Murray et al., 1983), and an unstructured home environment (Block, Block, & Keyes, 1988) appear to be more strongly associated with substance use among females. Both genders are influenced by parental and sibling substance use; however, there is some evidence that female adolescents are more likely than males to smoke if at least one parent (Charlton & Blair, 1989; Flay, Hu, & Richardson, 1998; Gritz, 1982; Murray et al., 1983; Nolte, Smith, & O'Rourke, 1983; Williams, 1973) or a sister smokes (Van Roosmalen & McDaniel, 1992). Similarly, parental drinking appears to influence adolescent daughters more than it affects sons (Forney, Forney, & Ripley, 1988; Thompson & Wilsnack, 1984).

Having friends who use drugs has consistently been shown to be the strongest predictor of adolescent substance use. Many studies find no gender differences in peer influences (Bodinger de Uriarte & Austin, 1991; Clayton, 1991), but several studies suggest that peers may have different influences on males and females at different ages (Chassin et al., 1986; Hu et al., 1995). For example, in a sample of students in 6th through 11th grade, Chassin and colleagues found that transitions to higher levels of smoking were predicted by an increased number of smoking friends for girls at younger ages and for boys at older ages.

Low attachment to school, including lower school performance, lower academic aspirations, less interest in school, and greater truancy, has been associated with cigarette (Krohn, et al., 1986) and other drug use (Ensminger et al., 1982; Newcomb et al., 1987; Paulson, Coombs, & Richardson, 1990) for both males and females. Few studies have looked at gender differences in exposure to drug use in the community, but one study suggests that community influences may have a stronger effect on females than on males (Feigelman et al., 1995).

Psychosocial and Intrapersonal Factors

In the smoking antecedents literature, there is a frequently mentioned hypothesis that males may smoke cigarettes as a mechanism to cope with social insecurity, while females who smoke are more socially advanced and self-confident (Clayton, 1991). Recent studies provide some evidence for this distinction. Cigarette use among female adolescents is more strongly associated with social competence (Lifrak et al., 1997), sociability, and lack of shyness (Allen et al., 1994). Although many smoking prevention programs are based on the assumption that adolescents begin to smoke because they lack the skills to obtain social approval in other ways, Gilchrist, Schinke, and Nurius (1989) found that resistance skills and resistance self-efficacy are positively associated with cigarette smoking among high-risk girls. Male substance use, on the other hand, is more strongly associated with high levels of self-derogation (Harlow, Newcomb, & Bentler, 1986), loneliness, hopelessness (Allen et al., 1994), alienation, and anxiety about social interactions (Thomas, 1996).

The literature on adolescent self-concept, self-worth, and self-image includes findings that are inconsistent with a profile of the female substance user as a self-confident individual. The relationship between substance use and self-concept, self-esteem, and self-image has long been debated due to conflicting findings (Bodinger de Uriarte & Austin, 1991). Furthermore, it is difficult to generalize about these relationships because of the different elements involved in self-concept and the different measurement approaches that are used. Nevertheless, many studies show that females have lower self-esteem and poorer self-concepts than males (e.g., Pederson, Koval, & O'Connor, 1997), and this puts them at greater risk for tobacco, alcohol, and other drug use (e.g., Block et al., 1988).

One element of self-image that puts females at risk for use of specific substances is concern about physical appearance and weight. Females tend to be more susceptible than males to society's emphasis on slenderness. Many perceive themselves as being overweight and diet more often than males do. Perceived unattractiveness, dieting, being moderately overweight, and weight concern (Camp et al., 1993; French et al., 1994; Halek et al., 1993) are more strongly associated with the use of cigarettes and amphetamines (Gritz & Crane, 1991) among females than among males. Some adolescent females appear to be using cigarettes and aphetamines as a weight-control strategy (Camp et al., 1993; French et al., 1994; Halek et al., 1993).

Depression, anxiety, and stress may also have different effects on substance use among males and females. Female adolescents have more symptoms of depression and anxiety than do male adolescents (Patton et al., 1996; Pederson et al., 1997; Pope et al., 1994). There is some evidence for a stronger relationship between depression and cigarette use in males (Malkin & Allen, 1980), but other evidence shows stronger relationships between depression and cigarette use (Patton et al., 1996) and depression and alcohol use in females (Deykin, Levy, & Wells, 1987; Windle & Barnes, 1988). Studies of adult women also document a strong relationship between substance use and depression (Cohen et al., 1991). During adolescence and adulthood, increases in difficult life events (Baer et al., 1987) and stress (Windle & Barnes, 1988; Sanders-Phillips, 1998) are predictors of smoking and drinking among females. More research is needed to determine the extent to which adolescent males and females differ in their use of substances to cope with stress, anxiety, and depression.

Attitudes and Cognitions

Several studies suggest that gender-role ideology, or one's attitudes about the proper social roles of men and women, account for sex differences in alcohol use. Females with traditional gender-role attitudes drink less, while males with conventional gender-role attitudes drink more than their nonconventional counterparts (Celentano & McQueen, 1984; Mosher & Sirkin, 1984). Among adolescents, those with conventional gender attitudes conform more closely to cultural norms that condone drinking among males but not among females (Huselid & Cooper, 1992; Thomas, 1996). Gender differences in other drug use among adolescents may also be attributed to conventional gender-role attitudes, which discourage use among females (Ferrence, 1980).

Adolescent beliefs about social norms for drug use may also differ by sex. Girls report less perceived approval of alcohol use from friends than do boys (Keefe, 1994; Pope et al., 1994), and it appears that females may be more susceptible than males to peer approval of drinking (Pope et al., 1994). In regard to perceived approval of alcohol use from parents, no differences between boys and girls have been found, and perceived parental approval is strongly associated with drinking for both groups.

There is also evidence that boys and girls differ in their beliefs about the consequences of alcohol, tobacco, and other drug use. For example, Chassin and colleagues (1985) found that adolescent boys believe that drinking enhances their social image among peers, while teenage girls do not view drinking as socially desirable (Chassin, Tetzloff, & Hershey, 1985). Overall, girls expect fewer benefits and more costs from alcohol use than do boys (Keefe, 1994). In addition, girls are more likely to hold attitudes that reinforce the health compromising properties of smoking (Pederson et al., 1997). Thomas (1996) reported that adolescent males have stronger beliefs about various positive physical and psychosocial effects of alcohol use than females do, and pro-alcohol beliefs have a direct effect on alcohol and other drug use among males but not among females.

In summary, these findings provide some support for gender differences in the pathways from risk factors to adolescent substance use and abuse. As early as first grade, boys and girls have been found to differ in aggressiveness, and there is evidence that aggressiveness is a strong predictor of increased substance use in adolescence by males but not by females (Kellam et al., 1983). Risk factors such as low attachment to parents, low parental monitoring, parental drinking and smoking, concern about physical appearance and weight, increases in depression and stress, and perceived peer approval for drinking appear to be stronger predictors for substance use among females than males. Risk factors such as poor social skills, loneliness, alienation, and greater pro-alcohol beliefs may be stronger predictors of substance use for males relative to females.

Gender differences in relationships between risk factors and substance use are also probably related to gender differences in developmental factors such as changes in social and cognitive processes during adolescence (e.g., parental and peer bonding) and the onset of puberty (Brooks-Gunn & Reiter, 1990). Although all adolescents experience changes in attachments to friends relative to parents, these processes may differ somewhat for males and females. Puberty, the series of biological changes that result in a reproductively mature individual, has been shown to exert small but consistent effects on the self-image and social relationships of young adolescents. These effects, in turn, may be related to drug use and other problem behaviors, and they may differ by sex. For example, the psychological effects of menstruation have been associated with increased consumption of alcohol among female adolescents (Lee, 1978).

GENDER ISSUES IN TREATMENT AND PREVENTION

Treatment Programs

Since males and females may begin using and abusing alcohol, tobacco, and other drugs at a different pace and through different etiological processes, it has been suggested that gender-specific treatment and prevention programs may be more effective than those that use a mixed-gender approach. Recent literature on alcohol and other drug treatment abounds with compelling aruguments for female-specific approaches. Researchers have documented barriers to treatment that affect females more than males, including lack of finances, the need for child care and transportation (Reed, 1987; Schliebner, 1994), perceived sexism of programs (e.g., predominantly male treatment staff) (Reed, 1985), and shame about substance use. In addition, it has been suggested that women have specific needs for treatment that males may not have, including parenting training, empowerment training, learning to cope with a history of sexual abuse and domestic violence, and the need for female-specific health services (e.g., gynecological, prenatal care) and mental health services (e.g., eating disorders, low self-esteem) (Kearney, 1997; Reed, 1987; Wald, Harvey, & Hibbard, 1995).

Although many female-specific treatment approaches have been tried in the United States, there have been few methologically sound evaluations of such programs (Moras, 1998). The strongest study of a gender-specific treatment intervention was conducted by Dahlgren and Willander (1989), who randomly assigned female alcohol users to either a female-specific or a mixed-gender treatment program. They found that women in the female-specific program had less alcohol consumption and better social adjustment at the 2-year follow-up than did women in the mixed-gender program. In another alcohol use treatment study in which randomization was not used, women in female-specific programs showed no better outcomes than did women in mixed-gender programs (Copeland & Hall, 1992). However, Copeland and colleagues (1993) and others (Reed & Liebson, 1981) report that women who enroll in female-specific programs differ demographically from those who enroll in traditional programs, suggesting that broader availability of female-specific programs may expand the population of female substance users who will enter treatment (Moras, 1998).

Few studies have examined gender differences in the efficacy of behavioral substance use treatments for alcohol and other drug use. Of the studies that have been conducted, no gender differences have been reported for semicomprehensive treatment approaches, contingency management methods, or relapse prevention treatments (Moras, 1998).

Prevention Programs

As with treatment, several prevention researchers have argued persuasively that female-specific prevention interventions may be more effective than mixed-gender approaches, particularly for smoking (e.g., Clayton, 1991; Gilchrist et al., 1989). Most prevention studies that target both sexes have not examined differential efficacy for males and females. Two of the studies that have looked at this question have reported that psychosocial-based programs are more effective in reducing the onset of alcohol, tobacco, and other drug use among female adolescents than among males (Botvin, Baker, Filazzola, & Botvin, 1990; Graham, Johnson, Hansen, Flay, & Gee, 1990). However, other studies show that such programs are less effective with females than males (DeJong, 1987; Gilchrist, Gillmore, & Lohr, 1990). In the study by Gilchrist and colleagues

(1989), girls at high risk for becoming smokers were the least responsive to a social skills building intervention, compared to low-risk girls and high- and low-risk boys. The authors conclude that substantial reductions in smoking among female adolescents may require a different approach than the social skill-building programs that are currently considered the state-of-the-art.

A review of the prevention literature found only a few drug use prevention studies that evaluated the efficacy of a gender-specific approach. Palinkas and colleagues randomly assigned high-risk females to either a social skills and empowerment training program or a control intervention with no skills training (Palinkas et al., 1996). They found that the social skills training had a negative effect; that is, the prevalence of alcohol and drug use increased significantly among females in the skills training group but not among those in the control group. Worden and colleagues (1996) tested the relative efficacy of a combined school-based smoking prevention program and media intervention that included separate media spots for males and females, but placed greater emphasis on the female-targeted ones, versus a school program alone. They found that weekly smoking among girls in the media-plus-school intervention communities increased less over a 4-year period than among girls in the school-only communities. Among boys, changes in weekly smoking followed the same pattern as for girls, but the difference was not statistically significant (Worden et al., 1996).

In summary, there is no clear research evidence that female substance users require gender-specific treatments. However, some findings suggest that gender-specific treatment interventions might be valuable for subtypes of female users (Moras, 1998). Less attention has been paid to the issue of gender-specific prevention interventions, but there is limited evidence to suggest that female-specific approaches may be more beneficial for females, particularly to reduce cigarette smoking.

Implications for Substance Use Prevention Interventions

Effective prevention programs address risk factors, such as social influences, normative beliefs, social skills, and expectancies regarding use, that are the strongest predictors of substance use and are most amenable to change (Tobler, 1986). Most of these programs are school based and are delivered to mixed-gender groups of students. However, research reviewed in this chapter suggests that males and females may develop patterns of drug use at different rates and by different etiological pathways. Current mixed-gender approaches may not be as valuable for both gender groups as approaches that include at least some gender-specific components.

Gender-specific approaches could be designed to place greater emphasis on the risk factors that appear to be more important for each gender group. For example, the role of female concerns about weight control should be addressed in a smoking prevention program and could be best addressed in a female-only setting. Similarly, discussion of issues regarding drug use during pregnancy, sexual abuse victimization, and menstruation, as well as skills training in coping with stress, may be more relevant to female than to male adolescents. It has also been suggested that, since female addicts often are initiated into drug use and supplied drugs by male partners, drug abuse prevention for females should directly address males' roles in the introduction to drugs (Amaro & Hardy-Fanta, 1995). For males, programs that place greater emphasis on changing pro-substance-use beliefs and building social competence and skills may achieve greater reductions in alcohol, tobacco, and other drug use.

Although the idea of structuring prevention programs differently for males and females is not new, few researchers and practitioners have experimented with this type of prevention approach. Perhaps it is because most substance use prevention programs are implemented in schools, and separation of students into single-gender groups is logistically difficult. However, students are often placed in ability groupings for teaching such subjects such as math and reading (Clayton, 1991). Future generations of substance use prevention research should begin to test these types of approaches. One model that may be effective is to provide some program components, such as those suggested previously, in gender-specific groupings, and others, such as factual information about social influences and the consequences of substance use, in mixed-gender groupings (Clayton, 1991).

CONCLUSION

Research on psychosocial determinants of alcohol, tobacco, and other drug use among adolescents should place greater emphasis on gender differences. Although many studies report the prevalence of specific determinants by gender, few have investigated whether these factors have differential predictive power for males and females. More etiological studies that utilize longitudinal designs are needed. Researchers should strive, in particular, to replicate studies on specific antecedents that have shown gender differences in associations with substance use. Research should also examine theory-derived combinations of antecedents using multivariate modeling techniques, such as structural equation modeling. Such techniques allow one to investigate the mechanisms of gender as a moderator (Baron & Kenny, 1986) by simultaneously evaluating separate models for males and females.

To increase our understanding of how well prevention interventions work for gender groups, intervention research that targets mixed-gender groups should report differential effectiveness for males and females. In addition, future intervention studies should focus on the efficacy of gender-specific prevention programs. Female- and male-specific approaches could be compared to mixed-gender programs. Component study designs could address the relative efficacy of a gender-specific versus mixed-gender setting for specific components such as skills training.

Acknowledgment.   This research was funded by a grant from the National Institute on Drug Abuse, in conjunction with the Office of Research on Women's Health (Ro3 DA 10560-01; Rohrbach, P. I.).

REFERENCES

Allen, O., Page, R. M., Moore, L., Hewitt, C. (1994). Gender differences in selected psychosocial characteristics of adolescent smokers and nonsmokers. *Health Values, 18*(2), 34–39.

Amaro, H., & Hardy-Fanta, C. (1995). Gender relations in addiction and recovery. *Journal of Psychoactive Drugs, 27*(4), 325–337.

Anthony, J. C., Warner, L. A., & Kessler, R. C. (1994). Comparative epidemiology of dependence on tobacco, alcohol, controlled substances, and inhalants: Basic findings from the National Comorbidity Study. *Experimental Clinical Psychopharmacology, 2,* 244–268.

Baer, P. E., Garmezy, L. B., McLaughlin, R. J., Pokorny, A. D., & Wernick, M. J. (1987). Stress, coping, family conflict, and adolescent alcohol use. *Journal of Behavioral Medicine, 10*(5), 449–467.

Baron, R. M., & Kenny, D. A. (1986). The moderator-mediator variable distinction in social psychological research: Conceptual, strategic, and statistical considerations. *Journal of Personality and Social Psychology, 51*(6), 1173–1182.

Battig, K., Buzzi, R., & Nil, R. (1982). Smoke yield of cigarettes and puffing behavior in men and women. *Psychopharmacology, 76,* 139–148.

Block, J., Block, J. H., & Keyes, S. (1988). Longitudinally foretelling drug usage in adolescence: Early childhood personality and environmental precursors. *Child Development, 59,* 336–355.

Blumenthal, S. J. (1998). Women and substance abuse: A new national focus. In Wetherington, C. L. & Roman, A. B. (Eds.), *Drug addiction research and the health of women* (pp. 13–32). NIH Publication No. 98-4290. Rockville, Maryland: U.S. Department of Health and Human Services, National Institutes of Health, National Institute on Drug Abuse.

Bodinger de Uriarte, C., & Austin G. (1991). *Substance abuse among adolescent females* (Prevention Research Update, No. 9). Portland, OR: Northwest Regional Educational Laboratory.

Botvin, G. J., Baker, E., Filazzola, A. D., & Botvin, E. M. (1990). Cognitive-behavioral approach to substance abuse prevention: One year follow-up. *Addictive Behaviors, 15*(1), 47–63.

Brook, J. S., Whiteman, M. M., & Finch, S. (1992). Childhood aggression, adolescent delinquency, and drug use: A longitudinal study. *Journal of Genetic Psychology, 153*(4), 369–383.

Brooks-Gunn, J., & Reiter, E. (1990). The role of perbertal processes. In Feldman, S. S., & Elliott, G. R. (Eds.), *At the threshold: The developing adolescent.* Cambridge, MA: Harvard University Press.

Camp, D. E., Klesges, R. C., & Relyea, G. (1993). The relationship between body weight concerns and adolescent smoking. *Health Psychology, 12*(1), 24–32.

Celetano, D. D., & McQueen, D. V. (1984). Alcohol consumption patterns among women in Baltimore. *Journal of Studies on Alcohol, 45,* 355–358.

Charlton, A., & Blair, V. (1989). Predicting the onset of smoking in boys and girls. *Social Science Medicine, 29*(7), 813–818.

Chassin, L., Presson, C. C., Montello, D., Sherman, S. J., McGrew, J. (1986). Changes in peer and parent influence during adolescence: Longitudinal versus cross-sectional perspectives on smoking initiation. *Developmental Psychology, 22*(3), 327–334.

Chassin, L., Tetzloff, C., & Hershey, M. (1985). Self-image and social-image factors in adolescent alcohol use. *Journal of Studies on Alcohol, 46,* 39–46.

Clayton, S. (1991). Gender differences in psychosocial determinants of adolescent smoking. *Journal of School Health, 61*(3), 115–120.

Cohen, S., Schwartz, J., Bromet, E., & Parkinson, D. (1991). Mental health, stress, and poor health behaviors in two community samples. *Preventive Medicine, 20,* 306–315.

Copeland, J., & Hall, W. (1992). A comparison of women seeking drug and alcohol treatment in a specialist women's and two traditional mixed-sex treatment services. *British Journal of the Addictions, 87,* 499–504.

Copeland, J., Hall, W., Didcott, P., & Biggs, V. (1993). A comparison of a specialist women's alcohol and other drug treatment service with two traditional mixed-sex services: Client characteristics and treatment outcome. *Drug and Alcohol Dependency, 32,* 81–92.

Dahlgren, L., & Willander, A. (1989). Are special treatment facilities for female alcoholics needed? A controlled 2-year follow-up study from a specialized female unit (EWA) versus a mixed male/female treatment facility. *Alcoholism: Clinical and Experimental Research, 13*(4), 499–504.

DeJong, W. (1987). A short-term evaluation of Project DARE: Preliminary indications of effectiveness. *Journal of Drug Education, 17*(4), 279–294.

Deykin, J. E., Levy, J. C., & Wells, V. (1987). Adolescent depression, alcohol, and drug abuse. *American Journal of Public health, 77,* 178–182.

Ensminger, M. E., Brown, C. H., & Kellam, S. G. (1982). Sex differences in antecedents of substance use among adolescents. *Journal of Social Issues, 38*(2), 25–42.

Feigelman, S., Xiaoming, L., & Stanton, B. (1995). Perceived risks and benefits of alcohol, cigarette, and drug use among urban low-income African-American early adolescents. *Bulletin of the New York Academy of Medicine, 72*(1), 57–75.

Ferrence, R. G. (1980). Sex differences in the prevalence of problem drinking. In O. J. Kalant (Ed.), *Research advances in alcohol and drug problems: Volume 5, Alcohol and drug problems in women.* New York: Plenum Press.

Flay, B. R., Hu, F. B., & Richardson, J. (1998). Psychosocial predictors of different stages of cigarette smoking among high school students. *Preventive Medicine, 27,* A9–A18.

Forney, P. D., Forney, M. A., & Ripley, W. K. (1988). Alcohol and Adolescents: Knowledge, attitudes, and behavior. *Journal of Adolescent Health Care, 9,* 194–202.

French, S. A., Perry, C. L., Leon, G. R., & Fulkerson, J. A. (1994). Weight concerns, dieting behavior, and smoking initiation among adolescents: A prospective study. *American Journal of Public Health, 84*(7), 1818–1820.

Frezza, M., di Padova, C., Pozzato, G., Terpin, M., Baraona, E., & Lieber, C. S. (1990). High blood alcohol levels in women: The role of decreased gastric alcohol dehydrogenase and first-pass metabolism. *New England Journal of Medicine, 322,* 95–99.

Gilchrist, L. D., Gillmore, M., & Lohr, M. (1990). Drug use among pregnant adolescents. *Journal of School Health, 59*(5), 181–188.

Gilchrist, L. D., Schinke, S. P., & Nurius, P. (1989). Reducing onset of habitual smoking among women. *Preventive Medicine, 18,* 235–248.

Graham, J. W., Johnson, C. A., Hansen, W. B., Flay, B. R., & Gee, M. (1990). Drug use prevention programs, gender, and ethnicity: Evaluation of three seventh-grade Project SMART cohorts. *Preventive Medicine, 19,* 305–313.

Gritz, E. R. (1982). The female smoker: Research and intervention targets. In J. Cohen, J. W. Cullen, & L. R. Martin (Eds.), *Psychological aspects of cancer.* New York: Raven Press.

Gritz, E. R., & Crane, L. (1991). Use of diet pills and amphetamines to lose weight among smoking and nonsmoking high school seniors. *Health Psychology, 10*(5), 330–335.

Gritz, E. R., Klesges, R. C., & Meyers, A. W. (1989). The smoking and body weight relationship: Implications for intervention and postcessation weight control. *Smoking Behavior and Weight Control, 11*(4), 144–153.

Halek, C., Kerry, S., Humphrey, H., Crisp, A. H., & Hughes, J. M. (1993). Relationship between smoking, weight, and attitudes to weight in adolescent school girls. *Postgraduate Medical Journal, 69,* 100–106.

Harlow, L. L., Newcomb, M. D., & Bentler, P. M. (1986). Depression, self-derogation, substance use, and suicide ideation: Lack of purpose in life as a mediational factor. *Journal of Clinical Psychology, 42*(1), 5–20.

Hawkins, J. D., Catalano, R. F., & Miller, J. Y. (1992). Risk and protective factors for alcohol and other drug problems in adolescence and early adulthood: Implications for substance abuse prevention. *Psychological Bulletin, 112,* 64–105.

Hill, S. Y. (1984). Vulnerability to the biomedical consequences of alcoholism and alcohol-related problems among women. In Wilsnack, S. C. & Beckman, L. J. (Eds.), *Alcohol problems in women.* New York: Guilford Press.

Hu, F. B., Flay, B. R., Hedeker, D., Siddiqui, O., & Day, L. E. (1995). The influences of friends' and parental smoking on adolescent smoking behavior; the effects of time and prior smoking. *Journal of Applied Social Psychology, 25*(22), 2018–2047.

Huselid, R. F., & Cooper, M. L. (1992). Gender roles as mediators of sex differences in adolescent alcohol use and abuse. *Journal of Health and Social Behavior, 33,* 348–362.

Johnson, S. (1991). Recent research: Alcohol and women's bodies. In P. Roth (Ed.), *Alcohol and drugs are women's issues.* Metuchen, NH: Scarecrow Press, 32–36.

Johnson, R. E., & Marcos, A. C. (1988). Correlates of adolescent drug use by gender and geographic location. *American Journal of Drug and Alcohol Abuse, 14*(1), 51–63.

Johnston, L. D., O'Malley, P. M., & Bachman, J. G. (1996). *National survey results on drug use from the Monitoring the Future Study, 1975–1995. Volume 1, Secondary School Students.* NIH Publication No. 96-4139. Rockville, MD: U.S. Department of Health and Human Services, Public Health Service, National Institutes of Health, National Institute on Drug Abuse.

Jones, B. M., & Jones, M. K. (1976). Women and alcohol: Intoxication, metabolism, and the menstrual cycle. In Greenblatt, M. & Shuckit, M. A. (Eds.), *Alcohol problems in women and children.* New York: Grune and Stratton, 1976.

Kandel, D. B. (1980). Drinking and drug use among youth. *Annual Review of Sociology, 6,* 235–285.

Kandel, D. B., Davies, M., Karus, D., & Yamaguchi, K. (1986). The consequences in young adulthood of adolescent drug involvement: An overview. *Archives of General Psychiatry, 43,* 746–754.

Kandel, D. B., & Logan, J. A. (1984). Patterns of drug use from adolescence to young adulthood: I. Periods of risk for initiation, continued used, and discontinuation. *American Journal of Public Health, 74*(7), 660–666.

Kandel, D. B., Warner, L. A., & Kessler, R. C. (1998). The epidemiology of substance use and dependence among women. In C. L. Wetherington & A. B. Roman (Eds.), *Drug addiction research and the health of women* (pp. 105–130). NIH Publication No. 98-4290. Rockville, Maryland: U.S. Department of Health and Human Services, National Institutes of Health, National Institute on Drug Abuse.

Kandel, D. B., & Yamaguchi, K. (1993). From beer to crack: Developmental patterns of drug involvement. *American Journal of Public Health, 83*(6), 851–855.

Kearney, M. H. (1997). Drug treatment for women: Traditional models and new directions. *Journal of Obstetrics Gynecologic and Neonatal Nursing, 26*(4), 459–468.

Keefe, K. (1994). Perceptions of normative social pressure and attitudes toward alcohol use: Changes during adolescence. *Journal of Studies on Alcohol, 55,* 46–54.

Kellam, S. G., Brown, C. H., Rubin, B. R., & Ensminger, M. E. (1983). Paths leading to teenage psychiatric symptoms and substance use: Developmental epidemiological studies in Woodlawn. In S. B. Guze, F. J. Earls, & J. E. Barrett (Eds.), *Childhood Psychopathology and Development.* New York: Raven Press.

Krohn, M. D., Naughton, M. J., Skinner, W. F., Becker, S. L., & Lauer, R. M. (1986). Social disaffection, friendship patterns and adolescent cigarette use: The Muscatine Study. *Journal of School Health, 56*(4), 146–150.

Lee, E. E. (1978). Female adolescent drinking behavior: potential hazards. *Journal of School Health, 48*(3), 151–156.

Lifrak, P. D., McKay, J. R., Rostain, A., Alterman, A. I., & O'Brien, C. P. (1997). Relationship of perceived competencies, perceived social support, and gender to substance use in young adolescence. *Journal of American Academy of Child Adolescence Psychiatry, 36*(7), 933–940.

Lukas, S. E., Sholar, M. B., Lundahl, L. H., Lamas, X., Kourie, E., Wines, J. D., Kragie, L., & Mendelson, J. H. (1996). Sex differences in plasma cocaine levels and subjective effects after acute cocaine administration in human volunteers. *Psychopharmacology, 125,* 346–354.

Malkin, S. A., & Allen, D. L. (1980). Differential characteristics of adolescent smokers and nonsmokers. *Journal of Family Practice, 10*(3), 437–440.

Moras, K. (1998). Behavioral therapies for female drug users: An efficacy-focused review. In C. L. Wetherington & A. B. Roman (Eds.), *Drug addiction research and the health of women* (NIH Publication No. 98-4290, pp. 197–222). Rockville, Maryland: U.S. Department of Health and Human Services, National Institutes of Health, National Institute on Drug Abuse.

Mosher, D. L., & Sirkin, M. (1984). Measuring a macho personality constellation. *Journal of Research in Personality, 18,* 150–163.

Murray, M., Swan, A. V., Bewley, B. R., & Johnson, M. R. D. (1983). The development of smoking during adolescence: The MRC/Derbyshire smoking study. *International Journal of Epidemiology, 12*(2), 185–192.

Newcomb, M. D., Maddahian, E., Skager, R., Bentler, P. M. (1987). Substance abuse and psychosocial risk factors among teenagers: Associations with sex, age, ethnicity, and type of school. *American Journal of Drug and Alcohol Abuse, 13*(4), 413–433.

Nolte, A. E., Smith, B. J., & O'Rourke, T. (1983). The relative importance of parental attitude and behavior upon youth smoking. *Journal of School Health, 53*(4), 265–271.

Palinkas, L. A., Atkins, C. J., Miller, C., & Ferreira, D. (1996). Social skills training for drug prevention in high risk female adolescents. *Preventive Medicine, 25,* 692–701.

Patton, G. C., Hibbert, M., Rosier, M. J., Carlin, J. B., Caust, J., & Bowes, G. (1996). Is smoking associated with depression and anxiety in teenagers? *American Journal of Public Health, 86*(2), 225–230.

Paulson, M. J., Coombs, R. H., & Richardson, M. A. (1990). School performance, academic aspirations, and drug use among children and adolescents. *Journal of Drug Education, 20*(4), 289–303.

Pederson, L. L., Koval, J. J., & O'Connor, K. (1997). Are psychosocial factors related to smoking in grade-6 students? *Addictive Behaviors, 22*(2), 169–181.

Pope, S. K., Smith, P. D., Wayne, J. B., & Kelleher, K. J. (1994). Gender differences in rural adolescent drinking patterns. *Journal of Adolescent Health, 15,* 359–365.

Reed, B. G. (1981). Women clients in special women's demonstration drug abuse treatment programs compared with women entering selected co-sex programs. *The International Journal of the Addictions, 16*(8), 1425–1466.

Reed, B. G. (1985). Drug misuse and dependency in women: The meaning and implications of being considered a special population or minority group. *International Journal of the Addictions, 20,* 13–62.

Reed, B. G. (1987). Developing women-sensitive drug dependence treatment services: Why so difficult? *Journal of Psychoactive Drugs, 19*(2), 151–164.

Reed, B. G., & Liebson, E. (1981). Women clients in special women's demonstration drug use treatment programs compared with women entering selected co-sex programs. *International Journal of the Addictions, 16*(8), 1425–1466.

Sanders-Phillips, K. (1998). Factors influencing health behaviors and drug abuse among low-income black and Latino women. In C. L. Wetherington & A. B. Roman (Eds.), *Drug addiction research and the health of women* (NIH Publication No. 98-4290 pp. 439–466). Rockville, Maryland: U.S. Department of Health and Human Services, National Institutes of Health, National Institute on Drug Abuse.

Saunders, J. B., Davis, M., & Williams, R. (1981). Do women develop alcohol liver disease more readily than men? *British Medical Journal, 282,* 1140–1143.

Schliebner, C. T. (1994). Gender-sensitive therapy. An alternative for women in substance abuse treatment. *Journal of substance abuse treatment, 11*(6), 511–515.

Substance Abuse and Mental Health Services Administration (1992). *National Household Survey on Drug Abuse: Population estimates 1992.* Washington, DC: U.S. Department of Health and Human Services, Public Health Service.

Substance Abuse and Mental Health Services Administration (1996). *Preliminary estimates from the 1995 National Household Survey on Drug Abuse.* Washington, DC: U.S. Department of Health and Human Services, Public Health Service.

Thomas, B. S. (1995). The effectiveness of selected risk factors in mediating gender differences in drinking and its problems. *Journal of Adolescent Health, 17,* 91–98.

Thomas, B. S. (1996). A path analysis of gender differences in adolescent onset of alcohol, tobacco, and other drug use (ATOD), reported ATOD use and adverse consequences of ATOD use. *Journal of Addictive Diseases, 15*(1), 33–52.

Thompson, K. M., & Wilsnack, R. W. (1984). Drinking and drinking problems among female adolescents: Patterns and influences. In S. C. Wilsnack & L. J. Beckman (Eds.), *Alcohol problems in women.* New York: Guilford Press.

Tobler, N. (1986). Meta-analysis of 143 adolescent drug prevention programs: Quantitative outcome results of program participants compared to a control or comparison group. *Journal of Drug Issues, 17,* 537–567.

U.S. Department of Health and Human Services (1989). *Reducing the health consequences of smoking: 25 years of progress. A report of the Surgeon General.* DHHS Publication No. (CDC) 89-8411. Washington, DC: U.S. Government Printing Office.

U.S. Department of Health and Human Services (1990). *Healthy People 2000: National health promotion and disease prevention objectives.* DHHS Publication No. (PHS) 91-50212. Washington, DC: Department of Health and Human Services, Public Health Service.

U.S. General Accounting Office (1996). *Drug and alcohol use: Billions spent annually for treatment and prevention activities.* Washington, DC: General Accounting Office.

Van Roosmalen, E. H., & McDaniel, S. A. (1989). Peer group influence as a factor in smoking behavior of adolescents. *Adolescence, 24*(96), 801–816.

Van Roosmalen, E. H., & McDaniel, S. A. (1992). Adolescent smoking intentions: gender differences in peer context. *Adolescence, 27*(105), 87–105.

Wald, R., Harvey, S. M., Hibbard, J. (1995). A treatment model for women substance users. *The International Journal of the Addictions, 30*(7), 881–887.

Williams, A. F. (1973). Personality and other characteristics associated with cigarette smoking among young teenagers. *Journal of Health and Social Behavior, 14,* 374–380.

Windle, M., & Barnes, G. M. (1988). Similarities and differences in correlates of alcohol consumption and problem behaviors among male and female adolescents. *International Journal of the Addictions, 23*(7), 707–728.

Worden, J. K., Flynn, B. S., Solomon, L. J., Secker-Walker, R. H., Badger, G. J., & Carpenter, J. H. (1996). Using mass media to prevent cigarette smoking among adolescent girls. *Health Education Quarterly, 23*(4), 453–468.

CHAPTER 18

Preventing Substance Use among Latino Youth

CHARLES R. MARTINEZ, JR.
J. MARK EDDY
DAVID S. DEGARMO

INTRODUCTION

The Hispanic/Latino population is the most rapidly growing sociodemographic group in the United States. The total U.S. population grew 13% from 1990 to 2000, but the Latino population grew by 58% during the same period (U.S. Census Bureau, 2001). According to the 2000 census, there were approximately 35 million Latino individuals residing in the United States (U.S. Census Bureau, 2001). This figure represents 12% of the total U.S. population, which makes the Latino group the largest ethnic minority in the country. The Latino population is relatively youthful compared with the total U.S. population. While 26% of the U.S. population was under 18 years of age in 2000, 35% of the Latino population was under 18. Latinos also had a lower median age (26 years) compared to that of the entire U.S. population (35 years).

Despite this relatively young age, substance use and abuse does not occur with greater frequency among Latino subgroups than among nonminority groups. However, there is evidence that lifetime drug use rates are increasing and pose a significant problem for the Latino community (Vega & Gil, 1999) and that Latino and other ethnic minority youth may be at greater risk for the co-morbid effects and consequences of substance use, including school failure, incarceration, and poor health (Wallace et al., 1995; Kandel, 1995; Pentz, 1995).

CHARLES R. MARTINEZ, JR., J. MARK EDDY, AND DAVID S. DEGARMO • Oregon Social Learning Center, Eugene, Oregon 97401

Given the significant threat that substance use and abuse poses to the Latino community, it is not surprising that there has been a call for increased efforts to advance our understanding of substance abuse in the Latino community. This chapter addresses methodological issues inherent in research with Latino and other minority populations and presents epidemiological data on the prevalence of substance use among Latino youngsters. It also discusses the etiology of substance use for Latino youngsters and its co-morbidity with other problem behaviors. Finally, it examines research on preventing substance use among Latino youngsters.

METHODOLOGICAL COMPLEXITIES

In many comparative cross-cultural studies on substance use and abuse, Anglo-Americans (who represent the numerical and cultural majority) often serve as the "control group" against which other (numerically smaller) ethnic groups are compared. Likely outcomes of such an ethnocentric comparative approach are (1) reinforcement of negative stereotypes about racial/ethnic subgroups and (2) minimal theory and conceptual development concerning substance use etiology and effective prevention (Collins, 1995). Such ethnocentric approaches are even more problematic when researchers fail to examine or measure putative mechanisms that may explain observed racial/ethnic differences, such as socioeconomic status (SES), acculturation, ethnic identity, and societal oppression (Betancourt & Lopez, 1993; Cauce, Coronado, & Watson, 1998; Foster & Martinez, 1995).

Problems in conducting multicultural research begin with definitions. Terms such as *race, ethnicity,* and *culture* are often used interchangeably (Betancourt & Lopez, 1993; Foster & Martinez, 1995). In fact, several of the studies discussed in this chapter compare ethnic groups that could include people of multiple races (e.g., Hispanic/Latino) to racial groups (e.g., White, Black). Definition problems also arise because racial or ethnic group classifications do not represent homogeneous groups of people but encompass variations in physical characteristics, social status, cultural background, language use, and other factors (Collins, 1995). In fact, within-group differences tend to account for more variance in both biological and psychological phenomena than do between-group differences (Zuckerman, 1990). In particular, most U.S. Latinos can trace their origins to one or more of 20 Latin American countries, each with different histories and cultural traditions. Latinos also vary greatly with regard to socioeconomic circumstances, immigration histories, ethnic identity, place of birth, acculturation levels, and language proficiencies.

This chapter uses a culturally variant framework to discuss and interpret comparative studies. Unlike the ethnocentric models that focus on cultural deviance, this approach emphasizes culturally rooted values, beliefs, and norms in explaining observed between-group differences and views such differences as an adaptation to largely external circumstances (Cauce et al., 1998; Szapocznik & Kurtines, 1993). Our approach emphasizes understanding the processes involved in substance use prevention within an ethnic population. It does not view ethnicity per se as a risk factor for substance use but views it as a marker for contextual factors (e.g., SES, assimilation, cultural adaptation, acculturation stress, ethnic identity) that may increase risk for some youngsters. Such an approach will not only improve knowledge of sources of within-group variability but also undermine inaccurate stereotypes about substance use among Latinos.

EPIDEMIOLOGY OF SUBSTANCE USE

The use and abuse of licit and illicit drugs has been implicated as a reason for high numbers of arrests and poor health for Latino and African-American youth (Wallace et al., 1995). Because Latino and other minority youth are at greater risk for the co-related and consequent problems of

TABLE 18.1. Proportion of Youngsters Indicating Past-Month Substance Use in National Epidemiological Studies: Comparisons among Ethnic Groups[a]

	National Household Survey on Drug Abuse (1999)			Monitoring the Future (combined data: 1999, 2000)								
				Hispanic			White			Black		
Age/grade:	Hispanic 12–17	White 12–17	Black 12–17	8th	10th	12th	8th	10th	12th	8th	10th	12th
sample size	3,516	16,901	3,297	4,000	3,100	2,200	18,900	18,200	17,700	4,800	3,100	3,300
Substance												
Any Illicit drug	11.4	10.9	1.7	15.2	23.7	27.4	11.2	23.0	25.9	10.8	17.0	20.3
Marijuana	7.4	8.0	7.3	12.7	20.5	24.6	8.4	20.2	22.7	9.3	15.8	19.0
Cocaine	0.8	0.6	0.0	2.7	3.0	3.6	1.1	1.8	2.5	0.4	0.3	0.8
Hallucinogens	1.2	1.3	0.2	2.0	2.0	3.8	1.2	2.9	3.2	0.5	0.5	0.9
Inhalants	2.5	1.9	1.2	5.6	2.3	3.1	5.2	2.9	2.1	2.3	1.1	1.3
Any alcohol	19.8	13.3	19.9	26.7	40.5	51.2	24.7	43.9	55.1	16.0	24.7	30.0
Cigarettes	12.1	17.1	8.6	16.6	19.6	27.7	17.7	28.2	37.9	9.6	11.1	14.3

[a]Only three ethnic subgroups are presented here, due to limitations in the MTF dataset. The NHSDA does provide additional details on other ethnic subgroups for interested readers.

substance abuse, one might expect that rates of substance use would be higher in these groups than among White youth. However, epidemiological studies consistently show that this is not the case. In fact, some studies of adolescents have shown that Latino youth use drugs at lower rates than do Whites (e.g., Kandel, 1995; Wallace et al., 1995). The most current data on substance use among Latino youth come from the two largest national epidemiological surveys of American youth, in which youngsters reported use of various substances within the past 30 days (see Table 18.1).

The first, the National Household Survey on Drug Abuse (NHSDA), began in 1971 as an epidemiological survey of drug use among the civilian noninstitutionalized U.S. population, 12 years of age or older. The survey is administered individually in face-to-face interviews in the homes of participants. The 1999 NHSDA found that 11.4% of Latino youth, ages 12 to 17, reported using illicit drugs within the past month, which was similar to the 10.9% rate of use for white youth (SAMHSA, 2000). The lowest rate of past-month illicit drug use was 8.4% for Asian youngsters. The highest rate was 19.6% for American-Indian youngsters. For recent alcohol use, 19.8% of Latino youth reported use within the previous month (the average alcohol use rate across ethnic groups was 29.4%). Thirty-four percent of Latino youngsters also reported that they had smoked cigarettes within the previous 30 days (compared to an average rate of 37.1% across ethnic groups). Many Latino youth (36.6%) also indicated that they smoked marijuana once per month. Similar to other findings (e.g., Wallace et al., 1995), no consistent gender differences in rates of substance use emerged in any ethnic group.

The ongoing Monitoring the Future project (MTF; Johnston, O'Malley, & Bachman, 2000), which began in 1975, surveys youngsters in the 8th, 10th, and 12th grades.

Questionnaires are administered to groups of youngsters in their classrooms. Recent MTF results showed prevalence rates similar to NHSDA rates for various ethnic groups, although youngsters who participated in that survey reported somewhat more use of substances across the board. Interestingly, differences in grade-related findings emerged between White, African-American, and Latino students. Specifically, Latino students in the 8th grade indicated greater use of most substances (except amphetamines) than did White and African-American 8th graders. For example, 7.3% of Latino 8th-graders indicated that they had used at least one illicit drug (other than marijuana) in the past month, compared with 5.8 and 2.3% for White and African-American

8th-graders, respectively. For marijuana use among 8th-graders, 12.7% of Latinos, 8.4% of Whites, and 9.3% of African-Americans indicated they had used within the past month. By the 12th grade, Latino-youth substance use rates tended to fall between White students (who were higher) and African-American students (who were lower). For example, among 12th-graders, 10.9% of Latino youngsters, 11.3% of White youngsters, and 3.2% of African-American youngsters reported past-month illicit drug use (other than marijuana).

One possible explanation for the findings that 8th-grade Latino students reported greater substance use relative to other racial/ethnic groups than did 12th-grade Latino students is that Latino youngsters may initiate use of substances at an earlier age (Johnston et al., 2000). Support for this is seen in data from another national-level epidemiological study which showed that a greater proportion of Latino high school students reported having tried alcohol (38%) and marijuana (13%) before age 13, than did White students (29 and 8%, respectively), or African-American students (33 and 11%, respectively; Snyder & Sickmund, 1999). Other researchers suggest that lower reported use of substances by Latino students is due to an under-representation of Latinos in high school-based surveys due to a higher dropout rate than that of other ethnic groups (Wallace et al., 1995).

Taken together, these national findings suggest that while the prevalence rates for substance use are not typically higher for Latino children, compared with the general population, they may initiate use earlier, starting an earlier trajectory toward more severe outcomes, including school dropout. Furthermore, the prevalence data show that the problem of substance use is not a minor one among Latino youth. Many Latino youth are affected. Moreover, as discussed in the following, Latino youth are more likely to experience deleterious consequences of substance use compared with the general youth population (Kandel, 1995; Pentz, 1995). Such issues become even more salient when one considers the rapid population growth of Latino families and the relative lack of effective interventions that target early substance use and its common precursors among these families.

ETIOLOGY OF SUBSTANCE USE

Numerous researchers have found that adolescent substance abuse correlates with academic difficulties, disruptive behavior, association with deviant peers, and early sexual behavior, both in the general population (Hawkins, Catalano, & Miller, 1992; Kellam et al., 1983) and across ethnic groups (Apospori et al., 1995; Newcomb, 1995; Vega et al., 1993). Jessor and Jessor (1977) refer to these behaviors as symptoms of a "problem behavior" syndrome.

Latinos are particularly vulnerable to the negative correlates and consequences of substance use. For example, in one study Latino sixth- and seventh-graders reported more delinquency-type problem behaviors than did White students (Vazsonyi & Flannery, 1997). Latino youngsters are also disproportionately represented in the juvenile corrections systems, making up more than 18% of juvenile offenders in residential placement (Bureau of Justice Statistics, 2000). Latino youngsters (especially those who are foreign born) are also markedly more likely to drop out of school than are their non-Latino peers; a recent study showed that Latinos drop out at about twice the rate of White students (National Center for Education Statistics, 2000). Given their greater vulnerability to concurrent and consequent problems linked to substance use, addressing and preventing substance use is particularly important for the well-being of Latino youngsters.

There is growing evidence that substance use and other problem behaviors unfold across childhood and adolescence in a predictable developmental sequence (e.g., Reid & Eddy, 1997). Most notably, a variety of studies indicate that child aggressive and antisocial behavior in the home often precedes such behavior in school (Patterson, Reid, & Dishion, 1992), and such behaviors predict adolescent substance use (Block, Block, & Keyes, 1988; Kellam et al., 1983). The following sections examine a developmental perspective that integrates the findings of various longitudinal studies and has demonstrated some promise with regard to prevention of problem behaviors, including substance use (e.g., Eddy, Reid, & Fetrow, 2000; Reid et al., 1999).

A Social Interaction Learning Perspective

Developmental models of the etiology of substance use have identified a number of risk and protective factors for substance use. Newcomb (1995) organizes these factors into four domains: (1) culture and society (e.g., social norms about drug use, availability of drugs, economic conditions), (2) interpersonal (e.g., family management practices, parental drug use, association with deviant peers), (3) psychobehavioral (e.g., early problem behavior, academic failure), and (4) biogenetics (e.g., inherited susceptibility to drug abuse, psychophysiologic vulnerability to drug effects). Social interaction learning theory is a developmental model that delineates which risk and protective factors are proximal and which are more distal influences on adolescent problem behaviors (see Reid, Patterson, & Snyder, in press).

Within a social interaction learning framework, family members and peers are presumed to influence each other's behavior in a bidirectional shaping process (e.g., parent to child and child to parent). Parent–child and peer–child interactions are hypothesized to directly shape child and adolescent adjustment. In contrast, contextual factors (e.g., SES, family stress, family structure transitions, parental adjustment, genetic factors, neighborhood, marital adjustment, and social support) are thought to exert their effects on a youngster's adjustment indirectly, most notably through their effects on parenting practices. If one or more negative contexts impinge on a family, many aspects of parenting practices can suffer and the adjustment of children and adolescents can be negatively affected. The effects of contextual factors on youngsters' substance use and negative adjustment are hypothesized to be mediated by parenting practices. This theoretical model, dubbed Coercion Theory (see Reid et al., in press) is illustrated in Figure 18.1. It is one version of the "ecological" models (Bronfenbfrenner, 1979) that is popular in prevention research today (e.g., Szapocznik & Coatsworth, 1999; Kellam & Van Horn, 1997).

A variety of studies support aspects of the social interaction learning model. For example, there is considerable evidence that parenting practices are a proximal focal point in the etiology of early- to mid-adolescence problem behaviors, including substance use (Dishion, Capaldi, & Yoerger, 1999; Dishion & Loeber, 1985), particularly in terms of mediating the impact of contextual factors on those behaviors. In several studies, coercive discipline practices mediated the relationship between parental stress and a youngster's antisocial behavior (Conger, Patterson, & Ge, 1995; Forgatch, Patterson, & Ray, 1996; Patterson, 1986). Similarly, lax monitoring, coercive discipline, and poor problem solving have been found to mediate the relationship between parental psychopathology (e.g., antisocial qualities, depression) and antisocial behavior in youngsters (Forgatch & DeGarmo, 1997; Patterson & Dishion, 1985).

We recently conducted two studies that tested the mediation of social context effects on youngster adjustment by parenting practices. Both studies used the Oregon Divorce Study (ODS-II) sample of divorcing mothers and their sons (grades 1 to 3). The first study showed that the effect of mothers' education on child academic achievement was mediated by parental academic skill building (DeGarmo, Forgatch, & Martinez, 1999). The second study showed that the effect of family structure transitions on child behavioral, emotional, and academic adjustment was mediated by positive and coercive parenting factors (Martinez & Forgatch, 2002).

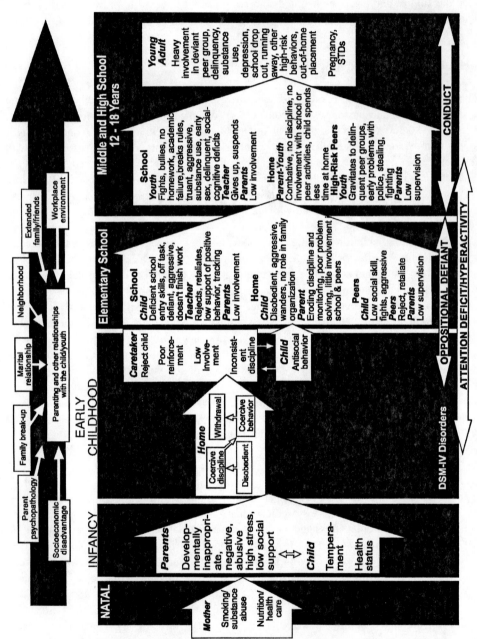

FIGURE 18.1. Social interaction learning: A developmental model for children's problem behavior.

Together, these studies suggest that contexts play an indirect role in a youngster's adjustment to the extent that they disrupt effective parenting practices. Unfortunately, few studies have explored the generalizability of these findings across ethnic subgroups. There is no reported study of actual parenting practices within a Latino family cultural context that includes measures of acculturation, acculturation stress, and structural barriers (e.g., discrimination, oppression). In contrast, there have been studies of parenting values, such as familism (e.g., cohesiveness, frequent direct interaction, reciprocity, pride, and respect) (Vega, 1990) in relation to acculturation and substance by youth use over time (Gil, Wagner, & Vega, 2000). Familism is negatively influenced by acculturation stress and is negatively related to approval by youth of antisocial behavior. The degree to which measures of perceptions, such as familism, are related to positive or coercive parenting, however, is unclear.

Acculturation and Related Issues

Acculturation is a multidimensional construct that describes phenomena resulting from continuous contact between groups of individuals from different cultures and subsequent changes in the cultural patterns of one or both groups (Berry, 1998). Because acculturation is multidimensional, including such factors as language proficiency, language use, nativity, culturally related behavioral preferences, and ethnic identity, no consistent or uniform definition or measurement strategy has been used in the literature (Escobar & Vega, 2000; Rogler, Cortes, & Malgady, 1991). In the United States, most acculturation researchers have assumed that increments of involvement in the American host culture entail corresponding decrements of involvement in traditional culture. However, some researchers argue the need to abandon this assumption and assess "Latinoness," "Americanism," and "biculturalism" separately (Szapocznik, Kurtines, & Fernandez, 1980).

In an attempt to summarize research on Latino acculturation, Rogler and colleagues (1991) conducted a review of studies examining the linkage between acculturation and mental health in Latino samples. Although lack of measurement uniformity made formal quantitative meta-analysis impossible, the authors cite numerous studies that found both linear positive and linear negative relationships between acculturation and psychological distress and other studies that show a curvilinear relationship in which biculturalism is associated with better mental health. Such divergence suggests that linear theories about acculturation are insufficient to account for the process of adjustment (Gil, Vega, & Dimas, 1994). Moreover, acculturation itself is a marker for other psychosocial processes (e.g., ethnic identity processes, experience of structural barriers) that should be measured as potential explicating variables that link acculturation with family outcomes (Escobar & Vega, 2000).

Acculturation factors have been shown to account for considerable within-group variation for Latino adolescent substance use and deviant behavior. A number of studies show that greater acculturation is associated with increased risk for substance use. For example, Ortega et al. (2000) examined lifetime risk for psychiatric illness and substance use disorders among three Latino groups (i.e., Mexican American, Puerto Rican, "other" Hispanic) using epidemiological data from the National Comorbidity Survey. They found that, even when controlling for age, income, and education, U.S.-birth status and English-language preferences were independent predictors of substance use disorders in the three groups. Amaro et al. (1990), using data from the Hispanic Health and Nutrition Evaluation Survey, found greater past-year cocaine and marijuana use among U.S.-born Latinos compared with foreign-born Latinos, controlling for age and SES. Vega et al. (1993) also showed that acculturation factors were positively associated with adolescent Cuban boys' reports of delinquent behavior, controlling for psychosocial and family protective variables.

Vega and Gil (1999) present an ecological model for etiology of Latino adolescent drug use which emphasizes that use among immigrant and U.S.-born Latino adolescents is affected by their and their families' different socialization experiences. For both U.S.- and foreign-born adolescents, the acculturation process is idiosyncratic and highly dependent on social context. Inculcation into minority status varies based on availability of Latino social, economic, and political infrastructure in the social areas in which Latino families live. This process is referred to as segmented assimilation (Portes & Zhou, 1993). Some areas in the United States (e.g., Miami) support more Latino infrastructure than do others.

When the social context is impoverished, with poor educational systems and few opportunities, acculturation and family stress are common outcomes. In this model, as in the social interaction learning model, family environment is the proximal predictor of substance use. In the words of Vega and Gil (1999):

> "When the Hispanic family is less effective in high risk, disorganized communities, the essential protective factor contributing to positive adolescent identity, resiliency, and adaptability is compromised. As researchers and preventionists, we have discovered that a central source in the prevention of delinquent and drug using behaviors among Hispanic children and adolescents, the family, is frequently the first 'victim' of Americanization for a sizable group of immigrants." (p. 65)

In a variety of studies, family and parenting factors have been shown to predict substance use and related problems for Latino adolescents. For example, Dumka, Roosa, and Jackson (1997) showed that immigrant and U.S.-born Mexican-American mothers' greater acculturation predicted more consistent discipline, which in turn predicted less depression and fewer conduct problems among their fourth-grade children. Vega et al. (1993) used self-report data to show that family and parenting protective factors (i.e., respect, pride, cohesion, parental support) contributed to a disposition to deviance for Cuban-American adolescents, controlling for psychosocial and acculturation variables. Similarly, Apospori et al. (1995) found that high family pride and support buffered the relationship between deviance and later drug use for Latino adolescent boys.

As noted previously, Gil et al. (2000) examined the longitudinal relationships between acculturation (i.e., language use, nativity), acculturation strain, familism, parental respect, and later disposition to deviance and alcohol use. Using structural equation modeling, they found that for both U.S.- and foreign-born Latinos, greater acculturation was associated with more language conflicts and acculturation stress. Acculturation stress was associated with lower familism and parental respect. Familism at the beginning of the study predicted lower disposition to deviance one year later. Greater parental respect also predicted less disposition to deviance for U.S.-born Latino adolescents, which was associated with less alcohol involvement one year later. Taken together, these findings underscore that parenting factors are important proximal predictors of Latino youth outcome. Factors such as acculturation are clearly important as well, but these are likely to operate as distal influences on adjustment, mediated through parenting.

A Convergent Perspective

Figure 18.2 shows an expansion of social interaction learning theory that includes culturally specific concepts relevant to Latino adolescent substance use and other problem behaviors. This model considers both social and acculturation contexts that may set the stage for disruptions in functioning for youngsters. Social contexts and acculturation factors are shown as covariates, with bidirectional influences. Both of these factors are shown to relate directly to family stress processes.

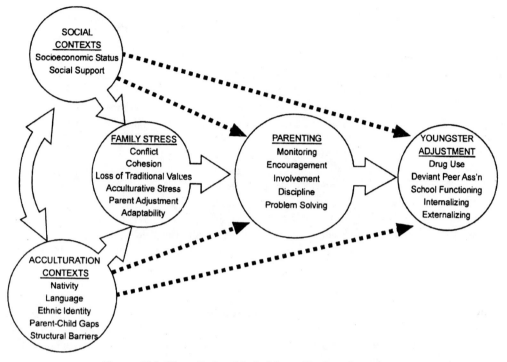

FIGURE 18.2. Theoretical model of etiology of Latino substance use.

We hypothesize that the subjective experience of stress and distress mediate potential influences of acculturation and social contexts on outcomes for families. In fact, variance in perceived stress and coping may explain why some families are resilient in the face of difficult life circumstances. For Latino families, the experience of acculturation strain and the loss of traditional Latino family values are particularly important outcomes of difficult social circumstances. The model illustrates that a family environment favoring stress predicts disruptions in parenting practices, which in turn predicts substance use and related outcomes for adolescents. Parenting practices are represented as the most proximal sphere of influence for youngsters. For our purposes here, we emphasize the importance of the flow of socialization from parent to youngster. However, the process is not that simple; a youngster's adjustment impacts both parenting and family stress processes (Patterson et al., 1992).

INTERVENTION STRATEGIES

The theoretical model we propose identifies the Latino family as a crucial intervention point for families with children at risk of substance use. Yet, few culturally specific and family-based intervention programs have been developed that target substance use and its precursors for Latino families. This section discusses how to foster community collaboration in developing, testing, and implementing culturally specified interventions relevant to Latinos, and looks at the few interventions with some empirical support that emphasize the Latino family and parents as agents of positive change.

Community Engagement

Preventive interventions aimed at ameliorating substance use and related problems take place within a larger community context. This is particularly true of culturally specified interventions. Furthermore, many prevention researchers suggest that intervention effects are maximized with high levels of community involvement (Fisher & Ball, in press; Weissberg & Greenberg, 1998). Pentz (1995) articulated a stepwise process for engaging communities in prevention research. Steps in this model include assessing background conditions, assessing and promoting community readiness, gaining support and collaboration, and organizing the community. Such steps are particularly important for intervention work with Latino families. Latino communities may have had past exposure to "hit-and-run" preventive intervention researchers who bring in an intervention for a brief period of time and then leave the community after "the sample" has been obtained. We suggest that implementation of prevention research and intervention technology in Latino communities is best conducted in the context of community empowerment (e.g., Fisher & Ball, in press; Fisher, Storck, & Bacon, 1997). In this approach, community members are actively involved in the construction, oversight, implementation, evaluation, and possible continuation of the prevention program.

Culturally Specified Latino Family Interventions

A number of promising empirical studies evaluated family-based interventions for Latino young-sters at risk for substance use and related problems. To date, however, only one research group in the United States has published in this area over a long period of time. Szapocznik and associates at the University of Miami have worked extensively to develop and test preventive interventions that address intergenerational conflict, acculturation stress, and family disorganization in Cuban families with youngsters at risk of substance use. One approach, known as Family Effectiveness Training (FET), or Brief Strategic Family Therapy, is grounded in a strategic structural systems family therapy model (Szapocznik, Rio, Perez-Vidal, Kurtines, & Santisteban, 1986; Szapocznik et al., 1989). Family sessions are used to deliver preventive psychoeducational material and as a context in which to intervene with maladaptive family interactions. As part of FET, parents learn effective parenting skills, including family communication, positive encouragement, problem solving, and conflict resolution. During the course of the program, interventionists also use Bicultural Effectiveness Training (BET) to help families address intergenerational and intercultural conflict arising from acculturation gaps between parents and youngsters (Szapocznik et al., 1989).

Randomized studies show that FET produces benefits to problem behavior of youngsters, as reported by parents and in youngster's reports of self-concept, relative to a minimum contact control condition (Szapocznik et al., 1989). In another study, the BET component of FET was evaluated independently in a comparison with structural family therapy (Szapocznik, Rio, Perez-Vidal, Kurtines, Hervis et al., 1986) and found to be as effective as structural family therapy in improving questionnaire-assessed family interaction patterns, adolescent behavior problems, and psychopathology. It was more effective in reducing acculturation and bicultural gaps for Cuban families. These findings suggest that family-focused preventive intervention can produce positive benefits for Latino youngsters at risk for substance use. The unique integration of parenting-effectiveness intervention strategies with strategies designed to address acculturation stress arising from intergenerational and intercultural conflict between parents and youngsters appears particularly important. Recent theoretical extensions of FET emphasize, even more strongly, the need for prevention interventions that strengthen parenting functions because parenting, especially for Latino families, is viewed as the bedrock of a youngster's social ecology (Szapocznik & Coatsworth, 1999).

Achievement for Latinos through Academic Success (ALAS) (Larson, Mehan, & Rumberger, 1998) is a more recent, culturally specified intervention program designed for middle school students. It targets school success, one of the key correlates of substance use for youngsters. The ALAS is school and family based. It emphasizes social and task-related problem-solving skills, student recognition activities, attendance monitoring, frequent teacher feedback to students and parents, and teaching parents effective school participation and teen-management skills. In a comparison of Latino students participating in the ALAS program with a matched group of non-participating Latino students, the ALAS produced positive short-term and one–year sustained outcomes, including school retention, credits earned, and grades.

Parent Training

Because family is a particularly powerful and salient source of influence and support for Latinos, family-based interventions are prime candidates for preventive intervention efforts. Reviews of the majority-population literature consistently show that parent-training interventions, in particular, can influence adjustment outcomes for children and youngsters across a broad spectrum of behavioral, social, and emotional problems (Kazdin, 1987; Lipsey & Wilson, 1993; Weisz et al., 1995). Several teams of researchers and clinicians were involved in developing parent training for families with troubled children (Hawkins et al., 1966; Patterson & Brodsky, 1966; Wahler et al., 1965). While applications of parent training have been developed and tested throughout the world, the focus here is on the parent-training model developed and tested at the Oregon Social Learning Center (OSLC) over the past 40 years (Reid et al., in press).

The core components of parent-training interventions are theoretically derived from the social interaction learning framework and emphasize teaching parents effective family-management strategies (e.g., monitoring, skill encouragement, positive involvement, appropriate discipline, problem solving) while simultaneously helping parents decrease their use of coercive tactics (Forgatch & Martinez, 1999). In a review of 82 studies on psychosocial treatment of children and adolescents with conduct disorders, the OSLC intervention model was one of only two interventions found to meet the stringent criteria for a "well-established" treatment (Brestan & Eyberg, 1998). The other treatment, that of Carolyn Webster-Stratton, is closely linked to the OSLC social learning perspective (Webster-Stratton, 1984, 1994).

OSLC researchers have delivered successful interventions in individual and group settings and in family, school, and foster-care environments. The parent-training interventions demonstrated efficacy in reducing problems, such as out-of-home placements, police contacts, days institutionalized (Chamberlain, 1990; Eddy et al., 2000), problem behaviors at school (Dishion & Andrews, 1995; Forgatch & DeGarmo, 1999), physical aggression on the playground (Reid et al., 1999), depression (Forgatch & DeGarmo, 1999), and substance use (Dishion & Andrews, 1995). Most recently, Martinez and Forgatch (2001) demonstrated efficacy in preventing child non-compliance, which is the building block of later more serious antisocial behavior. This study is particularly important because it showed that intervention benefits to child noncompliance were maintained for two years after completion of the intervention. Intervention benefits were mediated by intervention benefits to parenting practices. Similar mediational findings are seen in several other recent OSLC studies (e.g., Eddy & Chamberlain, 2000; Forgatch & DeGarmo, 1999).

Despite such promising results, parent-training intervention researchers at OSLC and elsewhere are just beginning to examine the generalizability of such efforts to communities that presumably could benefit most from them. In fact, numerous researchers have espoused the need to develop and evaluate the efficacy of culturally specified parent training intervention programs (Cheng Gorman & Balter, 1997; Forehand & Kotchick, 1996; Kumpfer & Alvarado, 1995). While a number of family-based intervention programs have been translated into Spanish (and other languages), the resulting programs remain essentially unchanged from the original programs (Cheng Gorman & Balter, 1997). On the other hand, a culturally-specified intervention model involves incorporating the values of the target population to facilitate successful parenting within a particular cultural group (Cheng Gorman & Balter, 1997). More culturally specified preventive interventions for Latino families are needed to address the complex issues faced by these families. Such interventions will need to be flexible enough to address the high level of variability in history, stress, and acculturation processes among Latino families.

A Comprehensive Approach

Prevention scientists frequently promote an ecological approach to ameliorating substance use (e.g., Newcomb, 1995; Vega & Gil, 1999). While many past prevention efforts have taken place in schools, most have failed to include the critical context of family environment and parenting (Kumpfer & Alvarado, 1995). It is likely that work in any single context will not address the problem completely. Rather, a multicontext, culturally specific approach is needed.

Along these lines, Szapocnik and colleagues (e.g., Pantin & Szapocznik, 1996; Szapocznik & Coatsworth, 1999) have been developing a Structural Ecodevelopmental Preventive Intervention that targets various aspects of the social interactions of parents, children, peers, and teachers that are linked to later substance use and abuse. The key concept, similar to that in parent training, is that all interventions are ultimately intended to strengthen parent and family functioning. In keeping with our earlier comments on the importance of community collaboration, we feel that preventive interventions, such as this, need to be part of a community-defined prevention plan that combines the strengths of established family-based intervention strategies with culturally specific strategies that address the unique challenges faced by Latino families.

CONCLUSION

The Latino population is the fastest growing ethnic subgroup in the United States. While Latino youth are at no greater risk for substance use than are other youth, there is considerable evidence that substance use represents a significant problem for many Latino families. Some data indicate that Latino youth might be at greater risk for the co-morbid effects and consequences of substance use (e.g., school failure, incarceration, poor health). However, despite the need for treatment and prevention services for Latino youngsters involved with substances, Latinos are much less likely to have access to mental health intervention than are White youngsters (DHHS, 2001). Perhaps even more importantly, when Latino youngsters do receive intervention services, they are less likely to receive the evidenced-based interventions that have been touted as "best practices" by prevention and treatment researchers (DHHS, 2001).

We believe that evidenced-based prevention provides an important foundation for culturally appropriate programs for Latino youngsters. While we think it is a mistake to assume that such interventions, which have been tested and implemented primarily in nonminority populations, are transportable without cultural adaptation, we think it is equally problematic to assume that such interventions have little or no generalizability.

Prevention efforts have identified a number of within-group contextual factors involved in the etiology of substance use among Latino youth, including family socioeconomic status, birth status, acculturation processes, acculturation stress, and structural barriers. Theoretical models suggest that such factors exert their effects on youngsters indirectly, by impacting more proximal variables. Parenting practices are the most proximal influence in child adjustment. While parent-training interventions have demonstrated efficacy in reducing substance use and its antecedents, these approaches have not been either developed or evaluated within culturally specific contexts. We need to develop and pilot test such interventions in order to advance our knowledge about the prevention of substance use and related problems among Latino youth.

REFERENCES

Amaro, H., Whitaker, R., Coffman, G., & Heeren, T. (1990). Acculturation and marijuana and cocaine use: Findings from HHANES 1982–84. *American Journal of Public Health, 80* (Suppl.), 54–60.

Apospori, E. A., Vega, W. A., Zimmerman, R. S., Warheit, G. J., & Gil, A. G. (1995). A longitudinal study of the conditional effects of deviant behavior on drug use among three racial/ethnic groups of adolescents. In H. B. Kaplan (Ed.), *Drugs, crime, and other deviant adaptations: Longitudinal studies* (pp. 211–230). New York: Plenum Press.

Berry, J. W. (1998). Acculturation and health. In S. S. Kazarian & D. R. Evans (Eds.), *Cultural clinical psychology: Theory, research, and practice* (pp. 39–57). New York: Oxford University Press.

Betancourt, H., & Lopez, S. R. (1993). The study of culture, ethnicity, and race in American Psychology. *American Psychologist, 48,* 629–637.

Block, J., Block, J. H., & Keyes, S. (1988). Longitudinally foretelling drug use in adolescence: Early childhood personality and environmental precursors. *Child Development, 59,* 336–355.

Brestan, E., & Eyberg, S. (1998). Effective psychosocial treatments of conduct-disordered children and adolescents: 29 years, 82 studies, and 5,272 kids. *Journal of Clinical Child Psychology, 27,* 180–189.

Bronfenbrenner, U. (1979). *The ecology of human development.* Cambridge, MA: Harvard University Press.

Bureau of Justice Statistics (2000). *Correctional populations in the United States, 1997.* Washington DC: U.S. Department of Justice.

Cauce, A. M., Coronado, N., & Watson, J. (1998). Conceptual, methodological, and statistical issues in culturally competent research. In M. Hernandez & R. Isaacs (Eds.), *Promoting cultural competence in children's mental health services.* Baltimore, MD: Brookes.

Chamberlain, P. (1990). Comparative evaluation of specialized foster care for seriously delinquent youths: A first step. *Community Alternatives: International Journal of Family Care, 2*(2), 21–36.

Chavez, J. M., & Roney, C. E. (1990). Psychological factors affecting the mental health status of Mexican American adolescents. In A. R. Stiffman & L. E. Davis (Eds.), *Ethnic issues in adolescent mental health* (pp. 73–91). Newbury Park, CA: Sage.

Cheng Gorman, J., & Balter, L. (1997). Culturally sensitive parent education: A critical review of quantitative research. *Review of Educational Research, 67*(3), 339–369.

Collins, R. L. (1995). Issues of ethnicity in research on the prevention of substance use. In G. J. Botvin, S. Schinke, & M. A. Orlandi (Eds.), *Drug use prevention with multiethnic youth* (pp. 28–45). Thousand Oaks, CA: Sage.

Conger, R. D., Patterson, G. R., & Ge, X. (1995). It takes two to replicate: A mediational model for the impact of parents' stress on adolescent adjustment. *Developmental Psychology, 66,* 80–97.

DeGarmo, D. S., Forgatch, M. S., & Martinez, C. R., Jr. (1999). Parenting of divorced mothers as a link between social status and boys' academic outcomes: Unpacking the effects of SES. *Child Development, 70*(5), 1231–1245.

DHHS (2001). *Mental Health: Culture, Race, and Ethnicity.* Washington, DC: Department of Health and Human Services, U.S. Public Health Services.

Dishion, T. J., & Andrews, D. W. (1995). Preventing escalation in problem behaviors with high-risk young adolescents: Immediate and 1-year outcomes. *Journal of Consulting and Clinical Psychology, 63*(4), 538–548.

Dishion, T. J., Capaldi, D. M., & Yoerger, K. (1999). Middle childhood antecedents to progression in male adolescent substance use: An ecological analysis of risk and protection. *Journal of Adolescent Research, 14,* 175–206.

Dishion, T. J., & Loeber, R. (1985). Adolescent marijuana and alcohol use: The role of parents and peers revisited. *American Journal of Drug and Alcohol Abuse, 11*(1–2), 11–25.

Dumka, L. E., Roosa, M. W., & Jackson, K. M. (1997). Risk, conflict, mothers' parenting, and children's adjustment in low-income, Mexican immigrant, and Mexican American families. *Journal of Marriage and the Family, 59,* 309–323.

Eddy, J. M., & Chamberlain, P. (2000). Family management and deviant peer association as mediators of the impact of treatment condition on youth antisocial behavior. *Journal of Consulting and Clinical Psychology, 68*(5), 857–863.

Eddy, J. M., Reid, J. B., & Fetrow, R. A. (2000). An elementary-school based prevention program targeting modifiable antecedents of youth delinquency and violence: Linking the interests of families and teachers (LIFT). *Journal of Emotional and Behavioral Disorders, 8*(3), 165–176.

Escobar, J. I., & Vega, W. A. (2000). Mental health and immigration's AAAs: Where are we and where do we go from here? *Journal of Nervous & Mental Disease, 188*(11), 736–740.

Fisher, P. A., & Ball, T. J. (2002). The Indian Family Wellness project: An application of the tribal participatory research model. *Prevention Science, 3*(3), 233–238.

Fisher, P. A., Storck, M., & Bacon, J. G. (1997). *Applying community empowerment research principles: A study of psychosocial adjustment among American Indian and Caucasian adolescents in a rural community sample.* Paper presented at the Society for Research in Child Development, Washington, D.C.

Forehand, R., & Kotchick, B. A. (1996). Cultural diversity: A wake-up call for parent training. *Behavior Therapy, 27*(2), 187–206.

Forgatch, M. S., & DeGarmo, D. S. (1997). Adult problem solving: Contributor to parenting and child outcomes in divorced families. *Social Development, 6*(2), 238–254.

Forgatch, M. S., & DeGarmo, D. S. (1999). Parenting through change: An effective prevention program for single mothers. *Journal of Consulting and Clinical Psychology, 67*(5), 711–724.

Forgatch, M. S., & Martinez, C. R., Jr. (1999). Parent management training: A program linking basic research and practical application. *Journal of the Norwegian Psychological Society, 36,* 923–937.

Forgatch, M. S., Patterson, G. R., & Ray, J. A. (1996). Divorce and boys' adjustment problems: Two paths with a single model. In E. M. Hetherington & E. A. Blechman (Eds.), *Stress, coping, and resiliency in children and families* (pp. 67–105). Mahwah, NJ: Erlbaum.

Foster, S. L., & Martinez, C. R., Jr. (1995). Ethnicity: Conceptual and methodological issues in child clinical research. *Journal of Clinical Child Psychology, 24*(2), 214–226.

Gil, A. G., Vega, W. A., & Dimas, J. M. (1994). Acculturative stress and personal adjustment among Hispanic adolescent boys. *Journal of Community Psychology, 22,* 43–54.

Gil, A. G., Wagner, E. F., & Vega, W. A. (2000). Acculturation, familism and alcohol use among Latino adolescent males: Longitudinal relations. *Journal of Community Psychology, 28*(4), 443–458.

Hawkins, J. D., Catalano, R. F., & Miller, J. Y. (1992). Risk and protective factors for alcohol and other drug problems in adolescence and early adulthood: Implications for substance abuse prevention. *Psychological Bulletin, 112*(1), 64–105.

Hawkins, R. P., Peterson, R. F., Schweid, E., & Bijou, S. W. (1966). Behavior therapy in the home: Amelioration of problem parent-child relations with the parent in a therapeutic role. *Journal of Experimental Child Psychology, 4,* 99–107.

Hough, R. L., Landsverk, J. A., Karno, M., Burnam, M. A., Timbers, D. M., Escobar, J. I., & Regier, D. A. (1987). Utilization of health and mental health services by Los Angeles Mexican Americans and Non-Hispanic whites. *Archives of General Psychiatry, 44,* 702–709.

Jessor, R., & Jessor, S. L. (1977). *Problem behavior and psychosocial development.* New York: Academic Press.

Johnston, L. D., O'Malley, P. M., & Bachman, J. G. (2000). *The monitoring the future national survey results on adolescent drug use: Overview of key findings, 1999.* Rockville, MD: National Institute on Drug Abuse.

Kandel, D. B. (1995). Ethnic differences in drug use: Patterns and paradoxes. In G. J. Botvin, S. Schinke, & M. A. Orlandi (Eds.), *Drug use prevention with multiethnic youth* (pp. 81–104). Thousand Oaks, CA: Sage.

Kazdin, A. E. (1987). Treatment of antisocial behavior in children: Current status and future directions. *Psychological Bulletin, 102*(2), 187–203.

Kellam, S. G., Brown, C. H., Rubin, B. R., & Ensminger, M. E. (1983). Paths leading to teenage psychiatric symptoms and substance use: Developmental epidemiological studies in Woodlawn. In S. B. Guze, F. J. Earls, & J. E. Barrett (Eds.), *Childhood psychopathology and development* (pp. 17–47). New York: Raven Press.

Kellam, S. G., & Van Horn, Y. V. (1997). Life course development, community epidemiology, and preventive trials: A scientific structure for prevention research. *American Journal of Community Psychology, 25*(2), 177–188.

Kumpfer, K. L., & Alvarado, R. (1995). Strengthening families to prevent drug use in multiethnic youth. In G. J. Botvin, S. Schinke, & M. A. Orlandi (Eds.), *Drug use prevention with multiethnic youth* (pp. 255–294). Thousand Oaks, CA: Sage.

Larson, K., Mehan, H., & Rumberger, R. (1998). Capturing Latino students in the academic pipeline. In P. Gandara (Ed.), CLPP Policy Report (pp. 7–16). Berkeley, CA: Chicano/Latino Policy Project.

Lipsey, M. W., & Wilson, D. B. (1993). The efficacy of psychological, educational and behavioral treatment: Confirmation from meta-analysis. *American Psychologist, 48*(12), 1181–1209.

Martinez, C. R., Jr., & Forgatch, M. S. (2001). Preventing problems with boys' noncompliance: Effects of a parent training intervention for divorcing mothers. *Journal of Consulting and Clinical Psychology, 69*(3), 416–428.

Martinez, C. R., Jr., & Forgatch, M. S. (2002). Adjusting to change: Linking family structure transitions with parenting and boys' adjustment. *Journal of Family Psychology, 16*(2), 107–117.

National Center for Education Statistics (2000). *Dropout rates in the United States: 1999.* Washington DC: Office of Educational research and Improvement, U.S. Department of Education.

Newcomb, M. D. (1995). Drug use etiology among ethnic minority adolescents: Risk and protective factors. In G. J. Botvin, S. Schinke, & M. A. Orlandi (Eds.), *Drug use prevention with multiethnic youth* (pp. 105–129). Thousand Oaks, CA: Sage.

Ortega, A. N., Rosenheck, R., Alegria, M., & Desai, R. A. (2000). Acculturation and the lifetime risk of psychiatric and substance use disorders among Hispanics. *Journal of Nervous & Mental Disease, 188*(11), 728–735.

Pantin, H., & Szapocznik, J. (1996). *Structural Ecosystems Prevention Intervention.* Unpublished manuscript, Center for Family Studies, Miami.

Patterson, G. R. (1986). Performance models for antisocial boys. *American Psychologist, 41,* 432–444.

Patterson, G. R. (1997). Performance models for parenting: A social interactional perspective. In J. Grusec & L. Kuczynski (Eds.), *Parenting and the socialization of values: A handbook of contemporary theory* (pp. 193–235). New York: Wiley.

Patterson, G. R., & Brodsky, G. (1966). A behaviour modification programme for a child with multiple problem behaviours. *Journal of Child Psychology and Psychiatry, 7,* 277–295.

Patterson, G. R., & Dishion, T. J. (1985). Contributions of families and peers to delinquency. *Criminology, 23*(1), 63–79.

Patterson, G. R., Reid, J. B., & Dishion, T. J. (1992). *Antisocial boys (Vol. 4).* Eugene, OR: Castalia.

Pentz, M. A. (1995). Prevention research in multiethnic communities: Developing community support and collaboration, and adapting research methods. In G. J. Botvin, S. Schinke, & M. A. Orlandi (Eds.), *Drug use prevention with multiethnic youth* (pp. 193–214). Thousand Oaks, CA: Sage.

Portes, A., & Zhou, M. (1993). The new second generation: Segmented assimilation and its variants. *The Annal of the American Academy of Political and Social Sciences, 530,* 74–96.

Reid, J. B., & Eddy, J. M. (1997). The prevention of antisocial behavior: Some considerations in the search for effective interventions. In D. M. Stoff, J. Breiling, & J. D. Master (Eds.), *The handbook of antisocial behavior* (pp. 343–356). New York: Wiley.

Reid, J. B., Eddy, J. M., Fetrow, R. A., & Stoolmiller, M. (1999). Description and immediate impacts of a preventive intervention for conduct problems. *American Journal of Community Psychology, 27*(4), 483–517.

Reid, J. B., Patterson, G. R., & Snyder, J. (Eds.). (2002). Antisocial behavior in children and adolescents: A developmental analysis and model for intervention. Washington, DC: American Psychological Association.

Rogler, L. H., Cortes, D. E., & Malgady, R. G. (1991). Acculturation and mental health status among Hispanics: Convergence and new directions for research. *American Psychologist, 46*(6), 585–597.

SAMHSA (2000). *Summary of findings from the 1999 National Household Survey on Drug Abuse.* Rockville, MD: SAMHSA, Office of Applied Studies.

Snyder, H. N., & Sickmund, M. (1999). *Juvenile offenders and victims: 1999 national report.* Washington, D.C.: Office of Juvenile Justice and Delinquency Prevention.

Szapocznik, J., & Coatsworth, J. D. (1999). An ecodevelopmental framework for organizing the influences on drug abuse: A developmental model of risk & protection. In M. Glantz & C. R. Hartel (Eds.), *Drug abuse: Origins and interventions.* Washington DC: American Psychological Association.

Szapocznik, J., & Kurtines, W. M. (1993). Family psychology and cultural diversity: Opportunities for theory, research and application. *American Psychologist, 48*(4), 400–407.

Szapocznik, J., Kurtines, W. M., & Fernandez, T. (1980). Bicultural involvement and adjustment in Hispanic-American youths. *International Journal of Intercultural Relations, 4,* 353–365.

Szapocznik, J., Rio, A., Perez-Vidal, A., Kurtines, W., Hervis, O., & Santisteban, D. (1986). Bicultural effectiveness training (BET): An experimental test of an intervention modality for families experiencing intergenerational/intercultural conflict. *Hispanic Journal of Behavioral Sciences, 8*(4), 303–330.

Szapocznik, J., Rio, A., Perez-Vidal, A., Kurtines, W., & Santisteban, D. (1986). Family effectiveness training (FET) for Hispanic families. In H. P. Lefley & P. B. Pedersen (Eds.), *Cross-cultural training for mental health professionals* (pp. 245–261). Springfield, IL: Charles C Thomas.

Szapocznik, J., Santisteban, D., Rio, A., Perez-Vidal, A., Santisteban, D., & Kurtines, W. M. (1989). Family effectiveness training: An intervention to prevent drug abuse and problem behaviors in Hispanic adolescents. *Hispanic Journal of Behavioral Sciences, 11*(1), 4–27.

Therrien, M., & Ramirez, R. R. (2000). *The Hispanic Population in the United States: March 2000.* Washington DC: Current Population Reports, P20-535, U.S. Census Bureau.

U.S. Census Bureau (2001). *The Hispanic Population: Census 2000 Brief.* Washington DC: U.S. Census Bureau.

Vazsonyi, A. T., & Flannery, D. (1997). Early adolescent delinquent behaviors: Associations with family and school domains. *Journal of Early Adolescence, 17,* 271–293.

Vega, W. A. (1990). Hispanic families in the 1980's: A decade of research. *Journal of Marriage and the Family, 52,* 1015–1024.

Vega, W. A., & Gil, A. G. (1999). A model for explaining drug use behavior among Hispanic adolescents. *Drugs & Society, 14*(1–2), 57–74.

Vega, W. A., Gil, A. G., Warheit, G. J., Zimmerman, R. S., & Apospori, E. A. (1993). Acculturation and delinquent behavior among Cuban American adolescents: Toward an empirical model. *American Journal of Community Psychology, 21*(1), 113–125.

Vega, W. A., Kolody, B., Aguilar-Gaxiola, S., Alderete, E., Catalano, R., & Caraveo-Anduaga, J. (1998). Lifetime prevalence of DSM-III-R psychiatric disorders among urban and rural Mexican Americans in California. *Archives of General Psychiatry, 55*(9), 771–778.

Vega, W. A., Kolody, B., Aguilar-Gaxiola, S., & Catalano, R. (1999). Gaps in service utilization by Mexican Americans with mental health problems. *American Journal of Psychiatry, 156*(6), 928–934.

Vega, W. A., & Rumbaut. (1991). Ethnic minorities and mental health. *Annual Review of Sociology, 17,* 351–383.

Vega, W. A., Zimmerman, R. S., Warheit, G. J., Apospori, E., & Gil, A. G. (1993). Risk factors for early adolescent drug use in four ethnic and racial groups. *American Journal of Public Health, 83*(2), 185–189.

Wahler, R. G., Winkle, G. H., Peterson, R. F., & Morrison, D. C. (1965). Mothers as behavior therapists for their own children. *Behaviour Research and Therapy, 3,* 113–124.

Wallace, J. M., Jr., Bachman, J. G., O'Malley, P. M., & Johnston, L. D. (1995). Racial/ethnic differences in adolescent drug use: Exploring possible explanations. In G. J. Botvin, S. Schinke, & M. A. Orlandi (Eds.), *Drug use prevention with multiethnic youth* (pp. 59–80). Thousand Oaks, CA: Sage.

Webster-Stratton, C. (1984). Randomized trial for two parent-training program for families with conduct-disordered children. *Journal of Consulting and Clinical Psychology, 52,* 666–678.

Webster-Stratton, C. (1994). Advancing videotape parent training: A comparison study. *Journal of Consulting and Clinic Psychology, 64,* 583–593.

Weissberg, R. P., & Greenberg, M. T. (1998). Prevention science and collaborative community action research: Combining the best from both perspectives. *Journal of Mental Health, 7*(5), 470–492.

Weisz, J. R., Weiss, B., Han, S. S., Granger, D. A., & Morton, T. (1995). Effects of psychotherapy with children and adolescents revisited: A meta-analysis of treatment outcome studies. *Psychological Bulletin, 117,* 450–468.

Zuckerman, M. (1990). Some dubious premises in research and theory on racial differences: Scientific, social, and ethical issues. *American Psychologist, 45,* 1297–1303.

CHAPTER 19

African-American Substance Use Epidemiology and Prevention Issues

WILLIAM L. TURNER
MICHAEL J. HENCH

INTRODUCTION

The problems associated with alcohol and other drug use and abuse in the United States present a pressing health and social crisis. The cost that substance abuse exacts, however, is not distributed equally across the population. Historically, its impact has been experienced disproportionately by African-Americans (Wallace, 1999). Some researchers (Nobles et al., 1987) blame the high prevalence of drug use and abuse in the African-American community, at least in part, on an erosion of Black cultural values; but one cannot ignore the lack of prevention efforts aimed specifically at African-Americans. And considering that the African-American population is expected to nearly double from 33.5 million to 61 million by 2050 (Day, 1996), the prevention of substance abuse among the nation's non-White population will be of escalating significance. This chapter examines drug abuse risk factors inherent in being African-American and protective factors that might help prevent drug abuse by Black youths and adults. It also discusses drug abuse prevention efforts aimed specifically at the Black community. It begins with an analysis of the epidemiology of alcohol and other drug use among African-Americans in an attempt to shed light on risk and protective factors.

WILLIAM L. TURNER • Department of Family Social Science, University of Minnesota—Twin Cities, St. Paul, Minnesota 55108
MICHAEL J. HENCH • Department of Family Studies, University of Kentucky, Lexington, Kentucky 40506

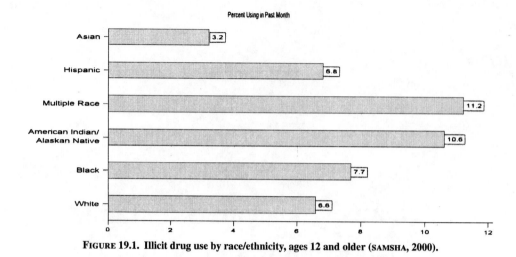

FIGURE 19.1. Illicit drug use by race/ethnicity, ages 12 and older (SAMSHA, 2000).

PREVALENCE OF SUBSTANCE USE AND ABUSE

It is estimated that 87.7 million Americans or 39.7% of the population age 12 or older has used an illicit drug at least once in their lives. The Black population falls slightly under this national average at 37.7% (SAMHSA, 2000). The current rate of illicit drug use is 7.7% among all African-Americans age 12 or older, which is the highest rate among racial/ethnic groups with the exception of the Native-Americans (see Figure 19.1). In recent years, past-month use of any illicit drug use has increased more among Black non-Hispanics than among other groups, and Blacks consistently report higher past-month usage of illicit drugs than do White and Hispanic groups (Sloboda, 1999).

Marijuana is the most widely used illicit drug by Black adults and youth. Marijuana use appears to be accelerating among all racial/ethnic groups, but a comparison of White, Black, and Hispanic populations from 1990 to 1997 showed that past-month prevalence of marijuana use was highest among Blacks (Sloboda, 1999). This trend also appears to hold for cocaine (Sloboda, 1999). Following marijuana and cocaine powder, the most frequently used illicit drugs by African-Americans are analgesics, hallucinogens, inhalants, and stimulants (SAMHSA, 2000) (Figure 19.2).

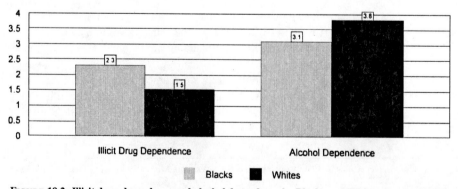

FIGURE 19.2. Illicit drug dependence and alcohol dependence by Blacks and Whites SAMHSA (2000).

Alcohol use by African-Americans is a different story. Their rates of alcohol use and dependence are also relatively low, especially in relation to whites (see Figure 19.2). Data on current, binge, and heavy use of alcohol among Blacks indicate that they have the lowest rate of reported use, except for Asian-Americans (SAMHSA, 2000).

As with alcohol, tobacco use by Blacks is among the lowest of any racial/ethnic group. Their lifetime use of cigarettes is 27.5%, with a current rate of 22.5%, both second only to Asian-Americans (SAMHSA, 2000).

Gender Differences

Gender studies show that Black males have a significantly higher rate of illicit drug use (12.6%) than do Black females (8.7%) (SAMHSA, 2000). This gender difference is particularly significant in relation to other racial/ethnic groups, particularly Whites. Additional research is necessary to clarify why such a gender disparity exists among African-Americans, but its existence strongly suggests a critical need for preventive measures targeted specifically at Black males.

Age Differences

In addition to gender differences, the epidemiology of alcohol and other drug use among African-Americans across the lifespan shows a great disparity between Black adolescents, with relatively low levels of drug use among adolescents and high levels among adults. This disparity is not found to the same extent in other racial/ethnic groups. When comparing Blacks and Whites in terms of drug usage at various age levels, Black youths have lower usage rates than do White youths. In early adulthood differences are smaller, and by middle adulthood the rates are often higher among Blacks (Bachman et al., 1991).

Drug surveys over the past 3 decades have consistently shown that Black youths have some of the lowest levels of drug use (especially alcohol and tobacco) relative to other groups (Johnston, O'Malley, & Bachman, 2000; Bachman et al., 1991). Illicit drug use by Black youths is lower than for all other major racial/ethnic groups with the exception of Asian-Americans (see Figure 19.3). The 30-day alcohol use prevalence rates are lower for Black 8th, 10th, and 12th-graders than for other groups (Wallace et al., 1999). African-American youths also have the lowest rates of smoking. In 1999, 14.9% of African-American high school seniors reported current smoking compared to 40.1% of White and 27.3% of Hispanic seniors (Johnston et al., 2000).

African-American adolescents ages 12 to 17 have significantly lower levels of drug dependence compared to other racial/ethnic groups. Black youths report the lowest percentage of alcohol or any illicit drug dependence of all major racial/ethnic groups (SAMHSA, 2000). In addition, Bachman et al. (1991) found that Black youths, in comparison to White and Hispanic youths, are more likely to disapprove of drug use and regard it as a high-risk activity.

Why is there such a disparity in drug use between Black adolescents and adults? This question has yet to be fully answered, but Wallace et al. (1999) suggest two possibilities. The first is that witnessing high rates of drug-related problems experienced by some Black adults may encourage Black adolescents to delay or avoid completely the use of alcohol and other drugs. A second explanation is that some Black parents and families, in an attempt to protect children from the difficult circumstances and realities often associated with being a Black adult, may be able to effectively shield youngsters from using drugs.

What makes the fact that the majority of African-American youth abstain from drugs even more astonishing is the large number of negative factors that confront the Black community in

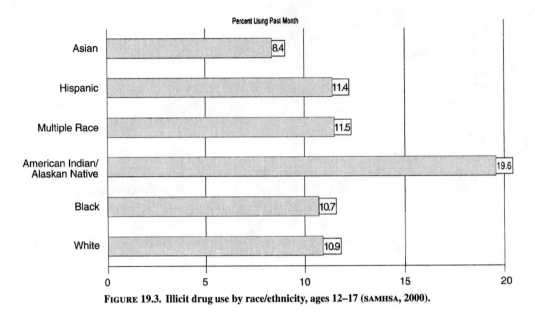

FIGURE 19.3. Illicit drug use by race/ethnicity, ages 12–17 (SAMHSA, 2000).

general. With regard to drug or alcohol education, for example, Blacks have fewer resources than do other racial/ethnic groups. Only 46.4% of Blacks report having talked to their parents about the dangers of alcohol and other drug use, compared with 59.1% of Whites. Black adolescents are also less likely to receive such information in school—50.7% as opposed to 63.1% for Whites (SAMHSA, 2000).

Disproportionate Adverse Consequences of Drug Use and Abuse

Despite lower levels of alcohol use and dependence than is seen among White Americans, Black youths and adults experience a disproportionately higher number of negative mental, social, and physical consequences of alcohol use (Wallace, 1999). Longitudinal analyses suggest that Blacks experience more chronic alcohol-related problems and that there has been an increase in the percentage and magnitude of such problems among African-Americans (Jones-Webb, Hsiao, & Hannon, 1995). Why is there such a disparity in adverse consequences between Black and White Americans? Wallace (1999) and Turner (2000) encourage researchers to look beyond individual and interpersonal risk factors toward factors relating to family, community, and the environment. Recently, researchers have begun testing empirical models which suggest that the disproportionate experience of substance-related problems among Blacks is associated with racial/ethnic differences in exposure to macrolevel risk factors and socioeconomic status.

National data indicate that although disadvantaged Black men experience more alcohol-related problems and consequences than do disadvantaged White men, Black men who have high socioeconomic status have significantly fewer alcohol-related problems than do White men of similar socioeconomic (Jones-Webb et al., 1995; Herd, 1989). Another study showed that Black women who complete 12 years of school are less likely than their White counterparts to be heavy users of alcohol and other drugs (Lille-Blanton, MacKenzie, & Anthony, 1991). Such studies strongly support the idea that the disproportionate experience by African-Americans of negative substance use outcomes is related to economic disadvantage.

Consider the environments in which many African-Americans live. Blacks are more likely to be poor and to live in urban areas of concentrated poverty. In fact, Blacks are four times more likely to live in poverty areas than outside of them (Wallace, 1999). These poverty areas are characterized by low family income, high unemployment, high population density, and greater numbers of liquor stores (Jones-Webb et al., 1997). The rate for current illicit drug use in metropolitan areas, compared to nonmetropolitan and rural areas, is nearly 3% higher: 7.1 versus 4.2% (SAMHSA, 2000). Census Bureau (2000) data show that 86.1% of the Black population lives inside or directly outside of a metropolitan area. This factor alone puts them at greater risk of alcohol and other drug use.

Blacks are more likely than members of other ethnic/racial groups to report that they have been approached by someone selling drugs. Compared to White youths, Black youths are more likely to report that illicit drugs are fairly easy or very easy to obtain in their community, to have seen someone selling drugs in their neighborhood occasionally or more often, and to report seeing people drunk or high occasionally or more often (SAMHSA, 2000). The physical, economic, and social availability of drugs clearly represent a contextual-level risk factor to which Black Americans are inequitably exposed. A full understanding of these and other risk factors is essential in designing drug use prevention programs. However, few preventive efforts have been developed specifically for African-Americans (Turner, 2000).

PREVENTION

While much is known about the prevalence and effects of drug use, less is known about how to prevent it. Reducing the risk that young people will use alcohol and other drugs typically involves school-based programs that focus on individual change. These school-based prevention programs have traditionally been designed for use with White, middle-class students (Elmquist, 1995) and are not generally appropriate or useful to African-Americans (John, Brown, & Primm, 1997; Crisp, 1980). As demonstrated by continued high rates of drug use and abuse among students, including African-Americans, school-based prevention programs have not been very successful. This is probably because no single generic prevention program is likely to be equally effective for all participants. One study, however (Rouse, 1989), did find that school-based drug education courses or lectures had a greater preventive impact on African-American youth than on White students. What is unfortunate is that African-Americans generally have less access to such programs (SAMHSA, 2000).

Despite the general ineffectiveness of school-based programs, vast resources and efforts have gone into their development and implementation, while little effort has focused on prevention programs that involve families and the community, even though there is a growing body of research showing that both play key roles in influencing how youth handle the temptations of alcohol and other drugs (Kumpfer, 1999). Oyemade and Washington (1990) argue that serious prevention efforts must consider the family and other systemic societal influences on later drug use. And many prevention researchers who work with minority families promote a focus on family involvement and family strengths (Beatty, 1994; Bierman & the Conduct Problems Prevention Research Group, 1997; Bry et al., 1999; Kumpfer, 1999; Oetting, Beauvis, & Edwards, 1988; Turner, 2000; Wallace, 1999). Researchers have also begun to consider the cultural appropriateness of such programs (Kumpfer, 1991). Understanding parenting styles and family assumptions of African-Americans, for example, and tailoring programs to them improves recruitment, retention, and effectiveness (Aktan, 1999; Kumpfer, 1999). In identifying the assumptions, however, it is crucial to acknowledge intragroup heterogeneity and the scope of variability in the African-American community. This variability can be to many factors, including geographic and regional differences, educational level, socioeconomic status, gender differences, religious affiliations, and age differences (Turner, 2000). It is imperative that we acknowledge them as broad generalizations only, so as not to perpetuate racial stereotypes.

Family and Community Prevention Efforts

Strengths- or competence-oriented theories of African-American families are the focus of recent prevention research. Both Turner (1995) and Boyd-Franklin (1989) recommend several strength-related concepts to be considered when working with African-American families. Foremost is the role of the extended family and the support it provides. The religious community offers an additional network of support. In addition, most African-Americans have a strong belief in the value of education and work and in the ability to implement and use coping skills in the face of economic hardship. Such family values can serve as the foundation for African-American drug abuse prevention programs.

Because empirically based prevention programs aimed specifically at African-Americans are few, Kazdin (1993) recommends modifying existing programs to take into account parenting, family, and cultural values of a specific ethnic group. Ho (1992) adds that cultural modifications to proven programs require a framework that is organized, culturally sensitive, and theoretically based. Family-based prevention programs for African-Americans should also pay close attention to religiosity, variations in child rearing practices, intragroup variations, and the disproportionate number of Black males who have drug-related problems (Turner, 2000). Nobles and Goddard (1993) further argue that such programs must be relevant to the needs and conditions of the community and must respond to problems that exist as defined by the community.

Unfortunately, few programs have been specifically modified for use in African-American communities. Kumpfer (1999), in a review of family prevention programs, lists several research-based exceptions, including Szapocznik's individual structural family therapy model (Santisteban, Szapocznik, & Rio, 1993), Family Effectiveness Training or Bicultural Effectiveness Training for high-risk pre-adolescents and adolescents (Szapocznik et al., 1989; 1986); Alvy's Effective Black Parenting Program (Alvy, 1987), and Kumpfer's Strengthening Families Program for rural and urban African-American families (Aktan, Kumpfer, & Turner, 1994). In addition, Lochman and Wells (1996) address cultural issues in the Duke Coping Power Program used with a largely urban African-American population. Turner (in press) addresses implementation of this program with rural African-American parents and children.

The objectives, content, and process of such programs need to be evaluated to determine if they are culturally significant for African-Americans. One such evaluation was undertaken with the Safe Haven Program, a substance abuse prevention program for African-American families in Detroit (Atkan, 1999). The Safe Haven Program is a modification of the Strengthening Families Program (Kumpfer, DeMarsh, & Child, 1989). The evaluation was conducted in the third and fifth years of the program. Participant feedback revealed that after modifications were made to the program, families were more dynamic and open and understood and identified with program materials to a greater extent. In addition, there was an increase in attendance by African-American men and fathers. Overall, the program was found to be effective in reducing childhood risk factors and increasing protective factors.

The Institute for African-American Mobilization, created in 1991 and sponsored by the Center for Substance Abuse Prevention's (CSAP) Community Partnership Training Program, also focuses on community-based substance abuse prevention efforts. The Center for Substance Abuse Prevention recognizes that in order to create, define, and shape prevention efforts in the

African-American community, it is critical to involve key members of the AfricanAmerican community. The Institute for African-American Mobilization uses community training workshops to facilitate African-American inclusion, mobilization, community development, and empowerment in efforts to increase prevention efforts.

African-American Parents for Drug Prevention was recently formed by colleagues representing key formal and informal organizations in the Black community including the Urban League, the NAACP, the National Council of Black Women, The Black Ministerial Alliance, and the African-American Panhellenic Association. The African-American Parents for Drug Prevention targets parents and other family members responsible for rearing children. Its mission is to provide parenting skills and education on how to shield children from the negative consequences of alcohol and other drug use. Its efforts are based on three elements: an African-American-centered module that includes a systematic and intentional process of acculturation and immersion in cultural traditions that is intended to provide a buffer against pressures to engage in self-destructive behavior; a family-centered module that is based on adult responsibility and community control for the welfare and well-being of African-American children; and a module that builds on adherence to spiritual values that have historically proved useful in the struggle to survive and triumph over destructive forces, such as drug and alcohol abuse.

A similar program, called to The Unity Project, was established by The Council on Alcohol and Drugs and AID Atlanta to reduce substance abuse and the incidence of HIV/AIDS in African-Americans. This 3-year initiative is funded by CSAP and is targeted at African-American youths age 11 to 18. Although the efficacy of the program has yet to be determined, The Unity Project is an example recently created programs that serve the needs of the African-American community exclusively.

Another example is the NTU (pronounced in-too, meaning "essence of life") project targeted at fifth- and sixth-grade African-American children considered to be at high risk for alcohol and other drug use. The NTU approach is based on African-American values and beliefs that are thought to help mediate or decrease risk factors and increase resiliency and protective factors among high-risk youth (Cherry et al., 1998). Although the analyses revealed no significant improvement (which is not surprising considering the young age of the participants and the fact that the majority of them reported negative attitudes toward drugs at pre- and post-test), gains in several protective factors among program participants should lead to reduced risk of alcohol and other drug use in later years.

Despite promising efforts to implement prevention programs specifically for African-American youths, messages communicated to these young people continue to be contradictory and confusing. The number of alcohol and tobacco advertisements targeted at African-Americans is astonishing. Messages present in the Black culture and popular media, especially rap music, movies, and cable television programs, often provide conflicting messages to youth regarding appropriate drug and alcohol use.

The National Clearinghouse for Alcohol and Drug Information (1995) and CSAP (1990) recommend several community-based strategies that promote healthy behavior among African-American youth, including:

- involving African-American adults as mentors and positive role models to help adolescents to find ways to resolve their problems without resorting to substance abuse;
- challenging myths about African-American youth involvement with alcohol and other drugs and celebrating the resilience and pride of young African-Americans;
- encouraging African-American churches to take a more active role in prevention efforts;
- creating bonds among churches, families, schools, law enforcement, businesses, and the media, and encouraging them to work together and share resources;

- encouraging African-American radio stations to promote prevention activities and cele-
  brate the accomplishments of youth in the community;
- conveying to young African-Americans the rich cultural heritage they share and bringing
  them together to use their talents and ideas to develop messages and communicate positive
  alternatives to alcohol and other drug use;
- mobilizing African-American communities to remove offensive alcohol and other drug
  related content from billboards and other media and encouraging them to promote pride
  in their neighborhoods by working together to fight drugs, crime, and violence;
- encouraging corporations and African-American businesses in particular to promote alcohol and other drug use prevention efforts and activities by donating space, materials, and
  resources;
- making information available at places, such as movie theaters and recreation centers,
  where African-American youths gather; and
- featuring African-American youths in materials such as billboards, brochures, ad campaigns, commercials, and movies that advocate the avoidance of alcohol and other drugs.

TREATMENT CONSIDERATIONS

African-Americans are twice as likely as White Americans to be in substance abuse treatment
(SAMHSA, 2000). But African-Americans, in general, have fewer treatment resources and are
an underserved population, compared with White Americans. Common barriers to treatment
that disproportionately affect the Black community include poverty and lack of health insurance.
According to Clark (1999), 22% of African-Americans, compared to 16% of all others, lack health
insurance, and 27% are below the poverty level, compared to 13% of all others. Furthermore,
only 26% of African-American household residents who reported a need for substance treatment
actually received such help.

Another problem for African-Americans is the Eurocentric orientation of most models of
addiction and addiction treatment. The literature does not indicate clearly whether African-
Americans fare better or worse than other ethnic/racial groups in substance treatment, so it is
difficult to determine whether more culturally specific treatment strategies will help deter relapse. However, African-Americans have specific needs that must be addressed to make treatment
more effective, and it is imperative that mental health professionals be well grounded in African-
American cultural values. It is equally important that they be aware of the heterogeneity that exists
within racial/ethnic groups. Boyd-Franklin (1989) makes it clear that there is no such thing as
the "Black family" and emphasizes that no particular set of values and beliefs is common to all
African Americans. It is important that those working in addiction treatment understand a person's
values and beliefs before hypotheses are drawn and interventions made. In order to compensate
for the beliefs, attitudes, and values that exist among African Americans individually and collectively, Wade (1994) recommends a multidimensional biopsychosocial model that appreciates the
cultural differences or concerns of such clients.

CONCLUSION

The disproportionate and devastating impact that alcohol and other drug use has had on the Black
community is becoming increasingly clear as is the need for rigorous research on the causes of
this inequity and ways to prevent it. As this chapter points out, researchers must first understand

the culture and diversity of the African-American community and identify ways to effectively involve families and communities in efforts to prevent substance abuse. Increased efforts must be made to understand and reinforce protective factors, such as religious and church activity, education, employment, family support, communal orientations, and ethnic pride. Additionally, the field of drug abuse prevention would be greatly enhanced by the increased involvement of African-American researchers and professionals who have a vested interest in the needs of the population and have a greater advantage in overcoming community barriers. In conclusion, the specific needs of the Black community must be understood and addressed if we are to overcome the disproportionate burden alcohol and other drug use imposes on this community.

REFERENCES

Aktan, G. B. (1999). A cultural consistency evaluation of a substance abuse prevention program with inner city African-American families. *The Journal of Primary Prevention, 19,* 227–239.

Aktan, G. B., Kumpfer, K. L., & Turner, C. W. (1996). Effectiveness of a family skills training program for substance use prevention with inner city African-American families. *Substance Use and Misuse, 31,* 157–175.

Alvy, K. T. (1987). *Black parenting: Strategies for training.* New York: Irvington.

Bachman, J. G., Wallace, J. M., O'Malley, P. M., Johnston, L. D., Kurth, C. L., & Neighbors, H. W. (1991). Racial/ethnic differences in smoking, drinking and illicit drug use among American High School seniors, 1976–1989. *American Journal of Public Health, 81,* 372–377.

Beatty, L. A. (1994). Issues in drug abuse prevention intervention research with African-Americans. In A. Cazares & L. Beatty (Eds.), *Scientific methods for prevention intervention research* (National Institute on Drug Abuse Publication No. 94-3631, pp. 171–202). Washington, DC: U.S. Department of Health and Human Services.

Bierman, K. L., & the Conduct Problems Prevention Research Group. (1997). Implementing a comprehensive program for the prevention of conduct problems in rural communities: The FAST Track Experience. *American Journal of Community Psychology, 25,* 493–514.

Boyd-Franklin, N. (1989). *Black families in therapy: A multi-systems approach.* New York: Guilford.

Brown, L. S. (1995). Substance abuse and HIV/AIDS: Implications of prevention efforts for Americans of African descent. In O. Amuleru-Marshall (Ed.), *Substance abuse treatment in an era of AIDS* (pp. 17–58). Rockville, MD: National Institute on Drug Abuse.

Bry, B. H., Catalono, R. F., Kumpfer, K., Lochman, J. E., & Szapocznik, J. (1999). Scientific findings from family prevention intervention research. In R. Ashery (Ed.), *Family-based prevention interventions.* Rockville, MD: National Institute of Drug Abuse.

Center for Substance Abuse Prevention (1990). Communicating about alcohol and other drugs: Strategies for reaching populations at risk. *CSAP Prevention Monograph, 5* (Serial No. BK170).

Cherry, V. R., Belgrave, F. Z., Jones, W., Kennon, D. K., Gray, F. S., & Phillips, F. (1998). NTU: An Africentric approach to substance abuse prevention among African-American youth. *The Journal of Primary Prevention, 18,* 319–339.

Clark, H. W. (1999). Treatment demand exceeds availability. *Center for Substance Abuse Treatment: Substance abuse in brief* (On-line). Available: http://www.samhsa.gov/csat/inbriefs/sept99.htm.

Crisp, A. D. (1980). Making substance abuse prevention relevant to low-income Black neighborhoods. *Journal of Psychoactive Drugs, 12,* 13–19.

Day, J. C. (1996). *Population projections of the United States by age, sex, race and Hispanic origin: 1995 to 2050* (U.S. Bureau of the Census Current Publication Reports No. P25-1130). Washington, DC: U.S. Government Printing Office.

Elmquist, D. L. (1995). Alcohol and other drug use prevention for youths at high risk and their parents. *Education and Treatment of Children, 18,* 65–88.

Harper, F. D. (1980). Research and treatment with Black alcoholics. *Alcohol Health and Research World, 4,* 10–16.

Herd, D. (1989). The epidemiology of drinking patterns and alcohol-related problems among U.S. Blacks. In National Institute on Alcohol Abuse and Alcoholism, *Alcohol use among U.S. ethnic minorities* (DHHS publication No. 89-1435). Washington, DC: U.S. Government Printing Office.

Ho, M. K. (1992). Differential application of treatment modalities with Asian American youth. In L. A. Vargas & J. D. Koss-Chioino (Eds.), *Working with culture: Psychotherapeutic interventions with ethnic minority children and adolescents* (pp. 182–203). San Francisco: Jossey-Bass.

John, S., Brown, L.S., & Primm, B. J. (1997). African-Americans: Epidemiologic, prevention and treatment issues. In J. H. Lowinson, P. Ruiz, R. B. Millman, & J. G. Langrod (Eds.), *Substance abuse: A comprehensive textbook* (3rd ed.) (pp. 94–113). Thousand Oaks, CA: Sage.

Johnston, L. D., O'Malley, P. M., & Bachman, J. G. (2000). *Monitoring the future national results on adolescent drug use: Overview of key findings, 1999* (National Institute on Drug Abuse Publication No. 00–4690). Washington, DC: U.S. Government Printing Office.

Jones-Webb, R., Hsiao, C., & Hannon, P. (1995). Relationship between socioeconomic status and drinking problems among Black and White men. *Alcoholism: Clinical and Experimental Research, 19,* 623–627.

Jones-Webb, R., Snowden, L., Herd, D., Short, B., & Hannan, P. (1997). Alcohol-related problems among Black, Hispanic and White men: The contribution of neighborhood poverty. *Journal of Studies on Alcohol, 58,* 539–545.

Kazdin, A. E. (1993). Adolescent mental health: Prevention and treatment programs. *American Psychologist, 48,* 127–140.

Kumpfer, K. L. (1991). How to get hard to reach parents involved in parenting programs. In D. Pines (Ed.), *Parent training prevention: Preventing alcohol and other drug problems among youth in the family* (DHHS Publication No. 91-1715). Washington, DC: U.S. Government Printing Office.

Kumpfer, K. L. (1999). *Strengthening America's families: Exemplary parenting and family strategies for delinquency prevention.* Rockville, MD: Office of Juvenile Justice and Delinquency Prevention.

Kumpfer, K. L., DeMarsh, J., & Child, W. (1989). *The Strengthening Families Program: Family training manual.* Salt Lake City, UT: University of Utah, Department of Health Education and Alta Institute.

Lillie-Blanton, M., MacKenzie, E., & Anthony, J. C. (1991). Black-white differences in alcohol use by women: Baltimore survey findings. *Public Health Reports, 106,* 124–133.

Lochman, J. E., & Wells, K. (1996). A social cognitive intervention with aggressive children: Prevention effects and contextual implementation issues. In R. De V. Peters & R. J. McMahon (Eds.), *Prevention of childhood disorders: Substance abuse and delinquency.* Thousand Oaks, CA: Sage.

National Clearinghouse for Alcohol and Drug Information. (1995). *Making prevention work: Actions for African-Americans* (On-line). Available: http:/www.health.org/govpub/mpw009/index.htm.

Nobles, W. W., & Goddard, L. (1993). *An African-centered model of prevention for African-American youth at high risk* (DHHS Publication No. 93-2015). Washington, DC: U.S. Government Printing Office.

Nobles, W. W., Goddard, L., Cavil, W. E., & George, P. Y. (1987). *In the culture of drugs in the Black community.* Oakland, CA: Black Family Institute.

Oetting, E. R., Beauvis, F., & Edwards, R. W. (1988). Alcohol and Indian youth: Social and psychological correlates of prevention. *Journal of Drug Issues, 81,* 87–101.

Oyemade, U., & Washington, V. (1990). The role of family factors in the primary prevention of substance abuse among high risk Black youth. In A. R. Stiftman & L. E. Davis (Eds.), *Ethnic issues in adolescent mental health* (pp. 267–284). Newbury Park, CA: Sage.

Rensnicow, K., Soler, R., Braithwaite, R. L., Ahluwalia, J. S., & Butler, J. (2000). Cultural sensitivity in substance use prevention. *Journal of Community Psychology, 28,* 271–290.

Rouse, B. (1989). *Drug abuse among racial/ethnic minorities: A special report.* Rockville, MD: National Institute on Drug Abuse.

Santisteban, D. A., Szapocznik, J., & Rio, A. T. (1993). Family therapy for Hispanic substance abusing youth: An empirical approach to substance abuse prevention. In R. S. Mayers, B. L. Kail, & T. D. Watts (Eds.), *Hispanic substance abuse* (pp. 157–173). Springfield, IL: Charles C Thomas.

Sloboda, Z. (1999). Drug patterns in the United States. In National Institute on Drug Abuse, *Epidemiologic trends in drug abuse* (National Institute of Health Publication No. 00–4530). Washington, DC: U.S. Government Printing Offices.

Substance Abuse and Mental Health Services Administration (SAMHSA) (2000). *Summary of findings from the 1999 National Household Survey on Drug Abuse* (DHHS Publication No. 00-3466). Washington, DC: U.S. Government Printing Office.

Szapocznik, J., Kurtines, W. M., Sanisteban, D. A., & Rio, A. (1989). *Breakthroughs in family therapy with drug-abusing and problem youth.* New York: Springer.

Szapocznik, J., Sanisteban, D. A., Rio, A., Perez-Vidal, A., Kurtines, W. M., & Hervis, O. (1986). Bicultural effectiveness training (BET): An intervention modality for families experiencing intergenerational/intercultural conflict. *Hispanic Journal of Behavioral Sciences, 6,* 303–330.

Turner, W. L. (2000). Cultural considerations in family-based primary prevention programs in drug abuse. *The Journal of Primary Prevention, 21,* 285–303.

Turner, W. L. (2002). Family and school-based drug abuse. *Family Relations, 52,* 302–306.

Turner, W. L. (1995). Healthy Black families: Protectors against substance abuse. *Employee Assistance Journal, 8,* 30–31.

U. S. Bureau of the Census. (2000). *Resident population estimates of the U.S. by sex, race, and Hispanic origin: April 1, 1990 to July 1, 1999, with short-term projection to September 1, 2000* (On-line). Available:http://www.census.gov/population/estimates/nation/intfile3-1.txt.

U. S. Census Bureau (2000). *Current population data, March 1999, racial statistics* (Online). Available: http://www.census.gov/population/socdemo/race/black/ tabs99/tab16.txt.

Valentine, J., Gottlieb, B., Keel, S., Griffith, J., & Ruthazer, R. (1998). Measuring the effectiveness of the Urban Youth Connection: The case for dose-response modeling to demonstrate the impact of an adolescent substance abuse prevention program. *The Journal of Primary Prevention, 18,* 363–387.

Wade, J. C. (1994). Substance abuse: Implications for counseling African-American men. *Journal of Mental Health Counseling, 16,* 415–433.

Wallace, J. M. (1999). The social ecology of addiction: Race, risk and resilience. *Pediatrics, 103,* 1122–1127.

Wallace, J. M., Forman, T. A., Guthrie, B. J., Bachman, J. G., O'Malley, P. M., & Johnston, L. D. (1999). The epidemiology of alcohol, tobacco and other drug use among Black youth. *Journal of Studies on Alcohol, 60,* 800–809.

CHAPTER 20

The Effectiveness of Alcohol and Drug Abuse Prevention among American-Indian Youth

FRED BEAUVAIS

JOSEPH E. TRIMBLE

INTRODUCTION

Misuse of alcohol is considered by most of America's indigenous populations to be their most serious and significant health problem, a problem that affects almost every facet of life. Discussions about drug use, mental and physical health, deviance, familial problems, and community structure and function among American-Indians and Alaska Natives must include, in some form or another, the influences of alcohol use and misuse. Therefore, it is reasonable to conclude that culturally resonant alcohol and drug use prevention strategies, if effective, would contribute to a significant reduction in illness, disease, deviance, and community disruption.

This chapter addresses prevention of alcohol and drug use and abuse in American-Indian and Alaska-Native communities. It provides information on the demographic characteristics of America's indigenous people then provides an overview of the field of substance use and misuse among American-Indian and Alaska-Native youth. It concludes with a discussion of specific ways to enhance drug abuse prevention research for these populations.

The terms American-Indian and Alaska Native are "ethnic glosses" (Trimble, 1991, 1995). They refer to the aboriginal populations of North America and are terms imbued with political

FRED BEAUVAIS • Tri-Ethnic Center for Prevention Research, Colorado State University, Fort Collins, Colorado 80523
JOSEPH E. TRIMBLE • Center for Cross-Cultural Research, Department of Psychology, Western Washington University, Bellingham, Washington 98226

and sociocultural considerations. In this chapter the terms "American-Indian" and "Indian" are used for the sake of brevity, but this is not meant to disregard the differences that exists among the many native tribes and villages.

DEMOGRAPHY OF AMERICAN-INDIANS AND ALASKA NATIVES

The physical, sociopolitical, and economic conditions that affect Indian youth vary from one locality to the next, but some common factors exist that relate directly to the problems of drug and alcohol abuse. The lands allotted to Indian people were typically of little economic value and usually in remote areas. In some places this is rapidly changing with the discovery of natural resources and other forms of economic development, but Indian reservations are still typically found in the poorest sectors of the country. Despite some changes for the better, poverty and its attendant ills of poor nutrition and inadequate health care affect all social structures, particularly the family. Inadequate housing, lack of transportation, and other basic support systems are still a daily reality in most reservation areas. Young (1994) summarized the health conditions of American-Indians as follows: "The recent epidemiologic history of Native American populations appears to be characterized by several key features: decline but persistence of infectious diseases, stabilizing at a level still higher than non-Native populations; rise in chronic diseases, but not quite rampant; and the overwhelming importance of social pathologies" (pp. 52–53).

Education on Indian reservations is another area marked by inadequacy and a lack of resources. Historical approaches to the education of Indian youth were extremely harsh and included use of boarding schools, which had an extremely deleterious effect on the family and other social institutions. It is only recently that Indian families have taken the opportunity to regain control of the educational systems and to have a central influence in the lives and development of their children.

Despite the negative picture that is generally drawn of Indian youth, there have been recent, dramatic changes in the social fabric of Indian communities that point to a much brighter future (Beauvais, 2000). Tribes have enthusiastically taken more and more responsibility for their affairs, and there is a sense that the coming generations will enjoy a much better quality of life. With respect to drug and alcohol abuse issues, Indian communities have been in the forefront of the development of prevention interventions, although as will be seen, the evaluation of these efforts has been sorely lacking.

Rates and Patterns of Substance Use

For more than 25 years it has been known that substance use and abuse is a significant problem for large numbers of Indian youth residing on reservations. Pinto (1973) was among the first to bring this to light and to argue for increased resources to address the problem. Subsequently, a variety of studies have demonstrated very high rates of use, although most of these studies have been conducted with geographically limited populations (e.g. Cockerham, 1975; Dick, Manson, & Beals; 1993; Longclaws et al., 1980). The studies of the Tri-Ethnic Center for Prevention Research at Colorado State University, however, have corroborated results of these local investigations and have shown higher rates of use for most drugs since 1974 for representative samples of Indian youth across the United States (Beauvais, 1992, 1996; Beauvais et al., 1989, 1996; Beauvais & LaBoueff, 1985; Beauvais & Oetting, 1988; Beauvais & Segal, 1992; Oetting & Beauvais, 1989;

Oetting et al., 1980; Oetting, Edwards, & Beauvais, 1989; Oetting & Goldstein, 1979). These higher rates have been found for lifetime, annual, and 30-day prevalence rates as well as for overall drug involvement (Oetting & Beauvais, 1983; Beauvais, 1996).

In 1992, the Tri-Ethnic Center had access to a large sample of adolescents from around the United States, including a substantial number of Indian youth who were not living on reservations. The data showed that non-reservation-Indian youth had levels of drug use lower than Indian youth living on reservations but higher than their non-Indian counterparts (Beauvais, 1992). The finding leads to the speculation that although reservation life has many positive aspects, there may be environmental variables, such as poverty and unemployment, that promote higher levels of substance use; Indian youth not living on reservations are not as subjected to these harsh conditions. Tri-Ethnic Center studies (Beauvais, 1992; Beauvais & Laboueff, 1985) and a recent study by Mitchell and Beals (1997) show only minor variations in drug use from one reservation to another, suggesting that the causative factors are common across groups and are not a result of cultural or geographic differences. However, boarding school students (May, 1982; Dick, Manson, & Beals, 1993) and high school dropouts (Beauvais et al., 1996) have been shown to have higher drug use than Indian youth in general.

Despite having higher rates of drug and alcohol use, the patterns of increases and decreases over time for Indian youth have paralleled those for other youth. Across the United States there was a substantial increase in drug use through the early 1980s and then a steady annual decline through 1992. At that point use began to rise again (Beauvais, 1996). The finding of recent increases has not been substantiated through epidemiological evidence for Indian youth, but numerous anecdotal reports from local prevention and treatment personnel on reservations and some preliminary survey data indicate that this is now occurring. The one exception to the pattern over the past 20 years is for Indian youth who use drugs at the most extreme levels. Tri-Ethnic Center researchers have identified a "high-risk" pattern (approximately 20% of Indian 7th- through 12th-graders) that has not changed substantially since 1980 (Beauvais, 1996).

This pattern suggests that there are a group of Indian youth who use drugs for much the same reason as other youth (i.e., they are subjected to the same secular influences that vary over time), but there is another group (i.e., those at high risk) whose drug use is rooted in extreme social and personal dysfunction. For the former, it is reasonable to conclude that prevention programs promoting pro-social values that work among youth in general will probably be effective for Indian youth. The high-risk youth, on the other hand, are likely to have a wide range of social dysfunction and will require more intense approaches.

Etiology and Correlates of Use

While not as extensive as that for other youth, there is a body of literature that examines the etiological and correlative factors in adolescent drug use among American-Indians. Some of these studies use a more broadly based theoretical perspective while others look at single or small groups of variables in a more descriptive approach. At the broader level are the studies of problem prone behavior theory (Mitchell & Beals, 1997), social learning theory (Winfree, Griffiths, & Sellers, 1989), and peer cluster theory (Oetting & Beauvais, 1987). The more limited studies have examined discrete sets of variables, such as emotional distress, self-esteem, anger and aggression, socialization variables, knowledge and attitudes, and demographic factors (Austin, Oetting, & Beauvais, 1993). The majority of these investigations have found a great deal of correspondence between the etiological factors in substance use for both Indian and non-Indian youth. One of the more general findings across all studies where it is included as a variable is that peer influence appears to mediate nearly all other psychosocial variables in the prediction of substance use (Oetting & Beauvais, 1987). While this conclusion regarding general similarity across ethnic groups is important, a number of studies have shown that there may be relative differences between cultural groups in the influence of peers. For example, a Tri-Ethnic Center study (Swaim et al., 1993) found that although peers were significant in predicting drug use among Indian youth, family influence was more substantial. This same analysis indicated that school had a smaller influence on decisions to use drugs for Indian youth than for other youth. These findings have important implications for designing prevention programs for Indian youth and suggest that the family, rather than the school, should be the main target for interventions.

Another difference often found between Indian and non-Indian youth is the influence of religion on levels of drug use (Austin et al., 1993); religious involvement appears to be a protective factor for non-Indian youth but has little effect on Indian youth. This may be a measurement problem since the meaning of religiosity differs greatly between the two groups, and scales used to measure this dimension in the general population may not be reliable with Indian groups.

Cultural or ethnic identification is also considered in the search for etiological factors. The prevailing belief is that Indian youth who have higher levels of identification with their culture will demonstrate lower drug and alcohol use. Despite this strong belief, the research data on this linkage have been extremely meager, not only for Indian youth but also for all other minority populations. (Oetting & Beauvais, 1990–1991; Beauvais, 1998; Trimble, 1991, 1995; Bates, Beauvais, & Trimble, 1997). Research to date on this issue has been aimed at finding a direct effect for cultural or ethnic identification, but the actual path may be indirect, operating through a number of other psychological and social variables. Given the strong investment among prevention and treatment professionals, examination of the relationship of cultural identification and substance abuse remains a fruitful and necessary area of inquiry. One hypothesis worth pursuing is that cultural identification may play a strong role in recovery from addiction problems later in life but that it has a reduced meaning for prevention among Indian youths who are struggling with adolescent developmental issues.

Regardless of the effects of culture on alcohol and drug use, there is a clear consensus among substance abuse researchers and practitioners that prevention programs must be designed to be culturally appropriate (Beauvais & LaBoueff, 1985; Fleming, 1992; May, 1995; Petroskey, Van Stelle, & De Jong, 1998; Trimble, 1992, 1995; Trimble, Padilla, & Bell-Bolek, 1987). Programs must include content and activities congruent with and which promote the values, beliefs, and practices of Native-Americans. The primary reasons for this are respect for the culture of American-Indian and Alaska-Native communities and to ensure that any program will be acceptable within those communities. Even though a particular approach may have been shown to be effective in reducing drug use among adolescents in other locations, it will have little chance of success in Indian communities if it is not accepted as being culturally relevant.

OVERVIEW OF PREVENTION ACTIVITIES

In 1982, the American-Indian anthropologist, Spero M. Manson, edited the first volume devoted exclusively to the subject of prevention among American-Indians and Alaska Natives. The book covered research, training, services, evaluation, and offered recommendations. It set an important and significant tone for a field that at that time had received little or no attention. Manson pointed out in his opening chapter that "relatively little prevention research has been conducted in the area of American-Indian mental health. Much of that which exists represents a very narrow focus" (p. 11). Considerable prevention research has been conducted since his work was published, but the works focus largely on commentary and recommendations and not on the science of prevention. However, many important and relevant etiological and epidemiological studies exist documenting over time the prevalence and use rates of alcohol and drugs.

In 1986, the United States Congress legislated the Anti-Drug Abuse Act. A major portion of the act led to creation of the Center for Substance Abuse Prevention (CSAP). CSAP's major mission is to promote the goal of no illicit drugs and no misuse of alcohol or other legal drugs. To accomplish this, CSAP focuses on youth and families living in high-risk settings (CSAP, 1991) and currently sponsors and promotes a variety of prevention activities and programs. These include demonstration grants for the prevention of alcohol and other drug abuse among high-risk youth, model projects for pregnant and postpartum women and their infants, and community partnership grants. In addition, CSAP sponsors communication programs that reach targeted populations with specific prevention messages and develops communication tools and materials that respond to the specific needs of certain audiences.

CSAP is also involved in compiling detailed information on the nature and effectiveness of the projects for specific ethnic minority and cultural groups. As part of that venture, CSAP asked several investigators to survey the project coordinators of the many ethnic specific projects. Results compiled from a survey of projects targeted for American-Indian and Alaska-Native communities illustrate the depth and range of the activities. By 1988, CSAP had awarded 18 grants that targeted communities with sizeable American-Indian and Alaska-Native populations; some 24 tribes and villages were represented in the prevention activities. Fleming and Manson (1990) conducted an extensive evaluation of the characteristics and effectiveness of the 18 programs.

Ninety-four percent of the community-based programs emphasized primary prevention activities designed to prevent a health-related problem from occurring among those who may be at risk. Some of the primary prevention activities involved the use of educational materials, promotion of Indian identity and building self-esteem through cultural events, and the use of self-help groups. Secondary and tertiary levels of prevention, which are intended to prevent a problem from intensifying or to alleviate the problem tend to emphasize counseling and psychotherapy. Individual and group therapy and counseling were found in 88% of the projects

Since the 18 programs were based at the community level, the opinions of local staff were important in shaping each project's design to fit local needs and cultural perceptions. Sixty-one percent of the projects reported that the success of the activities centered on improving relationships with their respective clients' families; 56% felt that it was important to support and maintain open communications across all levels of the project's operation.

Fleming and Manson (1990) asked their respondents to identify factors that place Indian youth at risk for using drugs and alcohol. Eighty-eight percent singled out poor self-esteem and parental abuse of alcohol as the greatest contributors to risk. The respondents also identified additional contributing factors including peer and friends use of drugs; abuse, neglect, and family conflict; sexual abuse and emotional and psychological difficulties; previous suicide threats or attempts; and alienation from the dominant culture's social values. The researchers also asked their respondents to identify factors that presumably prevent one from using and abusing drugs. Protective factors listed include having a well-defined spiritual belief system, a positive sense of self-worth, an ability to make good decisions about personal responsibilities, and the ability to act independently of others. The respondents also believed that one's friends and peers who act in healthy and responsible ways could serve as models for youth at risk. The majority of research conducted on Indian youth has focused on problem behaviors with very little emphasis on healthy or resiliency behaviors. At least two authors point out that unless further attention is paid to the factors involved in positive adolescent development among Indian youth, our knowledge of how to prevent negative behaviors will be seriously limited (Beauvais, 2000; Mitchell & Beals, 1997).

Basically, Fleming and Manson were able to demonstrate that some Indian community members have a good sense for social and psychological factors that contribute to drug use and seemed to recognize factors essential to preventing the problems from occurring or getting worse. More to the point, many Indian communities appear to have keen insight into drug and alcohol abuse problems and the commitment and knowledge necessary to intervene. Communities may require technical and expert assistance in certain phases of prevention and intervention programs, but such assistance is not an absolute necessity.

Another study (Owan, Palmer, & Quintana, 1987) surveyed nearly 420 schools from Head Start to the secondary school level with large American-Indian and Alaska-Native enrollments and 225 different tribal groups who were receiving grant support for alcohol and drug abuse projects from the Indian Health Service. Both the school and community respondents indicated that alcohol and drug abuse education was a major priority followed by a concern for building self-esteem and developing effective coping and decision-making skills. Owan et al. (1987) draw some important conclusions that emphasize the need for "early intervention to combat alcohol and substance abuse among Indian youths" (p. 71). They also emphasize that Indian youth need strong families in order to promote positive self-esteem, identity, and values. "Weak families," they argue, "produce uprooted individuals susceptible to 'peer clusters' prone to alcohol and substance abuse" (p. 71).

Over the past decade there have been numerous efforts to catalogue and summarize the nature of drug prevention activities among Indian youth (Breaking New Ground, 1990; Hayne, 1993, 1994; Owan et al., 1987). May and Moran, (1995) and May (1995) provided a comprehensive review of drug and alcohol prevention programs among Indian populations using the public health model of primary, secondary, and tertiary prevention. While it is clear that there is a tremendous amount of activity directed at preventing drug use in Indian communities, only a handful of studies have applied rigorous, scientific attention to determining program effectiveness. May and Moran (1995) concluded, "Few systematic outcome evaluations of either approach (primary and secondary prevention) have been completed in Indian communities. Thus, based on the work in the field to date, we believe that although these approaches have much promise, indications of success should be characterized as preliminary" (p. 297).

Social Skills

Among the few programs that have received some scientific scrutiny are those described by Schinke and Gilchrist and their colleagues (Gilchrist et al., 1987; Schinke, Botvin et al., 1988; Schinke et al., 1986; Schinke, Orlandi et al., 1988; Schinke, Schilling, & Gilchrist, 1986; Trimble, 1992). In the first of these studies (Gilchrist et al., 1987), a skills-enhancement program was developed to accommodate local tribal life-ways and administered to a group of young Indians in the Pacific Northwest. One-hundred two youth (mean age 11.34; 49% female) were screened, and half were randomly assigned to a program that included health education information about drugs and a series of exercises designed to identify values and improve decision-making skills regarding the future use of drugs and alcohol. Compared to the control group, youth in the experimental group exhibited lower rates of alcohol, marijuana, and inhalant use (but not tobacco) at both post-test and a 6-month follow-up. Also noted at both testing periods were reductions in self-perception as a drug user, an increase in knowledge about drugs, and an improved ability to refuse offers to use drugs. In a similar study involving problem solving, enhanced by the teaching and modeling of social-competence skills, Schinke et al. (1988) found reductions in alcohol, marijuana, inhalants, stimulants, and barbiturates at a 6-month follow up. Once again, random assignment to experimental and control conditions was used. The latter study is significant in that a "social-competence" component was derived from the theoretical notion that youth who can be trained in bicultural competence (i.e., can function comfortably in both Indian and Anglo society) should display better overall adjustment and lower substance use. This idea is discussed extensively by LaFromboise and Rowe (1983) and LaFromboise, Coleman, and Gerton (1993) and is consistent with the theoretical framework and empirical findings of Oetting and Beauvais (1990–1991) and Oetting (1993).

The idea of the efficacy of bicultural competence training should receive a great deal more attention in future research, given that it is one area in cross-cultural substance abuse research that is solidly theory based and has shown some promising empirical results. It is a general model that, if proven efficacious, will be applicable to other minority populations. However, not much has been done to follow up on the promising work of Schinke and Gilchrist in more than a decade.

Peers

In a pilot study with a group of highly alcohol-involved American-Indian youth, Carpenter, Lyons, and Miller (1985) found that the incorporation of peer counselors into a prevention program led to significant decreases in alcohol consumption at the end of the intervention and at 4-, 9-, and 12-month follow-ups. However, this was a very small ($n = 30$), uncontrolled study, and the results should be viewed with caution. In another small pilot study, Duryea and Matzek (1990) found some promising results using peer pressure resistance training with Indian elementary school students. While encouraging, the existing studies on peers and drug use among Indian youth are extremely limited. Given the centrality of peers in the etiology and maintenance of drug-using behavior in general and specifically within Indian populations, prevention programs incorporating peer dynamics need considerably more investigation.

Family

There is nearly universal agreement that the family is of paramount importance among and within all Indian groups (Fleming, 1992). While the centrality of the family in the development of children and adolescents is recognized by most cultures, the traditional kinship and extended family structure of Indian communities add importance to this source of socialization. With respect to influence on drug and alcohol use specifically, the previously cited study of Swaim et al. (1993) demonstrated that Indian families may take precedence over peers as the most proximal determinant of use or nonuse of drugs. This is contrary to the usual finding of the predominance of peer influence among non-Indian adolescents. (Oetting & Beauvais, 1986).

In general, family-based alcohol and drug use prevention programs have slowly grown in importance over the past decade. Kumpfer (1998), Dishion (1997), and Bry (1993), for example, present convincing evidence that family-based prevention strategies can reduce adolescent risk factors and alcohol and drug use rates. Kumpfer (1998) specifically maintains that "research has shown that parents play a major role in influencing their children's attitudes toward, and decisions about, alcohol and other drug use. When parents take an active role in their children's lives . . . they can address many of the root causes of drug use" (pp. 9–10).

Given the importance of the family, it is surprising that there is scant literature on prevention interventions that feature Indian and Native families. Hayne (1993, 1994) presented a review of more than 60 prevention programs on Indian reservations and at urban Indian centers. Less than

10% focus on the family as one of the more important intervention targets. Most of the programs list activities such as parent training skills, recreational activities to increase contact with the family, drug education for family members, and similar elements but only a few include the family as a central focus of the intervention. An exception is a recent project by Van Stelle, Allen, and Moberg (1998). It consists of a 24-week intervention that includes a family weekend retreat, a family drug abuse curriculum, home visits, family support groups, an elders resource council, and cultural activities that bring youth, parents, and elders together. The project enjoyed wide acceptance in the community and many of the existing service agencies participated. Unfortunately, no data were provided on behavioral outcomes, and there is no way to predict whether the program will continue beyond the 5 years allotted by federal funding.

School-Based Programs

By far, the majority of drug prevention programs in the United States are implemented in schools; the situation in Indian communities is not much different (Owan, Palmer, & Quintana, 1987). A further similarity is the lack of consistent assessment of effectiveness. A few programs have demonstrated specific, short-term gains (Bernstein & Woodall, 1987; Davis, Hunt, & Kitzes, 1989; Murphy & DeBlassie, 1984), but most lack any evidence that they can be generalized or that the gains are sustained over time. Particularly overlooked in school programs is the need for continued booster sessions over a period of years. The booster sessions seem to be the *sine qua non* of effective school-based programs (Botvin et al., 1995). Given the popularity of school-based interventions, it is imperative that more effort be placed on assessing their impact and on determining the dimensions required for effectiveness.

Policy

One area that has received virtually no attention in substance abuse prevention among Indian youth is policy. In an exhaustive overview of policy concerning alcohol reduction among Indian populations, May (1992) found few empirical studies, outside of those examining the effects of alcohol prohibition, that addressed policy topics. However, based on findings in the general literature and an analysis of policy options available in Indian communities, May listed 107 potential avenues for alcohol control. It is notable that, even as comprehensive as this list is, it did not include issues of school policies regarding drug and alcohol abuse among adolescents. This is a ripe and important area for research development and program opportunities. Policy options clearly overlap with legal approaches; but again, outside of the studies showing that prohibition has little effect on alcohol consumption in Indian communities, there are no studies showing how the police and courts can effectively address adolescent drug use prevention in Indian communities.

COMMUNITY-CENTERED PREVENTION

Countless studies of Indian and Native alcohol and drug use, including many of those reviewed previously, focus on the personality of the individual with the explicit reasoning that if one uncovers some deficiency all one has to do is to target prevention programs to prevent individual deviance from occurring, especially among youth who have been diagnosed as being at risk. Holder (1998), more pointedly, maintains that there is a common perception that "alcohol problems are seen as being caused by 'flawed people'—alcoholics, addicts, persons from broken families, incompletely socialized individuals, and psychologically damaged or genetically disadvantaged persons" (p. 7). Given the pattern of research and the emphasis on the "flawed character," there is an abundance of Indian and Native alcohol and drug abuse prevention research in the literature that focuses on low self-esteem, locus of control, acculturation stress, depression, deviance, alienation, anxiety, and related personality variables (Trimble, 1998).

Overall, however, prevention research findings based on an individual perspective are mixed and inconclusive. This is leading a few researchers to conclude that a paradigm shift must occur if we are to understand adolescent Indian substance use and misuse (see Grube, 1998; Oetting, Beauvais, & Edwards, 1988; Oetting, Donnermeyer et al., 1998; Oetting, Edwards, & Beauvais, 1989; Oetting, Swaim et al., 1989; Schroeder, Laflin, & Weis, 1993).

The cross-cultural psychologist, Harry C. Triandis, writing in a foreword to a text entitled, *Multiculturalism as a Fourth Force* (Pedersen, 1999), states that, "Humans see the world according to information that they sample from the environment. Members of different cultures sample different types of information. For example, members of Western, individualist cultures, when explaining what people do, sample mostly internal processes such as beliefs, attitudes, personality, personal goals, aspirations, and values. Members of the majority of the rest of the world sample mostly external processes, such as the in-group's goals, aspirations, and values" (p. xvii). The majority of alcohol and drug use researchers come from individualistic cultures in which the primary emphasis is on the individual; attention is given primarily to the goals and needs of the individual with an emphasis on discovering causal and correlative relationships among individual variables to explain substance use behavior, treatment, and prevention. The bulk of the substance use research on Indians and Natives also appears to have an individual-centered perspective.

It could be argued, however, that most American-Indians and Alaska Natives, especially those residing on reservations and in rural communities and villages, come from collectivist and situation-centered cultures. According to Triandis (1995) and Hofstede (1980), collectivism can be viewed as a social pattern of individuals who have strong ties with one another and regard themselves as part of one or more communities. Group goals take priority, and cohesiveness among community and family members is emphasized. If the majority of Indians and Natives represent a collectivist-centered orientation, then it makes sense to design and implement alcohol and drug use prevention research to fit a social ecological pattern rather than continuing to advocate approaches that center on an individualist perspective.

Research on drinking styles and patterns among Indians and Natives indicates that much of the drinking behavior occurs in group settings (see Mail & McDonald, 1980; Trimble & Bagwell, 1995). In addition, research findings on Indian youth indicate that strong influence on drinking and drug use is the peer group (Beauvais, 1992; Dinges & Oetting, 1993; Oetting, Donnermeyer et al., 1998; Oetting et al., 1991). Peer groups and friends are an intimate and influential segment of one's community. In turn, these groups are connected to their respective extended families, clans, and other forms of tribal and community-based organizational arrangements. Taken together, the social units form a network in which segments and units interact and subsequently influence one another. Multiple community influences can contribute to deviant behavior that in turn can contribute to alcohol and drug use behavior; such influences can include dysfunctional families, community disorganization, and poor school environments.

Communities are fluid, dynamic, and adaptive systems (Holder, 1998). Communities also consist of numerous resources "created by human activities and intentions, such as helping and healing (that) are intrinsically expanding and renewable" (Katz, 1983/84, p. 202). Communities are also synergistic and demonstrate a pattern through which human actions are related to one another and include the products of those interactions. Healing resources are activated by community members and are typically intended to be shared by others, especially those in need. A synergistic helping pattern of behavior is a renewable and expanding resource, and when communities are ready to focus their energies on a community problem, such as alcoholism, outcomes can be positive and long lasting.

Unfortunately, very few, if any, full-scale, community-centered Indian adolescent prevention programs have been implemented and carried out to their full conclusion (see Grube, 1998). There is some indication, however, that positions such as that espoused by Holder may be taking hold among those familiar with the needs of Indian communities. Certainly, the emphasis on community partnerships within CSAP is a reflection of this stance. May and Moran (1995) and May (1995) conclude from their reviews of prevention activities in Indian communities with a call for a more general, multifaceted, public health approach to drug abuse prevention (see also Rolf, 1995). Within the past 5 years, a major community partnership initiative, funded by the Robert Wood Johnson Foundation, has been undertaken by the American Indian and Alaska Native Mental Health Research Center at the University of Colorado Health Sciences Center. Called the Healthy Nations Project, this initiative led to the identification of 13 Indian urban and rural communities in which 5-year prevention projects are being developed. The projects are designed to be locally initiated and controlled efforts that are highly responsive to the cultural beliefs and needs of each location. Each project is expected to develop a variety of networking and intervention activities that address the problem of substance abuse across the continuum of needs through treatment, aftercare, and relapse prevention. Current descriptions of the progress in these communities reveal an impressive diversity of culturally grounded activities, but as yet there are no outcome results.

Many Indian community members talk about the need for community members to get fully involved in alcohol and drug prevention programs. If such an effort did occur, what should it emphasize? Holder (1998) suggests that a community systems perspective (1) considers a wide-ranging set of alcohol-involved problems instead of focusing on a single condition or problem; (2) studies the entire community rather than just individuals who are at risk; and (3) uses interventions that change the social, cultural, economic, and community conditions that influence alcohol use rather than rely on "single solutions" based on some social science theoretical principle. To accomplish such an undertaking synergy must be in place and community members must believe that they can control the outcome of a communitywide intervention.

A community-based alcohol and drug use prevention program must be sustainable, renewable, and built on the existing healing and helping resources present in the community (see Altman, 1995; Trickett, 1996, 1977; Trickett, Barons, & Buchanan, 1996). Community differences must be connected to adaptive strategies. Communities are not monolithic but socially and culturally split and sometimes fractured by age, gender, clan, camps, bands, and political districts; if the community problem is significant and potentially destructive, then fractured units must put aside differences to collaborate on the solution. Contextual and cultural differences also influence coping and adaptation and thus must be considered in designing and implementing interventions. Understanding behavior that occurs in one situation must also be understood when it occurs in other situations.

A community-centered approach to alcohol and drug use prevention does not mean that a few community members organize to deal with the problem. It does not mean that community members single out youth who may be potentially "flawed," "at risk," or otherwise prone to alcohol and drug use merely because they are youth and "treat" them with a "dosage" of educational materials that may impact their social and decision-making skills. Alcohol and drug use patterns and corresponding problems are much more complicated and involve numerous community, group, and individual-level factors. Holder maintains that, "Alcohol-involved problems are not simply the results of actions of a set of definable high-risk individuals; rather, they are the accumulative result of the structure and interactions of complex social, cultural, and economic factors within the community system" (p. 12). For prevention to occur effectively and for it to be sustained the total community—all segments—must be committed and involved. Rather than viewing communities as collections of at-risk youth and adults, perhaps it may prove useful to view them as "communities-at-risk," especially if there is an identifiable alcohol and drug use problem in the community. And, if communities are at risk, then it makes sense that the community approach the problem from a systematic perspective engaging all elements.

If an Indian or Native community is ready to recognize and subsequently respond to an alcohol and drug use problem it must first identify and use existing resources, build on its strengths, and educate others in the community about the nature of the resources. If the resources are not institutionalized, then procedures must be set in motion to weave them into the fabric of the community dynamic and make them part of the synergy. If research is called for, the community must carefully select consultants who are willing to collaborate with community leaders over lengthy periods of time following community traditions at each step. Research and preventive intervention occur at more than one level and thus can have synergistic effects that promote community ownership over time. Research and preventive-intervention strategies must be designed to serve the goals of community development and emphasize the importance of developing and enhancing local resources. And all along the way one must bear in mind that the community actually "owns" the data and the process; the researcher is an invited guest selected to assist in intervening and preventing a community problem.

Research Challenges

The problems involved in any scientific analysis of drug prevention efforts are only magnified when the arena of interest is expanded to encompass multiple community and individual activities and their interactions. Of particular concern is the unique nature of each community coalition and the interventions they define as being appropriate for their locale. The diversity precludes multiple applications of a standard approach that can be compared in an experimental design.

A second major problem is identification of a reasonable control community. American-Indian and Alaska-Native communities are heterogeneous, not only in their cultural makeup but also in structural characteristics, such as size, governance patterns, cultural lifeways and thoughtways, and economic bases. This heterogeneity creates major doubts as to whether external validity can be assured by any design.

A third issue is determining the actual level of exposure to any or all of the coalition efforts. While there may be a plethora of activities taking place in a particular community, it is often difficult to tell which ones, and to what degree, youth may have participated in them. In short, assessment of the effectiveness of community coalitions, or partnerships, usually entails fairly loose experimental designs and often equivocal results.

All of the previously cited problems were inherent in an effort to evaluate a community-based alcohol prevention program on a Western reservation by Cheadle et al. (1995). The initial plans for randomization and identification of comparable control communities were stymied by funding considerations. Consequently, the control communities were non-Indian locations in another state. Pre-, post-, and follow-up surveys of youth in the community did show reductions in alcohol and marijuana abuse over a 4-year period. However, similar, albeit smaller, reductions were seen in the "control" communities, and the research team was reluctant to attribute the reductions to the prevention program. Furthermore, the team was unable to document to what extent the youth had been exposed to prevention activities throughout the course of the program.

Community Readiness

In the past, interventions centered on the individual were accompanied by narrowly focused concepts and needs assessments. One consequence of this has been the promulgation of a seemingly endless succession of "new" drug prevention programs that are brought into communities, thrive while external funding is available, and then rapidly disappear when funding ends. It is likely that the individual pathology approach used by most of these programs is inappropriate and, consequently, communities never had an investment in the program from the beginning (Beauvais & Trimble, 1992). The need for such programs is often neither widely recognized nor accepted. The programs are usually designed by someone outside the community who is probably not fully aware of the culture of the community. Furthermore, many of the programs that are implemented are so ambitious that they overwhelm existing resources within the community. For example, a school-based program that requires a considerable financial investment in teacher training and materials will not work in a reservation school where both dollars and human capital are at the breaking point.

As a response to this mismatch between community needs, perceptions, and attitudes and the need for drug prevention interventions, an approach called "community readiness" has been developed that focuses on community dynamics, vis-à-vis the acceptance of needed interventions (see Plested et al., 1999). The underlying principle of this model is that communities are at different levels in their readiness and willingness to engage in prevention interventions. If the intervention is attempted before the community is ready, or if the intervention is too complex for the level of readiness, then implementation is likely to fail. Note that this model does not address the inherent value or quality of the intervention; an intervention may have been shown to be extremely effective in other locations but will misfire if the community is not ready to both accept and implement it.

The community-readiness model specifies nine stages of readiness in increasing order of complexity and the community's increasing willingness and ability to engage in prevention activities. Brief descriptions of three of the stages will help illustrate the model. The very lowest stage is "no awareness," a case in which a behavior is seen as normative or may even be encouraged; thus, there is no motivation to prevent the behavior. The following stage is "denial," in which there is recognition that substance abuse, for instance, is a problem but it is not something to be concerned about locally—"It is happening elsewhere but not here." Further along the continuum is the stage of "initiation." Here there is recognition of the problem, training has been initiated, and there is some form of prevention activity taking place. The ninth and final stage is "professionalization." At this point there is sophisticated programming, training, and evaluation, and the prevention activities are well-integrated into existing community structures.

A critical aspect of the community-readiness model is that it is prescriptive as well as descriptive. Descriptively, it can be used to objectively measure movement within the community, perhaps as a result of an intervention. Prescriptively, the model can be used to foster community development. At each stage there are interventions that can be undertaken to move the community along to the next stage. For example, early on, but not at the earliest stages, data, such as those from drug surveys, can be gathered to further inform and motivate a community to undertake prevention. It is important, however, that these interventions be timed appropriately and conform to what the community is ready to handle. It would be futile, and perhaps counterproductive, for instance, to collect drug survey data if the community was exhibiting tolerance toward drug use; data presented at this stage would be summarily ignored. Another aspect to the prescriptive nature of the model is that community members themselves provide the data and determine what steps are to be taken to increase readiness. A type of "self-study" is involved in which a census of local resources is taken and decisions made about how they can be used to move forward.

The community-readiness model is both qualitative and quantitative. Substantial amounts of interview data are collected in the process of specifying where a community is on the continuum. The result, however, is a numerical rating that can be used in statistical analyses to determine whether or not a community has changed in its level of readiness because of a community development intervention.

Once again, community readiness does not speak to the issue of the effectiveness of any drug prevention strategy. It does, however, provide an accurate gauge for determining at what point certain interventions can be introduced. Without attention to this critical timing, no program, no matter its demonstrated potency in similar communities, can be effective. Given the past history of a long procession of failed drug prevention programs in Indian communities, it would appear essential that more attention be paid to the community-readiness paradigm.

Cultural Sensitivity

In addition to developing new assessment and analytic approaches that allow for a focus on communities, there is a strong awareness that new programs need to adhere to the cultural norms of Indian communities. There are a number of requirements that must be recognized and attended to when the research enterprise crosses cultural boundaries. Failure to do so has led to failure of many research efforts, which for obvious reasons do not show up in the literature (See Manson (1989) for an exception.) Trimble (1977), Beauvais (1995), Rolf (1995), and Beauvais and Trimble (1992) discuss many of these requirements, including gaining access to research populations, gaining trust, collaboration in designing researchable ideas, collaboration in the research process, using measurements that capture concepts cross-culturally, and the interpretation and dissemination of results from a cultural perspective. Norton and Manson (1996) draw attention to a number of factors that must be addressed in conducting clinical research in American-Indian communities, including issues of confidentiality and anonymity of respondents and tribes, tribal participation and endorsement, and the benefits to be derived from the tribe through participation in the research. Confidentiality and informed consent, Norton and Manson argue, may present culturally unique problems for many tribal members, especially when consent forms must be translated and adjusted to fit tribal-specific world views.

Petrovsky et al. (1998) recently described a communitywide drug prevention program in an Indian community that not only had positive outcomes (substance use rates were lower than those of a comparison community) but also conformed to cross-cultural research requirements. Each of the four components of the intervention was designed after extensive discussions with community members; this took an extended period of time but was necessary to establish the legitimacy and relevance of the research project. In addition, community members were included as staff members. Interim project outcomes and problems were discussed with local people in an effort to adjust the goals to be not only scientifically rigorous but also to meet the needs of the local community. Results of the study included both quantitative and qualitative comparisons; the latter were most useful to the community in terms of determining the impact of the intervention.

CONCLUSION AND FUTURE DIRECTIONS

There are a few published articles about research findings on prevention programs for American-Indians and Alaska Natives, but there is need for more research on the topic. From the prevention and etiological literature, the following conclusions can be drawn with respect to designing effective prevention and intervention activities for American-Indian and Alaska Native youth.

1. The centrality of the extended family in Indian culture makes it imperative that families be involved in prevention approaches.
2. Peers exert a significant effect on drug using decisions, although to a lesser degree than among non-Indians.
3. As currently defined and measured, cultural identification is not directly related to substance abuse prevention, although it may be critical in treatment.
4. Many of the factors affecting youth in general also impact drug use among Indian youth.
5. Much more is known about risk than resiliency factors for Indian youth.
6. The evidence for the effectiveness of school-based programs is very limited, and
7. A community-based systems approach grounded in the unique and culturally specific lifestyles of Indian and Native communities is the most reasonable approach to preventing alcohol and drug use and abuse among adolescents.

As a consequence of Manson's 1982 seminal, Trimble (1984) posed a series of questions designed to advance prevention strategies, themes, and research among American-Indians and Alaska Natives. Even though they are more than 15 years old, they are still relevant for setting an agenda for future work. They include:

1. What forms of drug and alcohol use are thought to be preventable? By what indigenous and tribally specific means?
2. What are the models of human and transcultural competence—in terms of individuals, families, and communities—that account for the immense heterogeneity among American Indians and Alaska Natives? How can the models drive prevention and intervention strategies?
3. What are the characteristics of natural support systems and traditional ways of changing and strengthening them to promote and advance the prevention of substance use and abuse, illness, and individual and social deviance?
4. What culturally appropriate information about the causes and consequences of substance use and abuse, illness, and deviance is available for circulation and use in Indian and Native communities? What procedures are available to assist Indians and Natives in turning the cognitively based information into behavioral skills to assist them in coping with situations involving alcohol and drugs?
5. What are the psychosocial characteristics associated with the life-span predictors of substance use and misuse? What are the age-specific gender differences and characteristics?
6. What treatment modalities (indigenous and traditional) are available to effectively deal with substance use and misuse? What expectancy variables define treatment, the therapeutic relationship, and aftercare? From the Indian's point of view? From the intervenor's point of view?
7. Under what conditions and for what reasons are practices and techniques of traditional healers and shaman appropriate for dealing with Indian and Native substance use and misuse? What are the ethical issues associated with changing the shamanic traditions to accommodate conventional forms of health and wellness interventions including psychiatric and conventional psychological approaches?

REFERENCES

Altman, D. (1995). Sustaining interventions in community systems: On the relationship between researchers and communities. *Health Psychology, 14*(6), 526–536.
Austin, G., & Gilbert, M. (1989). Substance abuse among Latino youth. *Prevention Research Update, 3*. Los Alamitos, CA: Southwest Regional Laboratory.

Austin, G., Oetting, E., & Beauvais, F. (1993). Recent research on substance abuse among *American Indian youth. Prevention Reset Update (No. 11)*. Los Alamitos, CA: Southwest Regional Educational Laboratory.

Bates, S. C., Beauvais, F., & Trimble, J. E. (1997). American Indian adolescent alcohol involvement and ethnic identification. *Substance Use and Misuse, 32*(14), 2013–2031.

Beauvais, F. (1992). Drug use of friends: A comparison of reservation and non-reservation Indian youth. *American Indian & Alaska Native Mental Health Research, 5*(1), 43–50.

Beauvais, F. (Ed., 1992). Indian adolescent drug and alcohol use: Recent patterns and consequences (Special Issue). *American Indian and Alaska Native Mental Health Research, 5*(1), v–78.

Beauvais, F. (1995). Ethnic communities and research: Building a new alliance. In P. A. Langton (Ed.), *The challenge of participatory research: Preventing alcohol-related problems in ethnic communities* (CSAP Cultural Competence Series 3). Rockville, MD: Center for Substance Abuse Prevention.

Beauvais, F. (1996). Trends in drug use among American Indian students and dropouts, 1975–1994. *American Journal of Public Health, 86*(11), 1594–1598.

Beauvais, F. (1998). Cultural identification and substance abuse in North America—An annotated bibliography. *Substance Use and Misuse, 33*(6), 1315–1336.

Beauvais, F. (2000). Indian adolescence: Opportunity and challenge. In R. Montmeyer, G. Adams, & T. Gullotta (Eds.), *Advances in adolescent development: Vol. 9. Adolescent experiences: Cultural and economic diversity in adolescent development*. Newbury Park, CA: Sage.

Beauvais, F., Chavez, E., Oetting, E. R., Deffenbacher, J., & Cornell, G. R. (1996). Drug use, violence, and victimization among White American, Mexican American, and American Indian dropouts, students with academic problems, and students in good academic standing. *Journal of Counseling Psychology, 43*(3), 292–299.

Beauvais, F., & LaBoueff, S. (1985). Drug and alcohol abuse intervention in American Indian communities. *The International Journal of the Addictions, 20*(1), 139–171.

Beauvais, F., & Oetting, E. R. (1988). Inhalant abuse by young children. In R. A. Crider & B. A. Rouse (Eds.), *Epidemiology of inhalant abuse: An update* (NIDA Research Monograph No. 85). Rockville, MD: National Institute on Drug Abuse.

Beauvais, F., Oetting, E. R., Wolf, W., & Edwards, R. W. (1989). American Indian youth and drugs, 1976–1987: A continuing problem. *American Journal of Public Health, 79*(5), 634–636.

Beauvais, F., & Segal, B. (1992). Drug use patterns among American Indian and Alaskan Native youth: Special rural populations. *Drugs and Society, 7*(1/2), 77–94.

Beauvais, F., & Trimble, J. E. (1992). The role of the researcher in evaluating American-Indian alcohol and other drug abuse prevention programs. In M. Orlandi (Ed.), *Cultural competence for evaluators working with ethnic minority communities: A guide for alcohol and other drug abuse prevention practitioners* (pp. 173–201). Rockville, MD: Office for Substance Abuse Prevention, Cultural Competence Series 1.

Bernstein, E., & Woodall, W. (1987). Changing perceptions of riskiness in drinking, drugs, and driving: An emergency department based alcohol and substance abuse prevention program. *Annals of Emergency Medicine, 16*, 1350–1354.

Botvin, G., Baker, E., Dusenbury, L., Botvin, E., & Tracy, D. (1995). Long-term follow-up results of a randomized drug abuse prevention trial in a White middle-class population. *Journal of the American Medical Association, 272*, 1106–1112.

Breaking New Ground for American Indian and Alaska Native Youth: Program summaries (1990). Rockville, MD: Office for Substance Abuse Prevention.

Bry, B. (1993). *Research on family setting's role in substance abuse* (NTIS No. PB94-175692). Piscataway, NJ: Rutgers, The State University of New Jersey.

Carpenter, R., Lyons, C., & Miller, A. (1985). Peer-managed, self-control program for prevention of alcohol abuse in American Indian high school students: A pilot evaluation study. *International Journal of the Addictions, 20*, 299–310

Cheadle, A., Pearson, D., Wagner, E., Psaty, B., Diehr, P., & Koepsell, T. (1995). A community-based approach to preventing alcohol use among adolescents on an American Indian reservation. *Public Health Reports, 110*, 439–447.

Cockerham, W. (1975). Drinking attitudes and practices among Wind River Reservation Indian youth. *Quarterly Journal of Studies on Alcohol, 36*, 321–326.

CSAP (Center for Substance Abuse Prevention). (1991, Spring). OSAP mobilizes to combat a national crisis. *The fact is. . . .* Rockville, MD: National Clearinghouse for Alcohol and Drug Information.

Davis, S., Hunt, K., and Kitzes, J. (1989). Improving the health of Indian teenagers—A demonstration program in rural New Mexico. *Public Health Reports, 104*, 271–278.

Dick, R., Manson, S., & Beals, J. (1993). Alcohol use among male and female Native American adolescents: Patterns and correlates of student drinking in a boarding school. *Journal of Studies on Alcohol, 54*, 172–177.

Dinges, M., & Oetting, E. (1993). Similarity in drug use patterns between adolescents and their friends. *Adolescence, 28*(110), 253–266.

Dishion, T. (1997). *Advances in family-based interventions to adolescent drug abuse prevention*. Washington, DC: Paper presented at the National Institute on Drug Abuse Prevention Conference.

Duryea, E., & Matzek, S. (1990). Results of a first-year pilot study in peer pressure management among American Indian youth. *Wellness perspectives: Research theory and practice, 7,* 17–30.

Fleming, C. (1992). American Indians and Alaska Natives: Changing societies past and present. In M. Orlandi (Ed.), *Cultural competence for evaluators: A guide for alcohol and other drug abuse prevention practitioners working with ethnic/racial communities.* Rockville, MD: U.S. Dept. Health and Human Services (OSAP Cultural Competence Series #1, DHHS Pub. ADM 92-188492).

Fleming, C., & Manson, S. (1990). *Substance abuse prevention in American Indian and Alaska Native communities: A literature review and OSAP program survey.* Rockville, MD: Office for Substance Abuse Prevention.

Gilchrist, L., Schinke, S., Trimble, J., & Cvetkovich, G. (1987). Skills enhancement to prevent substance abuse among American Indian adolescents. *The International Journal of the Addictions, 22,* 869–879.

Grube, J. W. (1998). *Prevention of adolescent drinking and drinking problems: A review of research and recommendations.* Report submitted for the National Institute on Alcohol Abuse and Alcoholism, Prevention Research Branch Extramural Scientific Advisory Committee Review Meeting. Washington, DC: National Institute on Alcohol Abuse and Alcoholism.

Hartzberg, H. (1971). *The search for an American Indian identity: Modern Pan-Indian movements.* Syracuse, NY: Syracuse University Press.

Hayne, B. (1993). *An Eagle's View: Sharing successful American Indian/Alaska Native alcohol and other drug prevention programs (Vol I).* Portland, OR: Northwest Regional Educational Laboratory.

Hayne, B. (1994). *An Eagle's View: Sharing successful American Indian/Alaska Native alcohol and other drug prevention programs (Vol II).* Portland, OR: Northwest Regional Educational Laboratory.

Heath, D. B. (1978). Foreword. *Medical Anthropology, 2*(4), 3–8.

Hofstede, G. (1980). *Cultures' consequences.* Beverly Hills, CA: Sage.

Holder, H. (1998). *Alcohol and the community: A systems approach to prevention.* New York: Cambridge University Press.

Katz, R. (1983/84). Empowerment and synergy: Expanding the community's healing resources. *Prevention in Human Services, 3*(2/3), 201–225.

Kumpfer, K. (1998). Prevention works: On the front lines with CASP Director Karol Kumpfer. *Juvenile Justice, V*(2), 3–10.

LaFromboise, T., & Rowe, W. (1983). Skills training for bicultural competence: Rationale and application. *Journal of Counseling Psychology, 30,* 589–595.

LaFromboise, T., Coleman, H., & Gerton, J. (1993). Psychological impact of biculturalism. *Psychological Bulletin, 114,* 395–412.

Longclaws, L., Barnes, G., Grieve, L., & Dumoff, R. (1980). Alcohol and drug use among the Brokenhead Ojibwa. *Journal of Studies on Alcohol, 41,* 21–36.

Mail, P., & McDonald, D. (1980). *Tulapai to Tokay: A bibliography of alcohol use and abuse among Native Americans of North America.* New Haven, CT: HRAF Press.

Manson, S. (Ed., 1982). *New directions in prevention among American Indian and Alaska Native communities.* Portland, OR: National Center for American Indian and Alaska Native Mental Health Research, Oregon Health Sciences University.

Manson, S. (1989). *American Indian and Alaska Native Mental Health Research, 2.* Entire volume.

May, P. (1982). Substance abuse and American Indians: Prevalence and susceptibility. *International Journal of the Addictions, 17,* 1185–1209.

May, P. (1992). Alcohol policy considerations for Indian reservations and bordertown communities. *American Indian and Alaska Native Mental Health Research, 4,* 5–59.

May, P. (1995). The prevention of alcohol and other drug abuse among American Indians: A review and analysis of the literature. In P. Langton (Ed.), *The challenge of participatory research: Preventing alcohol related problems in ethnic communities* (pp.185–243). Rockville, MD: Center for Substance Abuse Prevention.

May, P., & Moran, J. (1995). Prevention of alcohol misuse: A review of health promotion efforts among American Indians. *American Journal of Health Promotion, 9,* 288–298.

Mitchell, C., & Beals, J. (1997). The structure of problem and positive behavior among American Indian adolescents: Gender and community differences. *American Journal of Community Psychology, 25,* 257–288.

Mitchell, C., O'Nell, T., Beals, J., Dick, R., Keane, E., & Manson, S. (1996). Dimensionality of alcohol use among American Indian adolescents: Latent structure, construct validity, and implications for developmental research. *Journal of Research on Adolescence.*

Moskowitz, J. (1989). The primary prevention of alcohol problems: A critical review of the review literature. *Journal of Studies on Alcohol, 50*(1), 54–88.

Murphy, S., & DeBlassie, R. (1984). Substance abuse and the Native American student. *Journal of Drug Education, 14,* 315–321.

Norton, I. M., & Manson, S. M. (1996). Research in American Indian and Alaska Native communities: Navigating the cultural universe of values and process. *Journal of Consulting and Clinical Psychology, 64*(5), 856–860.

Oetting, E. R. (1993). Orthogonal cultural identification: Theoretical links between cultural identification and substance use. In M. DeLaRosa & J. Adrados (Eds.), *Drug abuse among minority youth: Advances in research and methodology* (NIDA Research Monograph No. 130). Rockville, MD: National Institute on Drug Abuse.

Oetting, E. R., & Beauvais, F. (1983). A typology of adolescent drug use: A practical classification system for describing drug use patterns. *Academy Psychology Bulletin, 5,* 55–69.

Oetting, E. R., & Beauvais, F. (1986). Peer cluster theory: Drugs and the adolescent. *Journal of Counseling and Development, 65*(1), 17–22.

Oetting, E. R., & Beauvais, F. (1987). Common elements in youth drug abuse: Peer clusters and other psychosocial factors. *Journal of Drug Issues, 17*(1 & 2), 133–151.

Oetting, E. R., & Beauvais, F. (1989). Epidemiology and correlates of alcohol use among Indian adolescents living on reservations. In D. L. Spiegler, D. A. Tate, S. S. Aitken, & C. M. Christian (Eds.), *Alcohol use among U.S. ethnic minorities* (NIAAA Research Monograph No. 18) (DHHS Pub. No. (ADM) 89-1435, pp. 239–267). Washington, DC: U.S. Government Printing Office.

Oetting, E. R., & Beauvais, F. (1990–1991). Orthogonal cultural identification theory: The cultural identification of minority adolescents. *The International Journal of the Addictions, 25*(5A, 6A), 655–685.

Oetting, E., Beauvais, F., & Edwards, R. (1988). Alcohol and Indian youth: Social and psychological correlates and prevention. Special Issue: Alcohol problems and minority youth. *Journal of Drug Issues, 18*(1), 87–101.

Oetting, E., Donnermeyer, J., Trimble, J., & Beauvais, F. (1998). Primary socialization theory: Culture, ethnicity, and cultural identification. The links between culture and substance use. *Substance Use and Misuse, 33*(10), 2075–2107.

Oetting, E. R., Edwards, R. W., & Beauvais, F. (1989). Drugs and Native-American youth. *Drugs and Society, 3*(1/2), 5–38.

Oetting, E. R., Edwards, R., Goldstein, G. S., & Garcia-Mason, V. (1980). Drug use among adolescents of five southwestern native American tribes. *The International Journal of the Addictions, 15*(3), 439–445.

Oetting, E. R., & Goldstein, G. S. (1979). Drug use among Native American adolescents. In G. Beschner & A. Freidman (Eds.), *Youth Drug Abuse.* Lexington, MA: Lexington Books.

Oetting, E., Spooner, S., Beauvais, F., & Banning, J. (1991). Prevention, peer clusters, and the paths to drug abuse. In L. Donohew, H. Sypher et al. (Eds.), *Persuasive communication and drug abuse prevention* (pp. 239–261). Hillsdale, NJ: Lawrence Erlbaum Associates.

Oetting, E., Swaim, R., Edwards, R., & Beauvais, F. (1989). Indian and Anglo adolescent alcohol use and emotional distress: Path models. *American Journal of Drug & Alcohol and Abuse, 15*(2), 153–172.

Owan, T., Palmer, I., & Quintana, M. (1987). *School/community-based alcoholism/substance abuse prevention survey.* Rockville, MD: Indian Health Service.

Pedersen, P. (Ed., 1999). *Multiculturalism as a fourth force.* Philadelphia, PA: Brunner/Mazel.

Petroskey, E., Van Stelle, K., & De Jong, J. (1998). Prevention through empowerment in a Native American community. *Drugs and Society, 12,* 147–162.

Pinto, L. (1973). Alcohol and drug use among Native American youth on reservations: A growing crisis. In: National Commission on Marijuana and Drug Use. *Drug use in America: Problems in perspective* (pp. 1157–1178). Append. Vol. 1:Patterns and Consequences. Washington, DC: U.S. Govt. Printing Office.

Plested, B., Smitham, D., Jumper-Thurman, P., Oetting, E., & Edwards, R. (1999). Readiness for drug use prevention in rural minority communities. *Substance Use and Misuse, 34* (4, 5), 521–544.

Rolf, J. (1995). Methods to create and sustain cross-cultural prevention partnerships: The NAPPASA Project's American Indian-Anglo American example. In P. Langton (Ed.), *The challenge of participatory research: Preventing alcohol related problems in ethnic communities* (pp.149–181). Rockville, MD: Center for Substance Abuse Prevention.

Schinke, S., Gilchrist, L., Schilling, R., & Walker, D. (1986). Preventing substance abuse among American Indian and Alaska Native youth: Research issues and strategies. *Journal of Social Service Research, 9,* 53–67.

Schinke, S., Orlandi, M., Botvin, G., & Gilchrist, L. (1988). Preventing substance abuse among American-Indian adolescents: A bicultural competence skills approach. *Journal of Counseling Psychology, 35,* 87–90.

Schinke, S., Schilling, R., & Gilchrist, L. (1986). Prevention of drug and alcohol abuse in American Indian youths. *Social Work Research and Abstracts, 22,* 18–19.

Schroeder, D., Laflin, M., & Weis, D. (1993). Is there a relationship between self-esteem and drug use? Methodological and statistical limitations of the research. *Journal of Drug Issues, 23*(4), 645–664.

Snipp, C. M. (1989). *American Indians: The first of this land.* New York: Russell Sage Foundation.

Snipp, C. M. (1996). The size and distribution of the American Indian population: Fertility, mortality, residence, and migration. In G. Sandefur, R. Rindfuss, & B. Cohen (Eds.), *Changing numbers, changing needs: American Indian demography and public health* (pp.17–52). Washington, DC: National Academy Press.

Swaim, R. C., Oetting, E. R., Jumper Thurman, P., Beauvais, F., & Edwards, R. W. (1993). American Indian adolescent drug use and socialization characteristics: A cross-cultural comparison. *Journal of Cross-Cultural Psychology, 24*(1), 53–70.

Thornton, R. (1996). Tribal membership requirements and the demography of 'old' and 'new' Native Americans. In G. Sandefur, R. Rindfuss, & B. Cohen (Eds.), *Changing numbers, changing needs: American Indian demography and public health* (pp. 103–112). Washington, DC: National Academy Press.

Triandis, H. (1995). *Individualism and collectivism.* Boulder, CO: Westview.

Trickett, E. (1996). A future for community psychology: The contexts of diversity and the diversity of contexts. *American Journal of Community Psychology, 24*(2), 209–234.

Trickett, E. (1997). Ecology and primary prevention: Reflections on a meta-analysis. *American Journal of Community Psychology, 25*(2), 197–205.

Trickett, E., Barons, C., & Buchanan, R. (1996). Elaborating developmental, contextualism in adolescent research and intervention: Paradigm contributions from community psychology. *Journal of Research on Adolescence, 6*(3), 245–269.

Trimble, J. E. (1977). The sojourner in the American Indian community: Methodological concerns and issues. *Journal of Social Issues, 33,* 159–174.

Trimble, J. E. (1995). Toward an understanding of ethnicity and ethnic identification and their relationship with drug use research. In G. Botvin, S. Schinke, & M. Orlandi (Eds.), *Drug abuse prevention with multi-ethnic youth* (pp. 3–27). Thousand Oaks, CA: Sage.

Trimble, J. E. (1984). Drug abuse prevention research needs among American Indians and Alaska Natives. *White Cloud Journal, 3*(3), 22–34.

Trimble, J. E. (1992). A cognitive-behavioral approach to drug abuse prevention and intervention with American Indian youth. In L. A. Vargas and J. D. Koss-Chioino (Eds.), *Working with culture: Psychotherapeutic intervention with ethnic minority children and adolescents.* (pp. 246–275). San Francisco, CA: Jossey-Bass.

Trimble, J. E. (1991). Ethnic specification, validation prospects and the future of drug abuse research. *International Journal of the Addictions, 25*(2), 149–169.

Trimble, J. E. (1998). Social psychological perspectives on changing self-identification among American Indians and Alaska Natives. In R. H. Dana (Ed.), *Handbook of cross-cultural/multicultural personality assessment.* Mahwah, NJ: Lawrence Erlbaum Associates.

Trimble, J., & Bagwell, W. (Eds., 1995). *North American Indians and Alaska Natives: Abstracts of psychological and behavioral literature, 1967–1995* (No.15, Bibliographies in Psychology). Washington, DC: American Psychological Association.

Trimble, J. E., Padilla, A., & Bell-Bolek, C. (1987). *Drug abuse among ethnic minorities*, Office of Science Monograph Series, National Institute on Drug Abuse, Rockville, MD.

Trosper, R. (1981). American Indian nationalism and frontier expansion. In C. Keyes (Ed.), *Ethnic change* (pp. 247–270). Seattle: University of Washington Press.

United States Department of Education (1982). *A study of alternative definitions and measures relating to eligibility and service under Part A of the Indian Education Act.* Unpublished report, United States Department of Education, Washington, DC.

Van Stelle, K., Allen, G., & Moberg, D. (1998). Alcohol and drug prevention among American Indian families. *Drugs and Society, 12,* 53–60.

Winfree, L., Griffiths, C., & Sellers, C. (1989). Social learning theory, drug use and American Indian Youths: A cross-cultural test. *Justice Quarterly, 6,* 395–416.

Yee, A., Fairchild, H., Weizmann, F., & Wyatt, G. (1993). Addressing psychology's problems with race. *American Psychologist, 48*(11), 1132–1140.

Young, T. K. (1994). *The health of Native Americans: Toward a biocultural epidemiology.* New York: Oxford University Press.

CHAPTER 21

Drug Abuse Prevention Research for Asian and Pacific Islander Americans

W. William Chen

INTRODUCTION

Asian and Pacific-Islanders (APIs) are the fastest growing ethnic minority in the United States. The rates of growth were 142 and 107.8%, respectively, between 1980 and 1990. The total API population reached 8,451,000 or about 3.3% of total U.S. population in 1995, and it is estimated to reach 8.2% of the U.S. population in 2050 (U.S. Census Bureau, 1992). Ninety-five percent of APIs are Asian-Americans and 5% are Pacific-Islanders. Six subgroups make up almost 90% of the Asian-American population: Chinese (23.8%), Filipinos (20.4%), Japanese (12.3%), Asian-Indians (11.8%), Koreans (11.6%), and Vietnamese (8.9%). A majority of the APIs reside in only 10 states (CA, NY, HI, TX, IL, NY, WA, VA, FL, MA) and just over 50% live in the western United States (U.S. Census Bureau, 1992).

Despite their dramatic growth, APIs remain one of the least understood and most neglected ethnic minority groups. Due to lack of understanding and media influence, people often think of APIs as a "model minority" and a homogeneous group with few health problems. They are also perceived as being highly successful in educational attainment and socioeconomic status. In fact, APIs are a diverse group with different languages, cultures, levels of acculturation, and immigration histories. Almost three-quarters of APIs are foreign born, and many are recent immigrants or refugees.

An estimated 40% of APIs do not speak English fluently. Among Chinese and Koreans, 51% have limited English proficiency, and more than 60% of Southeast Asians have limited English proficiency (U.S. Census Bureau, 1990). Furthermore, a majority of Southeast Asian immigrants and refugees, particularly Hmong and Laotians, are generally poor, illiterate, and unfamiliar with

W. William Chen • Department of Health Science Education, University of Florida, Gainesville, Florida 32611

Western culture, which makes their adjustment to life in the United States very challenging (Zane & Kim, 1994). In addition, many APIs have numerous health problems, including drug use and abuse.

While the prevalence of substance use and abuse among U.S. adolescents is increasing, a general misconception is that these problems are relatively uncommon among API youth. Most prevention research literature also reports that adult APIs have fewer substance use and abuse problems than do other population groups. However, closer examination of the data reveals a different picture. For example, data now indicate that smoking among immigrant Southeast Asian men is significantly higher than among the general population (Centers for Disease Control and Prevention, 1992). Drug abuse, especially heroin abuse among Hmong and Laotians, is also a serious problem (Westermeyer, Lyfoung, & Neider, 1989).

To better understand the problems and issues related to prevention research on substance use and abuse among APIs, this chapter reviews the literature on (1) the extent of substance use and abuse, (2) factors affecting substance use and abuse, (3) prevention research targeted at APIs, and (4) methodological issues related to prevention research. Suggestions and recommendations are provided regarding substance use and abuse prevention research for APIs.

EXTENT OF SUBSTANCE USE AND ABUSE AMONG ASIAN AND PACIFIC-ISLANDERS

Existing data present an unclear and confusing picture of the extent of substance use and abuse among APIs. National epidemiological studies and some regional studies suggest that APIs are less likely to use and abuse drugs and alcohol than are other ethnic groups (Adlaf, Smart, & Tan, 1989; Bachman et al., 1991; DeMoor et al., 1989; Maddahian, Newcomb, & Bentler, 1985; NIDA, 1998). A report on prevalence of substance use among racial and ethnic groups in the United States, from 1991 to 1993, revealed that APIs had a relatively low prevalence of cigarette use, low prevalence of past-year illicit drug use (including marijuana and cocaine), low prevalence of past-year alcohol use, and low prevalence of heavy alcohol use and alcohol dependence (SAMHSA, 1998).

As shown in the Table 21.1, except for Central American Hispanics, APIs recorded the lowest prevalence on seven of the nine measures of substance use and abuse. However, the report indicates that given the extensive ethnic diversity of APIs and relatively small sample sizes, the results should be interpreted with caution. It also indicates that averages for the overall group may mask significant variations in the prevalence of substance use among subgroups. In a more recent report, based on the National Household Survey on Drug Abuse in 1996, APIs recorded the lowest prevalence of past-month illicit drug use, marijuana use, cocaine use, alcohol use, heavy alcohol use, and cigarette use (NIDA, 1998). Again, under-representation and limited access to high-risk groups of APIs were limitations of this study (Table 21.2).

Other regional studies examining the use and abuse of drugs and alcohol also reveal a low prevalence rate among APIs (Akutsu et al., 1989; Harford, 1992; Neumark-Sztainer et al., 1996; Newcomb et al., 1987). However, many recent studies reveal that drug and alcohol abuse among APIs are increasing, and certain API groups have equivalent or higher levels of alcohol and other drug abuse than do other population groups (Chin, Lai, & Rouse 1990–1991; D'Avanzo, 1997; Ja & Aoki, 1993; Kuramoto, 1994; McLaughlin et al., 1987; O'Hare & Van Tran, 1998; Varma & Siris, 1996; Weatherspoon, Danko, & Johnson, 1994; Wiecha, 1996). In a drug abuse needs assessment conducted in California, Sasao (1991) found a significant alcohol, tobacco, and other drug problem in many API subgroups. Marijuana and cocaine use were found in more assimilated APIs. In addition, Southeast Asians and other recent immigrants or refugees also had significant drug use and abuse problems (Yee & Thu, 1987).

TABLE 21.1. Percentage of Persons 12 and Older Using Cigarettes, Alcohol, Any Illicit Drugs, Marijuana, and Cocaine in the Past Year, Percentage in Need of Treatment, Percentage Reporting Dependence on Alcohol, Percentage Reporting Heavy Cigarette Use[a] in the Past Month, and Percentage Reporting Heavy Alcohol Use[b] in the Past Month.

Measures (Race/ethnicity)	By race/ethnicity (1991–1993)								
	Cigarette (past year)	Alcohol use (past year)	Illicit drug use (past year)	Marijuana (past year)	Cocaine (past year)	Need treatment	Alcohol dependence	Heavy cigarette use (past month)	Heavy alcohol use (past month)
All	30.9%	66.4%	11.9%	9.0%	2.5%	2.7%	3.5%	13.8%	5.1%
Non-Hispanic White	31.5	68.9	11.8	8.9	2.4	2.5	3.4	15.5	5.3
Non-Hispanic Black	29.9	55.4	13.1	10.6	3.1	3.9	3.4	9.1	4.7
Hispanic—Caribbean	21.2	60.8	7.6	5.6	1.5	1.6	1.9	3.6	2.5
Hispanic—Central America	17.9	51.1	5.7	2.7	1.1	1.5	2.8	2.3	2.2
Hispanic—Cuba	27.3	65.7	8.2	5.9	1.7	2.6	0.9	8.9	2.8
Hispanic—Mexico	29.1	63.7	12.7	9.1	3.9	3.6	5.6	4.7	6.9
Hispanic—Puerto Rico	32.7	59.5	13.3	10.8	3.7	3.7	3.0	11.8	4.0
Hispanic—South America	31.3	74.1	10.7	8.4	2.0	1.7	2.1	6.9	3.0
Hispanic—others	25.9	66.3	10.6	9.1	2.3	3.4	3.1	5.3	4.9
Asian/Pacific-Islanders	21.7	53.2	6.5	4.7	1.4	1.7	1.8	4.8	0.9

[a] Heavy cigarette use is defined as smoking a pack or more per day during the past 30 days.
[b] Heavy alcohol use is defined as drinking five or more drinks per occasion on five or more days during the past 30 days.

TABLE 21.2. Prevalence of Past-Month Drug Use in the United States by Race/Ethnicity, 1996[a]

Drugs race/ethnicity	Any illicit drug use (%)	Marijuana (%)	Cocaine (%)	Alcohol (%)	Heavy alcohol (%)	Cigarettes (%)
Total population	6.1	4.7	0.8	51.0	5.4	28.9
White	6.1	4.6	0.8	54.2	5.5	29.8
Black	7.6	6.6	1.1	41.9	5.3	30.4
Hispanic	5.3	3.7	1.1	43.2	6.2	24.7
American-Indian/ Alaskan Native	11.3	10.0	*t*	28.2	6.4	43.2
Asian/Pacific-Islander	3.7	2.7	*t*	36.9	1.3	12.8

[a]Low precision, no estimate reported. *Source:* National Household Survey on Drug Abuse, Substance Abuse and Mental Health Services Administration, Office of Applied Studies, 1998.

In a study of an epidemic of opium dependence among Asian refugees in Minnesota, Westermyer et al. (1989) reported that the Hmong population made up about 95% of the patient group for opium addiction at the University of Minnesota hospital and clinic. New evidence also indicates that opium use appears to be increasing among Southeast Asian immigrants and refugees (Westermyer et al., 1991). In a relatively large study conducted in New York, Welte and Barnes (1987) also showed that Asian-Americans consumed as much alcohol and drugs as did other ethnic groups in the study.

Studies conducted in the 1990s also indicate that smoking rates were higher for Asian-American men than for other ethnic groups (Austin, Prendergast, & Lee, 1989; Centers for Disease Control and Prevention, 1992b). For example, in a study of cigarette smoking among Chinese, Vietnamese, and Hispanics in California, researchers reported that both Chinese and Vietnamese adult men smoked more than did Hispanics (28.1 and 34.7% vs. 21.6%) (Centers for Disease Control and Prevention, 1992a). In a more recent study, the rate of smoking for Southeast-Asian men was reported to range from 34 to 43%, compared to 27.6% among Caucasian men (Jenkins et al., 1997). The susceptibility of Asian youths to smoking has also increased from 30 to 50%, and their smoking rates increased substantially by more than 50% in California from 1993 to 1996 (Asian and Pacific Islander Tobacco Education Network/Asian Pacific Partners for Empowerment and Leadership, 1998).

Inconsistency in the epidemiological data concerning the extent of substance use and abuse among Asian and Pacific-Islanders may be due to lack of comprehensive epidemiological data on specific API populations. Zane and Sasao (1992) point out that most studies conducted in the past tended to focus on the larger and more acculturated API groups (such as Chinese and Japanese), used primarily student populations, rarely examined API groups potentially at greater risk for drug and alcohol abuse, relied on disproportionately small sample sizes, seldom controlled for socioeconomic and other demographic differences that may be confounded with ethnicity, and failed to use appropriate measurement instruments that addressed language differences or conceptual differences in response to survey questions. Additionally, most survey instruments did not account for cultural differences that may affect the nature of self-report or self-disclosure concerning drug and alcohol use among Asian-Americans.

A majority of epidemiological studies on the extent of drug and alcohol use tended to derive data from two sources. One consisted of cases from treatment facilities or clinical settings. However, due to general underutilization of treatment services by APIs, a low prevalence of substance use and abuse is likely to be reported. Factors affecting underutilization of substance treatment facilities are discussed later in the chapter. The other main source of data came from noninstitutionalized populations and used self-report methods in questionnaires or interviews.

Again, under-reporting or unwillingness to disclose problems may lead to overall underestimates of actual substance use and abuse problems. More comprehensive epidemiological studies with designs that can assess different subgroups of APIs with different levels of acculturation and different immigration histories are needed to more accurately assess the full extent of the substance use and abuse problems among APIs.

FACTORS AFFECTING DRUG USE AND ABUSE AMONG ASIAN AND PACIFIC-ISLANDERS

Substance abuse prevention research that examines etiologic factors or risk factors associated with substance use and abuse can provide useful information for the development and implementation of prevention programs. The factors that influence the use and abuse of substances among Asian and Pacific-Islanders are complex and vary from study to study. Some studies suggested that the low rate of alcohol and drug use among APIs may result from genetic or biophysiological influences. Others show that ethnocultural factors may play a more important role in regulating the use of alcohol and other drugs. In addition, psychosocial factors related to social adjustment among APIs may also have an impact on the use and abuse of substances. An examination of each of these factors is important for the advancement of prevention research.

Biophysiological Influences

A large body of research indicates that genetic or biophysiological factors could play an important role in affecting substance use and abuse among APIs, particularly of alcohol consumption and dependence. One of the most frequently cited theories of biophysiological influences suggests that a significantly higher percentage of Asian-Americans display flushing after ingesting alcohol (ethanol-induced flushing) than do Caucasians, African-Americans, and Hispanics (Nakawatase, Yamamoto, Sasao, 1993; Straka et al., 1996; Sue, 1987; Tu & Isreal, 1995; Wall & Ethlers, 1995; Wall et al., 1997). Ethanol-induced flushing or hypersensitivity occurs as a result of the presence of high levels of acetaldehyde from alcohol metabolism and is characterized by facial flushing, tachycardia, and increased skin temperature. Seto et al. (1978) found that 60% of Chinese and 77% of Japanese had a visible flushing response to alcohol, but only 9% of Caucasians showed a mild flushing response. Studies further indicated that full-term babies of Asian-Americans show the same pattern of flushing after being exposed to alcohol. This biophysiological reaction experienced by APIs may be a deterrent to alcohol use (Akutsu et al., 1989; Parrish et al., 1990).

In addition to potential differences in alcohol metabolism, APIs have different metabolic responses to other drugs (Ho et al., 1988; Lin-Fu, 1993, 1994; Smith & Mendoza, 1996; Straka et al., 1996). For example, questions have been raised about the different acetylation rates of drugs such as procainamide and isoniazide among APIs, compared to other racial groups (Quock, 1992). One study found the effective weight-standardized dose of chlorpromazine for Asian-Americans to be only about half that for Caucasian Americans, and the dose at which extra pyramidal signs begin to appear was about two-thirds of Whites (Hui, Yu, & Kitazaki, 1992). Accordingly, genetic differences in pharmacokimetics should be considered when examining patterns of drug use and abuse among APIs.

Genetic or biophysiological factors alone, however, are not sufficient to explain the differences between Asian-Americans and other racial/ethnic groups (Johnson et al., 1990; Johnson & Nagoshi, 1990). Cheung (1993) found that within- and between-group differences in Asian-Americans appear to be large enough to place doubt on the impact of biophysiological factors.

For example, different levels of alcohol consumption between different generations of Asian-Americans with the same genetic make-up or biophysiological response cannot be fully explained by the flushing theory. Also, American-Indians whose levels of acetaldehyde and tendencies to flush have been shown to be high, exhibit higher levels of alcohol consumption and alcohol-related problems. It is clear that biophysiological factors do not fully explain the differences in alcohol and drug use between Asian-Americans and other ethnic groups.

Ethnocultural Influences

As previously mentioned, APIs living in the Unites States have diverse cultures, languages, immigration histories, and demographic characteristics. These differences in cultures and values can affect socialization patterns, use of leisure time, family network values, and intergenerational relationships and, therefore, can influence risk behaviors associated with use and abuse of alcohol and other drugs. Culturally patterned coping strategies and defensive behaviors can also play important roles in substance use and abuse.

Cheung (1993) suggested that differences between Chinese and American cultural values can account for differences in drinking styles. For example, Chinese culture is more "situation centered," which requires the individual to seek harmony with the social environment. Responsibility to others discourages the individual from getting drunk and exhibiting embarrassing behavior at social functions. The cultural influences of Confucianism and Taoism that stress the importance of moderation and harmony with the environment may also affect the use of alcohol among Asian-Americans. American culture tends to be "individual centered," which places emphasis on the self, on independence, and on assertiveness. These cultural values may be conducive to unrestrained individual freedom in drinking.

The situation-centered culture and values of moderation may provide a means of social control for excessive drinking. However, they may have a different effect on the use of other drugs. Yee and Thu (1987) suggest that the cultural values of moderation and desire for control may result in a preference for opium rather than alcohol for recent Southeast Asian immigrants because alcohol can result in loss of control over one's behavior. The increasing use and abuse of cigarettes, opiates, and other drugs could be a reflection of different cultural values among Southeast Asians in the United States.

Changing cultural values and other factors also appear to play a role in the way alcohol is used by Asian-Americans. Edwards, Thurman, & Beauvais (1995) indicate that as individuals become more acculturated, their alcohol use tends to resemble that of the majority culture, and in most cases this means an increase in alcohol use. Using acculturation measures, such as number of generations in the United States and loss of proficiency in speaking an Asian language, investigators have found that alcohol consumption varies directly with acculturation (Akutsu et al., 1989; Tsunoda et al., 1992). Some researchers even suggest that cultural factors exert a more powerful influence on substance use patterns than do physiological factors (Li & Rosenblood, 1994; Sue, 1987). One study of alcohol drinking patterns among Asian-Americans found that acculturated Japanese and Chinese students drink more than do their less acculturated counterparts (Sue, Zane, & Ito, 1979). Kitano (1989) also found that when the immigrants' traditional behavior comes in contact with the dominant culture, the traditional behavior will be modified over time.

The trend toward an increase in alcohol and other drug use is seen not only among Asian-Americans in the United States but among some Asians in their countries. Places like Korea, Japan, and Taiwan, which are the homelands of many Asian immigrants to the United States, have experienced rapid economic growth and social changes during the past several decades

(Cheung, 1993). Researchers have reported an 8-fold increase in alcohol use in Korea over a 20-year span and a 3-fold increase in consumption and a 100-fold increase in problem drinking in Taiwan over a 40-year span. Such findings suggest that ethnocultural factors alone cannot explain the complexity of substance use and abuse problems among APIs.

Psychosocial Influences

In addition to biophysiological and ethnocultural factors, psychosocial factors could also play an important role in affecting the use of alcohol and drugs among APIs. Yee and Thu (1987) find that use of drugs and alcohol as coping mechanisms is somewhat common among Southeast Asian refugees. They report that more than 40% of Vietnamese immigrants in Texas use alcohol as a means of coping with sorrows, and almost 12% use drugs for coping with psychological distress. Adjustment and mental health problems coupled with lack of social and institutional support may be major reasons APIs turn to psychoactive substances to alleviate their stress and forget their problems.

Chueung (1993) suggests that social adjustment problems are an important factor in excessive drinking and alcoholism among Asian Americans. Chin et al. (1990–1991) in a study of Asian-American alcoholics in New York concluded that (1) occupational constraints and ease of alcohol accessibility, (2) social isolation, and (3) family problems and role reversal challenges among recent immigrants are the main reasons that many Asian-American restaurant workers turn to alcohol and eventually developed drinking problems. In a study of Cambodian women on the east and west coasts, using structured interviews with a snowball sample method, D'Avanzo, Frye, and Froman (1994) found that more than 58% of the west coast sample used medications for self-treatment of conditions other than that for which the drug was prescribed. These include coping with stress, forgetting troubles, and dealing with physical discomforts. O'Hare (1995) also found significant differences in drinking patterns and level of associated problems between Asian-Americans and Caucasians. Asian-Americans tended to expect greater tension reduction from drinking, despite drinking less than Caucasian-Americans.

Other psychosocial risks include shame and shyness. McLaughlin et al. (1987) suggest that sensitivity to shame inhibits Asian-Americans from using drugs, while Caucasians use drugs to overcome shyness. However, Johnson et al. (1990) report that racial/ethnic differences in guilt and shame are almost nonexistent between persons of Chinese, Japanese, and Caucasian ancestry in Hawaii, despite the substantial differences in alcohol consumption between Chinese-Americans on the one hand and Japanese-Americans on the other.

Researchers also hypothesize that ethnic differences in alcohol use may be caused by differences in exposure to risk environments (Catalano 1992, 1993; Keefe & Newcomb, 1996; Newcomb & Bentler, 1986; Rowe, Vazsonyi, & Flannery, 1994). In general, Asian-American adolescents knew fewer adults who used drugs. They also reported fewer peer models of drug use than did their Caucasian peers (Newcomb & Bentler, 1986). Similar levels of exposure to risk factors for alcohol consumption were reported by Sue et al. (1979). Less exposure to psychosocial risk factors for drug and alcohol use eventually lead to fewer problems of substance use and abuse. This hypothesis was supported by a study conducted by Keefe and Newcomb (1996), who examined the influences of demographic, social, attitudinal, and intention variables related to actual drinking behavior among Asian and Caucasian populations. They concluded that ethnic differences in alcohol use between Asians and Caucasians were mainly due to different levels of exposure to risk factors. Asian students reported fewer drinking role models, perceived their parents and friends as being more negative toward their drinking, and expected more costs and fewer benefits from drinking. Asian students were also less likely to intend to drink in the future and engaged in less drinking than did Caucasian students.

Despite the mixed and inconclusive research findings regarding etiological and risk factors, APIS are still highly vulnerable and at risk for significant levels of substance use and abuse (Ja & Aoki, 1993). For example, Chi, Lubben, and Kitano (1989) found that heavy drinking is not uncommon among Asian-American males and that the pattern is influenced by social variables. In a study of drinking behavior among Chinese-, Japanese-, and Korean-Americans, Chi et al. (1989) reported that these three Asian-American ethnic groups have different patterns of alcohol consumption, though all had migrated from the same part of the world and are often perceived as having similar cultures. The social variables that significantly distinguished the groups included having a friend who drank, weekly worship, and going to bars or night clubs. The Asian-Americans who go to bars or night clubs and who have friends who drink are more likely to be heavier drinkers (Chi, Kitano, & Lubben, 1988; Chi, Lubben, & Kitano, 1988; D'Avanzo, 1997).

Although the factors that may affect the levels of substance use and abuse have been discussed separately, it is difficult to separate the potential effects of each when attempting to explain the ethnic differences of alcohol and drug use patterns. These factors are not necessary contradictory, and their influences may be correlated or interactive. More epidemiological studies are needed to examine the risk factors and causes of substance use and abuse specific to APIS.

PREVENTION RESEARCH TARGETED AT ASIAN AND PACIFIC-ISLANDERS

Although few prevention research studies have been conducted with APIS, several—using strong methodologies and vigorous control approaches and taking into account biophysiological, ethnocultural, and psychosocial variables—have been found to be effective. One such study was designed to reduce the prevalence of smoking and increase the rate of smoking cessation among Southeast Asian adults in Ohio. The program incorporated several prevention strategies: (1) It delivered the smoking prevention program to subjects in their native languages; (2) used trained bilingual, bicultural staff to implement linguistically appropriate and an ethnically approved approach; (3) incorporated level of acculturation in the research design; (4) offered complementary educational methodologies (for example, face-to-face oral explanations, lower literacy printed materials, videotaped instruction and encouragement); (5) provided different culturally appropriate motivational messages (for example, saving money, promoting good health and aesthetics rather than stopping smoking to avoid diseases); and (6) used the household as the unit of intervention rather than the individual smoker as the unit (Chen et al., 1993).

Preliminary data indicate that 17% of the Southeast-Asian smokers in the intervention group were able to quit smoking after completion of the program, compared to only 1% of smokers in the control group (Asian and Pacific Islander Tobacco Education Network/Asian Pacific Partners for Empowerment and Leadership, 1998). This was much better than the average 2.5% successful smoking cessation rate among the general population (Warner, 1993).

Another large community-based prevention program aimed at reducing smoking among Vietnamese-American men proved successful because it incorporated ethnoculturally appropriate intervention strategies. The media-led intervention used Vietnamese-language media and health education materials that were culturally appropriate and acceptable in assisting target populations to quit smoking. It lasted 39 months and targeted students and families. The post-test smoking rate of 33.9% in the intervention community (San Francisco) was significantly lower than the rate of 40.9% in the comparison community (Houston). The quitting rate was also higher in the intervention community than in the comparison community, and current smokers in the intervention community smoked significantly fewer cigarettes per day than did those in the comparison community (Jenkins et al., 1997).

Examining the impact of the Asian Youth Substance Abuse Project (AYSAP) in California, Zane & Kim (1994) suggest that the project was successful because it (1) linked peer- and family-oriented prevention approaches to the natural support systems of particular Asian and Pacific communities, (2) provided Asian-immigrant parents with the skills and experiences they needed to help their children adjust to American cultural norms and expectations, (3) developed programs that minimized shame and loss of face in Asian and Pacific families, and (4) provided programs that involved personalized contacts rather than relying on mass-media mechanisms.

Strategies using psychoeducation, role modeling, and coping skills to bolster self-efficacy to deal with stressful environmental challenges and to strengthen support networks within the family and community have been recommended for APIs for tertiary intervention programs (O'Hare & Van Tran, 1998). However, traditional treatment programs only can be applicable to APIs if they integrate appropriate cultural values into the treatment modalities. For example, Chin et al. (1991) found that principles of the Alcoholics Anonymous approach do not work with Chinese-American clients because they are extremely reluctant to discuss their drinking and personal problems in a group. In general, Chinese-Americans are unwilling to reveal their problems to people who are not members of their families or extended families because of cultural constraints.

In a study of social adjustment and alcoholism among Chinese immigrants in New York City, Chin and colleagues (1991) found that a traditional counseling approach is not the most effective treatment modality for clients with limited education and poor health and who have financial, employment, family, and adjustment problems. They conclud that somatic forms of treatment, medication, and problem-solving approaches are more effective for Chinese patients. Perez-Arce, Carr, and Sorensen (1993) also found that treatment approaches that treat all clients as peers regardless of age, occupation, or experience; that promote same-sex bonding as a support mechanism; and that uses a direct confrontational and feedback approach as their bases may not be appropriate for many API clients. They suggest that when adapting cognitive–behavioral therapy approaches for Southeast-Asian families, clinicians must be especially sensitive to factors such as guilt and shame and must enhance family communications, while also emphasizing respect for tradition, family hierarchy, and the importance of indigenous community supports that can be used to help reduce substance abuse.

The causes and risks of substance use and abuse and the need for prevention services are somewhat different for Asian Pacific-Islanders. To be effective, prevention and intervention programs need to be designed, based on the specific cultural characteristics and social environmental settings of Asian Pacific-Islanders. As a rule, strategies that include (1) delivering services from community-based sites, (2) incorporating community input into prevention delivery decisions, (3) using bilingual and bicultural staff, (4) linking services with indigenous formal and informal community support systems, and (5) developing intervention approaches that address culturally appropriate aspects of Asian Pacific Islanders' lives (such as family values, face concerns, survival related issues, flexibility in the use of time) have a better chance of being successful.

METHODOLOGICAL ISSUES RELATED
TO PREVENTION RESEARCH

Effective prevention programs must be based on comprehensive epidemiological research that defines the nature, scope, and progression of substance use, abuse, and addiction. Prevention programs for APIs must also consider biophysiological, psychosocial, and ethnocultural factors that affect the risk of drug use, abuse, and addiction. In addition, three important methodological issues, sample selection, data collection and survey instruments, must be considered.

Sample Selection

Prevention research focused on APIs has not been particularly helpful because it was unclear which population groups were being studied. This is a serious methodological issue because groups that appear to have the highest risk for substance use and abuse problems have seldom been studied. APIs are a heterogenous group and often this intergroup diversity has gone unrecognized or underappreciated. The level of specific risk factors, such as socioeconomic status, peer and family influences, school dropout rate, and other psychosocial variables, may be quite different. Other within-group differences, such as acculturation, ethnic identity, primary language, dialect, country of origin, immigrant history may also have a significant influence on the use and abuse of drugs and alcohol (Kuramoto, 1994). For example, a number of studies cite acculturation as a strong predictor of substance use among API groups (Akutsu et al., 1989; Chi et al., 1988b, 1989). In general, more acculturated Asian-Americans are more likely to consume alcohol and less likely to use cigarettes. Yet, recent immigrants and non-English-speaking Asians are more likely to be smokers than are those who speak English and are American born (Chen et al., 1993; Centers for Disease Control and Prevention, 1992a).

Because of the number of within-group differences among APIs, many researchers suggest that APIs cannot be considered a monolithic entity with simple data aggregation to indicate a particular pattern of substance use and abuse. Measures must be made within each ethnicity group to help determine true levels of drug use and abuse (Trimble, J. E., 1990–1991).

Data Collection

In addition to sample selection issues, data collection methods can also pose serious problems. For example, use of the telephone for data collection may yield biased samples because of low survey cooperation by APIs. In a study of race-ethnicity characteristics of participants lost to follow-up, Psaty et al. (1994) found that APIs had the highest rate of refusal in a telephone survey, compared to other ethnic groups. However, Sasao (1994) suggests that telephone surveys could be a reliable and cost-effective method of data collection for Asian-Americans if a list of phone numbers with clearly identifiable surnames were available.

Different levels of acculturation also affect the rate of response in prevention research among API groups. Zane and Sasao (1992) reporte that Japanese, born in Japan, had a higher rate of refusal to participate in a substance abuse study than did American-born Japanese. Household interviews based on the phone directories also present problems. This method may miss individuals at highest risk for substance use and abuse, such as single, recent immigrant males living either alone or in crowded communal arrangements with no private phone. They usually are not included in such samples.

Survey Instruments

Prevention research must also develop and apply reliable survey instruments that are conceptually sound and have construct validity for culturally diverse API populations. Measurements based on self-report present challenges for prevention research because of language barriers, difficulty of self-disclosure, different perceptions of substance use and abuse problems, and inconsistent patterns of response to survey questions due to sociocultural differences between and within API groups. Zane and Sasao (1992) point out that many studies fail to use bilingual surveys, administer translated surveys without evaluating conceptual equivalence, and do not account for cultural differences that may affect self-disclosure with respect to substance use and abuse. Cultural difficulty in openly acknowledging personal problems such as drug use and abuse is very common among API groups and often prevents self-reporting in an epidemiological study.

Differing perceptions of drug abuse due to different cultural views can also pose problems. Psaty et al. (1994) explain that social desirability or cultural influences could affect reports of smoking or dieting among Asian-Americans. In a study of substance abuse and mental health problems among Southeast Asians, Yee and Thu (1987) found that a significant number of the Southeast Asians viewed alcohol and smoking as acceptable ways for directly coping with stressful situations. It has also been reported that Japanese-born Japanese tend to reserve the term "substance abuse" for illicit drugs, such as marijuana, LSD, and heroin. Many APIs do not consider alcohol and cigarette use as problems (Johnson et al., 1987; Kitano et al., 1992). Finally, the way APIs respond to standardized surveys with Likert scales must be carefully examined before interpreting the results. For example, Asian-Americans tend to respond to a Likert scale survey by selecting the middle responses rather than the two extreme responses. This may be caused by cultural influences of moderation and modesty among Asian-Americans.

It is clear that methodological weaknesses in prevention research may have yielded a generalized underestimation of the level of substance use and abuse among APIs. Many of the epidemiological studies in the literature may have some methodological shortcomings, so interpretation of their results should be made with caution. More studies that use better sample selection, data collection methods, and culturally appropriate survey instruments are needed to further advance the substance abuse prevention research for APIs.

SUMMARY AND RECOMMENDATIONS

Many API communities are concerned about substance use and abuse problems, but research has not been adequate for guiding the development and implementation of effective prevention and treatment programs for these communities. More efforts are needed to examine the nature, extent, and scope of substance use and abuse among APIs. Studies are also needed to identify the biophysiological, psychosocial, and ethnocultural risk factors associated with substance use and abuse among APIs. Finally, studies that examine the design and implementation of effective prevention programs are needed to further advance the field of substance abuse prevention research for APIs.

Recommendations for Epidemiological Studies

Recent studies reveal that substance use and abuse are increasing in API groups, particularly among recent immigrants. The lack of quality national epidemiological data on API populations poses a continuing challenge for substance abuse prevention researchers. One solution involves over-sampling of APIs in national studies (Kuramoto, 1994; Zane & Sasao, 1992). Disaggregated and statistically significant samples are essential for identifying and understanding the nature, extent, and scope of the substance use and abuse among APIs. Specific recommendations for improving epidemiological studies include the following:

- Improve sampling techniques. (For example, use oversampling or snowballing.)
- Improve sensitivity of data-collection methods. (For example, use face-to-face outreach by indigenous workers rather than telephone surveys, design survey instruments sensitive to the issue of self-disclosure.)
- Improve epidmiological data by using precise measures of ethnic identification. (For example, use birth place, preferred language, ethnic society/organization, self-identification of a preferred ethnic group, country of origin, and length of residence in the United States.)
- Improve the quality of data by reducing the use of broad "ethnic gloss" to refer to APIs. (At least 32 distinct ethnic and cultural groups of APIs can be included under this designation, and differences between and among these groups are extraordinarily complex.)
- Enhance research participation by involving API community leaders and local organizations in all aspects of the epidemiological research. (This includes involving them in design the research, recruiting participants and interviewers, analyzing data, and disseminating the findings.)
- Improve the validity of survey instruments by determining the best questions to ask in the subjects' native languages. (Research questions and premises often do not translate well in API cultures.)
- Improve the quality of epidmiological research by matching interviewers to the research subjects' culture and preferred language. (When working with research subjects who may be anxious about their residency status or who may have experienced government persecution in their native countries, it is helpful that interviewers do not act like government officials and do speak the nature language.)

Recommendations for Primary Prevention Research

Few prevention programs have addressed the specific needs of all API subgroups because of significant diversity and geographic distribution. More research is needed to examine Asian Pacific-Islander groups, particularly the Southeast Asian refugees and Pacific-Islanders. Specific recommendations for improving primary prevention research include the following:

- Increase community and academic research to assist in developing effective prevention models. Most prevention research on substance use and abuse among APIs has been conducted without a strong theoretical basis and is not linked to mainstream substance abuse research.
- Develop effective local programs that can be distributed across the United States and the Pacific Islands.
- Establish a national center to coordinate local prevention research programs and to provide comprehensive technical assistance, training, and resources for communities that conduct programs for the API population.
- Focus on youth in the prevention effort. Reducing youth access and use will help reduce the overall rate of substance use and abuse among API populations. Based on the results of prevention research, programs aimed at API youth should attempt to alter their intentions to use drugs as adults. Also, programs aimed at parents of API children might focus special attention on changing their attitudes about substance use and abuse.

- Prevention programs need to be tailored to specific subgroups. For example, skills to resist peer influence are likely to be important for more acculturated API students, and should be included in prevention efforts.
- Effective prevention research needs to involve multiple program components that address risk factors across individual, family, peer group, and community (school, workplace, and local neighborhood).
- Develop and implement effective prevention programs by paying attention to different socioeconomic levels, educational backgrounds, nativity (foreign born versus U.S. born), and acculturation levels.
- Improve the quality of prevention research by using longitudinal designs and incorporating control groups.

Recommendations for Treatment/Tertiary Intervention

Availability of and access to effective treatment programs remain limited for APIs. Not only do linguistically and culturally competent services need to be considered when developing intervention programs, the subgroup, gender, generation, and socioeconomic factors must also be considered. Specific recommendations for treatment/tertiary intervention research include the following:

- Improve provision of substance abuse treatment services for API groups.
- Integrate substance abuse treatment services into other routine health care services.
- Develop and implement treatment programs that integrate a balance of cultural, linguistic, and socioeconomic needs for API populations.
- Facilitate formal and informal support systems, such as extended families, elders, and indigenous leaders, in the development and implementation of treatment programs.
- Involve APIs in ongoing intervention research to help develop effective methods of reaching all API populations, particularly underserved communities.
- Advance intervention research by assessing how ethnocultural factors can be better structured and strengthened to improve treatment effects throughout a variety of social interactions.

Recommendations for Protective Factor Research

To prevent substance use and abuse, effective programs need to focus on protective, or buffering, factors. If the prevalence and incidence of substance use and abuse are low among certain API groups, then prevention research that emphasizes the identification of protective factors needs to be developed and promoted. Potential protective factors important for API groups to resist substance use and abuse include family support and culturally relevant values inconsistent with the use of drugs, such as family relations, school achievement, and high level of self control. Recommendations for protective factor research include the following:

- Increase prevention research that focuses on identification of protective factors among Asians and Pacific-Islander groups.
- Increase prevention research that focuses on the evaluation of protective factors specific to ethnicity, immigration status, gender, and acculturation.
- Integrate the identified protective buffering factors in the development and implementation of prevention intervention programs in API communities.

REFERENCES

Adlaf, E. M., Smart, R. G., & Tan, S. H. (1989). Ethnicity and drug use: A critical look. *The International Journal of the Addictions, 24*(1), 1–18.

Akutsu, P. D., Sue, S., Zane, N. W., & Nakamura, C. Y. (1989). *Journal of Studies on Alcohol, 50*(3), 261–267.

Asian and Pacific Islander Tobacco Education Network/Asian Pacific Partners for Empowerment and Leadership (1998). *Asian American and Pacific Islander Blue Print for Tobacco Control.* pp. 1–7.

Austin, G. A., Prendergast, M. L., & Lee, H. (1989). Substance abuse among Asian American youth, *Prevention Research Update,* No. 5 (pp. 1–13). Portland, OR: Northwest Regional Educational Laboratory.

Bachman, J. G., Wallace, J. H., O'Malley, P. M., Johnston, L. D., Kurth, C. L., & Neighbors, H. W. (1991). Racial/ethnic differences in smoking, drinking, and illicit drug use among American high school seniors, 1976–89. *American Journal of Public Health, 81*(3), 372–377.

Catalano, R. F., Hawkins, J. D., Krenz, C., Gillmore, M., Morrision, D., Wells, E., & Abbott, R. (1993). Using research to guide culturally appropriate drug abuse prevention. *Journal of Consulting and Clinical Psychology, 61*(5), 804–811.

Catalano, R. F., Morrison, D. M., Wells, E. A., Gillmore, M. R., Iritani, B., & Hawkins, J. D. (1992). Ethnic differences in family factors related to early drug initiation. *Journal of Studies on Alcohol, 53*(3), 208–217.

Centers for Disease Control and Prevention (1992a). Cigarette smoking among Chinese, Vietnamese, and Hispanics— California, 1989–1991. *Morbidity Mortality Weekly Report, 41*(20), 362–367.

Centers for Disease Control and Prevention (1992b). Cigarette smoking among Southeast Asian immigrants—Washington State, 1989, *Morbidity Mortality Weekly Report, 41*(45), 854–855, 861.

Chen, M. S., Guthrie, R., Moeschberger, M., Wewers, M. E., Anderson, J., Kunn, P., & Nguyen, H. (1993). Lessons learned and baseline data from initiating smoking cessation research with Southeast Asian adults. *Asian American and Pacific Islander Journal of Health, 1*(1), 196–214.

Cheung, Y. W. (1993). Beyond liver and culture: A review of theories and research in drinking among Chinese in North America. *International Journal of Addition, 28*(14), 1497–1513.

Chi, I., Kitano, H. H., Lubben, J. E. (1988a). Male Chinese drinking behavior in Los Angeles. *Journal of Studies on Alcohol, 49*(1), 21–25.

Chi, I., Lubben, J. E., & Kitano, H. H. (1988b). Heavy drinking among young adult Asian males. *International Social Work, 31,* 219–229.

Chi, I., Lubben, J. E. & Kitano, H. H. (1989). Differences in drinking behavior among three Asian American groups. *Journal of Studies on Alcohol, 50*(1), 15–23.

Chin, K. L., Lai, T. F., & Rouse, M. (1990–1991). Social adjustment and alcoholism among Chinese immigrants in New York City. *International Journal of Addiction, 25*(5A, 6A), 709–730.

D'Avanzo, C. E. (1997). Southeast Asians: Asian Pacific Americans at risk for substance misuse. *Substance Use and Misuse, 32*(7–8) 829–848.

D'Avanzo, C. E., Frye, B., & Froman, R. (1994). Culture, stress, and substance use in Cambodian refugee women. *Journal of Studies on Alcohol, 55,* 420–426.

DeMoor, C., Elder, J. P., Young, R. L., Wildey, M. B., & Molgaard, C. A. (1989). Generic tobacco use among four ethnic groups in a school age population. *Journal of Drug Education, 19*(3), 257–270.

Edwards, R. W. Thurman, P. J., & Beauvais, F. (1995). Patterns of alcohol use among ethnic minority adolescent women. *Recent Development in Alcoholism, 12,* 369–386.

Gillmore, M. R. Catalano, R. F., Morrison, D. M., Wells, E. A., Iritani, B., & Hawkins, J. D. (1990). Racial differences in acceptability and availability of drugs and early initiations of substance use. *American Journal of Drug and Alcohol Abuse, 16*(3 & 4), 185–206.

Harford, T. C. (1992). Family history of alcoholism in the United States: prevalence and demographic characteristics. *British Journal of Addictions, 87*(6), 931–935.

Ho, S. B., DeMaster, E. G., Shafer, R. B., Levine, A. S., Morley, J. E., Go, V. L., & Allen, J. I. (1988). Opiate antagonist nalmefene inhibits ethano-induced flushing in Asians: A preliminary study. *Alcohol Clinical and Experimented Research, 12*(5), 705–712.

Hui, K. K., Yu, J. L., & Kitazaki, L. (1992). *How to avoid pitfalls in the drug treatment of the chinese patients.* In Proceedings of the sixth international conference on health problems related to the chinese in North America, June 1992; San Francisco, CA.

Ja, D. R., & Aoki, B. (1993). Substance abuse treatment: Cultural barriers in the Asian-American community. *Journal of Psychoactive Drugs, 25*(1), 61–71.

Jenkins, C. N. H., McPhee, S. J., Pham, A. G. Q., Ha, N. T., & Stewart, S. (1997). *American Journal of Public Health, 87*(6), 1031–1034.

Johnson, R. C., & Nagoshi, C. T. (1990). Asians, Asian Americans and alcohol. *Journal of Psychoactive Drugs, 22*(1), 45–52.

Johnson, R. C., Nagoshi, C. T., Ahern, F. M., Wilson, J. R., & Yuen, S. H. L. (1987). Cultural factors as explanations for ethnic group difference in alcohol use in Hawaii. *Journal of Psychoactive Drugs, 19*(1), 67–75.

Johnson, R. C., Nagoshi, C. T., Danko, G. P., Honbo, K. A., & Chou, L. L. (1990). Familar transmission of alcohol use norms and expectancies and reported alcohol use. *Alcohol Clinical and Experimental Research, 14*(2), 216–220.

Keefe, K., & Newcomb, M. D. (1996). Demographic and psychosocial risk for alcohol use: Ethnic differences. *Journal of Studies on Alcohol, 57*(5), 521–530.

Kitano, H. H. (1989). Alcohol and the Asian-American. In T. D. Watts & R. Wright (Eds.), *Alcoholism in minority populations* (pp. 143–156). Springfield, IL: Charles C Thomas.

Kitano, H. H., & Chi, I. (1985). Asian Americans and alcohol: The Chinese, Japanese, Koreans, and Filipinos in Los Angeles. In D. Spiegler, D. Tate, S. Aitken, & C. Christian (Eds.), *Alcohol use among U.S. ethnic minorities* (pp. 373–392). Rockville, MD: National Institute on Alcohol Abuse and Alcoholism.

Kitano, H. H., Chi, I., Rhee, S., Law, C. K., & Lubben, J. E. (1992). Norms and alcohol consumption: Japanese in Japan, Hawaii and California. *Journal of Studies on Alcohol, 53*(1), 33–39.

Kuramoto, F. H. (1994). Drug abuse prevention research concerns in Asian and Pacific Islander populations. *NIDA Research Monograph 139,* 249–272.

Leung, P., & Sakata, R. (1990). Drug and alcohol rehabilitation counseling with Asian Americans. *Journal of Applied Rehabilitation Counseling, 21*(3), 49–51.

Li, H. Z., & Rosenblood, L. (1994). Exploring factors influencing alcohol consumption patterns among Chinese and Caucasians. *Journal of Studies on Alcohol, 55,* 427–433.

Lin-Fu, J. S. (1993). Asian and Pacific Islanders: An overview of demographic characteristics and health care issues. *Asian American and Pacific Islander Journal of Health, 1*(1), 20–36.

Lin-Fu, J. S. (1994). Ethnocultural barriers to health care: A major problem for Asian and Pacific Islander Americans. *Asian American and Pacific Islander Journal of Health, 2*(4), 290–298.

Maddahian, E., Newcomb, M. D., & Bentler, P. M. (1985). Single and multiple patterns of adolescents substance use: Longitudinal comparisons of four ethnic groups. *Journal of Drug Education, 15*(4), 311–326.

McLaughlin, D. G., Raymond, J. S., Murakomi, S. R., & Goebert, D. (1987). Drug use among Asian Americans in Hawaii. *Journal of Psychoactive Drugs, 19*(1), 85–94.

Nakawatase, T. V., Yamamoto, J., & Sasao, T. (1993). The association between fast-flushing response and alcohol use among Japanese Americans. *Journal of Studies in Alcohol, 54*(1), 48–53.

National Institute on Drug Abuse (NIDA) (1998). *Drug use among racial/ethnic minorities* (NIH pub.) Rockville, MD: NIDA.

Neumark-Sztainer, D., Story, M., French, S., Cassuto, N., Jacobs, D. R., & Resnick, M. D. (1996). Patterns of health-compromising behaviors among Minnesota adolescents: Sociodemographic variations. *American Journal of Public Health, 86*(11), 1599–1606.

Newcomb, M. D., & Bentler, P. M. (1986). Substance use and ethnicity: Differential impact of peer and adult models. *Journal of Psychology, 120,* 83–95.

Newcomb, M. D., Maddahian, E., Skager, R., & Bentler, P. M. (1987). Substance abuse and psychosocial risk factors among teenagers: Associations with sex, age, ethnicity, and type of school. *American Journal of Drug and Alcohol Abuse, 13*(4), 413–433.

O'Hare, T. (1995). Differences in Asian and white drinking: Consumption level, drinking contexts, and expectancies. *Addictive Behavior, 20*(2), 261–266.

O'Hare, T., & Van Tran, T. (1998). Substance abuse among Southeast Asians in the U.S.: Implications for practice and research. *Social Work in Health Care, 26*(3), 69–80.

Parrish, K. M., Higuchi, S., Stinson, F. S., Dufour, M. C., Towle, L. H., & Harford, T. C. (1990). Genetic or cultural determinants of drinking: A study of embarrassment at facial flushing among Japanese and Japanese-Americans. *Journal of Substance Abuse, 2*(4), 439–447.

Perez-Arce, P., Carr, K. D., & Sorensen, J. L. (1993). Cultural issues in an outpatient program for stimulant abusers. *Journal of Psychoactive Drugs, 25*(1), 35–44.

Psaty, B. M., Cheadle, A., Koepsell, T. D., Diehr, P., Wickizer, T., Curry, S., Vonkorff, M., Perrin, E. B., Pearson, D. C., & Wagner, E. H. (1994). Race- and ethnicity-specific characteristics of participants last to follow-up in a telephone cohort. *American Journal of Epidemiology, 140*(2), 161–171.

Quock, C. P. (1992). Health problems in the Chinese in North America. *Western Journal of Medicine, 156,* 557–558.

Rowe, D. C., Vazsonyi, A. T., & Flannery, D. J. (1994). No more than skin deep: Ethnic and racial similarity in developmental process. *Psychological Review, 101,* 396–413.

Sasao, T. (1991). *Statewide asian drug service needs assessment: A multimethod approach.* Sacramento, CA: California Department of Alcohol and Drug Programs.

Sasao, T. (1994). Using the surname based telephone survey methodology in Asian-American communities: Practical issues and caveats. *Journal of Community Psychology, 22*(4), 283–295.

Seto, A., Tricomi, S. Goodwin, D. W., Kolodney, R., & Sullivan, T. (1978). Biochemical correlates of ethanol-induced flushing in Orientals. *Journal of Studies on Alcohol, 39,* 1–11.

Smith, M. W., & Mendoza, R. P. (1996). Ethnicity and pharmacogenetics. *Mount Sinai Journal of Medicine, 63*(5–6), 285–290.

Straka, R. J., Hansen, S. R., Benson, S. R., & Walker, P. F. (1996). Predominance of slow acetylators of Nacetyltransferase in a Hmong population residing in the United States. *Journal of Clinical Pharmacology, 36*(8), 740–747.

Substance Abuse and Mental Health Services Administration (SAMSHA) (1998). *Prevalence of substance use among racial and ethnic subgroups in the United States 1991–1993,* DHHS Publication No. (SMA) 98-3202.

Sue, D. (1987). Use and abuse of alcohol by Asian Americans. *Journal of Psychoactive Drugs, 19*(1), 57–66.

Sue, S., Zane, N., & Ito, J. (1979). Alcohol drinking patterns among Asian and Caucasian Americans. *Journal of Cross-Cultural Psychology, 10,* 41–56.

Trimble, J. E. (1990–1991). Ethnic specification, validation prospects, and the future of drug use research. *International Journal of the Addiction, 25*(2A), 149–170.

Tsunoda, T., Parrish, K. M., Higuchi, S., Stinson, F. S., Kono, H., Ogata, M., & Harford, T. C. (1992). The effective of acculturation on drinking attitudes among Japanese in Japan and Japanese Americans in Hawaii and California. *Journal of Studies on Alcohol, 53*(4), 369–377.

Tu, G. C., & Israel, Y. (1995). Alcohol consumption by orientals in North America is predicted largely by a single gene. *Behavioral Genetics, 25*(1), 59–65.

U. S. Bureau of the Census (1990). *Statistical abstract of the United States, 1990.* Washington, DC: US Government Printing Office.

U. S. Census Bureau (1992). *Population projections of the United States, by age, sex, race, and Hispanic origin: 1992–2050.* Washington, DC: US Government Printing Office.

Varma, S. C., & Siris, S. G. (1996). Alcohol abuse in Asian Americans: Epidemiological and treatment issues. *American Journal on Addictions, 5*(2), 136–143.

Wall, T. L., & Ethlers, C. L. (1995). Acute effects of alcohol on P300 in Asians with different ALDH2 genotypes. *Alcohol Clinical and Experimental Research, 19*(3), 617–622.

Wall, T. L., Peterson, C. M., Peterson, K. P., Johnson, M. L., Thomasson, H. R., Cole, M., & Ethlers, C. L. (1997). Alcohol metabolism in Asian American men with genetic polymorphisms of aldehyde dehydrogenase. *Annuals of Internal Medicine, 127*(5), 376–379.

Warner, K. E. (1993). Editorial: Profits for doom. *American Journal of Public Health, 83,* 1211–1213.

Weatherspoon, A. J., Danko, G. P., & Johnson, R. C. (1994). Alcohol consumption and use norms among Chinese Americans and Korean Americans. *Journal of Studies on Alcohol, 55*(2), 203–206.

Welte, J. W., & Barnes, G. M. (1987). Alcohol use among adolescent minority groups. *Journal of Studies on Alcohol, 48*(4), 329–336.

Westermeyer, J., Lyfoung, T., & Neider, J. (1989). An epidemic of opium dependence among Asian refugees in Minnesota: Characteristics and causes. *British Journal of Addiction, 84*(7), 785–789.

Westermeyer, J. C., Lyfoung, T. Westermeyer, M., & Neider, J. (1991). Opium addiction among Indochinese refugees in the United States: Characteristics of addicts and their opium use. *American Journal of Drug and Alcohol Abuse, 17*(3), 267–277.

Wiecha, J. M. (1996). Differences in patterns of tobacco use in Vietnamese, African American, Hispanic, and Caucasian adolescents in Worcester, Massachusetts. *American Journal of Preventive Medicine, 12*(1), 29–37.

Yee, B. W. K., & Thu, N. D. (1987). Correlates of drug use and abuse among Indochinese Refugees: Mental health implications. *Journal of Psychoactive Drugs, 19*(1), 77–83.

Zane, N., & Kim, J. H. (1994). Substance use and abuse. In N. W. S. Zane, D. T. Takeuchi, & K. N. J. Young (Eds.), *Confronting critical health issues of asian and pacific islander americans* (pp. 316–343). CA: Sage.

Zane, N., & Sasao, T. (1992). Research on drug abuse among Asian Pacific Americans. *Drugs and Society, 6*(3–4), 181–209.

PART VI

INTERACTIONS BETWEEN BIOLOGY AND SOCIAL CONTEXT—RISKS FOR MULTIPLE BEHAVIORAL AND MENTAL DISORDERS

CHAPTER 22

Basic Science and Drug Abuse Prevention: Neuroscience, Learning, and Personality Perspectives

MICHAEL T. BARDO

THOMAS KELLY

DONALD R. LYNAM

RICHARD MILICH

INTRODUCTION

This chapter examines contributions from the neurosciences, learning theory, and personality research, and their implications for drug abuse prevention. The behavior of primary interest is drug abuse, not simply drug use. This is an important distinction since most prevention programs with demonstrated effectiveness target the initiation of drug use. Epidemiologic data from the 1996 Monitoring the Future Study indicate that among adolescents, between 57 and 22% of those reporting ever having used drugs in their lifetime had not used the drugs in the year prior to survey. The highest noncontinuation rate was for inhalants and the lowest was for marijuana (National Institute on Drug Abuse, 1998).

The premise of this chapter is that some people are more vulnerable or susceptible to abusing drugs. Neurobiological mechanisms are suggested by the results of a number of related studies on the genetic bases for differential response to various drugs, on the biological responses due

MICHAEL T. BARDO, THOMAS KELLY, DONALD R. LYNAM, AND RICHARD MILICH • Department of Psychology, University of Kentucky, Lexington, Kentucky 40506

to environmentally stimulated experiences of stress and excitation, on behavioral pharmacologic conditioning, and on the biologic basis of personality and variation in personality structure. The chapter discusses how these disparate lines of investigation can be integrated to arrive at a more complete understanding of the problems of and solutions for drug abuse.

CONTRIBUTIONS FROM NEUROSCIENCE

Clinical evidence suggests that vulnerability to drug abuse can be predicted by the degree of positive reward derived from the initial drug experience. In a study by Haertzen, Kocher, and Miyasato (1986), drug abusers and nonabusers were asked to rate their first experience with various drugs, including stimulants, opiates, sedative-hypnotics, and hallucinogens. Drug abusers reported significantly greater positive feelings from their first experience. Although these data are retrospective, the study is important because it suggests that individuals differ in their initial reaction to drugs of abuse. Individual differences in the acute rewarding effect of various drugs reflects, at least in part, neuropharmacological differences related to both genetic and environmental factors. Basic animal and human research in the neurosciences supports this general conclusion.

Genetic Approaches

Perhaps one of the most profound advances in basic research over the past 2 decades stems from our ability to manipulate the genetic code of laboratory animals. Genetic studies of laboratory animals have provided a new tool to advance our knowledge about the biological basis of vulnerability to drug abuse. For a review of these genetic approaches, see Crabbe and Phillips (1998).

One particularly useful approach is the so-called "knockout" procedure in which a selected gene is replaced with a mutant allele in an otherwise normal organism, typically a mouse (see Lodish et al., 1995). By examining the phenotypic expressions that are altered in the knockout mouse, the function of the gene at the cellular and behavioral levels can be studied. For example, it is well known that psychostimulant drugs, such as amphetamine and cocaine, release dopamine in the brain due to their actions at the dopamine transporter (DAT). These neurochemical changes are greatly diminished in DAT knockout mice (Jones et al., 1998). Since dopamine release is thought to be a critical mechanism involved in the rewarding effect of psychostimulant drugs (Bardo, 1998), this neurochemical finding suggests that DAT knockout mice would be relatively immune to psychostimulant abuse. Contrary to this prediction, however, DAT knockout mice display cocaine conditioned place preference (Sora et al., 1998), suggesting that the cellular target for cocaine reward may involve more than dopamine neurotransmission. Such work illustrates how the knockout technique provides basic information about the connection between cellular and behavioral events that occur in response to drugs of abuse.

Another useful genetic approach is provided by recombinant inbred strains of mice. This approach involves inbreeding two parental strains in such a way that multiple inbred strains are produced, each with a unique pattern of recombinations of the parental chromosomes. A powerful analytic technique, referred to as the method of quantitative trait loci (QTL), is then used to link a potential gene of interest to a previously typed marker gene. For example, QTL analysis has been used to identify candidate genes that control sensitivity to the effects of alcohol (Crabbe et al., 1994). This work shows that sensitivity and tolerance to alcohol-induced hypothermia are polygenic traits. Interestingly, some identified QTL are associated with both sensitivity and tolerance to alcohol, suggesting that each is controlled by a similar nearby gene.

A host of genetic studies in humans also indicates that vulnerability to substance abuse is heritable. Most work in this area is based on data collected from alcoholics (Cloninger & Begleiter, 1990). In general, the strongest evidence for a genetic influence on alcoholism is obtained from the most severe alcoholic subtype (Johnson, van den Bree, & Pickens, 1996). With various drugs of abuse, including alcohol, considerable attention focuses on genes encoding membrane proteins involved in dopamine neurotransmission. This research indicates that gene markers for dopamine D_2 receptors are present more often in substance abusers than in control populations (Uhl et al., 1993). These findings corroborate work with laboratory animals showing that dopamine D_2 receptors in the brain, particularly in the nucleus accumbens and prefrontal cortex, play a critical role in drug reward (Bardo, 1998).

In some cases, genes may exert direct effects on how the body absorbs and eliminates drugs, either increasing or decreasing vulnerability to drug abuse. Recent work indicates that variation in expression of CYP2A6, a genetically polymorphic enzyme involved in the metabolism of nicotine into cotinine, may play an important role in vulnerability to tobacco dependence in cigarette smokers (Pianezza, Sellers, & Tyndale, 1998). In this work, individuals lacking a fully functional CYP2A6 allele were found to have reduced ability to metabolize nicotine. These individuals were also shown to smoke significantly fewer cigarettes than individuals with fully active CYP2A6 alleles. Genetic variation in the CYP2A6 enzyme may also play a role in the ethnoracial differences observed in nicotine metabolism and smoking-related disease risks among African-American, Hispanic, and White smokers (Carabello et al., 1998; Perez-Stable et al., 1998).

The association between different gene markers and vulnerability to substance abuse may also be mediated, at least in part, by various heritable personality traits. This type of mediational effect is seen in recent work showing that genetic encoding for dopamine D_4 receptors, which have considerable homology with the D_2 subtype, may be associated with high novelty seeking in humans (Benjamin et al., 1996; Ebstein et al., 1996; however, see Vandenbergh et al. (1997)). Importantly, novelty seeking is a trait that is positively correlated with use and abuse of drugs in different populations (Donohew, Lorch, & Palmgreen, 1991; Wills, Windle, & Cleary, 1998; Zuckerman, 1994). This suggests that high novelty seekers may have an enhanced sensitivity to the dopaminergic activation produced by rewarding drugs. Alternatively, high novelty seekers may simply be inclined to join social groups that engage in risky behaviors, such as drug use, and thus drug availability and peer pressure may play an important mediational role in the relationship between novelty seeking and drug use.

Environmental Approaches

Neuroscience research suggests that exposure to stress may be an important environmental factor that influences vulnerability to drug abuse. In rats, exposure to stressors either early or late in life increases the psychostimulant and rewarding effects of amphetamine (Dellu et al., 1996; Piazza et al., 1990). Similarly, cocaine-seeking behavior that has been extinguished can be reinstated if rats are exposed to stressful events (Ahmed & Koob, 1997). The increase in vulnerability to drug abuse evident with exposure to stress may involve several neurohormonal mechanisms, including those regulating corticosterone levels in blood and dopamine neurotransmission in the mesolimbic system (Kreek & Koob, 1998).

Vulnerability to drug abuse is also determined by the amount of exposure to novel environmental stimuli that occurs during development. Research over the past 40 years has shown that rats raised in an enriched condition (EC) show profound neural and behavioral changes relative to rats raised in an impoverished condition (IC). Environmental enrichment increases neocortical weight and thickness, primarily due to an increased density of glial and capillary endothelial cells

(Sirevaag & Greenough, 1988). Environmental enrichment also increases various neurochemical markers in the neocortex, including acetylcholinesterase activity (Rosenzweig et al., 1962), levels of norepinephrine and dopamine (Reige & Morimoto, 1970), and densities of dopaminergic terminals in the prefrontal cortex (Winterfeld, Teuchert-Noodt, & Dawirs, 1998). Correlated with these neocortical changes, EC rats are superior to IC rats in various learning tasks using either appetitive or aversive stimuli (Renner & Rosenzweig, 1987).

Environmental enrichment during the adolescent period may also potentiate the effects of amphetamine and related psychostimulant drugs that are administered during young adulthood. For example, acute administration of amphetamine increases locomotor activity more in EC rats than in IC rats (Bowling & Bardo, 1994; Bowling, Rowlett, & Bardo, 1993). EC rats also show greater amphetamine conditioned place preference than do IC rats (Bowling & Bardo, 1994). Using oral self-administration, EC rats also show greater initial consumption of cocaine (Hill & Powell, 1976). These acute behavioral changes may be related to alterations in activity of the mesolimbic dopamine reward system, as environmental enrichment potentiates the neurochemical effect of amphetamine in the nucleus accumbens (Bowling et al., 1993). Importantly, in contrast to the acute effects of amphetamine, the behavioral effects (e.g., locomotor activity) following chronic exposure to amphetamine are diminished by environmental enrichment (Bardo et al., 1995; Fowler et al., 1993; Smith, Neill & Costall, 1997). In a recent study conducted in our laboratory, we also found that intravenous self-administration of amphetamine was reduced in EC rats relative to IC rats (Bardo et al., 2001). Thus, while producing an initial increase in the acute psychostimulant effect, environmental enrichment seems to serve as a protective factor in reducing long-term stimulant self-administration.

It is not yet clear why environmental enrichment reduces self-administration of drugs. However, one intriguing possibility is that repeated exposure to novel environmental stimuli during development alters the mesolimbic dopamine reward pathway in a manner that reduces the relative impact of drugs on this neurobiological system. Considerable evidence has accumulated to indicate that, similar to drugs of abuse, exposure to novelty increases locomotor activity and produces reward (Bardo, Donohew, & Harrington, 1996). Approach to novelty is also known to activate the mesolimbic dopamine reward pathway. In a study conducted by Rebec et al. (1997), dopamine activity in the brain was monitored using *in vivo* voltammetry in rats during free-choice entry into a novel compartment from a familiar compartment. Upon entry into novelty, there was a brief, but pronounced, rise in dopamine activity. The response was apparent in the nucleus accumbens, a limbic-related area believed to play a critical role in reward, but not in the overlying neostriatum, an area involved in motor performance.

CONTRIBUTIONS FROM LEARNING THEORY

During the past century, research on the behavior of an individual organism within its environmental context has given rise to dramatic improvements in our understanding of factors that influence the behavior of individuals, including drug use behavior. The following is a brief description of the predominant theoretical perspectives (respondent and operant conditioning) that dominate research. These perspectives can be applied with remarkable precision to describe the variables controlling individual drug use behavior and can have implications for its prevention.

Conditioning Theories

Beginning with the efforts of Bekhterev (1932) and Pavlov (1927) at the start of the last century, research on the associations between environmental stimuli and behavior have led to the development of theoretical perspectives on behavior known as respondent and operant conditioning. A classic example of respondent conditioning is seen in Pavlov's work showing the ability of meat powder to control the probability of salivation in a hungry dog. Associations between stimuli, such as meat powder, and other behaviorally inactive stimuli, such as a bell or buzzer, can result in the formation of a new relationship in which the previously inactive, or neutral, stimulus (the bell or buzzer) acquires control over the probability of the behavior (salivation). Investigators have established a wealth of information regarding the parameters and conditions under which associations between stimuli lead to changes in the relationships between the stimuli and behavior (e.g., Rescorla, 1967).

Conditioning theories are not limited to reflexive stimulus-response relationships determined by the physiology of the individual organism. The work of Watson (1914) and Skinner (1938), among others, demonstrated the important role of environmental contingencies on voluntary, or operant, behavioral repertoires of individual organisms. Respondent conditioning theories focus on environmental stimuli that precede behavior. Operant conditioning theories extend the analysis to include environmental stimuli that follow behavior. A central tenet of operant conditioning theory is that the probability of a behavior is related to both antecedent and consequent stimulus events. Behavior is influenced by its consequences, such as reinforcement or punishment, but it is also influenced by prior environmental conditions. Unlike respondent conditioning, in which antecedent stimulus control is determined in part by the physiology of the organism, environmental control of voluntary behavior emerges over time based on a history of contingencies associated with the behavior occurring in the presence and absence of the environmental conditions. As such, voluntary behavior must be evaluated using three "terms," including antecedent environmental conditions (sometimes referred to as discriminative stimuli), behavior (sometimes referred to as the response), and consequent environmental conditions (sometimes called reinforcing and punishing stimuli).

A number of variations of conditioning theory have been formulated over the years, including some that have generated criticism from other fields of psychology (e.g., methodological behaviorism) (see Lee, 1988). However, it is important to note that there are substantial methodological and conceptual variations among theories of operant conditioning. It is now widely recognized, for example, that private events, including emotions and thoughts, have been subjected to experimental analysis and are clearly within the realm of the field of inquiry in some conditioning theory perspectives (e.g., radical behaviorism). It is also important to note that the application of these principles in drug treatment (e.g., Bickel & Kelly, 1997) has proved to be remarkably effective (e.g., Higgins et al., 1993; Silverman et al., 1996).

Behavioral Pharmacology

During the past 40 years, the experimental methodology developed for investigating voluntary behavior has been applied in studies of the effects of drugs on behavior. This specialized field, behavioral pharmacology (e.g., Thompson & Schuster, 1968), has shown that the interaction of drugs and behavior follows the same laws that were established in research on conditioning theory. For example, cocaine produces a reliable increase in heart rate and blood pressure in much the same way that meat powder produces a reliable increase in salivation. Furthermore, and of critical importance for the science of drug abuse prevention, associations between inactive environmental stimuli and cocaine can result in the formation of new relationships in which the previously inactive stimuli (e.g., razor, mirror, white powder) come to engender drug-like behavior similar to that observed following cocaine administration (e.g., increases in heart rate) (Newlin, 1992; O'Brien et al., 1992). The parameters and conditions under which associations between environmental stimuli and drug stimuli are formed is consistent with what has been reported in the respondent conditioning literature (e.g., Siegel, 1978; Wikler, 1948). Functional associations have been observed after as few as two drug-stimulus pairings in humans (e.g., Newlin, 1986).

There is an interesting complication with regard to respondent conditioning and drugs. It turns out that drug use can result in complex stimulus dimensions depending on the drug and on the parameters under which it is administered. Repeated administration of many sedative or analgesic drugs (such as alcohol, barbiturates, or opiates), for example, can lead to tolerance, with progressively higher doses being required to produce a standard effect. It can be argued that self-adjusting feedback mechanisms engender drug-opposite responses following drug use, and that these drug-opposite responses are associated with the development of tolerance (Siegel et al., 1982). For example, if alcohol produces an increase in skin temperature, self-adjusting feedback mechanisms are thought to initiate a drug-opposite reduction in skin temperature in order to maintain homeostasis. In addition, either the abrupt discontinuation of a drug following the development of tolerance or the administration of a pharmacological agent that antagonizes the pharmacological effects of the drug may result in the appearance of an adverse constellation of stimulus conditions known as an abstinence syndrome, or drug withdrawal. In the same manner in which an association between environmental stimuli and drug stimuli can result in the conditioning of drug-like behavior, associations between environmental stimuli and drug stimuli can also result in the conditioning of drug-opposite behavior, or behavior associated with drug withdrawal. Although many clinical and experimental demonstrations of these phenomena have been reported, the exact conditions by which stimuli become conditioned to engender drug-like, drug-opposite, and/or withdrawal behavior remains unclear, (e.g., O'Brien et al., 1992; Newlin, 1992).

Much of the behavior of relevance to drug abuse prevention falls within the domain of voluntary or operant behavior in that initial drug use is in large part voluntary. Fortunately, as with respondent conditioning, the laws of behavior established through operant research generalize effectively to the realm of drugs and behavior. Substantial research has shown that drugs function as antecedent stimuli controlling other behaviors, that drugs can function as reinforcing or punishing stimuli, thereby influencing the likelihood of future drug-seeking behavior; and that drug-taking behavior is itself influenced by antecedent and consequent stimuli (e.g., Thompson, 1984).

Drugs can also function as discriminative stimuli, controlling the probabilities of other behavior following drug use. This process has been demonstrated in humans and animals, and cross-species generality in the discriminative stimulus functions of drugs has been reported (e.g., Kamien et al., 1993; Preston & Bigelow, 1991). The methodology used to investigate the discriminative stimulus effects of drugs involves the use of differential reinforcement to train subjects to emit a specific response in the presence of one training dose and to emit an alternative response in the presence of a second training dose. Once differential responding to drug cues has been established, the functional elements of the drug cue that are associated with stimulus control can be evaluated using a variety of testing procedures. This technique has been effective for investigating biological factors (e.g., receptor mechanisms, neurotransmitter modulation) associated with the effects of drugs and for evaluating conditions (e.g., individual difference factors, potential pharmacological treatments) that might alter the cues associated with drug use. Equally important, this research demonstrates that drug use can influence the probability of other behavior. Drug use, for example, can serve as a cue for participation in other forms of behavior (e.g., membership in social groups, sexual behavior, aggressive behavior) (see Falk, 1983). Clearly, since drug use can trigger alternative behaviors, including highly reinforcing social behaviors, the discriminative stimulus effects of drugs have important implications for prevention efforts.

Drugs of abuse also function as reinforcers in that use of these drugs increases the probability of behavior preceding the use (e.g., Meisch & Stewart, 1999). As with drug discrimination, a substantial number of experimental demonstrations of drug reinforcement have been found (e.g., Griffiths, Bigelow, & Henningfield, 1980). For example, cocaine, alcohol, opiates, barbiturates, anesthetic agents, volatile solvents, and nicotine are all readily self-administered in experimental settings, while other centrally acting drugs, including antidepressant and antipsychotic drugs, do not maintain drug-taking behavior. In fact, given the remarkable overlap between drugs that function as reinforcers in experimental settings and drugs that are abused by humans, new drugs with purported clinical efficacy are now routinely tested in experimental self-administration models to assess their potential for abuse (Meisch & Stewart, 1999).

The reinforcing effects of a drug are related, in part, to the pharmacological properties of the drug and to the neurobiology of the organism (e.g., Ritz, 1999a,b). While many factors are clearly associated with drug abuse, it is important to recognize that one necessary cause of every clinical case of drug abuse is that an individual is exposed to a drug that functions as a reinforcer. Drug abuse does not occur if an individual takes only drugs that do not function as reinforcers (e.g., antipsychotic medications). Many factors must be taken into account when evaluating clinical issues associated with drug abuse. Many individuals use drugs with reinforcing effects, but only a few develop problems. Simple exposure to a drug with reinforcing effects is not a sufficient cause of drug abuse. However, it is not clear that there is any other single factor more integral to the development of drug abuse. Much of the current effort in development of medications for drug abuse treatment, for example, focuses on modification of the reinforcing efficacy of drugs of abuse (Tai, Chiang, & Bridge, 1997). As such, the development of procedures that could modify the reinforcing effects of drugs would have broad-ranging implications for prevention.

Finally, taking a drug also functions as a response that can itself come under discriminative stimulus control, and other reinforcing consequences can impact the future probabilities of drug-taking behavior. For example, drug self-administration can be achieved in both humans and animals in controlled settings by making delivery of alternative reinforcers, such as sweetened beverages, food, or money, contingent on drug-taking behavior (Samson, Pfeffer, & Tolliver, 1988). Over time, as the organism is repeatedly exposed to the reinforcing effects of the drug, the alternative reinforcer contingency can be eliminated and drug-taking behavior will remain intact, maintained only by the drug. Again, given that the etiology of drug use is an important concern for the development of a comprehensive science of prevention, issues associated with antecedents and consequences of drug-taking behavior deserve careful consideration.

THE CONTRIBUTION OF BASIC RESEARCH ON PERSONALITY

Personality traits are individual differences in the tendency to behave, think, and feel in certain consistent ways. Despite attempts to call the reality and utility of personality traits into question (Mischel, 1968), recent work provides little reason to doubt the existence or utility of personality traits. First, personality traits can be measured reliably (e.g., Epstein, 1979; Jackson & Paunonen, 1985), and different sources agree in their judgments of an individual's personality (e.g., Norman & Goldberg, 1963). For example, across the five dimensions of their personality inventory, Costa and McCrae (1992) found high average intraclass correlations between two peer raters ($r = 0.42$), between self- and peer ratings ($r = 0.46$), and between self- and spouse ratings ($r = 0.56$). Second, in studies of the basic structure of personality, similar traits are found in different ages, genders, and cultures. In a sample of more than 1,500 participants, Costa, McCrae, and Dye (1991) found extremely similar underlying structures in men and women, in older and younger adults, and in White and non-White participants; similar dimensions have been identified in children, adolescents, and adults (e.g., John et al., 1994). Results from cross-cultural studies in the Netherlands, Germany, Japan, and China are quite consistent with those using American samples (see John, 1990; Costa & McCrae, 1992). Third, personality traits are remarkably stable over time. In a sample of 398 men and women, Costa and McCrae (1988) found an average 6-year stability coefficient of 0.83 across the five broad domains measured by their personality inventory. In an earlier meta-analysis, Conley (1984) found that personality traits were almost as stable as intelligence across the life course; in fact, he found personality stability coefficients of 0.82 and 0.67 across 10- and 20-year time spans, respectively. Fourth, personality traits are substantially genetically influenced. In a study of twins reared apart and together, Tellegen et al. (1988) found that, on average, 51% of the variation in scores on three broad personality traits was due to genetic variation.

Personality traits are real and they are important in predicting developmental outcomes in multiple domains and in different age groups. Personality traits are related to measures of job performance (Barrick & Mount, 1991), and to risk- and health-promoting behaviors (Freidman et al., 1995). Knowledge of these traits can be used to design health and educational campaigns (Donohew, Palmgreen, & Lorch, 1994). Personality traits are robustly related to antisocial behavior in different countries, age cohorts, genders, and races (Caspi et al., 1994). Finally, personality traits are clearly related to substance use, both concurrently and prospectively (Chassin et al., 1996; Krueger et al., 1996; Masse & Tremblay, 1997; Shedler & Block, 1990; Trull & Sher, 1994). Accordingly, basic research on personality may help inform prevention science and substance abuse prevention efforts. Three areas of basic research are particularly important: (1) research on personality structure, (2) research on the biology of personality, and (3) research on the stability of personality.

The Structure of Personality

Much of the research on personality has been aimed at uncovering the underlying structure of personality, and researchers from several traditions have begun to converge on a common structure. There is good agreement on the number of basic traits (between 3 and 5) and on the nature of those traits (see John, 1990; Watson, Clark & Harkness, 1994). Most personality psychologists would agree on the existence of the "Big Two" (Wiggins, 1968): neuroticism, or negative emotionality, which refers to a dimension of emotional stability; and extraversion, or positive emotionality, which refers to the tendency of an individual to positively engage others in his or her environment. Individuals who score high on the neuroticism dimension experience various negative emotions more intensely and more frequently than do low scorers, blame themselves for problems, feel inadequate and inferior, are self-critical and overly sensitive to criticism, and experience high levels of stress. High scorers on the extraversion dimension seek out others, are forceful and assertive, feel lively and energetic, are cheerful, and enthusiastic, and seek out exciting and intense experiences. There is also some agreement on two other traits: agreeableness, which refers to an individual's interpersonal orientation and ranges from agreeable to antagonistic; and conscientiousness or constraint, which centers around the basic issue of impulse control. Individuals high in agreeableness are sincere, sympathetic, considerate, generous, believe that others are trustworthy, and seek to avoid conflict. Individuals high in constraint are deliberate, dependable, well-organized, traditional, capable of completing tasks when bored or tired, and tend to avoid dangerous or risky situations. The least agreed-upon trait is openness to experience, which involves curiosity and nonconformity.

The Biology of Personality

Basic research in personality also attempts to uncover the presumed underlying biological substrates of the major dimensions of personality (see Depue, 1996; Zuckerman, 1994). The basic assumption is that because dimensions of personality are genetically influenced, similar across cultures, and stable over time, they may be reflections of basic biological systems. Depue (1996) has put forth one of the most comprehensive and well-developed accounts. He argues that extraversion is a reflection of a behavioral facilitation system that is underpinned by two major ascending dopamine projection systems: (1) the mesolimbic system, discussed earlier, which arises from ventral tegmental area (VTA) and projects to limbic structures; and (2) the mesocortical system, which originates in the VTA and projects to the frontal areas of the cerebral cortex. He further suggests that constraint is related to functional activity in the central nervous system serotonin (5-HT) projections, which provide a tonic inhibitory influence over DA-mediated facilitatory effects (see Spoont, 1992). Finally, he offers more speculatively that noradrenergic activity in the locus ceruleus may modulate the affective system that underpins neuroticism. Using pharmacological challenge protocols in which agonists of DA and 5-HT are administered in order to assess individual differences in the reactivity of the systems, which are then correlated with personality measures, Depue and colleagues have generated good support for his propositions (see Depue et al., 1994).

This research on the neurobiology of personality also serves to inform prevention efforts and prevention science. First, the biology of personality, in conjunction with research on the relations between personality and substance use, can help identify particular etiologic pathways for future study. For example, research suggests that constraint is more strongly related to substance use than is extraversion (e.g., Sher & Trull, 1994). In fact, a longitudinal study of more than 1,000 participants found that constraint bore strong concurrent and predictive (across ten years) relations to all kinds of substance use and abuse in early adulthood (Flory et al., in press). In conjunction with Depue's analysis, these findings suggest that the etiology of substance use may have as much, if not more, to do with deficient serotonergic modulation of the DA system than with an overactive DA system. Second, the biology of personality may suggest certain pharmacologic treatments for different disorders. For example, if constraint is the most important dimension in relation to substance use and if constraint is a reflection of an underlying 5-HT system, then a pharmacologic intervention targeting the 5-HT system would be indicated.

The Stability of Personality

Some excellent basic research is being conducted on the stability of personality over long periods of time. Why personality is so stable, however, is an understudied and underappreciated question. However, the answer to this question has real implications for how we understand the effects of personality on behavior. The work being conducted in this area draws heavily on work in genetics and development, which suggests that genetic effects are environmentally mediated (Bouchard et al., 1990; Rutter et al., 1997; Scarr & McCartney, 1983). That is, genes may exert their effects indirectly by influencing the effective psychological environment experienced by an individual. Caspi (1997) has applied this idea to understanding the continuity of personality. Specifically, he argues that personality promotes its own continuity through three types of person–environment transactions: reactive, evocative, and proactive.

Reactive transactions occur when individuals exposed to the same environment experience it, interpret it, and react to it according to their preexisting tendencies. For example, aggressive children make hostile attributions in ambiguous situations, generate more aggressive responses, and are more likely to believe that aggressive responses will work. In contrast, depressed children pay more attention to negative cues, make internal stable and global attributions for negative events, and believe that assertive responses will be ineffective (Quiggle et al., 1992). Evocative transactions occur when individuals evoke distinctive reactions from their social environments on the basis of their personalities. For example, difficult-to-manage children evoke typical reactions from parents that include harsh and erratic parental discipline (Lytton, 1990), reduction of parental efforts at socialization (Maccoby & Jacklin, 1983), and increases in permissiveness for later aggression (Olweus, 1980). Finally, proactive transactions occur when individuals select or create social environments that are in line with their existing personalities. For example, individuals tend to choose similar people as friends and mates (Epstein & Guttman, 1984). In all of the above cases, these person–environment transactions tend to reinforce the existing personality.

This research informs prevention science in several ways. First, the continuity of personality provides information on how personality relates to drug use, which can inform our understanding of etiological mechanisms. That is, the previously cited account suggests that personality has broad and indirect effects on behavior. Specifically, personality probably affects drug use indirectly by influencing, among other things: (1) who one spends time with, (2) what one learns about drugs, (3) how one is responded to by others, (4) how one feels (level of stress), and (5) one's academic and occupational achievement. All of these variables have been repeatedly linked to drug use (Hawkins, Catalano, & Miller, 1992; Petratis, Flay, & Miller, 1995). Recent research is consistent with this theorizing (Chassin et al., 1996; Wills, DuHamel, & Vaccaro, 1995). In one study (Lynam et al., 2002), we found that more than 50% of the relation between 6th-grade sensation seeking and 10th-grade marijuana use is mediated by social/interpersonal (e.g., family conflict and peer use), cultural/attitudinal (e.g., social alienation and expectancies toward drugs), and intrapersonal (e.g., affective states and refusal skills) variables measured in the 7th and 8th grades. The research on continuity and the broad effects of personality also have implications for treatment. The mechanisms for the stability of personality are likely to be operative in promoting stability in substance use. That is, substance use may be stable because of the consequences it elicits. Finally, the previously cited research helps to indicate potential targets (e.g., peers, school achievement) for intervention that are presumably more malleable than the initial personality.

IMPLICATIONS FOR PREVENTION INTERVENTIONS

While genetic findings are important for understanding the biological mechanisms of drug abuse, there is also some potential application of this work for prevention scientists. At present, it does not seem prudent to suggest that a direct modification of the genome, so-called gene therapy, is a likely route for reducing the risk of drug abuse. However, mapping the genetic markers associated with vulnerability to drug abuse would provide an additional diagnostic tool for identifying those most at risk at an early age, prior to their first drug experience. When genetic markers are used in conjunction with psychosocial risk factors, such as sexual abuse, parental detachment, and academic failure, a more complete and accurate picture of the at-risk individual will be obtained. Children could be screened early on and be provided comprehensive and intensive services through late adolescence and young adulthood. There are several "pencil and paper" diagnostic tools available, such as the POSIT, developed by the National Institute on Drug Abuse, and the DUSI, created by Tarter and his associates at the University of Pittsburgh, that have been used effectively to refer children and adolescents for counseling and other supportive services.

Used in combination with genetic diagnostic tools they may increase the specificity and sensitivity of diagnosis (Tarter & Kirisci, 1997).

Findings from the studies of differential biological responses to the environment also suggest avenues for prevention intervention. In particular, if novelty activates the mesolimbic dopamine system in a manner similar to drugs of abuse, then novelty may substitute for drug reward. A recent study conducted by Koepp et al. (1998) illustrates this point. In that study, positron emission tomography was used to monitor dopamine activity in brains of human volunteers engaged in playing a highly novel video game. The game involved using a computer mouse to move a tank thorough a treacherous battlefield. The object of the game was to destroy enemy tanks and collect as many field flags as possible, with the difficulty level of the game being increased over time. The overall performance of subjects was rewarded with money. Data from the brain scan revealed that dopamine levels were increased during the video game, compared to baseline levels, and the increase was correlated with the difficulty level of the game. Importantly, the increase in dopamine was greatest in the brain region corresponding to the mesolimbic dopamine reward pathway. Thus, it appears that the dopamine release was responsible for the positive affect associated with the video game. Further work is necessary to determine if this novelty-evoked dopamine release may substitute for or reduce drug reward.

The substitution of a novel experience for drugs is the premise for what are termed "alternative" interventions. Most of these approaches offer activities that are challenging to the child or adolescent. Programs such as Outward Bound fall into this category. A meta-analysis conducted by Tobler (1992) found that these programs have promise as being successful. There has not, however, been extensive research on the effectiveness of these programs or for whom they are most successful.

Much of the current effort in prevention is designed to educate individuals on issues associated with drug use and problems associated with it. These programs are school-, family-, and/or community-based and focus on teaching effective strategies for countering factors associated with the initiation of drug use, such as peer influence, scholastic failure, and family disruption. Other programs focus on protective factors, such as social and scholastic skills training, leadership development, and self-esteem. Much of the work in conditioning theories of behavior, however, stresses the critical importance of proximal factors in the development and maintenance of behavior change. These dynamic behavioral processes occur during the initial exposure to drugs (e.g., Haertzen et al., 1986; Newlin, 1986) and continue during the repeated course of drug exposure. The most efficient method of changing drug-using behavior or reducing adverse consequences of drug use is to impact these dynamic processes by affecting the conditions in a more proximal manner (i.e., in settings in which drug-use occurs, or during times when drug use is occurring). Clearly, such an approach would be critical for effective drug treatment (e.g., Carroll et al., 1994; Higgins et al., 1993; Silverman et al., 1995; Wells et al., 1994). This is why the most effective prevention interventions, such as Life Skills Training and Project STAR, are so successful. They are designed to prepare children and adolescents for these "at-risk" times in their lives when they are in situations where tobacco, alcohol or drugs are offered (Botvin et al., 1995; Pentz et al., 1989). A significant challenge for those developing prevention interventions is to create realistic scenarios so that adolescents can practice communication, decision making, and resistance skills. Under these conditions, the likelihood of successful development and maintenance of efficacious behavior change can be maximized.

Finally, the research on the structure of personality has several implications for prevention science and prevention efforts. It points out the most basic dimensions of personality and provides a convenient taxonomy in which to organize the variety of research findings on personality and substance use. Although hundreds of personality traits have been described and dozens have been discussed in relation to substance use (e.g., sensation seeking, conformity, alienation, rebelliousness), it is possible to understand all of these traits as one of the five basic dimensions. These basic traits can also help us understand the high rates of co-morbidity between substance use and other mental health problems. Specifically, high levels of neuroticism are characteristic of all forms of psychopathology and, to the extent that high levels of neuroticism also characterize substance use disorders, this may explain the high rates of comorbidity. Similarly, the high comorbidity between substance use and antisocial behavior might be explained by low constraint. The structural model described previously may provide viable alternative explanations to some findings in the literature. For example, several theories of substance use posit that substance use occurs in the face of high levels of life stress in conjunction with an absence of available, active coping responses (Wills & Filer, 1996). The trait model suggests that high levels of stress and inadequate coping may both be manifestations of high neuroticism rather than separate factors.

These findings suggest that teaching coping strategies to children to prepare them for stressful life events or that the early identification and referral for support services for children who experience stress would reduce drug abusing behaviors. Researchers such as Kellam (Kellam et al., 1994) have found that shy aggressive children, particularly boys, are most at risk to abuse drugs in adolescence. For this reason, he and his colleagues designed a program for children in grades one and two, that address anti-social behavior and improves academic performance. A study was conducted in Baltimore where teachers were trained in the Good Behavior Game and Mastery programs. The results of this study are very promising in reducing substance abuse and other negative behaviors.

CONCLUSION: INTEGRATING BASIC SCIENCES RESEARCH WITH PREVENTION

This chapter has discussed three different research perspectives from the basic sciences, and attempted to show how each can inform our understanding of prevention science and practice. The final section of the chapter attempts to document that it is possible for investigators in such disparate areas of the basic sciences to infuence each other's research—as can be seen in research being undertaken at the Center for Prevention Research at the University of Kentucky, under the direction of Richard Clayton.

A guiding principle of the Center's research protocols is that sensation seeking is a starting point for designing more effective drug-abuse prevention programs. It appears to be the most widely studied personality trait in the area of substance abuse (Lynam et al., 2002), and a recent meta-analytic review (Derzon & Lipsey, 1999) found that it is among the most potent risk factors for substance use.

Although sensation seeking, as originally conceptualized by Zuckerman (1994), is a human personality trait, Bardo and his colleagues have demonstrated that this trait translates nicely into animal research and that neuroscientific studies can advance our understanding of human drug use and abuse. Specifically, Bardo has used an animal model to study the relation between novelty, or sensation, seeking and the rewarding effects of amphetamine. As Bardo et al. (1996) argue, novelty in the environment may operate similarly to stimulant drugs by activating the mesolimbic dopamine reward system. Such findings from the neuroscientific literature may help explain the increased risk of individuals with high scores in sensation seeking and may offer some insights into possible mechanisms of prevention. Specifically, if novelty-seeking and drug-seeking behavior involve a similar brain system, then novel stimuli might substitute for drugs.

Stimulated by the findings from Bardo's animal investigations of novelty seeking, Kelly and his colleagues have undertaken behavioral pharmacology studies of individuals scoring high or low in sensation seeking. The individuals being used in these ongoing studies, while having some history of exposure to stimulant drugs prior to the study, do not have a history indicative of a diagnosis for substance abuse disorder. The goal of these studies is to determine whether differences in sensation seeking may predict responses to various drugs of abuse. Results obtained thus far have shown that individuals high or low in sensation seeking differ significantly in their behavioral responses to both amphetamine and diazepam, as well as in drug discrimination trials. These results are consistent with the animal studies suggesting that sensation seeking may reflect differences in biological susceptibility to drugs of abuse.

Lynam and his colleagues have investigated how personality traits, such as sensation seeking, may be mediated by environmental factors in accounting for increased rates of drug use. Specifically, Lynam et al. (2002) have found that approximately half of the variance in the relation between sensation seeking and drug use is accounted for by more proximal cognitive and interpersonal risk factors, such as peer drug use, drug expectancies, and drug-refusal skills. What this means is that children and adolescents who are rated as high in sensation seeking are more likely to place themselves in situations or develop attitudes that are conducive to drug use. More importantly, it is these environmental mediators, rather than underlying biological mechanisms, that should be amenable to prevention interventions.

Finally, Donohew and his colleagues have focused their research on using messages in public service announcements (PSAs) to prevent or attenuate drug use among children and adolescents. Building on the research documenting a relation between sensation seeking and drug use, Donohew et al. (1991) argue that such messages should be targeted at high-sensation-seeking individuals, those most at risk for drug use or abuse. More importantly, the PSAs must be designed to capture the attention of and appeal to at-risk individuals. They need to be novel, arousing, unconventional, and fast paced, if they are to reach the target audience. In one study, Palmgreen et al. (1994) found that high sensation seeking individuals were more likely to call a telephone hotline number presented at the end of these PSAs. Field-based population studies are currently underway to determine whether the implementation and withdrawal of these PSAs systematically alter the rates of drug use in two different communities.

In this chapter, we have presented three distinct lines of basic science investigations, and the implications of each line for prevention science. Although each line has its preferred level of analyses, method of research, and explanatory constructs, we believe that our understanding of drug abuse and its treatment will be best advanced by investigators who are able to talk across these lines of inquiry. It seems unreasonable to believe that drug use has a single simple cause. Our theories and lines of investigation should acknowledge this.

REFERENCES

Ahmed, S. H., & Koob, G. F. (1997). Cocaine- but not food-seeking behavior is reinstated by stress after extinction. *Psychopharmacology, 132,* 289–295.

Bardo, M. T. (1998). Neuropharmacological mechanisms of drug reward: Beyond dopamine in the nucleus accumbens. *Critical Reviews in Neurobiology, 12,* 37–67.

Bardo, M. T., Bowling, Rowlett, J. K., Manderscheid, P., Buxton, S. T., & Dwoskin, L. P. (1995). Environmental enrichment attenuates locomotor sensitization, but not in vitro dopamine release, induced by amphetamine. *Pharmacology, Biochemistry & Behavior, 51,* 397–405.

Bardo, M. T., Donohew, R. L., & Harrington, N. G. (1996). Psychobiology of novelty seeking and drug seeking behavior. *Behavioural Brain Research, 77,* 23–43.

Bardo, M. T., Klebaur, J. E., Valone, J. M., & Deaton, C. (2001). Environmental enrichment decreases intravenous self-administration of amphetamine in female and male rats. *Psychopharmacology, 155,* 278–284.

Barrick, M. R., & Mount, M. K. (1991). The big five personality dimensions and job performance: A meta analysis. *Personnel Psychology, 44,* 1–24.

Bekhterev, V. M. (1932). *General principles of human reflexology.* New York: International Press.

Benjamin, J., Li, L., Patterson, C., Greenberg, B. D., Murphy, D. L., & Hamer, D. H. (1996). Population and familial association between the D4 dopamine receptor gene and measures of novelty seeking. *Nature Genetics, 12,* 81–84.

Bickel, W. K., & Kelly, T. H. (1997). Stimulus control processes in drug taking: Implications for treatment. In D. M. Baer, & E. M. Pinkston (Eds.), *Environment and behavior* (pp. 185–193). Boulder, CO: Westview Press.

Bouchard, T. J., Lykken, D. T., McGue, M., Segal, N. L., & Tellegen, A. (1990). Sources of human psychological differences: The Minnesota Study of Twins Reared Apart. *Science, 250,* 223–228.

Botvin, G. J., Baker, E., Dusenbury, L., Botvin, E. M., & Diaz, T. (1995). Long-term follow-up results of a randomized drug abuse prevention trial in a white middle-class population. *Journal of the American Medical Association, 273,* 1106–1112.

Bowling, S. L., & Bardo, M. T. (1994). Locomotor and rewarding effects of amphetamine in enriched, social and isolate reared rats. *Pharmacology, Biochemistry & Behavior, 48,* 459–464.

Bowling, S. L., Rowlett, J. K., & Bardo, M. T. (1993). The effect of environmental enrichment on amphetamine-stimulated locomotor activity, dopamine synthesis and dopamine release. *Neuropharmacology, 32,* 885–893.

Caraballo, R. S., Giovini, G. A., Pehacek, T. F., Mowery, P. D., Richter, P. A., Strauss, W. J., Sharp, D. J., Eriksen, M. P., Pirkle, J. L., & Maurer, K. R. (1998). Racial and ethnic differences in serum cotinine levels of cigarette smokers. *Journal of the American Medical Association, 280,* 135–139.

Carroll, K. M., Rounsaville, B. J., Gordon, L. T., Nich, C., Jatlow, P., Bisighini, R. M., & Gawin, F. H. (1994). Psychotherapy and pharmacotherapy for ambulatory cocaine abusers. *Archives of General Psychiatry, 51,* 177–187.

Caspi, A. (1997). Personality development across the life course. In W. Damon (Series Editor) & N. Eisenberg (Volume Editor), *Handbook of child psychology, Volume 3: Social, emotional, and personality development* (pp. 311–388). New York: Wiley.

Caspi, A., Moffitt, T. E., Silva, P. A., Stouthamer-Loeber, M., Krueger, R. F., & Schmutte, P. S. (1994). Are some people crime-prone? Replications of the personality-crime relationships across countries, genders, races, and methods. *Criminology, 32,* 163–195.

Chassin, L., Curran, P. J., Hussong, A. M., & Colder, C. R. (1996). The relation of parent alcoholism to adolescent substance use: A longitudinal follow-up study. *Journal of Abnormal Psychology, 105,* 70–80.

Cloninger, C. R., & Begleiter, H. (Eds., 1990). *Genetics and biology of addiction.* New York: Cold Spring Harbor Press.

Conley, J. J. (1984). The hierarchy of consistency: A review and model of longitudinal findings on adult individual differences in intelligence, personality, and self-opinion. *Personality and Individual Differences, 5,* 11–25.

Costa, P. T., & McCrae, R. R. (1988). Personality in adulthood: A six-year longitudinal of self-reports and spouse ratings on the NEO Personality Inventory. *Journal of Personality and Social Psychology, 54,* 853–863.

Costa, P. T., & McCrae, R. R. (1992). Four ways five factors are basic. *Personality and Individual Differences, 13,* 653–665.

Costa, P. T., McCrae, R. R., & Dye, D. A. (1991). Facet scales for Agreeableness and Conscientiousness: A revision of the NEO Personality Inventory. *Personality and Individual Differences, 12,* 887–898.

Crabbe, J. C., Belknap, J. K., Mitchell, S. R., & Crawshaw, L. I. (1994). Quantitative trait loci mapping of genes that influence the sensitivity and tolerance to ethanol-induced hypothermia in BXD recombinant inbred mice. *Journal of Pharmacology & Experimental Therapeutics, 269,* 184–192.

Crabbe, J. C., & Phillips, T. J. (1998). Genetics of alcohol and other abused drugs. *Drug and Alcohol Dependence, 51,* 61–71.

Dellu, F., Mayo, W., Vallee, M. Maccari, S., Piazza, P. V., Le Moal, M., & Simon, H. (1996). Behavioral reactivity to novelty during youth as a predictive factor of stress-induced corticosterone secretion in the elderly: a life-span study in rats. *Psychoneuroendocrinology, 21,* 441–453.

Depue, R. A. (1996). A neurobiological framework for the structure of personality and emotion: Implications for personality disorders. In J. F. Clarkin & M. F. Lenzenweger (Eds.), *Major theories of personality disorder* (pp. 347–390). New York: Guilford.

Depue, R. A., Luciana, M., Arbisi, P., Collins, P., & Leon, A. (1994). Dopamine and the structure of personality: Relation of agonist-induced dopamine activity to positive emotionality. *Journal of Personality and Social Psychology, 67,* 485–498.

Derzon, J. H., & Lipsey, M. W. (1999). What good predictors of marijuana use are good for: A synthesis of research. *School Psychology International, 20,* 69–85.

Donohew, R. L., Lorch, E. P., & Palmgreen, P. (1991). Sensation seeking and targeting of televised anti-drug PSAs. In L. Donohew, H. Sypher, & W. Bukoski (Eds.), *Persuasive communication and drug abuse prevention* (pp. 209–226). Hillsdale, CA: Lawrence Erlbaum.

Donohew, L., Palmgreen, P., & Lorch, E. P. (1994). Attention, need for sensation, and health communication campaigns. *American Behavioral Scientist, 38,* 310–322.

Ebstein, R. P., Novick, O., Umansky, R., Priel, B., Osher, Y., Blaine, D., Bennett, E. R., Nemanov, L., Katz, M., & Belmaker, R. H. (1996). Dopamine D4 receptor (D4DR) exon III polymorphism associated with the human personality trait of novelty seeking. *Nature Genetics, 12,* 78–80.

Epstein, E., & Guttman, R. (1984). Mate selection in man: Evidence, theory, and outcome. *Social Biology, 31,* 243–278.

Epstein, S. (1979). The stability of behavior: I. On predicting most of the people much of the time. *Journal of Personality and Social Psychology, 37,* 1097–1126.

Falk, J. L. (1983). Drug dependence: Myth or motive? *Pharmacology Biochemistry and Behavior, 19,* 385–391.

Flory, K., Lynam, D. R., Milich, R., Leukefeld, C., & Clayton, R. (in press). Personality correlates of substance use, anti-social behavior, and internalizing problems among young adults. *Experimental and Clinical Psychopharmacology.*

Fowler, S. C., Johnson, J. S., Kallman, M. J., Liou, J. R., Wilson, M. C., & Hikal, A. M. (1993). In a drug discrimination procedure isolation-reared rats generalized to lower doses of cocaine and amphetamine than rats raised in an enriched environment. *Psychopharmacology, 110,* 115–118.

Friedman, H. S., Tucker, J. S., Schwartz, J. E., Tomlinson-Keasy, C., Martin, L. R., Wingard, D. L., & Criqui, M. H. (1995). Psychosocial and behavioral predictors of longevity. *American Psychologist, 50,* 69–78.

Gauvin, D. V., Vanecek, S. A., Baird, T. J., Briscoe, R. J., Vallett, M., & Holloway, F. A. (1998). Genetic selection of alcohol preference can be countered by conditioning processes. *Alcohol, 15,* 199–206.

Griffiths, R. R., Bigelow, G. E., & Henningfield, J. E. (1980). Similarities in animal and human drug taking behavior. In N. K. Mello (Ed.), *Advances in Substance Abuse: Behavioral and Biological Research* (pp. 1–90). Greenwich, CT: Jai Press Inc.

Haertzen, C. A., Kocher, T. R., & Miyasato, K. (1986). Reinforcement from the first drug experience can predict later drug habits and/or addiction: Results with coffee, cigarettes, alcohol, barbiturates, minor and major tranquilizers, stimulants, marijuana, hallucinogens, heroin, opiates and cocaine. *Drug and Alcohol Dependence, 11,* 147–165.

Hawkins, J. D., Catalano, R. F., & Miller, J. Y. (1992). Risk and protective factors for alcohol and other drug problems in adolescence and early adulthood: Implications for substance abuse prevention. *Psychological Bulletin, 112,* 64–105.

Higgins, S. T., Budney, A. J., Bickel, W. K., Hughes. J. R., Foerg, F., & Badger, G. (1993). Achieving cocaine abstinence with a behavioral approach. *American Journal of Psychiatry, 150,* 763–769.

Jackson, D. N., & Paunonen, S. V. (1985). Construct validity and the predictability of behavior. *Journal of Personality and Social Psychology, 49,* 554–570.

John, O. P. (1990). The 'Big Five' factor taxonomy: Dimensions of personality in the natural language and questionnaires. In L. A. Pervin (Ed.), *Handbook of personality: Theory and research* (pp. 66–100). New York: Guilford.

John, O. P., Caspi, A., Robins, R. W., Moffitt, T. E., & Stouthamer-Loeber, M. (1994). The 'Little Five': Exploring the nomological network of the Five-Factor Model of personality in adolescent boys. *Child Development, 65,* 160–178.

Johnson, E. O., van den Bree, M. B. M., & Pickens, R. W. (1996). Subtypes of alcohol-dependent men: A typology based on relative genetic and environmental loading. *Alcoholism: Clinical and Experimental Research, 20,* 1472–1480.

Jones, S. R., Gainetdinov, R. R., Wightman, R. M., & Caron, M. G. (1998). Mechanisms of amphetamine action revealed in mice lacking the dopamine transporter. *Journal of Neuroscience, 18,* 1979–1986.

Kamien, J. B., Bickel, W. K., Hughes, J. R., Higgins, S. T., & Smith, B. J. (1993). Drug discrimination by humans compared to nonhumans: Current status and future directions. *Psychopharmacology, 111,* 259–270.

Kellam, S. G., Rebok, G. W., Ialongo, N., & Mayer, L. S. (1994). The course and malleability of aggressive behavior from early first grade into middle school: Results of a development epidemiologically-based preventive trial. *Journal of Child Psychology and Psychiatry, 35,* 359–382.

Koepp, M. J., Gunn, R. N., Lawrence, A. D., Cunningham, V. J., Dagher, A., Jones, T., Brooks, D. J., Bench, C. J., & Grasby, P. M. (1998). Evidence for striatal dopamine release during a video game. *Nature, 393,* 266–268.

Kreek, M. J., & Koob, G. F. (1998). Drug dependence: stress and dysregulation of brain reward pathways. *Drug and Alcohol Dependence, 51,* 23–47.

Krueger, R. F., Caspi, A., Moffitt, T. E., Silva, P. A., & McGee, R. (1996). Personality Qtraits are differentially linked to mental disorders: A multitrait-multidiagnosis study of an adolescent birth cohort. *Journal of Abnormal Psychology, 105,* 299–312.

Lee, V. L. (1988). *Beyond Behaviorism.* Hillsdale, NJ: Lawrence Erlbaum Associates.

Lodish, H., Baltimore, D., Berk, A., Zipursky, S. L., Matsudaira, P., & Darnell, J. (1995). *Molecular cell biology.* New York: Freeman.

Lynam, D. R., Milich, R., Miller, J. D., Flory, K., & Clayton, R. (2002). The indirect effects of sensation seeking on drug use. Submitted for publication.

Lytton, H. (1990). Child and parent effects in boys' conduct disorder. *Developmental Psychology, 26,* 683–697.

Maccoby, E. E., & Jacklin, C. N. (1983). The "person" characteristics of children and the family as environment. In D. Magnusson & V. L. Allen (Eds.), *Human development: An interactional perspective* (pp. 75–92). San Diego, CA: Academic Press.

Masse, L. C., & Tremblay, R. E. (1997). Behavior of boys in kindergarten and the onset of substance use during adolescence. *Archives of General Psychiary, 54,* 62–68.

Meisch, R. A., & Stewart, R. B. (1999). Animal research: Drug self-administration. In R. J. M. Niesink, R. M. A. Jaspers, L. M. W. Kornet, & J. M. van Ree (Eds.), *Drugs of abuse and addiction: Neurobehavioral toxicology* (pp. 64–97). Boca Raton, FL: CRC Press.

Mischel, W. (1968). *Personality and assessment.* New York: Wiley.

National Institute on Drug Abuse (1998). *National survey results on drug use from the monitoring the future study, 1975–1997. Volume 1: Secondary School Students.* NIH Publication No. 98-4345.

Newlin, D. B. (1992). A comparison of drug conditioning and craving for alcohol and cocaine. In M. Galanter (Ed.), *Recent developments in alcoholism: Alcohol and cocaine: similarities and differences, Vol. 10* (pp. 147–164). New York: Plenum Press.

Newlin, D. B. (1986). Conditioned compensatory response to alcohol placebo in humans. *Psychopharmacology, 88,* 247–251.

Norman, W. T., & Goldberg, L. R. (1963). Raters, ratees, and randomness in personality structure. *Journal of Personality and Social Psychology, 4,* 681–691.

O'Brien, C. P., Childress, A. R., McLellan, A. T., & Ehrman, R. (1992). A learning model of addiction. In C. P. O'Brien & J. H. Jaffe (Eds.), *Addictive States* (pp. 157–177). New York: Raven Press.

Olweus, D. (1980). Familial and temperamental determinants of aggressive-behavior in adolescent boys: A causal analysis. *Developmental Psychology, 16,* 644–660.

Palmgreen, P., Lorch, E. P., Donohew, L., Harrington, N. G., Dsilva, M., & Helm, D. (1994). Reaching at-risk populations in a mass media drug abuse prevention campaign: Sensation seeking as a targeting variable. *Drugs and Society, 8,* 29–45.

Pavlov, I. P. (1927). *Conditioned reflexes.* Oxford: Oxford University Press.

Pentz, M. A., Dwyer, J. H., MacKinnon, D. P., Flay, B. R., Hansen, W. B., Wang, E. Y., & Johnson, C. A. (1989). A multi-community trial for primary prevention of adolescent drug abuse: Effects on drug use prevalence. *Journal of the American Medical Association, 21,* 3259–3266.

Perez-Stable, E. J., Herrera, B., Jacob, P., & Benowitz, N. L. (1998). Nicotine metabolism and intake in black and white smokers. *Journal of the American Medical Association, 280,* 152–156.

Petraitis, J., Flay, B. R., & Miller, T. Q. (1995). Reviewing theories of adolescent substance use: Organizing pieces of the puzzle. *Psychological Bulletin, 117,* 67–68.

Pianezza, M. L., Sellers, E. M., & Tyndale, R. (1998). Nicotine metabolism defect reduces smoking. *Nature, 393,* 750.

Piazza, P. V., Deminiere, J. M., Le Moal, M., & Simon, H. (1990). Stress- and pharmacologically-induced behavioral sensitization increases vulnerability to acquisition of amphetamine self-administration. *Brain Research, 514,* 22–26.

Preston, K. L., & Bigelow, G. E. (1991). Subjective and discriminative effects of drugs. *Behavioural Pharmacology, 2,* 293–313.

Rahdert, E., Sloboda, Z., & Czechowicz, D. (1995). *Adolescent drug abuse: Clinical assessment and therapeutic interventions.* National Institute on Drug Abuse, Monograph 156.

Quiggle, N. L., Garber, J., Panak, W. F., & Dodge, K. A. (1992). Social information processing in aggressive and depressed children. *Child Development, 63,* 1305–1320.

Rebec, G. V., Christensen, J. R. C., Guerra, C., & Bardo, M. T. (1997). Regional and temporal differences in real-time dopamine efflux in the nucleus accumbens during free-choice novelty. *Brain Research, 776,* 61–67.

Reige, W. H., & Morimoto, H. (1970). Effects of chronic stress and differential environments upon brain weights and biogenic amine levels in rats. *Journal of Comparative & Physiological Psychology, 71,* 396–404.

Renner, M. J., & Rosenzweig, M. R. (1987). *Enriched and impoverished environments: effects on brain and behavior.* New York: Springer-Verlag.

Rescorla, R. A. (1967). Pavlovian conditioning and its proper control procedures. *Psychological Review, 74,* 71–80.

Ritz, M. C. (1999a). Molecular mechanisms of addictive substances. In R. J. M. Niesink, R. M. A. Jaspers, L. M. W. Kornet, & J. M. van Ree (Eds.), *Drugs of Abuse and Addiction: Neurobehavioral Toxicology* (pp. 150–189). Boca Raton, FL: CRC Press.

Ritz, M. C. (1999b). Reward systems and addictive behavior. In R. J. M. Niesink, R. M. A. Jaspers, L. M. W. Kornet, & J. M. van Ree (Eds.), *Drugs of abuse and addiction: Neurobehavioral toxicology* (pp. 124–149). Boca Raton, FL: CRC Press.

Rosenzweig, M. R., Krech, D., Bennett, E. L., & Diamond, M. C. (1962). Effects of environmental complexity and training on brain chemistry and anatomy: A replication and extension. *Journal of Comparative & Physiological Psychology, 55*, 429–437.

Rutter, M., Dunn, J., Plomin, R., Simonoff, E., Pickles, A., Maughan, B., Ormel, J., Meyer, J., & Eaves, L. (1997). Integrating nature and nurture: Implications of person-environment correlations and interactions for developmental psychopathology. *Development and Psychopathology, 9*, 335–364.

Samson, H. H., Pfeffer, A. O., & Tolliver, G. A. (1988). Oral ethanol self-administration in rats: Models of alcohol-seeking behavior. *Alcoholism: Clinical and experimental research, 12*, 591–598.

Scarr, S., & McCartney, K. (1983). How people make their own environments: A theory of genotype—Environment effects. *Child Development, 54*, 424–435.

Shedler, J., & Block, J. (1990). Adolescent drug use and psychological health: A longitudinal inquiry. *American Psychologist, 45*, 612–630.

Sher, K. J., & Trull, T. J. (1994). Personality and disinhibitory psychopathology: Alcoholism and antisocial personlaity disorder. *Journal of Abnormal Psychology, 103*, 92–102.

Siegel, S. (1978). Morphine tolerance: Is there evidence for a conditioning model? *Science, 200*, 343–344.

Siegel, S., Hinson, R. E., Krank, M. D., & McCully, J. (1982). Heroin 'overdose' death: Contribution of drug-associated environmental cues. *Science, 216*, 436–437.

Silverman, K., Higgins, S. T., Brooner, R. K., Montoya, I. D., Cone, E. J., Schuster, C. R., & Preston, K. L. (1996). Sustained cocaine abstinence, in methadone maintenance patients through voucher-based reinforcement therapy. *Archives of General Psychiatry, 53*, 409–415.

Sirevaag, A. M., & Greenough, W. T. (1988). A multivariate statistical summary of synaptic plasticity measures in rats exposed to complex, social and individual environments. *Brain Research, 441*, 386–392.

Skinner, B. F. (1938). *The behavior of organisms.* New York: Appleton–Cemtury–Crofts.

Smith, J. K., Neill, J. C., & Costall, B. (1997). Post-weaning housing conditions influence the behavioral effects of cocaine and d-amphetamine. *Psychopharmacology, 131*, 23–33.

Sora, I., Wichems, C., Takahashi, N., Li, X., Zeng, Z., Revay, R., Lesch, K., Murphy, D. L., & Uhl, G. R. (1998). Cocaine reward models: conditioned place preference can be established in dopamine- and in serotonin-transporter knockout mice. *Proceedings of the National Academy of Sciences USA, 95*, 7699–7704.

Spoont, M. R. (1992). Modulatory role of serotonin in neural information processing: Implications for human psychopathology. *Psychological Bulletin, 112*, 330–350.

Tai, B., Chiang, N., & Bridge, P. (1997). *Medication development for the treatment of cocaine dependence: Issues in clinical efficacy trials.* National Institute on Drug Abuse Research Monograph Series 175. Rockville, MD: U.S. Department of Health and Human Services, National Institutes of Health Publication No. 98-4125.

Tarter, R. E., & Kirisci, L. (1997). The Drug Use Screening Inventory for adults: psychometric structure and discriminative sensitivity. *American Journal of Drug and Alcohol Abuse, 23*(2), 207–219.

Tellegen, A., Lykken, D. T., Bouchard, T. J., Wilcox, K. J., Segal, N. L., & Rich, S. (1988). Personality similarity in twins reared apart and together. *Journal of Personality and Social Psychology, 54*, 1031–1039.

Thompson, T. (1984). Behavioral mechanisms of drug dependence. In T. Thompson, P. B. Dews, & J. E. Barrett (Eds.), *Advances in behavioral pharmacology, Vol. 4* (pp. 2–45). New York: Academic Press.

Thompson, T. T., & Schuster, C. R. (1968). *Behavioral Pharmacology.* Englewood Cliffs, NJ: Prentice-Hall.

Tobler, N. S. (1992). Drug prevention programs can work: Research findings. *Journal of Addictive Diseases, 11*(3), 1–28.

Trull. T. J., & Sher, K. J. (1994). Relationship between the five-factor model of personlaity and axis I disorders in a nonclinical sample. *Journal of Abnormal Psychology, 103*, 350–360.

Uhl, G., Blum, K., Noble, E., & Smith, S. (1993). Substance abuse vulnerability and D2 receptor genes. *Trends in Neuroscience, 16*, 83–88.

Vandenbergh, D. J., Zonderman, A. B., Wang, J., Uhl, G. R., & Costa, P. T. (1997). No association between novelty seeking and dopamine D4 receptor (D4DR) exon III seven repeat alleles in Baltimore longitudinal study of aging participants. *Molecular Psychiatry, 2*, 417–419.

Watson, D., Clark, L. A., & Harkness, A. R. (1994). Structures of personality and their revelance to psychopathology. *Journal of Abnormal Psychology, 103*, 18–31.

Watson, J. B. (1914). *Behavior: An introduction to comparative psychology.* New York: Holt.

Wells, E., Peterson, P., Gainey, J., Hawkins, J. D., & Catalano, R. (1994). Outpatient treatment for cocaine abuse: A controlled comparison of relapse prevention and twelve-step approaches. *American Journal of Drug and Alcohol Abuse, 20*, 1–17.

Wiggins, J. S. (1968). Personality structure. In P. R. Farnsworth, M. R. Rosenzweig, & J. T. Polefka (Eds.), *Annual review of social psychology, Vol 19*(pp. 293–350). Palo Alto, CA: Annual Reviews.

Wikler, A. (1948). Recent progress in research on the neurophysiological basis of morphine addiction. *American Journal of Psychiatry, 105*, 329–338.

Wills, T. A., DuHamel, K., & Vaccaro, D. (1995). Activity and mood temperament as predictors of adolescent substance use: Test of a self-regulation mediational model. *Journal of Personality and Social Psychology, 68,* 901–916.

Wills, T. A., & Filer, M. (1996). Stress-coping model of adolescent substance use. In T. H. Ollendick, & R. J. Prinz (Eds.), *Advances in clinical child psychology, Vol 18* (pp. 91–132). New York: Plenum.

Wills, T. A., Windle, M., & Cleary, S. D. (1998). Temperament and novelty seeking in adolescent substance use: convergence of dimensions of temperament with constructs from Cloninger's theory. *Journal of Personality & Social Psychology, 74,* 387–406.

Winterfeld, K. T., Teuchert-Noodt, G., & Dawirs, R. R. (1998). Social environment alters both ontogeny of dopamine innervation of the medial prefrontal cortex and maturation of working memory in gerbils (*Meriones unguiculatus*). *Journal of Neuroscience Research, 52,* 201–209.

Zuckerman, M. (1994). *Behavioral expressions and biosocial bases of sensation seeking.* Cambridge UK: Cambridge.

CHAPTER 23

Cross-National Comparisons of Co-Morbidities between Substance Use Disorders and Mental Disorders

Ronald C. Kessler

Sergio Aguilar-Gaxiola

Laura Andrade

Rob Bijl

Luiz Guilherme Borges

Jorge J. Caraveo-Anduaga

David J. DeWit

Bo Kolody

Kathleen R. Merikangas

Beth E. Molnar

William A. Vega

Ellen E. Walters

Hans-Ulrich Wittchen

INTRODUCTION

The majority of current substance abusers in the United States have one or more mental disorders, according to studies of diagnostic patterns in community samples (Grant & Harford, 1995; Merikangas et al., 1996; Regier et al., 1990) as well as in clinical samples (Allan, 1995; Mirin et al., 1991; Penick et al., 1994). Two separate patterns are involved. First, there are strong lifetime co-morbidities between substance use disorders and mental disorders in the United States (Kessler et al., 1996; Regier et al., 1990). Second, co-morbidity is associated with chronicity of both substance use disorders and mental disorders (Kranzler, Del Boca, & Rounsaville, 1996; Hirschfeld et al., 1990; Keitner et al., 1991), leading to higher rates of episode co-morbidity than of lifetime co-morbidity (Kessler, 1997).

Co-morbid mental disorders create problems for the treatment of substance use disorders, especially when the abused substances are used to self medicate dysphoric moods. In cases of this sort, recurrence of dysphoria can precipitate relapse of substance abuse (George et al., 1990). In addition, the substance use disorders are associated with high rates of relapse in substance use, aimed at avoiding withdrawal and self-medication of withdrawal symptoms. Furthermore, because of the greater burden of having two disorders, people with co-morbidity are typically more impaired and at greater risk of suicide than are patients with a pure substance use disorder (Hirschfield et al., 1990; Merikangas & Stevens, 1998; Sheehan, 1993).

Epidemiologic studies in the United States clearly show that mental disorders usually occur at an earlier age than do substance use disorders, that the median time interval between first onset of primary mental disorders and first onset of secondary substance use disorders is 5 years or more, that primary mental disorders predict the subsequent first onset of substance use disorders, and that the highest risk of severe secondary substance use disorders is found among people whose mental disorders begin during either childhood or adolescence (Kessler et al., 1996, 1997). These findings raise the interesting possibility that successful outreach and treatment of youth with primary mental disorders might help prevent the onset of substance use disorders (Kessler & Price, 1993).

Although the great majority of research on co-morbid substance and mental disorders has been carried out in the United States, two recent reports extend some of the results of that research to other countries. The first comes from a MacArthur Foundation task force that supports parallel reanalyses of epidemiological survey data from a number of countries (Merikangas et al., 1996) in order to study basic patterns of co-morbidity between substance use disorders and mental disorders. These analyses document consistently significant co-morbidity of lifetime substance use disorders with lifetime anxiety and depressive disorders in all countries studied. The second report,

RONALD C. KESSLER AND ELLEN E. WALTERS • Department of Health Care Policy, Harvard Medical School, Boston, Massachusetts 02115
SERGIO AGUILAR-GAXIOLA • Department of Psychology, California State University at Fresno, Fresno, California 93740
LAURA ANDRADE • Instituto de Psiquiatria, Universidate de Sao Paulo, Sao Paulo, Brazil 05403-010
LUIZ GUILHERME BORGES • Departamento de Investigaciones en Servicios de Salud, Calzada, Mexico
JORGE J. CARAVEO-ANDUAGA • Instituto Mexicana de Psiquiatria, Huipulco, Mexico
ROB BIJL • Netherlands Institute of Mental Health, Utrecht, Netherlands 3502 JC
DAVID J. DEWIT • Addiction Research Foundation, London, Ontario N6G 4X8
BO KOLODY • Sociology Department, San Diego State University, San Diego, California 92182
KATHLEEN R. MERIKANGAS • National Institute of Mental Health, National Institutes of Health, Bethesda, Maryland 20892-2670
BETH E. MOLNAR. • Havard School of Public Health, Harvard University, Boston, MA 02115
WILLIAM A. VEGA • Institute for Quality Research and Training, Robert Wood Johnson Medical School—UMDNJ, New Brunswick, NJ 08901
HANS-ULRICH WITTCHEN • Max Planck Institute of Psychiatry, Muënchën, Germany 80804

from the World Health Organization's International Consortium in Psychiatric Epidemiology (ICPE) (Merikangas et al., 1998), analyzed data from general population surveys in six countries to investigate age of onset distributions based on retrospective reports. The results clearly show that co-morbid mental disorders typically have ages of onset that predate the onset of substance use disorders (Merikangas et al., 1998).

This chapter builds on these two cross-national studies by presenting data on the associations between primary mental disorders and the subsequent first onset of substance use disorders. The analyses are based on ICPE surveys carried out in six countries: Canada, the United States, Mexico, Brazil, the Netherlands, and Germany. We begin by presenting aggregate data on the strength of associations between particular primary mental disorders and later substance disorders in a pooled data set that combines results from 11 countries. We then present country-specific results that estimate the proportion of all causes of substance use disorder that can be traced to prior mental disorders. The chapter closes with a discussion of clinical implications and future research needs.

METHODS

Samples

Seven surveys carried out in six countries are included in the analysis. The surveys were carried out in North America, Latin America, and Europe, with a total sample size of 28,658. All surveys were based on general population probability samples rather than on patient samples or quota samples of the general population. All interviews were carried out face to face rather than on the telephone or through mail questionnaires. See Table 23.1

FRESNO COUNTY. The Mexican American Prevalence and Services Survey interviewed a stratified, multistage clustered area probability sample of household residents of Mexican or Mexican-American origin residing in Fresno County, California (Vega et al., 1998). The age range was from 18 to 59. Separate strata with target sample sizes of 1,000 each were interviewed in the city of Fresno, in towns and villages elsewhere in the county, and in rural parts of the county, for a total sample size of 3,012. Fieldwork was carried out from 1995 to 1997. The 2,874 respondents between 18 and 54 years of age are included in this report. The response rate in screened eligible households was 90.0%.

TABLE 23.1. Sample Characteristics

	Age range	Sample size	Response rate (%)
Study site			
São Paulo (Brazil)	18–64	(1179)	65.2
Fresno (CA)	18–54	(2874)	90.0
Munich (Germany)	14–24	(3021)	71.1
Mexico City (Mexico)	18–54	(1734)	60.4
Netherlands	18–64	(7076)	70.0
Ontario (Canada)	15–54	(6902)	88.1
United States	15–54	(8098)	82.4

NOTE. From "Comorbidity of Substance Use Disorders with Mood and Anxiety Disorders: Results of the International Consortium in Psychiatric Epidemiology," by K. R. Merikangas, R. L. Mehta, B. E. Molnar, E. E. Walters, J. D. Swendsen, S. Aguilar-Gaziola, R. Bijl, G. Borges, J. J. Caraveo-Anduaga, D. J. Dewit, B. Kolody, W. A. Vega, H.-U. Wittchen and R. C. Kessler,1998, *Addictive Behaviors, 23* p. 895. Copyright 1998 by Elsevier Science Ltd. Adapted with permission.

MUNICH, GERMANY. The Early Developmental Stages of Psychopathology Study interviewed a stratified random sample of 3,021 residents of Munich between 14 and 25 years of age as the baseline of a three-wave prospective study (Wittchen et al., 1996). The sample was drawn from the official population registry of the greater Munich area, and stratification was based on demographic characteristics available in the registry. Predesignated respondents in the age range of 14 to 15 were oversampled. Fieldwork was carried out in 1995. The baseline response rate was 71.1%, with an additional 4% giving partial information.

MEXICO CITY, MEXICO. The Epidemiology of Psychiatric Co-morbidity Project interviewed a stratified multistage clustered area probability sample of household residents in a subsample of the 16 political divisions of the city (Caraveo, Martinez, & Rivera, 1998). The age range of the sample was from 18 to 65, with a total sample size of 1,932. Fieldwork was carried out in 1995. The 1,734 respondents between 18 and 54 years of age are included in the report. The response rate was 60.4%.

THE NETHERLANDS. The Netherlands Mental Health Survey and Incidence Study interviewed a nationally representative household sample as the baseline of a three-wave prospective study (Bijl et al., 1998). The sample was drawn using a multistage clustered area probability design. The age range was from 18 to 64. Fieldwork was carried out in 1996. The total sample size of the baseline survey was 7,076. The baseline response rate was 70.0%.

ONTARIO, CANADA. The Mental Health Supplement to the Ontario Health Survey interviewed a stratified subsample of 6,902 people residing in households that participated in the Ontario Health Survey (OHS) (Offord et al., 1994). The OHS was based on a stratified, multistage area probability sample of the Ontario household population. Residents of remote areas, aboriginal peoples living on reserves, long-term psychiatric patients, and prison inmates were excluded from the sample. The OHS response rate was 88.1%, while the conditional response rate of the MHS was 77.8%. Fieldwork was carried out in 1990 and 1991.

SÃO PAULO, BRAZIL. The Epidemiological Catchment Area Study in the City of São Paulo interviewed a stratified area probability sample of 1,464 residents of the catchment area of the University of São Paulo Medical Centre. Stratification was based on age with an oversampling of those aged 18 to 24 and older than 59. The design allowed for multiple respondents per household. The age range was from 18 to older than 80. Fieldwork was carried out from 1994 to1996. The 1,179 respondents in the age range of 18 to 64 are included in the report. The response rate was 65.2%.

UNITED STATES. The U.S. National Co-morbidity Survey interviewed a nationally representative household sample of the contiguous United States using a multistage area probability design (Kessler et al., 1994). The age range was from 15 to 54, with an oversampling of respondents in the age range of 15 to 24. A total of 8,098 respondents participated in the survey. The response rate was 82.4%. A subsample of 5,877 respondents, including all those who screened positive for a mental disorder, all respondents in the 15 to 24 age range, and a random subsample of other respondents, were also administered a risk-factor interview. Fieldwork was carried out from 1990 to 1992. The 5,872 respondents in the age range 15 to 54 are included in the current report.

Measures

All surveys used the World Health Organization's Composite International Diagnostic Interview (CIDI) (WHO, 1990) to make diagnoses. The CIDI is a fully structured diagnostic interview designed for use by trained interviewers who are not clinicians. Diagnoses for all but one site used DSM-III-R criteria. DSM-IV criteria were used in Munich. CIDI organic exclusion rules were imposed in making diagnoses, but diagnostic hierarchy rules were not. Prior studies have found acceptable reliability and validity for all the CIDI disorders considered here (Wittchen, 1994; Kessler et al., 1998).

The substance use measures included in the CIDI are lifetime use (ever had at least 12 drinks of alcohol in a single year and ever used any of the drugs assessed in the surveys at least five times), the lifetime occurrence of at least one DSM-III-R Criterion A symptom of alcohol or drug dependence, and the lifetime occurrence of dependence. Drug use included both nonmedical use of prescription medications (analgesics, tranquilizers, sedatives, and stimulants) and use of illegal drugs (marijuana-hashish, cocaine-crack, hallucinogens, and inhalants). The mental disorders in the assessment included mood disorders (major depression, dysthymia, and mania), anxiety disorders (panic attack without either panic disorder or agoraphobia, panic disorder, agoraphobia, social phobia, simple phobia, generalized anxiety disorder, post-traumatic stress disorder, and obsessive–compulsive disorder), conduct disorder, adult antisocial behavior, and antisocial personality disorder (the conjunction of conduct disorder and adult antisocial behavior).

Age at onset plays an important part in the current report. In three of the surveys (the United States, Fresno, and Mexico City), this age was assessed for mood and anxiety disorders by asking respondents if they could remember their exact age the very first time they had the disorder. Respondents who could not remember their exact age were asked about the earliest age they could clearly remember having the disorder. The response to this question was used as a conservative upper estimate of the age of onset of the disorder. A single question asking for age of onset was used for mood and anxiety disorders in the other surveys. A different approach to date onset was used for substance use disorders. In four of the surveys (Ontario; the United States; Fresno, CA; and Mexico), respondents were asked separately to date the age of onset of each of the nine Criterion A symptoms of dependence for each of the nine classes of substances assessed in the surveys (alcohol, four types of prescription medications, and four types of illicit drugs). Age of onset was defined as the age when the respondent first reported persistence of the disturbance for at least 1 month or repeatedly over a longer period of time. Age of onset of dependence was defined as the age at which the third qualifying symptom occurred. The other surveys used a more simple dating method in which respondents were simply asked to report on their age of first having any of the reported symptoms associated with alcohol use and separately for the age of first symptom associated with drug use. For purposes of carrying out survival analyses to predict first onset of dependence, age of onset of dependence was set to equal age of onset of the first symptom in these surveys.

Analysis Methods

Simple cross-tabulations were used to study patterns of lifetime co-morbidity between substance use disorders and mental disorders. Comparisons of retrospective age of onset reports were then used to classify respondents with lifetime co-morbidity into those having a primary mental disorder (i.e., their mental disorder was reported to have started at an earlier age than their substance use disorder), those having a primary substance use disorder, and those who reported that the two disorders started at the same age.

Discrete-time survival analysis was then used to analyze the effects of primary mental disorders in predicting the subsequent first onset of substance use and substance use disorders. This was done by using the retrospective age of onset reports to convert the person-level data file into a person-year file for each outcome disorder. Separate observational records were created in this data file for each year of each person's life up to and including the year of first onset of the outcome. A dichotomous outcome variable was then created to discriminate the year of first onset of the outcome disorder (coded 1) from years prior to the onset of the outcome disorder (coded 0). These data files were then analyzed using logistic regression models that included controls for person-year and cohort.

The mental disorders were treated as time-varying predictors of the subsequent onset of substance-use disorders. This was done by creating a set of two dichotomous variables ("active" and "remitted") to characterize the occurrence of each mental disorder. Each "active" disorder variable was coded 0 up to the retrospectively reported age of onset of the mental disorder and 1 thereafter through the reported age of offset of the mental disorder. In the year following age of offset, the "active" disorder variable was switched back to a code of 0 while the "remitted" disorder variable was changed from a code of 0 to a code of 1. The logits in these models can be interpreted as discrete-time survival coefficients for the associations of the mental disorders with the subsequent onset of substance use disorders in models that include a series of dichotomous control variables for each year of age represented in the data file (Efron, 1988). All models were estimated separately for men and women, based on evidence from previous studies indicating that there are significant gender differences in patterns of co-morbidity (Kessler et al., 1996).

Due to the complex sample designs and weighting of the surveys, standard errors of the survival coefficients were estimated using the Jacknife Repeated Replications (JRR) (Kish & Frankel, 1974), which adjusts for the clustering and weighting of cases. The survival coefficients were exponentiated and are reported below in the form of odds-ratios. The 95% confidence intervals of these coefficients are also reported and have been adjusted for design effects. Multivariate tests were based on Wald chi-square tests computed from coefficient variance–covariance matrices that were adjusted for design effects. When we speak of a result as being "significant" below, we are referring to statistical significance based on two-sided design-based tests evaluated at the .05 level.

The final step in the analysis was to carry out simulations based on the results of the survival models. The simulations began by computing cumulative predicted probabilities of lifetime substance use disorders for each respondent, based on the significant predictors in the survival models and then summing these totals to arrive at the predicted number of people with each substance use disorder. This set of calculations was then recomputed based on a series of revised models in which we assumed that the proportions of respondents with the mental disorders that predict substance-use disorders were zero. Population-attributable risk proportions were computed for each mental disorder using simulation methods. These estimates describe the proportion of all substance use disorders that could be attributed to the prior mental disorders.

RESULTS

Prevalences of Substance Use, Problems, and Dependence

Tables 23.2 and 23.3 show lifetime prevalence estimates for alcohol and drug use, problems among users, dependence among problem users, and dependence in the total samples of each survey, as well as in the pooled dataset that combines results across all surveys for alcohol (Table 23.2) and

TABLE 23.2. Lifetime Prevalences of Alcohol Use, Problems, and Dependence in the Seven Surveys by Gender

	Use in total sample		Problems among users		Dependence among problem users		Dependence in total sample	
	%	(se)	%	(se)	%	(se)	%	(se)
Alcohol—men								
São Paulo (Brazil)	92.8	(1.2)	47.8	(2.7)	17.4	(3.1)	7.7	(1.5)
Fresno (CA)	95.6	(0.8)	40.0	(2.0)	44.2	(3.0)	16.8	(1.3)
Munich (Germany)	93.8	(0.5)	38.0	(1.6)	28.1	(2.5)	10.0	(1.0)
Mexico City (Mexico)	97.1	(0.4)	35.8	(2.7)	40.7	(3.5)	14.1	(1.4)
Netherlands	96.7	(0.3)	46.8	(1.5)	19.7	(1.2)	8.9	(0.6)
Ontario (Canada)	95.8	(0.4)	36.9	(1.8)	40.6	(2.4)	14.3	(1.0)
United States	94.1	(0.7)	40.2	(1.2)	52.6	(1.7)	19.8	(0.7)
Total	95.4	(0.2)	40.9	(0.7)	35.1	(0.9)	13.7	(0.4)
χ^2_6	60.0^a		38.8^a		291.0^a		147.7^a	
Alcohol—women								
São Paulo (Brazil)	70.2	(1.8)	21.8	(1.8)	21.8	(4.3)	3.3	(0.6)
Fresno (CA)	73.6	(1.7)	17.2	(2.1)	37.7	(5.8)	4.8	(1.0)
Munich (Germany)	95.1	(0.5)	13.8	(0.9)	18.9	(3.3)	2.5	(0.5)
Mexico City (Mexico)	82.7	(1.9)	3.5	(0.6)	39.0	(9.1)	1.1	(0.3)
Netherlands	88.1	(0.7)	17.9	(1.4)	12.1	(1.4)	1.9	(0.3)
Ontario (Canada)	90.1	(1.4)	13.9	(0.6)	32.8	(3.1)	4.1	(0.4)
United States	90.7	(0.8)	22.5	(1.3)	42.7	(2.1)	8.7	(0.7)
Total	87.2	(0.5)	16.6	(0.5)	28.7	(1.2)	4.1	(0.2)
χ^2_6	300.3^a		175.6^a		153.3^a		203.6^a	

[a] Significant between site difference at the .05 level, two-sided test.

for drugs (Table 23.3). Users with substance "problems" were defined as having at least one of the DSM-III-R. A Criteria symptoms of substance dependence. There is substantial variation across the surveys in the prevalences of use and dependence as well as in the conditional prevalences of problems among users and in the conditional prevalences of dependence among problem users. However, there is also a good deal of consistency in the tables in three respects. First, the prevalences of alcohol use and dependence are consistently higher than the prevalences of drug use and dependence among both men and women in all seven surveys. Second, these prevalences are consistently higher among men than among women for both alcohol and drugs in all seven surveys. Third, the conditional risk of problems among users is consistently higher for alcohol than for drugs among men in all seven surveys, while this risk is higher for drugs than for alcohol among women in all seven surveys.

Cross-Sectional Bivariate Co-Morbidities

Merikangas et al. (1998) previously reported on lifetime bivariate co-morbidity between substance use disorders and broad classes of mental disorders (e.g., any mood disorder and any anxiety disorder) in six of the seven surveys analyzed here. They clearly show that the patterns of co-morbidity at this level of aggregation are quite similar across all the surveys. The results in Tables 23.4 through 23.7 provide more fine-grained information about these same comorbidities at the level of the individual mental disorders. Given the large number of data elements

TABLE 23.3. Lifetime Prevalences of Drug Use, Problems, and Dependence in the Seven Surveys by Gender

	Use in total sample		Problems among users		Dependence among problem users		Dependence in total sample	
	%	(se)	%	(se)	%	(se)	%	(se)
Drug—men								
São Paulo (Brazil)	33.3	(2.1)	40.0	(5.1)	27.1	(7.7)	3.6	(1.0)
Fresno (CA)	55.0	(1.9)	31.4	(1.9)	55.1	(3.9)	9.5	(1.0)
Munich (Germany)	39.4	(1.4)	24.1	(1.8)	25.9	(3.7)	2.5	(0.4)
Mexico City (Mexico)	19.7	(2.0)	8.7	(1.8)	64.5	(14.1)	1.1	(0.3)
Netherlands	16.8	(0.7)	44.8	(2.5)	27.4	(3.4)	2.1	(0.3)
Ontario (Canada)	50.1	(1.2)	23.6	(1.6)	38.4	(4.6)	4.5	(0.5)
United States	55.0	(1.5)	33.6	(1.5)	48.5	(2.0)	9.0	(0.6)
Total	39.9	(0.6)	30.0	(0.8)	41.2	(1.6)	5.0	(0.2)
χ^2_6	829.1[a]		117.4[a]		50.1[a]		241.1[a]	
Drug—women								
São Paulo (Brazil)	15.3	(1.4)	35.0	(5.0)	20.2	(7.1)	1.1	(0.5)
Fresno (CA)	32.1	(1.9)	25.4	(3.3)	49.1	(5.9)	4.1	(0.6)
Munich (Germany)	29.2	(1.4)	20.2	(2.2)	27.1	(5.7)	1.7	(0.4)
Mexico City (Mexico)	3.3	(0.7)	11.2	(3.9)	37.1	(12.0)	0.5	(0.2)
Netherlands	11.9	(0.5)	42.3	(2.7)	28.7	(3.1)	1.5	(0.2)
Ontario (Canada)	36.6	(1.3)	14.8	(1.3)	35.4	(6.8)	1.9	(0.4)
United States	47.9	(1.6)	26.0	(1.8)	47.7	(2.6)	6.0	(0.5)
Total	28.4	(0.6)	23.6	(0.9)	39.0	(1.9)	2.7	(0.2)
χ^2_6	1020.7[a]		109.7[a]		30.6[a]		107.4[a]	

[a] Significant between site difference at the .05 level, two-sided test.

involved, these results are presented for all seven surveys combined rather than separately for each survey.

Data concerning lifetime co-morbidity of alcohol use problems (at least one symptom of abuse or dependence) and dependence with the mental disorders assessed in the surveys are reported in Table 23.4 for men and in Table 23.5 for women. Results are presented in the form of odds ratios (ORs). Consistent with previous research, the overall pattern is overwhelmingly positive, with 99% of the ORs greater than 1.0 and 87% statistically significant. It is noteworthy that the ORs associated with conduct disorder, adult antisocial behavior, and antisocial personality disorder are generally stronger than those associated with mood disorders or anxiety disorders. Within the mood disorders, co-morbidity is generally stronger for mania than for dysthymia or major depression. In comparison, no individual anxiety disorders stand out as consistently having stronger ORs than the others. The ORs associated with alcohol dependence are generally larger than those associated with alcohol problems (in 83% of the comparisons), while the ORs associated with problems are generally larger than those associated with use (in 90% of the comparisons). Gender differences are neither large nor systematic.

Parallel results for lifetime co-morbidities of drug use, problems, and dependence with the same mental disorders are reported in Tables 23.6 (men) and 23.7 (women). The patterns in these tables are similar to, but stronger than, those for alcohol, with 90% of the ORs larger than the comparable ORs in Tables 23.4 and 23.5. All but one of the ORs in Tables 23.6 and 23.7 are

TABLE 23.4. Comorbidities of Lifetime Alcohol Use Disorders among Men

	Use			Problems			Dependence		
	%	OR	(95% CI)	%	OR	(95% CI)	%	OR	(95% CI)
Mood disorders									
Major depression	8.9	1.9	(1.2–2.9)	13.4	2.5	(2.2–2.9)	18.1	2.8	(2.4–3.3)
Dysthymia	3.3	1.5	(0.7–2.9)	5.1	2.5	(2.0–3.0)	8.4	3.7	(2.9–4.7)
Mania	1.4	3.4	(1.2–9.6)	2.3	3.2	(2.0–5.0)	3.8	4.2	(2.7–6.3)
Any mood disorder	11.1	2.2	(1.4–3.3)	16.7	2.6	(2.3–2.9)	23.6	3.2	(2.7–3.7)
Anxiety disorders									
Agoraphobia	3.4	1.0	(0.5–1.7)	4.9	2.0	(1.5–2.8)	7.7	3.0	(2.3–3.8)
GAD	2.1	1.3	(0.7–2.5)	3.4	2.8	(2.1–3.6)	5.2	3.4	(2.5–4.6)
Panic attack[a]	3.3	2.5	(1.2–5.2)	5.6	3.1	(2.3–4.1)	8.2	3.8	(2.8–5.0)
Panic disorder	1.3	1.7	(0.6–4.4)	2.1	2.6	(1.9–3.6)	3.4	3.6	(2.6–5.0)
OCD[b]	0.8	4.2	(3.1–5.7)	1.3	3.6	(1.8–7.1)	2.2	3.5	(1.7–7.4)
PTSD[c]	3.2	3.1	(0.8–12.2)	5.1	2.8	(1.7–4.5)	8.4	4.4	(2.8–6.7)
Simple phobia	5.5	1.6	(1.0–2.6)	8.1	2.3	(1.9–2.8)	11.9	3.0	(2.4–3.7)
Social phobia	7.7	1.1	(0.8–1.5)	11.1	2.1	(1.8–2.5)	16.2	2.9	(2.4–3.4)
Any anxiety disorder	15.9	1.4	(1.0–1.8)	22.3	2.2	(2.0–2.5)	30.7	2.9	(2.5–3.3)
Other disorders									
Conduct disorder[d]	21.0	2.3	(1.5–3.6)	34.9	3.9	(3.3–4.7)	44.7	4.4	(3.6–5.4)
Adult antisocial behavior[d]	14.3	3.6	(2.1–6.3)	29.0	7.7	(6.3–9.4)	41.7	8.0	(6.7–9.7)
Antisocial personality disorder[d]	9.1	2.5	(1.4–4.6)	19.0	7.7	(6.0–9.8)	27.9	7.3	(5.8–9.2)
Any other disorder (CD/AAB/ASP)	26.2	2.9	(1.9–4.4)	44.9	5.0	(4.2–5.8)	58.5	6.1	(5.0–7.4)
Numbers of disorders									
Exactly one disorder	16.8	1.6	(1.1–2.2)	20.9	1.7	(1.4–1.9)	22.2	1.5	(1.3–1.8)
Exactly two disorders	5.1	2.0	(1.1–3.4)	7.6	2.4	(2.0–2.9)	10.1	2.6	(2.1–3.2)
Three or more disorders	8.7	1.8	(1.2–2.7)	15.7	4.4	(3.8–5.2)	28.4	6.9	(5.9–8.1)
Any disorder	30.6	1.9	(1.5–2.4)	44.1	2.9	(2.7–3.3)	60.7	4.6	(4.0–5.3)

[a] Includes Fresno (CA), Munich (Germany), Mexico City (Mexico), Ontario (Canada), and United States.
[b] Includes São Paulo (Brazil), Munich (Germany), and Netherlands.
[c] Includes Munich (Germany) and United States.
[d] Includes Fresno (CA), Ontario (Canada), and United States.

greater than 1.0 (99%), and 98% are statistically significant. As in the analysis of alcohol, the ORs associated with conduct disorder, adult antisocial behavior, and antisocial personality disorder are generally stronger than those associated with mood disorders or anxiety disorders. Within the mood disorders, the ORs for mania are substantially stronger than those for dysthymia or major depression, while no individual anxiety disorders stand out as more important than the others. The ORs associated with drug dependence are generally larger than those associated with drug problems (in 93% of the comparisons), while the ORs associated with problems are generally larger than those associated with use (in 93% of the comparisons). Finally, no consistent gender differences can be seen across the tables.

Temporal Priorities

Merikangas et al. (1998) previously reported aggregate data on temporal priorities of first onset of substance use disorders compared to any co-morbid mood disorder and anxiety disorder in six

TABLE 23.5. Comorbidities of Lifetime Alcohol Use Disorders among Women

	Use			Problems			Dependence		
	%	OR	(95% CI)	%	OR	(95% CI)	%	OR	(95% CI)
Mood disorders									
Major depression	17.0	1.7	(1.4–2.1)	31.7	3.0	(2.6–3.3)	41.2	3.9	(3.2–4.8)
Dysthymia	6.2	1.0	(0.8–1.2)	11.7	2.4	(2.0–2.8)	16.9	3.3	(2.5–4.4)
Mania	1.2	2.3	(1.2–4.3)	3.5	5.6	(4.0–7.8)	3.7	4.0	(2.5–6.5)
Any mood disorder	19.9	1.6	(1.4–1.9)	37.5	3.2	(2.8–3.6)	46.4	4.0	(3.3–4.8)
Anxiety disorders									
Agoraphobia	7.0	1.1	(0.8–1.4)	12.0	2.1	(1.8–2.5)	18.9	3.4	(2.7–4.4)
GAD	4.1	1.1	(0.9–1.5)	8.0	2.5	(2.0–3.1)	11.1	3.3	(2.3–4.6)
Panic attack[a]	6.9	2.0	(1.4–2.9)	14.6	3.1	(2.6–3.8)	21.4	4.5	(3.4–5.9)
Panic disorder	3.5	1.3	(0.9–1.8)	7.3	2.8	(2.3–3.4)	10.7	3.8	(2.7–5.3)
OCD[b]	0.8	0.9	(0.4–2.2)	2.0	2.9	(1.7–5.2)	2.3	2.8	(0.8–10.3)
PTSD[c]	7.7	1.4	(0.6–3.2)	16.5	3.4	(2.7–4.3)	25.1	5.0	(3.9–6.5)
Simple phobia	11.3	1.2	(1.0–1.4)	20.8	2.5	(2.1–2.9)	25.7	3.0	(2.3–3.7)
Social phobia	11.5	1.4	(1.1–1.9)	23.2	3.0	(2.6–3.5)	30.1	3.8	(3.1–4.6)
Any anxiety disorder	26.8	1.3	(1.1–1.6)	45.9	2.9	(2.5–3.3)	57.5	4.1	(3.5–4.9)
Other disorders									
Conduct disorder[d]	7.8	2.2	(1.4–3.5)	20.9	5.3	(4.1–6.8)	29.3	6.7	(4.5–9.9)
Adult antisocial behavior[d]	5.4	3.7	(1.3–10.1)	19.2	10.1	(7.4–13.8)	29.4	11.9	(8.8–16.0)
Antisocial personality disorder[d]	2.4	4.2	(1.1–16.6)	8.9	10.8	(6.8–17.1)	15.0	13.2	(8.3–21.0)
Any other disorder (CD/AAB/ASP)	10.9	2.5	(1.6–4.0)	31.3	7.0	(5.5–8.8)	43.7	9.0	(6.7–12.3)
Numbers of disorders									
Exactly one disorder	19.1	1.4	(1.1–1.7)	23.6	1.4	(1.3–1.7)	22.7	1.3	(1.0–1.6)
Exactly two disorders	9.0	1.5	(1.1–1.9)	15.3	2.2	(1.8–2.7)	14.9	1.9	(1.4–2.6)
Three or more disorders	9.8	1.4	(1.1–1.8)	24.2	4.3	(3.7–5.0)	39.5	7.4	(6.1–8.9)
Any disorder	37.8	1.6	(1.4–1.8)	63.2	3.7	(3.3–4.1)	77.2	6.3	(5.0–8.0)

[a] Includes Fresno (CA), Munich (Germany), Mexico City (Mexico), Ontario (Canada), and United States.
[b] Includes São Paulo (Brazil), Munich (Germany), and Netherlands.
[c] Includes Munich (Germany) and United States.
[d] Includes Fresno (CA), Ontario (Canada), and United States.

of the seven surveys analyzed here. The results show that mood disorders typically begin after onset of alcohol and drug use and alcohol problems but prior to the onset of drug problems or substance dependence. Co-morbid anxiety disorders typically occur before first onset of alcohol problems, but not use, and before first use of drugs. However, these results were presented only for aggregate mood and anxiety disorders and for men and women combined. This high level of aggregation could be deceptive, based on the finding in the clinical literature that these temporal priorities differ substantially by type of disorder and by gender (Jaffe & Ciraulo, 1986; Lewis, Rice, & Helzer, 1983). The results in Tables 23.8 (men) and 23.9 (women) provide more fine-grained information about these temporal priorities at the level of the individual mental disorders by gender. Results are presented for all seven surveys combined rather than separately for each survey due to the large number of data elements.

There are 78 comparisons in each table—13 mood and anxiety disorders for each of 6 substance measures. No comparable results are reported for Conduct Disorder (CD), Adult Antisocial Behavior (AAB), or Antisocial Personality Disorder (ASPD) because age of onset of these disorders was not assessed. Approximately two-thirds of the comparisons in each table show that the proportion of respondents who reported that their mental disorder started before their substance

TABLE 23.6. Comorbidities of Lifetime Drug Use Disorders among Men

	Use			Problems			Dependence		
	%	OR	(95% Cl)	%	OR	(95% Cl)	%	OR	(95% Cl)
Mood disorders									
Major depression	12.5	2.1	(1.8–2.5)	18.9	2.9	(2.4–3.5)	21.2	3.0	(2.3–4.0)
Dysthymia	4.7	2.1	(1.7–2.6)	8.1	3.3	(2.5–4.4)	10.5	4.0	(2.8–5.6)
Mania	1.9	1.9	(1.3–2.7)	4.5	5.2	(3.5–7.7)	8.2	9.0	(5.7–14.2)
Any mood disorder	15.5	2.1	(1.9–2.4)	24.6	3.3	(2.7–3.9)	29.5	3.8	(3.0–4.8)
Anxiety disorders									
Agoraphobia	5.1	2.3	(1.8–3.0)	8.7	3.5	(2.7–4.5)	11.9	4.4	(3.2–6.1)
GAD	3.2	2.4	(1.7–3.2)	5.7	3.7	(2.7–5.1)	8.1	4.9	(3.3–7.1)
Panic attack[a]	5.2	3.9	(2.8–5.4)	8.3	3.6	(2.6–4.9)	10.0	3.8	(2.6–5.7)
Panic disorder	2.1	2.6	(1.8–3.6)	3.4	3.4	(2.4–4.9)	5.5	5.2	(3.4–8.0)
OCD[b]	1.6	3.4	(1.7–6.6)	2.7	4.9	(2.6–9.2)	5.4	8.7	(2.8–27.5)
PTSD[c]	4.5	2.7	(1.4–5.0)	6.6	2.8	(1.7–4.5)	11.7	5.2	(3.1–8.6)
Simple phobia	7.4	1.9	(1.6–2.3)	12.7	3.2	(2.5–4.0)	18.2	4.5	(3.3–6.0)
Social phobia	10.6	1.9	(1.7–2.3)	16.4	2.8	(2.4–3.4)	23.5	4.2	(3.3–5.3)
Any anxiety disorder	21.9	2.1	(1.9–2.4)	32.3	3.1	(2.6–3.6)	42.6	4.4	(3.6–5.5)
Other disorders									
Conduct disorder[d]	28.5	3.1	(2.5–3.8)	47.3	4.9	(3.9–6.0)	56.8	6.1	(4.7–7.9)
Adult antisocial behavior[d]	21.8	5.4	(4.1–7.1)	43.6	8.5	(7.0–10.2)	56.6	11.1	(8.7–14.2)
Antisocial personality disorder[d]	14.1	5.4	(3.8–7.6)	31.0	8.9	(6.8–11.5)	40.3	9.8	(7.2–13.4)
Any other disorder (CD/AAB/ASP)	36.2	3.7	(3.0–4.4)	59.9	6.3	(5.2–7.6)	73.1	9.8	(7.5–12.8)
Numbers of disorders									
Exactly one disorder	21.2	1.7	(1.5–1.9)	22.5	1.6	(1.3–1.8)	18.8	1.2	(0.9–1.5)
Exactly two disorders	7.2	2.1	(1.8–2.5)	9.1	2.2	(1.8–2.6)	11.5	2.7	(2.0–3.4)
Three or more disorders	16.3	5.5	(4.6–6.6)	31.9	8.2	(6.9–9.8)	46.6	12.3	(10.0–15.3)
Any disorder	44.7	3.1	(2.8–3.5)	63.5	5.1	(4.3–5.9)	76.9	8.7	(6.8–11.0)

[a] Includes Fresno (CA), Munich (Germany), Mexico City (Mexico), Ontario (Canada), and United States.
[b] Includes São Paulo (Brazil), Munich (Germany), and Netherlands.
[c] Includes Munich (Germany) and United States.
[d] Includes Fresno (CA), Ontario (Canada), and United States.

disorder differs significantly from the proportion who reported that their substance use disorder started before their mental disorder. The dominant pattern is for mental disorders to occur before substance less often for mood (0% of significant comparisons among men and 56% among women) than for anxiety (58% of significant comparisons among men and 78% among women) disorders, more often for dependence than for problems (90% of comparisons), and more often for problems than for use (64% of significant comparisons).

Focusing on men, we see that alcohol and drug use, problems, and dependence are all more likely to occur prior to the onset of mood disorders than after. Of the 15 significant differences in these proportions among men, 15 (100%) show substance-before-mental to be more common than mental-before-substance. The pattern is more complex for anxiety disorders. Alcohol and drug use and problems are more likely to occur prior to than after first onset of agoraphobia, generalized anxiety disorder (GAD), panic, and post-traumatic stress disorder (PTSD), but after rather than before first onset of other anxiety disorders. Alcohol and drug dependence are more likely to occur after than prior to first onset of all anxiety disorders. Of the 36 significant differences in proportions involving anxiety disorders among men, 58% show mental-before-substance to be more common, and the others show substance-before-mental to be more common.

TABLE 23.7. Comorbidities of Lifetime Drug Use Disorders among Women

	Use			Problems			Dependence		
	%	OR	(95% CI)	%	OR	(95% CI)	%	OR	(95% CI)
Mood disorders									
Major depression	25.1	2.3	(2.1–2.6)	40.1	4.0	(3.3–4.8)	43.3	4.2	(3.3–5.3)
Dysthymia	8.9	1.8	(1.5–2.1)	16.7	3.5	(2.9–4.3)	19.8	4.0	(3.0–5.3)
Mania	2.0	3.0	(2.1–4.3)	5.0	6.6	(4.4–9.8)	6.9	8.0	(5.4–11.9)
Any mood disorder	28.7	2.3	(2.0–2.5)	47.1	4.4	(3.7–5.2)	50.8	4.7	(3.7–5.9)
Anxiety disorders									
Agoraphobia	10.7	2.1	(1.8–2.5)	15.1	2.6	(2.2–3.2)	21.5	3.9	(2.9–5.3)
GAD	6.4	2.2	(1.8–2.7)	11.4	3.6	(2.7–4.8)	13.3	4.0	(2.8–5.6)
Panic attack[a]	11.3	3.1	(2.6–3.8)	22.2	5.1	(4.1–6.5)	25.8	5.6	(4.3–7.2)
Panic disorder	5.7	2.4	(1.9–3.0)	11.7	4.6	(3.6–6.0)	13.1	4.7	(3.4–6.4)
OCD[b]	1.6	2.3	(1.3–4.3)	3.4	4.8	(2.3–10.2)	4.4	5.6	(1.9–16.9)
PTSD[c]	12.1	3.1	(2.4–4.1)	24.3	5.5	(4.1–7.2)	29.9	6.2	(4.3–8.8)
Simple phobia	16.0	1.9	(1.7–2.2)	24.6	2.9	(2.5–3.4)	30.9	3.8	(3.0–4.8)
Social phobia	17.6	2.3	(2.0–2.7)	28.3	3.6	(3.0–4.4)	30.9	3.8	(2.9–4.9)
Any anxiety disorder	38.7	2.4	(2.2–2.6)	57.7	4.4	(3.7–5.2)	64.1	5.3	(4.1–7.0)
Other disorders									
Conduct disorder[d]	12.5	3.7	(2.8–4.9)	27.1	6.6	(4.9–8.7)	34.9	8.2	(5.7–11.9)
Adult antisocial behavior[d]	9.8	6.2	(4.4–8.8)	26.8	12.4	(9.5–16.2)	36.9	15.4	(11.3–21.0)
Antisocial personality disorder[d]	4.4	7.3	(4.5–11.8)	13.5	14.4	(9.7–21.6)	20.5	18.2	(11.3–29.1)
Any other disorder (CD/AAB/ASP)	17.9	4.3	(3.4–5.5)	40.5	8.8	(7.0–11.0)	51.2	11.5	(8.8–15.0)
Numbers of disorders									
Exactly one disorder	23.1	1.5	(1.3–1.7)	23.4	1.4	(1.1–1.7)	18.4	1.0	(0.7–1.4)
Exactly two disorders	12.2	1.8	(1.5–2.1)	18.5	2.6	(2.2–3.2)	17.7	2.4	(1.7–3.2)
Three or more disorders	18.5	3.7	(3.2–4.2)	35.9	6.9	(5.9–8.1)	47.5	9.9	(7.8–12.5)
Any disorder	53.7	2.8	(2.5–3.0)	77.8	7.0	(5.8–8.3)	83.6	9.4	(7.1–12.4)

[a] Includes Fresno (CA), Munich (Germany), Mexico City (Mexico), Ontario (Canada), and United States.
[b] Includes São Paulo (Brazil), Munich (Germany), and Netherlands.
[c] Includes Munich (Germany) and United States.
[d] Includes Fresno (CA), Ontario (Canada), and United States.

The mental-before-substance pattern is consistently more common among women than among men. As with men, alcohol and drug use among women tend to begin prior to the onset of mood disorders. However, unlike men, there is a clear trend for mood disorders to occur prior to the onset of alcohol dependence, drug problems, and drug dependence (in 100% of significant comparisons) among women. The mental-before-substance pattern is even clearer for anxiety disorders, in which 97% of the significant differences for substance problems or dependence show mental-before-substance to be more common than substance-before-mental.

Predicting Substance Use Problems and Dependence

Survival analyses were used to estimate the effects of mental disorders, considered one at a time, in predicting the subsequent first onset of substance dependence. In addition, disaggregated survival models were used to estimate the component effects on dependence due to effects of the mental disorders on subsequent initiation of substance use in the total sample, first onset of problem

TABLE 23.8. Temporal Ordering of Mental Disorders versus Substance Use, Problems, and Dependence[a] among Men

	Alcohol						Drug					
	Use		Problems		Dependence		Use		Problems		Dependence	
	%	(se)	%	(se)	%	(se)	%	(se)	%	(se)	%	(se)
Mood disorders												
Major depression first	12.6	(1.4)	32.0	(2.0)	39.7	(3.5)	26.1	(1.9)	39.1	(2.9)	44.6	(4.8)
Substance use disorder first	82.6	(1.6)	57.2	(2.4)	49.5	(3.9)	65.5	(2.1)	51.1	(3.0)	45.2	(5.3)
Major depression/substance same year	4.8	(1.1)	10.7	(1.2)	10.8	(1.7)	8.4	(1.1)	9.8	(2.3)	10.2	(2.5)
Dysthymia first	13.3	(2.4)	28.4	(3.3)	35.7	(4.9)	22.2	(3.4)	31.6	(5.7)	30.9	(6.2)
Substance use disorder first	81.8	(2.6)	57.7	(3.7)	46.4	(5.3)	67.8	(3.4)	52.9	(5.7)	54.4	(7.7)
Dysthymia/substance same year	4.9	(1.1)	13.9	(2.1)	17.9	(3.9)	10.0	(1.7)	15.5	(4.3)	14.6	(4.6)
Mania first	16.1	(4.7)	37.9	(5.4)	30.9	(7.1)	34.4	(6.6)	42.3	(8.6)	45.2	(10.3)
Substance use disorder first	76.9	(6.8)	46.0	(6.2)	48.5	(8.7)	61.1	(6.8)	53.2	(8.7)	34.8	(9.9)
Mania/Substance same year	7.0	(3.0)	16.2	(4.5)	20.6	(7.9)	4.5	(2.0)	4.6	(2.3)	19.9	(9.4)
Any mood disorder first	13.5	(1.4)	33.8	(1.9)	39.6	(3.2)	26.8	(1.8)	40.8	(2.9)	43.6	(4.3)
Substance use disorder first	81.3	(1.7)	53.9	(2.1)	46.5	(3.4)	64.4	(2.0)	50.0	(3.0)	43.6	(4.7)
Any mood/substance same year	5.2	(1.0)	12.3	(1.3)	13.9	(2.0)	8.8	(1.0)	9.1	(1.9)	12.8	(3.2)
Anxiety disorders												
Agoraphobia first	25.4	(3.1)	35.4	(3.6)	52.3	(5.1)	34.1	(4.0)	40.4	(6.3)	54.6	(8.9)
Substance use disorder first	70.2	(3.3)	56.8	(3.8)	43.3	(4.8)	59.0	(4.1)	51.1	(6.2)	37.5	(8.5)
Agoraphobia/substance same year	4.3	(1.2)	7.9	(2.0)	4.4	(2.1)	6.8	(1.7)	8.5	(2.6)	7.9	(3.7)
GAD first	12.2	(2.9)	33.9	(4.2)	46.2	(5.7)	28.0	(4.0)	41.5	(6.0)	52.0	(7.4)
Substance use disorder first	83.9	(3.1)	61.4	(4.4)	45.4	(5.8)	66.0	(4.2)	48.5	(6.1)	40.0	(7.4)
GAD/substance same year	3.9	(1.8)	4.7	(1.5)	8.4	(3.0)	6.0	(2.0)	10.0	(5.2)	7.9	(4.1)
Panic attack first	24.9	(3.2)	37.9	(3.7)	47.1	(5.4)	35.4	(4.2)	48.1	(7.4)	56.8	(7.5)
Substance use disorder first	68.6	(3.6)	54.1	(3.9)	44.1	(5.4)	54.6	(4.4)	37.8	(6.0)	38.4	(6.8)
Panic attack/substance same year	6.5	(2.4)	8.0	(2.8)	8.8	(3.5)	10.0	(2.7)	14.1	(5.3)	4.9	(2.3)
Panic disorder first	6.0	(2.2)	28.5	(4.9)	38.0	(7.5)	12.7	(3.6)	24.1	(6.0)	27.8	(7.6)
Substance use disorder first	93.2	(2.3)	66.3	(5.4)	53.2	(7.5)	76.7	(4.6)	66.7	(6.4)	60.6	(8.2)
Panic disorder/substance same year	0.8	(0.6)	5.2	(2.1)	8.8	(3.6)	10.5	(3.6)	9.2	(4.3)	11.6	(6.0)
OCD first	41.2	(21.2)	69.8	(8.0)	60.4	(13.7)	47.7	(13.7)	51.7	(17.9)	30.1	(11.4)
Substance use disorder first	58.8	(21.2)	27.8	(7.8)	33.0	(12.8)	32.7	(10.4)	31.6	(12.1)	39.0	(25.3)
OCD/substance same year	0.0	—	2.4	(0.4)	6.7	(2.0)	19.6	(10.9)	16.7	(13.0)	30.9	(24.9)
PTSD first	27.3	(4.3)	45.1	(6.1)	57.4	(6.7)	39.8	(5.5)	48.2	(7.8)	68.7	(6.0)
Substance use disorder first	67.7	(4.5)	48.5	(5.8)	36.4	(6.2)	53.0	(5.1)	46.1	(6.3)	26.7	(5.4)
PTSD/substance same year	5.0	(1.6)	6.4	(2.6)	6.2	(2.6)	7.2	(1.8)	5.6	(3.8)	4.6	(3.3)
Simple phobia first	55.9	(3.4)	71.1	(3.5)	74.1	(3.4)	63.6	(3.6)	70.5	(5.9)	72.4	(8.2)
Substance use disorder first	40.5	(3.4)	24.0	(3.1)	20.6	(3.4)	30.8	(3.6)	20.8	(5.3)	23.0	(8.0)
Simple phobia/substance same year	3.6	(0.9)	4.9	(1.6)	5.3	(1.6)	5.6	(1.2)	8.6	(3.1)	4.6	(2.2)
Social phobia first	55.8	(2.0)	71.2	(2.3)	74.5	(3.5)	70.2	(2.1)	71.7	(3.0)	75.2	(4.2)
Substance use disorder first	38.1	(1.9)	23.6	(2.1)	20.3	(3.4)	24.4	(2.1)	20.4	(3.3)	19.5	(4.1)
Social phobia/substance same year	6.2	(1.1)	5.1	(0.9)	5.2	(1.4)	5.5	(1.0)	7.9	(2.6)	5.3	(2.2)
Any anxiety disorder first	49.2	(1.4)	65.7	(1.6)	71.9	(2.6)	61.4	(1.7)	68.3	(2.5)	74.0	(2.9)
Substance use disorder first	45.0	(1.5)	28.8	(1.4)	22.6	(2.6)	32.8	(1.6)	23.3	(2.1)	20.7	(2.7)
Any anxiety/substance same year	5.8	(0.7)	5.6	(0.9)	5.5	(1.0)	5.8	(0.8)	8.4	(2.0)	5.2	(1.5)

[a] Among those with both mental and substance use disorders.

TABLE 23.9. Temporal Ordering of Mental Disorders versus Substance Use, Problems, and Dependence[a] among Women

	Alcohol						Drug					
	Use		Problems		Dependence		Use		Problems		Dependence	
	%	(se)	%	(se)	%	(se)	%	(se)	%	(se)	%	(se)
Mood disorders												
Major depression first	18.7	(1.5)	41.0	(2.4)	52.1	(4.3)	34.0	(1.9)	46.9	(3.0)	53.8	(4.2)
Substance use disorder first	75.5	(1.6)	46.5	(2.5)	34.1	(3.8)	54.6	(1.9)	38.1	(2.9)	27.4	(3.8)
Major depression/substance same year	5.8	(0.7)	12.5	(1.3)	13.9	(2.1)	11.3	(1.0)	15.0	(1.7)	18.7	(3.0)
Dysthymia first	21.9	(3.1)	47.6	(3.3)	57.3	(5.7)	39.5	(3.1)	49.8	(4.3)	46.8	(5.9)
Substance use disorder first	72.5	(3.0)	42.3	(3.2)	28.0	(4.6)	50.9	(2.9)	34.3	(3.9)	29.2	(5.5)
Dysthymia/substance same year	5.6	(1.6)	10.2	(1.9)	14.6	(3.7)	9.5	(1.5)	16.0	(3.0)	24.0	(5.4)
Mania first	21.4	(5.2)	43.0	(6.7)	41.3	(11.0)	40.5	(6.5)	54.6	(10.1)	58.3	(10.4)
Substance use disorder first	72.1	(5.7)	43.7	(6.7)	48.1	(11.1)	47.5	(6.6)	35.3	(10.5)	30.8	(9.9)
Mania/substance same year	6.4	(2.6)	13.3	(4.3)	10.6	(5.7)	12.0	(3.6)	10.1	(4.2)	11.0	(5.5)
Any mood disorder first	20.3	(1.5)	44.9	(2.1)	55.2	(3.9)	36.6	(1.7)	50.9	(2.9)	56.4	(3.8)
Substance use disorder first	73.7	(1.5)	43.7	(2.1)	30.9	(3.3)	52.3	(1.8)	35.9	(2.7)	27.5	(3.3)
Any mood/substance same year	6.0	(0.8)	11.3	(1.2)	13.9	(2.0)	11.0	(0.9)	13.1	(1.6)	16.2	(2.7)
Anxiety disorders												
Agoraphobia first	32.0	(2.6)	48.6	(3.8)	57.4	(5.5)	38.8	(2.9)	48.2	(4.4)	54.1	(5.4)
Substance use disorder first	63.5	(2.5)	45.3	(3.6)	36.2	(5.4)	52.8	(2.8)	42.1	(4.7)	34.2	(5.2)
Agoraphobia/substance same year	4.4	(0.9)	6.1	(1.7)	6.5	(2.2)	8.4	(1.7)	9.8	(2.5)	11.7	(3.9)
GAD first	20.7	(3.0)	34.5	(5.2)	46.8	(8.7)	29.5	(3.5)	56.3	(4.8)	61.9	(7.5)
Substance use disorder first	74.9	(3.2)	52.0	(5.2)	31.6	(7.1)	55.8	(3.8)	33.3	(4.6)	23.0	(6.7)
GAD/substance same year	4.4	(1.4)	13.5	(2.8)	21.6	(9.6)	14.6	(2.2)	10.3	(2.5)	15.0	(5.1)
Panic attack first	26.6	(2.1)	43.2	(4.7)	54.1	(5.9)	35.5	(2.7)	45.0	(4.7)	53.9	(5.3)
Substance use disorder first	67.2	(2.4)	50.2	(4.8)	34.2	(5.2)	58.4	(2.9)	49.2	(4.8)	36.9	(5.0)
Panic attack/substance same year	6.2	(1.1)	6.6	(1.6)	11.7	(4.1)	6.1	(1.2)	5.8	(1.6)	9.2	(3.0)
Panic disorder first	13.3	(2.7)	37.5	(4.9)	39.9	(7.9)	26.8	(3.6)	51.6	(5.1)	51.9	(6.6)
Substance use disorder first	81.4	(3.2)	51.0	(5.1)	50.0	(8.4)	65.2	(4.0)	44.7	(5.1)	41.0	(6.9)
Panic disorder/substance same year	5.3	(1.6)	11.5	(2.5)	10.1	(4.4)	8.0	(1.8)	3.7	(1.7)	7.1	(3.2)
OCD first	59.2	(16.8)	76.1	(10.0)	100.0	(0.0)	53.2	(12.8)	67.6	(14.3)	46.8	(27.3)
Substance use disorder first	40.8	(16.8)	20.3	(9.6)	0.0	(0.0)	22.6	(10.6)	24.2	(13.1)	53.2	(27.3)
OCD/substance same year	0.0	—	3.6	(3.4)	0.0	(0.0)	24.2	(11.2)	8.2	(7.4)	0.0	(0.0)
PTSD first	49.0	(3.5)	57.6	(4.1)	72.3	(5.5)	60.3	(3.2)	68.3	(3.3)	69.9	(5.8)
Substance use disorder first	46.0	(3.4)	32.6	(3.5)	24.1	(4.6)	36.0	(2.9)	24.5	(2.6)	23.6	(4.7)
PTSD/substance same year	4.9	(1.2)	9.7	(2.7)	3.6	(1.8)	3.6	(1.4)	7.2	(2.9)	6.5	(4.5)
Simple phobia first	71.0	(2.1)	81.8	(2.0)	88.5	(2.8)	75.0	(2.1)	80.5	(2.6)	85.3	(2.8)
Substance use disorder first	24.7	(1.9)	15.2	(1.8)	7.4	(2.0)	22.0	(2.1)	16.8	(2.5)	10.1	(2.6)
Simple phobia/substance same year	4.3	(1.0)	3.0	(0.8)	4.1	(2.3)	3.0	(0.8)	2.7	(1.0)	4.6	(2.9)
Social phobia first	66.5	(1.8)	77.4	(2.1)	79.0	(3.5)	70.8	(2.0)	76.1	(2.8)	78.1	(3.6)
Substance use disorder first	26.1	(1.5)	18.4	(1.9)	17.8	(3.3)	22.3	(1.7)	20.2	(2.8)	17.7	(3.5)
Social phobia/substance same year	7.4	(0.9)	4.3	(1.0)	3.1	(1.2)	6.9	(1.1)	3.6	(1.1)	4.2	(1.8)
Any anxiety disorder first	61.3	(1.4)	73.7	(1.6)	80.0	(2.1)	66.5	(1.5)	77.1	(1.8)	85.1	(2.2)
Substance use disorder first	33.0	(1.3)	20.9	(1.5)	15.1	(1.8)	27.1	(1.4)	18.3	(1.8)	12.0	(1.9)
Any anxiety/substance same year	5.8	(0.6)	5.4	(0.8)	4.9	(1.4)	6.4	(0.7)	4.6	(0.8)	2.9	(1.1)

[a] Among those with both mental and substance use disorders.

use among users, and first onset of dependence among problem users. Results are reported in Tables 23.10–23.13 in the form of exponentiated survival coefficients, which can be interpreted as ORs. Tables 23.10 (men) and 23.11 (women) show the results for alcohol. Tables 23.12 (men) and 23.13 (women) show the results for drugs.

Initial models examined the impact of both active and remitted mental disorders. Results of Wald chi-square tests suggest that remitted disorders are not significantly associated with subsequent initiation of substance use problems. Thus, all results presented here focus on the relationship between active mental disorders and subsequent initiation of substance problems.

Focusing first on alcohol, we see a clear pattern of statistically significant positive associations, with 91% of the ORs greater than 1.0 and 84% of these ORs statistically significant. Prior mental disorders consistently predict alcohol use (83% of ORs greater than 1.0, 56% significant), the transition from use to problem use (100% of ORs positive, 95% significant), and the transition from problems to dependence (95% of ORs greater than 1.0, 76% significant). The effects on the transition from use to problem use are generally stronger than the effects either on initial use (87% of comparisons) or on the transition from problem use to dependence (89% of comparisons).

It is noteworthy that the ORs in the far-right column of the tables, which estimate the effects of prior mental disorders on subsequent first onset of alcohol dependence in the total sample, are consistently larger than the ORs to the left, which look at effects on first use and on the transitions from use to problems and problems to dependence. This is because all of the component effects are significant and the total effects on dependence are cumulative functions of the component effects. These total effects are quite substantial: ORs ranging between 3.0 and 7.5 for mood disorders, between 2.4 and 7.7 for anxiety disorders, and between 4.1 and 13.2 for conduct disorder, adult antisocial behavior, and antisocial personality disorder. No individual mental disorders stand out as consistently more important than others within these three broad sets. The magnitude of the mood and anxiety effects on alcohol dependence are roughly comparable for both men (2.5–7.5) and women (2.4–7.7), although there is a weak trend for the ORs to be somewhat stronger among women than among men. In comparison, the effects of conduct disorder, adult antisocial behavior, and antisocial personality disorder are consistently and substantially higher among women (5.9–13.2) than among men (4.1–6.1).

Parallel results for the effects of mental disorders on the subsequent first onset of drug use, problems, and dependence are reported in Tables 23.12 (men) and 23.13 (women). The pattern here is similar to, but stronger than, the pattern seen for alcohol, with 98% of the ORs greater than 1.0 and 87% statistically significant. Unlike the situation with alcohol, the effects of mental disorders in predicting first use of drugs (ORs ranging between 1.6 and 7.5) are somewhat larger than the effects in predicting the transition from use to problem use (1.4–5.2) and the effects in predicting the transition from problem use to dependence (0.9–7.8) in the majority of comparisons (64% of comparisons of use versus problem use and 81% of comparisons of use versus dependence).

As with alcohol, the ORs in the right columns of Tables 23.12 and 23.13, which estimate the effects of prior mental disorders on subsequent first onset of drug dependence in the total sample, are consistently larger than the ORs to the left, which look at effects on first use and on the transitions from use to problems and problems to dependence. The majority of these effects (67%) are larger than those found for alcohol. The ORs range between 4.4 and 18.6 for mood disorders, between 3.3 and 14.0 for anxiety disorders, and between 5.5 and 14.8 for conduct disorder, adult antisocial behavior, and antisocial personality disorder. Mania stands out as consistently more important than the other mood disorders (with ORs of 11.4–18.6 for mania compared to 4.4–6.9 for other mood disorders). The phobias stand out as less important than the other anxiety disorders (with ORs of 3.3–4.2 for phobias compared to 4.2–14.0 for other anxiety disorders). There is a slight tendency for the ORs to be stronger among women than men (in 54% of the comparisons

TABLE 23.10. Mental Disorders Predicting the Subsequent First Onset of Alcohol Use, Problems, and Dependence among Men

	Use in total sample				Problems among users[a]				Dependence among problem users				Dependence in total sample			
	OR[b]	(95% CI)	OR[c]	(95% CI)	OR[b,d]	(95% CI)	OR[c,d]	(95% CI)	OR[b,e]	(95% CI)	OR[c,e]	(95% CI)	OR[b,e]	(95% CI)	OR[c,e]	(95% CI)
Mood disorders																
Depression	1.0	(0.5–2.0)	0.8	(0.4–1.6)	3.7	(2.7–5.1)	2.8	(2.0–4.0)	2.1	(1.4–3.1)	1.3	(0.9–1.8)	4.4	(3.1–6.1)	2.2	(1.5–3.2)
Dysthymia	1.6	(0.8–3.2)	1.6	(0.8–3.5)	2.7	(1.6–4.5)	1.4	(0.8–2.5)	11.2	(4.9–25.7)	5.0	(2.0–12.8)	6.0	(3.5–10.2)	2.3	(1.4–4.0)
Mania	0.4	(0.2–0.9)	0.3	(0.2–0.7)	2.4	(0.9–6.2)	1.3	(0.3–5.3)	1.1	(0.4–3.1)	0.8	(0.3–2.4)	3.0	(1.3–7.1)	1.2	(0.3–4.7)
Any mood disorder	1.1	(0.6–2.0)			3.6	(2.7–4.7)			2.5	(1.7–3.6)			4.8	(3.6–6.5)		
Anxiety disorders																
Agoraphobia	1.0	(0.5–1.9)	0.9	(0.5–1.6)	2.2	(1.4–3.5)	1.2	(0.6–2.3)	1.8	(0.9–3.7)	1.3	(0.6–2.6)	3.2	(2.1–4.9)	1.3	(0.7–2.5)
GAD	2.5	(0.2–36.6)	0.8	(0.1–8.5)	2.1	(1.2–3.7)	0.8	(0.4–1.8)	4.2	(1.6–11.4)	1.2	(0.4–3.5)	5.1	(2.6–10.1)	1.3	(0.6–2.8)
Panic attack	2.1	(0.9–4.6)	1.9	(0.8–4.2)	2.4	(1.2–5.0)	1.1	(0.6–2.2)	2.2	(1.2–4.0)	1.6	(0.9–2.9)	4.2	(2.7–6.6)	2.3	(1.1–4.8)
Panic disorder	0.2	(0.1–0.6)	0.1	(0.0–0.4)	N/E	N/E	N/E	N/E	N/E	N/E	N/E	N/E	7.5	(1.1–49.4)	2.0	(0.3–14.0)
OCD	N/E	N/E	N/E	N/E	N/E	N/E	N/E	N/E	N/E	N/E	N/E	N/E	3.7	(N/C–N/C)	1.8	(0.0–N/C)
PTSD	1.8	(0.8–4.1)	1.2	(0.4–4.2)	2.6	(1.6–4.4)	1.1	(0.7–1.8)	5.0	(2.7–9.2)	3.0	(1.5–6.0)	5.9	(3.3–10.4)	2.0	(1.0–4.2)
Simple phobia	1.4	(0.9–2.3)	1.3	(0.9–1.9)	2.1	(1.5–2.8)	1.3	(0.9–1.9)	1.4	(0.9–2.2)	1.0	(0.6–1.6)	2.8	(2.1–3.6)	1.2	(0.8–1.8)
Social phobia	1.0	(0.7–1.3)	0.8	(0.6–1.0)	2.0	(1.5–2.5)	1.4	(1.0–1.8)	1.6	(1.1–2.3)	1.2	(0.8–1.9)	2.5	(2.0–3.3)	1.4	(1.0–1.9)
Any anxiety disorder	1.3	(1.0–1.7)			2.2	(1.8–2.6)			1.6	(1.2–2.1)			2.9	(2.4–3.6)		
Other disorders																
Conduct disorder	2.1	(1.7–2.6)	1.6	(1.3–2.1)	2.6	(2.1–3.2)	2.4	(1.8–3.1)	1.5	(1.1–1.9)	1.3	(1.0–1.8)	4.1	(3.4–5.0)	3.2	(2.3–4.3)
AAB	2.8	(2.2–3.4)	2.1	(1.6–2.8)	3.5	(2.8–4.3)	3.9	(3.1–5.1)	1.6	(1.2–2.2)	1.6	(1.2–2.1)	6.1	(4.9–7.6)	6.0	(4.6–7.8)
ASP	3.2	(2.4–4.3)	1.1	(0.7–1.8)	3.1	(2.4–4.0)	0.4	(0.3–0.6)	1.6	(1.0–2.3)	0.8	(0.5–1.2)	5.6	(4.2–7.4)	0.4	(0.2–0.7)
Any other disorder	2.2	(1.8–2.6)			3.3	(2.7–4.0)			1.6	(1.3–2.1)			5.5	(4.6–6.7)		
Number of disorders																
Exactly one disorder	1.2	(1.1–1.4)			2.3	(1.9–2.7)			1.2	(1.0–1.5)			2.7	(2.2–3.3)		
Exactly two disorders	1.5	(1.2–2.0)			3.8	(3.0–4.9)			1.4	(1.1–1.8)			4.5	(3.6–5.7)		
Three or more disorders	2.6	(2.0–3.3)			4.3	(3.5–5.3)			2.3	(1.7–3.2)			8.8	(7.1–11.0)		
Any disorder	1.6	(1.4–1.8)			2.9	(2.5–3.4)			1.6	(1.3–1.9)			4.4	(3.7–5.2)		
$\Delta\chi^2_{12,14}$	153.3[f]				273.3[f]				65.0[f]				428.7[f]			

NOTE. N/E = Parameter not estimable due to small sample size; N/C = nonconvergent parameter estimates.
[a] São Paulo (Brazil) and Netherlands not included.
[b] From models with 1 psychiatric predictor at a time and controls (age, cohort, survey).
[c] From models with all 14 psychiatric predictors and controls.
[d] Also controls for age of alcohol use onset.
[e] Also controls for age of alcohol use onset and age of alcohol problem onset.
[f] Significant at the .05 level, two-sided test.

TABLE 23.11. Mental Disorders Predicting the Subsequent First Onset of Alcohol Use, Problems, and Dependence among Women

	Use in total sample[a]				Problems among users[a]				Dependence among problem users				Dependence in total sample			
	OR[b]	(95% CI)	OR[c]	(95% CI)	OR[b,d]	(95% CI)	OR[c,d]	(95% CI)	OR[b,e]	(95% CI)	OR[c,e]	(95% CI)	OR[b,e]	(95% CI)	OR[c,e]	(95% CI)
Mood disorders																
Depression	1.7	(1.1–2.5)	1.4	(1.0–2.1)	3.3	(2.5–4.5)	2.1	(1.5–2.9)	2.2	(1.4–3.3)	1.3	(0.9–2.1)	5.6	(4.2–7.4)	2.3	(1.6–3.4)
Dysthymia	1.0	(0.5–2.0)	0.7	(0.3–1.3)	4.3	(2.9–6.3)	2.3	(1.4–3.6)	3.7	(1.8–7.9)	2.7	(1.3–5.8)	5.6	(3.2–9.6)	1.9	(1.1–3.4)
Mania	6.9	(1.8–26.3)	3.9	(0.5–30.9)	5.2	(2.1–12.1)	3.5	(1.1–10.8)	0.9	(0.0–3.0)	0.5	(0.1–2.1)	7.5	(2.8–19.7)	1.7	(0.6–4.6)
Any mood disorder	1.7	(1.2–2.5)			3.7	(2.8–4.8)			2.2	(1.6–3.2)			6.0	(4.7–7.7)		
Anxiety disorders																
Agoraphobia	1.1	(0.7–1.7)	0.7	(0.4–1.3)	2.2	(1.5–3.1)	0.9	(0.5–1.5)	2.1	(1.3–3.4)	1.2	(0.6–2.5)	3.6	(2.5–5.1)	0.9	(0.4–1.8)
GAD	1.6	(0.9–3.0)	0.8	(0.4–1.7)	3.4	(2.0–5.9)	1.5	(0.7–3.2)	4.0	(1.9–8.6)	2.1	(0.9–4.9)	7.7	(4.3–13.8)	1.8	(0.9–4.0)
Panic attack	1.9	(1.3–2.6)	1.2	(0.8–1.8)	2.8	(2.1–3.8)	1.6	(0.9–2.6)	2.2	(1.3–3.8)	1.5	(0.7–2.9)	5.6	(3.9–8.2)	2.3	(1.0–5.2)
Panic disorder	3.9	(N/C–N/C)	3.1	(0.0–N/C)	3.7	(1.1–12.0)	1.4	(0.4–4.4)	N/E	N/E	N/E	N/E	2.4	(0.4–13.3)	0.6	(0.1–4.5)
OCD	0.6	(0.1–2.7)	0.5	(0.1–2.4)	1.5	(N/C–N/C)	0.6	(N/C–N/C)	N/E	N/E	N/E	N/E	N/E	N/E	N/E	N/E
PTSD	1.5	(0.9–2.3)	1.3	(0.8–2.9)	2.4	(1.7–3.4)	1.3	(0.9–1.9)	2.3	(1.3–3.8)	1.7	(0.9–3.2)	4.9	(3.4–7.2)	2.0	(1.1–3.8)
Simple phobia	1.4	(1.1–1.7)	1.1	(0.8–1.4)	1.9	(1.4–2.6)	1.1	(0.8–1.5)	1.7	(1.2–2.4)	1.4	(0.8–2.2)	2.7	(2.0–3.6)	1.4	(0.9–2.2)
Social phobia	1.7	(1.4–2.1)	1.5	(1.2–1.8)	2.5	(2.0–3.0)	1.7	(1.3–2.2)	1.0	(0.7–1.3)	0.6	(0.4–0.9)	2.9	(2.3–3.6)	1.2	(0.8–1.9)
Any anxiety disorder	1.5	(1.3–1.8)			2.3	(1.9–2.9)			1.6	(1.2–2.1)			3.6	(2.9–4.5)		
Other disorders																
Conduct disorder	2.4	(1.6–3.6)	1.8	(1.1–2.9)	3.1	(2.3–4.2)	2.5	(1.7–3.7)	1.5	(1.0–2.2)	1.0	(0.6–1.6)	5.9	(3.9–8.9)	3.5	(1.7–6.9)
AAB	4.0	(3.0–5.3)	3.2	(2.2–4.8)	4.6	(3.4–6.3)	3.6	(2.4–5.4)	2.2	(1.5–3.2)	1.4	(0.9–2.4)	11.0	(8.2–14.7)	5.7	(3.3–9.8)
ASP	4.4	(2.9–6.6)	0.7	(0.3–1.6)	4.5	(2.8–7.3)	0.5	(0.2–1.0)	2.6	(1.4–4.7)	1.7	(0.7–4.3)	13.2	(8.1–21.3)	0.7	(0.2–1.9)
Any other disorder	2.8	(2.0–3.9)			3.8	(2.9–5.0)			1.7	(1.2–2.4)			7.9	(5.8–10.7)		
Number of disorders																
Exactly one disorder	1.3	(1.1–1.5)			2.2	(1.8–2.7)			1.9	(1.3–2.8)			3.8	(2.7–5.3)		
Exactly two disorders	1.5	(1.3–1.9)			3.1	(2.4–4.0)			1.5	(0.9–2.3)			5.0	(3.6–7.0)		
Three or more disorders	1.8	(1.5–2.3)			4.5	(3.6–5.6)			2.7	(1.9–3.8)			11.1	(8.1–15.1)		
Any disorder	1.5	(1.3–1.7)			3.0	(2.5–3.5)			2.1	(1.5–2.8)			6.0	(4.6–7.9)		
$\Delta \chi^2_{12,14}$	115.1[f]				253.1[f]				70.5[f]				374.9[f]			

NOTE. N/E = Parameter not estimable due to small sample size; N/C = Nonconvergent parameter estimates.
[a] São Paulo (Brazil) and Netherlands not included.
[b] From models with 1 psychiatric predictor at a time and controls (age, cohort, survey).
[c] From models with all 14 psychiatric predictors and controls.
[d] Also controls for age of alcohol use onset.
[e] Also controls for age of alcohol use onset and age of alcohol problem onset.
[f] Significant at the .05 level, two-sided test.

TABLE 23.12. Mental Disorders Predicting the Subsequent First Onset of Drug Use, Problems, and Dependence among Men

	Use in total sample[a]				Problems among users[a]				Dependence among problem users				Dependence in total sample			
	OR[b]	(95% CI)	OR[c]	(95% CI)	OR[b,d]	(95% CI)	OR[c,d]	(95% CI)	OR[b,e]	(95% CI)	OR[c,e]	(95% CI)	OR[b,e]	(95% CI)	OR[c,e]	(95% CI)
Mood disorders																
Depression	3.5	(2.5–5.0)	1.9	(1.2–2.9)	2.4	(1.7–3.5)	1.4	(1.0–2.1)	1.4	(0.8–2.4)	0.9	(0.4–1.8)	4.4	(3.2–6.0)	1.4	(0.9–2.2)
Dysthymia	3.7	(2.1–6.4)	2.0	(1.1–3.6)	3.2	(1.6–6.4)	1.8	(0.9–3.9)	1.7	(1.0–3.0)	1.4	(0.6–3.0)	4.4	(2.8–6.7)	1.5	(0.8–3.1)
Mania	2.1	(1.3–3.6)	0.8	(0.4–1.6)	3.0	(1.6–5.6)	1.2	(0.5–2.6)	4.5	(1.9–10.3)	2.4	(0.7–8.4)	11.4	(7.0–18.6)	2.7	(1.2–5.7)
Any mood disorder	3.2	(2.4–4.2)			3.0	(2.1–4.3)			1.7	(1.1–2.7)			5.4	(4.1–7.2)		
Anxiety disorders																
Agoraphobia	2.5	(1.7–3.7)	1.3	(0.8–2.2)	1.7	(1.1–2.6)	0.8	(0.4–1.4)	2.9	(1.6–5.4)	1.0	(0.5–2.3)	4.2	(2.6–6.9)	1.0	(0.5–2.0)
GAD	5.7	(3.3–9.6)	2.4	(1.3–4.6)	3.1	(1.6–6.1)	1.4	(0.7–3.0)	2.9	(1.2–7.1)	1.5	(0.4–5.4)	7.3	(4.1–13.0)	2.3	(1.0–5.5)
Panic attack	4.7	(2.8–7.8)	2.4	(1.2–5.0)	1.8	(0.8–3.9)	1.3	(0.4–4.3)	2.3	(0.9–5.8)	0.7	(0.1–3.3)	4.2	(2.4–7.6)	1.0	(0.3–2.9)
Panic disorder	3.4	(1.3–9.1)	1.2	(0.4–3.6)	2.0	(0.5–8.6)	1.3	(0.3–5.7)	7.8	(3.1–19.8)	4.1	(1.2–14.7)	14.0	(5.4–36.0)	5.0	(1.6–15.2)
OCD	5.5	(2.0–14.8)	2.8	(0.8–9.5)	2.4	(0.7–8.3)	1.0	(0.2–4.8)	3.9	(0.2–85.5)	0.5	(0.0–12.4)	11.8	(1.5–92.9)	1.2	(0.1–17.2)
PTSD	5.0	(2.7–9.3)	1.9	(1.0–3.5)	1.5	(0.9–2.6)	0.8	(0.3–1.8)	5.8	(1.9–17.9)	2.9	(0.9–9.5)	5.5	(2.9–10.5)	1.4	(0.6–3.5)
Simple phobia	1.7	(1.3–2.3)	1.2	(0.8–1.6)	2.2	(1.6–3.0)	1.5	(1.1–2.1)	3.2	(1.9–5.3)	2.1	(1.1–4.0)	3.8	(2.6–5.4)	1.6	(0.9–2.6)
Social phobia	1.6	(1.3–2.0)	1.0	(0.9–1.3)	2.0	(1.6–2.6)	1.4	(1.0–1.9)	2.6	(1.6–4.1)	1.9	(1.1–3.3)	3.6	(2.7–4.9)	1.8	(1.1–2.8)
Any anxiety disorder	2.0	(1.7–2.4)			2.1	(1.6–2.7)			2.7	(1.9–3.9)			4.2	(3.3–5.3)		
Other disorders																
Conduct disorder	2.8	(2.4–3.4)	2.2	(1.7–2.8)	2.5	(1.9–3.2)	1.9	(1.4–2.6)	1.4	(1.0–2.0)	1.2	(0.7–2.0)	5.5	(4.1–7.2)	3.8	(2.5–5.8)
AAB	3.8	(2.9–4.8)	3.2	(2.5–4.2)	3.0	(2.4–3.8)	2.6	(1.9–3.6)	1.8	(1.2–2.6)	1.7	(1.1–2.5)	8.1	(6.3–10.3)	8.0	(5.3–12.1)
ASP	3.9	(2.9–5.2)	0.7	(0.5–1.0)	3.2	(2.4–4.2)	0.8	(0.5–1.2)	1.6	(1.0–2.5)	0.8	(0.4–1.7)	7.2	(5.4–9.5)	0.4	(0.2–0.6)
Any other disorder	3.2	(2.7–3.8)			2.9	(2.3–3.7)			1.7	(1.2–2.4)			8.4	(6.2–11.3)		
Number of disorders																
Exactly one disorder	1.8	(1.5–2.0)			1.8	(1.4–2.2)			1.0	(0.7–1.5)			2.9	(2.1–4.0)		
Exactly two disorders	2.4	(2.0–2.9)			2.9	(2.1–4.0)			2.1	(1.3–3.4)			6.8	(4.8–9.6)		
Three or more disorders	4.2	(3.4–5.2)			4.3	(3.3–5.6)			2.4	(1.6–3.4)			14.2	(10.9–18.6)		
Any disorder	2.4	(2.1–2.7)			2.6	(2.1–3.2)			1.7	(1.2–2.3)			6.3	(4.9–8.2)		
$\Delta\chi^2_{14}$	268.0[f]				113.2[f]				68.2[f]				434.4[f]			

[a] São Paulo (Brazil) and Netherlands not included.
[b] From models with 1 psychiatric predictor at a time and controls (age, cohort, survey).
[c] From models with all 14 psychiatric predictors and controls.
[d] Also controls for age of drug use onset.
[e] Also controls for age of drug use onset and age of drug problem onset.
[f] Significant at the .05 level, two-sided test.

TABLE 23.13. Mental Disorders Predicting the Subsequent First Onset of Drug Use, Problems, and Dependence among Women

	Use in total sample[a]				Problems among users[a]				Dependence among problem users				Dependence in total sample			
	OR[b]	(95% CI)	OR[c]	(95% CI)	OR[b,d]	(95% CI)	OR[c,d]	(95% CI)	OR[b,e]	(95% CI)	OR[c,e]	(95% CI)	OR[b,e]	(95% CI)	OR[c,e]	(95% CI)
Mood disorders																
Depression	3.2	(2.3–4.4)	2.2	(1.5–3.2)	2.8	(2.1–3.7)	1.8	(1.3–2.4)	2.1	(1.3–3.4)	1.1	(0.6–2.0)	6.6	(5.0–8.6)	2.5	(1.8–3.6)
Dysthymia	3.0	(2.0–4.6)	1.2	(0.7–1.8)	3.9	(2.6–5.8)	2.0	(1.3–3.0)	1.9	(1.0–3.7)	1.3	(0.6–2.8)	6.9	(4.5–10.7)	2.5	(1.4–4.2)
Mania	7.5	(3.9–14.4)	2.7	(1.3–5.6)	5.2	(2.4–11.5)	3.2	(1.3–8.2)	2.0	(0.8–5.1)	1.9	(0.4–9.3)	18.6	(10.4–33.3)	7.1	(2.5–20.3)
Any mood disorder	3.4	(2.5–4.5)			3.0	(2.3–4.0)			1.9	(1.2–2.9)			7.2	(5.4–9.4)		
Anxiety disorders																
Agoraphobia	2.1	(1.3–3.4)	1.1	(0.6–2.3)	1.8	(1.1–2.9)	1.0	(0.5–1.8)	1.9	(1.2–3.1)	1.5	(0.7–3.1)	4.2	(2.8–6.5)	1.4	(0.7–2.7)
GAD	4.8	(3.4–6.9)	2.2	(1.3–3.7)	3.7	(2.3–5.9)	1.4	(0.8–2.5)	2.2	(1.1–4.2)	2.1	(0.6–7.7)	7.7	(4.7–12.5)	1.4	(0.7–3.1)
Panic attack	3.2	(2.4–4.2)	1.9	(1.2–3.0)	3.1	(1.9–5.1)	2.0	(1.1–3.8)	1.6	(1.0–2.6)	1.1	(0.5–2.7)	6.8	(4.9–9.4)	2.1	(1.1–3.9)
Panic disorder	4.5	(2.8–7.2)	1.9	(1.1–3.1)	2.9	(1.6–5.2)	1.0	(0.6–1.9)	0.9	(0.3–2.4)	0.3	(0.1–1.3)	6.3	(2.8–14.3)	1.1	(0.4–3.3)
OCD	5.3	(1.9–15.2)	1.6	(0.5–5.4)	1.4	(0.2–7.3)	0.5	(0.1–2.0)	2.8	(0.7–11.3)	5.1	(0.8–31.6)	5.7	(1.5–21.6)	0.4	(0.1–1.5)
PTSD	2.7	(1.8–4.1)	1.6	(0.9–2.8)	3.1	(1.9–4.9)	2.0	(1.2–3.2)	2.2	(1.1–4.4)	1.5	(0.7–3.6)	6.1	(3.6–10.2)	2.2	(0.9–5.5)
Simple phobia	1.6	(1.3–1.9)	1.0	(0.8–1.3)	2.3	(1.7–2.9)	1.3	(1.0–1.8)	1.9	(1.2–3.0)	2.0	(1.2–3.2)	3.6	(2.7–4.7)	1.8	(1.2–2.7)
Social phobia	2.2	(1.8–2.6)	1.5	(1.2–1.8)	2.0	(1.4–2.8)	1.2	(0.8–1.9)	1.2	(0.8–1.7)	0.7	(0.4–1.2)	3.3	(2.6–4.3)	1.0	(0.6–1.5)
Any anxiety disorder	2.2	(1.9–2.5)			2.5	(1.9–3.2)			1.6	(1.2–2.2)			4.7	(3.7–6.1)		
Other disorders																
Conduct disorder	3.2	(2.2–4.6)	2.3	(1.4–4.0)	2.0	(1.4–2.8)	1.6	(1.0–2.4)	2.4	(1.5–4.0)	1.6	(0.8–3.3)	7.2	(4.9–10.4)	4.4	(2.0–9.8)
AAB	5.1	(3.9–6.7)	4.0	(2.6–6.1)	4.2	(2.8–6.2)	3.2	(1.8–5.5)	2.1	(1.3–3.4)	1.1	(0.6–2.2)	12.5	(9.1–17.2)	6.6	(4.1–10.6)
ASP	5.5	(3.5–8.5)	0.6	(0.3–1.4)	4.3	(2.4–7.8)	0.9	(0.4–2.0)	2.9	(1.5–5.5)	1.6	(0.6–4.3)	14.8	(9.3–23.6)	0.6	(0.2–1.8)
Any other disorder	3.7	(2.7–5.1)			2.7	(2.0–3.7)			2.3	(1.5–3.4)			9.7	(7.2–13.1)		
Number of disorders																
Exactly one disorder	2.0	(1.7–2.2)			2.0	(1.5–2.8)			1.0	(0.6–1.7)			3.6	(2.5–5.3)		
Exactly two disorders	2.3	(1.9–2.7)			3.4	(2.4–4.8)			1.2	(0.7–2.2)			7.1	(4.8–10.6)		
Three or more disorders	3.5	(3.0–4.2)			4.5	(3.4–5.9)			2.1	(1.3–3.3)			16.2	(11.7–22.4)		
Any disorder	2.4	(2.2–2.6)			3.1	(2.4–4.0)			1.5	(1.0–2.3)			7.8	(6.0–10.3)		
$\Delta \chi^2_{14}$	349.6[f]				138.0[f]				44.7[f]				406.9[f]			

[a] São Paulo (Brazil) and Netherlands not included.
[b] From models with 1 psychiatric predictor at a time and controls (age, cohort, survey).
[c] From models with all 14 psychiatric predictors and controls.
[d] Also controls for age of drug use onset.
[e] Also controls for age of drug use onset and age of drug problem onset.
[f] Significant at the .05 level, two-sided test.

TABLE 23.14. Population Attributable risk (PAR) Proportions of Substance Use, Problems, and Dependence Predicted by Prior Mental Disorders by Gender

	Alcohol				Drug			
	Use (%)	Problems among users (%)	Dependence among problem users (%)	Dependence in total sample (%)	Use (%)	Problems among users (%)	Dependence among problem users (%)	Dependence in total sample (%)
Men								
Mood disorder	0.0	2.5	3.7	6.4	1.9	4.5	3.0	9.6
Anxiety disorder	0.2	4.8	4.9	10.5	3.1	6.6	8.4	17.5
Conduct and antisocial personality disorders	1.4	19.4	16.2	38.7	11.5	24.9	12.8	51.2
All mental disorders	1.3	21.4	19.3	40.5	12.9	27.5	19.8	54.7
Women								
Mood disorder	0.5	10.7	11.2	22.8	5.9	12.9	10.7	27.0
Anxiety disorder	0.5	13.4	9.7	20.9	6.5	14.5	9.6	25.9
Conduct and antisocial personality disorders	1.2	17.1	10.7	33.5	7.2	16.0	7.8	34.8
All mental disorders	1.6	26.5	17.9	41.4	13.0	28.1	16.0	47.8

TABLE 23.15. Population Attributable Risk (PAR) Proportions of Substance Dependence Due to Prior Mental Disorders by Gender and Survey Site

	Men		Women	
	Alcohol dependence (%)	Drug dependence (%)	Alcohol dependence (%)	Drug dependence (%)
São Paulo (Brazil)	N/E	N/E	N/E	44.2
Fresno (CA)	60.7	76.9	63.1	74.2
Munich (Germany)	10.2	11.8	31.5	45.0
Mexico City (Mexico)	2.2	19.9	35.2	70.6
Netherlands	N/E	25.6	N/E	54.3
Ontario (Canada)	40.8	66.2	41.3	53.6
United States	46.5	58.4	43.5	46.8

NOTE. N/E = parameter not estimable due to small sample size.

versus 35% in which the ORs are stronger among men than among women and 11% in which the ORs are the same for men and women).

Population-Attributable Risks of Substance Disorders Due to Mental Disorders

The results in Tables 23.10 to 23.13 were used to estimate the proportion of all substance use disorders that would have been prevented by the successful treatment of prior mental disorders. As noted previously in the section on analysis methods, these population attributable risk (PAR) proportions were estimated using simulations, based on the assumptions that the results in Tables 23.10 to 23.13 are accurate reflections of population processes that are due to causal effects of the mental disorders on secondary substance use disorders. PAR estimates are shown in Table 23.14 separately for the effects of the three broad classes of mental disorders considered here in models that do not control for the other disorders as well as for the total effects of all these disorders combined. The results show that very large proportions of alcohol and drug dependence in the total sample are due to prior mental disorders: 40.5% of alcohol dependence among men, 41.4% of alcohol dependence among women, 54.7% of drug dependence among men, and 47.8% of drug dependence among women.

Comparing entries within a single row of the table shows that the PARs due to the impact of the mental disorders on initiation of alcohol use are consistently the smallest entries in the table and that the PARs associated with the transition from use to problem use are generally the largest. Comparing entries within a single column of the table shows that the PARs due to conduct disorder, adult antisocial behavior, and antisocial personality disorder are generally larger than those due to mood disorders or to anxiety disorders. The PARs due to mood and anxiety disorders are consistently larger for women than for men, while the PARs due to conduct disorder, adult antisocial behavior, and antisocial personality disorder are consistently larger for men than for women. These gender differences are largely due to differences in disorder prevalences rather than to differences in conditional risks by gender. The mood disorder PARs are consistently smaller than the anxiety disorder PARs among men, while the mood disorder PARs are roughly equivalent in magnitude to the anxiety disorder PARs among women.

Summary information on the consistency of these results across surveys is reported in Table 23.15. As can be seen, the PARs for alcohol dependence among men range from lows of 2.2%

in Mexico and 10.2% in Munich to highs between 40.8 and 60.7% in Ontario, the United States, and Fresno. In comparison, the PARs for alcohol dependence among women are more consistently high, ranging from a minimum of 31.5% in Munich to a maximum of 63.1% in Fresno. There is also more variability in the drug dependence PARs among men than among women, with three fairly low male PARs (11.8% in Munich, 19.9% in Mexico, and 25.6% in the Netherlands) and higher PARs (58.4–76.9%) in Ontario, the United States, and Fresno. The PARs are consistently high in all surveys among women (44.2–74.2%).

DISCUSSION

The results reported in this chapter are limited by the fact that they are based on cross-sectional data using retrospective age of onset reports to reconstruct temporal priorities between first onsets of substance use disorders and mental disorders. Recall failure could lead to bias in the estimated strength of associations between temporally primary mental disorders and the subsequent first onset of substance use disorders. An additional limitation is that many people are unwilling to admit substance use problems or mental disorders to survey interviewers (Turner et al., 1998). This could lead to distorted estimates of PAR, even if recall error in dating onset is absent in the subsample of respondents who are willing to disclose information about these disorders. A final limitation is that the PAR estimates cannot be interpreted as reflecting causal influences of mental disorders due to the fact that we cannot rule out the influences of unmeasured common causes.

Within the context of these limitations, we found lifetime prevalences of substance disorders consistent with those found in previous general population surveys (Gureje et al., 1996; Helzer et al., 1990). To the extent that these results are in error, they are likely to be underestimates, which means that the true population prevalences of these disorders are likely to be even higher than those reported here. We also found strong lifetime co-morbidities of substance use, problems, and dependence, with a wide range of DSM-III-R mental disorders. These are similar in magnitude to those found in previous general population surveys (Grant & Harford, 1995; Regier et al., 1990) and clinical studies (Hesselbrock, Meyer, & Keener, 1985; Penick et al., 1994). As the likelihood of conscious nondisclosure of disorders is likely to be much lower in clinical studies, where patients have voluntarily come for help, than in community surveys, this consistency of findings across the two types of samples is important.

In addition, consistent with results in previous community surveys (Kessler et al., 1996; Merikangas et al., 1996) and clinical studies (Hesselbrock et al., 1985; Jaffe & Ciraulo, 1986), we found that retrospective age of onset reports consistently date the first onset of substance dependence as occurring subsequent to the first onset of mood disorders in the majority of women but not of men, and subsequent to the first onset of co-morbid anxiety disorders in the vast majority of both men and women. Although we did not date the onset of conduct disorder, adult antisocial behavior, or antisocial personality disorder, DSM-III-R criteria require symptoms of conduct disorder to occur prior to age 15, and we asked respondents only about symptoms that occurred prior to this age. If we use age 14 as the upper age of onset of conduct disorder, we find that the vast majority of respondents with a history of both conduct disorder and substance dependence had a first onset of dependence after the onset of conduct disorder.

We have much less evidence from previous studies to use as a comparison in evaluating our findings regarding the effects of temporally primary mental disorders in predicting the subsequent first onset of substance use disorders. Only a few longitudinal community surveys have investigated this issue prospectively. There is consistent evidence in these studies that conduct disorder is a powerful risk factor for substance use disorders (Dembo et al., 1985; Lewis, Rice, & Helzer, 1983). The evidence is less consistent for similar effects of mood disorders or anxiety disorders, with some studies finding effects (Kranzler, Del Boca, & Rounsaville, 1996; Kushner, Sher, & Erickson, 1999) and others failing to find effects (Schuckit & Hesselbrock, 1994).

None of these earlier studies attempted to estimate the proportion of all substance dependence that could be attributed to earlier mental disorders. Our results are striking in this regard in suggesting that earlier mental disorders are enormously important, accounting for at least 40% of all cases of lifetime alcohol or drug dependence among men and women in each of the seven surveys analyzed. It is unclear whether associations as powerful as these would be found in longitudinal studies. Nor is it clear that such associations, if they could be documented, reflect causal influences of mental disorders, influences of unmeasured common causes, or methodological artifacts due to systematic measurement error. Given the potential importance of the results for policy and intervention purposes, it is clear that future research should attempt to adjudicate between these contending possibilities.

Two important points are worth noting as being of potential importance in arguing that the statistically significant survival coefficients reported here are due, at least in part, to a causal effect of primary mental disorders. The first is that the coefficients reported here represent the impact of active mental disorders rather than remitted disorders. As noted earlier, remitted disorders were not found to be significantly related to subsequent substance use problems. This finding is consistent with the possibility that something about mental disorders themselves, rather than about stable risk factors that persist beyond the remission of these disorders, is associated with risk of secondary substance use disorders. Although not proving that successful treatment of primary mental disorders will lead to a reduced risk of onset of substance use disorders, this important preliminary result certainly increases the plausibility of such an effect.

The second important point comes from an analyses, which is currently unpublished, involving self-medication, a process that is often proposed as the key causal pathway linking primary mental disorders with the subsequent onset of substance use disorders (Khantzian, 1997). Self-medication is the process of using alcohol or other drugs in a conscious effort to control dysphoric mood. Respondents in three of the seven surveys analyzed here (United States; Fresno, CA; and Mexico City) were asked explicit questions about self-medication linked separately to mood and anxiety disorders. Creation of separate mental disorder predictor variables that discriminate mood and anxiety disorders with self-medication from the same disorders without self-medication show that only the former are associated with elevated risk of subsequent substance use disorders. It is important not to over interpret this result, as it is based on retrospective data, and the self-medication might well have started after the onset of substance dependence. Nonetheless, this specification is consistent with our finding that the strongest effects of mental disorders are on the transition from use to problem use, and this, in turn, is consistent with the possibility that at least some part of the substantial PAR estimates found here are due to causal effects of mental disorders.

These results lead to obvious speculation about the possibility that early intervention and successful treatment of mental disorders might help prevent the onset of a substantial proportion of substance use disorders in the countries included in this investigation. With this possibility in mind, it is noteworthy that only a small minority of the respondents with co-morbid mental and substance disorders reported that they obtained professional treatment for their mental disorders prior to the age of onset of their secondary substance use disorders. It is also noteworthy that a comparison of age-of-onset reports for temporally primary mental disorders and subsequent substance use disorders shows a window of opportunity for preventive intervention (i.e., subsequent to the onset of the primary mental disorder and prior to the onset of the secondary substance use disorder) of between 5 and 8 years for most mental disorders. The bulk of this time interval for the vast majority of respondents is when they are still in school, which means that group screening in schools would be a feasible way of targeting people to receive the intervention. Schools might also be a practical location for delivery of the intervention.

Currently, high-risk preventive interventions for substance abuse among youth are almost entirely directed at youth with conduct problems. The results presented here show that this is a mistake. This is especially true among girls, in whom mood and anxiety disorders are associated with between one-fourth and one-fifth of all substance dependence. Only one-third of female substance dependence is associated with conduct disorder and adult antisocial behavior. It is uncertain whether early outreach and intervention to treat mood and anxiety disorders prior to the onset of secondary substance use disorders would be effective in preventing the latter disorders, but the results reported here certainly suggest that this may be a useful approach. This is an appealing possibility for a number of reasons (Kessler & Price, 1993). One is that there are accurate methods for identifying potential intervention subjects with mental disorders. A second is that there are well-established treatment technologies for implementing the preventive interventions. A third is that, unlike the situation with most prevention efforts, the subjects of the intervention efforts are already in pain and, therefore, presumably motivated to engage in prevention efforts. Based on these considerations, we believe the evidence warrants the initiation of open trials to evaluate the potential effectiveness of early outreach and treatment of mood and anxiety disorders among youth in an effort to prevent the onset of substance use disorders. If those trials are promising, there should be randomized effectiveness trials to evaluate the impact of such interventions as an adjunct to currently available school-based prevention programs.

REFERENCES

Allan, C. A. (1995). Alcohol problems and anxiety disorders-A critical review. *Alcohol and Alcoholism. 30,* 145–151.

Bijl, R. V., Van Zessen, G., Ravelli, A., de Rijk, C., & Langendoen, Y. (1998). The Netherlands Mental Health Survey and Incidence Study (NEMESIS): Objectives and design. *Social Psychiatry Psychiatric Epidemiology, 33,* 581–6.

Caraveo, J., Martinez, J., & Rivera, B. (1998). A model for epidemiological studies on mental health and psychiatric morbidity. *Salud Mental, 21,* 48–57.

Dembo, R., Allen, N., Farrow, D., Schmeidler, J., & Burgos, W. (1985). A causal analysis of early drug involvement in three inner-city neighborhood settings. *International Journal of the Addictions, 20,* 1213–1237.

Efron, B. (1988). Logistic regression, survival analysis, and the Kaplan-Meier Curve. *Journal of the American Sociological Association, 83,* 414–425.

George, D. T., Nutt, D. T., Dwyer, B. A., & Linnoila, M. (1990). Alcoholism and panic disorder: Is the co-morbidity more than coincidence? *Acta Psychiatrica Scandinavica, 81,* 97–107.

Grant, B. F., & Harford, T. C. (1995). Co-morbidity between DSM-IV alcohol use disorders and major depression: Results of a national survey. *Drug and Alcohol Dependence, 39,* 197–206.

Gureje, O., Vazquez-Barquero, J. L., & Janca, A. (1996) Comparisons of alcohol and other drugs: Experience from the WHO collaborative cross-cultural applicability (CAR) study. *Addiction, 91,* 1529–1538.

Helzer, J. E., Canino, G. J., Yeh, E.-K., & Bland, R. C. (1990). Alcoholism: North America and Asia: A comparison of population surveys with the Diagnostic Interview Schedule. *Archives of General Psychiatry, 47,* 313–319.

Hesselbrock, M. N., Meyer, R. E., & Keener, J. J. (1985). Psychopathology in hospitalized alcoholics. *Archives of General Psychiatry, 42,* 1050–1055.

Hirschfeld, R. M. A., Hasin, D., Keller, M. B., Endicott, J., & Wunder, J. (1990). Depression and alcoholism: Co-morbidity in a longitudinal study. In J. D. Maser & C. R. Cloninger (Eds.), *Co-morbidity of mood and anxiety disorders* (pp. 293–304). Washington, DC: American Psychiatric Press.

Jaffe, J. H., & Ciraulo, D. A. (1986). Alcoholism and depression. In R. E. Meyer (Ed.), *Psychopathology and addictive disorders* (pp. 293–320). New York: Guilford Press.

Keitner, G. I., Ryan, C. E., Miller, I. W., Kohn, R., & Epstein, N. B. (1991). 12-Month outcome of patients with major depression and co-morbid psychiatric or medical illness (compound depression). *American Journal of Psychiatry, 148,* 345–350.

Kessler, R. C. (1997). The prevalence of psychiatric co-morbidity. In S. Wetzler & W. C. Sanderson (Eds.), *Treatment strategies for patients with psychiatric co-morbidity* (pp. 23–48). New York: Wiley.

Kessler, R. C., Aguilar-Gaxiola, S., Andrade, L., Bijl, R., Borges, B., Caraveo-Anduaga, J. J., DeWit, D. J., Kolody, B., Merikangas, K. R., Molnar, B. E., Vega, W. A., Walters, E. E., Wittchen, H.-U., & Ustun, T. B. (2001). Mental-substance co-morbidities in the ICPE surveys. *Psychiatria Fennica, 32* (suppl. 2), 62–80.

Kessler, R. C., Crum, R. M., Warner, L. A., Nelson, C. B., Schulenberg, J., & Anthony, J. (1997). Lifetime co-occurrence of DSM-III-R alcohol abuse and dependence with other psychiatric disorders in the national co-morbidity survey. *Archives of General Psychiatry, 54,* 313–321.

Kessler, R. C., McGonagle, K. A., Zhao, S., Nelson, C. B., Hughes, M., Eshleman, S., Wittchen, H.-U., & Kendler, K. S. (1994). Lifetime and 12-month prevalence of DSM-III-R psychiatric disorders in the United States: Results from the National Co-morbidity Survey. *Archives of General Psychiatry, 51,* 8–19.

Kessler, R. C., Nelson, C. B., McGonagle, K. A., Edlund, M. J., Frank, R. G., & Leaf, P. J. (1996). The epidemiology of co-occurring addictive and mental disorders: Implications for prevention and service utilization. *American Journal of Orthopsychiatry, 66,* 17–31.

Kessler, R. C., & Price, R. H. (1993). Primary prevention of secondary disorders: A proposal and agenda. *American Journal of Community Psychology, 21,* 607–633.

Kessler, R. C., Wittchen, H.-U., Abelson, J. M., McGonagle, K., Schwarz, N., Kendler, K. S., Knäuper, B., & Zhao, S. (1998). Methodological studies of the Composite International Diagnostic Interview (CIDI) in the US National Co-morbidity Survey. *International Journal of Methods in Psychiatric Research, 7,* 33–55.

Khantzian, E. J. (1997). The self-medication hypothesis of substance-use disorders: A reconsideration and recent applications. *Harvard Review of Psychiatry, 4,* 231–244.

Kish, L., & Frankel, M. R. (1974). Inferences from complex samples. *Journal of the Royal Statistical Society, 36,* 1–37.

Kranzler, H. R., Del Boca, F. K., & Rounsaville, B. J. (1996). Co-morbid psychiatric diagnosis predicts three-year outcomes in alcoholics: A posttreatment natural history study. *Journal of Studies on Alcohol, 57,* 619–626.

Kushner, M. G., Sher, K. J., & Erickson, D. J. (1999). Prospective analysis of the relation between DSM-III anxiety disorders and alcohol use disorders. *American Journal of Psychiatry, 156,* 723–732.

Lewis, C. E., Rice, J., & Helzer, J. E. (1983). Diagnostic interactions: Alcoholism and antisocial personality. *Journal of Nervous and Mental Diseases, 171,* 105–113.

Merikangas, K. R., Angst, J., Eaton, W., Canino, G., Rubio-Stipec, M., Wacker, H., Wittchen, H.-U., Andrade, L., Essau, C., Kraemer, H., Robins, L., & Kupfer, D. (1996). Co-morbidity and boundaries of affective disorders with anxiety disorders and substance misuse: Results of an international task force. *British Journal of Psychiatry, 168*(Suppl. 30), 58–67.

Merikangas, K. R., Mehta, R. L.., Molnar, B. E., Walters, E. E., Swendsen, J. D., Aguilar-Gaxiola, S., Bijl, R., Borges, G., Caraveo-Anduaga, J. J., Dewit, D. J., Kolody, B., Vega, W. A., Wittchen, H.-U., & Kessler, R. C. (1998). Co-morbidity of substance-use disorders with mood and anxiety disorders: Results of the International Consortium in Psychiatric Epidemiology (ICPE). *Addictive Behaviors, 23,* 893–907.

Merikangas, K., & Stevens, D. E. (1998). Substance abuse among women: Familial factors and co-morbidity. In C. L. Wetherington & A. B. Roman (Eds.), *Drug addiction research and the health of women* (pp. 245–269). Bethesda, MD: National Institute on Drug Abuse.

Mirin, S. M., Weiss, R. D., Griffin, M. L., & Michael, J. L. (1991). Psychopathology in drug abusers and their families. *Comprehensive Psychiatry, 32,* 36–51.

Offord, D. R., Campbell, D., Cochrane, J., Goering, P. N., Lin, E., Rhodes, A., & Wong, M. (1994). *Mental health in Ontario: Selected findings from the Mental Health Supplement to the Ontario Health Survey.* Toronto: Queen's Printer for Ontario.

Penick, E. C., Powell, B. J., Nickel, E. J., Bingham, S. F., Riesenmy, K. R., Read, M. R., & Campbell, J. (1994). Co-morbidity of lifetime psychiatric disorder among male alcoholic patients. *Alcoholism: Clinical and Experimental Research, 18,* 1289–1293.

Regier, D. A., Farmer, M. E., Rae, D. S., Locke, B. Z., Keith, B. J., Judd, L. L., & Goodwin, F. K. (1990). Co-morbidity of mental health disorders with alcohol and other drug abuse. *Journal of the American Medical Association, 264,* 2511–2518.

Schuckit, M. A., & Hesselbrock, V. (1994). Alcohol dependence and anxiety disorders: What is the relationship? *American Journal of Psychiatry, 151,* 1723–1734.

Sheehan, M. F. (1993). Dual diagnosis. *Psychiatric Quarterly, 1193,* 107–134.

Turner, C. F., Ku, L., Rogers, S. M., Lindberg, L. D., Pleck, J. H., & Sonenstein, F. L. (1998). Adolescent sexual behavior, drug use, and violence: Increased reporting with computer survey technology. *Science, 280,* 867–873.

Vega, W. A., Kolody, B., Aguilar-Gaxiola, S., Alderete, E., Catalano, R., & Caraveo-Anduaga, J. (1998). Lifetime prevalence of DSM-III-R psychiatric disorders among urban and rural Mexican Americans in California. *Archives of General Psychiatry, 55,* 771–778.

Wittchen, H.-U. (1994). Reliability and validity studies of the WHO-Composite International Diagnostic Interview (CIDI): A critical review. *Journal of Psychiatric Research, 28,* 57–84.

Wittchen, H.-U., Zhao, S., Abelson, J. M., Abelson, J. L., & Kessler, R. C. (1996). Reliability and procedural validity of UM-CIDI DSM-III-R phobic disorders. *Psychological Medicine, 26,* 1169–1177.

World Health Organization (WHO) (1990). *Composite International Diagnostic Interview (CIDI, Version 1.0).* Geneva, Switzerland: World Health Organization.

CHAPTER 24

Drug Prevention Research for High-Risk Youth

LEONA L. EGGERT

BROOKE P. RANDELL

INTRODUCTION

Increasing numbers of adolescents are at high risk of abusing alcohol, tobacco, and other drugs, but some are at greater risk than others for a steady progression toward drug abuse. These high-risk youth also tend to have multiple interrelated problem behaviors, including aggression, depression, and suicidal behavior. In our studies, we find that the frequency and breadth of drug use, drug control problems, and adverse drug use consequences are significantly greater for high-risk youth than for typical high school students. Such findings accentuate the need for strategic prevention programs for high-risk adolescents.

High-risk youth are those who show early warning signs for alcohol and other drug abuse but who do not yet meet the diagnostic criteria for substance abuse, as defined by DSM-IV criteria (IOM, 1994). Research has shown that those most likely to abuse drugs are from 12 to 20 years of age and show signs of dysfunctional and antisocial behaviors, including truancy, academic failure, early and promiscuous sexual behavior, depression and suicidal behaviors, criminal behaviors, and deviant peer bonding (Eggert & Kumpfer, 1997; Elliott, Huizinga & Ageton, 1985; Hawkins et al. 1987; Kumpfer, 1989). High-risk youth not only manifest a significant number of the risk factors associated with drug abuse but also tend to have fewer of the protective factors known to guard against drug involvement. The greater the number of risk factors and the fewer the number of protective factors, the higher the risk status. In general, high-risk youth are poorly bonded to school, their families, and pro-social peers, and are beginning to demonstrate problem behaviors linked with substance use or abuse.

LEONA L. EGGERT AND BROOKE P. RANDELL • School of Nursing, University of Washington, Seattle, Washington 98195

Drug use and abuse among high-risk youth impose a heavy burden on public health: the leading causes of death among youth—motor vehicle accidents, unintentional injuries, homicides, and suicides—frequently involve alcohol and other drug use. Accordingly, reducing drug involvement may not only decrease the adverse consequences of drug use, such as school dropout, unemployment, criminal activity, and emotional disorders, but also decrease deaths due to accidents, homicide, and suicide. Few would argue that there is a pressing need for effective drug abuse prevention programs, especially for high-risk youth. Indeed, there is an increasing demand from policymakers, school administrators, and practitioners for proven prevention approaches.

In response to this need, prevention scientists have called for comprehensive drug abuse prevention programs that address multiple, interrelated problem behaviors. Such comprehensive approaches are called "indicated" prevention programs. Their goal is to identify high-risk individuals and intervene to address the personal and social factors that place these youth at greater risk of delinquency, drug experimentation, and other antisocial or problem behaviors. Unfortunately, few indicated drug abuse prevention programs for high-risk youth have been tested, and important questions remain to be answered: What works for high-risk youth? How does it work? And under what conditions? This chapter is an effort to begin to answer these questions.

INFLUENCES ON ADOLESCENT DRUG INVOLVEMENT

A great deal of evidence supports the assertion that high-risk youth often experience several common antecedent risk factors that must be considered as co-occurring dependent variables in indicated drug abuse prevention research.

Co-Occurring Drug Involvement, Aggression, Depression, and School Deviance

The problem behaviors that tend to cluster in high-risk youth are drug use, aggression, depression, and suicidal behavior.

- Drug involvement can be seen as existing on a continuum from nonuse to abuse (Eggert, Herting, & Thompson, 1996; Newcomb, 1992). A recent test of a hierarchical measurement model of drug involvement revealed that it is reflected by (1) increasing access to drugs; (2) frequency of alcohol, tobacco, and other drug use; (3) drug use control problems, and (4) adverse drug use consequences (Herting, Eggert, & Thompson, 1996).
- Aggression involves problems in controlling anger as well as assault on people or objects (Eggert, 1994; Spielberger et al., 1983).
- Depression refers to a combination of cognitive–behavioral indicators that include depressed affect, anxiety, hopelessness, and distorted thinking (Beck, Kovacs, & Weissman, 1975; Eggert, Thompson, & Herting, 1994).
- School deviance is defined as poor school performance (declining or failing grades, truancy) and school dropout.

The evidence that these problem behaviors tend to cluster in high-risk youth is strong (Jessor, 1993; Thompson, Moody, & Eggert, 1994). General literature reviews (Gans et al., 1990; Hawkins, Catalano & Miller, 1992; Osgood, 1991) indicate that drug abuse is linked with aggression, depression, and school deviance (Davidson & Linnoila, 1991; Kandel, Raveis, & Davies, 1991; Paton, Kessler, & Kandel, 1977) as well as depression and suicidal behaviors (Kandel et al., 1991;

Levy & Deykin, 1989; Thompson et al., 1994; Thompson, Mazza, & Eggert, 1999). Other studies show that youth who are chronic truants and/or school dropouts are more likely to be involved with drugs and/or delinquent behavior (Austin, 1992; Eggert & Nicholas, 1992; Kellam et al., 1983; Weng, Newcomb, & Bentler, 1988; Thompson et al., 1994).

We are only beginning to disentangle causal linkages among these variables (Thompson & Eggert, 1999; Thompson, Eggert, & Herting, 2000), but extensive research demonstrates that no one factor sufficiently explains and predicts adolescent drug abuse (e.g., Glants & Pickens, 1992; Goodstadt & Mitchell, 1990; Hawkins et al., 1987, 1992; Kandel, Kessler, & Margulies, 1978; Newcomb & Bentler, 1988; Newcomb & Harlow, 1986; Stein, Newcomb, & Bentler, 1987). Focusing only on reducing drug abuse and ignoring the co-occurring problem behaviors of aggression, depression, and school deviance would be both short-sighted and without theoretical support. Promoting change in each of these four problem behaviors should be the overall goal of drug-abuse prevention efforts with youth at high risk. However, it is also important to consider common antecedent risk factors.

Antecedent Risk Factors: Personal, School, Peer, and Family Influences

Personal characteristics, along with school, peer, and family contexts are known to be linked with drug abuse, violence, emotional distress, and school deviance (Brook et al., 1990; Kandel & Andrews, 1987; Resnick et al., 1997), and appear to be pervasive antecedent influences on adolescent problem behavior. Strain theory (Elliott et al., 1985) suggests that strain, or stress, emanates from intrapersonal factors (Newcomb & Earleywine, 1996) as well as from interpersonal networks—school, peers, and family (Anderson & Henry, 1994; Elliott et al., 1985; Rutter & Giller, 1983; Wills, 1985). Stress from these sources is common among high-risk youth (Powell-Cope & Eggert, 1994; Thompson et al., 1994), and there is evidence for links between these risk factors and alcohol, tobacco, and other drug use and abuse.

- Personal Risk Factors: Personal factors or characteristics linked with adolescent problem behaviors include perceived stress, anxiety, low personal control, and discrepancies between actual experiences and "wishful thinking." Indicators of personal strain, such as unmet needs and low outcome expectancies, are thought to influence drug involvement and school deviance (directly and indirectly) by weakening an adolescent's involvement with and commitment to pro-social groups and norms (Donovan, Jessor, & Costa, 1988; Elliott et al., 1985; Kaplan et al., 1984; Norem-Hebeisen & Hedin, 1981; Schinke, Botvin, & Orlandi, 1991; Watson & Friend, 1969; Weiner & Litman-Adizes, 1980). In addition, the lives of aggressive and depressed individuals tend to be void of caring, supportive relations (Dryden, 1981; Eggert, et al., 1996; Gotlib & Whiffen, 1991; LaGaipa & Wood, 1981). Consistent with the hypothesized effects of strain, high-risk youth report lower personal control, as well as greater drug involvement, depression, anxiety, violence, and victimization (Manscill & Rollins, 1990; Mechanic & Hansell, 1989; Newcomb & Bentler, 1988; Thompson et al., 1994; Wills, 1985).
- School Risk Factors: We know that high-risk youth have lower school bonding/support, which is linked with alcohol, tobacco, and other drug abuse (Eggert & Nicholas, 1992), as well as with aggression and depression (Eggert et al., 1994, 1996; Eggert, Thompson, Herting, & Nicholas, 1994; Resnick et al., 1997). High-risk youth also reveal two to three times as many negative feelings about and serious problems at school, including frequent quarrels with teachers, suspensions, and other disciplinary actions (Eggert & Nicholas,

1992; Garnefski & Okam, 1996; Powell-Cope & Eggert, 1994). Academic failure and low commitment to school, especially among youth in the higher grades, typically explain 10 to 20% of the variance in alcohol, tobacco, and other drug use and violence (Gabriel & Nickel, 1997). Having school problems, compared to problems at home or with peers, has the strongest independent relationship with both aggression and addiction-risk behaviors for boys (β = .34 and .32) and for girls, albeit somewhat less so (β = .23 and .24) (Garnefski & Okam, 1996).

- Peer Risk Factors: Peer relationships can be risk factors for adolescent drug involvement (Hansen & Graham, 1991). A deviant orientation—defined as attachment to deviant peers and involvement in risky, delinquent behaviors—increases the probability of drug involvement and other deviant behaviors (Dryfoos, 1991; Kandel et al., 1978; Newcomb & Bentler, 1988). This is consistent with strain, social control, learning theories (Elliott et al., 1985), and with substantial empirical evidence. Peer influences that correlate with alcohol, tobacco, and other drug use include having friends who encourage or pressure one to use drugs (Duncan, Duncan, & Hops, 1994; Eggert & Nicholas, 1992; Graham, Marks, & Hansen, 1991) and peer tolerance or approval of drug use (MacKinnon et al., 1991). When adolescents want to use drugs, they seek out peers known to be drug users or dealers (Eggert & Nicholas, 1992; Ennett & Bauman, 1994; Oetting & Beuvais, 1987). Moreover, in comparisons of peer versus parental influences, both family and peer influences predict adolescent drug involvement (Duncan et al., 1995; Randell et al., 1999); but peer influences are relatively more important than family influences during mid-adolescence (Biddle, Bank, & Marlin, 1980); and peer encouragement predicted increases in drug use over time as adolescents mature (Duncan et al., 1995). In studies reviewed, deviant peer bonding was usually the strongest predictor, accounting for the most variance in alcohol, tobacco, other drug use/abuse, and other problem behaviors (typically 30% to 50%).

- Family Risk Factors: An integrated model of strain, social control, and social learning theories indicates that certain family factors predict adolescent problem behaviors (Elliott et al., 1985; Wills et al., 1994). High levels of family conflict are known to increase the risk for alcohol, tobacco, other drug abuse, and other problem behaviors (Farrington et al., 1985 (as cited in Hawkins et al. (1992)); Hawkins et al., 1992; Rutter & Giller, 1983). Parenting characterized by unclear or unrealistic expectations, lack of praise, heightened criticism, and inconsistent discipline predicts adolescent drug use, aggression, and depression (Baumrind, 1991; Brook et al., 1990; Garnefski & Okam, 1996; Hawkins et al., 1992; Kandel & Andrews, 1987; Keitner & Miller, 1990; McCauley & Myers, 1992). Research also suggests that parental drug use has direct (Hawkins et al., 1992; Wills et al., 1994) and indirect effects (through deviant peer bonding, less control and coping) (Brook et al., 1990; Wills et al., 1994) on adolescent drug use. Moreover, high-risk youth, compared to typical high school students, evidence more family conflict, distress, greater parental drug use, and less family support for school (Powell-Cope & Eggert, 1994; Thompson et al., 1994; Gabriel & Nickel, 1997). In the studies reviewed, family risk factors typically explained from 10 to 40% of the variance in adolescent alcohol, tobacco, and other drug use, aggression/violence, school outcomes and emotional distress.

The previously cited evidence has implications for building an integrated theoretic model for preventing drug abuse among high-risk youth. First, it is clear that individual characteristics combine with school, peer, and family factors for some youth in a manner that results in multiple emotional and behavioral problems. Accordingly, individual and social network characteristics must be addressed in indicated prevention models for high-risk youth (Eggert & Kumpfer, 1997;

Hawkins et al., 1992; Kumpfer, 1987). Second, prevention models must be superimposed on an etiologic model of co-occurring problem behaviors.

COMPREHENSIVE INDICATED PREVENTION APPROACHES

It is currently acknowledged in the field of indicated drug abuse prevention that multiple strategies in different settings are necessary to decrease drug involvement among high-risk youth. We know from universal prevention approaches in middle schools that integrating multiple strategies in the home, school, and community reduces the incidence and prevalence of drug use (Pentz, et al., 1989). Similarly, we know that positive effects are stronger when both parents and young children are involved in family-oriented drug prevention programs (Kumpfer & DeMarsh, 1986). Integrating multiple strategies within multiple contexts is also recommended by the National Institute on Drug Abuse in their videotape, Coming Together on Prevention (1995) and in a set of drug abuse prevention research dissemination and application materials (1997). Recommendations from multiple sources suggest that indicated prevention approaches for high-risk youth should:

- attend to the multivariate correlates of adolescent drug involvement (Dryfoos, 1991; Eggert, 1998; Hawkins et al., 1992; Newcomb & Earleywine, 1996; NIDA, 1998);
- include a peer support component to test its effect on preventing the escalation of drug involvement and co-occurring problem behaviors (Botvin & Tortu, 1988; Brook et al., 1992, Eggert, Herting, et al., 1994; et al., 1995);
- be situated in schools, which are a logical environment for prevention activities (Eggert et al., 1994, 1997; Goodstadt & Mitchell, 1990; Hawkins et al., 1992); and
- be comprehensive—that is, include multiple interventions aimed at intrapersonal, interpersonal, and environmental risk and protective factors (Pentz, 1998; NIDA, 1998; Tobler, & Stratton, 1997; Wills et al., 1996).

Achieving these goals with youth at high risk poses major challenges. It involves (1) identifying and serving the most elusive and highest-risk youth; (2) matching theory-based preventive interventions to reduce specific, identified risk factors and enhancing assets of the high-risk individuals; and (3) integrating the proposed interventions into high schools and/or communities whose cultures are not always friendly toward research (Eggert & Kumpfer, 1997).

At least two research programs are currently testing indicated drug abuse prevention efforts for high-risk youth: Project Toward No Drug Abuse (Dent et al., 1995; Sussman et al., 1994; Sussman, 1996a, 1996b; Sussman et al., 1997; Sussman & Johnson, 1996) and Reconnecting Youth (Eggert, Nicholas, & Owen, 1995; Eggert Herting, et al., 1994; Eggert, Thompson et al., 1995; Eggert et al., 1997; Eggert, 1998).

Project Toward No Drugs (TND) is a nine-session curriculum for continuation (alternative) high school students designed to be self-administered or delivered by a teacher or health educator (Sussman, 1996). The curriculum consists of motivational activities, social skills training, and decision-making components. Preliminary data from 1,300 students indicate that those who received the intervention by either method of administration had increased knowledge of the central curriculum concepts when compared to students in control groups (Sussman et al., 1994). Follow-up studies specifically examining substance use will provide evidence to determine program efficacy. The developers of the program attribute initial success to (1) extensive testing and involvement of continuation high school students in curriculum development, (2) tailoring the curriculum to target risk factors specific to this high-risk population, and (3) selection of implementation strategies that are consistent with the structure of continuation high school educational programs.

Reconnecting Youth (RY) has as its core the Personal Growth Class, a semester-long class taught by highly trained, empathic teachers who foster the development of a mutually supportive peer group that encourages positive behaviors (Eggert, Thompson, Herting, & Nicholas, 1994; Eggert et al., 1995). RY specifically targets youth at high risk for school dropout. The class focuses on enhancing the student's self-esteem, improving decision-making and communication skills, and improving personal control—the ability to manage stress, anger, and depression. The ultimate goals of the program are to (1) decrease drug involvement, (2) increase school performance, and (3) increase emotional well-being. Embedded in the RY program is a social network bonding component. Initially, bonding activities are confined to the classroom, but as student's skills increase and the positive peer relationships are strengthened, students are coached to "reconnect" to school. Analysis of data from 600 participating students indicates that the program was effective in (1) curbing drug use progression and decreasing hard drug use, (2) decreasing drug use control problems and adverse drug use consequences, (3) increasing grade point average, and (4) decreasing depression and suicide-risk behavior. The program also influenced posited mediators of drug involvement; students demonstrated increased personal control, self-esteem, and school bonding, and decreased deviant peer bonding (Eggert, Thompson, Herting, & Nicholas, 1994; Eggert, Thompson et al., 1995).

The developers of the RY program attribute its success to (1) involving high-risk youth in shaping the curriculum; (2) targeting risk factors specific to this high-risk population; (3) careful teacher selection to ensure both competence with and caring for the high-risk population; (4) deliberate attention to creating a positive-peer culture, simultaneously addressing the need for group belonging while counteracting the potentially deleterious effects of deviant-peer bonding; and (5) selection of implementation strategies that can be delivered during the regular school day as part of the student's assigned course load.

What is immediately obvious about these two programs is that they each contain many of the essential elements for indicated prevention programs. Each is school based, attends to the multivariate correlates of adolescent drug involvement, includes a peer support component, and is comprehensive. That is, each targets environmental risk and protective factors common to the high-risk group. However, neither program directly addresses family risk factors. What is not known is whether integrating school-based and parent prevention strategies with identified, high-school-aged, high-risk youth will work to produce stronger effects than programs that target youth alone. To test this, we developed a comprehensive model called Parents and Youth with Schools (Project PAYS).

The PAYS indicated prevention model is designed to counteract important assumed risk factors (discussed earlier) and enhance mediating factors, those personal and social resources believed to serve a protective function. Project PAYS combines RY with Parents as Partners, combined individual home-based/small group experience for parents. Each PAYS component contributes uniquely to the posited effects of the prevention model on assumed risk and protective factors. Both these program elements are grounded in social network support theory.

Figure 24.1 is based on transactional–ecological models of risk and protective factors (Felner & Felner, 1989; Hawkins et al., 1992; Jessor, 1991; Newcomb & Earlywine, 1996; Scheier, Newcomb, & Skager, 1994; Wills, Pierce, & Evans, 1996). It also includes the interpersonal/sociocultural submodel in Huba, Wingard, and Bentler's (1980) framework of drug behavioral lifestyles that focuses on significant relationships in youths' interpersonal and school support networks. Transactional–ecological models permit the desired integration of etiologic and

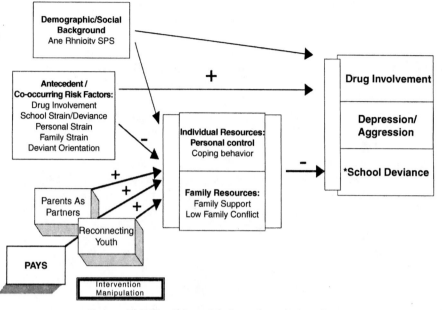

FIGURE 24.1. Heuristic model of PAYS intervention effects.

prevention dimensions because transactional processes refer to the interaction between individual and environmental factors. Such models posit common pathways to drug abuse, school deviance, aggression, and depression. In the simplest terms, stress and strain theories suggest that deviant behavior (e.g., drug abuse, school deviance) is the result of stresses and frustrated needs or wants. Social control theory assumes that stress and strain are universal; thus, the critical variable is the strength of social controls regulating the behavior and mediating strain. Importantly, from a prevention and social support perspective, support from significant network members (family, peers, and teachers) serves to mediate stress and decrease drug involvement and co-occurring problem behaviors. Figure 24.1 depicts a heuristic model that bridges what is known about the presumed causes of drug abuse in high-risk youth and preventive interventions that hold promise for changing these factors.

The Social Network Support Model

The approach to behavior change in the PAYS program assumes that adolescent behavior is influenced by the social support from various sources in their social networks. This social support and influence includes two central elements: (1) expressive support or bonding (caring, group belonging, positive reinforcement) and (2) instrumental support (concrete "aid," help, and advice). The extended benefits of social support are widely acknowledged (Anderson & Henry, 1994; Cauce & Srebnik, 1989; Cohen & Syme, 1985; Eggert, 1987). Studies of resiliency (Blaney & Ganellen, 1991; Jessor, 1993; Resnick et al., 1997) and social support (Cohen & Syme, 1985; Sarason, Pierce, & Sarason, 1991) indicate that persons with greater personal and social resources fare better than those without—for many health-related problems (Eggert, 1987; Kumpfer & Turner, 1991; Lin, Dean, & Ensel, 1986; Rainer & Slavin, 1992, Thompson, Eggert & Herting, in press). Thus, social support interventions have the potential of changing key mediating factors known to influence adolescent drug involvement, aggression, depression, and school performance. According to this model, instrumental social support interventions in the form of skills training can help adolescents acquire essential skills. Social support should work to create a reinforcing, interpersonal context that is crucial to acceptance of the skills training and altering the cluster of problem behaviors that are the foci of the PAYS prevention model.

Table 24.1 links the PAYS intervention strategies with assumed risk factors and theoretic mechanisms that detail the posited influence of the intervention strategies on four targeted mediators. Promising social support interventions (expressive and instrumental) (Cutrona & Russell, 1991; Dunkel-Schetter & Bennett, 1991; Eggert, 1987) in the four domains of family, school, peers, and the individual (Column 1) are described. Strategies delivered in the separate components of PAYS, RY, and Parents as Partners, are indicated by an "X" (columns 2, 3, and 4, respectively). Assumed etiologic risk factors (described previously) are also indicated in the table (column 5), as are the theoretic mechanisms for how the strategies are thought to influence key mediating factors (column 6).

Family-Focused Preventive Interventions

The parent support component of PAYS has the goal of engaging parents (or the primary adults in a youth's social network) in a "partnership" role with the school and the research team—to help their teens have a better experience in school. Based on a review of key empirically based strategies (Bry, 1988; Bry & Krinsley, 1992; Dishion, 1998; Ezekoye, Kumpfer, & Bukoski, 1986; Kumpfer & DeMarsh, 1986; Kumpfer et al., 1997; Moskowitz, 1988) specific approaches were designed to enhance:

- family communication and cohesion;
- the "parent-to-school" bond and, thus, parent commitment and support of their child's school-related goals and activities;
- family management and parenting competence in monitoring adolescent behavior, in applying consistent discipline and logical consequences, and in joint decision making by parents and children; and
- suitable modeling and communication of anti-drug-abuse norms (c.f., Table 24.1, column 1).

In prior research, both family support, which includes family bonding or cohesion and parental norms against drug involvement have been shown to moderate the risk of exposure to drug-using peers, a key predictor in adolescent drug involvement among high-risk youth (Brook et al., 1990; Dielman, 1994; Dielman et al., 1993; DiPrete & Forristal, 1994; Kaplan, Martin, & Robbins, 1984; Kraemer & Thiemann, 1987; Rohrbach et al., 1987). In addition, parental support and control and parental expectations for school achievement were associated with lower levels of risky behaviors (Barnes & Farrell, 1992; Resnick et al., 1997). Family bonding explained 14 to 15% of the variance in emotional distress and 8 to 9% of the variance in alcohol, tobacco, and other drug use among 9th- to 12th-graders. (Resnick et al., 1997).

Based on the previous findings, parental or family support (also called family attachment, bonding, or cohesion) is the major mediating factor to be influenced by the parent-focused interventions in PAYS. Family support is defined as communicated caring and help exchanged across close, interpersonal family ties. Theoretically, family support should work by fulfilling the high-risk youth's basic human needs for love and attachment and by reducing uncertainty about parents as a reliable source of help (Eggert, 1987). Parental support should be intrinsically rewarding,

TABLE 24.1. Prevention Domains/Strategies, Assumed Risk Factors, & Theoretic Mechanisms for How Prevention Strategies are Posited to Influence Four Mediators: Perceived Personal Control, Family Support, School Bonding and Conventional/Pro-Social Peer Bonding

Prevention domain and strategies	Parent & Youth (PAYS)	Youth focus (RY)	Parent focus (PAP)	Assumed antecedent risk factors	Theoretic mechanism for how the prevention strategies are posited to influence the targeted mediators
A. Family—skills training in					
1. Enhancing family communication/cohesion	X		X	Perceived family distress; conflicts with parents; poor family/school connections	Expressed parental support and caring increases parent-adolescent connectedness; this increases *perceived family support*
(a) Training in listening, in praising					
(b) Training in conflict negotiation with youth					
2. Enhancing parent support of youth's goals:	X		X		Parental expectations for school achievement and expressed support/help for school increases *school bonding*
(a) Becoming a partner with youth and school					
(b) Training in communicating support of goals					
3. Enhancing family management by training in:	X		X	Perceived coercive parenting; unclear &/or unfair rules	Authoritative parenting—highly demanding and highly responsive—generates the youth's *sense of personal control.*
(a) Parental monitoring					
(b) Consistent discipline/logical consequences					
(c) Decision making skills with youth					
4. Communicating normative drug use behaviors:	X		X	Parental drug use / abuse; non-con-ventional norms	Parental influence works via the youth's perceived normative standards promoting *conventional/prosocial peer bonding*
(a) Modeling conventional drug use norms					
(b) Training in reinforcing non-use with youth					
B. School					
1. Setting norms for and monitoring	X	X		Negative view of school experience norms of skipping classes and ATOD use at school; poor relations with teachers; low access to help; nonparticipation in school activities	Monitoring behaviors alone is known to increase competence; success in school increases sense of *personal control.*
(a) Attendance in all classes					
(b) Improved achievement in all classes					
(c) No drug involvement at school					
2. Improving school network support	X	X			Teacher support increases a sense of belonging, motivation, positive experiences in school, thus increasing *school bonding*
(a) Delivering consistent RY teacher support					
(b) Fostering teacher support in all classes					
(c) Providing individual case management					
3. Prosocial school bonding activities	X	X			

(cont.)

TABLE 24.1. (Continued)

Prevention domain and strategies	Parent & Youth (PAYS)	Youth focus (RY)	Parent focus (PAP)	Assumed antecedent risk factors	Theoretic mechanism for how the prevention strategies are posited to influence the targeted mediators
C. Peers					
1. Norm setting in the RY group of personal and group commitment to the program goals of (a) "Doing school"—attending & achieving (b) Managing moods (c) Decreasing drug involvement	X	X		Norms of "skipping" and using drugs; lack of personal goals	Personalizes perceptions of links between drug involvement, anger/depressed mood, and school achievement. Goal setting increases motivation, and thus, *a sense of personal control*
2. Adoption and daily reinforcement of norms related to a positive peer group culture—i.e., (a) Active support/help for each group member's progress toward goal achievement (b) Negative reinforcement of deviant norms, activities and relationships	X	X		Susceptibility to negative peer influences	The positive peer group culture reinforces prosocial norms and adoption of RY goals; perceived peer group support increases a sense of belonging; both increase *conventional/prosocial peer bonding*
3. Replacing deviant peer/group belonging with prosocial group belonging to in RY class	X	X		Deviant friends in peer network	
D. Individual—Social & life skills training in					
1. Decision making—learning to use STEPS and applying process to making healthy decisions about drug use, school, and mood management	X	X		Impulsiveness; poor decision-making skills	Personally relevant nonjudgmental feedback increases positive decisions and decreases deviant orientation/behaviors; Decreases
2. Personal control—learning stress, anger & depression management skills; practicing coping skills for "triggers" related to drug use, truancy and uncontrolled moods	X	X		Uncontrolled emotions; learned helplessness/poor coping skills	stress and uncontrolled emotions, therefore increasing *sense of personal control and competencies*
3. Self-esteem enhancement—learning to communicate esteem enhancing talk for self & others	X	X		Low self-worth; deviant self-image	Esteem enhancement and exchanging support and negotiation skills increases social competence and *pro-social peer and school bonding*
4. Interpersonal communication—learning to give and receive support with friends, and negotiation skills with teachers and parents	X	X		Poor social/interpersonal skills	

provide clear boundaries, and, thereby, influence reductions in the adolescents' drug involvement, aggression, depression, and school deviance. The parent-focused strategies in PAYS should work to increase the youth's perceived family support as well as influence personal control and pro-social peer and school bonding, countering negative influences (Sussman & Johnson, 1996) and linking family with school strategies.

School-Focused Preventive Interventions

Three key school environment prevention strategies are included in the PAYS model to enhance the overall school experience:

- setting norms for and monitoring non use of alcohol, tobacco, or other drug use at school, and attendance and achievement in all classes;
- improving the overall school network support—from all teachers and through individual case management; and
- facilitating pro-social school bonding.

These school-based strategies should motivate and provide social support from specific adults in the high-risk youth's school network, increasing access to help at school. Increasing access to help should reduce barriers and provide greater opportunities for school bonding, thereby enhancing self-efficacy skills acquisitions (Pentz, 1993, 1998; Weissberg et al., 1989). We know that when youth are involved in meaningful connections to school, they experience opportunities for school bonding and peer-group belonging (a central concern for adolescents). They also tend to experience less loneliness, healthy fun, and a greater purpose in life (Harlow, Newcomb, & Bentler, 1986; Newcomb & Harlow, 1986). These school environment strategies should dampen specific risk factors.

Social learning and social control theories link school risk factors with alcohol, tobacco, and other drug use and other problem behaviors of interest. Theoretically, providing youth with greater amounts of school network support—by shaping and monitoring opportunities for them to participate in meaningful relationships with caring adults, in pro-social school activities, and in community service—should influence specific behavior change. School network support should (1) directly increase students' personal competencies and control, thus reinforcing a positive view of school and teachers, and (2) directly increase conventional school bonding through a greater sense of belonging and purpose (Bandura, 1977; Botvin & Dusenbury, 1989; Catalano et al., 1991; Eggert, Thompson, & Herting, 1994; Schinke & Gilchrist, 1984; Schinke et al., 1991). With greater conventional school bonding and enhanced personal control, the desired reductions in the outcomes of interest should occur (Brendtro, Brokenleg, & Van Bockern, 1990; Eggert & Herting, 1993; Kellam et al., 1991; Kellam & Rebok, 1992; Thompson & Eggert, 1999; Thompson, Eggert, & Herting, 2000). These specific family and school strategies and theoretic mechanisms are closely linked to the peer-focused strategies.

Peer-Focused Preventive Interventions

For developmental and etiologic reasons, peers represent a critical context for delivering prevention strategies for high-risk youth. Several key strategies in PAYS are designed specifically to engage and motivate youth in an interactive peer-group approach—RY (Eggert, Nicholas et al., 1995; Eggert, 1997; Eggert et al., 2001). These strategies are also designed to counteract negative peer bonding/activities and include:

- setting and maintaining norms within the RY group for making personal commitments to the goals of "doing school," decreasing drug involvement, and improving mood management (Eggert, Nicholas, et al., 1995);
- adopting and reinforcing daily the norms of a positive peer group culture (Brendtro et al., 1990; Eggert, Nicholas et al., 1995; Tobler, 1992; Vorrath & Brendtro, 1985) while negatively reinforcing deviant norms and activities; and
- replacing deviant group bonding with pro-social group bonding in the RY class (cf., Table 24.1, column 1).

Peer-focused strategies involve developing and maintaining a positive peer-group culture (Brendtro et al., 1990; Vorrath & Brendtro, 1985) to counteract key antecedent risk factors. This pro-social culture is known to positively influence conventional peer bonding and reduce drug involvement, aggression, depression, and school deviance (Eggert & Herting, 1991; Eggert, Herting, Thompson, Nicholas, & Dicker, 1994; Thompson, Eggert & Herting, in press). Deliberately creating pro-social, interactional, and recreational contexts for high-risk youth is an essential intervention strategy. Daily provisions of these activities in the RY class and in multiple booster-group activities over a full school year were shown to be a necessary "dose" for bringing about behavior change (Brendtro, et al., 1990; Eggert, Thompson, et al., 1995; Thompson et al., 1997; Tobler, 1986, 1992; Vorrath & Brendtro, 1985).

The strategies of the RY peer-group approach were designed specifically in response to the culture and norms of "skippers"—potential dropouts (Eggert & Nicholas, 1992). The need for group belonging was a central dimension linked with skipping classes and abusing drugs on campus. Hence, prevention efforts must actively attenuate deviant peer bonding and risky behavioral lifestyles (Botvin & Dusenbury, 1989; Brook et al., 1992; Duncan et al., 1994; Elliott, 1994; Gabriel & Nickel, 1997; Hundleby & Mercer, 1987; Schinke et al., 1991).

The posited theoretic mechanisms for how the prevention strategies work are complex. Conventional, pro-social peer bonding is the primary mediator predicted to influence the desired outcomes. Positive-peer relationships are pivotal for healthy adolescent development (Cauce & Srebnik, 1989; Heller, Price, & Hogg, 1991; Moskowitz, 1988). In social influence models (Botvin & Dusenbury, 1989; Dorn, 1984), pro-social bonding counteracts deviant orientation (Elliott et al., 1985; Kellam et al., 1983). Hence, expressive and instrumental support from RY peers should fulfill an adolescent's needs for group belonging. It should also reinforce pro-social norms and provide opportunities for developing new non-drug-using friends (Cauce & Srebnik, 1989; Vorrath & Brendtro, 1985), thereby negatively influencing deviant peer bonding (Eggert et al., 1994; Eggert et al., 1995). The peer group should reinforce life skills acquisitions in the RY class and directly influence personal competencies and control (Bandura, 1977; Eggert, Thompson, Herting, & Nicholas, 1994; Eggert, Nicholas, & Owen, 1995). These outcomes are believed to occur because the RY teachers actively develop and maintain conventional peer group support in the class by modeling support, positively reinforcing it among group members, and negatively reinforcing deviant peer bonds and activities, as suggested in Vorrath and Brendtro's (1985) "positive peer culture" model. In fact, our previous work supports teacher and peer support as mechanisms by which the program worked. Specifically, teacher support influenced reductions in drug use control problems and consequences (Eggert & Herting, 1991). Similarly, personal control, enhanced by peer support, had direct effects on the reduction of suicide-risk behaviors. The observed changes in increased peer support were directly attributable to the RY teacher's role in fostering the positive-peer culture (Thompson, Connelly, & Eggert, in press). This approach to drug abuse prevention is unique; peer factors are usually viewed as risk factors, and it is rare to find program elements designed to develop and maintain positive peer influences for remaining drug free (Hansen & Graham, 1991).

The three program components discussed previously are all designed to influence specific sectors of the high-risk youth's social network—family, school, and peers—acting on external forces influencing the youth's behavior. The final program component is designed to change specific intrapersonal factors.

Individual-Focused Preventive Interventions

Social and life skills training is the primary preventive intervention in the individual-focused domain. This strategy involves coaching youth in specific monitoring, coping, and relapse prevention skills for enhancing self-efficacy and social skills linked with the outcomes of interest (Botvin & Dusenbury, 1989; Botvin & Tortu, 1988; Eggert, Nicholas, & Owen, 1995; Eggert et al., 1996). Central elements of this strategy are (1) providing personally relevant information and feedback related to each youth's skill building and (2) coaching youth in ways to apply the specific skills to improve school performance, mood management, and drug use control. Social and life skills training provides youth with daily opportunities for learning and practicing personal and interpersonal social skills necessary for effective coping and adaptation. The four skill areas are:

- making healthy decisions about drug use, school and mood management;
- exercising personal control by practicing stress, anger, and depression management skills to cope with "triggers" related to drug use, truancy, and uncontrolled moods;
- communicating self-esteem enhancing talk for self and others; and
- exchanging support with friends and negotiating with parents and teachers.

Personal competencies, or control, is a mediating factor that directly influences adolescent substance use, aggression, depression, and school deviance (Eggert, Thompson, Herting, & Nicholas, 1994; Eggert, Nicholas, & Owen, 1995). RY skills training, based on integrated social learning, control, and strain theories (Elliott et al., 1985), provides opportunities for learning important life skills within a supportive interpersonal and valued peer-group context via greater modeling, practice, and reinforcement for pro-social coping and activities. Moreover, RY skills training units specifically address key factors that influence the cluster of outcomes. Personally relevant feedback delivered in a nonjudgmental way has been linked with increased motivation (Janis, 1983) and with decreased denial and resistance and increased self-help motivation (Miller & Rollnick, 1991; Miller & Sanchez, 1993; Miller & Sovereign, 1989). The posited mechanism is that information and practice reduces uncertainty and increases skills competency and a sense of personal control. These, in turn, decrease negative outcomes (Botvin & Dusenbury, 1989; Dorn, 1984; Igoe, 1991; Thompson et al., in press).

FUTURE DIRECTIONS AND RECOMMENDATIONS

Because few comprehensive drug prevention models like PAYS have received rigorous empirical tests for their efficacy, this theory-based model could serve as a spring board for future research. Specifically needed are efficacy trials of indicated prevention programs involving high-risk youth who (1) are showing early warning signs of antecedent risk factors associated with drug involvement, (2) are engaging in drug use but do not meet the criteria of a drug abuse diagnosis, (3) are showing signs of multiple co-occurring problem behaviors, or (4) have participated in a prevention program and are at high risk of relapse. We propose a test of the PAYS program as an example of how the science of indicated prevention research might be advanced. It is anticipated that the PAYS model can be generalized to research efforts designed to test other indicated prevention programs.

PAYS was specifically designed for high-risk, high-school-aged youth. Therefore, youth drawn from categories 1, 2, or 3, previously cited, would be appropriate for efficacy tests of Project PAYS. Given our current knowledge and the public health burden of potential drug abuse among high-risk youth, we recommend the following:

- To test the overall efficacy of PAYS with high-risk youth (potential high school dropouts in regular high schools or youth in alternative school settings). Such tests would determine if the high-risk youth participants in PAYS, compared to control groups, would show significantly different changes over time in: decreased drug involvement, aggression, depression, and school deviance and increased personal control, family support, school bonding, and conventional, pro-social peer bonding.
- To test the efficacy the PAYS program components—RY Parents as Partners—to discover if PAYS is superior to RY alone and whether RY alone is superior to Parents as Partners alone in achieving the desired outcomes and immediate personal and social enhancements.
- To test the overall efficacy of PAYS and its separate components, would necessitate a four-group randomized experiment with a large number of high-risk youth (~ 200 per group). A repeated measures design would be needed and the appropriate unit of analysis would be the individual youth enrolled in the experiment (Kreft, 1998). Suitable analytic methods (e.g., trend analyses, Latent Growth-curve Modeling) would be used to examine the levels and shape of change in mediating and outcome factors over time.

Testing indicated preventive interventions in this manner will contribute to our understanding of program efficacy as well as enlighten us about the mechanisms by which the intervention works. As is the case with the PAYS experiment described above, we will be able to demonstrate how well the program works and identify the mechanisms by which it works. Finally, comparing across the comprehensive program components will further our understanding of the relative gains obtained when interventions are delivered to parents and youth combined, youth alone, or parents alone.

Generalization Studies

Carefully designed and implemented efficacy trials are essential to the advancement of prevention science. However, once an indicated prevention program has demonstrated efficacy under tightly controlled conditions, further testing is necessary to determine to which other populations of high-risk youth the program can be generalized. We have evidence that RY works when delivered as a regular high school class to potential high school dropouts. What we do not know is whether it would work for youth in alternative high schools, incarcerated youth, or street youth. We do not know in what ways the program would need to be altered to achieve the same outcomes in different populations and settings. Successful efficacy trials need to be followed by implementation or dissemination studies.

Prevention services research is concerned with testing efficacious programs under "real-world" conditions and the establishment of boundary conditions for these programs. Both Projects TND and RY were designed to be school-based, since schools are an ideal setting for prevention efforts, especially with high-risk youth. However, many high-risk youth are not reached if we confine our programming to schools. What is not known is what other settings would be suitable for implementation and delivery of these and other indicated prevention programs. For example, the developers of RY are currently receiving many requests to train others to implement RY. These requests come from a variety of providers and settings (including community agencies planning to deliver RY in alternative schools and law enforcement personnel in juvenile detention settings). Despite the fact that RY was not intended to be delivered in these settings or with these youth, the requests for science-based programs like RY come from individuals who claim that nothing else exists. Hence, the boundary conditions of RY and all indicated prevention programs need to be tested in these sites to determine what adaptations, if any, are needed in terms of increased dosage, delivery modality, and other implementation factors.

In addition, prevention services research must addresses issues of cost-effectiveness. Few, if any, indicated prevention programs have been studied for cost-effectiveness. But even though they may be more expensive than universal or selective programs in terms of costs per individual, they may actually save untold millions to society in the long run. The cost of community-based indicated prevention efforts, when compared with the costs of treatment and incarceration, should be modest.

Preintervention Studies

While we know a great deal about the etiology of drug use and abuse and feel confident about program content, little is known about what motivates youth to change their drug use behavior or what intervention strategies are best suited to bring about desired outcomes in various populations. Effective prevention efforts must be based on sound empirical evidence so that they are sensitive to the characteristics and needs of high risk students' lives in key domains of influence. Understanding this comprehensive picture is a crucial first step in furthering the testing and implementation of effective strategies to curb adolescent drug abuse.

Most work to date has informed us of processes and pathways that lead to drug use and abuse, its course, and consequences (e.g., Newcomb, 1992; Brook et al., 1990, 1992; Newcomb & Earleywine, 1996). A shift is now needed toward the study of pathways leading away from drug experimentation and abuse, especially among high-risk youth. It is not necessarily the case that knowing more about the pathways to disorder will logically inform us about how to change that course and motivate these youth to adopt drug-free lifestyles. Key questions we need to address in preintervention studies include the following.

MOTIVATION. What would motivate high-risk youth to change their course from drug abuse to reduced drug use or nonuse? We cannot assume that what would be motivating for some high-risk youth would be the same for others. Thus, the shift must be toward discovering common principles inherent in different motivational strategies and the identification of particular features that stimulate some youth, but not others, to quit using drugs and living high-risk lifestyles. Common principles and models of successful recruitment into indicated prevention programs are needed. The need for motivation toward change does not stop with program entry however. We need to understand the processes that bring about change, the basic mechanisms of biological, behavioral, and psychological change if we are to reverse the trajectory toward drug abuse and addiction and the adoption of healthier life styles.

CONTENT. Which program components work for which high risk behaviors? And what is a necessary and sufficient dose? The extensive research on risk and protective factors provides us with the information necessary to define and describe the content of indicated prevention programs. Before a program is ready for rigorous testing, the content needs to be fitted to the population of interest, carefully specified as to targeted risk and protective factors, and pilot tested.

PROCESSES. What would work to reverse drug use progression—what conditions, what strategies, for which high-risk youth, and under what conditions. When we understand the mechanisms that motivate and bring about change in high-risk youth and we have carefully specified the intervention content to fit the population and targeted risk and protective factors, then we will be ready to determine the strategies necessary to accomplish the task. Does the intervention need to be delivered one-on-one, in small groups, in the school, or at home? What medium is the best method of presentation?

Both Sussman and Eggert did pilot studies in an effort to answer some of these critical questions before undertaking full tests of projects TND and RY. Sussman and colleagues completed a series of preliminary studies to identify critical program components and determine the fit of the interventions for alternative high school students (Dent, et al., 1995; Sussman, 1996; Sussman et al., 1994; Sussman et al., 1997). Specifically, they examined the effects of program components on knowledge and belief changes, selected lessons based on highest ratings of perceived efficacy, and compared two different presentation styles. Eggert and colleagues (Eggert & Nicholas, 1992) conducted a series of ethnographic studies which indicated that youth who are at high risk of dropping out of school are disconnected from school and family and loosely connected with negative peers. These youth identified "skippin" and "usin" as a way to belong, a way to deal with the disconnection they were experiencing. This led Eggert and her colleagues to recognize the importance of having a peer group that would "invite" these youth back into school as a critical element in drug abuse prevention efforts with potential high school dropouts. Other program elements include a personal, motivational invitation to recruit youth into RY—because this is how skippers invited each other to belong to the group; and small group bonding and recreational activities as the medium for all other program elements—because this was the central appeal for belonging to the group.

We argue strongly for preintervention efforts as well as rigorous efficacy tests and large dissemination studies to advance drug abuse prevention science with high-risk youth.

CONCLUSION

Indicated prevention research with youth at high risk has the potential for extending the empirical base for preventive interventions that lead to accepted, sustained, and effective programs. Such research has great potential for directly improving public health and decreasing the enormous social costs incurred from drug abuse and its impact on the leading causes of death among our youth. The need for these programs is substantial: approximately 25% of adolescents lead high-risk lifestyles and fit the criteria for indicated drug abuse prevention efforts. Combining school, peer, and parent approaches appear to be necessary to reconnect high-risk youth to school and halt the progression from drug involvement to drug abuse and addiction. The goal of indicated prevention trials is to produce proven programs that reduce the occurrence and extent of drug abuse among high-risk youth. Much work remains to be done in this field. It will take concerted efforts, funding for preintervention studies, and complex, methodologically sound, indicated prevention efficacy trials to make reaching this goal possible.

REFERENCES

Adams, G. R., Dyk, P., & Bennion, L. D. (1990). Parent-adolescent relationships and identity formation. In B. K. Barber & B. C. Rollins (Eds.), *Parent-adolescent relationships* (pp. 1–17). Lanham, MD: University Press of America.

Anderson, A. R., & Henry, C. S. (1994). Family system characteristics and parental behaviors as predictors of adolescent substance use. *Adolescence, 29,* 405–420.

Austin, G. (1992). *School failure and alcohol and other drug use.* Madison, WI: Wisconsin Clearinghouse, U. Wisconsin-Madison.

Bandura, A. (1977). Self-efficacy: Toward a unifying theory of behavioral change. Psychological *Review, 84,* 191–215.

Barnes, G. M., & Farrell, M. P. (1992). Parental support and control as predictors of adolescent drinking, delinquency, and related problem behaviors. *Journal of Marriage and the Family, 54,* 763–776.

Baumrind, D. (1991). The influence of parenting style on adolescent competence and substance use. *Journal of Early Adolescence, 11,* 56–95.

Beck, A. T., Kovacs, M., & Weissman, A. (1975). Hopelessness and suicidal behavior. *Journal of the American Medical Association, 234,* 1146–1149.

Blalock, H. M., Jr. (1985). *Causal models in the social sciences* (2nd ed.). Chicago: Aldine.

Blaney, P. H., & Ganellen, R. J. (1991). Hardiness and social support. In B. R. Sarason, I. G. Sarason & G. R. Pierce (Eds.), *Social support: An interactional view* (pp. 297–318). New York: Wiley.

Botvin, G. J. (1998). Preventing drug abuse through the schools: Intervention programs that work. In NIDA, *National conference on drug abuse prevention research: Presentations, papers, and recommendations* (pp. 43–56). NIH Publication 98-4293. Rockville, MD: NIH.

Botvin, G. J., & Dusenbury, L. (1989). Substance abuse prevention and the promotion of competence. In L. A. Bond & B. E. Compas (Eds.), *Primary prevention and promotion in the schools* (pp. 146–178). Newbury Park, CA: Sage.

Botvin, G. J., & Tortu, S. (1988). Peer relationships, social competence and substance abuse prevention: Implications for the family. *Journal of Chemical Dependency Treatment, 1,* 145–173.

Brendtro, L. K., Brokenleg, M., & Van Bockern, S. (1990). *Reclaiming youth at risk.* Bloomington, IN: NES.

Brook, J. S., Brook, D. W., Gordon, A. S., Whiteman, M., & Cohen, P. (1990). The psychological etiology of adolescent drug use: A family interactional approach. *Genetic, Social and General Psychology Monographs, 116,* 111–267.

Brook, J. S., Whiteman, M., Cohen, P., & Tanaka, J. S. (1992). Childhood precursors of adolescent drug use: A longitudinal analysis. *Genetic, Social and General Psychology Monographs, 118,* 195–213.

Bruvold, W. H., & Rundall, T. G. (1988). A meta-analysis and theoretical review of school based tobacco and alcohol intervention programs. *Psychology and Health, 2,* 53–78.

Bry, B. H. (1988). Family-based approaches to reducing adolescent substance use: Theories, techniques and findings. In E. R. Rahdert & J. Grabowski (Eds.), *Adolescent drug abuse: Analysis of treatment research* (NIDA Research Monograph 77 (pp. 39–68). Department of Health and Human Services. Washington DC: U.S. Government Printing Office.

Bry, B., & Krinsley, K. E. (1992). Booster sessions and long-term effects of behavioral family therapy on adolescent substance use and school performance. *Journal of Behavior Therapy and Experimental Psychology, 23,* 183–189.

Bry, B., McKeon, P., & Pandina, R. J. (1982). Extent of drug use as a function of number of risk factors. *Journal of Abnormal Psychology, 91,* 273–279.

Bukoski, W. (1986). School-based substance abuse prevention: A review of program research. In S. Griswold-Ezekoye, K. Kumpfer, & W. Bukoski (Eds.), *Childhood and chemical abuse: Prevention and intervention* (pp. 95–115). New York: Haworth Press.

Catalano, R. F., Hawkins, J. D., Wells, E. A., Miller, J., & Brewer, D. (1991). Evaluation of the effectiveness of adolescent drug abuse treatment, assessment of risks for relapse and promising approaches for relapse prevention. *International Journal of the Addictions, 25,* 1085–1140.

Cauce, A. M., & Srebnik, D. S. (1989). Peer networks and social support. In L. A. Bond & B. E. Compas (Eds.), *Primary prevention and promotion in the schools* (pp. 235–254). Newbury Park, CA: Sage.

Center for Disease Control (1994). *Morbidity and Mortality Weekly Report, 43,* 40–43.

Cohen, S., & Syme, S. L. (Eds.), (1985). *Social support and health.* New York: Academic Press.

Coie, J. D., Watt, N. F., West, S. G., Hawkins, J. D., Asarnow, J. R., Markman, H. J., Ramey, S. L., Shure, M. B., & Long, B. (1993). The science of prevention. *American Psychologist, 48,* 1013–1022.

Costner, H. L. (1989). The validity of conclusions in evaluation research: A further development of Chen and Rossi's theory-driven approach. *Evaluation and Program Planning, 12,* 345–353.

Cutrona, C. E., & Russell, D. W. (1991). Type of social support and specific stress: Toward a theory of optimal matching. In B. R. Sarason, I. G. Sarason, & G. R. Pierce (Eds.), *Social support: An interactional view* (pp. 319–366). New York: Wiley.

Davidson, L., & Linnoila, M. (Eds., 1991). *Risk factors for youth suicide.* New York: Hemisphere.

Dent, C. W., Sussman, S., Stacy, A. W., Sun, P., Craig, S., Simon, T. R., Burton, D., & Flay, E. (1995). Two-year behavioral outcomes of Project Toward No Tobacco Use. *Journal of Consulting Clinical Psychology, 3*(4): 676–7

Dielman, T. E. (1994). School-based research on the prevention of adolescent alcohol use and misuse: Methodological issues and advances. *Journal of Research on Adolescence, 4,* 271–293.

Dielman, T. E., Butchart, A. T., & Shope, J. T. (1993). Structural equation model tests of patterns of family interaction, peer alcohol use and intrapersonal predictors of adolescent alcohol use and misuse. *Journal of Drug Education, 23,* 273–316.

DiPrete T. A., & Forristal J. D. (1994). Multilevel models: Methods and substance. *Annual Review of Sociology, 20,* 331–357.

Dishion, T. J. (1998). Advances in family-based interventions to prevent adolescent drug abuse. In NIDA, *National conference on drug abuse prevention research: Presentations, papers, and recommendations* (pp. 87–100). NIH Publication 98-4293. Rockville, MD: NIH.

Donovan, J. E., Jessor, R., & Costa R. M. (1988). Syndrome of problem behaviors in adolescence. *Journal of Consulting and Clinical Psychology, 56,* 762–765.

Dorn, F. J. (1984). The social influence model: A social psychological approach to counseling. *Personnel and Guidance Journal, 62,* 342–345.

Dryden, W. (1981). The relationships of depressed persons. In S. Duck & R. Gilmour (Eds.), *Personal relationships 3: Personal relationships in disorder* (pp. 191–214). New York: Academic Press.

Dryfoos, J. G. (1990). *Adolescents at-risk: prevalence and prevention.* New York: Oxford.

Dryfoos, J. G. (1991). Preventing high risk behavior. *American Journal of Public Health, 81,* 157–158.

Drug Strategies (1996). *Making the grade: A guide to school drug prevention programs.* Washington, DC: Author.

Drug Strategies (1998). *Safe schools, safe students: A guide to violence prevention strategies.* Washington, DC: Author.

Duncan, T. E., Duncan, S. C., & Hops, H. (1994). The effects of family cohesiveness and peer encouragement on the development of adolescent alcohol use: A cohort-sequential approach to the analysis of longitudinal data. *Journal of Studies on Alcohol, 55,* 588–599.

Dunkel-Schetter, C., & Bennett, T. L. (1991). Differentiating the cognitive and behavioral aspects of social support. In B. R. Sarason, I. G. Sarason, & G. R. Pierce (Eds.), *Social support* (pp. 267–296). New York: Wiley.

Eggert, L. L. (1987). Support in family ties: Stress, coping, and adaptation. In T. L. Albrecht & M. B. Adelman (Eds.), *Communicating social support* (pp. 80–104). Beverly Hills, CA: Sage.

Eggert, L. L. (1986). Psychosocial approaches in prevention science: Facing the challenge with high-risk youth. *Communicating Nursing Research, 29,* 73–85.

Eggert, L. L. (1994). *Anger management skills for training adolescents.* Bloomington, IN: NES.

Eggert, L. L. (1998). Reconnecting Youth: An indicated prevention program. In NIDA, *National conference on drug abuse prevention research: Presentations, papers, and recommendations* (pp. 57–72). NIH Publication 98-4293. Rockville, MD: NIH.

Eggert, L. L., & Herting, J. R. (1991). Preventing teenage drug abuse: exploratory effects of network social support. *Youth and Society, 22,* 482–524.

Eggert, L. L., & Herting, J. R. (1993). Drug exposure among potential dropouts and typical youth. *Journal of Drug Education, 23,* 31–55.

Eggert, L. L., Herting, J. R., & Thompson, E. A. (1996). The drug involvement scale for adolescents (DISA). *Journal of Drug Education, 26,* 101–130.

Eggert, L. L., Herting, J. R., Thompson, E. A., Nicholas, L. J., & Dicker, B. G. (1994). Preventing adolescent drug abuse and high school dropout through an intensive school-based social network development program. *American Journal of Health Promotion, 8,* 202–214.

Eggert, L. L., & Kumpfer, K. L. (1997). *Drug abuse prevention for at-risk individuals* (NIH Publication #97–4115). Rockville, MD: DHHS, National Institutes of Health, National Institute on Drug Abuse, Office of Science Policy and Communications.

Eggert, L. L., & Nicholas, L. J. (1992). Speaking like a skipper: 'Skippin' an' gettin' high.' *Journal of Language and Social Psychology, 11,* 75–100.

Eggert, L. L., Nicholas, L. J., & Owen, L. (1995). *Reconnecting Youth: A peer group approach to building life skills.* Bloomington, IN: NES.

Eggert, L. L., Seyl, C., & Nicholas, L. J. (1990). Effects of a school-based prevention program for potential high school dropouts and drug abusers. *International Journal of the Addictions, 25,* 772–801.

Eggert, L. L., Thompson, E. A., & Herting, J. R. (1994). Measure of adolescent potential for suicide (MAPS): Development and preliminary findings. *Suicide and Life-Threatening Behavior, 24,* 359–381.

Eggert, L. L., Thompson, E. A., Herting, J. R., & Nicholas, L. J. (1994). A prevention research program: Reconnecting at-risk youth. *Issues in Mental Health Nursing, 15,* 107–135.

Eggert, L. L., Thompson, E. A., Herting, J. R., & Nicholas, L. J. (1995). Reducing suicide potential among high-risk youth: Tests of a school-based prevention program. *Suicide and Life-Threatening Behavior, 25,* 276–296.

Eggert, L. L., Thompson, E. A., Herting, J. R., & Randell, B. P. (2001). Reconnecting youth to prevent drug abuse, school dropout, and suicidal behaviors among high-risk youth. In E. Wagner and H. B. Waldron (Eds.), *Innovations in adolescent substance abuse intervention* (pp. 51–84). Oxford: Elsevier Science.

Elliott, D. S. (1994). Health enhancing and health compromising life-styles. In S. G. Millstein, A. C. Petersen, & E. O. Nightingale (Eds.), *Promoting the health of adolescents: New directions for the 21st century.* New York: Oxford.

Elliott, D. S., Huizinga D., & Ageton, S. S. (1985). *Explaining delinquency and drug use.* Newbury Park, CA: Sage.

Ezekoye, S., Kumpfer, K., & Bukoski, W. (Eds., 1986). *Childhood and chemical abuse: Prevention and early intervention.* New York: Haworth Press.

Felner, R. D., & Felner, T. Y. (1989). Primary prevention programs in educational context: A transactional-ecological framework and analysis. In L. A. Bond & B. E. Compas (Eds.), *Primary prevention and promotion in schools.* Newbury Park, CA: Sage.

Gabriel, R. M., & Nickel, P. R. (1997). *Risk and protective factors associated with alcohol, tobacco and other drug use and violence: Secondary analysis of the 1995 WA State survey of adolescent health behaviors.* Olympia, WA: DSHS, Division of Alcohol and Substance Abuse.

Gans, J. E., Blyth, D. A., Elster, A. B., & Gaveras, L. L. (1990). *America's adolescents: How healthy are they?* Chicago, IL: American Medical Association.

Garnefski, N., & Okam, S. (1996). Addiction-risk and aggressive/criminal behavior in adolescence: Influence of family, school, and peers. *Journal of Adolescence, 19,* 503–512.

Glantz, M., & Pickens, R. (Eds., 1992). *Vulnerability to drug abuse.* Washington DC: American Psychological Association.

Goodstadt, M. S., & Mitchell, E. (1990). Prevention theory and research related to high-risk youth. In E. N. Goperud (Ed.), *Breaking new ground for youth at-risk* (DHHS Publication No. ADM 89-1658) (pp. 7–23). Washington, DC: U.S. Government Printing Office.

Gotlib, I. H., & Whiffen, V. E. (1991). The interpersonal context of depression: Implications for theory and research. In W. H. Jones & D. Perlman (Eds.), *Advances in Personal Relationships, 3* (pp. 177–206). London: J. Kingsley.

Government Accounting Office (1992). *Adolescent drug use prevention: Common features of promising community programs.* Report to the Chairman, Subcommittee on Select Ed, Committee on Education and Labor, House of Rep. Washington, DC.

Graham, J. W., Marks, G., and Hansen, W. B. (1991). Social influence processes affecting adolescent substance use. *Journal of Applied Psychology, 76,* 291–298.

Hansen, W. B. (1992). School-based substance abuse prevention: A review of the state of the art in curriculum, 1980–1990. *Health Education Research, 7,* 403–430.

Hansen, W. B. (1998). Prevention programs: What are the critical factors that spell success? In NIDA, *National conference on drug abuse prevention research: Presentations, papers, and recommendations* (pp. 27–42). NIH Pub. No. 98-4293. Rockville, MD: NIH. NIDA.

Hansen, W. B., & Graham, J. W. (1991). Preventing alcohol, marijuana, and cigarette use among adolescents: Peer pressure resistance training vs. establishing conservative norms. *Preventive Medicine, 20,* 414–430.

Hansen, W. B., & McNeal, R. B. (1997). The law of maximum expected potential effect: Constraints placed on program effectiveness by mediator relationship. *Health Education Research, 11,* 501–507.

Harlow, L. L., Newcomb, M. D., & Bentler, P. M. (1986). Depression, self-derogation, substance use, and suicide ideation: Lack of purpose in life as a mediational factor. *Journal of Clinical Psychology, 42,* 5–21.

Hawkins, J. D., Catalano, R. F., & Miller, J. Y. (1992). Risk and protective factors for alcohol and other drug problems in adolescence and early adulthood: The implications for substance abuse prevention. *Psychological Bulletin, 112,* 64–105.

Hawkins, J. D., Lishner, D. M., Jenson, J. M., & Catalano, R. F. (1987). Delinquents and drugs: What the evidence suggests about prevention and treatment programming. In NIDA, *Youth at high risk for substance abuse* (DHHS Publication No. ADM 87-1537) (pp. 81–131). Washington DC: U.S. Government Printing Office.

Heller, K., Price, R. H., & Hogg, J. R. (1991). The role of social support in community and clinical interventions. In B. R. Sarason, I. G. Sarason, & G. R. Pierce (Eds.), *Social support* (pp. 482–508). New York: Wiley.

Herting, J. R., Eggert, L. L., & Thompson, E. A. (1996). A multidimensional model of adolescent drug involvement. *Journal of Research on Adolescence, 6,* 325–361.

Huba, G. J., Wingard, J. A., & Bentler, P. M. (1980). Framework for an interactive theory of drug use. In D. J. Lettieri, M. Sayers, & H. W. Pearson (Eds.), *Theories on drug abuse.* Rockville, MD: NIDA.

Hundleby, J. D., & Mercer, G. W. (1987). Family and friends as social environments and their relationship to young adolescents' use of alcohol, tobacco, and marijuana. *Journal of Marriage and Family, 49,* 151–164.

Igoe, J. B. (1991). Empowerment of children and youth for consumer self-care. *American Journal of Health Promotion, 6,* 55–65.

Institute of Medicine. (1994). Reducing risk for mental health disorders: Frontiers for preventive intervention research. Washington, DC: National Academy.

Janis, I. L. (1983). *Short term counseling: Guidelines based on recent research.* New Haven, CT: Yale University.

Jessor, R. (1991). Risk behavior in adolescence: A psychosocial framework. *Journal of Adolescent Health, 12,* 596–605.

Jessor, R. (1993). Successful adolescent development among youth in high-risk settings. *American Psychologist, 48,* 117–26.

Johnson, L. D. (1996). Changing trends, patterns, and nature of marijuana use. In: *National conference on marijuana use: Prevention, treatment and research.* NIH Pub. No. 96-4106. Washington, DC: Supt. of Docs., U.S. Government Printing Office.

Johnson, L. D., O'Malley, P. M., & Bachman, J. G. (1996). *National survey results on drug use from the Monitoring the Future Study, 1975–1995: Vol. 1. Secondary school students.* NIH Pub. No. 96-4139, Rockville, MD: U.S. DHHS, NIH, NIDA.

Kandel, D. B., & Andrews, K. (1987). Processes of adolescent socialization by parents and peers. *International Journal of the Addictions, 22,* 319–342.

Kandel, D. B., Kessler, R. C., & Margulies, R. Z. (1978). Antecedents of adolescent initiation into stages of drug use: A developmental analysis. In D. B. Kandel (Ed.), *Longitudinal research and drug use: Empirical findings and methodological issues* (pp. 73–98). Washington DC: Hemisphere.

Kandel, D., Raveis, V. H., & Davies, M. (1991). Suicidal ideation in adolescence: Depression, substance use and other risk factors. *Journal of Youth and Adolescence, 20,* 289–307.

Kaplan, H. B., Martin, S. S., & Robbins, C. (1984). Pathways to adolescent drug use: Self-derogation, peer influence, weakening of social controls, and early substance use. *Journal of Health and Social Behavior, 25,* 270–289.

Kasen, S., Johnson, J., & Cohen, P. (1990). The impact of school emotional climate on student psychopathology. *Journal of Abnormal Child Psychology, 18,* 165–177.

Keitner, G. I., & Miller, I. W. (1990). Family functioning and major depression: An overview. *American Journal of Psychiatry, 147,* 1128–37.

Kellam, S. G., Brown, C. H., Rubin, B. R., & Ensminger, M. C. (1983). Paths leading to teenage use: Developmental epidemiological studies in Woodlawn. In S. B. Buze, F. F. Earls, & J. E. Barrett (Eds.), *Childhood psychopathology and development* (pp. 17–51). New York: Raven.

Kellam, S. G., & Rebok, G. W. (1992). Building developmental and etiological theory through epidemiologically based preventive intervention trials. In J. McCord & R. E. Tremblay (Eds.), *Preventing antisocial behavior: Interventions from birth through adolescence.* New York: Guilford Press.

Kellam, S. G., Werthamer-Larsson L., Dolan L. J., Brown, C. H., Mayer, L. S., Rebok, G. W., Anthony, J. C., Laudolff, J., & Edelson, G. (1991). Developmental epidemiologically based preventive trials: Baseline modeling of early target behaviors and depressive symptoms. *American Journal of Community Psychology, 19,* 563–584.

Kraemer, H. C., & Thiemann, S. (1987). *How many subjects? Statistical power analysis in research.* Newbury Park, CA: Sage.

Kreft, I. G. G. (1998). An illustration of item homogeneity scaling and multilevel analysis techniques in the evaluation of drug prevention programs. *Evaluation Review, 22,* 46–77.

Kumpfer, K. L. (1989). Prevention of alcohol and drug abuse: A critical review of risk factors and prevention strategies. In Shaffer, D., Philips, I., & Euzer, N. (Eds.), Prevention of Mental Disorders, Alcohol and Other Drug Use in Children and Adolescents (pp. 309–371). OSAP Monograph No. 2. Rockville, MD.

Kumpfer, K. L., & DeMarsh, J. P. (1986). Family-oriented interventions for the prevention of chemical dependency in children and adolescents. In S. Ezekoye, K. Kumpfer, & W. Bukoski (Eds.), *Childhood and chemical abuse: Prevention and intervention.* New York: Haworth.

Kumpfer, K., Rigby, D., Walsh, E. M., & Sorenson, S. L. (1997). *Substance abuse prevention theory and research-based programs: What works!* (NIH Publication No. 97-4110). Rockville, MD: Department of Health and Human Services, NIDA.

Kumpfer, K., & Turner, C. W. (1991). The social ecology model of adolescent substance abuse: Implications for prevention. *International Journal of the Addictions, 25,* 435–463.

LaGaipa, J. L., & Wood, D. H. (1981). Friendship in disturbed adolescents. In S. Duck & R. Gilmour (Eds.), *Personal relationships, 3: Personal relationships in disorder* (pp. 169–190). NY: Academic Press.

Levy, J., & Deykin, E. (1989). Suicidality, depression, and substance abuse in adolescence. *American Journal of Psychiatry, 146,* 1462–1467.

Lin, N., Dean, A., & Ensel, W. (1986). *Social support, life events, and depression.* Orlando: Academic Press.

Lorion, R. P. (1990). Basing preventive interventions on theory: Stimulating a field's momentum. In R. P. Lorion (Ed.), *Protecting the children: Strategies for optimizing emotional and behavioral development.* New York: Haworth.

MacKinnon, D. P., Johnson, C. A., Pentz, M. A., Dwyer, J. H., Hansen, W. B., Flay, B. R., & Wang, E. Y-I. (1991). Mediating mechanisms in a school-based drug prevention program: First-year effects of the Midwestern Prevention program: First-year effects of the Midwestern Prevention Project. Health Psychology, 10(3), 164–172.

Manscill, C. K., & Rollins, B. C. (1990). Adolescent self-esteem as an intervening variable in parental behavior and academic achievement relationship. In B. K. Barber & B. C. Rollins (Eds.), *Parent-adolescent relationships* (pp. 95–118). Lanham, MD: University Press of America.

McCauley, E., & Myers, K. (1992). Family interaction in mood-disordered youth. *Child and Adolescent Psychiatric Clinics of North America, 1,* 111–127.

Mechanic, D., & Hansell, S. (1989). Divorce, family conflict and adolescent well-being. *Journal of Health and Social Behavior, 30,* 105–116.

Miller, W. R., & Rollnick, S. (1991). *Motivational interviewing.* New York: Guilford.

Miller, W. R., & Sanchez, V. C. (1993). Motivating young adults for treatment and lifestyle change. In G. Howard (Ed.), *Issues in alcohol use and misuse by young adults.* Notre Dame, IN: University of Notre Dame Press.

Miller, W. R., & Sovereign, R. G. (1989). The check-up: A model for early intervention in addictive behaviors. In T. Loberg, W. R. Miller, P. E. Nathan, & G. A. Marlatt (Eds.), *Addictive Behaviors* (pp. 219–31). Amsterdam, Netherlands: Swets & Zeitlinger.

Moskowitz, J. (1988). Evaluating the effects of parent groups on the correlates of adolescent substance abuse. *Journal of Psychoactive Drugs, 17,* 173–178.

National Crime Prevention Council (1988). *Reaching out: School-based community service programs.* Washington, DC.

National Institute on Drug Abuse (1991). *Drug abuse and drug abuse research.* DHHS Publication No. ADM 91-1704. Washington DC: U.S. Government Printing Office.

National Institute on Drug Abuse (1998). *National conference on drug abuse prevention research: Presentations, papers, and recommendations.* NIH Publication 98-4293. Rockville, MD: NIH.

Newcomb, M. D. (1992). Understanding the multidimensional nature of drug use and abuse: The role of consumption, risk factors, and protective factors. In M. Glantz & R. Pickens (Eds.), *Vulnerability to drug abuse* (pp. 255–297). Washington DC: American Psychological Association.

Newcomb, M. D., & Bentler, P. M. (1988). The impact of family context, deviant attitudes, and emotional distress on adolescent drug use: Longitudinal latent-variable analyses of mothers and their children. *Journal of Research in Personality, 22,* 154–176.

Newcomb, M. D., & Earleywine, M. (1996). Intrapersonal contributors to drug use: The willing host. *American Behavioral Scientist, 39,* 823–837.

Newcomb, M. D., & Harlow, L. L. (1986). Life events and substance use among adolescents: Mediating effects of perceived loss of control and meaninglessness in life. *Journal of Personality and Social Psychology, 51,* 564–577.

Newcomb, M. D., McCarthy, W. J., & Bentler, P. M. (1989). Cigarette smoking, academic lifestyle, and social impact efficacy: An eight-year study from early adolescence to young adulthood. *Journal of Applied Social Psychology, 19,* 251–281.

Newcomb, M. D., Scheier, L. M., & Bentler, P. M. (1993). Effects of adolescent drug use on adult mental health: A prospective study of a community sample. *Experimental and Clinical Psychopharmacology, 1,* 215–241.

Norem-Hebeisen, A., & Hedin, D. P. (1981). Influences on adolescent problem behavior: Causes, connections, and contexts. In NIDA, *Adolescent peer pressure* (pp. 21–46). DHHS Publication No. ADM 86-1152. Washington, DC: U.S. Government Printing Office.

Osgood, D. W. (1991). *Covariation among health problems in adolescence.* Washington DC: Office of Technical Assistance.

Pandina, R. J. (1998). Risk and protective factor models in adolescent drug use: Putting them to work for prevention. In NIDA, *National conference on drug abuse prevention research: Presentations, papers, and recommendations* (pp. 17–26). NIH Publication 98-4293. Rockville, MD: NIH.

Paton, S., Kessler, R., & Kandel, D. (1977). Depressive mood and adolescent illegal drug use. *Journal of Genetic Psychology, 131,* 267–289.

Pentz, M. A. (1993). Benefits of integrating strategies in different settings. In A. Elster, S. Panzarine, & K. Holt (Eds.), *AMA state-of-the-art conference on adolescent health promotion: Proceedings* (pp. 15–33). Arlington, VA: National Center for Ed Mat/Child Health.

Pentz, M. A. (1998). Preventing drug abuse through the community: Multicomponent programs make the difference. In NIDA, *National conference on drug abuse prevention research: Presentations, papers, and recommendations* (pp. 73–86). NIH Publication 98-4293. Rockville, MD: NIH.

Pentz, M. A., Dwyer, J. H., MacKinnon, D. P., Flay, B. R., Hansen, W. B., Wang, E., & Johnson, A. (1989). A multicommunity trial for primary prevention of adolescent drug use. *JAMA 261*(22), 3259–3266.

Peterson, P. L., Hawkins, J. D., Abbott, R. D., & Catalano, R. F. (1994). Disentangling the effects of parental drinking, family management, and parental alcohol norms on current drinking by black and white adolescents. *Journal of Research on Adolescence 4,* 203–227.

Powell-Cope, G. M., & Eggert, L. L. (1994). Psychosocial risk and protective factors: Potential high school dropouts vs. typical youth. *National Dropout Center Yearbook I* (pp. 23–51). Lancaster, PA: Technomic.

Rainer, K. L., & Slavin, L. A. (1992). *Social support networks and stressful events of low-income African-American adolescents and their single mothers.* Presented at the Society for Research on Adolescence Meeting, Washington DC.

Resnick, M. D., Bearman, P. S., Blum, R. W., Bauman, K. E., Harris, K. M., Jones, J., Tabor, J., Beuhrin, T., Sieving, R. E., Shew, M., Ireland, M., Bearinger, L. H., & Udry, R. (1997). Protecting adolescents from harm: Findings from the national longitudinal study on adolescent health. *Journal of the American Medical Association, 278,* 823–865.

Rogosa, D., & Willett, J. B. (1985). Understanding correlates of change by modeling individual differences in growth. *Psychometrika, 50,* 203–228.

Rohrbach, L. A., Graham, J. W., Hansen, W. B., Flay, B. R., & Johnson, C. A. (1987). Evaluation of resistance skills training using multitrait-multimethod role play skill assessment. *Health Education Research, 2,* 401–407.

Rutter, M., & Giller, H. (1983). *Juvenile delinquency: Trends and perspectives.* New York: Penguin Books.

Sarason, B. R., Sarason, I. G., & Pierce, G. R. (Eds., 1991). *Social support: An interactional view.* New York: Wiley.

Scheier, L. M., Newcomb, M. D., & Skager, R. (1994). Risk, protection, and vulnerability to adolescent drug use: Latent-variable models of three age groups. *Journal of Drug Education, 24,* 49–82.

Schinke, S. P., Botvin, G. J., & Orlandi, M. A. (1991). *Substance abuse in children and adolescents: Evaluation and intervention.* Newbury Park, CA: Sage.

Schinke, S. P., & Gilchrist L. D. (1984). *Life skills counseling with adolescents.* Austin, TX: Pro-Ed.

Spielberger, C. D., Jacobs, G., Russel, S., & Crane, R. S. (1983). Assessment of anger. In J. N. Butcher and C. D. Spielberger (Eds.), *Advances in personality measurement, 2* (pp. 161–189). Hillsdale, NJ: Erlbaum.

Stein, J. A., Newcomb, M. D., & Bentler, P. M. (1987). An 8-year study of multiple influences on drug use and drug use consequences. *Journal of Personality and Social Psychology, 53,* 1094–1105.

Sussman, S. (1996a). Development of a school-based drug abuse prevention curriculum for high-risk youths. *Journal of Psychoactive Drugs, 28*(2), 169–182.

Sussman, S. (1996b). Drug abuse prevention programming: Do we know what content works? *American Behavioral Scientist, 39,* 868–883.

Sussman, S., Dent, C., Simon, T., Stacy, A., Galaif, E., Moss, M., Craig, S., Johnson, C. (1994). Immediate Impact of Social Influence-Oriented Substance Abuse. *Prevention Curricula in Traditional and Continuation High Schools. Drugs & Society, 8,* 65, 1994.

Sussman, S., Simon, T. R., Dent, C. W., Stacy, A. W., Galaif, E. R., Moss, M. A., Craig, S., & Johnson, C. A. (1997). Immediate impact of thirty-two drug abuse prevention activities among students at continuation high schools. *Substance Use and Misuse, 32*(3), 265–281.

Sussman, S., & Johnson, C. A. (Eds., 1996). Drug abuse prevention: Programming and research recommendations. *Special issue, American Behavioral Scientist, 39.*

Thompson, E. A., Connelly, C. D., & Eggert, L. L. Co-occurring problem behaviors among potential high school dropouts: Drug use, aggression, depression, and suicidal behaviors. Manuscript submitted for publication.

Thompson, E. A., & Eggert, L. L. (1999). Using the Suicide Risk Screen to identify suicidal adolescents among potential high school dropouts. *J. Am. Acad. Child Adolescent. Psychiatry,* 38(12), 1506–1514.

Thompson, E. A., Eggert, L. L., & Herting, J. R. (2000). Mediating effects of an indicated prevention program for reducing youth depression and suicide risk behaviors. Suicide and Life-Threatening Behavior, 30(3), 252–271.

Thompson, E. A., Horn, M., Herting, J. R., & Eggert, L. L. (1997). Enhancing outcomes in an indicated drug prevention program for high-risk youth. *Journal of Drug Education, 27,* 19–41.

Thompson, E. A., Mazza, J. J., Herting, J. R., & Eggert, L. L. (2002). The mediating roles of anxiety, depression, and hopelessness on adolescent suicidal behaviors. Manuscript submitted for publication.

Thompson, E. A., Moody, K., & Eggert, L. L. (1994). Discriminating suicide ideation among high-risk youth. *Journal of School Health, 64,* 361–367.

Tobler, N. S. (1986). Meta-analysis of 143 adolescent drug prevention programs. *Journal of Drug Issues, 16,* 537–567.

Tobler, N. S. (1992). Drug prevention programs can work: Research findings. *Journal of Addictive Diseases, 11,* 1–28.

Tobler, N. S., & Stratton, H. S. (1997). Effectiveness of school-based drug prevention programs: A meta-analysis of the research. *Journal of Primary Prevention, 18,* 71–128.

University of Michigan (1994). *Press release report on Monitoring the Future Study* (Dated 12/8/94). Update with a recent reports 1997–98.

U.S. Department of Health and Human Services (1994). *Preliminary estimates from the national household survey on drug abuse.* Rockville, MD: NIDA. UPDATE with 1997–98 reports.

Vorrath, H., & Brendtro, L. (1985). *Positive peer culture* (2nd ed.). Chicago: Aldine.

Watson, D., & Friend, R. (1969). Measurement of social-evaluative anxiety. *Journal of Consulting and Clinical Psychology, 33,* 448–457.

Weinberg, N. Z., Dielman, T. E., Mandell, W., & Shope, J. T. (1994). Parental drinking and gender factors in the prediction of early adolescent alcohol use. *International Journal of the Addictions 29,* 89–101.

Weiner, B., & Litman-Adizes, T. (1980). An attributional, expectancy-value analysis of learned helplessness and depression. In J. Garber & M. Seligman (Eds.), *Human helplessness: Theory and applications.* New York: Academic Press.

Weissberg, R. P., Caplan, M. Z., & Sivo, P. J. (1989). A new conceptual framework for establishing school-based social competence promotion programs. In L. A. Bond & B. E. Compas (Eds.), *Primary prevention and promotion in the schools* (pp. 255–296). Newbury Park, CA: Sage.

Weng, L. J., Newcomb, M. D., & Bentler, P. M. (1988). Factors influencing non-completion of high school: A comparison of methodologies. *Educational Research Quarterly, 12,* 8–22.

Wills, T. A. (1985). Stress, coping, and tobacco and alcohol use in early adolescence. In S. Shiffman & T. A. Wills (Eds.), *Coping and substance use.* New York: Academic Press.

Wills, T. A., Pierce, J. P., & Evans, R. I. (1996). Large-scale environmental risk factors for substance use. *American Behavioral Scientist, 39,* 808–822.

Wills, T. A., Schreibman, D., Benson, G., & Vaccaro, D. (1994). Impact of parental substance use on adolescents: A test of a mediational model. *Journal of Pediatric Psychology, 19,* 537–556.

CHAPTER 25

Research Designs for Family Studies

MICHAEL VANYUKOV
HOWARD MOSS
RALPH E. TARTER

INTRODUCTION

Research aimed at delineating the influence of the family on the etiology of drug abuse addresses three interrelated sets of issues. First, epidemiological research is conducted to determine whether the prevalence of substance abuse is greater among biologically related individuals compared to the general population. Second, comprehensive investigations into drug abuse etiology are directed at elucidating the relative contribution of genetic and unique individual and shared familial and extrafamilial environmental factors in the variation of the liability to drug abuse. And third, etiologic research in which the family system is conceptualized as a social unit, irrespective of the biological relationships, is directed at clarifying the intrafamilial environment. Specifically, the quality of interpersonal interactions, which predispose to drug abuse among family members, is investigated.

The ensuing discussion examines the paradigms that are commonly employed to investigate the impact of the family on drug abuse etiology. These paradigms are heuristic for clarifying the influence of familial factors on drug abuse etiology inasmuch as it has already been established that the rate of substance abuse is higher among family members where one member has this disorder compared to the rate of substance abuse among unrelated individuals in the general population (Cadoret et al., 1986). The family is a structure of kindred (biological) relationships as

MICHAEL VANYUKOV AND RALPH E. TARTER • School of Pharmacy, University of Pittsburgh, Pittsburgh, Pennsylvania 15261
HOWARD MOSS • Department of Psychiatry, University of Pennsylvania, Philadelphia, Pennsylvania 19104

well as of a social system. The kindred relationships reflect varying degrees of genetic similarity (e.g., 100% in identical twins, 50% in full siblings, and 25% in half siblings). Genetic factors contribute strongly to affective, behavioral, and cognitive functioning, thereby determining in part the congruity among family members on traits contributing to substance abuse etiology. Hence, the behavior of the family system is the product of the dispositions of its individual members. Ultimately, therefore, it is essential to understand the determinants of individual makeup comprising the family in order to understand the functioning of the family system. This discussion will be confined to an examination and review of paradigms which are applicable for clarifying the impact of parents on children with respect to revealing the influences of genetic lineage as well as the patterns of interpersonal interaction on drug abuse etiology. Undoubtedly, the quality of sibling relationships and the dyadic marital relationship are also important determinants of drug abuse etiology; however, these aspects of the family environment have not been investigated systematically and lie outside the scope of this chapter. The reader is referred to Barnes (1990), Bry (1983), and Kumpfer (1995) for a discussion of these latter topics.

DEFINITION OF FAMILY

The term *family* has a wide array of meanings. In biological classification, it refers to a category position located between an *order* and a *genus*. Its informal use in law enforcement refers to a locally independent unit of the Cosa Nostra. Among geneticists, the family is specified as a pedigree in which biological relationships are documented in the context of each member's relationship to common ancestry. Social scientists commonly adopt a broader perspective of the family which, unfortunately, has more ambiguous boundaries. For example, nonbiological and nonadoptive relationships (e.g., "godparent") are commonly included in the designation of family, based only on the fact that there is some degree of social closeness or identification with the nuclear unit.

Research on the impact of the family on any particular outcome requires explicit description of the structure and the relationships (biological and nonbiological) among the members comprising the family unit. In this regard, the spatial and temporal relationships among its members need to be specified.

Spatial Relationships among Family Members

This aspect of the family unit pertains to each member's domicile. For example, whether the whole nuclear family is living in the same household needs to be determined and controlled in research comparing families as well as members within a family. Also, whether siblings occupy the same bedroom or have separate rooms must be established as potential influences on outcome. For example, having either a shared or a separate bedroom impacts on the quality of the sibling relationship, exposure to drugs, and drug paraphernalia and has manifold other influences on each child's activities. Furthermore, the location of extended family members and biologically unrelated members (e.g., foster children in the same house as either risk-enhancing or risk-mitigating influences) needs to be ascertained in characterizing the spatial organization of the family. Clearly there are myriad variations of living arrangements that augment as well as attenuate the liability to a drug abuse disorder; these need to be explicitly documented and controlled in research directed at elucidating the role of the family on etiology as well as its moderating influence on prevention or treatment intervention.

Example of a pedigree with substance abuse

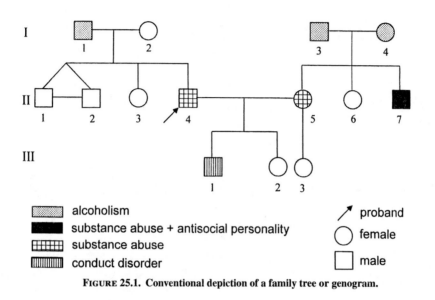

FIGURE 25.1. Conventional depiction of a family tree or genogram.

Temporal Relationships among Family Members

Whereas spatial relationships characterize the degree of environmental closeness, biological closeness is characterized by the ancestral relationships among family members. Figure 25.1 presents a typical example of a pedigree chart (family tree). As a standardized method of communication, generations are numbered with Roman numerals, and individuals within each generation are numbered according to birth order with Arabic numerals. The person who draws the researcher's attention to a family first is called the *proband* (propositus, index case); this person need not have any distinguishing characteristic or disorder. In this diagram, this person is numbered II-4. Marriage (or mating) is designated by a horizontal line directly connecting male and female symbols, and symbols representing children branch down from a horizontal attached to the marriage line. Individuals II-I and II-2 are monozygotic twins (if they were dizygotic or of an unknown zygosity, there would be no horizontal line connecting them or a question mark instead of the line.) Individuals III-I and III-2 are full siblings. As can be observed, a standard genogram communicates at a glance substantial information about the family.

There are two general strategies for researching families where clarifying ancestral relationships is pertinent to the goals of a study. A *bottom–up paradigm* is employed where children are ascertained as the probands to characterize lineage patterns. Alternatively, where a parent is the proband, a *top–down paradigm* is employed. In order to prevent sampling bias and confounds, it is essential that an investigation use *exclusively* one of these two ascertainment approaches, because the type as well as the location from which the proband is drawn determine to a large extent the pattern of findings. For example, antisociality is well known to increase the risk for substance use in the children. Families in which either the father or the mother is antisocial are different from families in which the child is antisocial. Thus, if the goal of a prevention trial or etiology study is directed at determining the role of the family on antisociality and drug abuse, it is not appropriate to employ more than one strategy for ascertaining the proband.

GENERAL MODEL

Figure 25.2 depicts a general model outlining the component factors involved in the risk for substance abuse at the individual level. Individual genotype (set of the genes that the person possesses) influences the choice of individual environments (e.g., peer affiliation, individual life experience) and contributes to the formation of the environment that the family members have in common (e.g., socioeconomic level, neighborhood). Genotype and environment, in their interaction, determine the individual phenotype for the trait termed the *liability to substance use disorder.* To fully understand the denotative meaning of this trait requires some elaboration.

Falconer (1965) introduced the concept of "liability" to human genetics. Liability is a latent trait which, if measured, "would give us a graded scale of the degree of affectedness or of normality and we should find that all individuals above a certain value exhibited the disease and all below it did not" (p. 52). The individual's value on this scale is his/her liability phenotype. Phenotypic values surpassing a certain point on the scale of the liability, the *threshold,* are ascribed a diagnostic label (e.g., "alcoholism" or "substance abuse"). Suprathreshold phenotypes in DSM-IV are collectively referred to as "substance use disorder." Within this affected state, three levels of severity are denoted; respectively, these are abuse, psychological dependence, and physical dependence. By definition, prevention is the process of reducing liability among individuals who have not surpassed the diagnostic threshold.

It is accepted that the variation in the liability to substance abuse is a complex function of manifold social, psychological, physiological, and biochemical variables which influence the initiation and maintenance of substance use and ultimately the development of a DSM substance use disorder. In keeping with the central limit theorem, these manifold variables, in aggregate, are describable by a Gaussian curve. It is noteworthy that, with respect to alcoholism, evidence has been obtained supporting the theoretical expectation of a Gaussian distribution of liability in studies of female twins (Kendler et al., 1992) and of older males and females (Prescott et al., 1994a,b).

Ontogenetic Perspective of Substance Abuse Etiology

The static model of liability determination shown in Figure 25.2, although heuristic, does not take into account the fact that individual phenotypes are changeable. Unlike, for example, eye color, the liability phenotypes for substance abuse develop and change concomitant to ongoing reciprocal interactions with manifold environments (e.g., family, school, work, neighborhood) during the course of the lifespan. A central goal in prevention practice is to minimize exposure

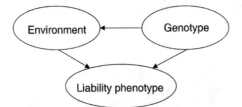

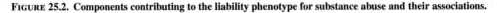

FIGURE 25.2. Components contributing to the liability phenotype for substance abuse and their associations.

to environments that are likely to produce the enhancing liability phenotypes among genetically predisposed individuals. For example, a child's temperament makeup (phenotype), influenced by both genetic and family environment factors, frequently leads to serious conduct problems by middle childhood. A major task is, therefore, to modify the quality of family interactions, particularly between parent and child, so that the precursor condition of drug abuse, namely, conduct problems, can be avoided. Figure 25.3 depicts a general framework for understanding substance abuse as the culmination of ontogenetic development. At the top of the figure, the Gaussian distribution represents the person's norm of reaction (the range of potential liability values) and age-specific outset behavior phenotype position (V_t) in its projection on the liability scale at the time of birth. As previously noted, the person's liability phenotype changes during ontogeny. Hence, the trajectory linking predisposition or risk status to outcome, mediated by events occurring during ontogeny, is not a straight line. As shown in Figure 25.3, shifts of the person's position on the liability scale depicted by the curving line across age, can occur bidirectionally. In other words,

Dynamic Model of the Liability Phenotype Determination

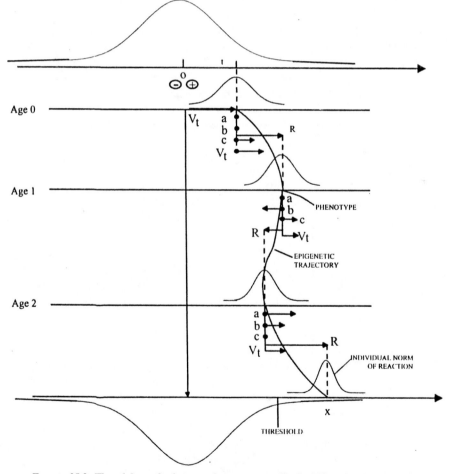

FIGURE 25.3. The etiology of substance abuse conceptualized within a developmental framework.

the person can either be oriented in the direction toward a deviant position on the liability trait (i.e., closer to a suprathreshold diagnosis indicated by the area on the right from the threshold in the lower Gaussian distribution) or, alternatively, be directed toward normative adjustment during the course of development (i.e., indicated by the area in the bottom distribution that is not shaded). Because the trajectory linking liability status at birth to a drug abuse outcome is not typically a straight line but fluctuates during development, it is important to implement interventions that are targeted to ameliorating the individually unique liability-enhancing characteristics which are particular to the person at various stages of chronological development. From the standpoint of etiology, it can be readily appreciated from this model how normal development can be shifted suddenly toward a substance abuse outcome and how substance use and abuse can rapidly remit.

The task in prevention is first to determine the basis for the person's high value on the liability trait. This entails disaggregating the genotypic and environmental contributions to the person's liability trait score. Next, by understanding the phenotype–environment interaction, a reorientation of the developmental trajectory toward more normative adjustment can be accomplished through effective intervention. Prevention, therefore, aims to avert the person from crossing the liability threshold, that is, manifesting a condition of such severity so as to warrant the diagnosis of Substance Use Disorder.

In this ontogenetic model, individuals end up as either affected (drug abuse) or nonaffected (zero use to diagnostic threshold of abuse) depending on events occurring throughout ontogeny. In effect, the quality of interaction between the person (having certain phenotypes) and the environment determines the acquisition of new phenotypes that promote drug abuse. Structuring the environment effectively provides the mechanism by which liability-enhancing phenotypes can be prevented (e.g., conduct problems). Up to the time of adolescence, the family is usually the most powerful environmental influence; thus, its importance in drug abuse prevention cannot be overemphasized. The powerful influence of the family on child development is thus crucial for understanding the emergence and augmentation of the liability to drug abuse during the formative stages of development.

During the course of development, the psychological makeup becomes, however, increasingly complex via interaction with the environment.

As shown in Figure 25.3, intermediary behavior phenotypes and multiple other factors, manifest prior to the outcome, are represented as vectors. In this manner, behavior has both force and direction in shaping the subsequent course of behavioral development. For example, conduct problems are a vector for early-age drug initiation concomitant to the social environment opportunities provided by a deviant pattern of adjustment. The point to be made is that the patterning of psychological development occurs in such fashion that behavior at each stage influences strongly the behavioral topography manifest at succeeding stages. The process by which phenotypes at one stage (e.g., temperament) influence the emergence of successive behavior (e.g., conduct problems) is referred to as *epigenesis*.

Figure 25.4 provides a concrete example of epigenesis based on published empirical findings. It can be seen that behavioral phenotypes are chained from infancy to young adulthood to culminate in a drug abuse outcome. At the outset, a deviation in the temperament trait, behavioral activity level, influences the quality of parent–child interactions. Importantly, children exhibiting a high behavioral activity level experience interactions which are characterized by low parental supervision and poor disciplinary practices (Webster-Stratton & Eyberg, 1982). These types of interactions influence the developmental trajectory toward a drug abuse outcome by first inculcating a deviant behavior style which then increases the risk for drug use in later life (Loeber, 1990). In this illustration, the child's liability to drug abuse is continuously modified during ontogeny to produce phenotypes which increasingly predispose to initiation of drug consumption. Also, in

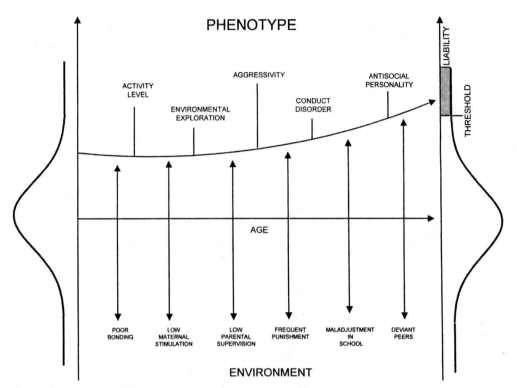

FIGURE 25.4. Example of behavioral epigenesis in which temperament phenotype in infancy, succeeded by a series of intermediary outcome phenotypes during childhood and adolescence, culminates in a suprathreshold disorder of substance abuse.

this example, it can be seen why drug consumption commonly begins early in life and, in many cases, when the youngster attains an age when first exposed to drug-using opportunities. However, it is emphasized that depending on the person's liability and developmental trajectory, both of which are unique to each person in the population, initiation of drug consumption can occur at any time in life. In this regard, the ontogenetic model described herein is equally appropriate for elucidating substance abuse in adolescents as well as in the elderly population.

In summary, there are three major components contributing to variation in the liability to substance abuse. These are genotypic variations, shared environmental effects, and unique or unshared environmental influences. The family is an especially important influence on the child's liability status for two main reasons: the genetic contribution to the phenotype of offspring (i.e., the characteristics associated with elevated risk for substance abuse) and the quality of the environment.

It is not possible to completely disaggregate genetic from environmental influences on drug abuse etiology when studying biologically related intact nuclear families. Research is limited to demonstrating associations on particular phenotypes and genotypes, explorations of familial transmission, and linkages between particular phenotypes and specific chromosomes. To date, emerging studies in this new area of inquiry have yielded encouraging findings regarding the association between drug abuse and a variety of phenotypes in family members (Blackson et al., 1994; Moss et al., 1992; Tarter & Vanyukov, 2001). Molecular genetic associational studies also have yielded encouraging findings (Smith et al., 1992; Vanyukov et al., 2001).

Six types of paradigms are commonly employed to clarify the relationship between alcohol and drug abuse, behavioral phenotypes, and environmental influences in families. These are the *high-risk paradigm,* the *twin paradigm,* the *cross-fostering* or *adoption paradigm,* the *twins reared apart in separate environments paradigm,* the *reconstituted family paradigm,* and the *incomplete nuclear family paradigm.* Each of these paradigms is reviewed in the following in relation to advantages and limitations as well as to information that has been accrued that informs about the etiology of substance abuse.

THE HIGH-RISK PARADIGM

In the high-risk paradigm, a family member who is recognized to be at elevated risk for developing drug abuse is studied. This high-risk person is compared to an individual from another family who is deemed to be at lower risk in the population to develop the outcome. High and low average risk status of individuals is usually ascribed according to the presence of particular characteristics in family members. Typically, either the presence or the absence of substance abuse in first- and second-degree adult family members has been used to ascertain high- and low-risk individuals. Inasmuch as offspring of alcoholics and drug abusers are more likely to develop these disorders themselves in adulthood compared to offspring of normal parents, it can be inferred that children of affected parents are, on average, at high risk. In order to prevent confounds concomitant to drug use behavior and its consequences, it is essential that individuals are investigated who do not have a history of drug abuse. For this reason, most studies employing the high-risk paradigm have focused on children. It is appropriate, however, to study adult relatives of substance abusers (e.g., siblings or offspring) provided that they have not consumed psychoactive substances or do not qualify for a substance use disorder diagnosis. Where adults are studied, it may not be feasible to accrue subjects who have had no exposure to psychoactive drugs (e.g., alcohol, nicotine); hence, it is necessary to set a threshold of substance involvement which would enable elucidating the liability to drug abuse while not yielding data which are confounded by a history of exposure.

The high-risk paradigm has proven to be heuristic for identifying numerous phenotypic characteristics in unaffected relatives which appear to comprise components of the liability to substance abuse. As previously discussed, children of alcoholic and drug-abusing parents are distinguishable from children whose parents do not have a substance use disorder with respect to a variety of physiological, biochemical, and psychological processes (see also Tarter & Mezzich, 1992; Tarter, Moss, & Vanyukov, 1995). These findings, because they reflect mean group differences (high- versus low-risk group status), cannot be generalized to the individual case. Nonetheless, an emerging empirical literature has revealed a variety of psychological deviations in high-risk children which, if modified, would attenuate the risk for a substance abuse outcome. Collectively, these deviations can be subsumed within the rubric of disinhibitory psychopathology (Gorenstein & Newman, 1980) and include most prominently impulsivity, antisociality, and risk taking. Affect and emotion dysregulation, evidenced as difficult temperament (Tarter & Vanyukov, 1994), irritability (Tarter et al., 1995), and depression (Chasin, Rogush, & Barrera, 1991) have also been observed in children at elevated risk for substance abuse. Executive cognitive functioning involving mental processes subserving goal-directed motivation (e.g., strategic thinking, attentional control, self-monitoring) has also been shown as being deficient in high-risk youth (Giancola et al., 1996). High-risk youth have additionally been shown to misinterpret the content of interpersonal interactions, forming instead misattributions of the intentions of others (Rolf et al., 1988). These latter findings, reflecting a core disorder of psychological dysregulation (Tarter et al., 1999), illustrate the range of deviant phenotypes in high-risk youth which, if deflected toward the normative segment of the liability distribution, would accordingly reduce the risk for substance abuse.

Heightened Familial Risk for Substance Abuse

Several methods for the delineation of familial risk have been utilized. These include affected parent designs (Schuckit, 1980; Sher et al., 1991; Sher & Levenson, 1982), measures of the lineality of familial influence (patrilineal, matrilineal, bilineal) (Stabenau, 1984), familial density of affected cases (Hill et al., 1990), multigenerational status (Volicer, Volicer, & D'Angelo, 1985), and the number of affected relatives multiplied by a coefficient indicative of their biological closeness to the proband (Alterman, 1988). Each method is predicated upon the supposition that elevated risk covaries with the number of affected individuals in the family. From a prevention standpoint, the familial aggregation of substance abuse underscores the need to treat affected family members as a method of diminishing substance abuse risk in children. In effect, terminating substance abuse among adults in the family has the potential benefit of increasing their involvement and improving their rapport with the children.

From a research design perspective, it should be noted that elevated risk may be manifest as either the extreme value of the risk variable itself (e.g., earlier age of onset) or as a disproportionate representation of cases arising among a typically lower prevalence group (e.g., elevated proportion of alcohol abuse cases among females) (Bale et al., 1984; Chakraborty et al., 1984). Early age of onset of substance abuse in parents has been found to be associated with greater deviancy in offspring; hence, it would appear that preventions need to be more intensive for those children whose parents developed a substance use disorder at a young age. Similarly, the available evidence suggests that although the prevalence of substance use disorder is lower in females than in males, the liability may actually be higher to develop the disorder. Even though not yet intensively investigated, there is sufficient suggestive evidence indicating that females may, therefore, require more concerted prevention intervention than males despite their lower prevalence rate for a substance use disorder.

A Categorical Approach to the Delineation of Elevated Familial Risk

In response to the previously described limitations for investigating risk status, it is noteworthy that a particularly useful quantitative approach to the categorical assessment of familial aggregation of alcohol and other drug use disorders has been proposed (Chakraborty et al., 1984). This approach involves determining whether there is an elevation of risk for alcohol or drug abuse in a given pedigree (family unit) that is ascertained through a single proband compared to randomly sampled pedigrees in the population with similar configurations. Prior probabilities of each member of the pedigree being affected are obtained using age- and gender-based cumulative incidence data for alcohol and other drug abuse disorders.

Employing this method, the data on substance abuse status of each member of the pedigree (excluding the proband) are represented as $X = (X_1, X_2, \ldots, X_N)$ which is a vector 1's and 0's of the dimension N. Under the null hypothesis of no significant familial aggregation, the expectation of X is $(p_1, p_2, \ldots, p_N)$, and its variance–covariance matrix is a diagonal matrix with elements $p_i(1 - p_i)$, $i = 1, 2, \ldots, N$; where p_i denotes the probability (derived from appropriate age- and gender-specific cumulative incidence estimates) that a randomly drawn individual from the population at large of the same age (x) and gender as the ith individual in the pedigree is affected by age X. The null hypothesis is thereby evaluated by the test statistic $T(X)$:

$$T(X) = \sum_{i=1}^{N} \frac{(X_i - p_i)^2}{p_i(1 - p_i)}.$$

In order to test the significance of an observed value of $T(X)$, it is necessary to evaluate the permutation distribution of $T(X)$ because its null distribution cannot be approximated by any known distribution. From this distribution of all possible values of $T(X)$, obtained from enumeration of all possible permutations of X, one can determine the upper $100\alpha\%$ values of $T(X)$. If the observed $T(X)$ value exceeds the 0.95 cumulative probability of the permutation distribution, then the null hypothesis is rejected. That is, there is significant familial aggregation of alcohol or drug abuse. Such families may then be selected for incorporation into a high-risk group. In effect, employing this computational method, an objective framework is available to preventionists for identifying high-risk youth who arguably comprise the segment of the population having the greatest need for intervention. However, if the null hypothesis is accepted, then such families may be considered to be at average risk for a substance abuse disorder even if there are some affected members in the pedigree.

A Dimensional Approach to the Delineation of Heightened Familial Risk

In a variant of the high risk paradigm, probands are ascertained according to their dimensional score on a continuous psychological trait (e.g., socialization, aggressivity, behavioral activity level) implicated to be associated with the risk for substance abuse. This paradigm has been used to study the subjective response to psychoactive drugs (Sher & Levenson, 1982) and to determine the aggregation of alcoholism and other drug abuse in the family (Moss, Majumder, & Vanyukov, 1994). Significant family aggregation on continuous measures may be tested using the maximum-likelihood pedigree approach (Hopper & Mathews, 1982, 1983). Briefly, for normally distributed dimensional scores, a log-likelihood value is estimated for each pedigree and summed across all pedigrees within the sample to be investigated. The formula is

$$\log(\mathrm{Li})_i = -1/2 \ln |\Sigma_i| - 1/2(X_i - \mu)'\Sigma_i^{-1}(X_i - \mu).$$

In this formula, the ith pedigree, Σ is the matrix of expected covariances among family scores based upon kinship relationships and the hypothesized shared environmental factors; X_i is the vector of observed family data for the ith pedigree; and μ represents the vector of expected means from the population at large. Log-likelihood values above 1.0 suggest that the values observed in the experimental pedigrees, for the continuous variable of interest, are in excess of those expected from pedigrees drawn from the general population. In order to either test the null hypothesis of no familial excess on a continuous variable of interest (e.g., aggressivity) or test for differences between samples (e.g., substance abusers versus normal controls), the two relevant log-likelihoods may be computed. Tests for significant differences may be accomplished by taking advantage of the observation that twice the difference between two log-likelihoods approximates a chi-square distribution with degrees of freedom equal to the difference in the number of parameters estimated in fitting the two models. This approach also permits the testing of specific etiologic models for substance abuse through the specification of alternative parameters.

Between-Group Comparisons

Figure 25.5 schematically depicts the rationale underlying group comparisons employing the high-risk paradigm. While at the time of sampling, none of the children studied may not have been affected yet, their liability distribution was shown as reflective of that at their parents age. As can be seen, subjects are recruited from two segments of the distribution of the population on a particular variable or dimension. The dividing point for establishing high versus low risk is operationally specified by the investigator. In the top–down paradigm, families are selected based upon the presence and absence of substance abuse in the child's paternal and maternal sides of the family. The high- and low-risk children are the target cases or the units of study, whereas the proband is a parent. A dichotomized distribution is then assessed, and the two groups of children (no parent or relatives versus one or more parent or relatives with the disorder of interest) are contrasted on the characteristics of interest. However, as previously noted, other approaches can be employed to explore not only lineage (maternal or paternal) but also density of family loading (e.g., number of affected family members in proportion to family size).

In the bottom–up paradigm, risk status is generally inferred according to the proband's scores on some dimension or trait. Employing a design to create a dichotomous distribution, families of probands can also be classified as either high or low risk, depending on whether or not the child proband qualifies for a suprathreshold diagnosis (e.g., conduct disorder) that is presumed to be associated with an augmented risk for substance abuse. As previously noted, risk status can be inferred by scores obtained by probands on a dimensional trait (e.g., aggressivity, self-esteem,

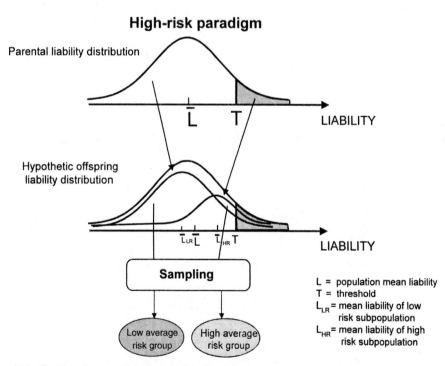

FIGURE 25.5. The high-risk paradigm. Putative high average risk and low average risk groups are composed based on ascertainment characteristics of family member, typically affected or nonaffected status for substance abuse. As can be seen from the shaded areas, proportionally more subjects in the high-risk group surpass the liability threshold.

platelet monoamine oxidase level). In this latter approach, individuals scoring above and below a designated value (e.g., 1, 2, or 3 SDs from the population mean) are segregated into high- and low-risk groups. Whether a top–down or bottom–up ascertainment strategy is employed, the aim is the same, that is, to partition the population distribution into two groups of which one has a putative high liability and the second has a presumed low liability. However, as can be seen in Figure 25.5, the low liability group usually is only moderately below the population mean on the liability trait.

By ascertaining subjects using the bottom–up approach according to a putative liability phenotype, it is possible to track subjects through the period of maximum risk to determine the impact of the particular trait on outcome. Comparing high- and low-risk youth at outcome provides the opportunity to demonstrate that subjects who manifest the characteristic as children are at elevated risk for substance abuse. Furthermore, a reduction of the characteristic induced by a prevention intervention in high-risk youth that is followed by a lower rate of substance abuse outcome, compared to control subjects, substantiates its integral etiologic importance.

Retrospective, Cross-Sectional, and Prospective High-Risk Studies

Once a risk classification schema is finalized, an investigation may be configured retrospectively, cross-sectionally, or prospectively. Valid causal inferences concerning substance abuse etiology cannot be drawn from either top–down or bottom–up studies which utilize retrospective or cross-sectional designs. However, relevant associations between phenotypic characteristics and risk group membership *can* be elucidated using these inexpensive efficient high-risk designs. Research findings generated through retrospective or cross-sectional designs must ultimately be subjected to prospective research designs for causal relationships to be confirmed.

Prospective studies of substance abuse etiology, although costly and difficult to accomplish, provide a direct estimate of the risk for developing a substance abuse disorder for a particular phenotypic value on a liability characteristic. In addition, prospective studies reduce several important sources of experimental bias, particularly the effects of selective recall and misclassification. Prospective research also allows for the analysis of factors which predict changes in substance use/abuse over time. For example, the relationship between intrafamilial transmissible influences and the age of onset of a substance use disorder can be studied. Likewise, remission of substance use consumption in relation to familial transmission can be investigated. Furthermore, the prospective high-risk paradigm not only permits investigation of the influence of the main risk characteristic on outcome (e.g., familial substance abuse) but also affords the opportunity to elucidate their effects on outcomes due to concurrent and influential co-morbidity such as antisocial personality or affective disorder. A disadvantage of the prospective high-risk design, however, is the possibility that study participation may be an intervention, thereby altering the natural course of the developmental trajectory. To control for this potential confound, the accrual of a prospective "no-contact" high-risk cohort allows for the estimation of research participation effects.

Family Resemblance and Transmission

Central to the conceptual framework of the "top–down" high-risk paradigm is the assumption that, within the high-risk group, there will be a significant degree of parent–offspring resemblance for the trait of interest. Complex traits, as previously noted, are multifactorial in that individual phenotype differences are influenced by variations in both genetic and environmental factors. The liability to substance abuse is one such complex trait that is postulated to be subject to intrafamilial

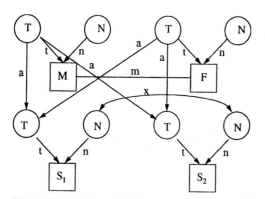

T = Transmissible component of phenotypic variance
N = Nontransmissible component of phenotypic variance
M = Matrix of maternal phenotypes
F = Matrix of paternal phenotypes
S = Matrix of offspring (siblings') phenotypes
m = The copath modeling homogamy
t = Transmissibility path coefficient
n = Nontransmissibility path coefficient
a = The tau path (the path coefficients measuring parental contribution into the offspring's variation)
x = The correlation between the nontransmissible components of siblings' phenotypes

FIGURE 25.6. Path model illustrates sources of family resemblance for investigating transmission of substance abuse.

transmission through the mechanism of multifactorial inheritance. The high-risk paradigm can, therefore, be employed to test for not only intrafamilial transmission but also other models which assume resemblance among family members.

A path diagram illustrating a model of multifactorial intrafamilial transmission is displayed in Figure 25.6. The nuclear family design does not provide the data necessary for partitioning phenotypic variance into its genetic and environmental components. Nevertheless, the two-generation material allows for estimating transmissible and nontransmissible contributions into the liability variation using the Tau model (Rice et al., 1980) and its modifications.

In this model, phenotypic variance is assumed to be composed of transmissible, T, and nontransmissible, N, components, caused, respectively, by the genetic and environmental sources of familial resemblance, and by the sources of variation that are not shared between the parental and offspring generations. M and F are matrices of parental phenotypes; S_1 and S_2 are offspring's (siblings') phenotypes; m is the copath modeling homogamy; a is the *tau* path (the path coefficients measuring parental contribution into the offspring's variation); x is the correlation between the nontransmissible components of siblings' phenotypes. The copath (conditional path [Carey, 1986]) allows modeling phenotypic assortment as mates' covariance without affecting variances of mates.

For substance use disorders, there are other salient models of intrafamilial transmission which can be tested using the high-risk paradigm. For example, a *purely genetic model of substance abuse etiology* would assume that environmental factors are noncontributory to variation in the liability to a substance abuse outcome. Thus, a purely genetic path model would show only genotypic influences on the offspring's phenotypic variation and the genotype–phenotype covariances would be high. For a *purely environmental or cultural model of substance abuse etiology,* all of the genotype–phenotype covariances would be low, such that genetic variation would contribute little to the phenotypic differences. The path coefficients for the environmental parameters, however, would have high values. This model, which describes nongenetic parental influences on variation in the liability for substance abuse among offspring, is termed "vertical cultural transmission." In cases where a parental trait directly influences the production of a similar trait in the offspring, the etiologic model is termed "direct vertical cultural transmission." For example, favorable attitudes toward drug use in parents may produce, through social factors, a favorable attitude toward drug use among offspring. However, a more complex phenomenon may also relate to outcome. Parental characteristics can contribute to phenotypic traits in the offspring which are quite distinct from those of the parents. For example, an inconsistent and violent parent may evoke adaptational responses in the offspring in the form of passivity, social anxiety, withdrawal, and ultimately alcohol or drug use. This form of nongenetic parental influence, termed "indirect vertical cultural transmission," is also testable using the high-risk paradigm (Kendler, 1988).

Contributions of the High-Risk Paradigm for Understanding Drug Abuse Etiology

Numerous investigations have been conducted to elucidate the extent to which children of alcoholics (high risk) can be discriminated from children of nonalcoholics (low risk). In the absence of longitudinal data demonstrating an association between the discriminating variables and a substance abuse outcome, it is not possible to infer that the features which distinguish high- from low-risk subjects either presage substance abuse or are merely interesting but essentially irrelevant epiphenomena. This caveat aside, it is noteworthy that differences in neurochemical, neurophysiological, psychophysiological, cognitive, and behavioral processes have been reported which distinguish high-risk children of alcoholics from lower risk children of nonalcoholics (Sher, 1991) and between children of other chemically dependent parents from normal parents (Johnson, 1991).

Comparatively less is known about the characteristics which discriminate children at high and low risk for substance abuse other than alcoholism. Indeed, one important and unresolved issue pertains to whether risk characteristics are specific to the abuse of particular psychoactive drugs (e.g., alcohol, opiates, benzodiazepenes) or whether there are common features associated with the risk for all types of drug abuse. Evidence supporting a shared liability is derived from the common observation of familial aggregation for abuse of different types of drugs. Although these latter findings are intriguing, the specificity of the liability to the abuse of psychoactive drugs still remains to be systematically investigated.

The issue of specificity of drug abuse liability aside, it is noteworthy that, to date, there has been a paucity of research conducted to identify the factors which distinguish individuals who are at high risk from those at average risk for substance abuse. Research currently ongoing at the Center for Education and Drug Abuse Research at the University of Pittsburgh has as one of its main objectives the goal of elucidating the features associated with elevated risk status across multiple levels of biological organization in the context of environmental influences. Findings emerging from this comprehensive research program indicate in particular that 10- to 12-year-old offspring of substance-abusing parents can be discriminated from children of normal parents on measures of temperament, aggressivity, affective distress, behavioral activity level, and neurophysiological functioning (Blackson, 1994; Brigham et al., 1995; Giancola et al., 1996). Moreover, phenotype similarity between parents and children has been demonstrated to mediate the relation between parental substance abuse and offspring's manifestation of risk characteristics (Blackson et al., 1994). These emerging results illustrate the importance of understanding family system functioning from the perspective of the psychological makeup of each family member. To date, drug abuse prevention directed at the family as the target unit has not addressed this crucial issue.

TWIN PARADIGM

The classical twin design is not generally considered within the rubric of family studies. Nonetheless, its inclusion herein in the framework of family research is relevant, as these paradigms include information about the sources of phenotypic variation that inform about the role of the family in substance abuse etiology.

Investigating twins is a central strategy in behavior genetics. Monozygotic (identical) twins (MZ) have 100% of their genes in common. Hence, all intrapair differences observed between MZ twins are due to environmental influences. In contrast, dizygotic (fraternal) twins (DZ) have, on average, 50% of their segregating genes in common. This is the same as non-twin siblings. The contemporaneous nature of twin rearing permits, however, the assumption, albeit somewhat controversial, that twins share exposure to a common family environment. Thus, the phenotypic correlation between monozygotic (MZ) twin pairs relative to dizygotic (DZ) twin pairs allows for the disaggregation of the components of phenotypic variance.

Using the notation previously introduced, the sources of phenotypic variation can be summarized in the form of estimates of heritability, that is, the influence of genotypic variation in the population on variation in phenotype:

$$h^2 = (V_a + V_d)/V_p.$$

Analogously, contribution of environmental influences in phenotypic variation (or environmentally) can be presented as

$$e^2 = (V_c + V_e)/V_p.$$

The sources of phenotypic covariance between twins of each type, given the *a priori* assumptions concerning genotypic similarity for each class of twin pairs, are

$$\mathrm{Cov(MZ)} = V_a + V_d + V_c$$
$$\mathrm{Cov(DZ)} = 0.5V_a + 0.25V_d + V_c.$$

In these formulae, Cov(MZ) and Cov(DZ) are expected covariances, respectively, of MZ and DZ twins reared together. Mathematically, it is not possible to obtain from these two formulae the estimates of the three parameters (V_a, V_d, V_c) included in the model. Hence, it is necessary to assume that one of them is fixed at 0. However, by using structural equation methods available in existing computer programs such as LISREL, EQS, and Mx, the best statistical fit for different models (e.g., specifying shared and unshared environmental and additive genetic components, additive genetic and unshared environmental components) can be investigated (Kendler et al., 1992).

It is important to point out what cannot be concluded from the results of twin studies. Despite assertions frequently encountered in the literature, *high or low estimates of heritability do not mean high or low contribution of heredity into a disorder, its etiology, or its severity.* Heritability estimates also do not imply that a disorder is more or less "genetic." In fact, heritability estimates do not implicate the *causes of a disorder.* Hence, even a hypothesized heritability estimate of 0 cannot be deduced to mean the absence of involvement of genes in the development of a disorder. Instead, the values of model parameters are related only to the *causes of differences between individuals in the particular population for the liability to the disorder at a particular point in time.* That is, heritability estimates describe proportions of the phenotypic variation corresponding to the contributions of genetic and environmental individual differences. Comparing the fit of the models specifying their different components enables the selection of the model which best accounts for observed covariations.

The parameters of the models are estimated under certain assumptions. These assumptions are necessary to make the computations possible and to make the model as inclusive as possible with respect to disaggregating the components of phenotypic variability. It is noteworthy that these assumptions may affect the generalizability of twin data as well as the precision of the obtained estimates. For instance, one assumption is that environmental correlations for the factors associated with the liability to the disorder in MZ and DZ twins are equal. However, in one study of alcoholism in females, this was found not to be the case: similar childhood environments were reported more by MZ twins than by DZ twins, although the similarity was not related to the liability to alcoholism (Kendler et al., 1992).

Results from twin studies investigating the etiology of substance abuse (other than alcohol abuse and tobacco abuse) are scarce. Significant differences in concordances between MZ and DZ twins for a diagnosis of the presence/absence of substance abuse have been shown for males but not for females; however, the absence of observed effects for females in this latter study may have been caused by insufficient statistical power (Pickens et al., 1991).

In the previous study, the genetic component of liability variance (heritability) was estimated at 0.31 in males and at 0.22 in females. Important gender differences in the composition of the liability variance were observed in the environmental components. While almost all phenotypic variation in females was determined by unshared environment (0.71), with the shared environmental component being negligible (0.07), environmental variation in males was caused mostly by shared environment (0.51).

Significant heritability (0.46) for the liability to drug abuse has been shown in a study of monozygotic twins reared apart (Grove et al., 1990). This cross-fostering design allows for a direct estimation of the genetic component of the phenotypic variance (as all of the resemblance between the co-twins is caused by their identical genes). That is, there is no contribution from common environment experienced by each co-twin, and there are no confounds caused by twin competition (Eaves, Eysenck, & Martin, 1989). Importantly, a high genetic correlation (0.78) between alcohol abuse and/or dependence and drug abuse was also found in this latter study, indicating that the variation in the liability to these different disorders shares a considerable proportion of genes.

Results from twin studies of alcoholism (Gabrielli & Plomin, 1985; Gurling, Murray, & Clifford, 1981; Hrubec & Omenn, 1981; Kaij, 1960; Kendler et al., 1992; McGue, Pickens, & Svikis, 1992; Partanen et al., 1966; Pickens et al., 1991) indicate that the concordance between MZ twins for alcohol use is significantly higher than that for DZ twins and *that the difference in concordances covaries with severity of the disorder.*

In a study of female twins (Kendler et al., 1992), in which liability phenotypes were classified into four categories of severity instead of the usual dichotomous affected/unaffected categorization, also gave empirical substantiation to the normally distributed liability model. In effect, the alcohol tolerance-dependence phenotype was at one extreme end of a dimension comprised of unaffected, problem-drinking, and alcoholism-without-tolerance/dependence phenotypes. Estimates of the heritability of the liability to alcoholism have been found to be 0.73 in males (McGue et al., 1992) and 0.61 in females (Kendler et al., 1992), However, as expected, estimates varied according to the definition of the threshold phenotype. These estimates were not different in an older age population (Prescott et al., 1994a,b), illustrating that a significant proportion of individual differences in the liability to alcoholism may be attributed to the differences between individual genotypes.

These findings have important implications for the role of sex-specific interventions in substance abuse prevention. For males, the shared environment of the family appears to play the more important role in substance abuse liability compared to that of unshared environmental influences. In contrast, among females, only unshared or unique environment contributed to phenotypic variation. Similar results have been obtained regarding alcohol consumption (Jardine & Martin, 1984). Among females, heritability was estimated at 0.56, with only unshared environment contributing to the phenotypic variation, while in males, the estimated heritability was 0.36, of which 20% of the phenotypic variance was accounted for by the shared environment of the family.

It should be noted that even though twin studies provide only a general understanding of the sources of the differences in the risk for substance abuse, these studies are heuristic in that they provide useful leads in the search for the specific factors that influence risk. By extension, as noted earlier, twin paradigms can assist in identifying specific prevention interventions for particular segments of the population (e.g., males and females). The investigation of twins also affords the opportunity to estimate the extent to which genetic variation contributes to biopsychological phenotypes associated with the shared family environment and risk for substance abuse. However, twins may not be considered representative of the general population considering their relatively low prevalence, atypical *in utero* environment, and socialization experiences. Nonetheless, they enable investigation of the liability to drug abuse where the degree of genetic similarity is known. Recognizing that twins are potentially not representative of the general population, it is important that the results of investigations are accommodated with findings obtained from studies of singlets in more typical families. In this fashion, a comprehensive understanding of drug abuse liability can be acquired.

CROSS-FOSTERING (ADOPTION) PARADIGM

The adoption design is capable of delimiting the genetic and environmental influences on the variation in the liability to substance abuse except for the contribution of anti- and early postnatal environmental factors. As with twins reared apart, all phenotypic resemblance between separated biological relatives is determined by the genes they have in common. In contrast, all similarity between adoptive relatives is determined by the environments they share. The adoption paradigm, especially involving extended families, allows for estimating all of the main parameters of the models of phenotypic variance, including genotype–environment correlation and interaction. Unfortunately, the utilization of the adoption paradigm is commonly mitigated by difficulties obtaining data on biological parents. Access to this information is restricted in many regions due to public or institutional policy. Consequently, only a few adoption studies investigating substance abuse have been conducted in the United States (e.g., Cadoret et al., 1986). Numerous investigations have, however, been carried out in Scandinavian countries. Beginning with the adoption studies conducted by Goodwin et al. (1973, 1974), it has been frequently found that the risk for alcoholism among adopted offspring of alcoholics is higher than that among children of nonalcoholics. Results from adoption studies have also indicated that a biologic background of alcohol problems is associated with an increased risk for drug abuse in adoptees (Cadoret et al., 1986). Furthermore, the abuse of nonalcoholic psychoactive substances is significantly greater among individuals who have a family history of drug abuse (Meller et al., 1988).

The studies conducted by Goodwin et al. (1973, 1974) on a Danish sample found that the risk for alcoholism in offspring of alcoholics is higher than that in children of nonalcoholics even when they are separated from their biological parents early in life. Interestingly, the data also revealed a trend toward a decrease in the frequency of alcoholism in sons who lived with their alcoholic fathers: 17% of them became alcoholics versus 25% of adopted-out sons of alcoholics. Results from another adoption study conducted on a Swedish sample (Bohman et al., 1987; Bohman, Sigvardsson, & Cloninger, 1981; Cloninger, Bohman, & Sigvardsson, 1981) showed that alcoholism frequency was higher in sons of alcohol-abusing fathers compared to normal fathers (22.8 versus 14.7%) as well as alcohol-abusing mothers compared to normal mothers (28.1 versus 14.7%). Alcohol abuse was not higher in daughters of alcoholic biological fathers compared to control fathers (3.5 versus 2.8%). However, in the absence of criminality in the fathers, and especially in daughters of affected mothers, the rate of alcoholism was significantly higher (10.3% versus 2.8%) (Bohman et al., 1981).

Using discriminant analysis allowed the authors of the previous study to distinguish in males two subtypes of alcohol abuse: "milieu limited" (type 1) and "male limited" (type 2) (e.g., Bohman et al., 1987). Among other characteristics, the subtypes differed most saliently with respect to age of onset, of the alcohol abuse. Typically, the type 2 variant had an earlier age onset, and fathers whose alcoholism was severe in contrast to the type 1 subjects whose onset was later and the father's alcoholism was either mild or severe. Heritability of the liability for type 2 alcohol abuse was about 90%, while for type 1 it was nonsignificant. The risk for alcoholism in offspring of type 1 fathers was *lower* than that in the general population if postnatal exposure to the "provocative" milieu was absent; however, the risk increased twofold in sons and threefold in daughters in the presence of a provocative milieu. These findings point to a nonadditive genotype–environment interaction (Bohman et al., 1987). In contrast, the risk for alcoholism was increased ninefold in sons of type 2 fathers regardless of environment. No effect was observed for daughters. Instead, the latter had an excess of complaints of headache, backache, and abdominal pains from an early age. However, "somatization" symptoms were observed only in women whose male relatives were characterized by criminal behavior with repeated violence and multiple registrations for alcohol abuse.

The two alcoholic types were also proposed to differ on certain personality dimensions described by Cloninger (1986). Type 1 was hypothesized to be associated with low novelty-seeking, high harm avoidance and high reward dependence, whereas type 2 exhibited opposite propensities on these dimensions. Subsequent research has not provided consistent empirical support for differences in the personality constellation of type 1 and type 2 alcoholics on these three traits (Irwin, Schuckit, & Smith, 1990). Indeed, a marked overlap is also observed between the symptom clusters employed to define the two subtypes (Irwin et al., 1990). However, in defense of Cloninger et al. (1981), it should be noted that this heterogeneity is consistent with the hypothesis of continuous variation in the liability to alcoholism as well as in personality traits associated with that liability. As the authors of the typology emphasize: "alcoholism is unlikely to be a discrete disease or even a set of discrete diseases with pathognomonic individual symptoms" (Cloninger et al., 1988, p. 567). The same conclusion can be confidently advanced for other types of psychoactive substance abuse.

Adoption studies, like twin studies, do not directly inform about etiology. Rather, estimates of genetic and environmental parameters reflect the relative contributions of different kinds of genetic and environmental influences to the variation of the liability to substance abuse. Consequently, these estimates do not implicate a genetic or environmental cause in the individual case. It should be noted that even for a monogenic disorder like phenylketonuria (PKU), where the heritability is 100%, a relatively simple environmental manipulation, such as a change in food consumption (amino acid composition), can prevent the disease.

TWINS REARED IN SEPARATE
ENVIRONMENT PARADIGM

A special case of the adoption design pertains to twins separated soon after birth and each twin is reared by an adoptive parent. Apart from immense logistic difficulties in conducting research of this type, and limitations regarding the generalizability of results obtained about such samples, this paradigm nonetheless provides invaluable information about the genetic influence on phenotypic expression where the degree of genetic similarity is known and different environment effects are investigated. In the largest study conducted to date, Bouchard and colleagues (Bouchard et al., 1990) have documented a significant genetic influence for a broad range of behaviors, attitudes, values, cognitive skills, and physical anthropometric characteristics. These studies are remarkable in having shown a genetic influence on psychological attributes and social behaviors which have been uncritically assumed to be determined entirely by socialization and experience.

RECONSTITUTED FAMILY PARADIGM

In reconstituted families, the members derive from a previous family unit. For example, divorce and remarriage introduce a new social environment for each adult member as well as for the children. This family structure is most useful for determining the impact of exposure to an affected parent on the risk for substance abuse. There are two basic variations on this paradigm. First, investigating reconstituted families enables determining the effects of a child's exposure to an affected parent prior to removal from that environment into a new family environment where the step-parent is normal. The most typical case is the child who is born into a family in which one parent is a substance abuser, and at some point during the child's development the parents divorce or separate and the child then domiciles with the normal parent and his/her new spouse. This paradigm is most useful for delineating whether there are critical periods during child development that are associated with augmented risk by determining whether there is a correlation between amount and duration of exposure to the affected parent on magnitude of risk for substance abuse. The results of a study conducted at the Center for Education and Drug Abuse Research (Moss, Clark, & Kirisci, 1997) suggest, for example, that the liability for substance abuse in male offspring is enhanced if the child is exposed to paternal substance abuse from age 6 onward.

In the second type of reconstituted family, exposure to an affected parent for the first time in the reconstituted family is investigated following an earlier period of development where neither biological parent was a substance abuser. Because the child is born to parents in which both parents are normal, it is possible to determine the degree to which this early experience can protect the child from developing a substance abuse disorder following parental divorce and subsequent remarriage by one partner to a person who already has, or develops, a substance abuse disorder. Thus, the impact of interaction patterns among family members (where a biologically unrelated parent has a substance abuse disorder) on substance abuse risk in children can be investigated.

There are myriad variations of reconstituted families. Hence, it is difficult to ascertain groups of families having a specific configuration in both the original and the reconstituted family. This is an important condition for between-group comparisons; namely, the family structure before and after reconstitution is similar in both control and experimental groups. Feasibility considerations notwithstanding, investigating reconstituted families affords the opportunity to elucidate the association between exposure of the child during specific stages of development to a substance abuse parent (biological or adoptive) and the child's risk for substance abuse.

INCOMPLETE NUCLEAR FAMILY PARADIGM

This family structure is operationally defined as a sibship living with only one biological parent. Researching the incomplete nuclear family enables addressing a number of important issues pertinent to substance abuse. For example, the extent to which a biological parent affected with substance abuse, but not living with the child for varying periods and duration during the child's development, influences the liability that can be determined. In one such study (Tarter, Schultz, & Kirisci, 2001) it was found that the risk for substance abuse in children was moderately increased if the child was domiciling with the unaffected mother compared to living with both the affected (substance abusing) father and the unaffected mother. The reasons for these differences are not readily apparent, but may reflect the possibility that there is a greater risk to offspring from diminished parenting resources than that caused by domiciling with a substance-abusing father. Thus, parental divorce or separation occurring during child development appears to augment the child's liability to substance abuse. Inasmuch as incomplete nuclear families are becoming increasingly common as the consequence of secular trends regarding personal choice for childbearing outside of a relationship, and through divorce, the special circumstances surrounding the development of drug abuse in such offspring with respect to the unique parameters of single parenting need to be explicated. From the standpoint of prevention, these findings suggest that the risk for substance abuse in children can be reduced by providing more supportive services to single mothers.

SUMMARY

The liability to substance abuse has a multifactorial basis. As described herein, family history and interaction patterns encompass, respectively, genetic and environmental sources of contribution to variation in this liability. Consequently, it is not surprising that familial factors have been consistently found to exercise a potent influence on the etiology of substance abuse. Whereas the influence of family dysfunction on severity of substance abuse in adolescents is widely recognized, it should be noted that it is not the only factor contributing to etiology for the majority of adolescents who qualify for a DSM-III-R diagnosis of Substance Use Disorder.

A comprehensive understanding of the impact of the family on drug abuse etiology requires elucidation of genetic and environmental sources of influence on liability variation. As described in this chapter, several well-established paradigms are capable of informing these two variance components on the liability. Emerging findings point to a genetic influence as determined from family and twin studies. Also, environmental influences have been long recognized as important; however, recent evidence implicates a greater contribution from the unshared environment compared to the shared intrafamilial environment.

Investigations of familial processes need to be conducted in the context of ontogeny of the individual members. Because the developmental trajectory culminating in a drug abuse outcome is changeable throughout the lifespan, it is essential to determine how changing environmental influences, including the family environment, exercise either a risk-enhancing or a risk-mitigating impact over time and across different stages of each child's psychosocial development. Considering psychological development as a succession of behavioral vectors in which each phenotype has force and direction, the quality of phenotype–family environment interactions that predispose to drug abuse is the cardinal focus of investigations aimed at clarifying familial influences on etiology. Toward this end, etiology research needs to elucidate how family influences shape ontogeny so that risk-enhancing interactional processes can be modified using preventions which effectively redirect high-risk youth toward normative development.

REFERENCES

Alterman, A. I. (1988). Patterns of familial alcoholism, alcoholism severity, and psychopathology. *Journal of Nervous and Mental Diseases, 176,* 167–175.

Bale, S. J., Chakravarti, A., & Strong, L. C. (1984). Aggregation of colon cancer in family data. *Genetic Epidemiology, 1,* 53–61.

Barnes, G. (1990). Impact of the family on adolescent drinking patterns. In L. Collins, K. Leonard, & J. Searles (Eds.), *Alcohol and the family: Research and clinical perspectives.* New York: Guilford.

Blackson, T. (1994). Temperament: A salient correlate of risk factors for drug abuse. *Drug and Alcohol Dependence, 36,* 205–214.

Blackson, T., Tarter, R., Martin, C., & Moss, H. (1994). Temperament mediates the effects of family history of substance abuse on externalizing and internalizing child behavior. *The American Journal on Addiction, 3,* 58–66.

Bohman, M., Cloninger, R., Sigvardsson, S., & von Knorring, A. L. (1987). The genetics of alcoholism and related disorders. *Journal of Psychiatric Research, 21,* 447–52.

Bohman, M., Sigvardsson, S., & Cloninger C. R. (1981). Maternal inheritance of alcohol abuse. *Archives of General Psychiatry, 38,* 965–968.

Bouchard, T. J., Lykken, D. T., McGue, M., & Segal, N. L. (1990). Sources of human psychological differences: The Minnesota Study of Twins Reared Apart. *Science, 250,* 223–228.

Brigham, J., Herning, M. R., Moss, H., Murrelle, L., & Tarter, R. (1995). Event related potentials and alpha synchronization in preadolescent boys at risk for substance abuse. *Biological Psychiatry, 37,* 834–846.

Bry, B. (1983). Empirical foundation of family based approached to adolescent substance abuse. In T. Clynn, C. Leukfeld, & J. Ladford (Eds.), *Preventing adolescent drug abuse* (Research Monograph No. 47, National Institute on Drug Abuse, pp. 154–171). Washington, DC: Government Printing Office.

Cadoret, R. J. (1986). Adoption studies: historical and methodological critique. *Psychiatric Developments, 4,* 45–64.

Cadoret, R. J, Troughton, E., O'Gorman, T. W., & Heywood, E. (1986). An adoption study of genetic and environmental factors in drug abuse. *Archives of General Psychiatry, 43,* 1131–1136.

Carey, G. A general multivariate approach to linear modeling in human genetics. American Journal of Human Genetics, 39: 775–786, 1986.

Chakraborty, R., Weiss, K. M., Majumder, P. P., Strong, L. C., & Herson, J. (1984). A method to detect excess risk of disease in structured data: Cancer in relatives of retinoblastoma patients. *Genetic Epidemiology, 1,* 229–244.

Chassin, L., Rogush, F., & Barrera, M. (1991). Substance use and symptomatology among adolescent children of alcoholics. *Journal of Abnormal Psychology, 100,* 449–463.

Cloninger, C. R. (1986). A unified biosocial theory of personality and its role in the development of anxiety states. *Psychiatric Developments, 4,* 167–226.

Cloninger, C. R., Bohman, M., & Sigvardsson, S. (1981). Inheritance of alcohol abuse: Cross-fostering analysis of adopted men. *Archives of General Psychiatry, 38,* 861–868.

Cloninger, C. R., Sigvardsson, S., von Knorring, A. L., & Bohman, M. (1988). The Swedish studies of the adopted children of alcoholics: A reply to Littrell. *Journal of Studies on Alcohol, 49,* 500–509.

Eaves, L. J., Eysenck, H. J., & Martin, N. G. (1989). *Genes, culture and personality. An empirical approach.* San Diego: Academic Press.

Falconer, D. S. (1965). The inheritance of liability to certain diseases, estimated from the incidence among relatives. *Annals of Human Genetics, 29,* 51–76.

Gabrielli, W. F., & Plomin, R. (1985). Drinking behavior in the Colorado adoptee and twin sample. *Journal of Studies on Alcohol, 46,* 24–31.

Giancola, P., Martin, C., Tarter, R., Pelham, W., & Moss, H. (1996). Executive cognitive functioning and aggressive behavior in preadolescent boys at high risk for substance abuse/dependence. *Journal of Studies on Alcohol, 57,* 352–359.

Goodwin, D. W., Schulsinger, F., Hermansen, L., Guze, S. B., & Winokur, G. (1973). Alcohol problems in adoptees raised apart from alcoholic parents. *Archives of General Psychiatry, 28,* 238–243.

Goodwin, D. W., Schulsinger, F., Moller, N., Hermansen, L., Winokur, G., & Guze, S. B. (1974). Drinking problems in adopted and nonadopted sons of alcoholics. *Archives of General Psychiatry, 31,* 164–169.

Gorenstein, E., & Newman, J. (1980). Disinhibitory psychopathology: A new perspective and model for research. *Psychological Review, 87,* 301–315.

Grove, W. M., Eckert, E. D., Heston, L., Bouchard, T. J., Segal, N., & Lykken, D. T. (1990). Heritability of substance abuse and antisocial behavior: a study of monozygotic twins reared apart. *Biological Psychiatry 27,* 1293–304.

Gurling, H. M. D., Murray, R. M., & Clifford, C. A. (1981). Investigation into the genetics of alcohol dependence and into its effects on brain function. *Twin research 3: Epidemiology and clinical studies* (pp. 77–87). New York: Alan R. Liss Inc.

Hill, S. Y., Steinhauer, S., Park, J., & Zubin, J. (1990). Event-related potential characteristics in children of alcoholics from high density families. *Alcoholism: Clinical and Experimental Research, 14,* 6–16.

Hopper, J. L., & Mathews, J. D. (1982). Extensions to multivariate normal models for pedigree analysis. *Annals of Human Genetics, 46,* 373–383.

Hopper, J. L., & Mathews, J. D. (1983). Extensions to multivariate normal models for pedigree analysis II: Modeling the effect of shared environment in the analysis of variation in blood lead levels. *American Journal of Epidemiology, 117,* 344–355.

Hrubec, Z., & Omenn, G. S. (1981). Evidence of genetic predisposition to alcoholic cirrhosis and psychosis: Twin concordances for alcoholism and its biological end points by zygosity among male veterans. *Alcoholism: Clinical and Experimental Research, 50,* 207–215.

Irwin, M., Schuckit, M., & Smith, T. L. (1990). Clinical importance of age at onset in type 1 and type 2 primary alcoholics. *Archives of General Psychiatry, 47,* 320–324.

Jardine R., & Martin, N. G. (1984). Causes of variation in drinking habits in a large twin sample. *Acta geneticae medicae et gemellologiae, 33,* 435–50.

Johnson, J. (1991). Forgotten no longer: An overview of research on chemically dependent parents. In T. Rivinus (Ed.), *Children of chemically dependent parents.* New York: Brunner/Mazel.

Kaij, L. (1960). Studies on the Etiology and Sequels of Abuse of Alcohol. Lund: Hakan Ohlssons Boktryckery.

Kendler, K. S. (1988). Indirect vertical cultural transmission: A model for nongenetic parental influences on the liability to psychiatric illness. *The American Journal of Psychiatry, 145*(6), 657–665.

Kendler, K. S., Heath, A. C., Neale, M. C., Kessler, R. C., & Eaves, L. J. (1992). A population-based twin study of alcoholism in women. *Journal of the American Medical Association, 268,* 1877–82.

Kumpfer, K. (1995). Strengthening families to prevent drug use in multiethnic youth. In G. Botvin, S. Schinke, & M. Orlandi (Eds.), *Drug abuse prevention with multiethnic youth* (pp. 255–294). Thousand Oaks, CA: Sage.

Loeber, R. (1990). Development and risk factors of juvenile antisocial behavior and delinquency. *Clinical Psychology Review, 10,* 699–725.

McGue, M., Pickens, R. W., & Svikis, D. S. (1992). Sex and age effects on the inheritance of alcohol problems: A twin study. *Journal of Abnormal Psychology, 101,* 3–17.

Meller, W. H., Rinehart, R., Cadoret, R. J., & Troughton, E. (1988). Specific familial transmission in substance abuse. *International Journal of the Addictions, 23,* 1029–1039.

Moss, H., Blackson, T., Martin, C., & Tarter, R. (1992). Heightened motor activity level in male offspring of substance abusing fathers. *Biological Psychiatry, 32,* 1135–1147.

Moss, H., Clark, D., & Kirisci, L. (1997). Timing of paternal substance use disorder cessation and the effect on problem behavior in sons. *American Journal on Addiction, 6,* 30–37.

Moss, H., Majumder, P., & Vanyukov, M. (unpublished manuscript). Familial resemblance for psychoactive substance use disorder: Behavioral profile of high risk boys.

Nixon, S. J., & Parsons, O. A. (1990). Application of the Tridimensional Personality Questionnaire to a population of alcoholics and other substance abusers. *Alcoholism: Clinical and Experimental Research, 14,* 513–517.

Partanen, J., Bruun, K., and Markkanen, T. (1966). Inheritance of Drinking Behavior: A Study of Intelligence, Personality and Use of Alcohol in Adult Twins. Helsinki: The Finnish Foundation for Alcohol Studies (Distributed by Rutgers Center of Alcohol Studies, New Brunswick, N. J.)

Pickens, R. W., Svikis, D. S., McGue, M., Lykken, D. T., Heston, L. L., & Clayton, P. J. (1991). Heterogeneity in the inheritance of alcoholism: A study of male and female twins. *Archives of General Psychiatry, 48,* 19–28.

Prescott, C. A., Hewitt, J. K., Heath, A. C., Truett, K. R., Neale, M. C., & Eaves, L. J. (1994a). Environmental and genetic influences on alcohol use in a volunteer sample of older twins. *Journal of Studies on Alcohol, 55,* 18–33.

Prescott, C. A., Hewitt, J. K., Truett, K. R., Heath, A. C., Neale, M. C., & Eaves, L. J. (1994b). Genetic and environmental influences on lifetime alcohol related problems in a volunteer sample of older twins. *Journal of Studies on Alcohol, 55,* 184–202.

Reich, T., Cloninger, C. R., Van Eerdevegh, P., Rice, J. P., & Mullaney, J. (1988). Secular trends in the familial transmission of alcoholism. *Alcoholism: Clinical and Experimental Research, 12,* 458–464.

Reis, D., Plomin, R., & Hetherington, M. (1991). Genetics and psychiatry: An unheralded window on the environment. *American Journal of Psychiatry, 148,* 283–291.

Rice J. P., Cloninger, C. R., and Reich, T. (1980). General causal models for sex differences in the familial transmission of multifactorial traits: An application to human spatial visualizing ability. Social Biology, 26, 36–47.

Robins, J., Johnson, J., Israel, E., Baldwin, J., & Chandra, A. (1988). Depressive affect in school aged children of alcoholics. *British Journal of Addiction, 83,* 841–848.

Robins, L. N., & Regieri, D. A. (Eds.) (1991). *Psychiatric Disorders in America. The Epidemiologic Catchment Area Study.* New York: The Free Press.

Rolf, J. E., Johnson, J. L., Israel, E., Baldwin, J., & Chandra, A. (1988). Depressive affect in school-aged children of alcoholics. British Journal of Addiction. 83: 841–848.

Schuckit, M. A. (1980). Self-rating of alcohol intoxication by young men with and without family histories of alcoholism. *Journal of Studies on Alcohol, 41,* 242–249.

Sher, K. (1991). *Children of alcoholics. A critical appraisal of theory and research.* Chicago, IL: University of Chicago Press.

Sher, L., & Levenson, R. (1982). Risk for alcoholism and individual differences in the stress-response dampening effect of alcohol. *Journal of Abnormal Psychology, 91,* 350–367.

Sher, K. J., Walitzer, K. S., Wood, P. K., & Brent, E. E. (1991). Characteristics of children of alcoholics: Putative risk factors, substance use and abuse, and psychopathology. *Journal of Abnormal Psychology, 100,* 427–448.

Smith, S., O'Hara, B., Persico, A., Gorelick, D., Newlin, D., Vahov, D., Solomon, L., Pickens, R., & Uhl, G. (1992). Genetic vulnerability to drug abuse. The D_2 receptor Taq 1B1 restriction fragment length polymorphism appears more frequently in polysubstance abusers. American *Journal of Psychiatry, 49,* 723–727.

Stabenau, J. R. (1984). Implications of family history of alcoholism, antisocial personality, and sex differences in alcohol dependence. *American Journal of Psychiatry, 141,* 1178–1182.

Tarter, R., Blackson, T., Brigham, J., Moss, H., & Caprara, G. (1995). Precursors and correlates for irritability. A two year follow-up at risk for substance abuse. *Drug and Alcohol Dependence, 39,* 253–261.

Tarter, R., Blackson, T., Loeber, R., & Moss, H. (1993). Characteristics and correlates of child discipline practices in substance abuse and normal families. *American Journal on Addictions, 2,* 18–25.

Tarter, R., & Mezzich, A. (1992). Ontogeny of substance abuse: Perspectives and findings. In M. Glantz & R. Pickens (Eds.), *Vulnerability to drug abuse.* Washington, DC: American Psychological Association Press.

Tarter, R., Moss, H., & Vanyukov, M. (1995). Behavior genetic perspective of alcoholism etiology. In H. Begleiter & B. Kissin (Eds.), *Alcohol and alcoholism, genetic factors.* New York: Oxford University Press.

Tarter, R., Schultz, K., & Kirisci, L. (2001). Does living with a substance abusing father increase substance abuse risk in male offspring? Impact on individual, family, school, and peer vulnerability factors. *Journal of Child and Adolescent Substance Abuse, 10,* 59–70.

Tarter, R., & Vanyukov, M. (1994). Alcoholism: A developmental disorder. *Journal of Consulting and Clinical Psychology, 62,* 1096–1107.

Tarter, R. E. & Vanyukov, M. M. (eds.). (2001). Etiology of Substance Use Disorder in Children and Adolescents: Emerging Findings from the Center for Education and Drug Abuse Research. The Haworth Press, Inc..

Tarter, R., Vanyukov, M., Giancola, P., Dawes, M., Blackson, T., Mezzich, A., & Clark, D. (1999). Etiology of early onset substance abuse: A maturational perspective. *Development and Psychopathology, 11,* 657–683.

Vanyukov, M. M., Maher, B. S., Ferrell, R. E., Devlin, B., Marazita, M. L., Kirillova, G. P., and Tarter, R. E. (2001). Association between the dopamine receptor D5 gene and the liability to substance dependence in males: A replication. Journal of Child and Adolescent Substance Abuse, 10: 55–63.

Volicer, L., Volicer, B. J., &. D'Angelo, N. (1985). Assessment of genetic predisposition to male alcoholism. *Alcohol and Alcoholism, 20,* 63–68.

Webster-Stratton, C., & Eyberg, S. (1982). Child temperament: Relationship with child behavior problems and parent-child interactions. *Journal of Clinical Child Psychology, 11,* 123–129.

PART VII

RESEARCH DESIGN, MEASUREMENT, AND DATA ANALYTIC ISSUES

CHAPTER 26

Design Principles and Their Application in Preventive Field Trials

C. Hendricks Brown

INTRODUCTION

It is the design of a trial that primarily determines the quality of any inferences we draw from the study. In a well-designed study, the possibility of intervention/control differences being caused by anything other than real differences is minute. On the other hand, a *flawed design* is one in which no analytic methods can be used to minimize the credibility of alternative explanations that could explain intervention/control differences. Over the last half of this century, scientists have developed rigorous standards for testing one intervention against another intervention or control condition (Meinert, 1986; Piantadosi, 1997), and these standards can and are being applied to evaluate prevention programs. Nevertheless, there is still a need to improve the overall quality of prevention designs. As is the case with trials involving medical treatments (Schulz, Chalmers, Hayes, et al., 1995; Schulz, Chalmers, Altman, et al., 1995; The Standards of Reporting Trials Group, 1994) it is still true that the majority of trials involving the prevention of behavioral disorders do not adhere to all of these rigorous standards (Mrazek & Brown, 1999). This paper is intended to enhance the quality of preventive trials by laying out standards for trial design.

While the design elements of a field trial are often selected based on detailed statistical and real-world criteria, the principles guiding the design choices are quite simple. Thomas Chalmers, MD, the former dean of the medical school at Harvard and one of the world's leading "trialists" in medical research, once provided a personal example which tells us exactly what we want from a trial design (Chalmers, 1995, 1996). Late in life he developed prostate cancer. When he went to the doctor for treatment, he asked his doctor a simple question: "Show me the written

C. Hendricks Brown • Department of Epidemiology and Biostatistics, University of South Florida, Tampa, Florida 33612

evidence that the treatment you suggest is best for me as a patient." It is not sufficient just to show that one group who received an intervention did better than another group who did not receive it. Any evidentiary argument must rule out to a sufficient degree alternative explanations besides intervention effectiveness. Starting from Chalmers' statement, we develop a framework for assessing the quality of a controlled trial study design and thereby identify the principles underlying good trial designs. In Chalmers' case, he was unconvinced by the evidence that his doctor provided. In fact, Chalmers urged his own doctor to get him into a randomized clinical trial for prostate cancer, and he in fact did enter such a trial as a patient. He was assigned a drug at random. To make the study as objective as possible, neither he nor his physician knew which treatment he received. Chalmers preferred the uncertainty of not knowing which of two treatments he received—since the treatment trial was blinded—to the administration of a drug that had not been tested in a trial.

The framework provided here is best suited for designs that have allocation of individuals or groups to intervention or a concurrent comparison condition. There are a number of preventive interventions, particularly those dealing with the law and/or policy, that are most often evaluated using historical controls, interrupted time series, or multiple baseline designs. We describe some of the features of these designs as well.

Evidence-based approaches to a range of health programs are now being developed (Chambless & Hollon, 1998; Evidence-Based Medicine Working Group, 1992; The Cochrane Controlled Trials Register, 1999). In prevention, this strategy involves (1) identifying effective programs by testing them in rigorous trials, (2) facilitating their adoption by practitioners or communities through dissemination strategies, and finally (3) ensuring that they are delivered to appropriate populations at the appropriate strength. While this evidence-based approach has a long history in medicine, a similar evidence-based perspective relying on the highest standard of randomized trials has begun in the drug prevention field (Sloboda & David, 1997). A hierarchy of evidence is now generally accepted for intervention studies, with the highest weight of evidence provided by multisite, repeated randomized trials and lower weight of evidence given to nonrandomized studies with control groups (Spitzer, 1979; 1996). Much less weight is given to studies which do not include an appropriate control group. However, we will see that automatic reliance on this hierarchy of evidence can lead to errors. Even some randomized trials are sufficiently flawed to be nearly useless for making inferences about the intervention effect.

With one exception (discussed in the following), the evidential standards for testing prevention programs with randomized trials can now be set as high as they are for testing medical treatments with traditional randomized clinical trials (RCT). Not only is it possible to random assign individuals, families, schools, or communities to prevention programs, but also there now exist many carefully designed randomized preventive trials in such diverse prevention areas such as drug and alcohol use and abuse [see reviews by Tobler & Stratton (1997) and best practices identified in Stoil and Hill (1996) and Grover (1998)], children's mental disorders [see Durlak & Wells (1997) for a review], HIV [see reviews by Kim et al. (1997) and Kalichman, Carey, & Johnson (1996)], intervention in the ages from 0 through 6 (see Mrazek & Brown, 1999), and delinquency, violence, and crime (see Tolan & Guerra, 1994; Sherman et al., 1997).

This chapter provides a framework for assessing the quality of a preventive field trial. Such a framework is useful for three purposes. First, research scientists can direct their attention to a limited number of essential elements in designing and implementing new preventive trials. Second, reviewers can concentrate their selection of prevention trials to those whose design involves a high level of standards. Third, advocates for prevention and consumers, i.e., communities and schools, need to be knowledgeable about what standards their prevention programs have met.

The evidentiary nature of controlled trials is most clearly described in the language of probability and statistics. However, in our presentation we will simply introduce the statistical concepts and use a bare minimum of statistical jargon, leaving the interested reader to individually pursue this chapter's references.

DIRECT AND INDIRECT ESTIMATION
OF A PREVENTION PROGRAM EFFECT

Here we define explicitly what we mean by prevention effect, both on an individual basis as well as on a sample and population basis. We define first the program effect on a single subject's outcome assessment. As this chapter relates to the prevention of drug use and abuse, we will use as our example an adolescent's frequency of marijuana use in the last year. Following Rubin's causal modeling approach (Brown, 1993; Rubin, 1974), we conceptualize that each person actually has two outcome measures. One measure we call Y is the frequency of marijuana use if the subject is assigned the intervention. The second measure Z is the frequency of marijuana use if the subject is assigned to control. The *individual intervention effect* for this subject is then defined as the difference Y − Z. We simply remark here that one cannot measure both Y and Z for an individual because a subject can only be assigned one intervention condition; we return to this point in the following. Similarly, let us define the *sample preventive effect* based on multiple subjects rather than on an individual. For each of the subjects in the sample, we identify a Y value to measure the frequencies of marijuana use under intervention and a Z value measuring the frequencies of marijuana use when assigned to a control condition. The sample preventive effect is the average of Y − Z over the entire sample.

Table 26.1 shows typical values for an intervention tested on six subjects. The first difference score of $Y - Z = 0 - 12 = -12$ is the individual preventive effect. It indicates that the first subject would smoke marijuana 12 times more that year without the intervention than with the intervention. The sample preventive effect is just the average of the differences Y − Z over the six subjects. Here this sample average is also −12 indicating that there is less marijuana use in this sample when they are all exposed to the intervention. We can also define the *population prevention effect* as the average of these Y − Z values over a complete population. As most experiments never measure everyone in a population but only sample subjects drawn from that population, this population average prevention effect is not computable. It is, however, one of the things we normally want a trial to estimate.

TABLE 26.1. Frequencies of Yearly Marijuana Use under Intervention and Control

Subject number	Intervention	Control	Difference
	Y	Z	Y − Z
1	0	12	−12
2	52	104	−52
3	2	7	−5
4	11	11	0
5	16	19	−3
6	0	0	0
Averages	13.5	25.5	−12.0

TABLE 26.2. Observed Frequencies of Yearly
Marijuana for Intervention and Control

Subject number	Intervention	Control	Difference
	Y	Z	Y − Z
1	?	12	?
2	52	?	?
3	2	?	?
4	?	11	?
5	16	?	?
6	?	0	?
Averages	23.2	7.7	15.6

Note that these definitions of intervention effect have nothing to do with who is assigned which intervention condition. It is this separation between the what we want to estimate and any design characteristics that allows us to determine which designs are appropriate.

Both the individual and the sample preventive effects we have calculated from Table 26.1 are what we call *direct* measures. They are based on individual but unobservable difference measures Y − Z of intervention impact. Because we can only observe either Y or Z for a single subject, we can never obtain a direct measure of intervention effect. There is, however, an alternative way to measure intervention effect. If we compute the average of the Y's for everyone and subtract from that the average of the Z's for everyone, the difference, $13.5 − 25.5 = −12$ is exactly the same as that which we obtained from the direct determination of intervention effect based on the individual difference scores. The use of this difference in column averages to measure the sample preventive effect with actual trial data is shown in Table 26.2.

In this table we have displayed the intervention assignments and scores for all six subjects and hidden those values that are not observed, i.e., the three Y values for intervention subjects 2, 3, and 5 and the three Z values for control subjects numbered 1, 4, and 6. In this form it is possible to obtain an average value of the Y's—for intervention subjects—and an average value of the Z's—for control subjects. The difference between these two averages, which in this sample is $23.3 − 7.7 = 15.6$, reflects what we call the *indirect* measure of the prevention impact.

This indirect value is exactly what we would ordinarily report for intervention versus control differences in a simple experiment such as this. It is not numerically the same as the direct measure of intervention impact. In this situation it happens that our estimator is 15.6, or larger than 0, suggesting that the prevention does not prevent marijuana use. Had we selected different subjects to receive the intervention, we would have obtained a different indirect estimator of the sample preventive impact.

Two conditions must hold for this indirect prevention effect to be an appropriate measure of the sample prevention effect. First the distribution of the Y values in the intervention group must be the same as the distribution of the Y values who did not get the intervention. Similarly, the distribution of the Z values in the control group must be the same as that of the Z values who received the intervention.[1] If one of these conditions were false, the averages of Y and Z in Table 26.2 would differ systematically from the corresponding averages in Table 26.1. When the assignment to the intervention condition is made randomly, and other good design characteristics are maintained, these two conditions (discussed in the following) are satisfied. However, when the

---

[1]Statisticians refer to these conditions as "strongly ignorable treatment assignment" (Brown, 1993a; Rosenbaum, 1984; Rubin, 1974, 1978).

assignment is nonrandom, no universal guarantee can be made about the validity of this indirect measure. This is a major reason why well-designed randomized trials have for the most part become the gold standard in prevention.

Most preventive field trials require more complex analysis than that indicated here. Baseline characteristics, for example, can be added to improve the prediction for each individual (Brown, 1993a). Multiple outcome measures can be added to examine developmental change (Muthen & Curran, 1997). Multiple levels of the environment can influence the individual (Bryk & Raudenbusch, 1992), and we can examine variation in impact as well (Brown, 1993a). Special handling of incomplete data may be needed as well (Brown, 1990; Schafer, 1997). All these factors lead us to develop a detailed statistical model to predict individual response. Regardless of how complex this model becomes, it can still be used to predict every individual's Y and Z responses in either the presence or the absence of an intervention. From this we can combine estimates over the entire sample to obtain an indirect measure of the sample preventive effect. If both the analytic model and the design of the trial are appropriate, then this quantity should be a good estimate of the population preventive effect.

SOURCES OF BIAS AND DESIGN THREATS

There are only a limited number of ways that our indirect estimate of preventive effect can fail to be a good estimator of the population preventive effect. In this section we discuss the major problems that occur in the design. Further details on their frequency of occurrence in preventive trials can be found in Brown, Berndt et al. (2000).

Selection Bias

The first reason for failure involves the sample selection. If the study sample is not representative of the population, the sample preventive effect will not be close to the population preventive effect. We use the term *selection bias* to refer to differences between the study sample and the target population. Thus, selection bias means that the sample preventive effect is systematically different from the population preventive effect one would like to estimate. In contrast, all of the other design problems discussed in the following refer to differences between the indirect sample preventive effect and the direct sample preventive effect.

Assignment Bias

There are numerous instances where the manner in which individuals are assigned to intervention or control conditions leads to systematic differences between the two groups. We call this situation *assignment bias* and give examples under Examples of Threats to Trial Integrity.

Statistical Power Threat

Even if there is no systematic or nonrandom assignment to the intervention, there may remain a large statistical variation between those assigned to intervention and those assigned to control. This type of difference is called *statistical power threat*. An increase in the sample size or the use of blocking and matching (Brown & Liao, 1999; Meinert, 1986; Piantadosi, 1997) can reduce this chance of a statistical anomaly but can never make it go away entirely.

Condition Bias

Another way for the indirect measure to differ from the direct measure is through what we call *condition bias*. Condition bias occurs when the intervention condition a subject actually receives is not the one assigned. For example, a child may be assigned to a control school but move to an intervention school. When an intervention is family based, condition bias can occur if one child in the family is assigned to intervention and another to control. Also, a teacher who is assigned to deliver the standard intervention may receive training in the intervention being tested, thereby providing this intervention to his or her students.

Implementation Threat

We use the term *implementation threat* to account for situations where the intervention is not delivered by the intervenors as intended. As we use the term (Brown & Liao, 1999), implementation involves the delivery of program components by intervention staff and the support structures provided by relevant institutions and organizations. Thus, training and supervision are also dimensions of implementation.

Participation Bias

Participation bias occurs when subjects assigned to the intervention drop out during the intervention period, take part in a limited amount of sessions, or do not participate fully in the intervention. These individuals or family units have low adherence and never receive the intended level of the intervention.

Measurement Threat

If the outcome measures that are used are inappropriate, invalid, or unreliable, or poorly administered, or if they used to assess a sample for which the measure was not designed, then we call this a *measurement threat*.

Assessment Bias

Assessment bias occurs when subjects assigned to intervention and control are either approached differently or assessed differently. Such bias if severe makes it impossible to attribute intervention/control differences to the intervention itself.

Attrition Bias

For the purposes of this chapter, we refer to loss to follow-up after the intervention period has ended as *attrition*. Attrition bias occurs if the subjects followed up in one or both of the intervention groups differ from those not followed up.

Analysis Threat

When improper statistical analyses are performed, or when there are errors in the management or organization of data, we say there is an *analysis threat*. Surprisingly, even papers that are published in our best journals sometimes contain statistical errors that invalidate whatever conclusions the authors make.

With a good design, we can reduce or even rule out all these design threats. When the design is successful then, one alternative remains to explain the observed difference between intervention and control group means: It reflects a real difference between the two groups. Naturally, we would like to limit all other possibilities to a minimum so that any observed difference can logically be attributable to an intervention effect.

We describe in this next section exactly where in the design of a trial these 10 threats occur.

EXAMPLES OF THREATS TO TRIAL INTEGRITY

We differentiate three distinct stages of a design based on the occurrence of two events (Brown & Liao, 1999), on the times when intervention is assigned, and on the completion of the intervention (see Table 26.3). The first stage is the *preintervention phase*. It consists of all the design activities occurring before the actual intervention assignment takes place. Starting with the target population, potential subjects proceed through certain steps before they are assigned to an intervention condition. Typically the order of these steps is the following. Each subject must be identified (or self-identify himself or herself) to the research staff, then be selected to be in the initial pool to be contacted. A subject must then be successfully contacted by the research staff, found to satisfy all eligibility criteria, and finally must consent to take part in the intervention trial. We identify the final group of subjects as the *consented sample*.

All the steps starting with the intervention assignment to the completion of the intervention period is defined to be the *intervention stage*. In addition to the design used to assign intervention condition, this stage also relates to the design used to implement the intervention and maintain a comparable control and to measure and/or control the level of implementation and participation by subjects.

The last stage is the *postintervention stage*. It consists of all the design considerations required to follow up the study sample. Sometimes there are multiple stages of follow-up data collection so that everyone is assessed on an inexpensive instrument and only a subset are selected for more extensive follow-up (Brown & Liao, 1999). The design for follow-up can sometimes provide an opportunity to correct for any already existing signs of imbalanced subject loss (Brown, Indurkhya, & Kellam, 2000).

Design Threats in the Preintervention Stage

There are two major threats in the preintervention stage. When major differences exist between the target population and the consented sample, there is selection bias (threat 3.1) and consequently there may be very low external validity (Cook & Campbell, 1979). An example of this was a recent study of preventing poor outcomes in children of alcoholics (Gensheimer, Roosa, & Ayers, 1990; Michaels, Roosa, & Gensheimer, 1992). The first attempt to identify such children involved a two-stage procedure, first inviting children who expressed concern and then screening their parents for alcohol abuse or dependence. The first stage was done in school classrooms where all children

TABLE 26.3. Phases of a Preventive Trial and Corresponding Threats

Trial events	Phase	Threats	Approaches to offset threat
Subject recruitment and consent	Preintervention	Selection bias	Population-based sampling, limited exclusion criteria, training in subject recruitment
		Statistical power threat	Increase sample size, covariate or multiple baseline adjustment
Assignment to intervention condition	Intervention	Assignment bias	Random concealed assignment, balanced concealed assignment when randomization not possible
Intervention delivered		Condition bias	Verify no previous exposure to the intervention; develop strong institutional base to maintain design
		Statistical power threat	Avoid imbalanced assignment to intervention conditions
		Implementation threat	Standardize training and supervision; institute accountability of intervenors
		Participation bias	Provide alternative times for intervention, child-care and transportation needs; use opinion leaders, culturally informed, and social influence principles
Follow-up after intervention period is complete	Postintervention	Measurement threat	Use valid outcome measures for population's age, language, and culture
		Assessment bias	Use interviewers who have no contact with subjects during intervention period
		Attrition bias	Divide follow-up sample into balanced replicates, completing interviews with each replicate before going on to next; analyze data with modern missing data methods
Data analysis		Analysis threat	Take into account group randomized designs, baseline covariates, multilevel modeling

viewed a videotape which portrayed out-of-control parenting. There was a general invitation to all children who "wanted to learn more about handling such problems" to attend a group meeting afterwards. About 40% of the children expressed interest. Nonetheless, very few of the parents who children actually consented had serious alcohol problems.

A second threat often encountered in the preintervention phase is too small a sample. When the number of sample subjects is low, so too is the chance of finding a significant intervention effect when the two intervention conditions are in actuality different (statistical power threat 3.3).

Another problem with small samples is that even under appropriate random assignment procedures, it is much easier to end up with intervention groups that differ substantively from one another on baseline characteristics. One example where this apparently occurred is a randomized trial of a developmental intervention in the Neonatal Intensive Care Unit (NICU). Als, Duffy, and McAnulty (1996) reported that her intervention improved neonatal development among infants in the NICU compared to controls. However, a review of her design (Ariagno et al., 1997; Merenstein, 1994) showed that one important risk factor, intraventricular hemorrhage, was much more prevalent in one group (10 of 18) than another (1 of 20). Such a difference at baseline on this important variable turned out to be an alternative plausible explanation to intervention effectiveness. If the study were larger, the probability of obtaining samples with the same degree of imbalance—already small for a total sample of 38—would have been lower.

Sample size need not refer only to the number of subjects. It may also pertain to the number of sites, for example, classrooms, schools, families, or communities where the intervention occurs. In such multilevel studies, the statistical power to test for an intervention effect is far more affected by the number of larger units, i.e., schools, than the number of subjects within the school (Brown & Liao, 1999; Murray, 1998).

One should also note that in preventive trials there are sometimes compelling reasons not to divide the subjects equally into the intervention conditions. This may at first be counterintuitive, since the statistical power of any test of the difference between two intervention conditions is always maximized when subjects are divided equally into the two groups. However, there are some designs where there is little drop in statistical power if instead of the same number of intervention and control subjects, there are twice as many controls as intervention, with the same number of subjects overall. If the intervention itself is costly, then the imbalanced design will be less expensive, a very real consideration of researchers who want to maximize statistical power for a fixed cost amount. A second reason why some researchers have chosen to maintain a larger control group than an intervention group is that the larger control group can provide a better opportunity to examine the natural growth trajectories in the absence of intervention (Kellam et al., 1991).

One reason that some preventive trials assign more subjects to intervention than control is because they anticipate that a sizable fraction of subjects assigned to the intervention will not participate (Vinokur, Price, & Caplan, 1991). Over assignment of subjects to intervention allows one to make more precise statements about the outcomes for participants. There now exist statistical adjustments to assess the true value of the intervention for participants (Little & Yau, 1998). However, a statistical comparison between participants and all controls is known to lead to erroneous conclusions about the intervention effect. Such a comparison should never take the place of a formal "intention to treat" analysis involving the full intervention and the full control group.

Design Threats in the Intervention Stage

We have described why random assignment is a general technique to minimize assignment bias (threat 3.2). Randomization schemes vary from the unsophisticated "coin-tossing" or "pick a number out of the hat" to the more sophisticated pseudorandom numbers generated by computer or the use of random number tables. A primary objective with all such procedures is to achieve what is called concealed assignment. That is, none of the parties involved in the intervention should be able to gain any knowledge about the assignment. Unfortunately, many experiments have been completely corrupted when assignment has not been concealed. For example, some trials have naively used an even–odd scheme to assign subjects. Such a systematic, nonrandom scheme is easy to decode, and it lays open the very real possibility that an intake worker could consciously or unconsciously delay the intake for some subjects in order for them to receive the "right" intervention. Under no circumstances should such a systematic scheme as even–odd assignment be used. Other systematic assignment schemes such as choosing all controls first can be even more disastrous. With all controls taken first, there is no way to distinguish the intervention effect from any change in intake or measurement procedures or personnel or system change that could occur midway during the experiment.

Referring back to nonsystematic procedures, many variations have been used in prevention trials. For example, Fast Track (Coie, 1998) and Project LIFT (Reid, Eddy, & Fetrow, 1999), both school-based interventions aimed at preventing conduct disorder and drug use, had the principals and other school officials draw their own school's intervention condition. Such a strategy, while not the most elegant or rigorous, can occasionally be preferred over computer-generated assignments, particularly when the number of draws is very small and there is advantage to having the schools participate in their own (nearly) random assignment. At the other extreme is the second Baltimore Preventive Trial conducted at Johns Hopkins. This classroom-based intervention trial was aimed at preventing aggression, drug use, and depression. It employed computer-generated random numbers to assign both children to first-grade teachers and those teachers to intervention condition (Ialongo et al., 1999).

Standards for random assignment have been established in the clinical trials field (Meinert, 1986). The best assignment procedures do two things. They make certain that no one can guess in advance which condition will be assigned. They also make certain to balance assignment across time, usually by making sure that within a sequence of six or eight subjects, an equal number are assigned to each group. These procedures should be followed, unless the active involvement of say school officials in "drawing from a hat" helps to provide school buy-in to the trial.

Some medical treatment trials, in particular those involving pharmaceuticals, adhere to a stronger condition than simply making sure that no one can guess which intervention will be assigned. In such trials both the medical staff and the patients, as well as all assessors, may be blinded or masked to the type of drug being given. Such complete masking is possible to achieve in most drug trials (by preparing placebo pills to look identical to treatment pills) but is nearly impossible to do in preventive trials. Because all individuals participating in a preventive trial are told during informed consent about all conditions to which they could be assigned, they will recognize whether they are getting the intervention condition or the control. Similarly, implementors of the intervention are clearly trained to deliver specific components, so they would necessarily know they are not delivering the control. Thus, preventive interventions are much closer in this regard to surgical trials where it is exceedingly rare for the surgeon and patient to be blinded to the identity of the procedure that was performed. From an extensive examination of more that 160 preventive trials examined by the author, there was not one intervention that could be termed blinded (Mrazek & Brown, 1999). It thus becomes extremely critical in preventive trials to ensure that assessors are unaware of the intervention status of the subject. Such procedures are described in a following section.

In field experiments, it is occasionally difficult or impractical to randomize subjects, although sometimes it is possible to randomize part of a study (Tolan & Brown, 1997). One example of this involves multicomponent preventive interventions. In some studies, it may not be feasible or ethical to offer a no-intervention condition. Instead, all subjects may be offered a universal intervention. Then subjects can be randomized to receive or not receive an additional selective or indicated intervention. This type of design is now being used in a field trial to prevent conduct disorder (Prinz, 1998).

Another way to incorporate randomization is in varying the timing of intervention. This type of design protects against situations where societal trends, say in drug availability, are increasing or decreasing within an area selected for study. A wait-listed control design, where the decision to offer the intervention to a subject immediately or to delay the intervention is decided by a randomization procedure, has been used in trials with children of divorce (Wolchik et al., 1993).

Community trials can also use this wait-list design. The Mpowerment Program (Kegels, Hays, & Coates, 1996) targets all young gay males in a city in an effort to reduce HIV seroconversion. Two communities are matched as carefully as possible and then one is selected randomly to receive the intervention first. The second community then receives the intervention a year later. The second community's payoff for waiting is that the program it receives in the second year can benefit from any program enhancements that are made in response to deficiencies found in the first community. While the information derived from comparing two communities in such a wait-listed design is relatively small, the intention is to continue selecting different pairs of communities and randomly assigning them to immediate or wait-listed intervention. By combining information across these separate studies, as one does in a meta-analysis, this pairwise randomized design will provide far more definitive information about prevention effect than a comparable nonrandomized community design, in which post-hoc comparison communities are likely to differ on community readiness and other salient characteristics.

The wait-listed control can also be used to implement a systemwide intervention, such as a drug prevention curriculum within a school district. If schools are selected randomly for intervention in the first or second year, the design will provide a rigorous test of short-term intervention effectiveness. To our knowledge, this type of design has not been used in school-based drug prevention testing despite its clear potential for providing an excellent evaluation opportunity.

Tolan and Brown (1997) describe common alternatives to assignment by randomization. Here we provide a list of several of the main alternatives, listed in ascending order by strength of evidence.

ASSIGNMENT BY SUBJECT SELECTION.   If subjects are completely free to choose for themselves whether they want the intervention condition or not, we cannot distinguish between an effect due to the intervention or an effect due to self-selection factors. One extreme example of this is involves the benefit of mental health services on women's psychiatric symptoms. From observational studies, it is apparent that women who choose mental health services have much poorer psychiatric symptoms later in life compared to women who choose not to use such services (Brown, Adams, & Kellam, 1981). The inference that services cause poorer psychiatric symptoms is not likely to be true; it is more credible that those who seek out services have more symptoms to begin with, a hypothesis supported by the data. This study design makes it virtually impossible to separate out causal effects of services from selection factors.[2]

HISTORICAL CONTROLS.   In this type of design subjects enrolled after the start of the intervention period are compared to subjects enrolled before the intervention begins. Historical controls are often used by school systems to evaluate a new drug prevention program. The problem with this design is that other changes may occur to affect the outcomes of one or both of these cohorts. One literature review that compared historical control designs with randomized designs for medical treatments found a profound difference between the two types of studies (Sacks, Chalmers, & Smith, 1983). They noted that interventions tested by historical controls were often judged to be successful by standard statistical methods whereas the same interventions tested in randomized trials were far less likely to be found efficacious. These authors attributed the different findings to a bias toward new interventions in historical control studies and ended by recommending against the use of historical controls whenever possible. Year to year variation has been noted in many epidemiologic studies [Johnston, O'Malley, & Bachman (1996) for drug

---

[2] One method that has been used is propensity scores (Rosenbaum & Rubin, 1983).

use rates among adolescents, and Kellam et al. (1991) for early risk factors for drug use]. While some of these variations are influenced by broad societal characteristics, such as the economy (Brenner, 1991), some have no clear explanation. For example, Kellam et al. (1975) showed high unexplained variability in teacher ratings of aggression in first-grade classrooms over a 3-year period. It would be completely inappropriate to use historical controls to test an intervention's impact on teacher ratings of aggression. The same caution is likely true in historical comparison of school suspensions, fights, or absences.

Sometimes a historical control design can be improved. Having a nonintervention cohort both precede and follow an intervention cohort protects against a general rising trend. Such a design was used in an HIV prevention program in Thailand (Celentano et al., 1998).

CONCURRENT CONTROLS.   In this type of design, two or more communities or groups are chosen for comparison. In one community subjects receive the intervention, while in the other they do not. The basic problem with this evaluation design is that the two communities are rarely comparable on all of the characteristics that may explain observed outcome differences. In one of Wagenaar's (1997) recent community intervention trials designed to test whether reducing alcohol availability lowered underage drinking, he noted that the community which received the intervention had higher community readiness at the beginning of the study. This preexisting difference could potentially explain any community differences just as well as could intervention condition. Unfortunately, few of the community intervention studies in which the comparison community is selected after the intervention community even bother to measure such important characteristics as community readiness or existing interventions.

One classic prevention trial used both a fully randomized design and a nonrandomized design using concurrent controls. The 1954 Salk Polio Vaccine Trial used over 400,000 second graders in its randomized trial. In addition, 725,000 first and third graders were used as an additional comparison group. The researchers concluded that even with this large number of subjects, the data from the randomized trial were superior for making inferences (Tanur, 1989).

PRE–POST DESIGN.   Unlike previous designs, this one does not have a true control group. In this design, each subject receives a pretest score followed by a post-test. The difference in scores reflects change attributed to the intervention. This type of design is often used in assessing whether knowledge, attitudes, or preexisting risk behaviors (i.e., unsafe sex practices) changed when a subject is assigned to the intervention. It is typically not helpful in evaluating the preventive effects of more distal outcomes because one cannot distinguish between changed due to the intervention or due to developmental course (Baltes & Nesselroade, 1973). In addition, there is grave danger that a pre–post design which starts with a worse than average sample will conclude erroneously that there is improvement at post-test due to the intervention when all that may be happening is regression to the mean. For example, a program to treat depressed patients should never use such a pre–post design without a comparison group since most depressed patients improve without treatment.

In preventive trials, subjects assigned to an intervention condition may not always receive the intervention condition they are assigned. We have termed this condition bias (threat 3.4). Those assigned to receive the intervention may move to a nonintervention school, for example. Similarly, consider the case of a classroom intervention trial where parents of children in one first-grade class receive a parent training intervention and parents in the other class do not (Ialongo et al., 1999). In the case of twins who are assigned to separate classes, both of the children will be exposed to the intervention because they share the same parents. This type of deviation from intervention assignment occurs in many field trials, but the rate of occurrence is usually small.

There can also be leakage of an intervention into neighboring control sites, another type of condition bias. For example, intervention teachers may share exercises and prevention strategies with their colleagues who do not receive the intervention unless care is taken to limit such interactions. Occasionally a design falls apart because implementers do not want people to get the control condition. In the Neonatal Intensive Care Unit (NICU), nurses believed so strongly in the merit of oxygen to support premature newborns that they waited until the doctors had left the unit to turn on the lights (Silverman, 1991).

Sometimes the intervention that is delivered is an attenuated version of that intended. This implementation threat (3.5) often occurs in effectiveness trials rather than in efficacy trials, since the former deliberately allows more variation in training, in selection of intervenors, and less supervision. Occasionally one finds trials that are otherwise well designed but fail to provide even the most basic information about whether an intervention was delivered as intended. For a recent example of how to examine the relationship between implementation and impact, see Ialongo et al. (1999).

Even more common in prevention trials is a failure to participate (threat 3.6). While intervening with the newly unemployed, Vinokur and colleagues (1991) found only about half those randomized to the intervention condition actually participated in the sessions. Because the standard analysis that one reports for intervention effect is based on the condition of assignment (i.e., intent to treat analysis) not just on those who participated, it is easy to see that low participation cannot help but diminish our measure of intervention impact. For designs to address participation directly, see Brown and Liao (1999).

Design Threats in the Postintervention Stage

Measurement threat (3.7) is high when the instrument used has low reliability or validity, particularly for the population being studied. The location and procedures used to ask sensitive questions are also important. This is especially true when assessing drug use by adolescents. Asking adolescents about drugs in their own homes, as done by the National Household Survey on Drug Abuse (NHSDA) yields prevalence rates that are half as large as similar school-based interviews such as that used by Monitoring the Future. These procedural differences can have serious effect on the conclusions of any preventive trial. Additionally, a measure may be of little value if applied to different population than that used to standardize the instrument.

Besides the choice of the measure, the assessment procedure itself may introduce a serious threat to making inferences (threat 3.8). If the assessor knows the assigned group, there is a great potential for introducing bias in the results. In fact, blindness of the assessor is critical for the integrity of the inferences. Even with assessor blindness, however, there are a few times when the rating process occurs differently for intervention and control subjects. Kitzman et al. (1997), for example, concluded that their home visiting intervention resulted in more reports of abuse than the controls because the workers had much more contact with the family. These differences in reported abuse were contrasted by substantial reductions in child hospitalizations for injuries, and even when hospitalized those children in the home visited group had far less serious injuries than those of the other group. Other behaviors, such as adolescent drug use, may also be subject to such surveillance bias in prevention programs which increase parental monitoring and supervision.

A final problem encountered in nearly all preventive trials is attrition (threat 3.9). Typically, the higher the amount of attrition in a study, the less confidence that we can generalize our inferences to the full population. However, the most problematic type of attrition for analytical purposes occurs when there is a different rate of missing data across intervention groups. It is often quite difficult if not impossible to be sure that intervention and control differences on the nonattrited sample reflect the same difference one would find for the entire population.

There has been some initial work on combining these threats into a single dimensional score. Brown, Berndt et al. (2000) developed a 4-point scale for each of these threats and obtained a weighted sum of the scores to represent a total threat to trial integrity. While this scale has not been validated nor have any reliability tests been done, the approach has merit in differentiating well-conducted from poorly conducted trials (Brown, Berndt et al., 2000).

COMPARISON OF DIFFERENT THREATS ACROSS DIFFERENT RESEARCH DESIGNS

A carefully controlled trial that has successfully avoided the 10 threats mentioned previously is very likely to provide definitive answers to the primary research questions. Some of the improvements in trial quality are quite easy to make. For example, replacing a systematic, unconcealed assignment procedure with a high-quality random assignment is not only easy but also no more expensive. There are other issues, however, that pose more difficult problems. Attrition is a major problem in all longitudinal research and especially so for preventive trials. In particular, attrition becomes a real problem in schools where turnover rates can be as high at 70% per year. The various sampling methods for dealing with attrition, i.e., randomly sampling a subset of hard to locate subjects from each intervention condition, are often useful in reducing the uncertainty around missing data.

Much of the important empirical results we will obtain on the effectiveness of prevention programs will in the future be based on carefully designed randomized trials. However, it would be remiss not to point out that such carefully designed trials are not able to address all questions of interest. The randomized clinical trial is not equipped to address a number of open-ended questions about the real-life application of such a program. Specifically, such trials, whether they are efficacy or effectiveness trials, fix the amount of training and supervision which is available and only address the benefit of a single program model. If and when such a program goes to scale, there may be substantial increases in caseload or supervision, there may be reductions in the program, or there may be similar restructuring. Since the preventive trial design attempts to hold all these factors fixed in order to answer one question, such important questions cannot be addressed in such an experiment. Other designs for implementation studies are in fact possible and indeed are quite useful as a follow-up to this more classic type of preventive trial.

The last category of threats involves analyses and data management (threat 3.10). An extensive examination of preventive trials in the first 6 years of life (Mrazek & Brown, 1999) found the following analytic problems to be the most frequent: treating a categorical variable as continuous in statistical analyses, using the wrong error variance term when randomization is at the group rather than at the individual level, failure to take account of significant baseline differences, and failure to report intent to treat analyses.

Multiple comparisons across different outcomes using the same subjects in a trial can sometimes lead to a misrepresention of significant findings. For example, if a large number of statistical tests are performed and all nonsignificant results are omitted from the discussion, the reported effect will appear more important than it really is. The problem of multiple comparisons can become substantial if one searches through all combinations of variables, planned and post-hoc comparisons, and interactions. Fortunately, such nondirectional searching for significance is generally frowned upon by reviewers and rarely found now in published papers.

COMBINING EVIDENCE ACROSS SIMILAR
INTERVENTION TRIALS

In its simplest form, evidence of an intervention effect within a single trial has to be based on two factors: the quality of the design and the strength of the finding on outcome(s). All systems in use involve these two types of evidence. We briefly describe three leading systems of evidence and suggest directions for improvement.

Guided by the work of the Canadian Task Force on the Periodic Health Examination (Spitzer, 1979), the U.S. Preventive Services Task Force (1989, 1996) formed a hierarchy of evidence to assess the degree of design rigor across related trials. The highest level in their system is multiple randomized field trials. The highest level of methodologic rigor used by the Blueprints Project, which identifies best programs for crime and delinquency prevention, requires two randomized trials with different researchers or a multicenter trial. Similarly, for an intervention to reach the highest level of evidence in CSAP's Prevention Enhancement Protocols System (PEPS), it must be tested in three different randomized trials, two of which are run by different researchers (Grover, 1998). The three grading systems capture two hallmarks of science, namely, the use of high-quality designs and the replication of research findings. However, there is still more effort needed to objectify these two criteria.

We suggest that these categorical grading systems need to be based on underlying scales that measure the quality of intervention design, rather than just its type, i.e., a randomized design. Not all randomized trials should receive the highest weight. A randomized trial with severely imbalanced intervention and control groups and high differential attrition would not appropriate for determining intervention impact. In fact, Brown, Berndt et al. (2000) provide evidence that one-quarter of self-proclaimed randomized or controlled preventive trials aimed at children before the age of 6 had so many threats that they could offer virtually no useful inferences. To date, however, it is not clear just where to set the criteria regarding sufficient design quality for inclusion in summary statements. These cutoffs now need to be determined empirically; as better designs become available we would typically be willing to raise the quality standards further. Thus, we propose measuring quality of a trial design using a scale rather than a categorical measure.

An early scale that quantified the quality of a trial was proposed by Chalmers et al. (1981). Oakley, Fullerton, and Holland (1995) have used a scale measure based on eight characteristics accepted by the Cochrane Collaboration as quality indicators of trials. Recently a 72-point scale called the Threats to Trial Integrity Score has been introduced (Mrazek & Brown, 1999) which shows some promise of achieving an appropriate level of reliability and validity. All 10 threats discussed earlier are assessed on a 4-point scale, and a weighted sum of these scores is then computed. With further development, such a tool could provide useful objective criteria to assess the quality of a preventive trial design among any number of prevention fields.

The second element of all the hierarchical systems used to combine evidence involved replicability. Here too there is need of careful operationalization of this term. It would be hard to find two preventive intervention trials that tested the exact same intervention, even if the intervention carried the same name. Specific criteria need to be developed to measure how replicable two intervention conditions are.

REFERENCES

Als, H., Duffy, F. H., & McAnulty, G. B. (1996). Effectiveness of individualized neurodevelopmental care in the newborn intensive care unit (NICU). *Acta Paediatrics Suppementl, 416*, 21–30.

Ariagno, R. L., Thoman, E. B., Boeddiker, M. A., Kugener, B., Constantinou, J. C., Mirmiran, M., & Baldwin, R. B. (1997). Developmental care does not alter sleep and development of premature infants. *Pediatrics, 100*, 9.

Baltes, P. B., & Nesselroade, J. R. (1973). The developmental analysis of individual differences on multiple measures. In J. R. Nesselroade & H. W. Reese (Eds.), *Life-span developmental psychology: Methodological issues.* New York: Academic Press.

Brenner, M. Harvey. (1991). Health, productivity, and the economic environment: Dynamic role of socioeconomic status. In Green, M. Gareth, Baker, & Frank (Eds.) Work, health, and productivity. New York: Oxford University Press. pp. 241–255.

Brown, C. H. (1990). Protecting against nonrandomly missing data in longitudinal studies. *Biometrics, 46,* 143–155.

Brown, C. H. (1993a). Statistical methods for preventive trials in mental health. *Statistics in Medicine,* 12, 289–300.

Brown, C. H. (1993b). Analyzing preventive trials with generalized additive models. *American Journal of Community Psychology, 21,* 635–664.

Brown, H., Adams, R. G., & Kellam, S. G. (1981). A longitudinal study of teenage motherhood and symptoms of distress: The Woodlawn Community Epidemiological Project. *Research in Community and Mental Health, 2,* 183–213.

Brown, C. H., Berndt, D., Brinales, J. M., Zong, X., & Bhagwat, D. (2000). Evaluating the Evidence of Effectiveness for Preventive Interventions: Using a Registry System to Influence Policy through Science. *Addictive Behaviors, 25,* 955–964.

Brown, C. H., Indurkhya, A., & Kellam, S. G. (2000). Power calculations for data missing by design with application to a follow-up study of exposure and attention. *Journal of the American Statistics Association, 95,* 383–395.

Brown, C. H., & Liao, J. (1999). Designs for randomized preventive trials in mental health: An emerging developmental epidemiology perspective. *American Journal of Community Psychology, 27,* 673–710.

Bryk, A. S., & Raudenbush, S. W. (1992). *Hierarchical linear models: Applications and data analysis methods.* New York: Sage.

Bukoski, W. J. (1997). Meta-Analysis of drug abuse prevention programs. U.S. Department of Health and Human Services, National Institutes of Health, National Institute on Drug Abuse, NIDA Research Monograph 170.

Carnine, D. (1998). The metamorphosis of education into a mature profession. Keynote Address, Society for Prevention Research Sixth Annual Meeting, Park City Utah.

Catania, J. A., Gibson, D. R., Chitwood, D. D., & Coates, T. J. (1990). Methodological problems in AIDS behavioral research: Influences on measurement error and participation bias in studies of sexual behavior. *Psychological Bulletin, 108,* 339–362.

Celentano, D. D., Nelson, K. E., Lyles, C. M., Beyrer, C., Eiumtrakul, S., Go, V. F., Kuntolbutra, S., & Khamboonruang, C. (1998). Decreasing incidence of HIV and sexually transmitted diseases in young Thai men: Evidence for success of the HIV/AIDS control and prevention program. *AIDS, 12,* 29–36.

Chalmers, T. C. (1995). Dr. Tom Chalmers, 1917–1995: The trials of a randomizer (Interview by Malcolm Maclure). *Canadian Medical Association Journal, 155,* 757–760.

Chalmers, T. C. (1996). Dr. Tom Chalmers, 1917–1995: The trials of a randomizer (Interview by Malcolm Maclure). *Canadian Medical Association Journal,* 155, 986–988.

Chalmers, I., Adams, M., Dickersin, K., & Hetherington, J. (1990). A cohort study of summary reports of controlled trials. *JAMA, 263,* 1401–1405.

Chalmers, T. C., Smith, H., Blackburn, B., Silverman, B., Schroeder, B., Reitman, D., & Ambroz, A. (1981). A method for assessing the quality of a randomized control trial. *Controlled Clinical Trials, 2,* 31–49.

Chambless, D. L., & Hollon, S. D. (1998). Defining empirically supported therapies. *Journal of Consulting and Clinical Psychology, 66,* 7–18.

Coie, J. (1998). Personal communication.

Cook, T. D., & Campbell, D. T. (1979). *Quasi-experimentation: Design and analysis issues.* New York: Houghton.

Cook, D. J., Sackett, D. L., & Spitzer, W. O. (1995). Methodologic guidelines for systematic reviews of randomized control trials in health care from the Potsdam Consultation on Meta-Analysis. *Journal of Clinical Epidemiology, 48,* 167–171.

Durlak, J. A., & Wells, A. M. (1997). Primary prevention mental health programs for children and adolescents: A meta-analytic review. *American Journal of Community Psychology, 25,* 115–152.

Dusenbury, L., Falco, M., & Lake, A. (1997). A review of the evaluation of 47 drug abuse prevention curricula available nationally. *Journal of School Health, 67,* 127–132.

Evidence-Based Medicine Working Group (1992). Evidence-based medicine: A new approach to teaching the practice of medicine. *JAMA, 268,* 2420–2425.

Gensheimer, L. K., Roosa, M. W., & Ayers, T. S. (1990). Children's self-selection into prevention programs: Evaluation of an innovative recruitment strategy for children of alcoholics. *American Journal of Community Psychology, 18,* 707–723.

Grover, P. L. (Executive Editor) (1998). Preventing substance abuse among children and adolescents: Family centered approaches. Reference guide, Second in the prevention enhancement protocols system (PEPS) series. Substance

Abuse and Mental Health Services Administration, Center for Substance Abuse Prevention, Division of State and Community Systems Development. DHHS Publication No. 3223-FY98.

Hetherington, J., Dickersin, K., Chalmers, I., & Meinert, C. L. (1989). Retrospective and prospective identification of unpublished controlled trials: Lessons from a survey of obstetricians and pediatricians. *Pediatrics, 84*, 374–380.

Hosman, C. M. H. (1995). Effectiveness and effect management in mental health promotion and prevention. In D. R. Trent & C. Reed (Eds.), *Promotion of mental health, Volume 4*. Aldershot: Avebury.

Ialongo, L. N., Werthamer, L., Kellam, S. K., Brown, C. H., Wang, S., & Lin, Y. (1999). Proximal impact of two first-grade preventive interventions on the early risk behaviors for later substance abuse, depression and antisocial behavior. *American Journal of Community Psychology, 27*, 599–641.

Johnston, L. D., O'Malley, P. M., & Bachman, J. G. (1996). *National survey results on drug use from the monitoring the future study, 1975–1995. Volume I, Secondary* school students. U.S. Department of Health and Human Services, National Institute on Drug Abuse, NIH Publication No. 96-4139.

Junker, C. A. (1998). Adherence to published standards of reporting: A comparison of placebo controlled trials published in English or German. *British Medical Journal, 280*, 247–249.

Kalichman, S. C., Carey, M. P., & Johnson, B. T. (1996). Prevention of sexually transmitted HIV infection: A meta-analytic review of the behavioral outcome literature. *Annals of Behavioral Medicine, 18*, 6–15.

Kegeles, S. (1997). Personal communication.

Kegeles, S. M., Hays, R. B., & Coates, T. J. (1996). The empowerment project: A community-level HIV prevention intervention for young gay men. *American Journal of Public Health, 86*, 1129–1136.

Kellam, S. G., Branch, J. B., Agrawal, K. C., & Ensminger, M. E. (1975). *Mental health and going to school: The Woodlawn program of assessment, early intervention and Evaluation*. Chicago, IL: University of Chicago Press.

Kellam, S. G., Werthamer-Larsson, L., Dolan, L., Brown, C. H., Mayer, L., Rebok, G., Anthony, J., Laudolff, J., Edelsohn, G., & Wheeler, L. (1991). Developmental epidemiologically-based preventive trials: Baseline modelling of early target behaviors and depressive symptoms. *American Journal of Community Psychology, 19*, 563–584.

Kim, N., Standon, B., Li, X., Dickersin, K., & Galbraith, J. (1997). Effectiveness of the 40 adolescent AIDS-risk reduction interventions: A quantitative review. *Journal of Adolescent Health, 20*, 204–215.

Kitzman, H., Olds, D. L., Henderson, C. R., Hanks, C., Cole, R., Tatelbaum, R., McConnochie, K. M., Sidora, K., Luckey, D. W., Shaver, D., Engelhardt, K., James, D., & Barnard, K. (1997). Effect of prenatal and infancy home visitation by nurses on pregnancy outcomes, childhood injuries, and repeated childbearing: A randomized controlled trial. *JAMA, 278*, 644–652.

Little, R. J. A., & Yau, L. (1998). Statistical techniques for analyzing data from prevention trials: Treatment of no-shows using Rubin's causal model. *Psychological Methods, 3*, 147–159.

Meinert, C. L. (1986). *Clinical trials: Design, conduct, and analysis*. New York: Oxford. Merenstein, G. B. (1994). Individualized developmental care: An emerging new standard for neonatal intensive care units? *JAMA, 272*, 890–891. Editorial.

Merenstein, G. B. (1994). Individualized developmental care. An emerging new standard for neonatal intensive care units? *Journal of the American Medical Association, 272*, 890–891.

Michaels, M. L., Roosa, M. W., & Gensheimer, L. K. (1992). Family characteristics of children who self-select into a prevention program for children of alcoholics. *American Journal of Community Psychology, 20*, 663–672.

Mrazek, P. J., & Brown, C. H. (1999). An evidence-based literature review regarding outcomes in psychosocial prevention and early intervention in young children. Final Report, Invest in Kids Foundation, Toronto Canada.

Murray, D. M. (1998). *Design and analysis of group-randomized trials. Monographs in epidemiology and biostatistics, volume 27*. New York: Oxford.

Oakley, A., Fullerton, D., & Holland, J. (1995). Behavioural interventions for HIV/AIDS prevention. *AIDS, 9*, 479–486.

Piantadosi, S. (1997). *Clinical trials: A methodologic perspective*. New York: Wiley.

Prinz, R. (1998). Personal communication.

Reid, J. B., Eddy, J. M., & Fetrow, R. A. (1999). Description and immediate impacts of a preventive intervention for conduct problems. *American Journal of Community Psychology, 27*(4), 483–517.

Rosenbaum, P. R. (1984). From association to causation in observational studies: The role of tests of strongly ignorable treatment assignment. *Journal of the American Statistical Association, 79*, 41–48.

Rosenbaum, P. R., & Rubin, D. B. (1983). The central role of the propensity score in observational studies for causal effects. *Biometrika, 70*, 41–55.

Rubin, D. B. (1974). Estimating causal effects of treatments in randomized and nonrandomized studies. *Journal of Educational Psychology, 66*, 688–701.

Rubin, D. B. (1978). Bayesina inference for causal effects: The role of randomization. *Annals of Statistics, 6*, 34–58.

Sacks, H. S., Chalmers, T. C., & Smith, H. (1983). Sensitivity and specificity of clinical trials: Randomized *v* historical controls. *Archives Internal Medicine, 143*, 753–755.

Schafer, J. L. (1997). *Analysis of incomplete multivariate data*. New York: Chapman Hall.

Schulz, K. F., Chalmers, I., Altman, D. G., Grimes, D. A., & Dore, C. J. (1995). The methodologic quality of randomization as assessed from reports of trials in specialist and general medical journals. *Online Journal of Current Clinical Trials,* Document Nl. 197.

Schulz, K. F., Chalmers, I., Grimes, D. A., & Altman, D. G. (1994). Assessing the quality of randomization from reports of controlled trials published in obstetrics and gynecology journals. *JAMA, 272,* 125.

Schulz, K. F., Chalmers, I., Hayes, R. J., & Altman, D. G. (1995). Empirical evidence of bias. Dimensions of methodological quality associated with estimates of treatment effects in controlled trials. *JAMA, 273,* 408–412.

Sherman, L. W., Gottredson, D., MacKenzie, D., Eck, J., Reuter, P., & Bushway, S. (1997). Preventing crime: What works, what doesn't, what's promising. A report to the United States Congress. U.S. Department of Justice Office of Justice Programs.

Silverman, M. (1991). Equipment requirements for community-based paediatric oxygen treatment. *Archives of disease in childhood, 66*(1), 1366.

Sloboda, Z., & David, S. L. (1997). *Preventing drug use among children and adolescents: A research-based guide.* National Institute on Drug Abuse, National Institutes of Health. NIH Publication No. 97-4212.

Spitzer, W. O. (Chairman) (1979). Report on the Task Force on the Periodic Health Examination. *Canadian Medical Association Journal, 121,* 1193–1254.

Stoil, M. J., & Hill, G. (1996). *Preventing substrance abuse: Interventions that work.* New York: Plenum Press.

Tanur, J. M. (1989). *Statistics: A guide to the unknown* (Third Edition). Pacific Grove, CA: Brooks Cole.

The Cochrane Controlled Trials Register. In *The Cochrane Library, Issue 1, 1999.* Oxford: Update Software. Updated quarterly.

The Standards of Reporting Trials Group (1994). A proposal for structured reporting of randomized controlled trials. *JAMA, 272,* 1926–1931.

Thornley, B., & Adams, C. (1998). Content and quality of 2000 controlled trials in schizophrenia over 50 years. *British Medical Journal, 317,* 1181–1184.

Tobler, N. S., & Stratton, H. H. (1997). Effectiveness of school-based drug prevention programs: A meta-analysis of the research. *Journal of Primary Prevention,18,* 71–128.

Tolan, P. H., & Brown, C. H. (1997). Evaluation research on violence interventions: Issues and strategies for design. In P. K. Trickett & C. Schellenbach (Eds.), *Violence against children in the family and community.* Washington, DC: American Psychological Association.

Tolan, P., & Guerra, N. (1994). What works in reducing adolescent violence: An empirical review of the field. Center for Study and Prevention of Violence, Institute for Behavioral Sciences, University of Colorado. U. S. Preventive Services Task Force (1989). *Guide to clinical preventive services: An assessment of 169 interventions.* Baltimore, MD: Williams & Wilkins.

U.S. Preventive Services Task Force (1996). *Guide to clinical preventive services,* (Second Edition). Baltimore, MD: Williams & Wilkins.

Vinokur, A. D., Price, R. H., & Caplan, R. D. (1991). From field experiments to program implementation: Assessing the potential outcomes of an experimental intervention program for unemployed persons. *American Journal of Community Psychology, 19,* 543–562.

Wagenaar, A. (1997). Personal communication.

Wolchik, S. A, West, S. G., Westover, S., & Sandler, I. N. (1993). The children of divorce parenting intervention: Outcome evaluation of an empirically based program. *American Journal of Community Psychology, 21,* 293–331.

CHAPTER 27

Major Data Analysis Issues in Drug Abuse Prevention Research

DAVID P. MACKINNON

JAMES H. DWYER

INTRODUCTION

Drug abuse prevention research often involves comparing groups of subjects exposed to a prevention program with subjects who were not exposed to the program and analyzing the differences between them to determine the effects of the program. This chapter examines some of the issues that arise in the statistical analysis of the effects of drug abuse prevention programs. They include (1) issues encountered in planning the study, (2) statistical techniques commonly applied in the evaluation of prevention programs, and (3) data analysis to assess how a prevention program achieves its effects. The chapter concludes with a discussion of future directions in data analysis in drug abuse prevention research.

PLANNING THE EXPERIMENT

Decisions made prior to the study can simplify and clarify statistical analysis of data from the project. Four major topics that must be considered when planning an experiment are: extrascientific issues, experimental design, data collection, and linking a theory of behavior change to components of the prevention program.

DAVID P. MACKINNON • Department of Psychology, Arizona State University, Tempe, Arizona 85287-1104
JAMES H. DWYER • UCLA Medical School, University of Southern California, Los Angeles, California 90089

Extra-Scientific Issues

Cost, ethics, and confidentiality are major extra-scientific issues that always have to be considered in prevention research. Costs include respondents' time and personnel for administration and data processing (laboratory analysis, keypunching, etc.). Ethical issues include rights of privacy, invasiveness of the procedure, and associated health risks. Confidentiality involves establishing procedures to ensure that information cannot be linked to individual subjects.

The importance of these issues can preclude the use of certain types of measures and experimental designs. The challenging question confronting prevention researchers is whether a measure or design with more potential for error or bias is adequate to achieve the goals of the study. Since there is always a degree of uncertainty in empirical studies, the goal is to strike a balance that minimizes uncertainty while addressing these extra-scientific factors.

Design

RANDOMIZATION.   Randomizing a large number of units to different conditions is a design strategy which ensures that subsequent differences between groups are due to the experimental manipulation rather than to differences in premanipulation characteristics of the two groups. Although randomization appears to be straightforward, it can actually be a complex process that should be documented thoroughly (Colton, 1974). For example, random assignment can lead to group imbalance when a small number of units are randomized.

The theory behind most commonly used statistical techniques assumes that units are randomly assigned, but there are situations in which randomization is not possible or is impractical. However, if the importance of the study outweighs the drawbacks presented by randomization, more elaborate statistical methods can be used to evaluate the effects of the program (Cook & Campbell, 1979; Sechrest & Hanna, 1990). For example, a statistical modeling procedure can be used to address the reasons for selection into the groups (Dwyer, 1981; Heckman, 1989; Virdin, 1992). Because the reason for the nonrandom assignment is not usually known, even statistical adjustments for nonrandomization may be insufficient.

COMPLEXITY.   An experimental design must be complex enough to test the hypotheses of the study and to address possible alternative interpretations of the results. On the other hand, a complex design with three different programs, independent samples of students over six time points, and varying numbers of pre- and postintervention measurements may overly complicate the data analysis task. If the major hypotheses can be answered with less complex designs, such as fewer experimental conditions, the statistical analysis will be simpler. Overall, more straightforward designs are easier to describe, understand (Cohen, 1990), and analyze.

STATISTICAL POWER.   Statistical power, the ability of a study to detect a real program effect, should be determined before a study begins. Statistical power calculations specify the required sample size needed to detect program effects based on effect size, Type I error rates (usually .05), and the desired power (usually .8) (Cohen, 1988; Kraemer & Thiemann, 1987; Meinert, 1986). For example, the required sample sizes for small, medium, and large effects for a two-group study with power equal to .8 and a two-tailed alpha of .05 are 393, 64, and 26 participants in each group, respectively (Cohen, 1988; p. 55). However, prevention studies often lack sufficient statistical power (Hansen, 1992), and power calculations are more complex because participants are often nested within social units such as schools (Murray, 1998). One drawback of prospective power calculations is that they are based on informed guesses about the expected size of the program effect and the variability of the dependent measure. But, even when the calculation of statistical power is based on very rough guesses regarding variance and likely effect sizes, such information is preferable to beginning a study without any estimates of required sample size.

The most common way to increase power is to add participants. Other approaches focus on reducing unexplained variability in the dependent variable. Adjusting post-test measures with the pre-test measures can reduce unexplained variability by removing consistent subject differences. More reliable dependent measures reduce unexplained variability (Cohen, 1988). In a randomized study, covariates that explain variability in the outcome measure are primarily used to reduce unexplained variability, which increases statistical power. When assignment is not random, these covariates also reduce some alternative explanations for the results of the study.

In general, the power and validity of conclusions from an experimental design can be enhanced by the inclusion of multiple measures prior to an intervention and multiple follow-ups. Such a design is advantageous because differences between units (such as schools or communities) in both the outcome and the time trend can be incorporated into the analysis. An experimental effect is then assessed in terms of a deviation from the trend of individual units rather than from a preintervention level. Such a design is especially important when randomization is not feasible or when only a small number of units can be assigned to conditions.

The availability of multiple measurements (whether postintervention or pre- and postintervention) has caused many experimenters to mistakenly assume that additional degrees of freedom can be extracted to increase the power of a statistical analysis. The misleading conclusions likely to arise from this approach have been demonstrated in a series of simulations (Murray et al., 1998). In general, any analytic strategy that yields degrees of freedom for the error term that exceed the number of units assigned to conditions can be a mis-specified statistical model with an actual Type I error rate that exceeds the nominal 5%.

ALTERNATIVE EXPLANATIONS. Control groups can rule out many alternative explanations for effects in the group receiving the program. It is possible, however, that mere exposure to any prevention program may encourage participants to answer questionnaire items in a way that favors the program. This is referred to as the "attention" alternative explanation. Comparison groups that receive some form of programming reduce the attention alternative explanation of program effects. In school-based, drug abuse prevention research, standard health education classes are often delivered to control groups. In drug abuse treatment evaluations, for example, clients who receive the new program are compared to clients who receive the standard treatment. More information on comparison groups to address alternative explanations of results can be found in Cook and Campbell (1979).

Another alternative explanation of drug abuse prevention results is potential bias in self-reports of drug use, but including biological, archival, or other types of measures in addition to self-reports can decrease the potential for bias. Generally, however, self-report measures have been found to be valid and reliable although accuracy can depend on the sample and context of measurement (Harrison & Hughes, 1997). Information regarding the measurement of drug abuse through self-report and biological measures of blood, hair, saliva, and urine should appear as studies currently underway are completed (Harrison & Hughes, 1997).

Data Collection

QUESTIONNAIRE DESIGN. Time and cost limit the number of constructs and items per construct that can be measured in questionnaires. Ideally, the reliability and validity of the measures in prevention research are determined prior to the study using methods such as those discussed by Campbell and Fiske (1959), Crocker and Algina (1986), and Dunn (1989). When psychometric properties are determined beforehand, the data analysis is simplified because the necessary scales are developed and the outcome measures are clear and relatively error free. If these analyses are not conducted prior to data collection, the development and assessment of the measurement properties substantially increase the data analysis load. Such issues are common in drug abuse prevention research because of the need to develop new scales. Fortunately, several widely used surveys now exist including the Monitoring the Future Study (Johnston, Bachman, & O'Malley 1997) and the American Drug and Alcohol Abuse scale (Oetting & Beauvais, 1990). Often copies of these questionnaires are available from the researchers.

IMPLEMENTATION DATA. Most prevention studies assume that program components are delivered as designed and consistently across different locations. This ideal situation rarely occurs (Pentz et al., 1990), so researchers should include a monitoring plan to measure the quality of the implementation (Basch, 1984). Uneven delivery will dilute the effects of the program. If implementation varies, then assessment of level of implementation will improve the ability of the data analysis to detect program effects. Implementation data are also useful because they provide information on the dose response effects of the intervention.

DATA QUALITY. Close monitoring of data collection is an essential part of research. Information on missing or absent subjects can be used in some statistical techniques. It will often be helpful to obtain a sample of subjects who are most difficult to measure so that more elaborate adjustments for missing data can be applied (Graham & Donaldson, 1993).

Data cleaning, such as finding outlier and out-of-range values, must be completed prior to data analysis. Consultation with the actual questionnaires is often required to resolve data-cleaning issues. The data-cleaning task is more complex when participants are merged across multiple waves because there will be some participants with data at only one or two measurement points. Participants may not merge because of keypunching and other errors that can only be resolved by examining the actual questionnaires and subject-tracking information.

COST-BENEFIT AND COST-EFFECTIVENESS DATA. Policymakers are increasingly asked to quantify the costs and benefits of prevention programs, or the extent to which the benefits of drug abuse prevention programs justify the costs. Policymakers are also asked to determine the least expensive program that will accomplish the program goal, or the cost-effectiveness of prevention programs. Researchers should try to document costs and benefits. Typically, costs are based on the per-pupil cost, including material and teacher fees to deliver the program. Benefits include reduced drug use, reduced absenteeism, and increases in self-esteem. More on potential economic measures can be found in Werthamer and Chatterji, (1999) and in Gold et al. (1996).

Definition of the Theoretical Basis of the Program

INTERVENTION DESIGN. Theoretical models forming the basis of intervention approaches are multidimensional. Consequently, prevention programs target several specific variables hypothesized to be causally related to the outcome measure. The variables that the programs are designed to change are called mediating variables or mediators. In school-based drug prevention, mediators include self-efficacy, social norms, and beliefs about consequences of drug use. [See Hansen (1992) for a comprehensive description of mediators targeted in prevention programs.]

Mediator analysis is used to increase understanding of the process or mechanisms by which these complicated prevention programs achieve their effects by linking program effects on mediators to program effects on outcomes.

Before a study is conducted, two important tasks should be completed. First, the links between the mediators targeted and the outcome variables should be elaborated, based on prior theoretical and empirical work. Second, the connection between the program components and the mediators targeted by each component should be summarized. Limitations of the program in changing drug abuse behavior are often clearly seen in this practical inquiry into the proposed prevention project. It is important to complete these tasks prior to the study, in order to increase the chances that measures of important mediators are in the questionnaire.

Although randomization of subjects to receive components targeting different mediators is ideal for some scientific purposes, it is often difficult to accomplish in prevention research because prevention programs are multidimensional. Experimental designs to study different mediation effects have recently been described (West & Aiken, 1997) and will increase as prevention research matures. Nevertheless, the best advice for the evaluation of a new prevention program is to pick an intervention with the largest possible effect, which usually means more components.

Moderating variables are also important (Baron & Kenny, 1986). Moderating variables interact with the prevention effects such that program effects differ across the levels of the moderator. Examples of moderators in prevention research are sex, age, ethnicity, and individual differences, such as risk-taking propensity or hostility (Aiken & West, 1991). Ideally, hypotheses regarding potential moderating variables are identified prior to the study to ensure that they are measured in the questionnaire. Federal initiatives requiring inclusion of both genders and minority groups in government-funded research should lead to more studies of differential effects across these subgroups.

Overall, when extra-scientific issues, experimental design, data collection, and linking a theory of behavior change to components of the prevention program are specified beforehand, data analysis is greatly simplified. More powerful statistical methods can be applied and alternative explanations of the study's results can be addressed. In many respects, the decisions made prior to study are more important than the analytical methods used to determine whether the prevention program was effective.

ANALYSIS ISSUES IN THE ESTIMATION OF PROGRAM EFFECTS

Mixed Model Analysis of Variance

The mixed design (Hays, 1988; Keppel, 1991; Keppel & Zedeck, 1989; Winer, Brown, & Michels, 1991) is the most common design in prevention studies. The simplest version of this design includes two components: exposure to the program (exposed or not exposed) and time of measurement (pre- and postprogram). In this two-by-two design, the interaction of the treatment "between-subjects" factor and the time "within-subjects" factor is the test of whether the program effect is statistically significant. The interaction tests whether the change over time is the same for both control and program conditions. The within-subjects factor reduces unexplained variability by using individuals as controls for themselves. The mixed design is summarized in the following equation:

$$Y_{ijk} = \mu_T + \alpha_i + \beta_j + \tau_k + (\alpha\beta)_{ij} + (\beta\tau)_{jk} + \varepsilon_{ijk},$$

where μ_T is the grand mean, α_i is the effect of the program, β_j is the effect of time of measurement, τ_k is the effect of the participants, $(\alpha\beta)_{ij}$ is the program by time of measurement interaction effect, $(\beta\tau)_{jk}$ is the interaction of time by participants, and ε_{ijk} is unexplained variability. The mean square for the interaction effect $(\alpha\beta)_{ij}$ is divided by the error term of subjects within time to obtain an F ratio with numerator degrees of freedom equal to $(n_i - 1)$ and denominator degrees of freedom equal to $n_i(n_j - 1)(n_k - 1)$, where n_i is the number of groups, n_j is the number of measurements, and n_k is the number of participants.

The statistical analysis of the mixed model is easily expanded for more than two groups and more than one measurement before and after the intervention by expanding the levels of the factors in the model and testing program effects with contrasts among measurements (e.g., by comparing measurements taken before the intervention to those taken after the intervention) and among groups (e.g., the comparison between the program group and the control group).

More than two within-subjects measurements require further assumptions regarding the covariances among the repeated measures. The repeated measures can be treated in a multivariate framework under the assumption that the covariances and variances among measures differ but the covariance matrix is common across subjects. If the repeated measures assumption of compound symmetry is correct, however, the repeated measures analysis of variance (ANOVA) will require fewer subjects for the same power as multivariate analysis of variance (Mulvenon, 1992). The effects in the model and the variations described previously can be estimated using existing computer programs, such as SAS or SPSS, or estimated in a regression format that requires the data analyst to specify the vectors associated with the effects in the model (Keppel & Zedeck, 1989; Kirk, 1982).

Analysis of Covariance

The ANOVA model can be recast as an analysis of covariance (ANCOVA) model with the pretest measure as a covariate. This model generally has more statistical power than the model described previously except when there are five or more repeated measurements from the same subjects (Maxwell, 1998). The ANCOVA model is summarized in the following equation:

$$Y = \beta_0 + \beta_1 X_1 + \beta_2 X_2 + \zeta_1,$$

where Y is the post-test score, β_0 is the intercept, β_1 codes the relationship between the pretest (X_1) and the post-test, β_2 codes the program effect (X_2), and ζ_1 is unexplained variability. If more than two groups are evaluated, then contrasts among the groups are additional predictor variables.

Growth Models

Growth models are one of the most popular ways to estimate intervention effects because differential growth and trends among subjects are explicitly modeled in the analysis. The models require at least three and preferably more repeated measures from the same subjects (Bryk & Raudenbush, 1992; Stoolmiller et al., 1993; Willett & Sayer, 1994). Typically, an intercept and linear slope are modeled, although it is likely that many developmental phenomena require higher level trends, such as the quadratic trend. Each participant is allowed to have different growth model coefficients (e.g., a different value for the linear trend coefficient). In these models, the program effect is evaluated as the effect on the slopes of participants in the program group compared to the slopes of participants in the control group as described in the following equations:

$$Y_{ti} = \beta_{0i} + \beta_{Li}X_{Lt} + \beta_{Qi}X_{Qt} + \zeta_{1ti}$$
$$\beta_{0i} = \lambda_{00} + \lambda_{P0}X_{Pi} + \zeta_{2i}$$
$$\beta_{Li} = \lambda_{0L} + \lambda_{PL}X_{Pi} + \zeta_{3i}$$
$$\beta_{Qi} = \lambda_{0Q} + \lambda_{PQ}X_{pi} + \zeta_{4i}$$

where β_{0i} is the intercept in the level 1 (within-individual level) equation for participants, β_{Li} codes the linear trend for each participant, β_{Qi} codes the quadratic trend for each participant, and ζ_{1ti} is unexplained variability in the individual-level model, and λ_{00} codes the average intercept across individuals and λ_{P0} codes the effect of the program on the intercept, λ_{0L} codes the average linear slope across the participants, and λ_{PL} codes the effect of the program on the linear slope, λ_{0Q} codes the average quadratic coefficient, and λ_{PQ} codes the effect of the program on the quadratic coefficient. The ζ_{2i}, ζ_{3i}, and ζ_{4i} code error variances.

The growth curve model can be easily changed to code other time-dependent effects that correspond to different hypotheses about program effects, such as a permanent change in level at the first post-test measure that maintains at all follow-up measures. The growth curve approach can also include a measurement model for the constructs, thereby adjusting for unreliability.

Categorical Dependent Variables

ANOVA-like models for categorical dependent measures are available using the generalized linear model (Koch, Singer, & Stokes, 1992; Zeger, Liang, & Albert, 1988). Tests of symmetry and marginal homogeneity and tests specific to the categorical dependent variable case are also available. More on these tests can be found in Agresti (1990); Bishop, Fienberg, and Holland (1975); and Woodward, Bonett, and Brecht (1990). The parameters of these models can be estimated with SAS CATMOD (SAS/STAT Guide, 1987) and GENLOG (Bonett, Brecht, & Woodward, 1985).

Logistic regression can be used to estimate the corresponding ANCOVA model for a categorical outcome variable, such as drug use in the past month. A benefit of the logistic regression model is that the exponent of the logistic regression coefficient is an odds ratio (Hosmer & Lemeshow, 2000). Similar technology now exists to estimate growth curve models with a categorical dependent variable (Hedecker, Gibbons, & Flay, 1994; Murray, 1998; Muthén & Muthén, 1998).

Survival analysis is an important and underused statistical method for categorical outcomes in prevention research. Survival analysis is a set of statistical methods developed to model the time until an event occurs, such as time to drug use onset or time to relapse among heroin addicts (Hosmer & Lemeshow, 1999). The method has rarely been used in prevention research with some exceptions (Siddiqui, Flay, & Hu, 1996; Wells-Parker et al., 1995). Application of these models requires data collection strategies to document the time when an event occurs, which may be unfamiliar to drug abuse prevention researchers.

Attrition

Analysis of attrition and its potential impact on internal and external validity has been discussed by several authors (Biglan et al., 1987; Graham et al., 1997; Hansen et al., 1985). One consistent finding in drug abuse prevention studies is that those who drop out of prevention studies are generally found to be more likely to use drugs at earlier measurements. An important test is whether there is an association between attrition and program assignment (Biglan et al., 1987; Hansen et al., 1985). Graham and Donaldson (1993) discuss when such differential attrition is a problem for internal and external validity.

Methods to adjust program effect estimates for missing data, including attrition, are now beginning to appear in the literature (Graham & Donaldson, 1993; Graham et al., 1997; Little & Rubin, 1987, 1989; Rindskopf, 1992; Schafer, 1997), and statistical software is now widely available to accomplish this task. For example, the SAS MIXED program can easily be adapted to include all data, even partially missing data (Murray, 1998). Several covariance-structure modeling programs, such as AMOS (Arbuckle, 1995) and Mplus (Muthén & Muthén, 1998), now include such estimations. The assumption of the majority of these methods is that the data are missing at random (MAR), which means that whether a variable is missing or not is related to variables used in the analysis. If the MAR assumption is violated, these methods may also be inaccurate. Little and and colleagues (Little & Rubin, 1987; Little & Yau, 1996) discuss alternative models for the violation of MAR assumption. In the future, it is likely that prevention researchers will learn much more about the missing-data mechanism and have accurate ways to estimate program effects in the presence of attrition.

Nested Effects

The analysis models described previously are complicated in drug abuse prevention studies when there is nesting of individuals within clinics, schools, or classrooms (Barcikowski, 1982; deLeeuw & Kreft, 1986; Hopkins, 1981; Murray, 1998; Murray & Hannan, 1990). Although prevention studies randomize these social units to conditions, analysis is typically at the individual level. The standard errors derived from analyses of individuals in nested designs may be too small, increasing the chance of finding a significant effect due to chance beyond the specified Type I error rate. Using schools as an example, such errors can occur when variability between schools exceeds that within schools. This situation is more likely to occur if students in schools are in general more similar to each other than to students in other schools or if interaction among students in a school increases homogeneity. The extent to which analyzing individuals will lead to incorrect results is determined by the extent to which the students in the same school are more similar compared to students in other schools. A quantitative measure of this effect is the intraclass correlation (Haggard, 1958). Fortunately, statistical methods to incorporate the nesting of subjects in units are now widely available.

By viewing repeated observations as nested within participants, and participants as nested within schools, it is possible to conduct statistical analyses at multiple levels. The Hierarchical Linear Model (HLM), including nesting of participants, is identical to the model previously described for the growth curve, except that the coefficients in the second level model reflect intercepts and slopes in schools rather than intercepts and slopes among individuals. The HLM formulas can be expanded to include both nesting of participants in schools and nesting of repeated observations within participants, which provides a comprehensive model for program effects (Bryk & Raudenbush, 1992). These methods also allow for the incorporation of partially complete data under the MAR assumption.

Incomplete Randomization

In drug abuse prevention studies, politically sensitive units, such as communities or schools, are often randomized to different conditions. In these situations, it is common for randomization to be incomplete. Administrators may not cooperate with plans or budget problems and other extra-scientific factors may preclude complete randomization. When randomization is incomplete, it is helpful to estimate program effects under alternative assumptions about the causal process that led to baseline differences between program and control groups. Statistical models provide an estimate of program effects within the context of assumptions about what would have occurred in the absence of an intervention effect. When a large number of units have been successfully randomized, the researcher can have some confidence about these assumptions. Two alternative models are suggested: one is the ANCOVA model that is conditional on baseline measures; the other is the unconditional or repeated measures model. The conditional model is appropriate when preintervention differences between groups are due to random sampling variability as with randomization of large numbers of units. The unconditional model is an alternative model in which baseline nonequivalencies are presumed to arise because of factors that continue after the intervention commences.

The conditional and unconditional models are summarized in the following equation:

$$Y_{1i} = \beta_0 + \beta_1 Y_{Oi} + \beta_2 X_P + \zeta_1,$$

where X_P is a dichotomous dummy variable indicating experimental condition (treatment or control), Y_{0i} is the baseline measure of the outcome variable, β_0 is the intercept, and ζ_1 is error variance. The constraints $E(\zeta) = \sigma_{x\zeta} = \sigma_x = 0$ specify the conditional version of the model. The constraints $\beta_1 = 1$, $E(\zeta) = \sigma_{x\zeta} = 0$ specify the unconditional version. The value of β_1 reflects the speed with which the dependent variable regresses to an equilibrium level. When $\beta_1 = 1$, the dependent variable does not regress to mean levels and the model is equivalent to regression on the difference dependent variable, $Y_{1i} - Y_{0i}$, which is the unconditional or repeated measures ANOVA model. When program and control groups are equivalent at baseline, the conditional and unconditional models yield identical estimates of program effects. Applications of conditional and unconditional models in drug abuse prevention research including the estimation of conditional and unconditional logistic regression models are described by Dwyer et al. (1989). The unconditional model may also be specified as a multiple dependent variable regression for two or more follow-up measurements.

When the study design allows two or more observations prior to the prevention program, it is possible to use the information from pretreatment time trends to estimate the extent to which baseline nonequivalencies remain constant or regress toward zero (Dwyer, 1981). This important design is not commonly used in prevention studies.

STATISTICAL ANALYSIS OF MEDIATING VARIABLES

The primary focus of all prevention studies is estimation of the effect of a prevention program on an outcome variable. Prevention researchers often stop data analysis at this point, even though further analysis can reveal additional information. As described earlier, the prevention program is designed to change mediators hypothesized to be causally related to the outcome variable. Mediator analysis is a set of analyses used to determine how the program had (or did not have) its effects on the outcome variable. These analyses are important even when the overall program effect is not significant, because it is possible for mediated effects to exist even when the overall program effect is zero. This can occur when effects via different pathways are in opposing directions, so that they cancel each other. Models that include positive and negative mediation (suppression) effects are sometimes called inconsistent models. [See Blalock (1969), Davis, (1985), and MacKinnon, Krull, & Lockwood (2002) for a discussion of these models.] Also, when a program does not work as planned and actually produces adverse results, mediator analyses may uncover explanations for the unexpected effects.

Mediation Analysis

The parameter estimates and standard errors in three regressions provide the necessary information to test for mediator effects (Judd & Kenny, 1981; MacKinnon & Dwyer, 1993):

$$Y_O = \beta_1 X_P + \zeta_1$$
$$Y_O = \beta_2 X_P + \beta_3 X_M + \zeta_3$$
$$Y_M = \beta_4 X_P + \zeta_2.$$

The symbols in the equations are the following: Y_O is the outcome variable, Y_M is the mediator as an outcome variable, X_P is the independent variable (prevention program), X_M is the mediator as an independent variable, β_1 codes the relationship between the program and the outcome, β_2 is the coefficient relating the program to the outcome adjusted for the effects of the mediator, β_3 is the coefficient relating the mediator to the outcome adjusted for the effects of the program, β_4 codes the relationship between the program and the mediator, and ζ_1, ζ_2, and ζ_3 code unexplained variability. The intercept is assumed to be zero, so scores are in deviation form. To be consistent with the mixed model and the unconditional model described previously, X_M and Y_M are the difference between time 2 and time 1 measures of the mediator, and Y_O is the difference between the outcome measure at time 2 and the outcome measure at time 1.

PROGRAM EFFECTS ON MEDIATORS. If the program effect on the mediators is not significant, then the prevention program was not effective in changing these mediators or the mediators may not have been measured well. If there are not program effects on the mediators, it may be that the program was not effective and is unlikely to have any effect on the outcome variable (if the mediation hypothesis is correct).

MEDIATOR EFFECTS ON THE OUTCOME MEASURE. The decision to target a mediator in the prevention program should be based on theory and prior empirical work demonstrating a relationship between the mediator and the outcome variable. As a result, the test of whether the mediator is significantly related to the outcome variable is a test of the theory behind the prevention program as well as a replication of past research demonstrating such relationships. If the mediator is related to the outcome variable, the effect of the mediator on the outcome variable (β_3) will be statistically significant when controlling for the effect of the prevention program variable (β_2).

MEDIATED EFFECT. If the program effect adjusted for the mediator (β_2) is zero when both the mediator and the program exposure variable are included in the model, there is evidence for complete mediation (Baron & Kenny, 1986; Judd & Kenny, 1981). It is unlikely that a single mediator would completely explain prevention program effects (Baron & Kenny, 1986). When the adjusted program effect (β_1) is larger than the program effect adjusted for the mediator (β_2), then there is some evidence of mediation. The value of the mediated or indirect effect equals the difference in the program effect without and with the mediator ($\beta_1 - \beta_2$) (McCaul & Glasgow, 1985). The mediated effect is also equal to the product of the β_3 and β_4 parameters. The rationale behind this calculation is that mediation depends on the extent to which the independent variable changes the mediator (β_4) and the extent to which the mediator affects the outcome variable (β_3).

The coefficient relating the independent variable to the outcome adjusted for the mediator (β_2) is the nonmediated or direct effect. The following formulas summarize the effects:

$$\text{Total Effect} = \beta_1 = \beta_4\beta_3 + \beta_2$$
$$\text{Mediated Effect} = \text{Indirect Effect} = \beta_4\beta_3 = \beta_1 - \beta_2$$
$$\text{Direct Effect} = \beta_2$$

The large sample standard error of the indirect or mediated effect was derived by Sobel (1982, 1986) using the multivariate delta method and is equal to

$$\sigma_{\beta_4\beta_3} = \sqrt{\beta_4{}^2\sigma^2{}_{\beta_3} + \beta_3{}^2\sigma^2{}_{\beta_4}}.$$

Ninety-five percent confidence limits for the mediated effect can be constructed by adding and subtracting 1.96 times the standard error computed in the previous formula from the mediated effect estimate (MacKinnon, Warsi, & Dwyer, 1995).

More Complicated Mediation Models. The single mediator models described previously can be easily extended to multiple mediators by expanding the mediators in the second mediation equation (MacKinnon, 2000). Several complications arise in the evaluation of multiple mediators that are related. The mediated effects are adjusted for other mediators that may provide a more accurate model for the mechanism by which the program works. Because the mediators were not randomly assigned to conditions, interpretation of differential mediation effects are qualified by the correlational relationship among mediators.

An additional application of the mediation model is in the analysis of implementation data. The implementation data can be viewed as a mediating variable such that the assignment to conditions increases exposure to the program which in turn affects the outcome measure. In one approach, all control schools are given a value of zero on implementation, and the program schools are given some nonzero value.

Mediation analyses have also been incorporated in other statistical methods. The procedures to estimate the mediated effect and its standard error described previously do not directly apply in logistic or probit regression because error variances are not fixed in these analyses (Winship & Mare, 1983). One solution is to standardize logistic and probit regression estimates and standard errors and then to calculate mediated effects as described previously (MacKinnon & Dwyer, 1993). Methods to assess mediation in the multilevel model have recently been described (Krull & MacKinnon, 1999).

FUTURE DIRECTIONS

Prevention research has been a driving force behind the development of new statistical methods, and the trend is likely to continue. During the past 10 years, growth curve modeling, survival analysis, hierarchical modeling, adjustments for missing data, cost-benefit analysis, and mediation analysis have been developed and applied in the evaluation of prevention programs. It is expected that these new methods will be refined and routinely applied in prevention research and that future methodological advancements will combine these approaches.

The ideal model for evaluation of prevention studies includes accurate measurement of multiple mediators and multiple outcomes, mixtures of categorical and continuous variables, missing data, hierarchical data, and repeated measurements to estimate growth over time. Statistical adjustments for violations of the assumptions of ANOVA and regression methods described in this chapter will likely continue (Wilcox, 1987). The use of computer-intensive methods, such as bootstrap and jackknife estimators (Efron, 1982) that do not require extensive assumptions about the data, will be further developed and applied in the statistical analysis of drug abuse prevention studies. Covariance structure modeling (Bentler, 1980; Bollen, 1989; Hayduk, 1987) approaches already address many of these methodological issues. With covariance structure models, measurement errors in the indicators of the constructs can be modeled (Fuller, 1987), parameter estimates among constructs can be adjusted for other variables in the model, longitudinal models can be estimated, missing data adjustments are available, and a measure of the entire fit of the model to the data can be obtained. When combined with the randomized experimental manipulation common in prevention research, these models are quite powerful for understanding the effects of prevention programs. Computer programs for the estimation of these models have become sophisticated and include options regarding the calculation of standard errors of mediated effects, analysis of both categorical and continuous measures, multiple groups analysis, adjustments for nonnormal data, and adjustments for missing data (Arbuckle, 1995; Bentler, 1989; Berk, 1988; Joreskog & Sorbom, 1988; Muthén & Muthén, 1998). It is expected that these programs will become even more powerful in the future, including many alternative estimation approaches for normal and nonnormal data, bootstrap estimation, adjustments for different patterns of missing data, and efficient estimation of models with both continuous and categorical measures.

Application of the statistical methods will also inform theory. The continued focus on mediational processes, both in terms of experimental studies to change mediators and in terms of the relationships between change in the mediators and outcomes, have the potential to provide the scientific results to guide theory and practice in prevention science. Understanding the critical components and constructs in prevention programs reduces the costs of programs while increasing their effectiveness. Greater understanding of the types of missing data in drug abuse prevention studies will lead to more accurate models to adjust for missing data. Theory regarding effects at different levels of observation will evolve from application of growth and hierarchical modeling.

Computer and other technical advances are likely to improve prevention methodology. Advances in the measurement of drug use with body fluids and hair will continue, leading to improved drug use measurement and more accurate assessment of self-report measures. The influence of the Internet is likely to increase, both as a resource to learn about methodological developments and as a place to download new software. One important internet site is the prevention research methodology web site organized by Hendricks Browne at the University of South Florida (http://yates.coph.usf.edu/research/psmg/index.html), which includes publications, a program to compute power for multilevel data, and a series of videotaped lectures. The Internet will also make it easier to use new software. Donald Hedecker at the University of Illinois now offers his multilevel software for categorical outcomes, MIXOR, for downloading from the Internet (http://www.uic.edu/~hedecker/mix.html). It is possible that ongoing prevention research data will be sent to experts in different advanced methodological disciplines for a thorough analysis. Of course, such analysis should not occur unless the methodologist has a detailed understanding of the planning and data collection for the project.

SUMMARY

This chapter has provided an overview of some of the data analysis issues confronting prevention researchers. Several decisions made prior to the study clarify the data analysis, including randomization of units to conditions, refinement of measures of relevant constructs, linking of program components to potential mediators, and strategies to reduce confounding of program effect estimates due to attrition. The mixed design with one between- and one within-subjects factor is complicated in actual prevention research when there are multiple levels of possible analyses and when there are missing data. New techniques based on hierarchical models adequately model differential growth among participants, the nesting of participants within schools, and inclusion of partially missing data. Such analyses now reflect state-of-the-art prevention evaluation. Conditional and unconditional models can be used to estimate program effects when there is incomplete randomization. The analysis of mediating variables which was described is likely to increase understanding of the mechanisms of program effects. Finally, future developments in statistical analyses of drug prevention studies were considered. In the discussion of the new statistical advances, it is important to keep in mind that the usefulness of statistical methods rests on the quality of the data collected, the research design, and on the truth of the substantive theory.

REFERENCES

(1999). http://www.vic.edu/~hedecker/mix.html.

(1999). http://yates.coph.usf.edu/research/psmg/index.html.

Agresti, A. (1990). *Categorical data analysis.* New York: Wiley.

Aiken, L. S., & West, S. G. (1991). *Multiple regression: Testing and interpreting interactions* Newbury Park, CA: Sage Publications.

Arbuckle, J. L. (1995). *Amos user's guide.* Chicago: Small Waters.

Barcikowski, R. S. (1982). Statistical power with group mean as the unit of analysis. *Journal of Educational Statistics, 6,* 267–285.

Baron, R. M., & Kenny, D. A. (1986). The moderator-mediator distinction in social psychological research: Conceptual, strategic, and statistical considerations. *Journal of Personality and Social Psychology, 51,* 1173–1182.

Basch, C. E. (1984). Research on disseminating and implementing health education programs in schools. *Journal of School Health, 54,* 57–66.

Bentler, P. M. (1980). Multivariate analysis with latent variables: Causal modeling. *Annual Review of Psychology, 31,* 419–456.

Bentler, P. M. (1989). *Theory and implementation of EQS: A structural relations program.* Los Angeles: BMDP Statistical Software.

Berk, R. A. (1988). Causal inference for sociological data. In N. J. Smelser (Ed.), *Handbook of sociology* (pp. 157–172). Newbury Park, CA: Sage.

Biglan, A., Severson, H., Ary, D. V., Faller, C., Gallison, C., Thompson, R., Glasgow, R., & Lichtenstein, E. (1987). Do smoking prevention programs really work? Attrition and the internal and external validity of an evaluation of a refusal skills training program. *Journal of Behavioral Medicine, 10,* 159–171.

Bishop, Y. M. M., Fienberg, S. E., & Holland, P. W. (1975). *Discrete multivariate analysis.* Cambridge, MA: MIT Press.

Blalock, H. M. (1969). *Theory construction: From verbal to mathematical formulations.* Englewood Cliffs, NJ: Prentice–Hall.

Bollen, K. A. (1989). *Structural equations with latent variables.* New York: Wiley.

Bonett, D. G., Brecht, M. L., & Woodward, J. A. (1985). GENLOG II: A general log-linear model program for the personal computer. *Educational and Psychological Measurement, 45,* 617–621.

Bryk, A. S., & Raudenbush, S. W. (1992). *Hierarchical linear models. Applications and data analysis methods.* Newbury Park, CA: Sage.

Campbell, D. T., & Fiske, D. W. (1959). Convergent and discriminant validation by the multitrait multimethod matrix. *Psychological Bulletin, 56*(2), 81–105.

Cohen, J. (1988). *Statistical power analysis for the behavioral sciences.* Hillsdale, NJ: Lawrence Erlbaum.

Cohen, J. (1990). Things I have learned (so far). *American Psychologist, 45,* 1304–1312.

Colton, T. (1974). *Statistics in medicine.* Boston: Little, Brown.

Cook, T. D., & Campbell, D. T. (1979). *Quasi-experimentation: Design and analysis issues for field settings.* Chicago: Rand McNally.

Crocker, L., & Algina, J. (1986). Introduction to classical and modern test theory. New York: Harcourt Brace Jovanovich.

Davis, M. D. (1985). *The logic of causal order. Series: Quantitative applications in the social sciences.* Beverly Hills, CA: Sage.

deLeeuw, J., & Kreft, I. G. G. (1986). Random coefficient models for multilevel research. *Journal of Educational Statistics, 11,* 57–86.

Dwyer, J. H. (1981). The excluded variable problem in non-randomized control group designs. *Evaluation Review, 8,* 559–572.

Dwyer, J. H., MacKinnon, D. P., Pentz, M. A., Flay, B. R., Hansen, W. B., Wang, E., & Johnson, C. A. (1989). Estimating intervention effects in longitudinal studies. *American Journal of Epidemiology, 130*(4), 781–795.

Dunn, G. (1989). *Design and analysis of reliability studies.* New York: Oxford.

Efron, B. (1982). *The jackknife, the bootstrap, and other resampling plans.* Philadelphia, PA: SIAM.

Fuller, W. A. (1987). *Measurement error models.* New York: Wiley.

Gold, M. R., Siegel, J. E., Russell, L. B., & Weinstein M. C. (1996), *Cost-effectiveness in health and medicine.* New York: Oxford University Press.

Graham, J. W., & Donaldson, S. I. (1993). Evaluating interventions with differential attrition: The importance of nonresponse mechanisms and use of follow-up data. *Journal of Applied Psychology, 78*(1), 119–128.

Graham, J. W., Hofer, S. M., Donaldson, S. I., MacKinnon, D. P., & Schafer, J. L. (1997). Analysis with missing data in prevention research. In K. J. Bryant, M. Windle, & S. G. West. *The science of prevention: methodological advances from alcohol and substance abuse research.* Washington, DC: American Psychological Association.

Haggard, E. A. (1958). *Intraclass correlation and the analysis of variance.* New York: Dryden Press.

Hansen, W. B. (1992). School-based substance abuse prevention: review of the state of the art in curriculum, 1980–1990. *Health Education Research, 7*(3), 403–430.

Hansen, W. B., Collins, L. M., Malotte, C. K., Johnson, C. A., & Fielding, J. E. (1985). Attrition in prevention research. *Journal of Behavioral Medicine, 8,* 261–275.

Harrison, L., & Hughes, A. (1997). The validity of self-reported drug use: Improving the accuracy of survey estimates. *NIDA Research Monograph 167,* Rockville, MD: National Institutes of Health.

Hayduk, L. A. (1987). *Structural equation modeling with LISREL: Essentials and advances.* Baltimore: The John Hopkins University Press.

Hays, W. L. (1988). *Statistics* (4th edition). New York: Holt, Rinehart, & Winston.

Heckman, J. J. (1989). Causal inference and nonrandom samples. *Journal of Educational Statistics, 14,* 159–168.

Hedecker, D., Gibbons, R. D., & Flay, B. R. (1994). Random effects regression models for clustered data with an example from smoking prevention research. *Journal of Consulting and Clinical Psychology, 62,* 757–765.

Hopkins, K. D. (1981). The unit of analysis: group means versus individual observations. *American Education Research Journal, 19,* 5–18.

Hosmer, D. W., & Lemeshow, S. (2000). Applied logistic regression analysis. New York: Wiley.

Hosmer, D. W., & Lemeshow, S. (1999). Applied survival analysis: Regression modeling of time to event data. New York: Wiley.

Johnston, L. D., Bachman, J. G., & O'Malley, P. M. (1997). *Monitoring the future: Questionnaire responses from the nation's high school seniors, 1995.* Ann Arbor, MI: Institute for Social Research.

Joreskog, K. G., & Sorbom, D. (1988). *LISREL VII.* Chicago: SPSS Inc.

Judd, C. M., & Kenny, D. A. (1981). *Estimating the effects of social interventions.* New York: Cambridge University Press.

Keppel, G. (1991). Design and analysis: A researcher's handbook. Englewood, NJ: Prentice Hall.

Keppel, G., & Zedeck, S. (1989). *Data analysis for research designs.* New York: Freeman.

Kirk, R. E. (1982). *Experimental design: Procedures for the social sciences.* Belmont, CA: Brooks/Cole.

Koch, G., Singer, J., & Stokes, M. (1992). Some aspects of weighted-least-squares analysis for longitudinal categorical data. In J. H. Dwyer, P. Lippert, & H. Hoffmeister (Eds.), *Statistical models for longitudinal studies of health.* New York: Oxford University Press.

Kraemer, H., & Thiemann, S. (1987). *How many subjects?* Newbury Park, CA: Sage.

Krull, J., & MacKinnon, D. P. (1999). Multilevel mediation modeling in group-based intervention studies. *Evaluation Review, 23*(4), 418–444.

Little, R. J. A., & Rubin, D. B. (1987). *Statistical analysis with missing data.* New York: Wiley.

Little, R. J. A., & Rubin, D. B. (1989). The analysis of social science data with missing values. *Sociological Methods and Research, 18,* 292–326.

Little, R. J. A., & Yau, L. (1996). Intent-to-treat analysis for longitudinal studies with drop-outs. *Biometrics, 52*(4), 1324–1333.

MacKinnon, D. P. (2000). Contrasts in multiple mediator models. In J. Rose, L. Chassin, C. C. Presson, & S. J. Sherman (Eds.), *Multivariate applications in substance use research*: New methods for new questions (pp. 141–160). Mahwah, NJ: Erlbaum.

MacKinnon, D. P., & Dwyer, J. H. (1993). Estimating mediated effects in prevention studies. *Evaluation Review, 17*(2), 144–158.

MacKinnon, D. P., Johnson, C. A., Pentz, M. A., Dwyer, J. H., Hansen, W. B., Flay, B. R., & Wang, E. (1991). Mediating mechanisms in a school-based drug prevention program: First year effects of the Midwestern Prevention Project. *Health Psychology, 10,* 164–172.

MacKinnon, D., Krull, J. L., & Lockwood, C. M. (2000). Equivalence of the mediation, confounding, and suppression effect. *Prevention Science, 4,* 173–181.

MacKinnon, D. P., Warsi, G., & Dwyer, J. H. (1995). A simulation study of mediated effect measures. *Multivariate Behavioral Research, 30*(1), 41–62.

Maxwell, S. W. (1998). Longitudinal designs in randomized group comparisons: When will intermediate observations increase statistical power? *Psychological Methods, 3*(3), 275–290.

McCaul, K. D., & Glasgow, R. E. (1985). Preventing adolescent smoking: What have we learned about treatment construct validity? *Health Psychology, 4,* 361–387.

Meinert, C. L. (1986). Clinical trials: Design, conduct, and analysis. *Monographs in Epidemiology and biostatistics 8.* New York: Oxford.

Mulvenon, S. W. (1992). *Analytic formula for power analysis in repeated measures designs.* Arizona State University: Unpublished doctoral dissertation.

Murray, D. M. (1998). *Design and analysis of group-randomized trials.* New York: Oxford University Press.

Murray, D. M., & Hannan, P. J. (1990). Planning for the appropriate analysis in school-based drug-use prevention studies. *Journal of Consulting and Clinical Psychology, 58,* 458–468.

Murray, D. M., Hannan, P. J., Wolfinger, R. D., Baker, W. L., & Dwyer, J. H. (1998). Analysis of data from group-randomized trials with repeat observations on the same groups. *Statistics in Medicine, 17,* 1581–1600.

Muthén, L. K., & Muthén B. O. (1998). *Mplus: Analysis of linear structural equations with a comprehensive measurement model.* Mooresville, IN: Scientific Software.

Oetting, E. R., & Beauvais, F. (1990). Adolescent drug use: Findings of national and local surveys. *Journal of Consulting and Clinical Psychology, 58*(4), 385–394.

Pentz, M. A., Trebow, E. A., Hansen, W. B., MacKinnon, D. P., Dwyer, J. H., & Johnson, C. A. (1990). Effects of program implementation on adolescent drug use behavior: The Midwestern Prevention Project (MPP). *Evaluation Review, 14*(3), 264–289.

Rindskopf, D. (1992). A general approach to categorical data analysis with missing data, using generalized linear models with composite links. *Psychometrika, 57*(1), 29–42.

SAS/STAT Guide for personal computers, Version 6, (1987). Cary, NC: SAS Institute Inc.

Schafer, J. L. (1997). *Analysis of incomplete multivariate data.* New York: Chapman & Hall/CRC Press.

Sechrest, L., & Hanna, M. (1990). The critical importance of nonexperimental data. In L. Sechrest, E. Perrin, & J. Bunker (Eds.), *Research methodology: Strengthening causal interpretations of nonexperimental data* (pp. 1–7). Washington, DC: U.S. Department of Health and Human Services.

Siddiqui, O., Flay, B. R., & Hu, F. B. (1996). Factors affecting attrition in longitudinal smoking prevention study. *Preventive medicine, 25*(5), 554–560.

Sobel, M. E. (1982). Asymptotic confidence intervals for indirect effects in structural equation models. In S. Leinhardt (Ed.), *Sociological methodology* (pp. 290–293). Washington, DC: American Sociological Association.

Sobel, M. E. (1986). Some new results on indirect effects and their standard errors in covariance structure models. In N. Tuma (Ed.), *Sociological methodology* (pp. 159–186). Washington, DC: American Sociological Association.

SPSS Advanced Statistics V2.0 (1988). Chicago: SPSS, Inc.

Stoolmiller, M., Duncan, T., Bank, L., & Patterson, G. R. (1993). Some problems and solutions in the study of change: Significant patterns in client resistance. *Journal of Consulting and Clinical Psychology, 61,* 920–928.

Virdin, L. (1992). A test of the robustness of estimators that model selection in the non-equivalent control group design. Arizona State University, Unpublished doctoral dissertation.

Wells-Parker, E., Bangert-Drowns, R., McMillen, R., & Williams, M. (1995). Final results from a meta-analysis of remedial interventions with drink/drive offenders. *Addiction, 90,* 907–926.

Werthamer, L., & Chatterji, P. (1999). *Preventive intervention cost-effectiveness and cost benefit literature review.* National Institute on Drug Abuse's Resource Center for Health Services Research.

West, S., & Aiken, L. (1997). Toward understanding individual effects in multicomponent prevention programs: Design and analysis strategies. In K. J. Bryant, M. Windle, & S. G. West (Eds.), *The science of prevention: Methodological advances from alcohol and substance abuse research* (pp. 167–209). Washington, DC: American Psychological Association.

Wilcox, R. R. (1987). *New statistical procedures for the social sciences: Modern solutions to basic problems.* Hillsdale, NJ: Erlbaum.

Willett, J. B., & Sayer, A. G. (1994). Using covariance structure analysis to detect correlates and predictors of individual change over time. *Psychological Bulletin, 116,* 363–381.

Winer, B. J., Brown, D. R., & Michels, K. M. (1991). *Statistical principles in experimental design* (3rd edition). New York: McGraw–Hill.

Winship, C., & Mare, R. D. (1983). Structural equations and path analysis for discrete data. *American Journal of Sociology, 89,* 54–110.

Woodward, J. A., Bonett, D. G., & Brecht, M. L. (1990). *Introduction to linear models and experimental design.* New York: Harcourt, Brace, Jovanovich.

Zeger, S. L., Liang, K.-Y., & Albert, P. S. (1988). Models for longitudinal data: A generalized estimating equation approach. *Biometrics, 44,* 1049–1060.

CHAPTER 28

Methodological Considerations in Prevention Research

LINDA M. COLLINS
BRIAN P. FLAHERTY

INTRODUCTION

Methodology, the study of research design, measurement, and statistical analysis, is an important area of prevention science. And like the rest of the field, prevention methodology is interdisciplinary. It embraces two distinct traditions: the social sciences, in which theory and a priori prediction are of paramount importance, and epidemiology, in which careful sampling in order to achieve representativeness is a prime concern. This chapter explores a number of methodological considerations spanning prevention methodology's dual traditions. It is not an exhaustive survey of methodological issues but does raise some issues that are particularly important and should be thought about by anyone doing prevention intervention research. It addresses the importance of theory in prevention research, issues surrounding the measurement of a single variable, and the measurement of and relationships among multiple variables.

THE ROLE OF THEORY AND MODELS

Researchers undertaking a prevention intervention project have many decisions to make, including how many subjects to sample, how to measure key constructs, and how frequently and when to

LINDA M. COLLINS AND BRIAN P. FLAHERTY • The Methodology Center and Department of Human Development, The Pennsylvania State University, University Park, Pennsylvania 16802

collect data. These decisions will have profound implications for how the study will be conducted and, in some cases, on what kinds of results are likely to be found. Perhaps nothing is more important than ensuring that these decisions be guided by a single, consistent set of operating principles and that these principles stem from the fundamental research questions that motivated the study in the first place. This can be accomplished by allowing a model of the process to guide these decisions, as described in Collins (1994).

All good prevention intervention research is theory driven. A researcher starts with a theory about how the problem behavior, say drug use, comes about. That is, the theory details the specific risk factors that increase the probability of drug use and the specific protective factors that decrease the probability of drug use. A researcher then elaborates on the theory to include details of how an intervention with certain specific components acts on the risk and protective factors to reduce risk of drug use. A model is an operational definition of a theory. Collins (1994) lists some of the issues that should be addressed by a model of the drug abuse onset process and how a prevention program impacts it:

- Which levels are involved in the process. (The term "level" refers to a cluster of study participants that has its own characteristics, such as a family, school, or classroom. Usually, the individual is considered a level.)
- The levels at which the intervention is expected to show effectiveness, and why.
- The levels that are expected to interact with the intervention or other variables.
- Whether change is characterized by continuous, quantitative growth is either expressed better in terms of discrete stages or incorporates features of both.
- Whether growth is steadily upward or downward, or not steadily in either direction.
- Whether the process of growth is the same for all subjects, or whether there are subgroups that exhibit different characteristics of growth.
- How quickly or slowly the process unfolds, and the interindividual heterogeneity in these rates.
- The exact relationship between putative causal variables and substance use.
- Whether causation is instantaneous or whether the effect takes place after a period of time.
- Whether there is a certain point in the process at which an effect can take place, for example, a developmental window of some kind.
- Whether important causal variables differ across groups, particularly naturally occurring groups, such as gender or ethnicity.
- The exact mechanism or mechanisms by which the intervention operates.
- How each variable is to be measured.

In other words, all the specifics of a theory about substance use and how it can be prevented should be specified in the model associated with the theory. Once the model has been developed, other decisions stem directly from it. For example, hypotheses stem from theory. However, the choice of analytic techniques and of specific variables required to test each hypothesis follows from the model. [For examples of prevention-related analyses closely guided by theory, see Donaldson, Graham, and Hansen (1994); Hansen et al., (1988); Hansen and Graham (1991).] In the sections that follow, a number of methodological considerations are raised, some of which require decisions on the part of the investigator. A clearly specified model can be an enormous help in making these decisions.

MEASUREMENT OF A SINGLE VARIABLE

Reliability and Validity

This section reviews some basic concepts of measurement and discusses more advanced issues. First, it is necessary to define the term "construct." Vogt (1993, p. 44) defines a construct as "something that exists theoretically but is not directly observable." Every measurement instrument is intended to measure a particular construct, such as adolescent alcohol use, psychological distress, or perceived norms about substance use. The two criteria by which a measure is evaluated are validity, the extent to which it measures the construct it is intended to measure, and precision. Precision can be operationalized in different ways depending on the measurement theory framework being used. In most cases, a classical test–theory framework or a related framework is used, and precision is operationalized as measurement reliability (Lord & Novick, 1968).

Within the classical test–theory framework, every observed score is made up of two components: a true score and random error. These two components are uncorrelated, so the observed variance of a measure is made up solely of true score variance and random error variance, with no term needed for the covariance of the two:

$$\sigma_X^2 = \sigma_T^2 + \sigma_E^2$$

The idea of a true score stems from the notion of a propensity distribution, a hypothetical distribution of an individual's scores that would be obtained if the individual took a test over and over an infinite number of times, with absolutely no carry-over effects of any kind and no learning over time. The average for an individual across this distribution is the true score. Reliability is defined as the proportion of observed score variance in a measure that is attributable to true score variance:

$$Reliability = \frac{\sigma_T^2}{\sigma_X^2}$$

This formula shows that reliability depends partly on the amount of true score variance. Thus, reliability is not solely a property of an instrument. Rather, it is a property of an instrument *in relation to a target population,* a property that can and will vary across populations. Given a fixed error variance, an instrument will be less reliable in a population with less true score variance than it will be in a population with more true score variance. Researchers should keep this in mind when assessing reliability. It is important to base a reliability study on a sample of the population in which the instrument is to be used.

Researchers often want to know if there is a minimum acceptable reliability. As is so often the case in statistics and in methodology, this is a judgment call. Nunnally and Bernstein (1994) point out that the standard varies depending on the use to which the instrument is to be put. For an instrument that is to be used in research, they recommend a reliability of at least .70 during the formative stages of the project. If the line of research appears promising, they recommend trying to improve the instrument to bring it up to a reliability of at least .80. An instrument that is to be used to make decisions about individuals, such as which individuals should be referred to a remedial reading program, should have a reliability of not less than .90.

However, it is a mistake to evaluate an instrument solely in terms of reliability. Validity is equally important. It is possible for an instrument to be highly reliable, even perfectly reliable, and to have no validity. To see why, consider the meaning of the term "true score," which is a bit of a misnomer. The score is not true in the sense that it is necessarily a true reflection of the construct it is intended to measure. In fact, true score variance is composed of valid variance, and invalid variance:

$$\sigma_T^2 = \sigma_{VALID}^2 + \sigma_{INVALID}^2$$

Valid variance is true score variance that is shared with the construct that the instrument is intended to measure. Invalid variance is true score variance, but it is not shared with the construct of interest. For example, consider an instrument intended to measure adolescent alcohol use. In this case, the instrument's valid variance is that variance shared with actual adolescent alcohol use. An example of invalid variance would be variance shared with perceptions of friends' use of alcohol. To the extent that the instrument is measuring perceptions of friends' use of alcohol, it is invalid, even if it is measuring the perceptions well, because this is not the construct that the instrument is intended to measure.

Because high reliability is no guarantee of validity, it is essential to demonstrate validity empirically. Depending on the situation, there are numerous ways to demonstrate validity. [For a discussion of this, see Pedhazur & Schmelkin (1991).] The strongest argument is made by demonstrating validity in a variety of contexts and by a variety of means. *Concurrent validity* is demonstrated by showing that the instrument correlates with another measure of the construct taken at the same time; *predictive validity* is demonstrated by showing that the instrument can be used to predict some meaningful quantity measured in the future; *convergent validity* is demonstrated by showing that the instrument correlates with other measures of the same construct that use very different methods; and *discriminant validity* is demonstrated by showing that the instrument does not correlate with measures of different constructs that use the same methods (Campbell & Fiske, 1959; Pedhazur & Schmelkin, 1991). A particularly strong argument for validity can be made if *construct validity* is demonstrated. Construct validity is demonstrated by making *a priori* theoretical predictions about a construct and then showing empirically that the instrument's behavior is consistent with the prediction. For example, if an instrument is intended to measure growth in a construct, then the instrument should show change over time.

Validity and Reliability across Cultural Groups

One consideration in prevention research is measurement in cross-cultural contexts, specifically whether instruments are reliable and, in particular, valid for different cultural groups. Unfortunately, there are no clear-cut answers in this important area. In order for measurement of any psychological or sociological construct to make sense, we have to make a fundamental assumption that the human experience, although it is in part unique to each individual, is structured the same for all individuals so that comparisons can be made. For example, when we measure rebelliousness in two adolescents, we are implicitly assuming that even if the adolescents differ in the *amount* of rebelliousness they have, rebelliousness is *the same thing* for each adolescent, and, therefore, it makes sense to compare their scores on rebelliousness. When we find that one has a high score and the other has a low score, we assume the scores are along the same continuum. Cross-cultural measurement tests the limits of this assumption. It asks: How much of the human experience is structured essentially the same for all humanity, how much of it is structured the same within groups but differently across groups, and how much of it is completely individual?

One issue arises when a single instrument is used in different cultural groups, ethnic groups, or even genders. The question is whether the instrument is equally valid for all groups or, put another way, whether the construct measured by the instrument is the same across groups. If the construct is the same, it is said that *factorial invariance* holds. This issue is usually addressed by using factor analysis to examine the data for evidence of the degree of factorial invariance (or lack of invariance). There is a long literature on procedures for establishing factorial invariance (Cunningham, 1991; Horn, 1991; Meredith, 1964a,b, 1965; Widaman & Reise, 1997). The most convincing evidence for factorial invariance is when the number of factors, factor loadings, and correlations among factors are identical across groups. Then it can be assumed that the structure is essentially the same across groups. It becomes clear that the factor structure is different across groups when a factor analysis suggests different numbers of factors across groups, or if the factor loadings are very different across groups. Under these conditions, it is difficult to know what to do. The choices are to try either to find enough common ground so that a single instrument can be selected that measures the same construct across groups or to abandon the idea of measuring the same construct across groups and develop different instruments.

If there is a core set of items that appears to define the construct for both groups, and other items that appear to figure differently in the construct across groups, one option is to remove the items that behave differently across groups and go with a reduced set of items. If the number of items to be removed is small, this can be a good strategy. However, in some cases so many items are removed that the construct that has little meaning for either group. In other words, this approach can trade validity for cross-group comparability.

Another approach is to give up on the idea of finding a single construct that has the same meaning across groups. Instead, instruments can be tailor-made for each group. The advantage of this approach is that it is possible to arrive at highly valid and reliable instruments within each group. The disadvantage is that it is almost impossible to make comparisons across groups. Whether this is a reasonable strategy depends on how important direct comparisons across groups are in a particular research setting.

Although the idea of tailoring measures to particular ethnic groups has some appeal, it may be a futile effort, at least in the United States. For example, while Latinos are often lumped together as a single group, within this group there are Mexicans, Central Americans, South Americans, Cubans, etc. There are many important cultural differences among these groups. Add to this the issue of acculturation, and a separate instrument may be needed for individuals born in the United States as opposed to those who immigrated here. Many Latinos born in the United States identify strongly with their parents, country, but have only limited ability to speak Spanish. For them it is necessary to have an English version of any instrument. Another problem is that many individuals in the United States identify with more than one ethnic group. It would be impossible to maintain enough versions of an instrument to accommodate each of these groups, even if it were desirable to do so. So the question comes back to the one posed at the beginning of this section: What is common across the human experience, and what is not? Only when this question is answered will it be possible to arrive at procedures for effective cross-cultural measurement.

DEALING WITH THE COMPLEXITIES
OF CHANGE OVER TIME: MEASUREMENT

This section discusses the idea of measurement reliability as an operational definition of measurement precision. This idea is based on a concept of the true score as *static,* or unchanging. This made sense in the context of intelligence and achievement testing in which these ideas were originally developed. However, it makes less sense in much of today's drug abuse prevention research. Prevention research frequently needs to measure changing, or *dynamic,* constructs. Examples of dynamic constructs abound in drug abuse research and include adolescent attitudes toward substance use, beliefs about normative trends in substance use, and substance use itself. In general, when researchers set about to measure dynamic constructs, they use traditional, mostly classical test-theory-based approaches. However, Collins and Cliff (1990; Collins, 1996) point out that there are serious shortcomings associated with using classical test-theory-based approaches to developing instruments to measure dynamic constructs. A major issue is that the formula for reliability (see previous) is based solely on within-time, interindividual variability. Yet when dynamic constructs are measured, the researcher is interested either in across-time, intraindividual variability, or in how each individual varies across time. This quantity does not enter into the traditional definition of reliability at all. Thus, this definition of reliability is poorly suited to measures of change over time. In fact, in cases in which there is little interindividual variability within each time, but measurable intraindividual variability across times, it is possible for a highly precise measure of change to be unreliable according to the traditional definition (see Collins & Cliff, 1990).

Unfortunately, there are still no widely used procedures for developing instruments specifically for measuring change across time. One avenue that appears promising is use of item-response-theory approaches to measurement of change (Embretson, 1991a,b; Fischer & Ponocny, 1994). With this approach it is possible to build in the idea of a changing true score, or "theta," as it is referred to. Another approach is growth curve modeling. Willett (1989) discusses how to assess the reliability of an instrument that measures a growth curve. Researchers who continue to use classical test-theory approaches for developing measures of change should remember to interpret their results with caution.

Another important issue in measurement of dynamic constructs comes up when aspects of the construct itself change over time. There are many constructs relevant to drug abuse prevention that change in how they manifest themselves over time. Temperament is one. This is a fairly stable characteristic of individuals, yet the same measure of temperament cannot be used from infancy to adulthood. How to develop a series of instruments that links age-appropriate measures of characteristics across the life span is a fascinating challenge for the field of drug abuse prevention and the social sciences in general.

RELATIONSHIPS AMONG CONSTRUCTS AND OVER TIME

Statistical Power

Statistical power is the probability of finding significant results, given that there truly is an effect to be detected. This is a critically important consideration in all prevention intervention research. For example, suppose a researcher proposes a new drug abuse prevention approach and requests a large sum of money to carry out an evaluation of the approach. Further, suppose that a power analysis shows that the probability of detecting the effect of this new approach, if the approach is in fact effective, is .20. Now suppose that the money is spent to carry out the study, and the difference between the program and the control groups is insignificant. Can it be concluded that the program is truly ineffective? Or, should it be concluded that even if the prevention approach were effective, the study had a slim chance of detecting this, and so no conclusion is possible? In a case like this, it might be better not to invest money until measures are taken to increase statistical power.

Statistical power is a function of three considerations, only two of which are really under the influence of the experimenter. One consideration is the alpha level of the statistical test. All else being equal, an increase in alpha will increase statistical power. Theoretically, a researcher can choose any alpha, but nobody ever increases alpha larger than the highly arbitrary .05 level, so realistically this is not a factor that will be changed by the experimenter in most cases. The second consideration is sample size, with a larger sample size increasing statistical power. This is usually under the direct control of the researcher. However, sometimes financial or practical considerations limit the sample size, or certain kinds of study participants may be in short supply, such as individuals suffering from rare diseases.

Effect Size

The third consideration is effect size, with larger effects associated with greater statistical power. Most researchers do not think of effect size as something that is under their direct control. However, a researcher can exert considerable influence on effect size, thereby increasing statistical power without increasing sample size (Hansen & Collins, 1994). For a simple two-group ANOVA-type design, effect size is defined as

$$Effect\ Size\ =\ \frac{\mu_A - \mu_B}{\sigma}$$

The numerator of the previous equation is the difference between the population mean for Group A and that for Group B. The denominator is the population variance. Strategies to increase effect size usually focus on increasing the difference between groups or reducing population variance. As Hansen and Collins (1994) discuss, the magnitude of group differences can be maximized by careful theory-driven targeting of appropriate mediators in prevention studies, by maintaining program integrity throughout the research project, and by appropriate timing of follow-up observations in a longitudinal study. Population variance can be minimized by careful sampling procedures and by increasing measurement reliability, provided that reliability is increased by reducing measurement error and not by increasing true score variance (see Zimmerman & Williams, 1986). The important point to remember is that even if the sample size has a strict upper limit due to finances, logistics, or sheer availability of subjects, it is still possible to take measurements that will help increase statistical power.

Significance and Effect Size

Sometimes a particular effect is significant, but it is not meaningful because it is very small. This can occur when the sample size is very large, and it is possible for a relatively small effect size to attain significance. A distinction is sometimes drawn between statistical significance and clinical significance. For example, a prevention program might be shown to produce a statistically significant delay in the onset of alcohol use, but if the delay is only 1 month, this is unlikely to be of any clinical significance in terms of later alcohol abuse and dependence problems. It is important always to evaluate a statistically significant effect for clinical or real-world significance, particularly when a large sample size is involved.

A related problem is that when very large sample sizes are involved, statistically significant results are almost inevitable, or that significance is reached merely because of the size of the sample. In thinking through this, it is important to draw a distinction between Type I and Type II errors. It is true that given a fixed alpha level and a NONZERO effect size, the probability of detecting the effect is greater for a larger sample size. In other words, the probability of a Type II error, failing to detect a true effect, decreases. However, increasing the sample size does not increase the probability of a Type I error, i.e., of mistakenly concluding that there is an effect when in reality there is none. In short, a larger sample size will produce significant effects based on smaller effect sizes, but it does not increase the probability of spurious significant findings.

DEALING WITH THE COMPLEXITIES
OF CHANGE OVER TIME: DATA ANALYSIS

Traditionally, the most widely used approach for dealing with change over time has been repeated measures ANOVA, but there are exciting alternatives that have conceptual appeal. Three such alternatives are growth curve modeling, survival analysis, and latent transition analysis.

Growth Curve Modeling

Growth curve modeling is suitable when three or more observations in time are obtained. Growth curve modeling addresses questions such as: Is overall growth characterized as linear or quadratic? Is growth related to individual differences, such as beliefs about social norms concerning substance use? Is growth related to group-level variables, such as experimental treatment condition? Growth curve modeling (Bryk & Raudenbush, 1987; Collins & Sayer, 2000; Curran, Harford, & Muthen, 1997; Duncan, Duncan, & Hops, 1996; Willett & Sayer, 1994) provides an alternative to repeated measures ANOVA and is much more congruent with the way most researchers think about change. In growth curve modeling, variables are modeled as a function of time. In other words, if the data are plotted, time is the X axis and the variable being modeled is the Y axis. In growth curve modeling, the occasions of measurement do not have to be equally spaced. With time itself an explicit part of the model, variability in the spacing of occasions of measurement is taken into account. In some approaches to growth curve modeling, the number and spacing of occasions of measurement can even vary across individuals.

In the growth curve framework, a growth curve is modeled for each individual. One overall model must be chosen, but the parameters of this model can vary for individuals. For example, if the overall model is linear, then a slope parameter and an intercept parameter are estimated for each individual. These slope and intercept parameters then can be related to other individual and group level variables. Suppose the onset of drug use is modeled as an individual level growth curve using a linear model. The intercept represents where the individual is at whatever time point is coded as zero. This is arbitrary to an extent, but suppose the initial time point is coded as zero. Then the intercept represents an individual's level of drug use at the outset, and the slope represents the rate of linear change over time. Now, suppose this is part of an intervention study in which there are treatment and control groups. Pretest differences between groups can be examined by looking at the intercepts. Program effectiveness can be examined by looking at slope differences. In a prevention intervention study, we would expect that the slope for the experimental treatment group would be smaller than the slope for the control group, indicating that the experimental group is taking up drug use at a slower rate than is the control group.

A question that often comes up in longitudinal research is whether there is a relationship between initial status and growth. This can be examined in a growth curve framework by looking at the correlation between the intercept parameter and the slope parameter. If this correlation is large and positive, it means that initial status is associated with more growth—a rich-get-richer scenario. If this correlation is large and negative, it means that those who start low on the dependent variable tend to grow more. Although this can represent a genuine effect, as when a deprived group gains more from an enrichment program than do those who are better off initially, it can also be caused by ceiling effects. If the correlation is small or zero, it suggests that there is little or no relationship between initial status and growth.

Two approaches for growth curve models are in wide use. One is latent growth curve modeling, in which a growth curve is fit with a statistical package, such as LISREL. The model is set up so that the slope and intercept parameters are estimated as factor scores. The other approach is to use a program for hierarchical models such as HLM. In this approach, the measures across time are considered nested within the individual. For many applications, these two approaches are identical. For others, which approach is better depends upon the exact application. In particular, HLM can handle designs in which individuals have been measured at different times and/or a different number of times.

For examples of the use of growth curve modeling in prevention research, see Duncan et al. (1998, 1991), Duncan and Duncan (1996), Curran, Harford, and Muthen (1997), and Sayer and Willett (1998).

Survival Analysis

Survival analysis may be appropriate when there are research questions about a discrete event, such as using a drug for the first time, relapsing after quitting, and so on. This approach addresses questions such as: On average, did the experimental treatment group try alcohol later than the control group? Did the age at which alcohol was tried relate to other individual or group-level variables? Survival analysis (Willett & Singer, 1991) has been widely used for years in epidemiology and is starting to gain more attention in prevention research (Bacik, Murphy, & Anthony, 1998; Siddiqui, Flay, & Hu, 1996; Stevens & Hollis, 1989). Survival analysis models the length of time until some event takes place. For example, survival analysis can be used to model the length of time until a first experience with tobacco. Independent variables, such as experimental condition, reported intentions to try tobacco, and so on, can be included. The independent variables may be time-varying. Survival analysis produces an extremely useful function known as the hazard function, which estimates the probability of the event as a function of time, given that the event has not already occurred. In a prevention study, a hazard function might provide the probability of a child trying tobacco for the first time as a function of age. The information contained in the hazard function can help in fine-tuning prevention programs. For example, if the hazard function shows that there is an age that is particularly risky for some type of substance use, it may be possible to use this information to schedule a booster session at that age.

Latent Transition Analysis

Latent transition analysis (LTA) is suitable for discrete variables that can be cross-tabulated and that have been measured at two or more times. It allows the user to develop models of stage sequences over time, for example, sequences of substances, and to examine whether progress through a sequence differs for an experimental treatment group compared to a control group. There are times when it makes sense to think of prevention-related variables as stage sequential. For example, the beginning of the substance use onset process can be thought of as a series of stages, with each substance being a stage (e.g., Collins et al., 1997). LTA (Collins & Wugalter, 1992) is a method for estimating and testing stage-sequential latent variable models. LTA takes as input categorical longitudinal data. In a model-testing framework, it allows the user to estimate the prevalence of stages and the incidence of stage transitions, adjusted for measurement error. It also allows the user to examine group differences in prevalence and incidence. For example, Hyatt and Collins (2000) modeled a stage-sequential onset process in which young adolescents first tried either tobacco or alcohol. From tobacco, adolescents next tried alcohol; from alcohol they tried either tobacco or had a first experience with drunkenness. Adolescents who progressed from there went on to try marijuana and then cocaine. Hyatt and Collins (2000) examined differences between adolescents who perceived their parents as permissive toward adolescent alcohol use and those who did not perceive their parents as permissive in this way. They found that adolescents who perceived their parents as permissive were more likely to have tried every substance.

LTA offers several features that are helpful to the prevention field. Because it takes a stage-sequential approach, it is possible to take a very fine-grained look at change over time, by examining change in terms of movement from one stage to another. This can reveal subtle differences that are important in prevention research, such as the finding by Graham et al. (1991) that adolescents who started their substance use experience with tobacco moved into the next stage of the onset process relatively quickly and were unaffected by a prevention program that showed otherwise significant results. LTA can help prevention researchers pinpoint where in the onset process a program is effective and where it is not, and also where in the onset process risk factors have their effects. LTA also has the advantage of examining change conditional on status at the previous time, eliminating the need for partialing out or controlling this. (Software to perform LTA analyses, called WinLTA, is available at http://methodology.psu.edu/)

THE TRAIT-STATE DISTINCTION

For more than 6 decades (Allport & Odbert, 1936), psychologists have attempted to disentangle relatively stable, enduring personal characteristics (called traits) and transitory, situational feelings and behaviors (called states). The trait–state distinction has been critical in many areas of psychological research, such as anxiety and emotion. Recently, structural equation models (SEM) employing the trait–state distinction have surfaced in the prevention literature (Dumenci & Windle, 1996; Windle, 1997) and elsewhere.

Distilling many years of work, Fridhandler (1986) describes four factors that differentiate traits and states. The first is their duration. Traits are always considered long term; states are short term. The second distinction is that states are continuous while traits are discontinuous. A state is an uninterrupted period of time. For example, if a state of joy is momentarily interrupted with a period of sorrow, three states are experienced: the first period of joy, the period of sorrow, and then the second period of joy. On the other hand, traits are exhibited repeatedly over time, but their expression is not constant. The third factor distinguishing traits from states is that states are observable or experienced, whereas traits are inferred. If a person is happy, he or she knows it because it is directly experienced; it is the current state of the person's feelings. However, a person for whom happiness is a trait is expected to be happy across many situations and times. The trait is inferred from many states. The final distinction between traits and states concerns their source. States are typically considered to be situationally caused, whereas traits are rooted in an individual's psychology. A person may be happy because something good happened earlier in the day. A trait of happiness is a person's tendency to be happy, an aspect of personality. These four distinctions have, in many instances, led to separate sets of measures for traits and states of the same construct. For example, there are separate trait and state anxiety scales.

Recent applications of trait–state ideas in prevention and elsewhere have involved a shift from using separate trait and state measures to decomposing the variance among a collection of items measured longitudinally into trait variance and state variance components via SEM (e.g., Dumenci & Windle, 1996; Windle, 1997). The distinctions between traits and states as outlined by Fridhandler (1986) are less evident using this method. In these current SEM applications, trait variance is defined as interitem covariance, which is stable longitudinally (across measurement periods), and state variance is defined as shared variance at a single measurement period. In other words, a trait is defined as the average of a behavior over time, and a state is defined as a deviation from this average at a particular time. Thus, from the SEM point of view, it is unnecessary to use separate trait measures for traits and state measures for states. To our knowledge, it has not been determined whether this approach yields validity comparable to that obtained when separate trait and state measures are used.

The trait–state distinction is useful to prevention researchers because many behaviors of interest may have both trait and state components. For example, substance use undoubtedly is caused by both personal characteristics (traits) and situational motivations (states). The relative influence of traits and states may be different for different people and at different developmental stages in the life course. Behaviors that are primarily evoked by traits may require a different prevention strategy than behaviors that are primarily evoked by states. Very little is known about the relative influence of trait and state components on substance use. Development of reliable and valid measures of trait substance use and state substance use is the first step to determining whether or not both components exist. If the SEM approach to trait–state research is to become prominent, it is important to establish whether a single instrument can be valid for measuring both a trait and a state.

MISSING DATA

Missing-data problems confront most researchers from time to time. There are two main sources of missing data in prevention research. One is when an individual fails to answer a question on a questionnaire, which may happen because the person does not have sufficient time to answer all the questions, because the question is on a sensitive subject, because the respondent accidentally skipped the question, or for some other reason. The other source of missing data is when an individual is not present for one or more data collection sessions.

Until fairly recently, methodology for dealing with missing data was crude, at best. The most commonly used approach was simply to jettison any respondents with incomplete data, in a procedure often called casewise deletion or listwise deletion. This approach does not have much to recommend it. Throwing out respondents because they have missing data can seriously bias results based on the remaining data, and the reduced sample size can lead to dramatic reductions in statistical power. Many statistical packages offer other approaches to missing data, such as mean substitution, an *ad hoc* procedure with no statistical foundation. Neither casewise deletion (except for trivial amounts of missing data) nor mean substitution has any place in contemporary prevention research.

Thanks to the pioneering work of statisticians, such as that by Little and Rubin (1987) and by Schafer (1997), there are now excellent procedures for dealing with missing data. Although these procedures are commonly called missing data analysis, this is a bit of a misnomer. The term makes people uncomfortable, because it appears to imply that replacements for missing data are somehow being created out of thin air. Although it is probably too late to change the terminology, it would be more accurate to call such procedures partial data analysis. These procedures do not create data where none exist, but make it possible for researchers to use all data contributed by each individual, even individuals who contribute only partial data.

The two main missing-data procedures in use today are maximum-likelihood procedures and multiple imputation. Maximum-likelihood procedures are almost invisible to the user. They automatically adjust parameter estimates for missing data and return unbiased, or considerably less biased, estimates. Multiple imputation is a more general procedure that can be used with any statistical procedure. With multiple imputation, the missing data are predicted based on information in the data that are present. Then, several new data sets are imputed, reintroducing uncertainty into the imputed data by adding a random error component to each imputed observation. In most cases, no more than five imputed data sets are required. Whatever statistical analysis was planned is carried out on each of the imputed data sets. The results from each data set are combined using rules provided by Rubin (1976).

Maximum likelihood and multiple imputation give virtually identical results under most circumstances. Maximum likelihood is the easier of the two procedures from the user's point of view because it requires doing the analysis only once and usually requires no special additional procedures to be conducted. Multiple imputation requires the user to repeat any analyses several times, once for each imputation. However, maximum likelihood missing data procedures have not been implemented for every statistical procedure. When maximum likelihood cannot be used, multiple imputation can. Although multiple imputation is a bit more demanding logistically, its flexibility is a tremendous asset.

The missing-data procedures described previously entail some assumptions. Data can be missing in one of three ways. Data can be missing completely at random (MCAR)—when the absence of data is unrelated to any variable of interest in a study. This can occur because either the absence is truly random (for example, a random lottery was held to remove children from class so that they could be interviewed by a newspaper reporter at the time they were supposed to complete the questionnaire) or it is caused by something that has nothing to do with the study (school district lines are redrawn, and the newly formed district refuses to participate in the study). Data are missing at random (MAR) when the absence is related to variables that have been measured. For example, an item on rebelliousness is near the end of the questionnaire and is not reached by the slower readers. The missing rebelliousness item can be modeled by other data, such as reading test scores and rebelliousness as measured on a previous data collection occasion. Data are not missing at random (NMAR) when their absence is caused primarily by the variable itself, and this cannot be modeled by other variables in the data set. One example would be when absence of data on a drug use item is caused because the respondent is using drugs and is absent from the measurement session.

It is an assumption of all missing data procedures that the data are MCAR or MAR. Maximum-likelihood procedures and multiple imputation will produce unbiased estimates under these circumstances. They will not produce unbiased estimates when the data are NMAR.

How can a researcher tell whether this assumption is met? Most of the time, this cannot be determined with any degree of certainty. But this should not stop researchers from using missing-data procedures. Most data sets are a mixture of MCAR, MAR, and NMAR missing data mechanisms. To the extent that the absence of data in a particular data set is the result of MCAR or MAR processes, the missing data procedures will result in unbiased parameter estimates. If a certain proportion of the missing data is the result of a NMAR procedure, the resulting estimates will be biased, but they will be less biased than they would have been with casewise deletion. In other words, a researcher is always better off using either maximum likelihood or multiple imputation rather than the traditional approaches, like casewise deletion, even if the assumptions for the newer procedures are not completely met.

For examples of the use of missing data procedures in prevention research, see Donaldson et al. (1994), Graham et al. (1996), and Hawkins et al. (1997). For an in-depth empirical example of missing data procedures, see Graham and Hofer (2000). For a more technical and thorough description of missing data procedures, see Schafer (1997).

MEDIATION

Mediation models play a central role in prevention research. Typically, an intervention or prevention program is designed not to operate directly on the outcome of interest but to change a mediator which, in turn, is theoretically linked to an outcome of interest. For example, substance use prevention programs are often targeted at personal characteristics, such as knowledge, perceptions of peer use, or resistance skills. These psychological constructs are then hypothesized to affect an individual's substance use behavior. In order to demonstrate program effectiveness, the program must be shown to affect the mediator, and that mediator, in turn, must have an effect on the outcome of interest (such as lowering the rate of substance use). Hansen et al. (1988) demonstrated that different school-based drug abuse prevention programs operate on different mediating variables.

The standard method of analyzing mediated relations, as presented by Judd and Kenny (1981), Baron and Kenny (1986), and Kenny, Kashy, and Bolger (1997) is to perform a series of regressions. First the outcome of interest, e.g., substance use, is regressed on the independent variable, e.g., a program variable. This first regression must show a significant relation between the independent variable and the outcome in order to merit continuation of the procedure. So, before proceeding to the next step of testing the mediated model, the prevention program must be shown to affect substance use. Once a significant correlation between the independent variable and the outcome has been shown, the hypothesized mediator is regressed on the independent variable. This regression shows that the program affects the hypothesized mediator, for example, that the prevention program is correlated with high drug-refusal skills. The final step is to regress the outcome on the mediator, while controlling for the presence of the independent variable. This is to demonstrate that the effect of the independent variable on the outcome diminishes in the presence of the mediator, and so, ostensibly, the effect the program has on the outcome (as found in the first regression computed) actually occurs through the mediator. Mackinnon and collaborators (Finch, West, & Mackinnon, 1998; Mackinnon & Dwyer, 1993; Mackinnon, Warsi, & Dwyer, 1995) have made many important contributions in the theory of mediation, statistical analysis of mediation, and the estimation of key quantities.

Although the previous method has been standard for many years, when it is applied to prevention data some questions are raised (Collins, Graham, & Flaherty, 1998). First, when we think of mediation in prevention we are usually thinking of a chain of events, where first a program is delivered; the mediator is affected by the program, and then the outcome is affected by the mediator. Clearly this chain takes place over time. However, there is no requirement to use longitudinal data in the Baron and Kenny procedure. Without longitudinal data, it is possible to determine that, for example, the mediator and outcome are related, but it is impossible to tell the order in which the events unfold. In fact, Collins et al. (1998) argue that a minimum of three waves of longitudinal data are needed to test mediation models. Thus, a pretest–post-test study is not sufficient. Second, when we think of mediation in prevention, we are typically thinking of an intrainidividual process. In other words, the chain of events occurs within each person. There is no provision in the standard procedure for examining the data for evidence for or against the idea that a preponderance of individuals in a sample are going through the treatment to mediator to outcome process. Collins et al. (1998) present a set of criteria for defining stage-sequential intraindividual mediation and discuss the ideas presented here in more detail.

RECIPROCAL CAUSATION

Although in our models we usually express causation as a unidirectional phenomenon, in many instances causation is reciprocal, where A influences B which then in turn influences A. Like mediation models, reciprocal causation models are of substantial value to prevention researchers. For example, consider personality and substance use (Stein, Newcomb, & Bentler, 1987). Does starting to use a substance affect one's personality, and does this change in personality in turn affect subsequent substance use? Conversely, are some personality types predisposed toward substance use, and does initiating substance use further exacerbate those personality traits? In another example, Sher et al. (1994) look at reciprocal influences between alcohol and tobacco use disorders prospectively in a college student sample. Does alcohol use influence subsequent tobacco use and vice versa? Finally, interpersonal influence (such as peer influence) is often thought of as reciprocal. This is different from the prior two examples, in that the hypothesized causal influence occurs within a dyad, not within an individual. The common feature among these three hypothesized processes is that there are reciprocal influences between two constructs of interest.

In order to study reciprocal causation effectively, longitudinal data are required. This has implications for both research design and analysis. In much the same way as longitudinal data are needed to detect a mediated relation, longitudinal data are also needed to detect a reciprocal relation. In fact, just as in the case of mediation, three times of measurement are required. For example, consider a potential reciprocal relation between tobacco and alcohol use during the onset process. In order to observe a reciprocal relation between alcohol use and tobacco use, an individual must be observed at three times:

1. A person must first be observed experimenting with or using only alcohol or tobacco.
2. Following the initial observation of the use of one substance, experimentation with the other substance must be observed without a concurrent escalation in the first substance. For example, if at the first time of measurement an individual drank alcohol regularly, then at the second time point he or she would need to have initiated tobacco use but not concurrently increased his or her alcohol use.
3. Following the initiation of the second substance, an escalation in the first substance must then be observed. So, after the time two observation of the person's tobacco initiation, at time three his or her alcohol use would increase.

This pattern of three sequential observed states of an individual offers support for a hypothesized reciprocal relation between alcohol and tobacco use during the onset process. Because the within-person changes follow one another, this lends support to the idea that they impact one another. If the changes co-occurred, it would be more difficult to attribute reciprocal causality.

Another aspect of reciprocal causation, apparent in the previous example, is that it occurs within the most basic unit of analysis, the individual or dyad. Therefore, it should be modeled on that level. In fact, looking at sample level statistics does not provide the information that modeling at the unit of analysis provides. If, in a sample of adolescents, we saw that alcohol use was associated with tobacco use, and that, conversely, tobacco use was associated with alcohol use, we would have no way of knowing if it is a reciprocal relation occurring within the individual or if these two constructs are related in the sample but are not reciprocally contingent. It could be that for some people only alcohol use leads to tobacco use, whereas for others tobacco use leads to alcohol use. Based on the sample level evidence alone, without examining individual-level data over time, it is impossible to determine which type of process is taking place. This means that traditional covariance structure modeling approaches cannot be used to test models of reciprocal causation as it is defined here. Flaherty (1997) provides a set of guidelines and a method for examining data for evidence of a reciprocal process at the level of the unit of analysis.

SUMMARY

This chapter discussed a number of methodological considerations that face prevention research. It examined the central importance of theory in design and analysis of prevention studies. It considered the role of factorial invariance in developing culture-specific measures. It discussed the importance of statistical power and how it is dependent on factors other than sample size. It considered growth curve models, survival analysis, and LTA, all relatively new procedures for dealing with change over time. It also discussed two approaches to the trait–state distinction and looked at missing data procedures and how important they are for prevention research. Finally, it discussed two general types of models that frequently arise in prevention research, mediation models and models of reciprocal causation, and how the customary ways of testing these models should perhaps be reconsidered.

REFERENCES

Allport, G. W., & Odbert, H. S. (1936). Trait-names: A psycho-lexical study. *Psychological Monographs, 47,* 1–171.

Bacik, J. M., Murphy, S. A., & Anthony, J. C. (in press). Drug use prevention data, missing assessments and survival analysis. *Multivariate Behavioral Research, 33,* 573–588.

Baron, R. M., & Kenny, D. A. (1986). The moderator-mediator variable distinction in social psychological research: Conceptual, strategic, and statistical considerations. *Journal of Personality and Social Psychology, 51,* 1173–1182.

Bryk, A. S., & Raudenbush, S. W. (1987). Application of hierarchical linear models to assessing change. *Psychological Bulletin, 101,* 147–158.

Campbell, D. T., & Fiske, D. W. (1959). Convergent and discriminant validation by the multi-trait multi-method matrix. *Psychological Bulletin, 56,* 81–105.

Collins, L. M. (1994). Some design, measurement, and analysis pitfalls in drug abuse prevention research and how to avoid them: Let your model be your guide. In A. Cazares & L. A. Beatty (Eds.), *Scientific methods for prevention intervention research.* National Institutes of Health: National Institute on Drug Abuse Research Monograph 139.

Collins, L. M. (1996). Measurement of change in research on aging: Old and new issues from an individual growth perspective. In J. E. Birren & K. W. Schaie (Eds.), *Handbook of the psychology of aging, Fourth edition.* San Diego, CA: Academic Press.

Collins, L. M., & Cliff, N. (1990). Using the Longitudinal Guttman Simplex as a basis for measuring growth. *Psychological Bulletin, 108,* 128–134.

Collins, L. M., Graham, J. W., & Flaherty, B. P. (1998). An alternative framework for defining mediation. *Multivariate Behavioral Research, 33,* 295–311.

Collins, L. M., Graham, J. W., Rousculp, S. S., & Hansen, W. B. (1997). Heavy caffeine and the beginning of the substance use onset process: An illustration of latent transition analysis. In K. Bryant, M. Windle, & S. West (Eds.), *The science of prevention: Methodological advances from alcohol and substance abuse research* (pp. 79–99). Washington, DC: American Psychological Association.

Collins, L. M., & Wugalter, S. E. (1992). Latent class models for stage-sequential dynamic latent variables. *Multivariate Behavioral Research, 27,* 131–157.

Collins, L. M., & Sayer, A. G. (2000). Modeling growth and change processes: Design, measurement, and analysis for research in social psychology. In H. T. Reis & C. M. Judd (Eds.), Handbook of Research Methods in Social Psychology (pp. 478–495). Cambridge: Cambridge University Press.

Cunningham, W. R. (1991). Issues in factorial invariance. In L. M. Collins & J. L. Horn (Eds.), *Best methods for the analysis of change.* Washington, DC: American Psychological Association.

Curran, P. J., Harford, T., & Muthen, B. (1997). The relation between heavy alcohol use and bar patronage: A latent growth model. *Journal of Studies on Alcohol, 57,* 410–418.

Donaldson, S. I., Graham, J. W., & Hansen, W. B. (1994). Testing the generalizability of intervening mechanism theories: Understanding the effects of adolescent drug use prevention interventions. *Journal of Behavioral Medicine, 17,* 195–216.

Dumenci, L., & Windle, M. (1996). A latent trait-state model of adolescent depression using the center for epidemiologic studes-depression scale. *Multivariate Behavioral Research, 31,* 313–330.

Duncan, S. C., & Duncan, T. E. (1996). A multivariate latent growth curve analysis of adolescent substance use. *Structural Equation Modeling, 3,* 323–347.

Duncan, T. E., Duncan, S. C., Alpert, A., Hops, H., Stoolmiller, M., & Muthen, B. (1991). Latent variable modeling of longitudinal and multilevel substance use data. *Multivariate Behavioral Research, 32,* 275–318.

Duncan, S. C., Duncan, T. E., Biglan, A., & Ary, D. (1998). Contributions of the social context to the development of adolescent substance use: A multivariate latent growth modeling approach. *Drug and Alcohol Dependence, 50,* 57–71.

Duncan, S. C., Duncan, T. E., & Hops, H. (1996). Analysis of longitudinal data within accelerated longitudinal designs. *Psychological Methods, 1,* 236–248.

Embretson, S. E. (1991a). A multidimensional latent trait model for measuring learning and change. *Psychometrika, 56,* 495–515.

Embretson, S. E. (1991b). Implications of a multidimensional latent trait model for measuring change. In L. M. Collins & J. L. Horn (Eds.), *Best methods for the analysis of change: Recent advances, unanswered questions, future directions.* Washington, DC: American Psychological Association.

Finch, J. F., West, S. G., & Mackinnon, D. P. (1998). Effects of sample size and nonnormality on the estimation of mediated effects in latent variable models. *Structural Equation Modeling, 4,* 87–107.

Fischer, G. H., & Ponocny, I. (1994). An extension of the partial credit model with an application to the measurement of change. *Psychometrika, 59,* 177–192.

Flaherty, B. P. (1997). *Assessing stage-sequential reciprocal influence with latent transition analysis.* Unpublished master's thesis, The Pennsylvania State University, University Park.

Fridhandler, B. M. (1986). Conceptual note on state, trait and the state-trait distinction. *Journal of Personality and Social Psychology, 50,* 169–174.

Graham, J. W., Collins, L. M., Wugalter, S. E., Chung, N. K., & Hansen, W. B. (1991). Modeling transitions in latent stage-sequential processes: A substance use prevention example. *Journal of Consulting and Clinical Psychology, 59,* 48–57.

Graham, J. W., & Hofer, S. M. (2000). Multiple imputation in multivariate research. In T. D. Little, K. U. Schnabel, & J. Baumert (Eds.), *Modeling longitudinal and multiple-group data: Practical issues, applied approaches, and specific examples* (pp. 201–218). Hillsdale, NJ: Erlbaum.

Graham, J. W., Hofer, S. M., Donaldson, S. I., MacKinnon, D. P., & Schafer, J. L. (1996). Analysis with missing data in prevention research. In K. J. Bryant, M. Windle, & S. G. West (Eds.), *The science of prevention: Methodological advances from alcohol and substance abuse research* (pp. 325–365). Washington, DC: American Psychological Association.

Hansen, W. B., & Collins, L. M. (1994). Seven ways to increase power without increasing N. In L. M. Collins & L. A. Seitz (Eds.), *Advances in data analysis for prevention intervention research.* National Institutes of Health: National Institute on Drug Abuse Research Monograph 142.

Hansen, W. B., & Graham, J. W. (1991). Preventing alcohol, marijuana, and cigarette use among adolescents: Peer pressure resistance training versus establishing conservative norms. *Preventive Medicine, 20,* 414–430.

Hansen, W. B., Graham, J. W., Wolkenstein, B. H., Lundy, B. Z., Pearson, J. L., Flay, B. R., & Johnson, C. A. (1988). Differential impact of three alcohol prevention curricula on hypothesized mediating variables. *Journal of Drug Education, 18,* 143–153.

Hawkins, J. D., Graham, J. W., Maguin, E., Abbott, R., Hill, K. G., & Catalano, R. F. (1997). Exploring the effects of age of alcohol use initiation and psychosocial risk factors on subsequent alcohol misuse. *Journal of Studies on Alcohol, 58,* 280–290.

Horn, J. L. (1991). Comment on issues in factorial invariance. In L. M. Collins & J. L. Horn (Eds.), *Best Methods for the analysis of change* (pp. 114–125). Washington, DC: American Psychological Association.

Hyatt, S. L., & Collins, L. M. (2000). Using latent transition analysis to examine the relationship between parental permissiveness and the onset of substance use. In J. Rose, L. Chassin, C. Presson, & S. Sherman (Eds.), *Multivariate applications in substance use research* (pp. 259–288). Hillsdale, NJ: Erlbaum.

Judd, C. M., & Kenny, D. A. (1981). Process analysis: Estimating mediation in treatment evaluations. *Evaluation Review, 5,* 602–619.

Kenny, D. A., Kashy, D. A., & Bolger, N. (1997). Data analysis in social psychology. In D. Gilbert, S. T. Fiske, & G. Lindzey (Eds.), *Handbook of social psychology* (4th edition, pp. 233–265). New York: McGraw–Hill.

Little, R. J. A., & Rubin, D. B. (1987). *Statistical analysis with missing data.* New York: Wiley.

Lord, F. M., & Novick, M. R. (1968). *Statistical theories of mental test scores.* Reading, MA: Addison–Wesley.

Mackinnon, D. P., & Dwyer, J. H. (1993). Estimating mediated effects in prevention studies. *Evaluation Review, 17,* 144–158.

Mackinnon, D. P., Warsi, G., & Dwyer, J. H. (1995). A simulation study of mediated effect measures. *Multivariate Behavioral Research, 30,* 41–62.

Meredith, W. (1964a). Notes on factorial invariance. *Psychometrika, 29,* 177–185.

Meredith, W. (1964b). Rotation to achieve factorial invariance. *Psychometrika, 29,* 187–206.

Meredith, W. (1965). A method for studying differences between groups. *Psychometrika, 30,* 15–29.

Nunnally, J. C., & Bernstein, I. H. (1994). *Psychometric Theory (3rd edition).* New York: McGraw–Hill.

Pedhazur, E. J., & Schmelkin, L. P. (1991). *Measurement, design, and analysis: An integrated approach.* Hillsdale, NJ: Elrbaum.

Rubin, D. B. (1976). Inference and missing data. *Biometrika, 63,* 581–592.

Sayer, A. G., & Willett, J. B. (1998). A cross-domain model for growth in adolescent alcohol expectancies. *Multivariate Behavioral Research, 33,* 509–543.

Schafer, J. L. (1997). *Analysis of incomplete multivariate data.* London: Chapman & Hall.

Sher, K. J., Gotham, H. J., Erickson, D. J., & Wood, P. K. (1996). A prospective, high-risk study of the relationship between tobacco dependence and alcohol use disorders. *Alcoholism: Clinical and Experimental Research, 20,* 485–492.

Siddiqui, O., Flay, B. R., & Hu, F. B. (1996). Factors affecting attrition in a longitudinal smoking prevention study. *Preventive Medicine, 25,* 554–560.

Stein, J. A., Newcomb, M. D., & Bentler, P. M. (1987). Personality and drug use: Reciprocal effects across four years. *Personality and Individual Differences, 8,* 419–430.

Stevens, V. J., & Hollis, J. F. (1989). Preventing smoking relapse, using an individually tailored skills-training technique. *Journal of Consulting and Clinical Psychology, 57,* 420–424.

Vogt, W. P. (1993). Dictionary of statistics and methodology: a non-technical guide for the social sciences. Newbury Park, CA: Sage.

Widaman, K. F., & Reise, S. P. (1997). Exploring the measurement invariance of psychological instruments: Applications in the substance use domain. In K. J. Bryant, M. Windle, & S. G. West (Eds.), *The science of prevention: Methodological advances from alcohol and substance abuse research* (pp. 281–324). Washington, DC: American Psychological Association.

Willett, J. B. (1989). Some results on reliability for the longitudinal measurement of change: Implications for the design of studies of individual growth. *Educational and Psychological Measurement, 49,* 587–601.

Willett, J. B., & Singer, J. D. (1991). How long did it take? Using survival analysis in educational and psychological research. In L. M. Collins & J. L. Horn (Eds.), *Best methods for the analysis of change: Recent advances, unanswered questions, future directions* (pp. 310–327). Washington, DC: American Psychological Association.

Windle, M. (1997). Alternative latent variable approaches to modeling change in adolescent alcohol involvement. In K. Bryant, M. Windle, & S. G. West (Eds.), *The science of prevention: Methodological advances from alcohol and substance abuse research* (pp. 43–78). Washington, DC: American Psychological Association.

Zimmerman, D. W., & Williams, R. H. (1986). Note on the reliability of experimental measures and the power of significance tests. *Psychological Bulletin, 100,* 123–124.

CHAPTER 29

Prevention Program Implementation

STEVEN SCHINKE
KRISTIN COLE

INTRODUCTION

Prevention programs, no matter how they are conceived and designed, vary according to situational factors in the school, community, or other context in which they are delivered. They occur in a context particular to each target site (McIntyre et al., 1996; Schinke & Botvin, 1999; Smith, Schinke & Springer, 2001). This is one reason that many important and effective prevention programs fail to find markets of acceptability even though they have been shown to be effective (Donaldson, Graham, Piccinin, & Hansen, 1995; Parcel, Perry, & Taylor, 1990). Investigators have discovered that prevention programs once developed and tested do not naturally diffuse themselves. Diffusion is the process by which new knowledge is "communicated through specific channels over time among members of a social system" (Rogers, 1995; p. 5). Rogers proposes that diffusing health behavior interventions, such as drug abuse prevention programs, involves four stages: dissemination, adoption, implementation, and maintenance. Dissemination occurs when communities are introduced to programs and encouraged to adopt them. Adoption is when the community agrees to accept and implement the program. Implementation is the program's actual delivery. Finally, in the maintenance stage, the community continues to use the program over time. This chapter focuses on the implementation issues and presents a case study that highlights major methodological procedures associated with implementation.

STEVEN SCHINKE AND KRISTIN COLE • School of Social Work, Columbia University, New York, New York 10025

IMPLEMENTATION ISSUES

Too often, drug abuse prevention programs that prove successful in clinical trials fail to move beyond the adoption stage in real-world settings. Several factors contribute to this. The decision to adopt a program is usually made by administrators, rather than by the program's implementers. Without the total commitment of its implementers, the program is likely to fail.

Implementing a program in another setting poses many dilemmas. Drug abuse prevention programs are often developed under the unusual conditions of good funding, skilled staff, and rich participant incentives. Translating an empirically tested preventive approach into a practical success for a larger market requires resources and attention to organizational functioning. Few program developers have access to such resources, or to a sophisticated understanding of the implementation process.

Program implementation refers to both the quantity and the quality of implementation. The number of program lessons, objectives, or components determines the quantity of the program. Quality refers to program integrity or fidelity (Parcel et al., 1990). Research suggests that implementation quantity and quality determine drug abuse prevention program outcomes (Pentz et al., 1990). Both the quantity and the degree to which program delivery adheres to the original program design jointly influence outcomes.

The value of program fidelity is controversial in implementation and diffusion research. Some argue that altering a program reduces its effectiveness (Calsyn, Tornatzky, & Dittman, 1977). Others say that program change is inevitable and that such "reinvention" is necessary to match the program with its audience (Berman & McLaughlin, 1978; Blakely et al., 1987). Reinvention proponents suggest that as long as the theory behind the program is not altered, or the "mezzo" level of the program is left intact, microlevel changes are permissible (Bauman, Stein, & Ireys, 1991). Research shows, for example, that when implementing school-based drug abuse prevention programs, teachers are more likely to use programs that afford them flexibility in delivery but also provide clear and specific directions (Hall & Hord, 1987).

Some sites make hospitable settings for a new program. Characteristics of the site (staff experience, availability, etc.), the cultural and political context, and population characteristics all influence program implementation (Bauman et al., 1991). In particular, such factors as high teacher morale, active support of principals or administrators, high degree of implementer involvement, and a good "fit" between the program and the community appear to facilitate implementation (Gold et al., 1991; Smith et al., 1995). Indeed, studies of drug abuse program implementation in schools find that principals significantly facilitate, or inhibit, implementation (Huberman & Miles, 1984). Other studies suggest the importance of implementer training (Basch, 1984; Levenson-Gingiss & Hamilton, 1989; Parcel et al., 1991). Yet another factor in successful implementation is the use of a "change agent" (Rogers, 1995). A change agent provides the links between program developers and program users. Finally, research has shown that program outcomes are enhanced if the program's objectives are consistent with the local community's goals (Butterfoss, Goodman, & Wandersman, 1996; Elias & Weissberg, 1991; Oetting et al., 1995).

The case study described in this chapter, albeit a demonstration project, illustrates the myriad issues involved in implementing a drug abuse prevention program in a southwestern U.S. community. Because the four stages of diffusion research demand the longitudinal perspectives of not only program developers and researchers but also program adopters and users, the chapter's case study is necessarily limited to the implementation stage.

CASE STUDY

This case study involves a prevention program aimed at reducing problems of tobacco and alcohol use among Mexican-American early adolescents. Expressly designed for the urban target site in south central Texas, the program combined cognitive–behavioral skills to help individuals acquire prevention knowledge, attitudes, and behaviors with community-oriented strategies to engage not only adolescents but also their parents, teachers, and key referents in supporting their application of prevention skills. The study had two goals: to reduce substance use among targeted adolescents and to conduct the study in a manner that would maximize its effectiveness and meaningfulness to the host community. In striving to achieve its goals, the study illustrates three elements of implementation research. These processes are enhancing programmatic sociocultural relevance, ensuring community ownership, and assessing implementation integrity.

Enhancing Sociocultural Relevance

In addition to scientific justification, clinical wisdom and common sense point out the need to design prevention programs that meet the needs of their target communities and populations and that reflect the sociocultural attributes of recipient groups. Social marketing research also suggests that the characteristics of specific consumer groups should guide the design and implementation of programs. Kotler (1982), for example, makes frequent reference to the need for social programs to address the prerogatives of consumers rather than those of developers. Implementation and diffusion research also show that culturally sensitive interventions have enhanced chances of subsequent adoption.

Consequently, for our intervention to engage youth from the Mexican-American community, we needed strategies compatible with the community's sociocultural framework. To develop such compatibility, we involved members of the Mexican-American community in the review, development, implementation, and administration of preventive intervention strategies. At the study's onset, we engaged the full-time services of an on-site project director who had been with a health promotion project in the same community. He also had a leadership position with a Mexican-American civil rights organization, edited a local newspaper aimed at Mexican-American readers, and was well respected in the community. The project director not only significantly influenced the development of the prevention program but also guided the selection of a community advisory board.

The board was composed of representatives from health and human services organizations, schools, churches, businesses, and voluntary organizations. Board members met regularly with the study team to design strategies that had a strong likelihood of at least being accepted by youth in the target community, if not ultimately proving efficacious as well. Within scientifically accepted conventions and also under the project director's supervision and advisory board's oversight, we convened and conducted a series of youth focus groups.

At first, focus groups were composed of heterogeneous samples, distributed by gender and ethnic–racial background about equal to their representation in the target community's school system. Quickly, however, patterns emerged in which nonminority youth and males were more likely to comment on stimulus material and appeared to influence minority youth and females. Despite their relatively small numbers, nonminority youth in particular seemed to skew focus group discussions toward ideas and topics that may or may not have been of common interest. For example, when asked about their favorite rock and roll musicians (to identify potential role models), focus group members regularly concurred with nonminority youth preferences.

To avoid such obvious peer influence problems, later focus groups were composed of homogeneous ethnic–racial groups and only one gender. Qualitatively, these groups appeared to generate diverse ideas with greater depth of content than the initial, more heterogeneous, groups. We then conducted a relatively long series of focus groups, asking youth to estimate the extent and nature of drug use and other substance use problems among their peers, suggested means of addressing these problems, and recommended motivators and potential delivery means for prevention intervention.

Operating in parallel with youth focus groups, the study's project director and advisory board were developing ideas for intervention aimed at Mexican-American youth in the target community. Material from both sources provided considerable guidance to increase the cultural sensitivity of program content as well as to improve the fit of evaluation mechanisms aimed at documenting intervention processes and outcome.

Ensuring Community Ownership

Community-based efforts that fail to address the surrounding sociopolitical context are unlikely to succeed. They are particularly apt to fail at any, or all, of three stages: initial outreach and community entry, implementation, and maintenance.

Initial outreach and community entry should begin with needs-assessment data. Following Rothman's (1979) community organization model, our study generated needs-assessment data from the community's planning meetings and informal discussions. These discussions, along with input from the focus groups and advisory board meetings, as well as key informant interviews with community members not on the board but interested in the study's goals, yielded information on the nature and manifestations of substance use among youth in the target community.

For example, nearly all information sources in the small, tightly knit community reported that weekend beer parties, often held in isolated areas on the outskirts of town, were a major source of youthful substance use and abuse. Needs assessments also revealed that youth parties were sometimes sanctioned by parents who apparently viewed heavy drinking during adolescence as a normal *rite de passage*. A few parents allegedly went so far as to purchase beer for parties and lend their rural property for the party site. Such qualitative data formed the foundation for a broad-based prevention effort that was aimed jointly at youth, parents, and community norms.

Rothman's model also seeks to specify potential barriers to initial entry, implementation, and institutionalization as part of a feasibility analysis. Our feasibility analysis attempted to assess the likelihood of a successful collaboration between the community and agency representatives and the research team. Here, advisory board members, key informants, and such official community gatekeepers as police officers, court officials, and school administrators suggested ways to overcome anticipated problems.

Regarding the allegedly parent-sanctioned drinking parties, for example, the feasibility analysis sought to determine whether families might impede rather than facilitate intervention delivery. Additional interviews were conducted with community and neighborhood representatives who might shed light on the issue. For example, besides interviewing clergy and lay leaders of the Mexican-American target group, we sought the opinions and the advice of members of the Anglo community.

A day-long meeting of church leaders was held in an effort to solicit responses from the surrounding community. In addition to the Catholic priest from a church that served the community's Mexican-American neighborhood, others in attendance at the meeting were an Episcopal priest from the community's largely White neighborhood and ministers from other denominations who could comment upon parental support, opposition, and leadership matters regarding youthful drinking. Church leaders, as the needs-assessment portion of the study emerged, proved to be reliable and highly accurate about issues of interest to the planning of a responsive substance abuse prevention program.

Further guided by Kotler's (1982) social marketing perspective, we involved the community in prevention–intervention program planning, implementation, and maintenance. We agree with Kotler that community ownership is a prerequisite for true institutionalization. Kotler's approach begins by including community representatives in all planning groups. This required our willingness and dedication to allow community needs and perspectives to drive our planning process. For example, many referents—including youth—called for increased programming, facilities, and support for the community's young people. From our meetings, we learned that a favored swimming pool had been closed and that there were few alternative recreational facilities for young people. Although not directly related to the provision of substance abuse prevention services, the reestablishment of recreational activities for youth could at least give the community tangible evidence of the project's positive intent and, at best, provide youth with positive alternatives to substance use.

Our experience taught us that when planning meetings are viewed as an opportunity for expert linkage—researchers as experts on the state-of-the-science, and community representatives as experts on the cultural, economic, and political dynamics of their community—interventions that evolve are more likely to be successful. When community involvement is perceived as meaningful and necessary, rather than as an exercise in tokenism, the potential failure points related to entry, implementation, and institutionalization are likely to be avoided.

Our approach to community involvement was also informed by Green's public health education model (1979). Green recommends adopting distinct planning phases that include a start-up phase in which community organizational structures are analyzed and opinion leaders are identified, an initial involvement phase in which a community advisory board is established and meetings are held both with the advisory board and with key individuals, an installation of change phase in which the educational intervention is implemented and community advisory board input is used for continued formative evaluation purposes, and a maintenance of change phase in which institutionalization in the initial demonstration sites and dissemination is sought.

For short-term, project-centered community involvement activities to be salient, potential long-term benefits for the community must also be assured. Otherwise, "community involvement" is justifiably seen as a means to an end defined entirely by a research agenda—an orientation that is not likely to elicit either community acceptance or support, much less involvement. In practical terms, maximizing the involvement of community members in this substance use prevention program meant establishing an administrative and planning structure that functioned through expert linkage rather than through top–down or researcher-based decision making. The community advisory board proved effective for this purpose.

Instead of the investigators designing prevention approaches based on their prior data and experience, the team relied on community members to direct the use of program resources. Communitywide events, for example, featuring music, food, and games were viewed by our referents as necessary to draw in youth. At first we were skeptical of such an allocation of intervention program resources, but then we were persuaded of the wisdom of hosting community events. Had we not been attuned to the potential value of drawing upon the background and perspective of our community advisors, decisions about resource allotments would have been vastly different and may not have produced positive outcomes.

Gaining the community's trust before initiating their involvement was crucial to our intervention. Members of the community needed to believe in both the integrity and the sincerity of the project before they would commit their time. The process of community organization began with the convening of a scientific advisory committee, the appointment of a local project director, a series of town meetings to elicit community involvement and to appoint a local agency to house the project, and a series of focus groups to determine the needs and preferences of the community's youth. During this process, the locus of the project changed (from school to community), resulting in a more mobile and flexible identity for the study. As a result, community ownership altered the study's original concept of its function and place in the community. Elements of the community organization process are described in more detail in the following.

ADVISORY COMMITTEE.   A scientific advisory committee of experts in the fields of cross-cultural affairs, prevention research, health behavior, and urban affairs was convened at the beginning of the study. The advisory committee had a significant impact on project operations, especially in the first year. Among other things, the committee recommended modifications to make the planned program more culturally specific and recommended keeping detailed process notes to chronicle the development of the study. That recommendation led to a subcontract with ethnographers at a nearby university.

Over time, and as local staff gained experience, the study became increasingly autonomous. In keeping with the goals of community ownership, the role of the research team changed. While our staff assumed primary responsibility for developing a community network and for determining the site and nature of community events, members of the community reallocated funds, proposed new venues for community intervention, and wrote grant applications for follow-on funding for the study.

VOLUNTEERS.   We also enlisted volunteers from the community to help spread the study's messages on substance use prevention. Trained volunteers learned the following skills: (1) to contact other persons and tell them about television and other programs including role models for behavior change; (2) to encourage attention to the role models; and (3) to encourage and reinforce positive imitative behaviors. These simple skills were modeled by staff and learned through brief role-plays during the staff's regular contact with the volunteers.

Our plans for recruiting volunteers (approaching institutions, eliciting interest, and having interested parties fill out a volunteer sheet and get trained) proved too formal and thus inappropriate for the Mexican-American community we were working with. Our original plan relied far too much on the Anglo-controlled institutions in the community. We had planned to have volunteers operating in neighborhoods, business settings, government agencies, and social clubs. These categories of social networks were chosen to be inclusive, not exclusive. Yet, we discovered through contacts with local leaders that the Mexican Americans in our study community had a set of social networks entirely distinct from those we had identified. One respondent suggested, for example, that the most effective volunteer enlistment would use the Mexican-American familialism and networks associated with the folk healers, or *curanderas*.

RESULTS OF COMMUNITY ORGANIZING.   The community-organization component, launched with the convening of a scientific advisory committee, a series of focus groups, and a series of town meetings to elicit community involvement, gradually became the central component of our intervention due to its influence on the intervention design. Efforts to develop community participation and ownership of the intervention strategy led to a realignment of priorities and a restructuring of the study. Because the goal of this project was to empower members of the local community to implement an effective drug abuse preventive intervention, we made every effort to work through the natural structures of the community.

The study established strong ties with a number of agencies, businesses, and individuals in the community, and yielded a network of organizations in the community dedicated to implementation of the project. Since the study's formal funding conclusion, the project director has continued in a leadership role within the community. He attributes this influence and visibility within the community to his experience in our study, which introduced him to the webs of influence in the community.

The flexibility implicit in the concept of a community-based program adapted to the needs of a community had advantages and disadvantages in implementation. Despite the success of our study in mobilizing community resources, particularly Hispanic participation in community issues, we did not find any significant change in the general rates of substance use as measured in the school-based survey instrument.

One explanation for our failure to discern statistically meaningful differences between youth who took part in the prevention program and those who did not was the relatively small statistical power of the study design. Originally slated as a demonstration study rather than as a rigorous outcome evaluation project, the field trial had one intervention and one control site. As such, comparisons using the site as the unit of analysis were not possible. Yet, assumedly high levels on nonindependence among study youth vitiate the power of using individuals as analytic units. The resulting low power may have exerted a deleterious influence on our ability to detect differential outcomes among study subjects.

Another potential reason for the absence of significant outcome differences is that intervention efforts may have improved not only the overall community in which the project was based but also the adjacent community that several as a control. The southcentral Texas region in which the research was conducted is comprised of tightly knit communities that share cultural identifications, youth related events, and resources. For example, youth from one town regularly ventured to the neighboring town for dances, concerts, and parties. The contagion of the experimental community events may, therefore, have affected somewhat those in the control arm, further eroding our ability to find outcome differences.

Less likely, though plausible, as explanations for clear statistical evidence in favor of the prevention program are the potency of the intervention strategies—since youth were exposed to many and varied activities—and the inconsistent delivery of intervention—since that was measured carefully during the study's focus on implementation. Without considerable additional investigaton, the true reasons for nonsignificant differences may never be known. Still, given a long history of prevention programs that, albeit highly worthwhile, often fell short of achieving startling outcomes, the present project's lack of causal effects is neither terribly surprising nor disappointing.

In the process of implementing this community-based and community-owned study, we uncovered many entrenched political issues and social networks in the community. This experience has relevance to future researchers at the community level. In the following, we discuss in more detail the benefits and challenges of closely involving the community in an intervention.

BENEFITS OF COMMUNITY PARTICIPATION.   Aside from the obvious ethical and theoretical advantages of involving the community in an intervention, there are a number of practical benefits of involving the community in any implementation. With community participation, the study requires less staff, is more likely to have relevance to the community, and is more likely to be a lasting force within the community.

Working through community networks can minimize the formal resources required to disseminate preventive interventions. Though it is beyond the resources of most interventions to hire staff who can make daily personal contact with community members, intervention teams working at the community level can mobilize volunteers for this function. Volunteers extend the intervention into homes, places of business, and social networks in the community, thus making it part of the informal as well as the formal experience of the community.

By involving the community in implementing an intervention, community members learn to more effectively organize themselves. This can be applied to other community-based efforts. In our study, each program was designed to be a supporting unit for other local prevention efforts. The League of United Latin American Citizens Council, for example, viewed our study as an opportunity to test new approaches of community outreach and as a method of delivering much needed education to the community.

As the project progressed, community ownership was cultivated by maintaining a diverse circle of contacts who gave us regular input regarding the cultural sensitivity of the project, using the media to announce public events and to invite support for those events, and seeking and establishing collaborative relationships with local agencies and relevant social programs.

After participating in our study, the community used networks established by the study's community advisory board to approach another pressing problem: the high dropout rate among Hispanic adolescents. Our study's project director was the keynote speaker at an initial meeting of parents and educators about the dropout problem.

Hiring a local and prominent bicultural member of the community significantly helped to nurture community ownership of the project. Having grown up in the community, the project director had a keen sense of the political, economic, and social stressors in the community. He had previous experience in an intervention conducted in a nearby urban community, where a parallel set of media and community prevention activities had been organized. That effort provided a source of comparison and methodological support for our project.

Because he was interested in redistricting the community so that the Hispanic citizens could elect a representative to public office, and because of his own political aspirations, the project director was invested in extending and strengthening community communication. His multifaceted involvement in the politics, media, and culture of the community uniquely equipped him for negotiating the ideals of the project throughout the community's sociocultural framework.

Without community input, researchers are at risk for overlooking existing programs. Community contributions during the needs-assessment phase of the intervention helped guide our research to provide needed services. During the community needs-assessment phase, we found that the community's priorities were skills training for high-risk youth and the need for substance-free alternative activities for local youth. Also, a number of substance use prevention programs were extant in the local schools and because recent research indicated the need for new strategies for implementing skills training in less formal environments and outside school (Schinke, Cole, & Poulin, 2000; Schinke, Tepauac, & Cole, 2000), our research activities emphasized implementation and coordination of efforts already in place. Accordingly, the project nicely illustrates the value of implementation research as a stage in the diffusion process.

DRAWBACKS OF COMMUNITY PARTICIPATION.   The community-assessment phase of the project had considerable influence on the conduct of our project. We tailored our intervention for the community we learned about through town meetings and subsequent qualitative observations and ethnographic study. However, deferring to community power can hamper the operations of the researcher in the community. First, researchers are bound to perceive communities and their problems differently from how communities perceive themselves. Researchers will view certain problems as more significant than community members may see them. Second, once the research team elicits the opinions and recommendations of the community, those recommendations must be heeded to preserve community confidence in the research team.

Deciding which sections of the community to target is also important. At first, we planned to target the entire community, including all of its schools and major mass media. We did not subdivide the community into various cultural subgroups. But in this racially and ethnically segregated community, the geographically defined community had little in common with the cultural community. Thus, the significance of hiring a bicultural Hispanic project director was exaggerated. Despite the intervention's intent to address the whole community, the project gradually became identified as an exclusively Hispanic project. As a result, preexisting social networks in the community were often negative rather than positive forces.

Needing a central site of operations, we decided to base our study in an existing community organization. The scientific advisory team recommended affiliation with a new rather than with an established organization so that we would have more freedom to innovatively mobilize the community. But the organization selected as a host agency withdrew during the community mobilization phase. Concurrently, participants in town meetings and advisory groups recommended that we base ourselves in a variety of locations, rather than at one site. As a result, the project's goals changed from one central drug prevention program to that of an enabling and coordinating force in the community.

The relocation of the center of operations posed a challenge and an unusual opportunity for the project. On one hand, the project had to work harder to establish its visibility in the community. Though housing a project in a host agency runs the risk of competing with that agency or alienating individuals who may have conflicts with that agency, research (Schinke, Orlandi, & Cole, 1992) has shown that affiliation with an existing agency improves service delivery and community acceptance of a new program.

Commensurate with our plans to include the community as much as possible, we provided a full explanation of the project's goals and theory through the mass media. But the project director's candor in publishing details regarding the intervention backfired when a school reacted negatively to the publication of survey results implying that the school's students used drugs. Here we encountered a major difficulty of sharing research results with the study community. We saw the data as information, but the schools saw it as bad press for their neighborhood, not an unjustified concern.

Assessing the Integrity of the Implementation

Through quantitative and qualitative measures, we assessed the quality of our substance use prevention program delivery.

QUANTITATIVE EVALUATION. Formal and informal process evaluation activities were conducted periodically during all intervention development and implementation activities to further ensure both the cultural relevance and the sensitivity of the intervention. This ongoing evaluation allowed us to make necessary adjustments while the intervention was still in the preliminary design stage. Process evaluation also identified unforeseen barriers to intervention delivery. Besides those already mentioned, other barriers to intervention discovered by process evaluation measures included access to youth in nonschool settings; finding a common curriculum that appealed to youth in different age cohorts and having varying experiences with drugs, alcohol, and other substances; and securing the commitment of qualified intervention agents in both school and community settings.

Anticipating necessary changes to intervention, we monitored the study's initial implementation and examined available process data from ongoing focus groups with youth involved in prevention activities (Schinke et al., 1992). With these data, we modified intervention procedures as needed. We also tried to identify, collect, catalogue, and evaluate new or existing intervention approaches that had potential applicability to alcohol and tobacco use prevention. Once identified, promising strategies with relevance to our own were discussed, evaluated, and, as appropriate, incorporated into our intervention.

At regular intervals, we conducted formal student surveys in both intervention and control schools. Student surveys yielded initial prevalence and attitudes of alcohol and tobacco use and the progressive effect of the intervention. The surveys also served as an incentive for involving the schools in the program. In addition to surveys, key informant interviews, and focus groups, unobtrusive measures and existing record analyses helped document and monitor the overall implementation and operation of the intervention program.

QUALITATIVE EVALUATION.   Annual in-depth interviews conducted with key informants from each focus group provided qualitative data. Key informants were asked to describe their observations of alcohol, tobacco, and drug-related behavior among youth and youths' reactions to program activities. These interviews supplied important feedback for prevention activity planning and dissemination. Also, the recorded interviews serve as a historical document of the changes in community norms and practices in the study locations.

To add depth and insight to the process and outcome evaluation of the drug abuse prevention program, we conducted ethnographic research. Because adolescents who regularly engage in substance use may prove difficult to find through schools or other community organizations, we needed an alternative strategy for reaching them. Also, studies on the etiology of substance abuse reveal that young people who are unhappy at school are at greater risk for threats to their health and well-being. Poor performance at school is an early predictor of substance use and other problem behaviors. Other studies show that substance use is negatively correlated with school attendance (Pirie, Murray, & Luepker, 1988). Youth under the age of 18 who are not in school are much more likely than their in-school peers to smoke or to use other drugs.

Clearly, we needed strategies for reaching and engaging youth who did not attend school regularly (or at all) or who were not in the habit of cooperating with school programs. The ethnographic component of our study was designed to fulfill three functions: contribute to the evaluation of the drug abuse prevention program, provide information about youth in both study and control communities who are disengaged from youth-serving institutions, and illuminate the attitudes and activities that form the lifestyle of those who spend considerable amounts of their time "hanging out."

The ethnographic component of the research was instructive. Although the study community was big enough to have a variety of ethnic, educational, business, and community viewpoints, it was sufficiently small to be captured holistically. Using contacts made earlier in the study, the ethnographers interviewed members of the community such as the priest of the largest Hispanic church in town, the assistant police chief, and the principal of the local high school to determine key observation sites.

Observational sites were then used by ethnographic team members to gather qualitative data on youth behavior patterns within the community. Of particular interest were patterns among Mexican-American adolescents related to substance use, alternative recreational activities, and social and peer interactions. Drawing from ethnographic data, we were able to further confirm the transfer of preventive intervention effects to study youth and, in an iterative fashion, to improve the focus of intervention strategies.

For example, a major source of ethnographic data were observations made of youth in community settings where underage drinking regularly took place and where smoking was commonplace. Serendipitously made by trained ethnographers, these observations revealed stark differences in patterns of deviant youth activity throughout the course of the study. Following intervention, rather than early in the intervention delivery process, fewer youth were engaged in fewer instances of drinking and smoking. What is more, other ethnographic data collections substantiated the potentially salubrious effects of community activities to encourage alcohol- and tobacco-free events aimed at members of the intervention community. Noncomparable ethnographic data from the control community did not permit across-condition evaluations to determine intervention effects on study outcomes.

CONCLUSIONS AND RECOMMENDATIONS

Our twin goals of targeting minority adolescents at the community level and of working through the natural structures of the community to foster a sense of community responsibility had both unexpected benefits and unexpected consequences. The project was revised to focus on the particular needs of Hispanic youth. Yet under the community's direction, the issue of substance abuse was frequently overshadowed by other community concerns. As the project director grew increasingly involved in community politics, several issues stole focus from the original intent to prevent substance use among the community's adolescents. Without specifically intending to, the project director and the study became involved in a number of other projects, including community redistricting, a parent literacy program, a dropout prevention committee, a peer leadership program, and an educational program based in a housing project.

The current program includes a network of supportive community organizations, a media campaign featuring positive role models, a team of volunteers trained to promote program awareness and to encourage role-model imitation, community events designed to attract high-risk youth to participate in skills-training contests, a specialized, small-group curriculum for social skills training of high-risk youth referred by local sources (e.g., juvenile probation, alternative schools), teacher training for adoption of school-based curricula, and environmental policy initiatives selected by local volunteers. These elements represent the bulk of the program objectives, though the overall structure and emphasis of the program changed as it proceeded.

Clearly, even in the demonstration stages, a prevention program may be subject to adaptation by the target community. The challenge for social scientists is to develop drug abuse prevention programs that are flexible yet robust. Programs need to both anticipate and allow for implementer modifications. Such modifications can facilitate a sense of ownership, which in turn may contribute to the success and the maintenance of the prevention program.

That research in prevention needs significant resources allocated for the transfer of innovative programming to the larger community is just as important. Murray (1986) has called dissemination "the neglected phase of the development and distribution cycle" (p. 375). If we are committed to preventing drug abuse among our nation's youth, we must insist that funding not only be provided for development of prevention programs but also for their diffusion.

REFERENCES

Basch, C. E. (1984). Research on disseminating and implementing health education programs in schools. *Journal of School Health, 54,* 57–66.

Bauman, L. J., Stein, R. E. K., & Ireys, H. T. (1991). Reinventing fidelity: The transfer of social technology among settings. *American Journal of Community Psychology, 19,* 619–639.

Berman, P., & McLaughlin, M. W. (1978). *Federal programs supporting educational change: Implementing and sustaining innovations* (Vol. 8). (Contract #R-1589/7). Washington, DC: U.S. Department of Education.

Blakely, C. H., Mayer, J. P., Gottschalk, R. G., Schmitt, N., Davidson, W. S., Rotiman, D. B., & Emshoff, J. G. (1987). The fidelity-adaptation debate: Implications for the implementation of public sector programs. *American Journal of Community Psychology, 15,* 253–268.

Butterfoss, F. D., Goodman, R. M., & Wandersman, A. (1996). Community coalitions for prevention and health promotion: Factors predicting satisfaction, participation, and planning. *Health Education Quarterly, 23*(1), 65–79.

Calsyn, R., Tornatzky, L. G., & Dittman, S. (1977). Incomplete adoption of an innovation: The case of goal attainment scaling. *Evaluation, 4,* 127–130.

Donaldson, S. I., Graham, J. W., Piccinin, A. M., & Hansen, W. B. (1995). Resistanceskills training and onset of alcohol use: Evidence for beneficial and potentially harmful effects in public schools and in private Catholic schools. *Health Psychology, 14*(4), 291–300.

Elias, M. J., & Weissberg, R. P. (1991). School-based social competence promotion as a primary prevention strategy: A tale of two projects. In *Protecting the children* (pp. 177–200). New York: Haworth Press.

Gold, R. S., Parcel, G. S., Walberg, H. J., Luepker, R. V., Portnoy, B., & Stone, E. J. (1991). Summary and conclusions of the THTM evaluation: The expert work group perspective. *Journal of School Health, 61,* 39–42.

Green, L. W. (1979). National policy in the promotion of health. *International Journal of Health Education, 12,* 161–168.

Hall, G., & Hord, S. (1987). *Change in schools: Facilitating the process (p. 122).* Albany: State University of New York Press.

Huberman, A. M., & Miles, M. B. (1984). Innovation Up Close: How School Improvement Works. New York: Plenum Press.

Kotler, P. (1982). Social marketing. In *Marketing for nonprofit organizations (2nd ed.).* Englewood Cliffs, NJ: Prentice–Hall.

Levenson-Gingiss, P., & Hamilton, R. (1989). Determinants of teachers' plans to continue teaching a sexual education course. *Family & Community Health, 12,* 40–53.

McIntyre, L., Belzer, E. G., Manchester, L., Blachard, W., Officer, S., & Simpson, A. C. (1996). The Dartmouth Health Promotion Study: A failed quest for synergy in school health promotion. *Journal of School Health, 66*(4), 132–137.

Murray, D. M. (1986). Dissemination of community health promotion programs: The Fargo-Moorhead Heart Health Program. *Journal of School Health, 56,* 375–381.

Oetting, E. R., Donnermeyer, J. F., Plested, B. A., Edwards, R. W., Kelly, K., & Beauvais, F. (1995). Assessing community readiness for prevention. *International Journal of the Addictions, 30,* 659–683.

Parcel, G. S., Perry, C. L., & Taylor, W. C. (1990). Beyond demonstration: Diffusion of health innovations. In N. Bracht (Ed.), *Health promotion at the community level.* Newbury Park, NJ: Sage.

Parcel, G. S., Ross, J. G., Lavin, A. T., Portnoy, B., Nelson, G. D., Winters, F. (1991). Enhancing implementation on the Teenage Health Teaching Modules. *Journal of School Health, 61,* 35–38.

Pentz, M. A., Trebow, E. A., Hansen, W. B., MacKinnon, D. P., Dwyer, J. H., Johnson, C. A., Flay, B. R., Daniels, S., & Cormack, C. (1990). Effects of program implementation on adolescent drug use behavior: The Midwest Prevention Project (MPP). *Evaluation Review, 14,* 264–289.

Pirie, P. L., Murray, D. M., & Luepker, R. M. (1988). Smoking prevalence in a cohort of adolescents, including absentees, dropouts, and transfers. *American Journal of Public Health, 78,* 176–179.

Rogers, E. (1995). *Diffusion of innovations* (4th edition). New York: The Free Press.

Rothman, J. (1979). Three models of community organization practice. In F. M. Cox, J. L. Erlich, J. Rothman, & R. E. Tropman (Eds.), *Strategies of community organization.* Itasca, IL: Peacock.

Schinke, S. P., & Botvin, G. J. (1999). Life skills training. *Contemporary Pediatrics, 16*(5) 108–117.

Schinke, S. P., & Tepavac, L. (1995). Substance abuse prevention among elementary school students. *Drugs & Society, 8*(3/4), 15–27.

Schinke, S. P., Cole, K. C., & Poulin, S. R. (2000). Enhancing the educational achievement of at-risk youth. *Prevention Science, 1,* 51–60.

Schinke, S. P., Orlandi, M. A., & Cole, K. C. (1992). Boys and girls clubs in public housing developments: Prevention services for youth at risk. *Journal of Community Psychology,* (OSAP Special Issue), 118–128.

Schinke, S. P., Orlandi, M. A., Vaccaro, D., Espinoza, R., McAlister, A., & Botvin, G. J. (1992). Substance use among Hispanic and non-Hispanic adolescents. *Addictive Behaviors, 17,* 117–124.

Schinke, S. P., Tepavac, L., & Cole, K. C. (2000). Preventing substance use among Native American Youth: Three-year results. *Addictive Behaviors, 25,* 387–397.

Smith, D. W., Steckler, A., McCormick, L. K., & McLeroy, K. R. (1995). Lessons learned about disseminating health curricula to schools. *Journal of Health Education, 26,* 37–43.

Smith, T. E., Schinke, S. P., & Springer, D. W. (2001). Single-system evaluation of child protective services training. *Professional Development, 3*(2), 33–39.

CHAPTER 30

Family Management Practices: Research Design and Measurement Issues

THOMAS J. DISHION
BERT BURRASTON
FUZHONG LI

INTRODUCTION

What do parents do to establish, maintain, or alter the developmental course of their teenager? Which dimensions of parenting lead to maladaptive outcomes in children? These are among the most perplexing questions in research on adolescent problem behavior. The two most studied variables in this area are parental family-management strategies (Patterson, 1982; Patterson, Reid, & Dishion, 1992) and the affective connection between parent and child, described as either the attachment relationship or the parent–child bond (Bowlby, 1969; Elliott, Huizinga, & Ageton, 1985; Hirschi, 1969). The family-management perspective emphasizes minimizing coercive and conflicted parent–child exchanges that contribute to antisocial and other problem behaviors. Researchers who emphasize the parent–child relationship consider it to be the key to an adolescent's success in other relationships throughout the life span. A more comprehensive view integrates multiple dimensions of parenting on child and adolescent social development. Baumrind (1985) considers parenting to have two dimensions: warmth (relationship quality) and control

THOMAS J. DISHION • Child and Family Center, University of Oregon, Department of Psychiatry, Eugene, Oregon 97401
BERT BURRASTON • Oregon Social Learning Center, Eugene, Oregon 97401
FUZHONG LI • Oregon Social Learning Center and Oregon Research Institute, Eugene, Oregon 97401

(behavior management). Hawkins and colleagues (1986) and McCord (1991) view the parent–child bond as a separate but correlated feature of the family environment, distinguishable from family management. Longitudinal studies suggest that this integration of family-management and relationship theories has promise in accounting for adolescent delinquent behavior. For example, McCord (1992) has reanalyzed the Cambridge–Somerville data and found that both dimensions of parenting can predict adolescent delinquency.

Despite these and other advances in understanding the contributions of parents to adolescent substance abuse, the field would benefit from a set of constructs and a model that delineates developmental processes leading to adolescent problem behavior and provides a target for intervention. A useful step in this process is to conduct construct validation studies that clarify the interrelation among parenting constructs and measurement issues that affect predictive validity. Careful examination of the measurement properties and validity of diverse approaches to conceptualization and assessment of parenting practices can lead to enhanced understanding of developmental processes and inform intervention science, as can be seen in the study described in this chapter.

THE STUDY

The goal of this study was to conduct a confirmatory factor analysis (CFA) of multiple measures of parenting practices in a sample of 224 families with high-risk, young adolescents (11 to 14 years of age). The families were involved in a series of intervention studies conducted to reduce escalating trends in problem behavior (Andrews, Soberman, & Dishion, 1995; Dishion & Andrews, 1995). Building on the work of Patterson and colleagues (1992), we collected measures from child, parent, and staff impressions of five family-management constructs: limit setting, monitoring, problem solving, positive reinforcement, and relationship quality. A significant advance in research on parenting practices is the use of multitrait–multimethod (MTMM) data. By combining measures, the fallibility of any individual strategy can be reduced, and the possibility of single-method bias can be avoided (Cook & Campbell, 1979; Dwyer, 1983). We used an MTMM measurement strategy to address construct validation questions: To what extent are these parenting constructs intercorrelated and at what level? The level of correlation among the parenting trait constructs addresses the issue of whether these practices either are part of a general parenting style or reflect distinct dimensions. To what extent does the measurement method (i.e., reporting agent—parent, child, or staff rater) account for covariation among the observed data?

Bank et al. (1990) discuss method problems in the context of structural equation modeling (SEM). A method problem exists when the most highly correlated indicators in a model are derived from the same measurement method. In an MMTM analysis, method constructs can be operationalized and studied along with parenting-trait constructs. In the context of SEM, competing models (e.g., trait versus method) can be compared using model fit indices as well as differences in the chi-square goodness-of-fit test (Bentler & Bonnett, 1980).

The parenting constructs (trait or method) were also evaluated with respect to criterion and predictive validity. In this analysis, measures of criterion and predictive validity were objective and independent of measures used to define the parenting constructs. Direct observations of negative parent–child exchanges form a valid criterion measure of parenting (Patterson, 1982; Patterson et al., 1992) as well as provide a target for intervention (Dishion & Andrews, 1995; McMahon & Peters, 1990; Patterson, 1974; Webster-Stratton & Hammond, 1990). As an index of problem behavior, we used official school and police records of an adolescent's conflicts with authority in the 2-year period after the initial assessment.

Participants

The participants were recruited for a series of studies underlying the development of the Adolescent Transitions Program, designed to help prevent adolescent drug and alcohol use. Participants were recruited in seven cohorts, from 1988 to 1992. All were considered to be at-risk. Cohorts 1 through 5 were referred by parents and were in grades 6, 7, and 8. Cohorts 6 and 7 were recruited through the schools and were all in grade 7. Baseline data for all participants were combined in the models tested.

The 224 participants included 111 boys and 113 girls who were predominantly (90%) European American. At baseline, they ranged in age from 10 to 14 years of age, with an average age of 12.2 years. The family status included 42.9% from single-family households (mostly single mothers), 36.2% from two-parent families in which one of the parents was a step-parent, and 21% from intact two-parent families. The families tended to be economically disadvantaged, with 48.2% receiving some sort of financial aid; 60% had a gross annual income less than $20,000; 80% of the mothers and 74% of the fathers had completed high school; and 17% of mothers and fathers had graduated from college. Assessment data included questionnaires, interviews, telephone interviews, videotaped observations, and official records.

Procedures

Prior to the start of treatment (baseline) and again shortly after completion of treatment (termination), the teens and their parents were interviewed separately for approximately 45 minutes. Afterward, the interviewer was asked to fill out an impressions form containing 25 questions covering a broad range of characteristics, ranging from each child's social skills to how likely it would be for the child to get in trouble with the police. Prior to the interview, the parent (or parents) and child were asked to complete several questionnaires. Questionnaires, including the Peer Involvement and Social Skill Questionnaire (Walker & McConnell, 1988) and the teacher Child Behavior Checklist (Achenbach, 1991), were also sent to the child's teacher.

At baseline, termination, and at yearly follow-up intervals, the parents and teens were contacted for a series of six brief telephone interviews, conducted at 3-day intervals. An attempt was made to conduct both the parent and the child telephone interviews on the same day when possible. The telephone interview included an assessment of the child's involvement in substance use, deviant peer groups, and other delinquent behaviors as well his or her impressions of the parents' monitoring and discipline practices.

Research staff members retrieved adult and juvenile court records. School records included standard test scores, transcripts of grades, attendance, and discipline contacts. Records were also kept of out-of-home placements to juvenile corrections facilities, group homes, and special schools for children with problem behavior.

The formation of constructs was hypothesis driven. Items from the interviews and staff impressions were generated to measure constructs within a general model of antisocial behavior (Patterson et al., 1992). In the analysis, the measurement method refers to the reporting agent. Table 30.1 identifies the construct, the reporting agent, the instrument used, and the 3-month retest stability. All constructs were formed from data collected prior to the start of treatment. Three-month retest stability scores were formed by correlating baseline measurements with like measurements taken shortly after termination.

TABLE 30.1. Family Management Constructs: Composition and 3-Month Retest Reliability

	Monitoring			Limit setting			Relationship quality			Positive reinforcement			Problem solving		
	n	α	s	n	α	s	n	α	s	n	α	s	n	α	s
Total construct			.70[a]			.54[a]			.67[a]			.51[a]			.47[a]
Total child report	8	.68	.63[a]		—	.47[a]			.61[a]			.47[a]	5	.87n	.46[a]
Child interview	—	—	.68[a]	—	—	.47[a]	—	—	.49[a]	—	—	.40[a]			
Child daily report	—	—	.48[a]	—	—	.33[a]	—	—	.67[a]	—	—	.40[a]			
Total parent report			.51[a]			.64[a]			.63[a]			.59[a]	7	.79mn	.43[a]
Parent interview	13	.81m	.70[a]	11	.81m	.65[a]	5	.85m	.65[a]			.57[a]			
Parent daily report	5	.38	.42[a]		—	.29[a]		—	.60[a]			.42[a]			
Family activity report							28	c	.48[a]						
Total staff impressions			.33[a]			.15[a]			.43[a]			.35[a]			.43[a]
FPC coder impression		—	.20[b]	5	.73	.15[c]	5	.86m	.22[b]		—	.31[a]		—	.32[a]
PEN-P coder impression		—	.26[a]			.32[a]	5	.86m	.38[a]		—	.20[b]	8	.86	.32[a]

NOTE. Dashes indicate that the scales consisting of fewer than five items were not reported; s = stability; m = values for the mother responses; n = separate alphas computed for the parent and child problems; c = scale was formed as a count of the number of items endorsed. [a] $p < .001$. [b] $p < .01$. [c] $p < .05$.

CONSTRUCTS

Monitoring

The definition of this construct relies on measures used in previous studies (e.g., Patterson & Dishion, 1985). Parent monitoring involves assuring that the child is in settings that are supervised by adults, articulation and enforcement of rules that track the child's whereabouts (e.g., leaving the phone number of friends with whom the child is visiting), and professional impressions of the parental supervision of the child.

A child report score was based on a personal interview and a series of telephone interviews in which the child was asked: "Do your parents know if you play with kids who get in trouble?", "Do your parents let you go anywhere without asking?", "How often do you tell your parents when you will return?" and "How often do you leave a note for your parents?" In the telephone interviews, the child was asked: "How much time have you spent with your parents in the previous 24 hours?" and "How often do you talk with your parents about what you have done or are going to do?"

The parent report was also based on personal and telephone interviews covering the previous 24 hours. In the personal interview, the parent was asked: "How often does your child go to forbidden places?", "How difficult is it to know where your child is?", "How often is there adult supervision when your child is away from home?", "How often is your child home by the set time?", and "How often is your child at a friend's house when they say they will be?" In the telephone interview the parent was asked: "How much time have you spent with your child in the previous 24 hours?" and whether or not the child was out after 7:00 p.m. without an adult.

Staff impressions included two separate impression inventories. Staff members using the Family Process Code (FPC) (Dishion et al., 1983) were asked to rate how well the parent (or parents) seemed to monitor the child. FPC intercoder reliability was .55, $p < .001$. Staff members using the Pencil-and-Paper Code (PEN-P) (Dishion & Soberman, 1994) were asked to rate how well informed the parents were about their child's whereabouts and whether or not the parents avoided intervening with the child. The intercorrelation between two raters was .38, $p < .05$.

Limit Setting

This construct (referred to as discipline in previous research) (Patterson, 1982; Patterson Dishion, & Bank, 1984, 1992) was expanded to include the parents' tendency to articulate clear and consistent rules. Skillful limit setting is firm, consistent, nonabusive, and used sparingly.

A child report was based on the personal interview that asked: "How often do your parents punish you after threatening punishment?", "How often can you get out of your parent's punishment?", "How often do your parents agree on punishment?", and "How often do your parents punish fairly?"

The parent interview assessed limit-setting skills: "How often do you follow through on punishment?", "How often does your punishment depend on mood?", and "How often can your child get out of a punishment?"

After coding the family's videotaped interactions using the FPC, staff members rated the parents' limit-setting abilities: "Did the parent (or parents) use ineffective discipline?", "Did the parent seem to lack parental discipline?", and "Did the parent give rationales?" FPC intercoder reliability was .61, $p < .001$.

Relationship Quality

The quality of the parent–child relationship in early adolescence has three theoretical dimensions: (1) the extent to which the parent and child are positive with one another when discussing family issues, (2) the extent to which the parent and child are involved in one another's lives in terms of shared activities, and (3) the sense of mutual acceptance and lack of rejection.

In the personal interview the child was asked, "How well do you get along with each of your parents?" In the telephone interview the child was asked, "Do your parents hug, kiss, or show affection to you?"

Parent reports were based on personal and telephone interviews and the Family Activities Checklist (1984), which contains 28 activities that previous groups of parents and children have identified as pleasurable events (e.g., going to a movie together). Parents were asked to indicate if any of the activities occurred within the past week. In the personal interview the parent was asked, "How easy is it to spend time with your child?" and "How difficult is it to be patient with your child?" In the telephone interview the parent was asked, "How often do you hug, kiss, or show affection to your child?"

After coding the family's videotaped interaction using the FPC, staff members were asked to rate the relationship each parent had with the child, how often each parent engaged in various behaviors with the child (e.g., "How often was mom/dad verbally affectionate with child?", "How often was mom/dad hostile to child?"), and how often the child engaged in various behaviors with each parent (e.g., "How often was the child friendly to mom/dad?", "How often did the child seem detached from mom/dad?"). FPC intercoder reliability was .69, $p < .001$. Staff members using the PEN-P were also asked, "How often did mom/dad/child show expressions of affections?", "How often did mom/dad/child use humor to lighten the situation?", and "How much does each family member enjoy spending time with the family?" The correlation among PEN-P coders was .66, $p < .001$.

Problem Solving

This construct reflects the parents' skill in actively resolving points of conflict or other family problems. The construct was first specified in Patterson's (1982) discussion of family management. Research by Forgatch (1989) studied the problem-solving process in detail, finding that expressed negative emotion disrupted problem-solving discussions and outcomes.

After a structured problem-solving task in which the family was asked to solve one problem the parents chose and one the child chose, the child was asked: "How well did you understand the problem?", "Do you think the problem was solved during the discussion?", and "How satisfied are you with the discussion?"

After the structured problem-solving task, the parents were asked: "How much did you agree on a solution?" and "Did the family decide to take some action?"

After coding the structured problem-solving task using the FPC, staff members were asked to rate how much each parent provoked the child to argue. FPC intercoder reliability was .64, $p < .001$. Staff members using the PEN-P were asked to rate how much of an emotional topic the problem was for the family and how well the family solved the problem (e.g., "What was the quality of the proposed solution?", "How likely is the family to follow through with the proposed solution?", and "Did the family discuss the advantages and disadvantages of the proposed solution?"). PEN-P intercoder reliability was .52, $p < .001$.

Positive Reinforcement

Positive reinforcement reflects the parents' skill in praising or complimenting their child, as well as their use of giving extra privileges for desired behaviors.

In the personal interview, the child was asked: "How often does your parent reward or praise you daily?" and "How often is your parent hard to please?" In the telephone interview the child was asked: "Did your parent praise or compliment you in the previous 24 hours?" and "Did your parent give you extra privileges?"

In the personal interview, parents were asked: "How often did you praise your child for a good job?" and "How often did you give something extra because you were pleased with your child?" In the telephone interview, they were asked: "Did you praise or compliment your child in the previous 24 hours?" and "Did you give something extra to your child in the previous 24 hours?"

After coding the family's videotaped interaction using the FPC, staff members were asked to rate each parent on whether or not they used sarcasm and if they were positive and reinforcing. FPC intercoder reliability was .62, $p < .001$. PEN-P coders were asked to rate each parent on whether they suggested using a social learning strategy for behavior management or if they suggested behavior management strategies that are hard to carry out. The correlation among PEN-P coders at .27 was not significant.

Authority Conflict

This construct indicates how often the child was either disciplined at school or had contact with police for problem behavior in the 2 years following intervention. It was measured using three scores created from public records. From juvenile court records, the number of offenses were counted and split into four scores: $0 =$ no offenses; $1 = 1$ offense; $2 = 2$ offenses; and $3 = 3$ or more offenses. The next measurement was the child's school status: $0 =$ in public school; $1 =$ in a special school because of behavioral problems or court mandate; and $2 =$ dropped out or expelled from school. Finally, a score was created from school records based on the number of discipline contacts the student received: $0 =$ no discipline contacts; $1 =$ below the 50th percentile of those receiving discipline contacts; $2 =$ between the 50th and 75th percentile; and $3 =$ above the 75th percentile. The three scores were added together to create the authority–conflict score.

Substance Use

This construct indicates how often the child used drugs, alcohol, and tobacco in the previous year. It was measured using two methods—a child self-report and a carbon monoxide breath test. All the variables were transformed into standardized values (z scores) so they would have equal variance and be on the same scale. Child drug use was the average of four child-report variables and the one breath-test variable. Factor analysis and scale reliability analysis indicated that the five variables formed an excellent factor, with an alpha of .84.

RESULTS

The first step in considering the relative contribution of trait and method variance in accounting for covariation in these measures of parenting is to inspect the correlation matrix (Campbell & Fiske, 1959). Specifically, visual inspection of the pattern of correlations (see Table 30.2) suggests larger issues with respect to the discriminant and convergent validity of these data.

TABLE 30.2. Pearson Product–Moment Correlations among Measures of Parenting Practices (Monitoring, Relationship Quality, Problem Solving, and Positive Reinforcement as Measured by Child Report, Parent Report, and Staff Impression)

	1	2	3	4	5	6	7	8	9	10	11	12	13	14	15
Monitoring															
1. Parent	1.00														
2. Child	.37	1.00													
3. Staff	.39	.31	1.00												
Limit setting															
4. Parent	.34	.13	.29	1.00											
5. Child	.21	.37	.18	.19	1.00										
6. Staff	.24	.27	.58	.25	.15	1.00									
Positive reinforcement															
7. Parent	.26	.09ns	.09ns	.23	.09ns	.09ns	1.00								
8. Child	.19	.40	.13	.10ns	.24	.09ns	.26	1.00							
9. Staff	.30	.12ns	.51	.23	.14	.50	.15	.06ns	1.00						
Relationship quality															
10. Parent	.52	.28	.22	.48	.22	.19	.35	.22	.24	1.00					
11. Child	.29	.43	.30	.22	.33	.16	.09	.53	.18	.42	1.00				
12. Staff	.32	.18	.49	.29	.19	.49	.14	.17	.67	.35	.36	1.00			
Problem solving															
13. Parent	.13ns	.15	.32	.38	.19	.27	.15	.14	.28	.28	.26	.34	1.00		
14. Child	.14	.23	.26	.22	.30	.19	.11ns	.16	.27	.16	.38	.38	.67	1.00	
15. Staff	.22	.14	.42	.23	.15	.37	.08ns	.01ns	.64	.26	.24	.66	.42	.37	1.00

NOTE. $N = 218$.

Parenting Trait

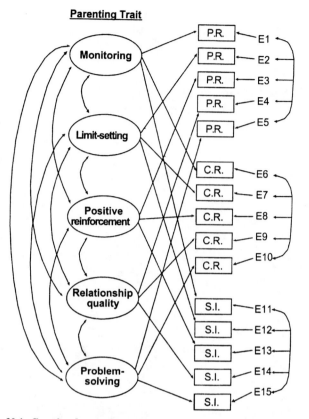

FIGURE 30.1. Correlated parenting traits and correlated uniqueness model (CTCU).

Correlations within the diagonals (right angles) represent convergent validity, or variation due to the specific parenting traits being measured. Ideally, convergent validity correlations are statistically reliable and large in magnitude (among the largest within matrix). As evident in Table 30.2, all but one convergent validity correlation was statistically reliable; however, nearly all correlations were moderate to weak in magnitude ($M = .31$). The average convergent validity coefficient was modestly higher than other remaining correlations in the matrix ($M = .26$), making evidence for convergent validity modest, based on visual inspection. In particular, the positive reinforcement construct shows the lowest convergent validity of all five parenting constructs. Parent report of positive reinforcement is reliably correlated with both child report and staff impressions, but child report and staff impressions are uncorrelated. This pattern of covariation results in parent report defining the factor (the highest factor loading) within the context of either an exploratory or CFA.

The magnitude of the method effects can be seen by examining the heterotrait–monomethod correlations (different traits, same method correlations). The larger the correlations, the more substantial the measurement method in accounting for covariation within these data. We found moderate-to-weak method effects ($M = .39$). The average method effect was slightly larger than the average trait effect ($M = .39, .31$, respectively).

A more rigorous approach to hypothesis testing, regarding the relative contribution of measurement method and parenting traits in accounting for these data, is the use of SEM as a format for testing confirmatory factor models. Marsh and Grayson (1995; Marsh, 1989) articulated the array of methodology issues, as well as optimal strategies for applying an SEM–CFA framework. An assumption underlying maximum likelihood estimation is that the data are multivariate normal. As a preliminary step, the distributional properties of the 15 indicators used in the MTMM analysis were examined. Skewness and kurtosis measures suggested that the marginal distributions of the data set were normal; skewness values averaged $-.38$, with a range of -1.18 to $.17$, and kurtosis values averaged $.44$ (absolute value), with a range of $-.54$ to 2.66.

The Marsh strategy (1989) was designed to be appropriate for all MTMM studies that have at least four traits and three methods factors. Marsh proposed examining a minimum of four SEM–CFA models in the analysis of MTMM (also, see Marsh & Grayson, 1995). The authors examined Marsh's four models and examined a fifth model, due to the result of the four prior models. In order to evaluate the discriminant validity of the parenting constructs, all four models allowed for correlations among the five traits.

The first SEM–CFA, correlated traits only (CTO), contains only trait factors and allows for no method effects. The other four models contain both trait factors and method effects: (1) correlated traits with correlated uniqueness or correlated errors (CTCU), (2) correlated traits with uncorrelated method factors (CTUM), (3) correlated traits with correlated method factors (CTCM), and (4) correlated traits with partially correlated method factors (CTPCM).

The CTO model is nested in the other four models, so that a comparison of fit with other models provides an indication of the size of the method effects (Marsh & Grayson, 1995). Any increase in the goodness-of-fit from the CTO model to the other models can be attributed to method effects (Joreskog, 1971). In all models, large and statistically significant trait factor loadings are an indication of convergent validity; small trait factor correlations are an indication of discriminant validity. Trait factor correlations approaching 1 are a sign of a lack of discriminant validity.

The CTCU model is identical to the CTO model, with one exception: In the CTCU, the error variances or uniqueness are correlated by methods (see Figure 30.1 and Table 30.3). The method effects are inferred by the correlated error variances. Those from the parents are uncorrelated with the method effects from the child or the staff, and the method effects associated with the

TABLE 30.3. Summary of Goodness-of-Fit Indexes for MTMM Model of Parenting Practices

Model	χ^2	df	TLI NNFI	CFI	Proper
1. Trait only (CTO)	417.924	80	.536	.646	No
2. Five correlated trait with correlated method errors (CTCU)	84.408	50	.937	.970	Yes
3. Five correlated traits; three uncorrelated methods (CTUM)	132.556	65	.905	.941	Yes
4. Five correlated traits; parent, child correlated methods (CTPCM)	120.459	64	.919	.951	Yes
5. Five correlated traits; three correlated methods; three correlated methods (CTCM)	102.745	62	.940	.964	No

NOTE. TLI = Tucker–Lewis index; CFI = comparative fit index.

child are uncorrelated with the method effects from the staff. Method effects are inferred by large correlated errors by methods. Therefore, if all the parent variable errors are significantly correlated with each other, we have parent–method effects. The same can be said about the child or staff variable errors.

In contrast, the CTUM, CTPCM, and CTCM models contain trait and method factors. They differ from each other in that CTUM assumes the method factors are uncorrelated with each other, and CTCM assumes the method factors are correlated with each other. The CTPCM assumes that only some of the method factors are correlated (Figure 2). Thus, comparing their fit indexes will test whether or not the method effects are correlated. The CTUM, CTPCM, and CTCM models assume that all the method effects from the parent can be explained by the parent–method factor, all the method effects from the child can be explained by the child–method factor, and all the method effects from the staff can be explained by the staff-method factor. Comparing the fit indexes between the CTCU model to the CTUM and CTCM models tests whether or not there is a unidimensionality of method effects. Method effects are inferred by large and statistically significant method factor loadings.

Caution should be used in analyzing the CTUM and the CTCM models because they often result in improper solutions. A solution is improper if it is not identifiable or if the estimated parameters fall outside the permissible range. For example, solutions with negative or zero variances are improper, and extreme caution should be used in interpreting them. Marsh and Bailey (1991) examined 435 MTMM matrices and found that 77% of the CTCM models resulted in improper solutions; the CTUM models fair a little better. The CTCU model almost always results in a proper solution (98% of the time). Marsh and Bailey also found that the matrices became stable when sample size was 250 or larger and as the number of traits and methods increased. They recommend as a minimum, testing four traits and three methods.

The tests of the five models are presented in Table 30.3, along with the goodness-of-fit indexes (chi-square statistic, TLI, CFI) derived from comparing the model-generated covariation coefficients to the observed covariation among the 15 indicators. The CTPCM model was run because the CTCM model resulted in an improper solution, but it fit the data well. As stated earlier, ill-defined solutions occur frequently in the CFA application to MTMM analysis. Researchers are encouraged to place their emphasis only on those models that result in proper solutions (Bagozzi, 1993; Marsh, 1989; Marsh & Grayson, 1995). In these analyses, only CTCU, CTUM, and CTPCM models resulted in proper, identified solutions.

Examination of the models' goodness-of-fit indicated that all models containing method effects were superior in fit to the trait-only model (CTO), indicating substantial method effects. The goodness-of-fit of the CTO model is not adequate. The best fitting models were the CTCM and CTCU models, with fits found to be almost identical. However, the CTCM model resulted in an improper solution. Therefore, we will not attempt to interpret this model past its goodness-of-fit index. It is unclear if unidimensionality of methods effects is supported because both the CTUM and the CTCM models fit the data well (TLI = .905 and .940, respectively), but the CTCU model fits the data equally well (TLI = .937). When comparing the CTCM model to the CTUM model, it appeared that the method factors were correlated with each other. However, because the CTCM model resulted in an improper solution, we were not able to interpret the CTCM model. The Lagrange Multiplier (Modification Index) indicated that the parent and child factors were correlated. Therefore, we ran a fifth model identical to the CTUM model, but with the parent- and child-method factors correlated (CTPCM), which resulted in a more superior fit than that of the CTUM model and a proper solution. We will interpret the CTCU and the CTPCM models.

Beginning with the CTCU model, which resulted in the best fitting model with a proper solution, the standardized loadings for each trait construct in the CTCU model are shown in

TABLE 30.4. Parameter Estimates for Best-Fitting Models: CFA–CTCU Model

Traits and methods		Trait factor loading	Squared multiple correlation	Uniqueness	Uniqueness correlations				
					MO	LS	PR	RQ	PS
MO	PR	.67	.45	.55	1.00				
LS	PR	.53	.28	.72	−.11	1.00			
PR	PR	.47	.22	.78	.18	.15	1.00		
RQ	PR	.63	.40	.60	.41	.35	.31	1.00	
PS	PR	.94	.88	.12	−.36	.27	−.03	.10	1.00
MO	CR	.50	.25	.75	1.00				
LS	CR	.38	.14	.86	.28	1.00			
PR	CR	.51	.26	.74	.38	.17	1.00		
RQ	CR	.64	.40	.60	.30	.20	.52	1.00	
PS	CR	.72	.52	.48	.16	.23	.08	.32	1.00
MO	CR	.54	.30	.70	1.00				
LS	CR	.33	.11	.89	.50	1.00			
PR	CR	.26	.07	.93	.45	.44	1.00		
RQ	CR	.42	.17	.83	.37	.40	.64	1.00	
PS	CR	.31	.10	.90	.33	.28	.62	.60	1.00

Trait correlations

	MO	LS	PR	RQ	PS
MO	1.00				
LS	.81	1.00			
PR	.52	.56	1.00		
RQ	.69	.77	.58	1.00	
PS	.43	.59	.42	.50	1.00

NOTE. See Table 30.5 for key to acronyms.

Table 30.4. Convergent validity is reflected in the magnitude of the trait loadings. Although most were moderate in size ($M = .52$), all loadings on the parenting trait factors were statistically significant. Problem solving, monitoring, and relationship quality have moderate factor loadings ($M = .66, .57,$ and $.56$, respectively), and limit setting and positive reinforcement had the lowest average factor loading ($M = .41$) for each. This constitutes evidence of convergent validity in the sense that different methods measuring the same trait are all statistically significant and appear to converge.

In the CTCU model, method effects are found in the uniqueness correlations among the different variables assessed by the same method. The method effects are mostly low with a few moderate correlations. Staff impressions has the highest average uniqueness correlation ($M = .46$.) Parent and child reports, on average, had small uniqueness correlations ($M = .23$ and $.26$, respectively). The trait effects are highest for the parent-report method and lowest for the staff-impressions methods ($M = .65$ and $.37$, respectively).

In the CTCU model, discriminant validity is assessed by examining the level of correlations between the different trait factors. The higher the correlations between the trait, the lower the discriminant validity. The traits most correlated with each other are monitoring and limit setting ($r = .81$), indicating that they are separate factors, but highly related to each other. The traits least correlated with each other are positive reinforcement and problem solving ($r = .42$), indicating that they are separate factors, but moderately related to each other. Overall, we do find discriminant validity, in that each trait forms a unique factor. However, as one would expect, these parenting traits are highly correlated to each other.

TABLE 30.5. Trait and Method Loadings for CTPCM Model

	MO	LS	PR	RQ	PS	PR	CR	SI
Parent report (ParR)								
Monitoring (MO)	.46					.48		
Limit setting (LS)		.43				.40		
Positive reinforcement (PO)			.24			.35		
Relationship quality (RQ)				.40		.85		
Problem solving (PS)					.87	.10ns		
Child report (CR)								
Monitoring (MO)	.41						.52	
Limit setting (LS)		.29					.37	
Positive reinforcement (PO)			.26				.63	
Relationship quality (RQ)				.49			.66	
Problem solving (PS)					.77		.18	
Staff impression (SI)								
Monitoring (MO)	.78							.23
Limit setting (LS)		.59						.32
Positive reinforcement (PO)			.52					.69
Relationship quality (RQ)				.62				.61
Problem solving (PS)					.47			.70
Mean factor loading	.55	.44	.34	.50	.70	.44	.47	.51

The advantage of the CTUM, CTPCM, and CTCM models is in the ease of comparing the magnitude of the trait effects to the magnitude of the method effects. The standardized loadings for each method and trait construct based on the CTPCM model are shown in Table 30.5. Convergent validity is reflected in the magnitude of the trait loadings. Although most of them were moderate in size ($M = .51$), all loadings on the parenting trait factors were statistically significant. This constitutes evidence of convergent validity in the sense that different methods measuring the same trait appear to converge. Note, however, that the magnitude of the loadings varied considerably across parenting constructs. For instance, loadings on the problem-solving factor were shown to be the highest in size ($M = .70$), whereas loadings on the positive reinforcement factor were the lowest ($M = .34$).

Loadings on the method factors were, on average, lower than those on the trait factors, but were also moderate in magnitude ($M = .47$); all but one were statistically significant, indicating moderate method effects. Moderate loadings on the method factors suggested that unique aspects of the reporting perspectives of the parent, child, and staff were an important source of covariation in these data. Not surprising, the method effects were minimal on the problem-solving construct, where the trait loadings were relatively high.

When discussing the magnitude of method and trait effects within each indicator, it is important to consider the proportion for which variance is accounted. The proportion of variance of an indicator accounted for by a trait or method factor is equal to the square of the standardized factor loading. These partitioned variances are summarized in Table 30.6.

Inspection of the proportion of variance in each indicator, accounted for by trait and method variance, revealed a mixed pattern. In general, the trait variance was small, ranging from a high of .76 to a low of .06. The method variance exceeded that of trait variance for 8 of the 15 variables, with 3 of the variances being almost identical; only parent report of relationship quality resulted in high method variance (SMC $= .72$). All three methods' measurement procedures showed a considerable amount of uniqueness (i.e., variance that was not explained by either the trait or

TABLE 30.6. Variance Components Due to Trait, Method, and Uniqueness for CTPCM Model

	Trait	Method	Uniqueness
Parent report			
Monitoring (MO)	.22	.23	.55
Limit-setting (LS)	.18	.16	.66
Positive reinforcement (PR)	.06	.13	.81
Relationship quality (RQ)	.16	.72	.12
Problem-solving (PS)	.76	.01	.23
Child report			
Monitoring (MO)	.17	.27	.56
Limit-setting (LS)	.09	.14	.77
Positive reinforcement (PR)	.07	.40	.53
Relationship quality (RQ)	.24	.43	.33
Problem-solving (PS)	.60	.03	.37
Staff impression			
Monitoring (MO)	.61	.08	.31
Limit-setting (LS)	.34	.10	.56
Positive reinforcement (PR)	.27	.47	.26
Relationship quality (RQ)	.38	.37	.25
Problem-solving (PS)	.22	.48	.30

the method factors). For example, the error variances exceed or are equal to the sum of the trait and method variances in 7 of the 15 observed variables. These results suggest that both method and error variance within each indicator combine to attenuate the level of variation within each indicator that can be attributed to the parenting traits. For example, only parent report of problem solving, child report of problem solving, and staff impressions of monitoring resulted in trait variances that exceeded the sum of the method and error variances (SMC = .76, .60, and .61, respectively). Whether or not we used Campbell and Fisk's method or any of the CFA models we found similar results. The method effects are slightly larger than are the trait effects, but both effects are moderate to weak.

As in the CTCU model, discriminant validity can be evaluated in the CFA models that include method factors, such as the CTUM, CTCM, and CTPCM, by inspection of the correlations among the trait and method latent-factor scores. Conceptually, correlations among traits should be negligible in order to satisfy evidence of discriminant validity. Inspection of Table 30.7 reveals that correlations among the traits were all significant and moderate to very high ($M = .70$), with the highest correlation between limit setting and monitoring ($r = .94$) and the lowest between monitoring and problem solving ($r = .45$).

Predictive Validity

The external validity models were a simple extension of the CTCU and CTPCM models, with the inclusion of two objectively measured external variables (authority conflict, substance use). Because of incomplete data in the external variables, the authors utilized EQS multisample procedures to test the assumption that the pattern of missingness is random (Little & Rubin, 1987).

The advantage of the CFA models that include method factors, such as CTUM, CTPCM or CTCM (when they result in a proper solution), is being able to test the level of covariance between the

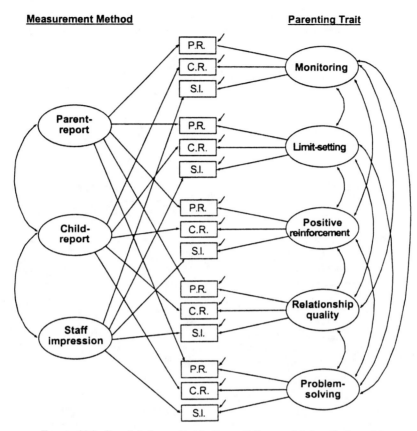

FIGURE 30.2. Correlated parenting traits, partially correlated methods model.

method effects and the outcome variables. In the CTPCM model, both trait and method factors were correlated with authority conflict and substance use 2 years later.

Generally, expectations regarding the predictive validity of the parenting traits were supported. Twelve out of 15 correlations specifying relationships between the parenting practice constructs and the external validity criteria were found to be statistically significant ($p < .05$). Table 30.8 contains the correlations between the trait factors and method factors with both authority conflict and drug use. Results of the CTPCM model revealed that monitoring was negatively related to authority conflict and drug use, indicating that high levels of parental monitoring were associated with low levels of conflicts with authority and drug use.

This further supports Dishion and colleagues' (Dishion & Loeber, 1985; Dishion & McMahon, 1998; Dishion, Reid, & Patterson, 1988) earlier findings about the importance of parental monitoring. We also found support for those who conceptualize parenting as multidimensional (Baumrind, 1985; Conger et al., 1992; Hawkins et al., 1986; McCord, 1991). Relationship quality and problem solving were found to be negatively related to drug use, indicating that parents' good relationship with their children and the ability to solve problems are associated with low levels of drug use. All the method factors are significantly related to authority conflict, with parent report being the highest ($ss = -.43$) and child report and staff impressions the lowest ($ss = -.21$ and $-.22$, respectively). Conversely, only the parent method factors is associated with drug use ($ss = .18$).

TABLE 30.7. Trait and Method Correlations for MTMM Model

Measures	Parenting traits					Methods		
	MO	LS	PO	RQ	PS	PR	CR	SI
1. MO	1.00							
2. LS	.94	1.00						
3. PO	.70	.83	1.00					
4. RQ	.64	.78	.73	1.00				
5. PS	.45	.63	.62	.67	1.00			
6. PR						1.00		
7. CR						.35	1.00	
8. SI						—	—	1.00

NOTE. MO = monitoring; LS = limit-setting; PR = positive reinforcement; RQ = relationship quality; PS = problem-solving; ParR = parent report; CR = child report; SI = staff impression.

Associations between the parenting factors and the two outcome variables, authority conflict, and drug use, were found to be stronger in the CTCU model. In the CTPCM model, only monitoring was found to be statistically significant. In contrast, monitoring, limit setting, and relationship quality were all found to be significantly negatively associated with authority conflict. Similarly, all the parenting variables were found to be significantly negatively associated with drug use. Monitoring had the highest associations with drug use of −.35 and positive reinforcement, and problem solving had the lowest associations of −.22 each.

Both the CTCU model and the CTPCM model produced similar associations between parenting factors and drug use. However, the two models produced very different associations between the parenting factors and the authority conflict. Adding a fourth method, such as direct observation, would solve the problem of one method defining a factor. Replacing staff impressions (a global rating system) with direct observations should also solve the problem. This is probably due to a combination of two conditions. First, the parent report factor is the factor most associated with authority conflict in the CTPCM model. Second, the CTCU model parent report defines or loads highest on four of the five traits. Therefore, the association that monitoring, limit setting, and

TABLE 30.8. Correlations among Parenting Practices and External Validity Factors of Adolescent Problem Behavior

	Authority conflict		Drug use	
Trait effect				
Monitoring	.16[a]	(−.44[b])	−.25[b]	(−.35[b])
Limit-setting	−.05	(−.27[b])	−.14	(−.22[b])
Positive reinforcement	.17	(−.06)	−.19	(−.22[a])
Relationship quality	−.03	(−.37[b])	−.25[b]	(−.33[b])
Problem-solving	−.00	(.00)	−.22[b]	(−.22[b])
Method effect				
Parent report	−.43[b]		−.18[b]	
Child report	−.21[b]		−.14	
Staff impressions	−.22[b]		−.11	

NOTE. Values in parentheses are from CTCU models; all other values are from CTPCM model; $n = 190$. [a]$p < .10$. [b]$p < .05$.

relationship quality have with authority conflict may be an artifact of the relationship between parent report and authority conflict.

DISCUSSION

The idea that parenting practices contribute to adolescent problem behavior has been around for some time (McCord, 1992). The scrutiny of parenting practices within a scientific paradigm has a much shorter history. However, much of the literature on the effects of parenting on adolescent delinquency and substance use is based exclusively on child, parent, or staff impressions, as these are the most economical measures. This report is the first example of using a CFA approach to MTMM data on parenting to rigorously evaluate the relative importance of traits versus methods in accounting for covariation.

Results from this study provide support for the construct validity of the parenting constructs. The five family management constructs showed reasonable convergent and discriminant validity within the MTMM framework. The correlations among the four constructs were quite high ($M = .70$, based on CTPCM), suggesting that parents who scored high on one dimension tended to score high on all dimensions of the parenting constructs. In fact, the level of correlation suggests a "G-factor" for parenting. If so, the debates in the literature regarding the specific parenting practices and family experiences that give rise to socialization outcomes such as antisocial behavior are not warranted, since one parenting practice appears to be equal to another.

There is a limited sense in which this conclusion is valid. Skillful parenting certainly requires attention to relationship issues in daily family life. Although parent training interventions do not often couch the intervention procedures in the language of relationships, if one looks closely at the actual parenting skills, relationship skills are essential to short- and long-term success. For example, when advising parents on limit setting, parents should avoid personal criticism, lecturing, or expressions of contempt (Dishion & Patterson, 1996; Forgatch & Patterson, 1989; Patterson & Forgatch, 1990).

When it comes to the field of family intervention, the debate regarding the optimal targeting of parenting practices is more than academic. Recommending that parents express more love to their child is not the same as suggesting different behavior management practices. A family management intervention model hypothesizes that the pattern of parent–child interactions needs revision vis-à-vis the issue of contingency (Dishion & Kavanagh, 1995; Patterson et al., 1992). Based on the pattern of convergent and external validity, we speculate that parent monitoring is a construct that has potential as an intervention target. It has repeatedly been shown to correlate with adolescent problem behavior and substance use, and these findings have been extended to multiethnic and urban samples (Chilcoate, Anthony, & Dishion, 1995; Dishion & McMahon, 1998). Inspection of the level of correlation between parent monitoring and relationship quality ($r = .63$) reveals that effective supervision requires a positive relationship between parents their teenager.

Methodological Implications

There were substantial method effects in the CFA that must be taken into account when modeling these 15 indicators. In this study, the method effects were conceptualized simply as those accompanying the reporting agent. Thus, each reporting agent brings an internal coherence to the global ratings that is not attributable to the behavior they are being asked to rate. Combining the method and trait constructs was referred to as the relativisitic theory of measurement. The central idea is that the variation within each indicator is attributable to both the behavioral phenomenon and the measurement tool (in this instance, reports of the participating parents and children and those of the research assistants).

The problem of method effects has been acknowledged and discussed in previous research (Bagozzi & Yi, 1990; Bank et al., 1990; Fiske, 1986, 1987). From a traditional psychometric perspective, measurement–method effects are interpreted in terms of sources of systematic bias (Fiske, 1987) or criterion contamination (Brogden & Taylor, 1950). Bagozzi and Yi's (1990) definition is typical of this position: "As an artifact of measurement, method variance can bias results when researchers investigate relations among constructs measured with the common method" (p. 547). The same argument was made in Cook and Campbell's (1979) discussion of monomethod bias. Bank et al. (1990) extended this discussion to the MTMM data (when one method tends to dominate across constructs), referring to it as the "glop problem" in structural equation modeling.

The findings from the current study raise questions of how to interpret these measurement–method effects. One interpretation is that they reflect different overall perspectives on parenting practices. Each agent has expectations based on his or her life experience, unique context, or reporting biases. For example, parents' interpretation of the self-report items may well depend on their own parenting practices or their own response style (e.g., high social desirability). By the same token, staff scores may be biased with respect to broadband personality attributions made about the parents, as well as behavior observed in the assessment setting. In either case, this aspect of method bias can be considered "noise" when studying the relation between parenting and adolescent problem behavior.

An alternative view of the method effects depicts the variance as theoretically meaningful. The fact that the child and parent methods correlated, as did the parent and staff impressions (while child and staff methods did not), suggests that shared perspectives yield similar reporting tendencies. If, for example, it was found that the child's perceptions of parenting practices had long-term predictive utility over and above the observed parenting practices, this would suggest that a child's positive reporting bias is developmentally significant, perhaps an indicator of the quality of the parent–child relationship.

CONCLUSION

Research scientists in the field clearly state that construct development is an iterative process (Nunnally, 1978). Patterson and colleagues (1992) link advances in psychometric studies and model development to intervention trials. The authors suggest that reliance on global reports of parenting practices will lead to highly intercorrelated parenting constructs, with a good percentage of their covariation attributable to method variance. When aggregating method and trait variance, the theoretical meaning of each is confused in subsequent modeling. These analyses suggest that continued study of the interrelation between measurement method and parenting practices is needed.

In general, direct observations are underutilized in developmental and intervention research. One of the critical advantages of observational data in developmental research is the ability to study the microsocial processes underlying socially significant child and adolescent outcomes (Patterson, 1982). Laboratory assessments of parent–child interaction may be particularly useful to this end. The advantage of structured assessments is that sequences of interest can be elicited by the design of the task. The parenting constructs studied in this report are better suited for direct assessments rather than by global reports (e.g., limit setting, positive reinforcement, problem solving, and perhaps monitoring).

The key idea in limit setting is that the parent does not contribute to the coercion process by using aversive tactics to set limits but consistently follows through with consequences when limits are violated (Patterson, 1982).

Positive reinforcement is potent when it contingently matches either new behaviors that a child is learning or positive behavior that is replacing previous bad habits. Problem solving has been successfully measured in a laboratory setting by Forgatch and Stoolmiller (1994), who report an assessment of problem solving that has considerable content validity and is based on the participant's ratings of how well the parent and child solved specific problems. Similarly, parent monitoring is a process of establishing procedures and rules regarding norms of behavior, along with supervising, to assure that those norms are followed. It may also be that staff impressions of monitoring are useful because of the complex set of skills required to supervise adolescents, which vary from family to family. A single parent may use a different approach to supervising a young adolescent, compared to a two-parent family, where one parent is available to supervise after school. However, children in both families may be equally monitored. Because of the high level of predictive validity of the monitoring construct and the importance of the parenting practice it measures during adolescence, this construct is critical for developmental and intervention science. In contrast, the relationship quality construct may best be measured by the participants' global impressions. Positive indications of a healthy parent–child relationship are that the child feels the parents are fair, the parents are satisfied with the child's level of cooperation, and the family enjoys recreational time together.

In this sense, all measures are not equal in the assessment of parenting practices—method and trait variance are conceptually related. We concur with Fiske (1987) that the construct validation process is crucial and not an inconvenient annoyance to be surmounted in a quick pilot study to evaluate whether a single measure of parenting has internal consistency or predictive validity.

Understanding the full range of validity issues, including criterion and predictive validity is critical, not only to advances in our understanding of the influence of families on adolescent problem behavior but also to advances in intervention science. A particularly relevant problem in intervention science is the measurement of change. Measures that accurately reflect the ebb and flow of human behavior are needed in the course of natural development, as well as change that occurs in response to interventions (Eddy, Dishion, & Stoolmiller, 1998).

Direct observations are one solution to this problem (Reid, 1978). In addition, any assessment that includes the temporal dimension to behavior is relevant to the issue of change. Over reliance on the personality assessment strategy has had a deleterious impact on the measurement strategies of sensitivity to change. For example, many of the measures included in this report provided the typical response format "always" through "never." Whether these are measured on a 5-point or 10-point scale, this assessment strategy lacks a temporal specificity. It would be difficult for anyone to tell when there has been meaningful change from one assessment probe to another. Based on the analyses in this report, as well as the body of research on adolescent problem behavior, we suggest that measures of parent monitoring sensitive to change need to be further developed.

The solution to these problems, as suggested by Fiske (1987), is to be more specific in the conceptualization and instrumentation of parenting constructs. Given this perspective and the findings from these analyses, we hope to be part of a new movement in the behavioral sciences that invests more energy, talent, and resources in the conceptualization and measurement of independent and dependent variables in the study of social development.

REFERENCES

Achenbach, T. M. (1991). *Manual for the Child Behavior Checklist/4-18 and 1991 profile.* Burlington: University of Vermont, Department of Psychology.

Allison, P. D. (1987). Estimation of linear models with incomplete data. In C. Clogg (Ed.), *Sociological methodology* (pp.71–103). San Francisco: Jossey-Bass.

Andrews, D. W., Soberman, L. H., & Dishion, T. J. (1995). The Adolescent Transitions Program: A school-based program for high-risk teens and their parents. *Education and Treatment of Children, 18,* 478–484.

Bagozzi, R. P. (1993). Assessing construct validity in personality research: Applications to measures of self-esteem. *Journal of Research in Personality, 27,* 49–87.

Bagozzi, R. P., & Yi, Y. (1990). Assessing method variance in multitrait-multimethod matrices: The case of self-reported affect and perceptions at work. *Journal of Applied Psychology, 75,* 547–560.

Bank, L., Dishion, T. J., Skinner, M., & Patterson, G. R. (1990). Method variance in structural equation modeling: Living with "glop". In G. R. Patterson (Ed.), *Depression and aggression in family interaction* (pp. 247–279). Hillsdale, NJ: Lawrence Erlbaum Associates, Inc.

Baumrind, D. (1985). Familial antecedents of adolescent drug use: A developmental perspective. In C. L. Jones & R. J. Battjes (Eds.), *Etiology of drug abuse: Implication for prevention* (pp. 13–44). National Institute on Drug Abuse Research Monograph 56. Washington, DC: Superintendent of Documents, U.S. Government Printing Office.

Bentler, P. M., & Bonett, D. G. (1980). Significance tests and goodness of fit in the analysis of covariance structures. *Psychological Bulletin, 88,* 588–606.

Bowlby, J. (1969). *Attachment and loss. Vol. 1. Attachment.* New York: Basic Books.

Brogden, H. E., & Taylor, E. K. (1950). The theory and classification of criterion bias. *Educational and Psychological Measurement, 10,* 159–186.

Campbell, D. T., & Fiske, D. (1959). Convergent and discriminant validation by the multitrait-multimethod matrix. *Psychological Bulletin, 56,* 81–105.

Chilcoate, H., Anthony, J., & Dishion, T. J. (1995). Parent monitoring and the incidence of drug sampling in multiethnic urban children. *American Journal of Epidemiology, 141,* 25–31.

Conger, R. D., Conger, K. J., Elder, G. H., Jr., Lorenz, F. O., Simons, R. L., & Whitbeck, L. B. (1992). A family process model of economic hardship and adjustment of early adolescent boys. *Child Development, 63,* 526–541.

Cook, T. D., & Campbell, D. T. (1979). *Quasi-experimentation: Design and analysis issues for field settings.* Boston: Houghton Mifflin Company.

Dishion, T. J., & Andrews, D. W. (1995). Preventing escalation in problem behaviors with high-risk young adolescents: Immediate and 1-year outcomes. *Journal of Consulting and Clinical Psychology, 63,* 538–548.

Dishion, T. J., Gardner, K., Patterson, G. R., Reid, J. B., & Thibodeaux, S. (1983). *The Family Process Code: A multi-dimensional system for observing family interaction.* Unpublished coding manual. (Available from Oregon Social Learning Center, 160 East 4th Avenue, Eugene, OR 97401-2426.)

Dishion, T. J., & Kavanagh, K. (1995, July). *Cognitive-behavioral intervention strategies for high-risk young adolescents: A comparative analysis of 1-year outcome effects.* Paper presented at the World Congress of Behavioural and Cognitive Therapies, Copenhagen, Denmark.

Dishion, T. J., & Loeber, R. (1985). Male adolescent marijuana and alcohol use: The role of parents and peers revisited. *American Journal of Drug and Alcohol Abuse, 11,* 11–25.

Dishion, T. J., & McMahon, R. J. (1998). Parental monitoring and the prevention of child and adolescent problem behavior: A conceptual and empirical formulation. *Clinical Child and Family Psychology Review, 1,* 61–75.

Dishion, T. J., & Patterson, S. G. (1996). *Preventive parenting with love, encouragement, and limits: The preschool years.* Eugene, OR: Castalia Publishing.

Dishion, T. J., Reid, J. B., & Patterson, G. R. (1988). Empirical guidelines for a family intervention for adolescent drug use. *Journal of Chemical Dependency Treatment, 1,* 189–222.

Dishion, T. J., & Soberman, L. (1994). *PEN-P.* Unpublished training manual. (Available from Oregon Social Learning Center, 160 East 4th Avenue, Eugene, OR 97401-2426.)

Duncan, T. E., & Duncan, S. C. (1995). Modeling the process of development via latent variable growth curve methodology. *Structural Equation Model, 2,* 187–213.

Dwyer, J. H. (1983). *Statistical models for the social and behavior sciences.* New York: Oxford University Press.

Eddy, J. M., Dishion, T. J., & Stoolmiller, M. (1998). The analysis of change in children and families: Methodological and conceptual issues embedded in intervention studies. *Journal of Abnormal Child Psychology, 26,* 53–69.

Elliott, D. S., Huizinga, D., & Ageton, S. S. (1985). *Explaining delinquency and drug use.* Thousand Oaks, CA: Sage.

Family Activities Checklist (1984). Unpublished assessment instrument. (Available from Oregon Social Learning Center, 160 East 4th Avenue, Eugene, OR 97401-2426.)

Fiske, D. W. (1986). Specificity of method and knowledge in social science. In D. W. Fiske & R. A. Shweder (Eds.), *Metatheory in social science* (pp. 61–82). Chicago: University of Chicago Press.

Fiske, D. W. (1987). Construct invalidity comes from method effects. *Educational and Psychological Measurement, 47,* 258–307.

Forgatch, M. S. (1989). Patterns and outcome in family problem solving: The disrupting effect of negative emotion. *Journal of Marriage & Family, 51,* 115–124.

Forgatch, M. S., & Patterson, G. R. (1989). *Parents and adolescents living together: II. Family problem solving.* Eugene, OR: Castalia Publishing.

Forgatch, M. S., & Stoolmiller, M. (1994). Emotions as contexts for adolescent delinquency. *Journal of Research on Adolescence, 4,* 601–614.

Hawkins, J. D., Lishner, D. M., Catalano, R. F., & Howard, M. O. (1986). Childhood predictors of adolescent substance abuse: Toward an empirically grounded theory. *Journal of Children in a Contemporary Society, 8,* 11–47.

Hirschi, T. (1969). *Causes of delinquency.* Berkeley: University of California Press.

Jöreskog, K. G. Statistical analysis of sets of congeneric tests. *Psychometrika, 36,*(2), 109–133.

Little, R. J. A., & Rubin, D. B. (1987). *Statistical analysis with missing data.* New York: Wiley.

Marsh, H. W. (1989). Confirmatory factor analyses of multitrait-multimethod data: Many problems and a few solutions. *Applied Psychological Measurement, 13,* 335–361.

Marsh, H. W., & Bailey, M. (1991). Confirmatory factor analyses of multitrait-multimethod data: A comparison of alternative models. *Applied Psychological Measurement, 15*(1), 47–70.

Marsh, H. W., & Grayson, D. (1995). Latent variable models of multitrait-multimethod data. In R. H. Hoyle (Ed.), *Structural equation modeling: Concepts, issues and applications* (pp. 177–198). Thousand Oaks, CA: Sage.

McCord, J. (1991). Family relationships, juvenile delinquency, and adult criminality. *Criminology, 29,* 397–416.

McCord, J. (1992). The Cambridge-Somerville Study: A pioneering longitudinal-experimental study of delinquency prevention. In J. McCord & R. Tremblay (Eds.), *Preventing antisocial behavior: Interventions from birth to adolescence* (pp. 196–209). New York: Guilford Press.

McMahon, R. J., & Peters, R. DeV. (1990). *Behavior disorders of adolescence: Research, intervention, and policy in clinical and school settings.* New York: Plenum Press.

Muthén, B., Kaplan, D., & Hollis, M. (1987). On structural equation modeling with data that are not missing completely at random. *Psychometrika, 52,* 431–462.

Nunnally, J. C. (1978). *Psychometric theory* (2nd edition). New York: McGraw–Hill.

Patterson, G. R. (1974). Interventions for boys with conduct problems: Multiple setting, treatments, and criteria. *Journal of Consulting and Clinical Psychology, 42,* 471–481.

Patterson, G. R. (1982). *Coercive family process.* Eugene, OR: Castalia Publishing.

Patterson, G. R., & Dishion, T. J. (1985). Contributions of families and peers to delinquency. *Criminology, 23,* 63–79.

Patterson, G. R., Dishion, T. J., & Bank, L. (1984). Family interaction: A process model of deviancy training. In L. Eron (Ed.) [Special issue]. *Aggressive Behavior, 10,* 253–267.

Patterson, G. R., & Forgatch, M. S. (1990). Initiation and maintenance of processes disrupting single-mother families. In G. R. Patterson (Ed.), *Depression and aggression in family interaction* (pp. 209–245). Hillsdale, NJ: Lawrence Erlbaum Associates.

Patterson, G. R., Reid, J. B., & Dishion, T. J. (1992). *A Social learning approach to family intervention: IV. Antisocial boys.* Eugene, OR: Castalia Publishing.

Reid, J. B. (1978). The development of specialized observation systems. In J. B. Reid (Ed.), *A social learning approach to family intervention. II. Observation in home settings* (pp. 43–49). Eugene, OR: Castalia Publishing.

Rubin, D. B. (1976). Inference and missing data. *Biometrika, 63,* 581–592.

Stanton, M. D., & Todd, T. C. (1982). *The family therapy of drug abuse and addiction.* New York: Guilford Press.

Szapocznik, J., & Kurtines, W. M. (1989). *Breakthroughs in family therapy with drug-abusing and problem youth.* New York: Springer.

Walker, H. M., & McConnell, S. R. (1988). *Walker-McConnell scale of social competence and school adjustment.* Austin, TX: Pro-Ed, Inc.

Webster-Stratton, C., & Hammond, M. (1990). Predictors of treatment outcome in parent training for families with conduct problem children. *Behavioral Therapy, 21,* 319–337.

CHAPTER 31

Power Analysis Models and Methods: A Latent Variable Framework for Power Estimation and Analysis

TERRY E. DUNCAN
SUSAN C. DUNCAN
FUZHONG LI

INTRODUCTION

Researchers have become increasingly sophisticated in applying tests for statistical significance in intervention research, but few are aware of the power of these tests. If a particular test is not statistically significant, it may be because there is no effect in the population or because the study design makes it unlikely that an effect, even if one did exist, would be detected. Power estimation can distinguish between these alternatives and is, therefore, a critical component of designing intervention experiments and testing their results. This chapter reviews the use of power estimation techniques typically used in prevention research and presents an extension of the power estimation paradigm within the latent-variable framework, specifically latent growth-curve modeling. The issues raised in this chapter are not new, but it is important that researchers consider them. Exactly how they handle these issues will depend on the questions asked, the resources available, and other considerations.

TERRY E. DUNCAN, SUSAN C. DUNCAN • Oregon Research Institute, Eugene, Oregon 97401
FUZHONG LI • Oregon Social Learning Center and Oregon Research Institute, Eugene, OR 97401

ERRORS IN HYPOTHESIS TESTING

The nature of longitudinal designs, subject attrition, nonequivalent groups, and nonnormally distributed outcomes all pose challenges when attempting to make inferences about the utility of a particular intervention protocol. Traditionally, the effectiveness of an intervention has been assessed in terms of group level means and variances of the behaviors of interest. True random assignment attempts to equate the treatment and control groups prior to the intervention, and the treatment effect is typically measured as the difference between the mean values of the two groups on the outcome behavior following the intervention. The hypothesis tested, the null hypothesis, assumes that the means of the treatment populations are equal. The alternative hypothesis is a mutually exclusive statement asserting that some population treatment means are not equal, that is, treatment effects are present. Commonly used analytic techniques to test the null hypothesis include t-tests, analysis of variance (ANOVA), analysis of covariance (ANCOVA), multivariate analysis of variance (MANOVA), multivariate analysis of covariance (MANCOVA), multiple regression, and multiple-sample structural equation modeling methods. Once the data are collected and analyzed, a statement is made regarding the null hypothesis on the basis of whether the test statistic falls into the established critical region. The inferential process involves a decision (regarding the null hypothesis) in which there are two options: reject or fail to reject.

Unfortunately, the procedures followed in hypothesis testing do not guarantee that a correct inference will be made. Regardless of whether the researcher decides to reject the null hypothesis (H_0), the decision will either be correct or incorrect depending on the state of affairs in the real world. The two types of errors that the researcher can commit are defined in Table 31.1. In Table 31.1 it can be seen that there are two states that the "real world" can take: Either the null hypothesis is true or it is false. There are also two decisions that the researcher can make: either reject or not reject H_0. The four possible combinations of states of reality and the types of decisions available to the researcher are listed in the table and discussed in the following section in relation to hypothesis testing within an intervention context.

1. Claiming the intervention was successful when it was not (reject H_0 when H_0 is true). This is called a Type I error, and in many intervention settings could be very costly. The probability of this type of error is α, also called the significance level, and is directly controlled by the experimenter who sets the value of α before the experiment begins. When the cost of committing a Type I error is high, the value of α would be set low, perhaps lower than the usual value of .05.

TABLE 31.1. Errors in Hypothesis Testing

	Reality	
Decision	H_0 true (no effects) H_1 false	H_0 false (real effects) H_1 true
Reject H_0, Fail to reject H_1	Incorrect decision Type I error Probability $= \alpha$	Correct decision Probability $= 1 - \beta$ "Power"
Fail to reject H_0, Reject H_1	Correct decision Probability $= 1 - \alpha$	Incorrect Decision Type II error Probability $= \beta$

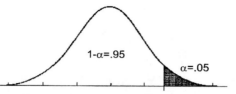

FIGURE 31.1. The relationship between the probability α and $1 - \alpha$ using the sampling distribution when the null hypothesis is true.

2. Deciding the intervention failed when it did fail. This is a correct decision made with probability $1 - \alpha$. The relationship between these probabilities can be illustrated using the sampling distribution when the null hypothesis is true. The decision point is set by alpha, the area under the tail or tails of the distribution. Setting alpha smaller moves the decision point further into the tail or tails of the distribution (see Figure 31.1).
3. Claiming the intervention did not work when it did. This is called a Type II error and is made with probability β. The value of β is not directly set by the experimenter but is a function of a number of factors including the size of α, the size of the effect, the size of the sample, and the variance of the original distribution. The value of β is inversely related to the value of α; the smaller the value of α, the larger the value of β. Setting α to a small value is not done without cost, as the value of β is increased.
4. Claiming that the intervention was successful when it was successful. This is the cell in which experimenters would generally like to be. The probability of making this correct decision is $1 - \beta$ and is called "power". A decision to set α low would result in a higher value of β, and subsequently $1 - \beta$ would be low. With substantially reduced power, it would be unlikely that the researcher would detect that the intervention was a success even if in reality it was successful. The relationship between the probability of a Type II error, β, and power, $1 - \beta$, is illustrated in Figure 31.2.

The relationship between α and β can be illustrated by overlapping the two previous sampling distributions, as seen in Figure 31.3. The size of the effect is the difference between the center points, the means, of the two distributions. If the effect size is increased, the relationship between the two probabilities of the two types of errors, Type I and Type II, is changed. Furthermore, when the error variance of the scores is reduced, the probability of a Type II error is decreased (assuming all else remains constant), as seen in Figure 31.4.

A major source of this error variance is individual variability. The size of the increase or decrease in β is a complex function of changes in many other values. For example, although the choice of sample size is the primary means by which power is controlled in an experiment,

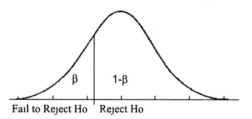

FIGURE 31.2. The relationship between the probability β, and power, $1 - \beta$, using the sampling distribution when there actually was an effect due to the intervention.

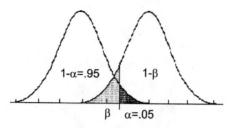

FIGURE 31.3. Size of the effect.

changes in the size of the sample may have either large or small effects on β depending on other aspects of the experiment. If a large treatment effect and small error are present in the experiment, then changes in the sample size will make little difference. The setting of α is not automatic but depends on an analysis of the relative costs to the two types of errors. The probabilities of Type I and Type II errors are inversely related. If the cost of a Type I error is high relative to the cost of a Type II error, then the value of α should be set relatively low. If the cost of a Type I error is low relative to the cost of committing a Type II error, then the value of α should be set relatively high.

In intervention research, it is often difficult to evaluate the relative costs of Type I and Type II errors. Both may be equally important, especially in exploratory research. Some argue that too much emphasis is placed on the level of significance of a test and too little on the power of the test. In many cases where H_0 is not rejected, were the power of the test taken into consideration, the decision might more appropriately have been that the intervention design did not provide an adequately sensitive (powerful) test of the hypothesis.

The sensitivity of an experiment, formally expressed as power, should be of critical importance to researchers contemplating an intervention study. Although most researchers implicitly take steps to increase power through their choice of experimental design and by their attempts to reduce error variance, comparatively few take advantage of the procedures available for evaluating the degree of sensitivity before the experiment is undertaken. Power analysis is most useful when planning a study. Such "prospective" power analyses are usually exploratory in nature, investigating the relationship between the range of sample sizes that are deemed feasible, effect sizes thought to be of practical importance, levels of variance that could exist in the population (generally estimated from the literature or from pilot data), and desired levels of α and statistical power. The result is a decision about the sample size and α level that will be used in the study and the target effect size that will be "detectable" with the given level of statistical power. Power estimates obtained in the planning stages of intervention force consideration of design sensitivity at a point when something can be done about it. According to Winer (1971):

> If experiments were conducted in the best of all possible worlds, the design of the experiment would provide adequate power for any predetermined level of significance that the experimenter were to set. However, experiments are conducted under the conditions that exist within the world in which one lives. What is needed to attain the demands of the well-designed experiment may not be realized.

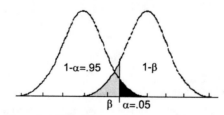

FIGURE 31.4. The probability of a Type II error as a function of error variance.

Cohen (1965) also argues that it is unwise to expend the time and money required to conduct a carefully planned and relevant intervention if the researcher's ability to reject a false null hypothesis is too low. See recent work by Allison et al. (1997) for design methods that simultaneously consider power and cost in the context of a randomized clinical trial.

After the study is completed and the results are analyzed, a "retrospective" power analysis can also be useful if a statistically nonsignificant result was obtained (e.g., Thomas, 1996). Here the actual sample size and α level are known, and the variance observed in the sample provides an estimate of the variance in the population. These values are used to calculate power at the minimum effect size thought to be of practical significance, or alternatively the effect size detectable with the minimum desired level of power. Note that calculating power using the effect size actually observed in the sample tells nothing about the ability of the test to detect scientifically or practically meaningful results (Thomas, 1997).

Cohen (1962) presented data to support the conclusion that in several areas of social science research, researchers are operating with less than adequate power, well under 40% power assuming a medium effect size, which suggests a small probability of rejecting a false null hypothesis despite a moderate effect size. In the conventions suggested by Cohen (1988), a small effect size = .20, a medium = .50, and a large effect size = .80. It should be noted that there is no statistical answer to the meaningfulness of these effect size statistics. They should be judged based on clinical significance, which may vary based on what is considered important by a particular research field. For example, an effect size of .05 (change of less than 5%) would be considered trivial in many psychology studies but could represent an important effect in medical research (e.g., studying the effect of experimental drug). For a complete discussion concerning empirical approaches to measuring clinical significance, see Jacobson and Truax (1991).

Sedlemeyer and Gigernzer (1989), using Cohen's (1965) pioneering work as a model, found that between 1965 and 1989 the power for published studies had changed. They suggested that in a majority of studies, the issue of power had been largely ignored, with only 2 of 64 studies even mentioning power. Such values imply that, in many studies, the likelihood of the researcher rejecting a false null hypothesis was extremely low. As a general standard, power is generally set at a level of at least 80%, although researchers argue whether this is adequate. For any given study, the appropriate level of power should be decided on the basis of the potential harm of a Type I error, the determination of a clinically important effect, and the importance of identifying an effect should one exist.

SAMPLE SIZE, EFFECT SIZE, LEVEL OF SIGNIFICANCE, AND DETERMINATION OF POWER

As a practical matter, the evaluation of statistical power requires the researcher to establish a level of significance, sample size, magnitude and direction of the anticipated treatment effects, and the within-class variance associated with the observations. This variation is, among other things, a function of the nature and reliability of the dependent outcome and the nature of the experimental design. Therefore, the question of power is often couched in terms of the sample size necessary to detect deviation from the null hypothesis.

Because treatment effects are defined in terms of parameters and estimated from sample statistics, sample size determines the accuracy by which the estimation proceeds. All things being equal, sample size determines the precision with which the parameters can be estimated. These four parameters—α, n, effect size, and statistical power—are so related that when any three of them are fixed, the fourth is exactly determined. However, even when α and n are known, the investigator does not usually know power since the magnitude of the effect size in the population is typically unknown. Thus, specifying the effect size is often the hardest part of conducting an appropriate power analysis.

Common Analytical Procedures for Power Estimation

t-TEST FOR INDEPENDENT SAMPLES.   This procedure is used to test the mean difference in two independent groups where the two groups share a common within-group standard deviation. The effect size for t-tests is the standardized difference, d, which is defined as the mean difference between groups divided by the common within-groups standard deviation, s. In theory, the effect size index (i.e., $(M_1 - M_2)/s$) extends from zero (indicating no effect) to infinity. In practice, d is limited to a substantially smaller range as reflected in the conventions suggested by Cohen (1988) for research in the social sciences: small ($d = .20$), medium ($d = .50$), and large ($d = .80$). The noncentrality parameter (NCP) is computed as

$$d^*\sqrt{2^*(N_1{}^*N_2)/(N_1 + N_2)}/\sqrt{2}$$

Power is then given by the centrality parameter (λ) of the noncentral t distribution (i.e., when the null hypothesis is false), the t-value required for significance given by the central t distribution, and the degrees of freedom.

ONE-WAY ANALYSIS OF VARIANCE.   An extension of the independent t-test is the one-way analysis of variance (ANOVA). The procedure allows the evaluation of the null hypothesis among two or more group means (e.g., $M_1 = M_2 = M_3 \ldots = 0$) with the restriction that the groups are levels of the same independent variable. The effect size (f) used in ANOVA is an extension of the effect size (d) used for a t-test. Similarly, f is based on the dispersion between groups divided by the dispersion within groups ($f = s_{between}/s_{within}$). This f is a "true" measure of effect size and should not be confused with the F statistic which takes into account both sample size and effect size. The noncentrality parameter (NCP) is computed as $f^{2*}(N_{total} - DF_{other})$, where DF_{other} represents the degrees of freedom associated with factors or interactions other than the currently specified factor or interaction. Power is given by the noncentral F distribution for NCP, the F-value required for significance, DF_1 and DF_2, where DF_1 represents the degrees of freedom for the current factor or interaction, and DF_2 is given by $DF_2 = N_{total} - DF_{factor} - DF_{other\ factors} - DF_{interactions} - DF_{covariates}$.

MULTIPLE REGRESSION.   Multiple regression is used to study the relationship between sets of independent (predictor) variables and a single dependent variable. Typically, sets of variables are entered into the multiple regression in a predetermined sequence. At each point in the analysis the researcher may test the significance of the increment (the increase in R^2 for the new set over and above all prior sets of variables) or the significance of all variables in the regression equation. Effect size for multiple regression is given by f^2, defined as a ratio of explained variance/error variance. This is similar to the index (f) used for ANOVA, except that f is based on the standard deviations, while f^2 is based on the variances. When used for a single set of variables, f^2 is equal to $R^2/(1 - R^2)$. When used for more than one set of variables, R^2 in the numerator is the increment to R^2 for the current set, while R^2 in the denominator is the cumulative R^2 for all sets in the regression. Cohen suggests the following conventions for research in the social sciences: small ($f^2 = .02$), medium ($f^2 = .15$), and large ($f^2 = .35$). Using a single set of variables, these would correspond to R^2 values of about .02, .13, and .26, respectively. The noncentrality parameter (NCP) is computed as $f^{2*}(\text{DF}_1 + \text{DF}_2 + 1)$ where DF_1 is the number of variables in set 1 and DF_2 is defined as N_{cases} — number of variables in set 2 — number of variables in set 2 — 1. Power is then given by the noncentral F distribution for NCP, the F-value required for significance, DF_1, and DF_2.

PROPORTIONS IN TWO INDEPENDENT GROUPS. The two-group test of proportions can be used to test the hypothesis that the proportion of cases meeting some criterion is identical in the two groups. If, for example, individuals are assigned to one of two intervention protocols and the null hypothesis that the interventions are equally effective is tested, the effect size for the two-sample test of proportions is based on the difference between the two proportions. Unlike the t-test, where a difference of 10 versus 20 is equivalent to a difference of 30 versus 40 (i.e., a 10-point difference in both cases), with the test of proportions the absolute values of the two proportions are relevant because a difference of 10 versus 20% represents a larger effect than a difference of 30 versus 40%. Cohen (1988) suggests the following conventional values: small (40 versus 50%), medium (40 versus 65%), and large (40 versus 78%). Although there are a number of computational formulae for power, the most accurate is the estimate given by Fisher's exact test, involving an iterative approach to power estimation. See Fisher (1955) for a complete discussion of this strategy.

CORRELATION IN TWO GROUPS. The two-sample correlation procedure is used to test the null hypothesis that the correlation between X and Y is identical in two populations. The effect size used is based on the difference between the two correlation coefficients. The effect size, r, is computed as $r = Z_{r1} - Z_{r2}$, where Z_{r1} is the Fisher-Z transformation for the first correlation and Z_{r2} is the Fisher-Z transformation for the second correlation. Power is computed as the area under the normal distribution curve to the left of Z_{req} (the Z required for significance) which is computed as

$$r^* \sqrt{(N' - 3)/2) - Z_{\text{req}}},$$

where $N' = ((2^*(N_1 - 3)^*(N_2 - 3))/(N_1 + N_2 - 6)) + 3$.

Power calculations can be done using the tables or charts provided in many articles and texts (e.g., Cohen, 1988; Kraemer & Thiemann, 1987; Lipsey, 1990). However, these often require some hand calculations before they can be used, including interpolation between tabled values. For example, Cohen (1988) presents an excellent discussion of the relations among α, n, effect size, and statistical power. He provides an extensive treatment of statistical power, presenting tables wherein power is estimated given values of the level of significance, α, measures of effect size (f), the sample size (n), and the degrees of freedom in the numerator of F ratios. Specifying the highest tolerable Type I error rate and the desired power, the researcher can use charts to discover the sample size. For a more comprehensive treatment of power using these approaches, see Borenstein (1994, 1997), Cohen (1965, 1988, 1992, 1994), and Kraemer and Thiemann (1987).

Computer software has the potential to make power analysis more accurate, interactive, and easy to perform. Thomas and Krebs (1997) provide a list of software capable of performing power or sample size calculations. Two Windows-based programs reviewed [NQUERY ADVISOR (Elashoff, 1995), POWER AND PRECISION (Borenstein, Rothstein, & Cohen, 1997)] provide on-screen guide windows that are displayed alongside the input menus as well as an extensive help system and on-line examples. For users unsure of how to present the results, both NQUERY ADVISOR and POWER AND PRECISION can produce grammatically correct summaries of analyses and produce quality graphs for publication (additional information on Nquery Advisor can be found at http://www.statsol.ie/nquery/nquery.html and on the Power and Precision program at http://www.PowerAndPrecision.com.)

Even though it is possible to determine power for a given level of significance, effect size, and sample size, there are many situations with sample size limitations. In other situations there may be a limit to how many subjects can be used based on the cost of the intervention, not to mention other real-world problems such as subject availability, attrition, and incomplete data. If the sample needed to achieve a desired level of power turns out to be larger than the available sample size, most researchers return to their initial set of decisions and make adjustments. Usually, original plans concerning the target population, instruments, statistical test, and level of significance are left unchanged. Rather than tinker with any of these facets, more often the researcher will lower power or increase effect size. Either of these adjustments (or a combination of the two) will allow the investigator to proceed despite the limited sample size.

A LATENT-VARIABLE FRAMEWORK FOR ANALYSES AND POWER ESTIMATION

Longitudinal prevention studies can be expensive and time consuming, particularly with a large number of subjects. Therefore, it is critical to know the minimum number of subjects needed to answer the research questions. One tactic not generally considered by researchers to increase power for a given sample size (or alternatively to decrease sample size for a given power) is to change statistical tests. The statistical techniques most often used in intervention research have both strengths and weaknesses. The strengths are that they draw on well-studied estimation procedures and that most applied researchers are sufficiently trained to implement these techniques. A serious weakness is that modeling with these techniques has generally been limited to a single response variable, which does not accommodate the analytic needs of many developmental theories. In addition, the assumption of homogeneity of variance between groups, usually required with traditional techniques, may be unrealistically restrictive in large intervention research (e.g., community-based experiments) in which variance effects may be attributed to varying degrees of program implementation and heterogeneity of individuals under study. Also, such techniques typically can not account for measurement error, which may attenuate the true effect sizes and decrease the power.

In the psychometric latent-variable tradition, the strengths and weaknesses are reversed. The estimation procedures are currently not well developed for sufficiently general cases, but the modeling framework has much more flexibility to answer research questions. As Muthén and Curran (1997) point out, however, questions remain about power for modeling growth in general, and intervention effects in particular, although several researchers have developed methods for power estimation for latent-variable models (for examples, see MacCallum, Browne, & Sugawara, 1995; Satorra & Saris, 1985).

In many intervention settings, the level of a behavior at a particular point in time is not as interesting as the trajectory of the behavior across multiple time points. Frequently, targeted behaviors change systematically over time. Therefore, the goal of the intervention is to alter the normative growth trajectory for the targeted behavior over time. To recast prevention evaluation in terms of growth, the effectiveness of an intervention is the extent to which it alters the normative growth trajectory that exists without the prevention regimen. Although typical analytic approaches can be useful for evaluating prevention effects under rather restrictive assumptions, they are limited in their ability to study systematic change. Limitations include reduced statistical power, inability to model individual differences in change, and an unnecessary restriction of inferences that can be drawn from the observed data (Rogosa, 1988; Rogosa & Willett, 1985). These limitations are particularly salient when attempting to assess the degree to which an intervention program influences the rate of change over time.

Extension of the Basic Growth Model for an Intervention Context

An alternative methodology for modeling change as a factor of repeated observations over time is called a latent growth model, or LGM. See Figure 31.5 (Muthén & Curran, 1997).

Growth-curve methodology can be thought of as having two stages. In the first stage, a regression curve, not necessarily linear, is fit to the repeated measures of each individual in the sample. In the second stage, the growth parameters (e.g., means and variances of the constant and linear trends) for an individual's curve become the focus of the analysis rather than the original measures.

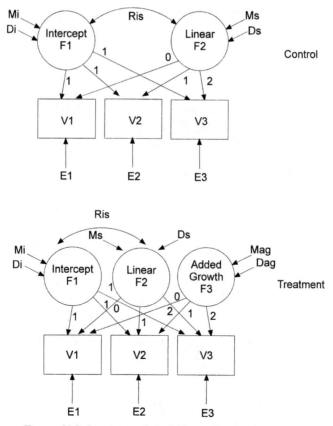

FIGURE 31.5. Latent growth model for an Intervention Context.

LGMs strongly resemble the classic confirmatory factor analysis. However, because they use repeated measures raw-score data, the latent factors are actually interpreted as chronometric common factors representing individual differences over time (McArdle, 1988). Meredith and Tisak (1990) demonstrated that repeated measures polynomial ANOVA models are actually special cases of LGMs in which only the factor means are of interest. In contrast, a fully expanded latent growth analysis takes into account both factor means and variances. This combination of the individual and group levels of analysis is unique to the procedure.

An important facet of multivariate LGMs, and an advantage over repeated measures polynomial ANOVA techniques, is that they enable associations to be made among the individual differences parameters. These associations are analogous to the synchronous structural equation model's correlation coefficient (Meredith & Tisak, 1990). They are crucial to any investigation of development because they indicate influences on development and, thus, are correlates of change.

Latent growth-curve methodology not only describes a single individual's developmental trajectory but also captures individual differences in the collection of trajectories over time. Another important attribute of LGMs is the ability to study predictors of those individual differences to answer questions about which variables exert important effects on the rate of development. At the same time, LGMs capture the important group statistics in a way that allows the researcher to study development at the group level.

The LGM approach is laid out in more technical detail in Meredith and Tisak (1990), Muthén (1991), and Willett and Sayer (1994). See also Duncan et al. (1999) for various issues related to applications of LGM. Examples of applications may be found in Duncan, Duncan, and Stoolmiller (1994), Duncan and Duncan (1995), Stoolmiller, et al. (1993), McArdle (1988), and McArdle and Epstein (1987). Other approaches to growth modeling can be found in Bryk and Raudenbush (1987), Duncan et al. (1995), Raudenbush, Brennan, and Barnett (1995), and Willet, Ayoub, and Robinson (1991).

The statistical basis for LGM estimation and testing is developed from general structural equation methodology. However, the LGM approach requires that the model be fitted to both means and variances/covariances. The LGM approach depicted in Figure 31.5 is based on repeated-measures data collected at three points over a 3-year period, although the procedure is applicable to any number of repeated observations and various temporal spacings.

Consider an intervention study in which individuals are randomly assigned to either treatment or control conditions. The control group represents the normative set of individual growth trajectories that would have been observed in the intervention group without treatment. The treatment effect is assessed by comparing the set of growth trajectories in the treatment population to that in the control population. In Figure 31.5, the top group represents the control condition and the bottom group represents the treatment group.

As can be seen in Figure 31.5, the first common factor in both groups is labeled the intercept and represents individual differences in the level of a particular attribute. The intercept is a constant for any individual across time and represents information in the sample concerning the mean, represented by M_i, and variance, represented by D_i, of the collection of individual intercepts that characterize each individual's growth curve. The second factor in both groups, labeled linear, represents the linear trend or slope of an individual's trajectory determined by the repeated measures. The slope factor has a mean, M_s, and variance, D_s, across the whole sample, and, like those associated with the intercept, can be estimated from the observed data.

How the factors are interpreted is determined by the fixed values of the factor loadings. In latent growth-curve methodology the factor loadings carry the information about the underlying time metric. In Figure 31.5, the factor loadings (0, 1, 2) represent linear growth coefficients. While the values selected for these loadings are somewhat arbitrary, in that various growth forms could be tested using different loadings, fixing the loadings at 0, 1, and 2 scales the growth metric to allow an unambiguous interpretation of the initial level and linear trends of the repeated measures. [See Duncan and Duncan (1995) for a complete discussion on this issue.]

Also shown in Figure 31.5 is an additional growth factor for the treatment population. While the first two factors (i.e., intercept and slope) are the same in both groups, a third factor in the treatment group represents incremental/decremental growth that is specific to that group. The treatment effect, therefore, is expressed in this added growth factor (Muthén & Curran, 1997).

A variety of growth models can be generalized to the simultaneous analysis of data from multiple populations. To some extent, population differences can be captured in single-population analyses by representing the different groups with dummy vectors as time-invariant covariates. However, to achieve more generality in modeling, as well as specificity in the examination of population differences, the multiple-population approach should be used.

As a first step, growth can be studied by a separate analysis of each group. Previous research may have established *a priori* hypotheses about the form of the growth trajectories. Inspection of individual and overall growth patterns may also inform the choice of growth forms to be tested in the analyses. In the second step, an analysis with two or more groups is performed in which the growth factors found in the single-sample analyses are simultaneously fit to all populations.

For illustration, longitudinal data were generated as part of a Monte Carlo study to show how latent growth modeling techniques can be extended to analyses involving multiple populations. The developmental model was based on a sample of 300 (150 treatment and 150 control). The covariance matrix and observed means generated for the two sample groups are presented in Table 31.2. The EQS structural equation modeling program (Bentler & Wu, 1995) was used for all model tests. Parameter estimates for the model are shown in Table 31.3. The model yielded a significant slope mean across the two groups, indicating that significant growth occurred. Also found were significant variances around the intercept and slope means, indicating that substantial variation existed in individual differences regarding initial status and trajectory. In addition, the added growth factor mean, .254, was significant, $t = 2.712$, $p < .05$, indicating a significant treatment effect for the intervention.

TABLE 31.2. Descriptive Statistics for the
Repeated Measures

	V1	V2	V3
Treatment			
	1.854		
	.957	2.200	
	.882	1.493	2.685
	1.510	1.684	1.858
Control			
	1.854		
	.957	2.378	
	.882	1.849	3.397
	1.510	1.938	2.366

NOTE. Covariances are in the triangle; means are presented in bottom rows of the matrix.

TABLE 31.3. Parameter Estimates for the
Intervention Growth Model

Parameter	Effect	t-value
Control group		
Means		
Intercept	1.510	19.838
Slope	.174	2.681
Variance		
Intercept	1.032	5.303
Slope	.343	2.952
Covariance	−.075	−.676
Intervention group		
Means		
Intercept	1.510	19.838
Slope	.174	2.681
Added growth	.254	2.712
Variance		
Intercept	1.032	5.303
Slope	.343	2.952
Added Growth	.178	1.647
Covariance	−.075	−.676

Statistical Power Estimation

Questions of statistical power naturally arise when testing and interpreting treatment effects. Researchers need to know whether they have any realistic chance of rejecting a null hypothesis or discriminating between one model and another. Suppose, for example, we wanted to evaluate post hoc the power of detecting our treatment effect (.254) as significantly different from zero at the 5% level of significance. Or prospectively, we assumed the added growth parameter estimates were reasonable, and we wanted to design an intervention to detect the effect of maximizing power while minimizing cost. There are numerous ways to approach this, including latent-variable modeling strategies based on the work of Satorra and Saris (1985) and Satorra (1989).

The estimation of power to detect misspecified latent-variable models is discussed by Satorra and Saris (1985), Saris and Satorra (1993), and Saris and Stronkhorst (1984). In principle, power can be estimated for any model by carrying out a Monte Carlo study that records the proportion of replications rejecting the incorrect model. The method proposed by Satorra and Saris, however, offers a great simplification over this resampling technique and is well suited to intervention research, given that power estimates are desired for very specific model misspecifications concerning the absence of treatment effects. Focusing on a single parameter (i.e., an effect with a unit degree of freedom), the following illustrates the Satorra and Saris (1985) two-step power estimation procedure, using the likelihood ratio (LR) chi-square test and estimation procedures based on model modification strategies: Lagrange multiplier (LM) test (Bentler, 1986) or, equivalently, the modification index (MI; Sörbom, 1989) and the Wald (W) test (Lee, 1985).

TWO-STEP ESTIMATION USING THE LR TEST.   Satorra and Saris (1985) show that when the hypothesized structural model is incorrect but not highly missspecified, power can be approximated using a two-step procedure. This involves two models, one that is assumed to be correctly specified and the other, more restrictive, assumed to be misspecified. Parameter values for both models must be explicitly stated, and may come from previous theory, previous experimentation, or some other rationale. The procedure outlined by Satorra and Saris (1985; see also Saris & Stronkhorst, 1984) is summarized as follows:

1. Specify a complete model under the alternative hypothesis, H_1. The model contains parameters of a given model along with parameter restrictions to be tested. For our example, we set the values of all parameters for this alternative model to those presented in Table 31.3, then computed the implied covariance matrix under H_1 from these parameter values using any input covariance matrix. The covariance matrices for the intervention and control groups are those displayed in Table 31.2.

2. Estimate the model under H_0 using the implied covariance matrix obtained in Step 1 with the same sample size. Specification of H_0 involves vectors of free and fixed parameters. In our example, means and variances/covariances for the intercepts and slopes of both groups represent free parameters, and the added growth factor mean represents the fixed parameter. The chi-square statistic obtained from this test corresponds to the noncentrality parameter (NCP) for the noncentral chi-square distributions.

As can be seen, the estimation of power using this procedure is based on estimation of an incorrect model (H_0) on the correct implied covaraince matrix for the alternative model. Because the two models are nested, the discrepancy index between the correct and incorrectly specified models, H_1 versus H_0, is reflected in the LR chi-square estimate, except that the value corresponds to the NCP in a statistical power analysis. Given the value of the NCP obtained, the degrees of freedom, and the probability level of the test chosen, the power of the test can be determined using the tables (e.g., Haynam, Govindarajulu, & Leone, 1973)for the noncentral chi-square distribution.

An SPSS utility program that calculates power for a given NCP using NCDF.CHISQ(x, df, ncp) function is presented below. The function computes the cumulative probability that an x value from the noncentral chi-square distribution, with degrees of freedom (df) and the specified NCP (ncp), will fall below the x value given.

Data List Free
    /x df ncp.   /* noncentrality parameter   */
Compute power $= 1-$ ncdf.chisq(x, df, ncp).   /* x equals a chi-square critical ratio value   */
                                                /* df equals degrees of freedom   */
                                                /* ncp equals noncentrality parameter   */
Begin Data.
End Data.
Formats power (f8.4).
Title "Power value."
List power.

For example, assume one has a NCP of 7.264 for a 1 df chi-square. Assuming a .05 level (two-tailed) test, the power is calculated as

$$\text{Power} = 1 - \text{ncdf.chisq} (3.841, 1, 7.264),$$

where the arguments in the parentheses are the 5% alpha level (a critical ratio of 3.841 with 1 degree of freedom) and the NCP value of 7.264. This returns a power value of .77. The program can be easily translated into SAS with the PROBCHI (x, df, nc) function.

In our example, model-fitting procedures for the test of the H_0 model fixing the added growth factor mean to zero resulted in the following test statistics: $\chi^2(9, N = 300) = 7.264$, $p = .60$, nonnormed fit index (NNFI) $= .968$, comparative fit index (CFI) $= 1.000$. (The EQS input program to accomplish these tests for this example can obtained from the authors). The difference in chi-square values from the two models provides an estimate that corresponds to the noncentrality parameter of the noncentral chi-square distribution, which is the distribution of chi-square when the null hypothesis is false. For our example, we obtained a chi-square difference of $\chi^2(1, N = 300) = 7.264$. This value, when cross-referenced in the noncentral chi-square table under 1 degree of freedom, provides an estimate of statistical power that exists to detect mis-specification given the estimated sample size. Given the χ^2 difference of 7.264 with 1 degree of freedom and $\alpha = .05$, power is estimated at approximately 77%.

ESTIMATION BASED ON LM AND W TESTS.   An alternative to the two-step power estimation procedure outlined earlier is the use of model modification strategies (Satorra, 1989). Instead of specifying an alternative value to be tested, the LM- and W-based test statistics can be used to approximate the NCP for each restriction in the model (Satorra, 1989). For a given fixed parameter or an equality constraint in a model, a modification index (LM in EQS, MI in LISREL) can be computed to predict the change in the model's chi-square that would accompany the freeing of the fixed parameter or the release of the equality constraint. Similarly, for a freely estimated parameter there is an associated test statistic, commonly referred to as a t-value, which, when squared, is equivalent to the W test (Lee, 1985). Unlike the LM test, the W test concerns eliminating a set of one or more unnecessary parameter estimates from a model.

Both LM and W statistics are asymptotically distributed as noncentral chi-square statistics, which are 1 degree of freedom NCPs. The LM, W, and LR tests are asymptotically equivalent (Buse, 1982; Satorra, 1989), and the use of these test statistics for power approximation has been shown to be asymptotically similar to the Saris–Satorra (1985; also Saris & Stronkhorst, 1984) approach demonstrated previously under the two-step estimation procedure.

Application of LM and W test statistics for power approximation is relatively straightforward. To obtain an LM test, one tests a model in which the parameter of interest is constrained to zero. To obtain a W test, one tests a model in which the parameter of interest is freely estimated. In our example, constraining the added growth factor mean to zero results in an LM value of 7.196. Similarly, the squared t-value for the freely estimated factor mean is 7.355. The NCPs for all three procedures are very close (7.264 for LR, 7.196 for LM, and 7.355 for W). With df $= 1$, $\alpha = .05$, $N = 300$, and an NCP of about 7, the power of the test of null hypothesis with the added growth factor mean is .77. Under these conditions there is a .77 probability of detecting a false null hypothesis when the alternative parameterization (i.e., the restriction imposed on the added growth factor mean) is true.

Computing power for a comparable factorial repeated measures ANOVA model resulted in an estimated power of approximately .61 for the same group by linear trend interaction (e.g., differences in mean level growth between treatment and control groups). In this case, resorting to the more traditional ANOVA approach to power analysis reduced the power of the test. To achieve a power of .77, as was obtained from the LGM analysis, utilizing the ANOVA method, one would have to increase the sample size ($N = 300$) to 436. This can be shown by taking the NCP value of 7.264 generated by the LGM procedure and substituting it into the following formula (Saris & Stronkhorst, 1984; p. 212):

$$\frac{the\ required\ value\ of\ noncentral\ parameter}{the\ obtained\ value\ of\ noncentral\ parameter} \times the\ sample\ size\ used = the\ required\ sample\ size.$$

Substituting the appropriate values into the equation provides the following result:

$$\frac{7.264}{5.00} \times 300 = 436.$$

Thus, a sample of at least 436 subjects would be required for a power of .77 to detect a misspecification in the added growth factor mean, assuming a .05 level of significance. These findings suggest that the LGM model had substantially greater power to detect the very same effect compared to the repeated-measures ANOVA model, and required 30% fewer subjects. These findings are similar to those reported by Curran and Muthén (1999), who found that to detect a small effect size at a power of .80, the LGM model they tested required 28% fewer subjects than required for the same effect size and power in a comparable ANCOVA model. The practical significance of increasing power from .66 to .77 can be considerable. If, for example, a community trial expects the cost of the intervention to be approximately $500 per intervention subject per t measurement (t_1, t_2, t_3), then up to $204,000 (3 × 136 × $500) would be saved by using the LGM procedure instead of the traditional ANOVA procedure. Other benefits would include less time and lower risk to the subjects.

CONCLUSION

Under the latent-variable approach to growth modeling, it is possible to separate normative growth from the growth due to the intervention. Power estimation within the latent-variable modeling framework is directly related to the parameter values of a specified model. The relations among values of the level of significance (α), measures of effect size (e.g., χ^2_{diff}), the sample size (n), and the degrees of freedom are identical to those presented in earlier sections. Within the latent-variable framework, a number of competing models and relationships can easily be assessed, providing important guidance for design decisions.

Power estimation is readily available through standard latent-variable techniques. Kaplan (1995) provides a comprehensive review of statistical power in structural equation modeling and calculations for power assessment of the overall model as well as for associated tests of individual parameters. McArdle (1994) discusses the possibility of incorporating planned missing data into designs and then estimating the parameters to be tested with maximum likelihood methods. In this chapter, we illustrated power estimation techniques in the context of evaluating treatment or intervention effects. As such, the calculation of power involves a unit of df assessment (i.e., added growth factor mean). There are, however, situations where one may wish to evaluate the power for an overall model which includes multiple parameters of interest. Recent work by MacCallum, Browne, and Sugawara (1996) provides a simple procedure for hypothesis testing and power analysis in the assessment of fit for latent-variable models. The method allows direct power estimation by testing a hypothesis of "close fit" of the population covariance matrix in terms of a null and alternative value of the root mean square error of approximation fit index proposed by Steiger and Lined (1980). The procedure can be easily applied in practice. Examining power simultaneously for multiple parameter systems in structural equation models is discussed by Saris and Satorra (1993). The procedure allows, without the need to specify alternative parameter values, evaluation of the power of a model test for multiple parameter restrictions, taking into account simultaneous misspecification. Unfortunately, the procedure is not readily available in standard computer software packages such as EQS or LISREL.

Ideally, power analysis should be integrated within the same statistical framework researchers use for their regular analyses. From a statistical point of view, the best procedures for power estimation should (1) employ the same statistical model for power and sample size estimation as that used for the desired analysis (for example, if the final model of interest is a latent-variable model, the best approach for power estimation would also use a latent-variable model), (2) cover the situations most commonly encountered by researchers, (3) be flexible enough to deal with new or unusual situations, (4) allow easy exploration of multiple values of input parameters, and (5) allow estimation of sampling variance from pilot data and from the statistics commonly reported in the literature.

The covariance structure approach demonstrated here differs from more traditional analytical approaches in at least three important ways. First, the use of the basic LGM requires formal specification of a model to be estimated and tested. Second, and perhaps the most compelling characteristic of LGM, is the capacity to estimate and test relationships among latent variables. The isolation of concepts from uniqueness and unreliability of their indicators increases the potential for detecting relationships and obtaining estimates of parameters close to their population values. Third, the LGM approach allows for a more comprehensive and flexible approach to research design and data analysis than any other single statistical model for longitudinal data in standard use by social and behavioral researchers. The basic latent-variable growth-curve approach advocated here allows for an integrated approach to modeling growth and development that includes both multiple measures and multiple occasions. The approach makes available to a wide audience of researchers an analytical framework for a variety of analyses of growth and developmental processes. The potential for integrating typical causal modeling features found in a majority of SEM applications and the dynamic features of the latent growth method described here make possible a more precise understanding of the influence various competing intervention modalities have on the development of substance use and other related deviant behaviors.

REFERENCES

Allison, D. B., Allison, R. L., Faith, M. S., Paultre, F., & Pi-Sunyer, F. X. (1997). Power and money: Designing statistically powerful studies while minimizing financial costs. *Psychological Methods, 2,* 20–33.

Bentler, P. M. (1986). *Lagrange Multiplier and Wald tests for EQS and EQS/PC.* Los Angeles: BMDP Statistical Software.

Bentler, P. M., & Wu, E. (1995). *EQS structural equations program manual.* Encino, CA: Multivariate Software Inc.

Borenstein, M. (1994). The case for confidence intervals in controlled clinical trials. *Controlled Clinical Trials, 15,* 411–428.

Borenstein, M. (1997). Hypothesis testing and effect size estimation in clinical trials. *Annals of Allergy, Asthmà, and Immunology, 78,* 5–16.

Borenstein, M., Rothstein, H., & Cohen, J. (1997). *Power and precision program manual.* Teaneck, NJ: Biostat.

Bryk, A. S., & Raudenbush, S. W. (1987). Application of hierarchical linear models to assessing change. *Psychological Bulletin, 101,* 147–158.

Buse, A. (1982). The likelihood ratio, Wald, and Lagrange Multiplier tests: An expository note. *The American Statistician, 36,* 153–157.

Cohen, J. (1962). The statistical power of abnormal-social psychological research: A review. *Journal of Abnormal and Social Psychology, 65*(3), 145–153.

Cohen, J. (1965). Some statistical issues in psychological research. In B. B. Wolman (Ed.), *Handbook of clinical psychology* (pp. 95–121). New York: McGraw–Hill.

Cohen, J. (1988). *Statistical power analysis for the behavioral sciences* (2nd edition). Hillsdale, NJ: Lawrence Erlbaum Associates, Inc.

Cohen, J. (1992). A power primer. *Psychological Bulletin, 112,* 155–159.

Cohen, J. (1994). The earth is round ($p < .05$). *American Psychologist, 49,* 997–1003.

Curran, P., & Muthén, B. (1999). Testing developmental theories in intervention research: Latent growth analysis and power estimation. *American Journal of Community Psychology, 27,* 567–595.

Duncan, T. E., & Duncan, S. C. (1995). Modeling the processes of development via latent variable growth-curve methodology. *Structural Equation Modeling, 2,* 187–213.

Duncan, T. E., Duncan, S. C., Hops, H., & Stoolmiller, M. (1995). Analyzing longitudinal substance use data via generalized estimating equation methodology. *Multivariate Behavioral Research, 30,* 317–339.

Duncan, T. E., Duncan, S. C., & Stoolmiller, M. (1994). Modeling developmental processes via latent growth structural equation methodology. *Applied Psychological Measurement, 18,* 343–354.

Duncan, T. E., Duncan, S. C., Strycker, L. A., Li, L., & Alpert, A. (1999). *An introduction to latent-variable growth-curve modeling: Concepts, issues, and applications.* Mahwah, NJ: Lawrence Erlbaum.

Elashoff, J. D. (1995). *Nquery Advisor user's guide.* Los Angeles, CA: Dixon Associates.

Fisher, R. A. (1955). Statistical methods and scientific induction. *Journal of the Royal Statistical Society, 17,* 69–78.

Haynam, G. E., Govindarajulu, Z., & Leone, F. C. (1973). Tables of the cumulative non-central chi-square distribution. In H. L. Harter & D. B. Owen (Eds.), *Selected tables in mathematical statistics* (Vol. 1, pp. 1–78). Providence, RI: Mathematical Statistical Society.

Jacobson, N. S., & Truax, P. (1991). Clinical significance: A statistical approach to defining meaningful change in psychotherapy research. *Journal of Consulting and Clinical Psychology, 59,* 12–19.

Kaplan, D. (1995). Statistical power in structural equation modeling. In R. H. Hoyle (Ed.), *Structural equation modeling: Concepts, issues, and application* (pp. 100–117). Thousand Oaks, CA: Sage.

Kraemer, H. C., & Thiemann, S. (1987). *How many subjects?* London, UK: Sage.

Lee, S.-Y. (1985). On testing functional constraints in structural equation models. *Biometrika, 57,* 239–251.

Lipsey, M. W. (1990). *Design sensitivity: Statistical power for experimental research.* Newbury Park, CA: Sage.

MacCallum, R. C., Browne, M. W., & Sugawara, H. M. (1996). Power analysis and determination of sample size for covariance structure modeling. *Psychological Methods, 1,* 130–149.

McArdle, J. J. (1988). Dynamic but structural equation modeling of repeated measures data. In R. B. Cattel & J. Nesselroade (Eds.), *Handbook of multivariate experimental psychology* (2nd edition) (pp. 561–614). New York: Plenum Press.

McArdle, J. J. (1994). Structural factor analysis experiments with incomplete data. *Multivariate Behavioral Research, 29,* 409–454.

McArdle, J. J., & Epstein, D. (1987). Latent growth curves within developmental structural equation models. *Child Development, 58,* 110–133.

Meredith, W., & Tisak, J. (1990). Latent curve analysis. *Psychometrika, 55,* 107–122.

Muthén, B. O. (1991). Analysis of longitudinal data using latent-variable models with varying parameters. In L. C. Collins & J. L. Horn (Eds.), *Best methods for the analysis of change* (pp. 1–17). Washington, DC: American Psychological Association.

Muthén, B. O., & Curran, P. (1997). General growth modeling with interventions: A latent-variable framework for analysis and power estimation. *Psychological Methods, 2,* 371–402.

Raudenbush, S. W., Brennan, R. T., & Barnett, R. C. (1995). A multivariate hierarchical model for studying psychological change within married couples. *Journal of Family Psychology, 9,* 161–174.

Rogossa, D. (1988). Myths about longitudinal research. In K. W. Schaie, R. T. Campbell, W. Meredith, & S. C. Rawlings (Eds.), *Methodological issues in aging research.* New York: Springer.

Rogossa, D., & Willett, J. B. (1985). Understanding correlates of change by modeling individual differences in growth. *Psychometrika, 50,* 203–228.

Saris, W. E., & Satorra, A. (1993). Power evaluations in structural equation models. In K. A. Bollen & J. S. Long (Eds.), *Testing structural equation models* (pp. 181–204). Newbury Park, CA: Sage.

Saris, W. E., & Stronkhorst, H. (1984). *Causal modeling in nonexperimental research.* Amsterdam: Sociometric Research Foundation.

Satorra, A. (1989). Alternative test criteria in covariance structure analysis: A unified approach. *Psychometrika, 54,* 131–151.

Satorra, A., & Saris, W. (1985). Power of the likelihood ration test in covariance structure analysis. *Psychometrika, 51,* 83–90.

Sedlemeyer, P., & Gigerenzer, G. (1989). Do studies of statistical power have an effect on the power of studies? *Psychological Bulletin, 105,* 309–316.

Sörbom, D. (1989). Model modification. *Psychometrika, 54,* 371–384.

Steiger, J. H., & Lined, J. M. (1980, June). *Statistically based tests for the number of common factors.* Paper presented at the Annual Meeting of the Psychometric Society, Iowa City, IA.

Stoolmiller, M., Duncan, T. E., Bank, L., & Patterson, G. R. (1993). Some problems and solutions in the study of change: Significant patterns in client resistance. *Journal of Consulting and Clinical Psychology, 61,* 920–928.

Thomas, L. (1996). Monitoring long-term population change: Why are there so many analysis methods? *Ecology, 77,* 49–58.

Thomas, L. (1997). Retrospective power analysis. *Conservation Biology, 11,* 276–280.

Thomas, L., & Krebs, C. J. (1997). A review of statistical power analysis software. *Bulletin of the Ecological Society of America, 78*(2), 128–139.

Willet, J. B., Ayoub, C. C., & Robinson, D. (1991). Using growth modeling to examine systematic differences in growth: An example of change in the function of families at risk of maladaptive parenting, child abuse, or neglect. *Journal of Consulting and Clinical Psychology, 59,* 38–47.

Willet, J. B., & Sayer, A. G. (1994). Using covariance structure analysis to detect correlates and predictors of individual change over time. *Psychological Bulletin, 116,* 363–381.

Winer, B. J. (1971). *Statistical Principles in Experimental Design.* New York: McGraw–Hill.

PART VIII

DRUG ABUSE PREVENTION: A LOOK INTO THE FUTURE

CHAPTER 32

Application of Computer Technology to Drug Abuse Prevention

Kris Bosworth

INTRODUCTION

In the 1970s, when personal computers began to give students access to computing technology at both school and home, some educators, including health educators, saw an opportunity to revolutionize the educational process. Although some of the predictions made in those early days have not come to pass, technology has radically altered how we locate and distribute knowledge (Gustafson et al., 1987; Lieberman, 1992; Orlandi, Dozier, & Marta, 1990). However, despite the tremendous promise of computer technology, very few computer-based drug abuse prevention programs are currently available. A review of the literature yields only a short list of programs that are theory based, are grounded on research in the field, use sound instructional design principles, and have been assessed for effectiveness in changing behavior.

This chapter discusses state-of-the-art computer technology in education; identifies and describes specific programs in the area of health promotion, specifically drug abuse prevention; and highlights barriers to the wider use of technology in prevention.

TECHNOLOGY UPDATE

Computer technology, defined as any technology involving or controlled by computers, appears to have the most powerful impact of all technology teaching tools, including film, radio, television, and the telephone. It allows students and teachers to interact in ways that are almost impossible with other types of technology. This section describes several applications of computer technology that are appropriate for prevention settings.

KRIS BOSWORTH • College of Education, University of Arizona, Tucson, Arizona 85721

The use of the computer as a teaching/learning tool is generically referred to as computer-assisted learning (CAL). It has three primary approaches: computer-assisted instruction (CAI), computer-managed instruction (CMI), and computer-enriched instruction (CEI).

In CAI, students interact with the material through computer-based lessons. This generally involves drill and practice, tutorials, and demonstration activities. Generally, the goal of such practice is to reinforce concepts previously introduced by a teacher. With tutorial programs, concepts are introduced and reinforced via computer. In demonstration lessons, the computer presents lessons and practice exercises.

In CMI, the computer acts as an electronic file manager. The curriculum is task based, and students are tested for mastery after completing each unit of instruction. Once students have passed a criterion test on a unit, they move to the next level. The computer keeps records of student responses and directs students to mastery through units of instruction.

CEI makes learning richer and more meaningful through simulation and instructional games. In simulations, students are presented with problems related to realistic situations and must use newly acquired skills to solve them. CEI offers students who already understand a concept entertaining and challenging practice sessions to achieve mastery or automaticity.

With increases in speed and memory, video animation and sound can be added to traditional CAL lessons to produce a multimedia presentation that can provide multiple avenues for presenting instruction. This is especially appealing to school-age children who spend on average three to four hours a day watching television and five to seven hours a week playing video games. Although the internal structure of the software is usually no different from other CAL programs, multimedia features enhance interest and engage learners. Multimedia components can also provide additional modeling of skills and opportunities to practice those skills.

When CAL presents content based on instructional design theories that identify steps or prerequisites for the learning process—as do performance engineering, performance technology, or structural learning theory—and is thoughtfully designed based on solid instructional design principles (Dede & Fontana, 1995; Dick & Carey, 1996; Street & Rimal, 1997), it has many unique features that enhance the prospect for learning and retention:

1. The branching capabilities of software allow information to be presented to specific users based on their previous responses to queries. Unlike print or video, the information can be tailored to the needs or desires of individuals.
2. Users can control the pace of learning. Well-designed software allows users to spend as much time as needed on a particular screen or section of the software, to repeat sections, or to return to previous sections. In making these choices, the user has the chance to practice decision-making skills.
3. Users receive immediate relevant feedback to questions or quiz items so that misconceptions can be easily corrected and further learning can be built on a more solid base.
4. Student decision-making skills are enhanced when an immediate response is demanded in a particular situation. In contrast, when a teacher poses questions, usually only a few students have the chance to respond immediately.
5. CAL software is always available, while classroom intervention may be a one-time event. This accessibility enhances the likelihood that students will receive the information they need when they have to make decisions about various risk-taking behaviors, not when the teacher or curriculum decides to present the information. This feature facilitates making up missed classes.
6. CAL provides current information in a consistent format and does not rely on the instructor having the knowledge or time to keep current on the issues. In addition, information can be easily updated, in contrast to text or video formats, which are relatively fixed.

7. Confidentiality gives users access to software that is most relevant to them without fear of embarrassment or judgment about their choices. Even the fact that a user has concern in a particular health area can be kept confidential.

Since the mid-1980s meta-analyses have identified positive knowledge gains from CAI (Kulik, Kulik & Bangert-Downs, 1985; Kulik & Kulik, 1991; Niemiec & Walberg, 1987). In the most recent study, Kulik and Kulik (1991) used findings from 254 controlled evaluation studies and found that CAL usually produces positive effects on students. These studies covered learners from kindergarten through adult. CAL programs raised examination scores by 0.30 standard deviations on average. The researchers deemed this a moderate but significant effect and noted that the size of the effect varied as a function of the study feature. For example, effects were larger in published than unpublished studies and in studies in which different teachers taught experimental and control classes. CAL also produced small but positive changes in student attitudes toward learning and computers.

In addition, use of CAL substantially reduced the amount of time needed for instruction. Kulik and Kulik (1991) conclude that CAL is "not only a cost effective alternative to traditional instruction but that it is far more cost effective than nontechnological innovations such as tutoring" (p. 91). Several studies have also shown that CAL statistically increases academic achievement scores when used to deliver instruction to learners with disabilities (Fletcher-Flin & Gravatt, 1995; Niemiec et al., 1996).

In the past decade researchers and instructional designers have identified two areas of problem solving and concluded that technology needs to be designed differently depending on the characteristics of the problem to be solved (Jonassen, 1997). A structured problem is one that has a specific outcome or answer, such as long division. Although the processes for determining the answer to such problems may be complex, the number of paths to the solution are known and can be predetermined. To solve such a problem, traditional instructional designers used technology to teach the rules and component skills that are deemed necessary to solve the problem (Gagné, 1985). An ill-structured problem, on the other hand, is one in which the learner must identify the characteristics of the problem as well as an acceptable solution and process by which the solution can be reached (Jonasson, 1997). Instructional design for ill-structured problems uses the assumptions and methods from constructivism and situated cognition, which purport that learning in these cases is both domain and context dependent (Bransford, 1994b). Clearly, from a youth's perspective, the decision to use or not to use a drug presents an ill-structured problem in which many conditions and information from multiple sources must be considered. For ill-structured problems, the medium is less relevant than the content and the design (Carr, 1997).

Accordingly, most current research on development and use of technology takes two theoretical learning approaches: learner-centered instruction and constructivism. In a learner-centered classroom, teachers work with students to generate questions and seek solutions in an environment that supports intellectual risk, tolerates ambiguity, and allows flexibility. The result is empowerment of students to manage their own learning (Anderson, 1997; Astuto, 1995; Erickson, 1997; McCombs & Whisler, 1997; Wolcott, 1996). A constructivist approach focuses on how people construct individualized understandings of the world. Each person makes sense of the world by synthesizing new experiences into what was previously understood. In a constructivist classroom, students frame their own questions and issues and then go about answering and analyzing them (Grennon-Brooks & Brooks, 1993; Gruender, 1996; Hannafin, Hannafin & Land, 1997).

The branching capabilities of computers and the multiple information sources that can be accessed through the Internet can facilitate and provide resources for a constructivist learning process, and CAL designers in the 1990s began exploring ways to use the computer as a tool for learning rather than for routine drill and practice (Jonassen, 1997). In classrooms, teachers are facilitators of learning and organizers of environments that enable students to search for answers. Similarly, designers of instructional software use more powerful technology to create learning environments that are complex enough to provide meaning and practical applications for information to give students a reason for learning. Problems anchored in this complex context are rich enough to provide students problem situations in a real-world context (Savery & Duffy, 1995). An example of such "situated instruction" can be found in the Jasper Woodbury Series for mathematical instruction at Vanderbilt University (Bransford, 1994a,b). In this series, the character Jasper is faced with situations, such as how to navigate a river or fly a hand glider, in which complex mathematical skills are needed.

In summary, CAL designs have evolved from a simple drill-and-practice format with limited applications to a more complex, sophisticated format with unlimited possibilities for engaging students in learning. The following sections describe several applications for drug abuse and prevention.

Interactive Voice Response Technology

The capacity of computers has been further enhanced by the addition of interactive voice response (IVR) technology, which allows computers to respond with either synthesized or prerecorded voice and to record the voices of users. Users dial a dedicated number and are asked to respond to a series of short questions by pushing the appropriate numbers on the keypad of a touch-tone phone. Access is usually controlled by an identification number and a password to protect the confidentiality of users. Data are then stored on the computer for analysis or are used to identify resources that might be helpful given the user profile.

Researchers at the Vermont Alcohol Research Center have been studying the validity of IVR technology in reporting drinking data and daily behavior (Lester et al., 1995; Mundt et al., 1995). The branching capabilities of the technology are exploited to expedite the reporting process. In one protocol, subjects are initially asked about their consumption of beer, liquor, and wine. If they did not drink any alcohol in the past day, they automatically receive questions from the computer about their reasons for not drinking. If they report any alcohol use, they are branched to another set of questions. The studies found high compliance rates, but the rates did deteriorate somewhat over time. In addition, a correlation of 0.72 was obtained between objectively measured breath alcohol concentrations and self-reported use. The researchers also found that the technology was flexible enough to permit changing questions throughout the data-collection period in order to probe any maladaptive behaviors or occurrences of relatively rare events. This gave the researchers opportunities to investigate potential relationships between these events and the development of detrimental habits. This might not have been possible with traditional reporting methods. This method gave the researchers the ability to obtain data quickly and inoffensively without either disrupting the behaviors under study or drawing inordinate attention to possible consequences.

The researchers identified a number of features of the technology that may have contributed to maintaining subject involvement. First, the flexibility of the system allowed subjects to integrate their reporting into normal daily routines with little effort. Second, providing subjects with a toll-free number allowed them to report behaviors even while traveling. Finally, IVR allowed actions to be taken quickly in order to secure data that would have been lost using more traditional reporting methods.

However, the researchers caution that the volume and complexity of such data require sophisticated and well-organized data-management systems that allow efficient flow of data with thorough error checking and immediate access to data through summary reports generated daily.

Alemi and Higley (1995) developed a computerized telephone interview system for assessing and advising callers about their health risks—AVIVA. The employees at Cleveland State University phoned the computer and listened to prerecorded (not synthesized) questions and answered by pressing keys on touch-tone phones. During the interview, AVIVA provided advice and, when appropriate, referred callers to other sources of information, such as risk-reduction programs or videotaped health information at a local library.

AVIVA was used by 70% of employees who had access to it. More than 60% of the users believed the AVIVA to be accurate, current, easy to understand, convenient, affordable, easy to use, and accessible. On all of these measures, AVIVA was statistically significantly rated higher than the users' current source of health education. One measure of the impact of AVIVA was the users' intentions to obtain additional information. Fifty-seven percent identified at least one risk factor, and 80% reported planning to change their health behavior in at least one health area. Eighty-three percent reported alcohol risks, and 86% reported smoking risks. However, the intent to change difference between the control group and the users of AVIVA was not statistically significant. Fourteen percent of AVIVA users planned to get videotaped information from the library, but no video tapes were checked out.

The researchers suggest three reasons for AVIVA use: (1) the computer interview provided callers with an opportunity to receive immediate feedback; (2) the interview was a novelty; (3) the interview maintained confidentiality. Because of the lack of change in intent or behavior, the researchers suggest that computerized risk assessment may play a more effective role when combined with other educational interventions. The ease of use and low cost allowed telephone interviews to be conducted in circumstances that have not heretofore been tried and that go beyond the traditional health-risk appraisal (Alemi et al., 1996).

Thomas, Cahill, and Santilli (1997), at the New York State Department of Health, developed an interactive computer game to serve as a tool for enhancing adolescent sense of self-efficacy in HIV/AIDS prevention programs. A form of IVR was used in a standard CAL format based on a Hollywood game show called "Risk of Love." Users were randomly given one of three tasks: (1) say no to sex if no condom is used, (2) ask a long-time partner to start using condoms, (3) ask a partner to get an HIV test. They recorded their answers on a microphone in the computer and could then listen to what they had said and revise their statements. Users could also listen to responses from other teens who modeled appropriate options.

The program, called Life Challenge, was delivered in computer kiosks that were field tested in 13 sites serving high-risk adolescents. In a pre- post-test design, statistically significant learning gains were demonstrated on knowledge items and self-efficacy scores, with the greatest improvement for those who had low baseline self-efficacy rates.

The researchers did not intend Life Challenge to be used as a stand-alone intervention. It was created as a "new and somewhat unique tool in the armamentarium of interventions available for use in HIV/AIDS education programs" (Thomas et al., 1997, p. 82). Life Challenge was promoted as a tool to reinforce knowledge and skills acquired in existing education and to offer practice in communication in dating relationships. Its major strength was the opportunity for confidential practice. The researchers warned that while developmental costs for the computer programs are high ($60,000 for two kiosks), dissemination costs via electronic media can be very low.

IVR allows for two-way interaction that mimics human conversation and can be used in a variety of ways: data collection, skills practice, or referral. In this way, common technology, such as the telephone, provides access points for more sophisticated technology.

Computer-Mediated Communication

In its simplest form, Computer-Mediated Communication (CMC) is a mode of written communication made possible by communications software driving the Internet, or the World Wide Web. CMC makes it possible for communication to occur between groups or individuals. Through computer networks, people can exchange, store, edit, broadcast, and copy any written document. They can send data and messages instantaneously, easily, at low cost, and over long distances.

CMC is like written discourse with some features that simulate spoken communication. Direct and simultaneous (synchronous) communication is much like spoken communication in that two or more people are simultaneously at computers carrying on a written "conversation." The communication tends to be sequential with transactions addressing the immediately preceding message.

Delayed, or asynchronous, communication is much more like written discourse. The person receiving the communication can respond (or not) at his or her leisure. A disadvantage is that such systems eliminate the nonverbal cues that generally enrich relationships and information exchanges. In the absence of such cues, users' perceptions of the communication context and its participants may constrain or alter the interpretation of messages (Walther, 1992).

Several groups of researchers in the health-promotion and -prevention fields have used CMC successfully to achieve various prevention goals. Among the first to report use of CMC for providing support were Schneider and Tooley (1986). They argue that asynchronous technologies, which they refer to as "computer conferencing," could play a useful role in health promotion. Their evaluation of the effectiveness of an online behavioral smoking-cessation program found that discussions on the electronic bulletin board have all the characteristics of a self-help group. Ultimately, many members were able to quit smoking while using computer conferencing. Due to the lack of a control group, no determination can be made of the role computer conferencing played in the treatment outcome. In a follow-up study, two versions of the smoking-cessation program were evaluated on a private Internet service. Subjects who had access to the computer conferencing in addition to a behavioral intervention were more likely to complete the treatment and succeed in quitting, compared with subjects who had access to the computer-based behavioral intervention only (Burling, Burling, & Latini, 2001).

In the early 1990s, Brennan and her colleagues conducted a series of studies of a computer program for delivering nursing services called Computer Link. The Computer Link system had three components: (1) an electronic encyclopedia, (2) a decision-making system, and (3) an electronic bulletin board. In separate studies, Brennan's group looked at caregivers of people with Alzheimer's disease or HIV/AIDS. The electronic bulletin board was the most frequently used feature by both groups. However, in a randomized control study of the effects of long-term participation in Computer Link, they found that although participants regularly used the electronic bulletin board, that usage did not increase their self-reported level of social support in other settings (Brennan, Moore, & Smyth, 1991, 1995; Brennan & Ripich, 1994).

Gustafson and his colleagues have developed a complex computer system to provide information and support to people facing HIV/AIDS, breast cancer, academic crisis, sexual assault, and substance abuse. CHESS (Comprehensive Health Educational Support System) consists of an integrated set of services to provide information, referral, skills training, decision support, and social support to users. CHESS is accessed via personal computers in users' homes and linked by a modem through a host computer.

The discussion group was the most frequently accessed service and was used much like an in-person support group. Users asked questions and received answers as well as gave and received support. Participants reported several advantages to use of CMC. First, they were not limited by time or location and could access the system to receive information or support at any time of the day or night. They could remain anonymous by giving code names and disclosing as little or as much as they wished. A final advantage was that the interaction was based solely on what someone wrote. The users were not influenced by prejudices, such as race, dress, sex, or other factors. The researchers conclude that "computer mediated support cannot, of course, replace in-person support. However, for rural people, shut-ins and those with issues about confidentiality and anonymity, CHESS provides a powerful adjunct opportunity for obtaining information and support" (Boberg et al., 1995, p. 300; Bosworth & Gustafson, 1991; Gustafson et al., 1992).

In a randomized control trial, CHESS computers were placed for 3 to 6 months in the homes of people diagnosed with HIV/AIDS. Investigators found that while CHESS was in the home, its users reported quality of life improvements, such as a more active lifestyle, fewer negative emotions, higher levels of cognitive functioning, and more social support and participation in health care. They also reported spending less time during ambulatory care visits, making more phone calls to providers, and having fewer and shorter hospitalizations.

An important finding of this study relates to the differences in outcomes based on the length of time the CHESS computers remained in the homes. For those who had CHESS for 3 months, no benefits remained and one (cognitive functioning) was significantly reversed after CHESS was removed. The group that kept the CHESS for 6 months continued to reap the benefits of the system in terms of participation in health care, additional social support, and less negative emotion, which were all maintained at a nine-month follow-up.

In terms of reporting fewer and shorter hospitalizations, the research team calculated that people with HIV/AIDS who used the CHESS system had a $720 per month lower hospital bill than did control subjects during implementation and a $222 lower hospital bill after implementation. They conclude "the estimated cost savings would be more than sufficient to support the purchase of computers and pay staff to run CHESS as a service for their HIV patients" (Boberg et al., 1995; p. 12).

Decision Support Systems

A Decision Support System (DSS) is an interactive, computer-based system that provides decision makers with easy access to data and models to support semi-structured or unstructured tasks. A DSS usually contains several subsystems that include assessments, access to data bases, and the ability to compare localized data with larger data sets or mathematically generated models. DSS is usually developed for decision makers, but some applications have been reported to help the general public or targeted populations make decisions about risk taking.

Several types of DSS are reported to have been used in drug abuse prevention. Holder (1996) reports on the SIMCOM (Simulated Community) model, which has been successfully simulating the effects of alcohol-prevention policy. This computer model was able to simulate how an intervention designed to change perceived risk of arrest while driving under the influence would affect the rate of alcohol-related crashes involving injury. It was also able to generate fresh estimates for 1993 to 1995 that closely matched the actual data later collected for this time period. Use of this tool can help decision makers understand and forecast likely outcomes of proposed prevention programs, thus providing information to allow more cost-effective decisions about implementation. This computer modeling is a unique tool that expresses the causal relationship between variables in a complex system. Holder cautions "although the complexity of computer models may present many more data-collection, communication, and technical challenges than traditional policy research, with further refinement computer simulations are likely to become vital components of prevention efforts to reduce alcohol-related problems" (p. 252).

Another DSS system for schools is DIADS (Drug Information, Assessment and Decisions for Schools; Bosworth & Yoast, 1991), which helps schools evaluate the probable effectiveness of their current prevention efforts using an expert-generated school assessment model containing 14 factors. Feedback from this assessment provides suggestions for improvement in current prevention programming. Currently DIADS is available on the World Wide Web at http://www.drugstats.org and links are provided to other Web resources to facilitate planning.

"Looking at Binge Drinking" (LBD) is a software program designed for school administrators and prevention specialists based at colleges and universities who are concerned about the rate of binge drinking among their students. By varying the basic data entered into the LBD program, school officials can explore how certain changes in their school or student body might affect the rate of binge drinking at the school (DeJong, 1996).

Based on a system for adults developed by Velicer and colleagues (1993, 1999), Aveyard and Cheng (1999) tested a three-session computer-based expert system. The system was based on the trans-theoretical model of behavior change with a goal of reducing smoking among students ages 13–14 in England.

On-line questionnaires were used to determine the appropriate stage of change of the user. Feedback as well as helpful strategies to increase confidence, resist temptation, and "think about smoking in the correct way" (p. 948) were given to help the user move to the next stage of change. Thus, the program was personalized for each student. However, based on a pre–post evaluation, the authors found no effect on the prevalence of regular smoking.

Games

Computer games are an engaging approach to reaching children and adolescents who are attracted to this venue during their free time. Games offer unlimited amount of rehearsal time for new skills. Lieberman (1998) reports found that over 70% of homes in the United States with children have video game systems, and children who play video games spend an average of 1.5 hours at play each day. Gaming attracts children who might not be attentive to or seek out health information from other, more conventional sources.

In the health area, Lieberman and colleagues have developed and evaluated three adventure games for children in the areas of asthma, diabetes, and smoking prevention. The smoking prevention game, Rex Ronan, vividly illustrates the detrimental effects of smoking by taking players on a microscopic journey through a smoker's body. Studies found that after playing the game, children ages 10 and 11 were able to provide more concrete and physiological reasons for resisting smoking. Users were also more like to have strengthened their resolve not to start smoking. The game was very appealing to youth ages 10–16 and they played it often (Lieberman, 1997; Tingen et al., 1997).

The World Wide Web (Internet)

Travel along the information superhighway has exploded in recent years. Internet access, which was once restricted to academic and government programs and scientists, is now available in schools, libraries, and homes to virtually everyone in the world. The Internet offers access to heretofore difficult to obtain resources, but it also has spawned many resources that have questionable prevention value or are detrimental to prevention. For example, advertisements for beer and liquor distributors, pornography, and pro-marijuana chat rooms are as accessible to first graders as they are to the adults for whom they are designed. A major challenge for prevention is teaching young people to assess and evaluate both the source and the quality of information. The many possibilities for using the Internet in prevention have just begun to be explored and refined within the prevention science community (Izenberg & Lieberman, 1998).

Many state and federal agencies have established web sites that provide important information and resources for teachers, students, and families (Silverman, 2000). Additionally, many publishers of drug prevention curricula, software, or programs have web sites that provide information about their products.

APPLICATIONS FOR PREVENTION

Computer-based technology has been used successfully in several prevention efforts. Although these approaches have been used in specialized areas, such as social stress training, AIDS prevention, contraception, and violence, they provide models for potential applications in drug abuse prevention. This section describes selected examples of these applications. [For additional applications, see Binik, Meana, and Sand (1994); Burling, Burling, and Latini (2001); Litman (1995); Paperny (1997); and Pomeroy and Detweiler (1995)].

Reis and Tymchyshyn (1992) completed a longitudinal evaluation of computer-assisted instruction on student contraceptive use. The program consisted of a personal computer-based instructional lesson covering facts about appropriate use of oral contraceptives and barrier methods and myths about sexuality and sexually transmitted diseases. At a 6-month follow-up, the 58 White female students who used the program, compared to 171 control subjects, showed evidence of long-term knowledge gains on several key pieces of information, including appropriate contingencies for missing 2 days of the pill, danger signs associated with contraceptives, and health risks of using oral contraceptives.

Noell and colleagues (Noell, Biglan, Hood, & Britz, 1994; Noell, Ary, & Duncan, 1997) developed a series of interactive video disks designed to reduce HIV/STD risk behaviors. These interventions were unique in that separate programs were developed for African Americans, Hispanics, and Caucasians at two age levels (middle school and high school). The disks used scenarios with extensive story lines to teach decision-making skills and socially appropriate responses to potentially risky sexual situations. The programs were presented by a teacher in a classroom with a remote control so the teacher could control the video disk. At the branching points, students made decisions directing program flow. A 30-day follow-up with 827 students in a randomized experiment found three of the four measures to be significant:

1. belief that a single incident of unprotected sex can result in STD or pregnancy,
2. positive intentions and attitudes toward use of condoms,
3. self-efficacy in remaining abstinent.

The researchers report that interactive video is successful in holding interest at a level that ultimately leads to effectiveness. Specific characteristics that are important include interactivity and matching video materials to the students' race/ethnicity. The use of a branching story line compelled student attention and was popular with the students. "The use of screens presenting discussion items at key points in the program proved to be an effective way to prompt student participation in discussions even when teachers were not entirely comfortable talking about sexual behavior" (p. 99). In addition, the fact the students got to choose in which direction they wanted the scenario to go appeared to increase attention and enthusiasm.

Stanton and colleagues (1996) provided AIDS risk-reduction information on the "Culturally and Developmentally Risk Assessment Tool" administered with "talking" computers. In a longitudinal study of the 383 African American young adolescents in a convenience sample of attendees at city recreation centers, the researchers found that contraceptive practices were stable over the 18 months of the study. After receiving the intervention, more than 80% of those who used oral contraceptives also used condoms. Knowledge about AIDS was positively associated with the use of more effective contraception methods.

As previously mentioned, Life Challenge is an interactive computer program for enhancing adolescents' sense of self-efficacy in an HIV/AIDS prevention program (Thomas, Cahill, & Santilli, 1997). Students accessed the software in kiosks that were field tested in certain sites serving high-risk students. Statistically significant learning gains were identified on knowledge and in self-efficacy scores. Students with the lowest baseline self-efficacy levels showed the greatest improvement.

Kritsch, Bostow, and Dedrick (1995) developed an interactive video disk providing AIDS information and tested recall of the information using three different formats. The first format was "click to continue," the second was passive observation, and the third required students to answer questions or fill in a blank before they were able to continue. In two experiments the researchers concluded that active construction (e.g., the condition in which the students had to type in a response) promoted recall and that programmed instruction such as this was appropriate for students at all ability levels.

Kumar and colleagues (1993) found similar results when they tested 92 undergraduates on computer-delivered nutrition education focusing on cancer prevention. Students were randomly assigned to a group that used an interactive computer, another group that used a noninteractive computer, and a group that read materials from brochures and handouts. The subjects in the interactive group took nearly twice as long to complete the program because they were required to respond to questions in the software. This group produced significantly greater knowledge gains when tested 3 weeks later. In addition, they lowered their fat intake by 42%, compared to a 26% reduction in the noninteractive computer group and a 19% reduction in the passive reading group. There were no significant changes in fiber, vitamin A, or vitamin C intake. The researchers conclude, "The present research confirmed the importance of constructive student responses when interacting with computer instructional programs. The fact that actively instructive responses at the computer resulted in the most significant reductions in reports of what students said they ate and what they actually ate suggests this form of instruction can be an important adjunct to health care and disease prevention programs" (p. 210).

SMART Team (Students Managing Anger and Resolution Together) uses multimedia to teach middle school students skills to resolve conflicts peacefully (Bosworth et al., 1996, 2000; Bosworth, Espelage, & DuBay, 1998). SMART Team contains eight modules and uses games, simulations, graphics, cartoons, animation, and interactive interviews with celebrities and peer role models to teach and model prosocial approaches to anger management and problem solving. Each module is designed as a separate program, so adolescents do not have to use them sequentially to receive the full prevention benefit.

In a randomized control study in a middle school in a midwest urban center, students who were exposed to SMART Team were more likely to have greater self-knowledge about how their behaviors might contribute to a conflict situation, to be less inclined to see violence as an appropriate way to solve conflicts, and to plan on using nonviolent strategies in conflict situations than nonusers. No significant pre–post test differences were found in confidence in being able to use nonviolent strategies or in number of aggressive acts reported.

SMART Team has been designated as an Exemplary Model Program by the Center for Substance Abuse Prevention (CSAP) in 1999 and as a Promising Model Program by the U.S. Department of Education in 2000.

COMPUTER-BASED DRUG ABUSE PREVENTION

In a thorough review of the literature, several computer-based programs aimed at drug abuse prevention were identified. Table 32.1 describes those computer-based interventions for drug abuse prevention.

"If You Drink: A Guide to Alcohol Education" (Meier & Sampson, 1989) was designed to take advantage of the ability of CAI to interest elementary, high school, and college students. It includes several modules:

1. the alcohol quiz—an assessment of alcohol knowledge and attitudes;
2. breathalyzer—a graphics program illustrating how blood alcohol content is affected by weight, number of drinks, and time period of consumption;
3. alcohol and drugs—a database describing interactions between alcohol and 15 commonly prescribed medications;
4. party—a simulation that allows users to make decisions about how to handle typical party situations involving alcohol and that provides feedback on the consequences of the user's decision.

Although the researchers are enthusiastic about the potential for this intervention, no formal evaluation is described.

Rickerd and his colleagues (1993) compared adolescent knowledge about alcohol risks as a result of receiving either computer-assisted instruction, physician-delivered anticipatory guidance, or no intervention. No description of the content of the CAI intervention or the physician-delivered guidance is provided. Eighty-nine adolescents presenting at a clinic for routine care were randomly assigned to one of the three groups. At post-test, adolescents from both intervention groups were significantly more knowledgeable than those in the control group. Males had higher knowledge scores than females. This study suggests that use of computer technology during routine adolescent health-care visits is effective and efficient in transmitting drug-related information.

Kinzie and colleagues (1993) report on development and testing of a computer-based multimedia prenatal alcohol education program designed for poor rural pregnant women, a majority of whom were African American. The program, The Healthy Touch, provides factual information about alcohol and pregnancy in a culturally relevant format and in a fashion that has the potential for enhancing learning and bringing about subsequent behavioral changes. In creating the program, open-ended interviews and focus groups were held with pregnant women who attended a prenatal clinic. This information guided not only the content of the program but also the types of scenarios and response options presented. The design used three concepts that have been essential in the development of successful educational programs: personal control, self-efficacy, and stimulation of curiosity. A young African American television personality hosted the program. The menu topics included (1) how babies eat and drink, (2) the effects of alcohol on babies, (3) healthy activities for moms, and (4) how to cope with difficult situations.

The researchers describe two cycles of field testing for this 20-minute program. In the first test, user satisfaction and suggestions for changing the program were elicited. In the second field test, preinput measures asking for selections of preferred leisure-time activities, snack foods, entertainment, and drinks while in social situations were elicited from participants. There were no control groups. On the premeasure, 39% of the women indicated they would select an alcoholic beverage in a social situation. After completing the program, that figure dropped to zero, with all participants indicating they would select a nonalcoholic beverage. In addition, 96% enjoyed using the program and thought it was easy to use. These preliminary results indicate that interactive multimedia can be useful for a relatively difficult-to-reach population.

TABLE 32.1. Prevention Interventions—Drug Abuse

Reference	Name	Description	Target population	Evaluation
Meier & Sampson (1989)	If You Drink: A Guide to Alcohol Education (IYD)	5 modules: The alcohol quiz, breathalyzer, database describing interaction between alcohol and 15 prescribed medicines, party simulation	Students (elementary, high school, college)	None
Rickerd et al. (1993)		Purpose: to compare adolescents' alcohol knowledge and satisfaction after receiving either CAI or physician-delivered anticipatory guidance or no intervention	Adolescents	Increased knowledge pre to post in both interventions
Kinzie et al. (1993)	The Healthy Touch	Multimedia prenatal alcohol education program for poor rural pregnant women	Pregnant patients	Formative evaluation—well accepted by this population.
Hawkins et al. (1987); BARN Research Group (1994)	BARN (Body Awareness Resource Network)	Provides teens with information, skills building and decision support in AIDS, AOD, body management, sex, smoking, stress management through games, simulations, interactive interviews, and graphics; currently being revised in a multimedia format adding animation and sound	Adolescents	Pre-test & 2-yr follow-up found students with previous use most likely to select topic of risk, more risk reduction in younger students, slowed the progression of alcohol use & problems.
Gropper et al. (1995)	Say No with Donny	Poor Israeli 5th/6th graders; 10 consecutive 90-min sessions; What are drugs/why people use? Stop and think of consequences; Id pro-drug pressures—peer, media and comm.; problem solving	5th and 6th grades	Formative evaluation–widely accepted by all users.
Shulman et al. (1995)		College students typed dilemmas about drugs into a prewritten computer program that followed a game format	College students	Students using computers structured more complex responses to dilemmas. No behavioral data collected.
Bryson (1999)	Alcohol 101	Multifaceted, comprehensive for college students. Three interactive video scenarios model safe decision-making skills and show consequences of poor decisions	College students	Short-term input on knowledge and intentions
Reis et al. (2000)	Refusal challenges	Students role play. 12 high-risk simulations with computer-simulated peers and feedback until correct response is given	Middle school	Pre-post-test and 6-month follow-up

Since the mid-1980s, Gustafson and his colleagues (BARN Research Group, 1994; Hawkins et al., 1987) have continually updated a comprehensive health-promotion program for adolescents. The Body Awareness Resource Network (BARN) is designed to provide adolescents with nonjudgmental health information, behavior-change strategies, and sources of referral in the context of responsible decision making in real-life situations. The programs cover five critical adolescent health issues: alcohol and other drugs, smoking prevention and cessation, human sexuality, stress management, diet management, and HIV/AIDS prevention. The alcohol and other drugs program includes:

1. two simulations in which users are confronted with situations (a party and a drinking-and-driving situation) in which they need to make decisions for characters in the simulation,
2. a quiz of critical information related to alcohol and other drugs,
3. an assessment of the seriousness of a potential drug problem and an interactive role-play session on resistance skills, and
4. several programs with information about alcohol and other drugs and consequences of use.

The smoking program presents:

1. an assessment of values and beliefs about smoking,
2. information about media influences on smoking, and
3. a self-assessment of smoking behavior that leads into an individually designed cessation program.

Orlandi and colleagues (1990) describe BARN as "utilizing that some of the more innovative aspects of computer learning systems" (p. 428). An evaluation of the BARN software using a pre- post-test control group design shows that among students who use BARN there is a slowing of progression from no use to experimental use to problem use. Whereas light smokers who used BARN were more likely to stop smoking, BARN had little impact on those who were already heavy smokers when they started using the system (BARN Research Group, 1994).

Gropper and colleagues (1995) targeted fifth- and sixth-grade children growing up in a poverty-stricken urban community in Israel. The program, "Say No with Donny," is based on social learning theory and uses an attractive cartoon-illustrated program that combines games, role playing, and group work techniques aimed at teaching resiliency skills. The program has 10 consecutive 90-minute sessions designed to be given on a weekly basis. It is highly structured and sequential, with a manual to give leaders a clear guide for running the session. After a brief review of the previous session, two children work together on the computer for 30 to 40 minutes. This is followed by a role-playing game that helps reinforce and integrate the material. In the final part of the session, the children are prepared for the next session. No evaluation data are reported.

Shulman, Sweeney, and Gerler (1995) describe a unique use of technology with Smith College students in a general health education class. One treatment group was guided through a series of discussions about dilemmas they had faced in their teen years and how those might have influenced their handling of similar dilemmas in college. The second group was involved in similar discussions but was asked to type their dilemmas into a computer using a series of guided questions so that students in the next class might benefit from their experience in dealing with these dilemmas. The investigator hypothesized that this process would facilitate growth in the students' ability to make healthier choices about their current alcohol use. Analysis of variance using pre- and postdifference scores indicated that students in the computer group increased their ability to structure more complex and higher-order thinking responses to dilemmas after going through the program. No behavioral or attitudinal data about alcohol or other drugs were collected. The group using discussion as the mode of intervention showed no change.

Refusal Challenges (Bryson, 1999) focuses on the skills needed to refuse alcohol, tobacco, and other drugs. This program uses several social skills training techniques including written instruction, modeling, cueing, rehearsal, corrective and instructive feedback, and reinforcement of correct responses. Students are introduced to 12 high-risk situations such as holding stolen goods, ditching school, writing graffiti, drinking alcohol, stealing alcohol, smoking cigarettes, using marijuana, etc. Students are asked to role-play these situations with a computer-simulated peer. The peer challenger attempts to convince the user to do something risky. As the user progresses, the situations become progressively more challenging, and the software offers fewer cues to the appropriate response.

Refusal Challenges was evaluated with 182 eighth-grade students in a rural California middle school. Randomly assigned students used Refusal Challenges in pairs in a computer-lab setting without adult intervention, although the computer teacher was in the room. Students were tested pre- and postintervention and 6 months after the intervention. There were significant differences in the refusal skill test scores between treatment and control groups both at post-test and at follow-up. Eighty-eight percent of the treatment group scored higher at post-test compared to 46% for the control group. In the treatment group, 83% scored higher at 6-month follow-up compared to their pretest score, while in the control group 56% scored higher.

Reis and her colleagues (Reis & Tymchyshyn, 1992, Reis et al., 2000) evaluated some interactive multimedia software programs for preventive alcohol education for college students. Three factors related to behavioral change are addressed in the software: (1) self-efficacy and maintaining personal control and safety while using alcohol, (2) expectations regarding the physiological and behavioral consequences of alcohol consumption, and (3) peer norms regarding alcohol consumption. The short-term impact of the software lesson was evaluated with 643 undergraduate students, of whom 248 received the computer-based intervention; 207, a didactic educational presentation; and 186, no education. The results of pre- post-test self-reports for the groups show that students who used the computer lessons reported learning more about dose response and ways to intervene with friends in peril. They were also more likely to try to change their behavior to become more safe and in control at either a party or other situation where alcohol was being served. The researchers conclude that "the software offers a flexible tool to address a range of learning needs and to trigger different dialogues within student groups regarding personal responsibility and decision making" (p. 415). Overall, this technology offers learning opportunities that extend beyond the few hours of use with the software. Another plus is that the students found it very engaging on a topic about which they would not usually seek information. The researchers conclude that "selective use of interactive technology may prove cost-effective in addressing issues such as alcohol education" (p. 415).

LESSONS LEARNED

A review of the literature raises many questions about the future use of technology in the field of prevention in general, and in drug abuse prevention specifically. The field of prevention traditionally relies on empirical research to guide use and practice. The research to date in the field of technological approaches to prevention is not strong enough to make a convincing argument for the application of technology to change either mediating variables or behavioral outcomes themselves. In drug abuse prevention specifically, few studies exist. Those that do exist show the strongest changes in knowledge, which is a necessary but not sufficient condition for behavior change. When looking at the broader field of health, including AIDS, cancer, nutrition, etc., studies indicate that the use of technology has potential for changing behaviors and helping people make better decisions about their health. Stronger effects are found when the technology is interactive and/or coupled with classroom or group discussion of the topics. In other words, computer technology appears to be most effective when used in a supportive role rather than as an isolated intervention.

Many studies to date have focused on user satisfaction and overcoming a real or perceived bias that people have against learning about health and/or other sensitive issues from a computer. In nearly all of the studies in which actual drug information was presented, user satisfaction was high even when a participant had negative perception of CAI prior to use. Kinzie, Schorling, and Siegel (1993) feel that personal control was a key factor in user satisfaction. This control was enhanced by frequent opportunities to choose the sequence of program content, the pacing of the program, and behavioral responses to situations. Moncher, Parms, and Orlandi (1989) suggested that interactive computer media may heighten user self-efficacy by letting users control their learning and "by showing them they can exert independent decision making about drugs, alcohol, and other personal choices" (p. 80). Reinforcing the feeling of control is inherent in computer software that is designed to maximize user control.

Another feature that is unique to the medium and may enhance user satisfaction is immediate individual feedback. Feedback on responses is essential in both coaching and learning, and is virtually impossible in most group-based prevention activities. With immediate feedback, individuals can modify their behavior, have erroneous ideas challenged, and better understand the material presented. This enables users to manipulate concepts directly and to explore results, which may be key factors in reducing the time taken to understand difficult concepts.

Multimedia technology utilizing audio, video, and graphics may be particularly helpful for users with either poor literacy skills or physical or learning disabilities. In this way, standard techniques that rely heavily either on print or on one-way communications can be formatted more effectively to meet the needs of special audiences.

DESIGN AND DEVELOPMENT ISSUES

Many formative evaluations identify the importance of a clearly articulated design process. A critical factor in the design of any intervention is a strong theoretical approach. Other formal behavioral theories and models attempt to explain why people behave as they do and can provide a conceptual framework to guide the development and evaluation of computer packages. Theory is essential not only to identify essential content, but also to guide in the presentation of information. The program goals and behavioral objectives can be used to guide the selection of an appropriate theoretical framework (Rhodes, Fishbein, & Reis, 1997).

A second component essential to creating good software is the involvement of representatives of the target population at several stages in development. Initially, developers need to understand the language and perspective on the target behaviors from the users themselves. This information can be elicited either through survey data or in focus groups. Some development teams create groups that are involved in the development process on a regular basis. Bosworth and her colleagues (1996), for example, formed an advisory committee of adolescents that met biweekly to evaluate scripts, graphics, and videos. At the very minimum, prototypes of the program need to be reviewed by representatives of the target population prior to full-scale implementation and/or evaluation.

A third component of well-designed software is a systematic process of formative evaluation, both by members of the target population and by experts in behavior change and prevention.

At the prototype stage, review of written scripts, storyboards, or drafts of the actual programs themselves allows changes to be made relatively easily and inexpensively. Formative evaluation should measure satisfaction with program mechanics as well as with the content. In addition, outcome measures should be obtained to determine whether the content is being assimilated by the learner in the intended way.

Finally, once the pilot implementation and evaluation have been successfully conducted with indications of behavioral impact, full-scale summative evaluations are essential. Such evaluations are needed to provide evidence of the role of the technology in preventing drug abuse.

To integrate theory-based principles and maximize the capabilities of the technology, a team approach must be taken in the development of software (Hardin & Reis, 1997). Any strong development team includes three specific disciplines: instructional design, prevention content experts, and computer programmers. Experts from these three fields need to work together from the beginning of the project so they can build on each other's skills. The content-area expert provides the theoretical background and approach as well as examples of successful strategies that have been used in other non-technology-based interventions. The computer programming expert has command of the possibilities of the technology and is able to integrate various forms of media into a final product. The instructional design expert has a strong background in learning theory and is able to translate content-area expertise into lessons and activities that are sensitive to the particular technology platform, the environment in which the program will be used (e.g., schools, clinics, or homes), and the target population.

The complexity of the design process and the necessity for including professionals from three different disciplines may be seen as major barriers to the design and implementation of high-quality software. Youth are accustomed to games and other interactive multimedia that cost millions of dollars to develop. For software in the drug abuse prevention area to hold interest, it must be of similar graphic and action quality and must contain realistic, nonjudgmental, compelling, and challenging information situated in authentic contexts. Interactivity is critical. On the other hand, the greater the interactivity the greater the time needed for development and consequently the greater the cost of the developmental process.

Many studies find that using software in conjunction with other activities, such as group interaction, traditional classroom activities, or clinic visits or referrals, creates an effective combination (Carr, 1997). Using the software alone usually produced short-term gains that led investigators to theorize that the most beneficial aspect of using computer-based technology was efficacy— i.e.; human interaction produces the same outcome but requires more time. As Barber (1993) concludes, the primary advantage of CAL lies in its capacity to accelerate learning.

One of the barriers to developing innovative applications of technology is cost. When an innovation is introduced, the cost of the equipment and the skill needed to manipulate the software are both high. As more development occurs, those prices are reduced and more experimentation becomes feasible. For example, when CD-ROMs were first introduced, making a master for a CD-ROM disk cost more than $50,000. Currently, equipment is available at a reasonable cost that allows users to duplicate CDs from office and home computers. Several developers note that although software development costs are beyond the means of most agency or school budgets, once the program has been developed, duplication costs are minimal (Kinzie et al., 1993).

CONCLUSION

Since the late 1970s, when computers were first introduced into classrooms, health educators and health-promotion scientists have attempted to harness this technology and its inherent appeal to youth for prevention purposes. Unfortunately, few of those efforts have been sustained to the point where efficacy can be shown through summative evaluation. While advances in the technology offer new frontiers for drug abuse prevention, few rigorous evaluations have been conducted. Those evaluations that have been conducted indicate, however, that there are some definite advantages and very few risks to using the technology. Because of its inherent appeal to youth, researchers and others developing drug prevention interventions should explore how their interventions might take advantage of the unique features that computer-based technologies offer. Researchers who have explored uses of technology need to be assertive in reporting the results of their studies. The prevention community needs to be attentive to the lessons that can be learned from less than perfect evaluation designs.

The past decade has seen tremendous advances in computer technology, allowing for more powerful prevention interventions. Prevention researchers have explored innovative uses of the technology and have identified several exciting opportunities to reach media-savvy generations. Over the next decade, the challenge to program developers and evaluators will be to integrate these promising technologies into existing programs and to identify, through rigorous evaluation, appropriate and effective applications.

REFERENCES

Alemi F., & Higley P. (1995). Reaction to "talking" computers assessing health risks. *Medical Care, 33,* 227–233.

Alemi, F., Stephens, R. C., Javalghi, R. G., Dyches, H., Butts, J., & Ghadiri, A. (1996). A randomized trial of a telecommunications network for pregnant women who use cocaine. *Medical Care, 34*(10 Suppl S), OS 10–OS 20.

Anderson, O. R. (1997). A neurocognitive perspective on current learning theory and science instructional strategies. *Science Education, 81,* 67–89.

Astuto, T. A. (1995). Activators and impediments to learner centered schools. *Theory into Practice, 34,* 243–249.

Aveyard, P., & Cheng, K. K. (1999). Cluster randomised controlled trial of expert system based on the trans-theoretical model for smoking prevention and cessation in schools. *British Medical Journal, 7215,* 948–954.

Barber, J. G. (1993). Computer-assisted drug prevention. *Journal of Substance Abuse Treatment, 7,* 125–131.

BARN Research Group (Bosworth, K., Gustafson, D. H., & Hawkins, R. P.). (1994). The BARN system: Use and impact of adolescent health promotion via computer. *Computers in Human Behavior, 10,* 467–482.

Binik Y. M., Meana, M., & Sand, N. (1994). Interaction with a sex-expert system changes attitudes and may modify sexual behavior. *Computers in Human Behavior, 10,* 395–410.

Boberg, E., Gustafson, D. H., Hawkins, R. P., Chan, Y., Bricker, E., Pingree, S., Berhe, H., & Peressini, A. (1995). Development, acceptance, and use patterns of a computer-based education and social support system for people living with AIDS/HIV infection. *Computers in Human Behavior, 11,* 289–311.

Bosworth, K. (1996). DIADS assessment. *Drug Stats* [Online]. Available: http://www.drugstats.org/diads/diads.html.

Bosworth, K., Espelage, D., & DuBay, T. (1998). A computer-based violence prevention intervention for young adolescents: A pilot study. *Adolescence, 33,* 785–795.

Bosworth, K., Espelage, D., DuBay, T., Dahlberg, L., & Daytner, G. (1996). Using multimedia to teach conflict resolution skills to young adolescents. *American Journal of Preventive Medicine, 11,* 65–74.

Bosworth, K., Espelage, D., DuBay, T., Daytner, G., & Karageorge, K. (2000). A preliminary evaluation of a multimedia violence prevention program for early adolescence. *American Journal of Health Behavior, 24,* 268–280.

Bosworth, K., & Gustafson, D. H. (1991). CHESS: Providing decision support for reducing health risk behavior and improving access to health services. *Interfaces, 21,* 93–104.

Bosworth K., & Yoast, R. (1991). DIADS: Computer-based system for development of school drug prevention programs. *Journal of Drug Education, 21,* 231–245.

Bransford, J. (1994a). The learning technology center at Vanderbilt University. *Educational Media and Technology Yearbook, 20,* 44–48.

Bransford, J. (1994b). Who ya gonna call? Thoughts about teaching and problem solving. In P. Hallinger, K. Lithwood, & J. Murphy (Eds.), *Cognitive Perspectives on Educational Leadership.* New York: Teacher's College Press.

Brennan, P., Moore, S., & Smyth, K. (1991). Computer link: Electronic support for the home caregiver. *Advances in Nursing Science, 13,* 14–27.

Brennan, P., Moore, S., & Smyth, K. (1995). Use of home-care computer network by persons with AIDS. *International Journal of Technology Assessment in Health Care, 10,* 258–272.

Brennan, P., & Ripich, S. (1994). Use of a home-care computer network by persons with AIDS. *International Journal of Technology Assessment in Health Care, 10*, 258–272.

Bryson R. (1999). Effectiveness of refusal skills software. *Journal of Drug Education, 29*, 359–371.

Burling, T., Burling, A., & Latini, D. (2001). A controlled smoking cessation trial for substance-dependent inpatients. *Journal of Consulting and Clinical Psychology, 69*, 295–304.

Burling, T., Seidner, A., & Gaither, D. (1994). A computer-directed program for smoking cessation treatment. *Journal of Substance Abuse, 6*, 427–431.

Carr, A. (1997). User-design in the creation of human learning systems. *Educational Technology Research and Development, 45*, 5–22.

Dede, C., & Fontana, L. (1995). Transforming health education via new media. In L. Harris (Ed.), *Health and the new media: Technologies transforming personal and public health.* Mahwah, NJ: Lawrence Erlbaum Associates.

DeJong, W. (1996). *Looking at binge drinking at 4-year colleges: Software user's guide.* Education Development Center.

Dick, W., & Carey, L. (1996). *The systemic design of instruction* (4th ed.), New York: HarperCollins.

Erickson, J. (1997). Building a community of designers: Restructuring learning through student hypermedia design. *Journal of Research in Rural Education, 13*, 5–27.

Fletcher-Flin, C. M., & Gravatt, B. (1995). The efficacy of computer assisted instruction (CAI): Meta-analysis. *Journal of Educational Computing Research, 12*, 219–241.

Gagné, R. M. (1985). *The conditions of learning* (4th edition). New York: Holt, Rinehart and Winston.

Grennon-Brooks, J., & Brooks, M. (1993). *In search of understanding: The case for constructivist classrooms.* Alexandria, VA: Association for Supervision and Curriculum Development.

Gropper, M., Liraz, Z., Portowicz, D., & Schindler, M. (1995). Computer integrated drug prevention: A new approach to teach lower socioeconomic 5th and 6th grade Israeli children to say no to drugs. *Social Work in Health Care, 22*, 87–103.

Gruender, C. D. (1996). Constructivism and learning: A philosophical appraisal. *Educational Technology, 36*, 21–29.

Gustafson, D. H., Bosworth, K., Chewning, B., & Hawkins, R. P. (1987). Computer-based health promotion: Combining technological advances with problem-solving techniques to effect successful health behavior changes. *The Annual Review of Public Health*, 387–415.

Gustafson, D. H., Bosworth, K., Hawkins, R. P., Boberg, E., & Bricker, E. (1992). CHESS: A computer-based system for providing information, referrals, decision support and social support to people in medical and other health-related crises. *Proceedings of the 16th Annual Symposium on Computer Applications in Medical Care* (pp.161–165).

Hannafin, M. J., Hannafin, K. M., & Land, S. M. (1997). Grounded practice and the design of constructivist learning environments. *Educational Technology Research and Development, 45*, 101–117.

Hardin, P., & Reis, J. (1997). Interactive multimedia software design: Concepts, process, and evaluation. *Health Education & Behavior, 24*, 35–53.

Hawkins, R., Gustafson, D., Chewning, B., & Bosworth, K. (1987). Reaching hard-to-reach populations: Interactive computer programs as public information campaigns for adolescents. *Journal of Communication, 37*, 8–28.

Holder, H. (1996). Using computer models to predict prevention policy outcomes. *Alcohol Health & Research World, 20*, 252–260.

Izenberg, N., & Lieberman, D. A. (1998). The web, communication trends, and children's health. *Clinical Pediatrics, 37*, 335–341.

Jonassen, D. H. (1997). Instructional design models for well-structured and ill-structured problem-solving learning outcomes. *Educational Technology Research and Development, 45*, 65–94.

Kinzie, M. B., Schorling, J. B., & Siegel, M. (1993). Prenatal alcohol education for low-income women with interactive multimedia. *Patient Education and Counseling, 21*, 51–60.

Kritsch, K. M., Bostow, D. E., & Dedrick, R. F. (1995). Level of interactivity of videodisc instruction on college students' recall of AIDS information. *Journal of Applied Behavior Analysis, 28*, 85–86.

Kulik, C. C., & Kulik, J. A. (1991). Effectiveness of computer-based instruction: An updated analysis. *Computers in Human Behavior, 7*, 75–94.

Kulik, J., Kulik, C. C., & Bangert-Downs, W. (1985). Effectiveness of computer-based education in elementary schools. *Computers in Human Behavior, 1*, 59–74.

Kumar, N. B., Bostow, D. E., Schapira, D. V., & Kritsch, K. M. (1993). Efficacy of interactive, automated programmed instruction in nutrition education for cancer prevention. *Journal of Cancer Education, 8*, 203–211.

Lester, L., Mundt, J., Perrine, M., & Searles, J. (1995). Validation of daily self-reported alcohol consumption using interactive voice response (IVR) technology. *Journal of Studies on Alcohol, 56*, 487–490.

Lieberman, D. A. (1992). The computer's potential role in health education. *Health Communication, 4*, 211–225.

Lieberman, D. A. (1997). Interactive video games for health promotion: Effects on knowledge, self-efficacy, social support and health. In R. L. Street, W. R. Gold, & T. Manning (Eds.), *Health promotion and interactive technology: Theoretical applications and future directions.* Mahwah, NJ: Lawrence Erlbaum Associates.

Lieberman, D. A. (1998). The researcher's role in the design of children's media and technology. In A. Druin (Ed.), *The design of children's technology.* San Francisco: Morgan Kaufmann.

Litman, R. E. (1995). Suicide prevention in a treatment setting. *Suicide and Life-Threatening Behavior, 25,* 134–142.

McCombs, B. L., & Whisler, J. S. (1997). *The learner-centered classroom and school: Strategies for increasing student motivation and achievement.* San Francisco, CA: Jossey-Bass.

Meier, S., & Sampson, J. (1989). Use of computer-assisted instruction in the prevention of alcohol abuse. *Journal of Drug Education, 19,* 245–256.

Moncher, M. S., Parms, C. A., & Orlandi, M. A. (1989). Microcomputer-based approaches for preventing drug and alcohol abuse among adolescents from ethnic-racial minority backgrounds. *Computers in Human Behavior, 5,* 79–93.

Mundt, J. C., Perrine, M. W., Searles, J. S., & Walter, D. (1995). An application of interactive voice response (IVR) technology to longitudinal studies of daily behavior. *Behavior Research Methods, Instruments, & Computers, 27,* 351–357.

Niemiec, R., Schmidt, M., Weinstein, J., & Walberg, H. (1996). Learner-control effects: A review of reviews and a meta-analysis. *Journal of Educational Computing Research, 15,* 157–174.

Niemiec, R., & Walberg, H. (1987). The effects of computer based instruction in elementary schools: A quantitative synthesis. *Journal of Research in Computing in Education, 20,* 85–103.

Noell, J., Ary, D., & Duncan, T. (1997). Development and evaluation of a sexual decision-making and social skills program: The choice is yours—preventing HIV/STDs. *Health Education & Behavior, 24,* 87–101.

Noell, J., Biglan, A., Hood, D., & Britz, B. (1994). An interactive videodisc-based smoking cessation program: Prototype development and pilot test. *Computers in Human Behavior, 10,* 347–358.

Orlandi, M. A., Dozier, C. E., & Marta, M. A. (1990). Computer-assisted strategies for substance abuse prevention: Opportunities and barriers. *Journal of Consulting and Clinical Psychology, 58,* 425–431.

Paperny, D. (1997). Computerized health assessment and education for adolescent HIV and STD prevention in health care settings and schools. *Health Education & Behavior, 24,* 54–70.

Pomeroy, E., & Detweiler, M. (1995). Compact disc interactive (CD-i) multimedia project. *The Journal of Biocommunication, 22,* 7–13.

Reis, J., Riley, W., Lokman, L., & Baer, J. (2000). Interactive multimedia preventive alcohol education: A technology for higher education. *Journal of Drug Education, 30,* 399–422.

Reis, J., & Tymchyshyn, P. (1992). A longitudinal evaluation of computer-assisted instruction on contraception for college students. *Adolescence, 27,* 803–811.

Rhodes, F., Fishbein, M., & Reis, J. (1997). Using behavioral theory in computer-based health promotion and appraisal. *Health Education & Behavior, 24,* 20–34.

Rickerd, V. I., Graham, C. J., Fisher, R., Gottlieb, A., Trosclair, A., & Jay, M. S. (1993). A comparison of methods for alcohol and marijuana anticipatory guidance with adolescents. *Journal of Adolescent Health, 14,* 225–230.

Savery, J., & Duffy, T. (1995). Problem based learning: An instructional model and its constructivist framework. *Educational Technology, 35,* 31–38.

Schneider, S., & Tooley, J. (1986). Self-help computer conferencing. *Computers and Biomedical Research, 19,* 274–281.

Shulman, H. A., Sweeney, B., & Gerler, E. R. (1995). A computer-assisted approach to preventing alcohol abuse: Implications for the middle school. *Elementary School Guidance & Counseling, 30,* 63–77.

Silverman, S. (2000). Health and safety sites. *Technology & Learning, 21,* 50.

Stanton, B. F., Li, X., Galbraith, J., Feigelman, S., & Kaljee, L. (1996). Sexually transmitted diseases, human immuno-deficieny virus, and pregnancy prevention. *Archives of Pediatrics and Adolescent Medicine 150,* 17–24.

Street, R. L., & Rimal, R. N. (1997). Health promotion and interactive technology: A conceptual foundation. In R. L. Street & W. R. Gold (Eds.), *Health promotion and interactive technology: Theoretical applications and future directions.* Mahwah, NJ: Lawrence Erlbaum Associates.

Thomas, R., Cahill, J., & Santilli, L. (1997). Using an interactive computer game to increase skill and self-efficacy regarding safer sex negotiation: Field test results. *Health Education & Behavior, 24,* 71–86.

Tingen, M. S., Gramling, L. F., Bennett, G., Gibson, E. M., & Renew, M. (1997). A pilot study of preadolescents using focus groups to evaluate appeal of a video game smoking prevention strategy. *Journal of Addictions Nursing, 9,* 118–124.

Velicer, W. F., Prochaska, J. O., Bellis, J. M., Diclementi, C. C., & Rossi, J. S. (1993). An expert system intervention for smoking cessation. *Addictive Behavior, 18,* 269–290.

Velicer, W. F., Prochaska, J. O., Fava, J. L., & Laforge, R. G. (1999). Interactive versus non-interactive and dose-response relationships for staged-matched smoking cessation programs in managed care. *Health Psychology, 18,* 21–28.

Walther, J. (1992). Impression development in computer-mediated interaction. *Western Journal of Communication, 57,* 381–398.

Wolcott, L. (1996). Distant, but not distanced: A learner-centered approach to distance education. *Tech Trends, 41,* 23–27.

CHAPTER 33

Putting Science into Practice

GALE HELD

INTRODUCTION

One of the greatest challenges to prevention researchers and practitioners is the accurate and timely application of prevention research and knowledge. Significant barriers continue to block timely application of prevention science, but an increased demand for accountability is fueling efforts to facilitate the application of sound scientific research. The Department of Education's (DOE) Safe and Drug Free Schools Program and the Center for Substance Abuse Prevention's (CSAP) State Incentive Cooperative Agreements, for example, require that effective, science-based programs be funded. States and communities are looking for clear guidance on the key characteristics of scientifically sound research and on prevention programs proven to be effective. But all too often a disconnect between research and practice delays the application of promising or even proven methodologies. On the other hand, evidence from the practice field is sometimes ignored or discounted by researchers, rather than used to guide the direction of future research.

This chapter focuses on ways to infuse state-of-the-art science into practice. It discusses a variety of approaches, such as knowledge synthesis, application, and dissemination and research design and scope.

DIFFUSION AND KNOWLEDGE APPLICATION THEORY

There is a strong body of research on knowledge application that helps explain how and by whom innovation is adopted. This knowledge drives—or should drive—how we transfer prevention

GALE HELD • MPA, Independent Consultant, Kensington, Maryland 20895–3823

research and knowledge. Since 1962, Everett Rogers's model for the practical application and integration of research—the diffusion system—has been the basis for much of the work done in knowledge application (Rogers, 1995a). Rogers describes an optimal change system that includes five stages through which an individual or organization must pass in the "innovation-decision" process. They are knowledge (exposure to, and some understanding of, the innovation), persuasion (forming a favorable or unfavorable attitude toward the innovation), decision (to adopt or reject the innovation), implementation (putting the innovation to use), and confirmation (seeking reinforcement for a decision). As a result of this process an innovation may be adopted, reinvented (modified), or possibly discontinued due to dissatisfaction with the innovation or through replacement by a new innovation.

Rogers also identifies factors that can affect the rate of adoption of an innovation—the innovation itself, the communication channels used to diffuse the innovation, the social system in which the innovation is being considered, and the strength of change agents for implementation. Other key factors are the degree to which the innovation is viewed as an improvement and compatible with existing values, how complex or difficult to understand the innovation is, the degree to which it can be tried on a limited basis, and the degree to which the results are visible to others. Networks are also critical to diffusion of innovations since individuals typically learn from each other. With regard to drug abuse prevention programs, specifically, Rogers (1995b) observes that perceptions of the relevance of the programs to the national or local agenda are important and can be a great stimulus for their adoption.

A completed, strong evaluation is optimal before diffusion, but this does not always happen. Spontaneous diffusion often occurs long before the evaluation is completed. In this process, successful drug abuse prevention programs are often reinvented (Rogers, 1995a), and reinvention may actually aid in the diffusion process. In fact, Rohrback, Graham, and Hansen (1993), in reviewing diffusion of school-based programs, suggest that encouraging teachers to deliver a program "as written" may decrease the likelihood that they will adopt it.

Building on the early work by Rogers, Backer lists four fundamental conditions that must be met in order for technology-transfer activities to result in change. They are:

1. Dissemination: Information about new scientific knowledge must be communicated effectively, in user-friendly and easily accessible formats.
2. Evaluation: There must be credible evidence that the program will lead to cost-effective, improved practice without undesirable side effects and that evidence must be communicated effectively.
3. Resources: There must be personnel, funds, and materials to implement the new practice.
4. Human dynamics of change: There must be active interventions to create an environment where those who will be implementing the innovation are involved and feel ownership (Backer, 1995a, 1997, 2000; Backer & David, 1995).

Backer (1995b) also refers to the essential need for "contextual engineering." Changing practice requires "setting the process of change itself into a larger context" with complex behavioral interventions at the micro- and macrolevels operating simultaneously through strategic planning focused on human issues.

Backer indicates that readiness for innovation can be assessed for both individuals and organizations. Readiness is often more a factor of perception than fact; the lack of readiness is not the same as resistance. Readiness, however, can be enhanced through social marketing, a management framework for market research that applies systematic efforts to understand the characteristics of the audience being targeted for change. Readiness for change is influenced by attitudes and beliefs about the larger context in which new ideas or technology are being implemented, product development, and incentives to facilitate voluntary adoption of the innovation or product (Backer, 1995a; Walsh et al., 1993).

Biglan and Hayes expand on this concept in their arguments for a functional contextualist framework for research and for community interventions (Biglan, 1993, 1995; Biglan & Hayes, 1996). This approach seeks to "develop an organized system of empirically based verbal concepts and rules that allow behavioral phenomena to be predicted and influenced with precision, scope, and depth" (Biglan, 1993). The focus is on identifying variables that predict and influence behavior—the behavior of both individuals and the environment and organizations within which they function. Biglan (1995) indicates a critical problem with many policies and programs is that they do not always specify the links between policies and programs and the desired behavior of individuals. All too often, information is provided about problems and possible solutions without specific guidance on how to effect the proposed change. At the core of Biglan's approach is recognition that an analysis of a unique case may or may not be generalizable to other cases; an act must be analyzed within its own context. Biglan also emphasizes the importance of "cultural materialism," which points to the importance of examining the economic consequences of any proposed change to see what effects it will have on the economic interests of that community. Last, he notes that to bring about change it is important to mobilize social contingencies on "behalf of the targeted practice." The incidence or prevalence of a behavior should increase to the extent that there is an increase in social reinforcement for that behavior. He cites three steps integral to changing cultural practices: (1) specifying the targeted practices and targeted populations, (2) analyzing the context for the targeted practices, and (3) analyzing the context for practices that support or oppose the targeted practice(1995).

Finally, NIDA identifies six key strategies for knowledge application in its monograph, *Reviewing the Behavioral Science Knowledge Base on Technology Transfer*, that reflect the views of many experts in dissemination. They are

1. personal contact between the innovation developers and the adopters,
2. strategic planning on how the technology or innovation will be adopted in new settings,
3. outside consultation on designing and implementing the change process,
4. translating information into language understood by the potential users, focusing on whether the innovation works and how it can be replicated,
5. convincing opinion leaders (potential adopters) to champion the cause, and
6. involving potential users in planning for innovation adoption (Backer, 2000; Backer, David, & Soucy, 1995).

Knowledge transfer is about identifying new best practices and programs, spreading information about them, and using technical assistance, training, and other means to help individuals and organizations implement them (Backer & Newman, 1995). Perhaps most important is that knowledge transfer must be carefully and strategically planned—actions to promote it should be intentional. Underlying all of these is the nature of drug abuse prevention technology itself—it is often considered "soft" science, not tied to medical interventions, and much of the scientific research is relatively new (Backer, 1991).

POTENTIAL BARRIERS TO APPLYING SCIENCE
TO PRACTICE

Bridging the gap between science and practice is not always easy. Barriers can be related to the innovation itself; failure to accurately and effectively communicate the information or innovation; tradition and resistance to change; potential adopters not valuing the innovation; and lack of incentives to implement the innovation (Laflin, Edmundson, & Moore-Hirschl, 1995; Shaperman & Backer, 1995). The barriers are related to the differing views and interests, as well as to the different "languages" used by scientists and practitioners; the different timetables of researchers and practitioners in applying prevention research and, relatedly, the different criteria used to determine that research is "ready" to be applied in the field; the readiness of policymakers, prevention practitioners, and communities to implement new research and ideas; and the lack of tested efficacy of some popular, widely adopted prevention approaches and programs and the difficulties in making change.

Different Interests/Different Jargon

Scientists and practitioners/policymakers have very different professional views of the world. The scientist lives comfortably with the "tentative and hypothetical," while the practitioner/ policymaker wants to "act with confidence" (Glaser, Abelson, & Garrison, 1983). Consequently, practitioners often view research as irrelevant, while scientists often view many attempts to apply research to real-world situations as inappropriate. Most information about current research comes from scientific journals or papers presented at conferences. This serves researchers well but not practitioners or policymakers. The language used is often unfamiliar to practitioners, and the articles and presentations frequently provide great detail on the methodology of the research project and pay less attention, if any, to the broader applicability of the project (Lipton, D., 1992; Mattick & Ward, 1992; Shanley, Lodge, & Mattick, 1996). Perhaps researchers could be trained to write their material in more understandable terms, or even more useful might be an "interpreter" or a "translator"—someone who can take the research material and translate it into a language and format that is meaningful and understandable to people in the field. Such material would minimize jargon, show clearly the relevance of the research to policy, program, and resource decisions, and provide the technical material in appendixes or through referrals to other documents.

The failure to communicate is more than a language issue. Researchers and practitioners need to be aware of the potential policy implications of the research finding, the relationship of the research finding to existing programs and the potential impact on those programs, the likelihood that a state or community would embrace the finding, and the conditions that must be met to ensure that the research finding can be understood and fully considered by a state or community when planning their prevention activities. They also need to recognize the very real potential for adaptation of programs to fit state and community needs, norms, and resources.

Timeliness

A key concern in the knowledge-application process is the timeliness of the release of scientific information to the practice field. Brown (1995) points out that research, by its very nature is reactive; it is a response to an identified problem, one that is usually present long before the research is completed. Accordingly, policymakers and practitioners are looking for answers long before the research is completed. Careful research, review, and analysis take time, but there needs to be prompt transfer of the knowledge once promising findings are made or the peer-review validation process is complete. This is equally applicable to knowledge synthesis activities—synthesis of peer-reviewed research. Several efforts have been tried or are underway, such as CSAP's Prevention Enhancement Protocols System (PEPS) and CSAP's National Center for the Advancement of Prevention (NCAP), which were designed to review and synthesize research and make it more understandable and usable to policymakers and practitioners. However, much of the work completed under these two programs remains unpublished long after the scientific review has been completed, reducing the value of the material. One consideration for future knowledge-application efforts is to develop a system that will facilitate timely processing of material so that it is available quickly (Backer, 1991).

Readiness

One significant issue for any prevention program is the readiness of those at whom the program is targeted and of those responsible for implementing it (Backer, 1995a, 2000; Biglan, 1993; 1995; Brown, 1995; Edwards et al., 2000; National Institute on Drug Abuse (NIDA), 1997a). Backer (1995a) describes readiness as "a state of mind about the need for an innovation and the capacity to undertake technology transfer." Individual and community readiness is frequently cited as an important factor for implementing programs, yet often little is said about what that actually means.

Backer (1995a) identifies several keys to readiness, including the interpersonal and social dynamics of the organization or community and change agents—opinion leaders in the organization who are often successful in assessing and developing readiness. He also notes that readiness can be enhanced by persuasive communication, getting people involved early to define what change is needed and how technology transfer can help, and management of external sources of information, such as the media (Backer, 1995a).

Biglan (1995) cites three principles that might guide action: (1) organizing to achieve and maintain substantial change in cultural practices; (2) using media advocacy; and (3) direct intervention, including reinforcing the targeted practice, punishing opposing practices, training in the behaviors needed for the targeted practices, providing services that support or promote the practice, and creating a community in which the practices are assured.

Edwards and others describe a community readiness model developed by the Tri-Ethnic Center for Prevention Research at the Colorado State University that cites several stages of community readiness and proposes that specific strategies be used to address them focusing on the ethnic and cultural beliefs and values of the community. In this model, community readiness to adopt a new innovation goes through nine stages—no awareness, denial, vague awareness, preplanning, preparation, initiation, stabilization, confirmation/expansion, and, finally, professionalism. These stages move a community from raising awareness of an issue to maintaining the momentum of their efforts and continued growth and enable a community not only to develop specific strategies but also to reassess their community readiness to move forward with the innovation (Edwards et al., 2000).

Several authors emphasize the need for early involvement of the potential user of the innovation as critical both in terms of ownership and in terms of ensuring the usefulness and relevance of the innovation (Backer, 1995 a,b; 1997; Biglan, 1995; Glaser et al., 1983; Laflin et al., 1995; Lipton, 1992). However, there has been little emphasis on how to ensure the readiness of the prevention professionals who must implement the programs or the appropriate role of technology,

including whether either the target group or the community has both the hardware/software availability and the computer literacy necessary to implement the new technology.

From Ineffective Practice to Science-Based Practice

One major barrier to putting science into practice is the widespread support in many states and
communities for popular prevention programs that have not been shown to be supported by science.
The popularity of such programs, the support they receive by funding agencies and legislatures,
the need for training in new approaches, and poor marketing of research-based approaches are
among the factors that keep states and communities from abandoning their current programs in
favor of science-based programs.

Perhaps the best example of this problem is seen in a recent DOE study of drug prevention
curricula in the schools. It found that, "Drug prevention approaches that have been shown to be
effective are not widely used, while approaches that have not shown evidence of effectiveness or
have not been evaluated properly are the most common approaches currently in use" (Planning and
Evaluation Service, 1997). The study found only one school district among the 19 examined had
a drug abuse prevention program that yielded positive effects on drug use over the 4 years of the
study. The DOE indicates that teaching children resistance skills and altering their misperceptions
of peer drug use are the most effective ways of affecting drug use. However, these are not the
approaches most schools use. Moreover, it appears that few school districts "know about or
consider research findings when planning their prevention programs," and few of them conduct
formal evaluations of the effectiveness of their programs (Planning and Evaluation Service, 1997).

The DOE study specifically cites the Drug Abuse Resistance Education (DARE) program
as a prime example of this problem. DARE, a school-based drug prevention program, has been
adopted by approximately 75% of the school districts nationwide, even though several analyses
suggest that the program is not effective in reducing substance abuse, except for tobacco use
(Ellickson, 1995; Ennett et al., 1994; Ennett, Ringwalt, & Flewelling, 1993; Minnesota Institute
of Public Health, 1997; Planning and Evaluation Service, 1997; Tobler, 1993). In fact, the DOE
report found that "participation in the DARE program was associated with more reports of student
drug use and more tolerant views toward drugs" (Planning and Evaluation Service, 1997). Other
approaches also found to be ineffective in reducing or preventing drug use or which have not been
adequately tested are those that teach self-esteem, decision-making skills, stress management,
and goal setting.

There are serious questions about DARE's effect on substance abuse prevention, but it has
served several useful purposes. Dunn (1993) argues that DARE is effective as a means of bridging
the gap between law enforcement and the schools. He found that DARE makes a difference by
providing essential information to young people, reinforcing self-esteem, providing a positive
experience with law enforcement, helping law enforcement view itself as part of the social service
system, helping policy officers better understand how and why children behave the way they do
on the streets, and delivering a strong no-use message.

DARE has enjoyed widespread popularity for many years and clearly has elements that appeal to policymakers and communities. Careful study of these elements and how they might be
incorporated into other, research-based, prevention programs could be useful. By identifying the
key elements responsible for its popularity, we can also learn about how to change from an ineffective practice to a science-based practice. This may mean modifications to an existing program
or replacing a program all together; the DARE experience offers us an opportunity to learn more
about how to influence prevention practice.

OVERCOMING BARRIERS

Barriers between science and practice are significant, but they are surmountable. In fact, a number of efforts that address them are underway. In 1996, CSAP conducted a structured evaluation of the different approaches used to reduce drug abuse. The resulting report to Congress, *Alcohol and Other Drug Abuse Prevention: The National Structured Evaluation* (U.S. Department of Health and Human Services (USDHHS) 1996), identified and defined core approaches to substance abuse prevention and made recommendations for future research. It specifically recommended research on outcomes, impact, cost-benefit and cost-effectiveness of prevention programs and on identifying risk and protective factors most "potent and capable of being affected by prevention efforts."

In an effort to facilitate the transfer of science to practice, the USDHHS, in collaboration with the DOE, the Department of Justice (DOJ), and the Office of National Drug Control Policy (ONDCP) developed a paper to describe the key characteristics of effective substance abuse prevention programs, based upon current research (USDHHS, 1999). This paper was shared with the field on several occasions to promote comment and discussion toward a final draft, and in 2000, ONDCP issued *Evidence Based Principles for Substance Abuse Prevention* as an insert with *The National Drug Control Strategy: 2000 Annual Report* (ONDCP, 2000).

Research Design and Scope

An entire area of study is devoted to understanding how best to disseminate knowledge so that it can be applied in practice. Policymakers at the national, state, and local levels are particularly concerned with dissemination. They want answers to specific questions and want a policy rationale for implementing any research or innovation (Backer, 1991; Glaser et al., 1983; Lipton, 1992). They need to know how the research can be applied in real-world situations and what the cost is likely to be (Holder, 1997; Schinke & Orlandi, 1991). They are faced with problems demanding immediate solutions and must make program and funding decisions with the best information available. It is incumbent on researchers to address this political context if they are going to maximize the value of their research.

The job of disseminating science and enabling the application of sound research is made much easier if research projects involve policymakers, practitioners, and the target community from the beginning of the project. Involvement facilitates their acceptance and "buy in" to the research and helps ensure that the research design takes into consideration the policy level, cultural and other interests and concerns of policymakers, practitioners, and communities. This involvement improves the likelihood that the ultimate findings will reflect the situation in the community. The findings are more likely to be transferable to other communities if the research has been clearly grounded in an understanding and appreciation of the real-world problems faced when implementing a prevention program (Backer, 1995a, 1997; Glaser et al., 1983; Laflin et al., 1995; Lipton, 1992; Shanley et al., 1996).

Two examples of research design and diffusion efforts that include active involvement of policymakers, practitioners, and the community are Hawkins and Catalano and associates' *Communities That Care* (1992) and an alcohol abuse program focused on children of substance abusers (Laflin et al., 1995). Each of these research projects involved community leaders very early in the design stage. With the *Communities That Care* approach, the community is actively involved in team-building, risk assessment, identification of prevention strategies, and the creation and implementation of an action plan. Collaborative efforts with local leaders are a critical first step and greatly enhance successful recruitment of hard-to-reach families (Harachi et al., 1996; Hawkins,

1995). In implementing an alcohol abuse prevention program, Laflin et al. (1995) noted that it is critical to involve the user in development of the program in order to maximize the sense of community ownership and to facilitate translation of the research findings into practice.

Disseminating research is as important as the initial research effort. Research that is neither made public nor is understandable to policymakers, prevention practitioners, and community leaders is of little value. Requiring explicit dissemination plans as part of research projects (Backer, 1991) or providing supplemental research funding tied to technology transfer (Brown, 1995) would help bridge the gap between research and application of research. Identifying research findings for early release would increase the likelihood of more rapid diffusion in sync with the needs of policymakers and prevention practitioners (Backer, 1991; Lipton, 1992; Rohrbach et al., 1996). Interim findings could be shared through journal articles, workshops, technical assistance, training, and the internet, rather than waiting for formal publication of guidelines or monographs. Greater attention to the feedback loop in research might also result in technology transfer influencing the research agenda by encouraging development of programs that might yield quick results and be more responsive to public-policy needs (Backer, 1991). Holder and others (1995) argue for a research model that moves research through several stages—basic research, preintervention research, efficacy testing, effectiveness testing, and demonstrations—and reports on the findings and progress at each phase.

Nothing is more unsettling to policymakers, prevention practitioners, and community leaders trying to make policy, program, and resource decisions than to hear that we "don't know what works in prevention." Yet all too often this is what they are told. While further research may be warranted, we already know a lot about what works in prevention, and that knowledge base is ever-increasing; we should not be afraid to say so. The great increase in prevention research, demonstrations, and knowledge has provided us with some sound, theory-based research and principles upon which to base prevention policy and program decisions. It is incumbent on researchers to identify what is known early in the research and to push to have that information disseminated to the field.

Two good examples of the impact of making prevention research available to policymakers in a timely manner are DARE and the reauthorization in the mid-1990s of the Department of Education's Drug Free Schools and Communities program. Rogers (1995b) describes how a 1987 evaluation by DeJong showing that DARE had some effects, although minimal, on preventing drug abuse was widely distributed to every chief of police in the country by the DOJ. The political climate was right for this widespread distribution of the findings, and DARE quickly became seen as a solution to the problem. Rogers notes that the socially constructed priority on the national agenda, the evidence of a problem, the evidence of a program that might solve the problem, and funding from the federal government all served as impetus for the rapid diffusion of the DARE program.

Similarly, just as Congress was considering eliminating the Drug Free Schools and Communities Act, supporters of the program were able to point to Gilbert Botvin's Life Skills Training as a prime example of successful school-based prevention programs. That evidence reportedly contributed to saving the program.

Knowledge Dissemination

Dissemination of scientific research is the first step in knowledge transfer and application, and there are a variety of dissemination channels, such as associations, federal and state agencies, and universities. Peer-reviewed journals can also be invaluable sources of information, though they are not necessarily routinely read by policymakers and practitioners. However, many journal publishers maintain websites that include abstracts and/or the full text of research reports, which makes access to the information easier for decision makers. And for practitioners who use the internet, there are enormous resources readily available through a variety of searchable databases—csap's PrevLine, the NIAAA (ETOH) alcohol and alcohol problems database, the Department of Education's ERIC database, the National Library of Medicine's Medline and Grateful Med, and NIDA's searchable database. In addition, we are seeing more Internet sites including abstracts of prevention research. Three examples are the *Research Briefs* included on PrevLine (www.health.org/research/res-brf), the Prevention Knowledge Base conducted by Tanglewood Research (2001) and supported by NIDA (http://www.tanglewood.net/kb.htm), and DOE's ERIC Digest (http://www.ed.gov/databases/ERIC_Digests/index/).

The Federal agencies most focused on drug abuse prevention, NIDA and CSAP, have taken the lead in bridging the gap between research and practice and transferring state-of-the-art science to practice. The National Institute on Alcohol Abuse and Alcoholism (NIAAA) has also recently begun greater efforts to link research and practice. NIDA has a multifaceted technology-transfer program (National Institute on Drug Abuse (NIDA) 1997c), consisting of print and audiovisual materials, in-service training courses and workshops, computerized self-teaching programs, and technical assistance in implementing new models. The program also involves a variety of strategies designed to ensure adoption of new technologies stemming from NIDA research. A key NIDA research dissemination program is Drug Abuse Prevention: Research, Dissemination and Applications (RDA). The prevention RDA includes four manuals that provide extensive practical information on prevention research, community readiness, and at-risk populations (NIDA, 1997b). NIDA also disseminates information on research through conferences, *NIDA Notes*, and *NIDA InfoFax*, and publications such as "Preventing Drug Use among Children and Adolescents: A Research-Based Guide" (NIDA, 1997d).

While NIAAA does not have a specific technology transfer program, it does provide information on its research through *Alcohol Health and Research World* and *Alcohol Alerts*. NIAAA also recently conducted a special research seminar for the National Association of State Alcohol and Drug Abuse Directors. It provided them with information on a variety of alcohol research projects, including prevention. Both NIDA and NIAAA support publications through the Association for Health Services Research on linking research and practice—*Connection,* on drug abuse services research, and *Front Lines*, on alcohol services research.

The CSAP knowledge-application program includes a broad array of information and education projects, including media campaigns, the National Clearinghouse for Alcohol and Drug Information (NCADI), the Regional Alcohol and Drug Awareness Resource Network (RADAR), training and technical assistance, knowledge synthesis, and guideline development. NCADI maintains and distributes a vast amount of print and multimedia prevention material from several federal agencies. NCADI maintains a large database of both public and private research and materials and regularly publishes *Prevention Pipeline*, which includes research highlights. Lastly, CSAP has established the internet-based, Substance Abuse Prevention Institute for Training and Technology Transfer (http://p2001.health.org), which contains a range of training resources from the former CSAP National Training System, including a library of prevention-related training courses and tools to assist in using the resources and assessing the needs for training and career development.

The DOJ maintains a clearinghouse and information system that includes material from the Office on Juvenile Justice and Delinquency Prevention (OJJDP). Much of the work in OJJDP is based on the Hawkins–Catalano risk- and protective-factor model and specifically addresses the substance abuse connection to juvenile delinquency. OJJDP has also widely disseminated a parenting strategy document, Kumpfer's (1993) *Strengthening America's Families*, that addresses the family's influence on delinquency and provides descriptions of promising parenting and family programs. The website, www.strengtheningfamilies.org, devotes considerable attention to this program and includes a literature review and model programs. Material on the OJJDP programs can be obtained through the National Criminal Justice Reference Service, which publishes a bimonthly catalog that includes abstracts of available research and program documents for distribution as well as information on how to access various DOJ bureaus and offices.

Another major effort supported by OJJDP was the development of "Blueprints" of 11 model and 21 promising violence prevention programs (2002) by the University of Colorado at Boulder, Center for the Study and Prevention of Violence. For each of the model programs they have developed comprehensive guides for communities to implement the programs. Many of the model programs have an effect on substance abuse, and 7 of the programs are recognized by the CSAP as effective programs—Bullying Prevention Program, Incredible Years, Life Skills Training, Midwestern Prevention Project, Multisystemic Therapy, Nurse Home Visitation and PATHS. Information on the Blueprints can be found at http://www.colorado.edu/cspv/blueprints.

As federal agencies are demanding greater accountability and implementation of science-based prevention programs, they are also trying to develop tools to assist states and communities in doing so. For example, in its *Guidelines for Effectiveness* (DOE, 1998), the DOE Safe and Drug Free Schools and Communities Program outlines the expectations for future funding under this program. DOE also asked the New England Comprehensive Assistance Center to develop a resource guide to operationalize that guidance and include descriptions of effective programs. The draft guide, *Applying Effective Strategies To Prevent or Reduce Substance Abuse, Violence, and Disruptive Behavior among Youth* (Scattergood et al., 1998) has been widely distributed and used by many states and communities. While DOE did not issue this guide in final, it did release a list of exemplary and promising programs in January 2001 (DOE, 2001).

Similarly, as CSAP has required that the State Incentive Cooperative Agreements fund science-based programs, they, too, have been developing further guidance on programs which meet their requirements. These include *A Catalog from CSAP's Findings Bank of Science-Based Prevention Practices* (1998), which describes effective programs from among CSAP's grantees, a monograph, *Understanding Substance Abuse Prevention: Toward the 21st Century: A Primer on Effective Programs* (CSAP, 1999), which provides a description of the theory behind the reviews of prevention programs, along with information on the first seven programs to pass the model program criteria and a three-part series, *Guide to Science-Based Practices,* including *Science-Based Substance Abuse Prevention: A Guide* (CSAP 2001e), *Promising and Proven Substance Abuse Prevention Programs* (CSAP, 2001d), and *Principles of Substance Abuse Prevention* (CSAP, 2001c). An additional resource, *Achieving Outcomes,* which was released in 2002, covers the range of topics associated with implementing research-based programs, including needs assessment, community readiness and capacity, program selection, program implementation, training and technical assistance, and evaluation.

CSAP also has two other major sources of information and guidance on science-based programs and practice—the prevention Decision Support System (DSS) and the Model Programs Dissemination Project. The DSS promotes scientific methods and programs for substance abuse prevention for use within communities and state prevention systems and provides guidance on selecting and implementing science-based programs (CSAP, 2000a). The DSS also includes a range of training resources from the former CSAP National Training System, including a library of prevention-related training courses and tools. The CSAP Model Programs Dissemination Initiative (2000b) identifies and disseminates information on effective substance abuse prevention programs based on a thorough review by CSAP's National Registry of Effective Prevention Programs (NREPP).

The NREPP is a formal process that reviews programs against stringent criteria to determine their effectiveness, including a review of theory, fidelity of interventions, process evaluation, data, outcome measures, analysis, replications, dissemination capability, and cultural and age appropriateness. All programs receive a summative score for utility and integrity of the research, and those passing the NREPP review process are described in the Model Programs website (www.modelprograms.samhsa.gov). However, those programs identified through NREPP which have also agreed to work with CSAP's dissemination program are listed as models, described in detail on the website and in hard copy, and actively promoted with states, communities, and national organizations. Through this program, CSAP also is engaged in ongoing discussions with states and national organizations about the issues associated with taking model programs to scale and developing tools and training to assist in the selection and implementation of model programs.

A key issue that is beginning to get greater attention is that of adaptation. While most researchers would prefer to see their programs implemented with fidelity, large-scale diffusion of research-based programs requires addressing adaptation. More and more there is recognition that adaptation will happen, so the focus is shifting more to how to guide that adaptation so that program content is not damaged (CSAP, 2001b). There are now efforts to identify the key components of successful, research-based programs. NIDA has issued a new request for applications, "The Next Generation of Drug Abuse Prevention Research," designed to address the questions of "when drug abuse prevention programs work, what accounts for their success?" (NIDA, 2001). CSAP, through its National Center for the Advancement of Prevention (NCAP), is conducting a core components analysis of effective programs to provide policymakers and practitioners better guidance on what is critical to the success of these programs so, if they make modifications, they can do so within the context of the core components.

CSAP also recently released initial findings from a literature review of fidelity and adaptation, *Finding the Balance: Program Fidelity and Adaptation in Substance Abuse Prevention* (CSAP, 2001b). This document concludes "that attention to BOTH fidelity and adaptation is essential for successful implementation of evidence-based substance abuse prevention programs" (CSAP, 2001b; p. 13). Many research-based programs have been developed with substantial funding, often through government or foundation dollars, and special circumstances that are not easily replicated in many communities. Communities make adaptations to fit their local needs, norms, and resources as well as to have a stronger sense of ownership of the program. The CSAP document offers guidelines for balancing program fidelity and adaptation and raises issues for consideration by researchers and program developers, program implementers, and funders and policymakers so that each can better address their respective activities to clarify program content and implementation issues. A full literature review will be available in 2002.

Last, much of the material described above, as well as other substance-abuse prevention related material, can be accessed and/or ordered through agency websites. NIDA, NIAAA, CSAP, SAMHSA, the DOE, and the DOJ all maintain websites through which much of this information can be downloaded. Website addresses are NIDA, www.nida.nih.gov; CSAP's NCADI, www.health.org; SAMHSA, www.samhsa.gov; NIAAA, www.niaaa.nih.gov; DOE, www.ed.gov; NCJRS, www.ncjrs.org; OJJDP, www.ojjdp.gov.

Guidelines and Knowledge Synthesis

Two methods developed to address the problem of translating scientific research into language and formats more likely to be used by policymakers and practitioners have been the development of guidelines and knowledge synthesis. The two structured guideline activities most relevant to drug abuse prevention are CSAP's Prevention Enhancement Protocols (PEPS) and the Agency for Health Care Research and Quality's (AHRQ) Practice Evidence Centers. However, neither has yet been evaluated, and the PEPS program was discontinued. Companion treatment guidelines developed by the Center for Substance Abuse Treatment, Treatment Improvement Protocols (TIPS) are developed as consensus documents and have undergone limited evaluation, primarily focusing on client use. A more expansive evaluation of TIPS is underway. Knowledge synthesis is conducted through literature reviews and meta analyses, but in the knowledge-application arena synthesis is more evident in the Public Health Service's Put Prevention into Practice program and CSAP's NCAP.

The CSAP Prevention Enhancement Protocol System (PEPS), a substance abuse prevention guideline program, was a CSAP initiative that began in 1992 and was designed to be the prevention counterpart to the TIPS. The PEPS guidelines are targeted at the state alcohol, tobacco, and other drug abuse agencies, substate agencies, local programs, individual practitioners, and collaborating agencies outside the substance abuse field. They were developed in response to the expressed need of these groups for help in identifying the best known science and practices to guide policy and program decision making. They selected and synthesized the strongest state-of-the-art prevention research and practice knowledge and made that information available in a format that is easy to read and understand. These documents were developed by experts in prevention research and practice, submitted for field review, and were revised as necessary to reflect input from both the scientific and the practice communities. The guideline package includes an implementation guide for policymakers and practitioners and a community guide for the general public.

Three PEPS were released, *Community Approaches to Reducing Youth Use of Tobacco* (1997a), *Preventing Substance Abuse among Children and Adolescents: Family-Centered Approaches* (1998b), and *Preventing Problems Related to Alcohol Availability: Environmental Approaches* (2000). Two others, *Media Approaches to Preventing Substance Abuse* and *School-Based Approaches to Preventing Substance Abuse* were under development when the program was discontinued. Evaluation of the completed products will be necessary to determine their ultimate effectiveness.

Similar to PEPS, the CSAP National Center for the Advancement of Prevention (NCAP) was created specifically to bridge the gap between prevention research and practice. The primary mission of NCAP is to "translate prevention science into creative, practical, and timely applications" (CSAP, undated a) and develop products that would be useful to policymakers and prevention practitioners at the national, state, and community levels. NCAP has developed a large number of documents, including *Guidelines and Benchmarks for Prevention Programming* (1995); reviews of the science involved in the six CSAP prevention strategies; an overview of the science and prevention models, guidelines, and implementation manuals related to youth access to tobacco products; implementation of the Synar Amendment and "Acheiving Outcomes". These documents undergo review by a panel of prevention scientists, as well as a field review of primarily state practitioners, but do not duplicate the expanded process used in developing PEPS guidelines. However, as with PEPS, while the NCAP work holds promise, at this time few of them have been formally released to the field. Hence, evaluation of their usefulness remains to be seen.

The Centers for Disease Control and Prevention (CDC) is currently developing the *Guide to Community Preventive Services* to address population-based approaches to public health services, focusing on community-based prevention and control strategies. This guide will summarize what is known about effective population-based interventions and, where data exist, include information on cost effectiveness. Need for the guide was identified in a feasibility study by the Council on Linkages between Academia and Public Health Practice, in collaboration with federal, state, and local public health agencies and with support from the Kellogg Foundation. The primary audiences are people involved in planning, funding, and implementinga population-based services and policies (U.S. Department of Health and Human Services, 1997). The Guide will include chapters on tobacco and alcohol. A chapter on tobacco has been completed and the chapter on the prevention of alcohol use and misuse is scheduled for completion in the Spring of 2002. The Guide is posted online at http://www.thecommunityguide.org/home_f.html.

The Agency for Healthcare Research and Quality's (AHRQ) Evidence-Based Practice Centers (EPCs), first funded in June 1997, are designed to conduct comprehensive reviews and rigorous analyses of the scientific literature to help clinicians, providers, and health plans improve clinical practice and decision making based on the best scientific knowledge available. The EPCs will "critically appraise, synthesize, and translate the existing evidence into information" (Atkins et al., 1998) that can be used by practitioners. Thirteen centers, including several of the original centers, were established in 2001 in institutions in the United States and Canada, when the contracts for the EPC were re-completed. As the information is developed, it is widely disseminated, using the Internet as a primary tool at www.ahrq.gov/clinic/epc. Topics for the centers are solicited routinely through the *Federal Register.* The only substance-abuse-related topic completed to date is the pharmacotherapy of alcohol dependence, which was completed by the EPC at the Research Triangle Institute and University of North Carolina at Chapel Hill (AHRQ, 1998b) and may be found on the AHRQ website.

These centers build on the long-standing AHRQ guidelines development program that was discontinued in the Fall of 1996. Like the guidelines, the reports and assessments produced by these Centers will be the result of careful review of the literature and peer review (Atkins et al., 1998). While AHRQ did not develop guidelines specifically directed at drug abuse, it did address tobacco cessation. The AHRQ guidelines (available on the AHRQ website, www.ahrq.gov) were developed in several forms for different audiences. They include the technical Guideline Report, a Quick Reference Guide for Clinicians for daily reference, and a Patient's Guide (AHRQ, 1993). A significant aspect of the AHRQ guideline program was the monitoring of the use of its guidelines. AHRQ funded several projects to study implementation of individual guidelines. Going beyond the most common evaluation methods of guideline development–client satisfaction or client use— AHRQ has attempted to evaluate the cost effectiveness of some of their guidelines, e.g., the Smoking Cessation Guideline.

In January 1999, AHRQ, in collaboration with the American Association of Health Plans and the American Medical Association, launched the National Guidelines Clearinghouse, an Internet-based source for evidence-based clinical guidelines (AHRQ, 1999b). The Clearinghouse, at www.guideline.gov, is designed to promote widespread access to guidelines for health professionals and others (AHRQ, 1998d). AHRQ, in collaboration with the Robert Wood Johnson Foundation, also uses Guideline Dissemination Grants to help professional groups and organizations develop training programs and other methods to adapt AHRQ guidelines for use by various provider groups.

AHRQ also administers Put Prevention into Practice (PPIP), a program first released in 1994, which is designed to address clinician and patient barriers to delivery of clinical preventive services. AHRQ relies on the creation of public–private partnerships with medical professional organizations, advocacy groups, community and business coalitions, managed care organizations and others to promote, disseminate, implement, and evaluate the PPIP materials (Griffith & Dickey, 1997). Implementation of the program has occurred in managed-care organizations, federal agencies (e.g., the Department of Defense) and in state and county agencies in at least four states. There have been seven separate evaluations of the PPIP, of the materials and of the program's effects on preventive services and practices, most showing increased awareness and/or use of the materials and positive preventive health care effects (AHRQ, 1999a).

The PPIP program is a good example of a comprehensive effort to take research, translate it into practical clinical guidance, and provide tools to help ensure that the guidance is applied in daily practice. The manual used by the program, *Clinicians Handbook of Preventive Services*

(AHRQ, 1998c), provides guidance on how to deliver preventive services and provides a summary discussion of the material included in the *Guide to Clinical Preventive Services* (U.S. Preventive Services Task Force, 1996). The package of materials that accompanies the *Handbook* goes beyond that developed with the PEPS and includes a variety of office and clinic system materials designed to serve as a guide to clinicians regarding preventive services and prompts for consumers to request services.

PPIP was created to be the implementation vehicle for the U.S. Preventive Services Task Force (USPSTF) recommendations, which were published in 1996 as the second edition of the *Guide to Clinical Preventive Services.* The *Guide* is based on a careful review of the evidence regarding clinical implementation of various preventive services; it addresses screening for drug abuse, problem drinking, and family violence, and also includes a chapter on counseling to prevent tobacco use. The *Guide* provides a full review of the data related to each condition, the effectiveness of early detection, recommendations from other groups, such as the American Medical Association and the American Academy of Family Physicians, and findings about the evidence to recommend for or against screening for the condition under review. Interestingly, for drug abuse the Task Force found insufficient evidence to recommend for, or against, routine screening, but did make recommendations regarding informing pregnant women of the potential adverse effects of drug use and advising clinicians to be alert to signs and symptoms of drug abuse and make referrals to treatment. The third edition, "Guide to Clinical Preventive Services, 2000–2002" (AHRQ, 2002) has been released but included no new topics related to substance abuse prevention (AHRQ, 1998a).

Application

There has been a national level effort to synthesize and transfer prevention knowledge, but there is a need for additional tools to assist practitioners apply that knowledge. Among efforts to do so are regional and state prevention resource centers, training, research application activities, and workforce development.

One of the early efforts was the DOE's Safe and Drug Free Schools regional centers that were charged with providing information, training, and materials to school systems in the states they served. However, in 1995 these centers were merged into the new DOE Comprehensive Regional Assistance Centers designed to cover a number of DOE programs beyond Safe and Drug Free Schools. Some of the centers have survived in the new center system and/or became Centers for the Application of Prevention Technologies (CAPTS).

The most recent national attempt at developing regional centers is the CAPTS. These six centers were first funded in September 1997; they are designed to assist states in applying "on a consistent basis, the latest research-based knowledge to their substance abuse prevention programs, practices, and policies" (CSAP, 1997b). The CAPTS are expected to transfer knowledge through both conventional and electronic means, establish a technical assistance network using local experts, provide skills development activities, and use electronic media innovatively—including teleconferencing, online events, videoconferencing, and database transfer. A large portion of their activity builds on other research and knowledge-synthesis work and repackages that research and practice knowledge into content and formats applicable to the states and communities in their regions. Each of them provide some guidance on implementing science-based programs and many of them include listings of specific programs. For example, the Central and Northeastern CAPTS developed several publications on such topics as science-based programs, levels of effectiveness, using science-based prevention strategies, and characteristics of science-based substance abuse prevention. The Western CAPT has developed an extensive, searchable electronic database of best practices that includes almost 40 programs. It provides information on program content, risk and protective factors, target populations, evaluation, and research findings. Information on the CAPTs may be found at www.captus.org.

While full evaluation of the CAPT program is not completed, some early reports of their experiences offer some lessons for successful diffusion. They reinforce the notion that how we present the science is often more the problem than practitioners understanding science. They caution against focusing too much of our efforts on computer technology in lieu of networking and personal contact in diffusion. They urge proceeding incrementally and addressing the systems issues around communication, resources, and readiness for change. Last, they highlight the importance of helping policymakers, practitioners, and citizens anticipate barriers and unintended spin-offs in implementing science-based programs (CSAP, 2001a).

Prevention-resource centers provide information-dissemination and training services designed to ensure that prevention professionals have the most current information and to facilitate application of prevention technology. Several states have implemented prevention resource centers, including Arizona, Illinois, Indiana, Kansas, Minnesota, Massachusetts, and Wisconsin. These resource centers provide a wide range of services, including clearinghouses, newsletters, journals, prevention materials, seminars and workshops, technical assistance and evaluation, and research. These centers have proven to be very popular, and the number of states establishing them has been expanding.

One of the most common methods used to transfer scientific knowledge to practitioners is training. Workshops and conferences, varying in length from 1 to perhaps 5 days, are well accepted as a method for transmitting prevention information. While these approaches are useful as part of a larger, systematic approach to knowledge application, there is little evidence that they alone affect practice. However, some training approaches that are coordinated with other activities are worthy of note.

One long-standing program sponsored by AHRQ, the User Liaison Program (ULP) Dissemination Support program, is specifically designed to transmit health-services research findings and descriptive and programmatic information through user workshops to a "broad spectrum of selected public and private users of health-services research," minimizing jargon and technical language (AHRQ, 1997). Since the 1970s, this program has focused on state and local officials and is expanding to include consumers, purchasers, practitioners, and policymakers. AHRQ also operates a national publications clearinghouse and publishes a variety of documents that help researchers and practitioners disseminate successful, science-based programs.

NIDA also provides materials to practitioners to help them apply science-based research in their prevention programs. The RDA program, cited earlier, provides substantial guidance on prevention programs for the general population as well as on community readiness and programs for at-risk individuals and groups. Other packages include the "Community-wide Drug Abuse Prevention Model," based on the Midwestern Prevention Project, which provides handbooks and intervention training materials for schools, parents, media, community leaders, and policymakers. Another package, the "School-Based High-Risk Youth Prevention Program," provides a curriculum for a high school course on skill-building in self-esteem, decision making, personal control, and interpersonal communications.

As noted earlier, the PPIP program looks beyond individual training events and develops materials to guide clinicians and individuals to provide and ask for services. Some examples of these materials are preventive care flowsheets, patient reminder postcards, posters, and wall charts. The manuals and other materials were developed through the PPIP program, but actual implementation of the program is carried out independently in both public and private clinical settings. PPIP program creators identify four essential principles for PPIP implementation: (1) having support from the top of the implementing organization, (2) having the health-care delivery team feel ownership of the program, (3) designating responsibility for implementation to a staff member, and (4) providing constant feedback to all staff involved in the program. One example of the application of this program is a skill-building course by the American College of Preventive Medicine that focuses on primary-care prevention and is designed to help physicians learn behavior-change counseling, how to design office systems to improve delivery of preventive services, understand the science behind the preventive services guidelines, and assess the quality of preventive services (American Medical Association, 1995).

An expanded concept of training being explored by csap in its work with the state alcohol and drug abuse agencies is Workforce Development, which builds on the former csap National Training System. More and more, it has become apparent that skill building, through follow-up technical assistance, mentoring, and coaching, is needed to help bring science to practice. Simple one-shot workshops or training are insufficient. Workforce development is a planned, integrated process and system through which structured learning experiences are tied to the knowledge or skill being transferred (Center for Substance Abuse Prevention, undated b). A major purpose of workforce development is to "integrate current research and best practices into state and community planning and implementation." Theory and research is one of the four foundational elements—the others being the state prevention plan, program standards, and certification. Two states—Arkansas and Colorado—are actively expanding their prevention-training systems to develop workforce development systems in which multiple knowledge-transfer approaches are used.

As noted previously, certification is one of the foundational elements of a workforce development system. While certification of prevention professionals has been under discussion and implemented to some extent in a few states, there is no uniform agreement on what it should entail and who should be included. We are, however, coming to recognize the importance of developing and maintaining a professional level of prevention practitioners. Some level of core competencies is essential so that there is a cadre of prevention professionals who understand and recognize the elements of science appropriate for their programs, how to critically analyze the prevention science presented to them, and how to apply that science to their own policy and program needs. Application will require adaptation within a given state or community, and we will need a prevention workforce capable of critically examining new research to ensure the appropriate application of science to their state or community. In response to this need, the International Certification Reciprocity Consortium (icrc) has identified core competencies that prevention professionals must have to be most effective in conceptualizing, developing, and implementing prevention programs. The competency domains include Program Coordination, Education and Training, Community Organization, Public Policy, Professional Growth and Responsibility, and Planning and Evaluation (Henderson & Heavner, 1994; Columbia Assessment Services, 1997).

Beyond the establishment of prevention resource centers, several states are taking more creative steps to promote the application of science to practice. For example, Iowa and Washington have required that at least 50% of the substance abuse prevention programs funded through the Substance Abuse Prevention and Treatment (sapt) Block Grant be science based. A growing number of other states are considering similar approaches. Washington also convenes a group of researchers to review new knowledge and offer advice to the state on developing and enhancing its programs. This level of attention to research demonstrates a strong commitment to developing sound, defensible programs that incorporate science into effective prevention programming. One outcome of this effort has been the formal adoption of the risk and protective factor model developed by J. David Hawkins, Richard F. Catalano, Jr., and associates (1992) for state planning and program implementation.

Another state, Arizona, is trying to make the "science and policy connection" by developing a system to enhance communication between scientists, improve the science–policy interface by multi-stake-holder dialogues, and developing a systemic communication process (Brown, 1997). At the explicit direction of the governor, the Governor's Drug and Gang Policy Council has been examining effective practices in prevention and treatment across multiple state departments and considering the appropriate policy direction to promote movement away from ineffective to effective programs. The state has developed a best practices guide and conducted a statewide best practices conference. They took a major step forward in March 2000, when they hosted a symposium to promote a dialogue among researchers, practitioners, and funders. Researchers from around the country met with Arizona funders, policymakers, and community practitioners in facilitated discussions to address the major issues associated with implementing science-based programs, including those around adaptation of those programs. A report on the symposium is under development.

Minnesota has taken a different approach. Working with a core group of prevention practitioners, the Minnesota Prevention Resource Center asked authors of four major research studies conducted in the state to identify the 10 most important recommendations from their research. The authors were asked to group those recommendations by schools, communities, and families/caregivers. An even larger group of prevention practitioners then prioritized the recommendations and developed some sample strategies for implementation. The end result was a guide, *Pulling It All Together*, to serve as a tool for sharing this information and promoting discussion within organizations and communities throughout the state (Minnesota Prevention Resource Center, 1993).

In 1970, New York established the Research Institute on Alcoholism (RIA) to study the use and abuse of alcohol, its causes, treatment, and prevention. RIA expanded its focus to include drugs in 1992. While research is the major focus of the institute, it has also implemented a communication strategy designed promote a continuous dialogue between the community and researchers. This strategy includes publishing a newsletter three times a year with findings from its research, conducting seminars and reporting on various research, and providing workshops that help research scientists improve their oral communication skills. Much of their work and their newsletter are readily available on the internet (www.ria.org) (RIA Report, 1996, 1997).

One prime example of moving research to practice has been a six-state consortium (Kansas, Maine, Oregon, South Carolina, Utah, and Washington), which, in 1992 working with the Social Development Research Group (SDRG) of the University of Washington, began implementing the Hawkins/Catalano model collaboratively, using a CSAP needs-assessment contract to facilitate collaboration. This is a stellar example of researchers working with states and communities to implement essentially the same model while making accommodations to reflect regional differences. These states have implemented needs assessments and, using those assessments, planned their programs using the risk- and protective-factor model. Their work has inspired other states to adopt a similar approach. Four of the six states continue to work collaboratively through a second needs-assessment contract with CSAP. In addition, SDRG and five of the original six (Kansas, Maine, Oregon, Utah, and Washington), joined by Colorado and Illinois, have a research grant from NIDA to study diffusion of the risk- and protection-focused prevention approach and examine its relationship to improving prevention outcomes (SDRG, 1997).

Foundations are also taking steps to enhance dissemination and utilization of research findings. Backer and Koon (1995) describe a variety of foundation efforts to improve information dissemination. For example, the Ford and Robert Wood Johnson foundations publish regular newsletters describing the results of their funded programs. The Robert Wood Johnson Foundation (RWJ) Foundation also hosted a symposium in the fall, 2000, "Prevention 2000: Moving

Effective Programs into Practice." At this symposium, researchers, policymakers and practitioners addressed the principles, marketing, technical assistance, and adaptation issues around bringing research to practice (RWJ, 2000). The report on the symposium is available on the Foundation's Website, www.rwjf.org.

The Ewing M. Kauffman Foundation has identified dissemination as a priority and expanded its staff to promote dissemination of its programs and linkages with national leaders around public policy on youth development. The Mitsubishi Electric America Foundation provides guidelines and technical assistance on dissemination and may also offer supplemental grants for dissemination to its grantees conducting service programs for young people with disabilities (Mitsubishi, 1997). The Better Homes Fund develops and markets nationwide training products on the best current knowledge and practices related to services for homeless families. Beyond their individual grant and dissemination efforts, foundations have recognized the need for greater learning from one another and collaborating on future programs to expand information networks (Mahoney, 1995).

Well over a dozen foundations support the work of Drug Strategies, an organization focused on reducing the demand for drugs and promoting more effective approaches to drug problems. Drug Strategies has issued a variety of publications addressing crime, welfare reform, the workplace, and schools, as well as profiles for individual states. Two of those publications are particularly good examples of efforts to bridge research and practice—*Making the Grade: A Guide to School Drug Prevention Programs* (Drug Strategies, 1997) and *Safe Schools, Safe Students: A Guide to Violence Prevention Strategies* (1998b). They provide a simple, nontechnical discussion of the major research findings on what works in prevention, identify key elements of successful programs, describe a variety of programs that include ratings on the key elements, and provide contacts for additional information. Another publication, *Keeping Score: We Can Reduce Drug Abuse* (Drug Strategies, 1998a), is a review of the impact of federal drug control spending on the country's drug problems. This report also highlights promising programs but notes that only a few have undergone rigorous evaluation due to limited prevention-research funding.

CONCLUSION

Prevention science and knowledge have clearly developed to a stage that prevention policymakers and professionals can confidently apply them in the conceptualization, development, and implementation of prevention policies and programs at the national, state, and community levels. However, all too often prevention science and knowledge are left in professional journals and at conferences and are not applied in the field in a timely manner. The reasons are many—the differences in priorities for researchers and policymakers and practitioners, the lack of agreement of what constitutes "enough" science to move forward and begin to design programs, the considerable complexity of the language often used to relate research findings, and differences in communicating research to the wide range of community professionals and volunteers who implement programs.

Successful transfer of science to practice requires information in repackaged or customized formats, seeking out innovators and early adopters, engaging in relationship building, problem solving, coaching, technical assistance, and facilitating networks at the national, state, and local level. While we are making progress in identifying approaches that facilitate the transfer of prevention science to practice, many of these approaches are in fledgling stages and are not yet evaluated. However, these approaches do address many of the concerns of previous efforts to transfer science to practice. Information alone is not enough; research reported in scientific journals is not enough; "one-shot" workshops and training are not enough.

REFERENCES

Agency for Healthcare Research and Quality (1993). *AHCPR program note: Clinical practice guideline development.* Rockville, MD: Author.

Agency for Healthcare Research and Quality (1997). *User Liaison Program (ULP) Dissemination support: Request for proposals.* Electronic, 9/97.

Agency for Healthcare Research and Quality (1998a). *AHCPR Announces New U.S. Preventive Services Task Force,* Rockville, MD: Author.

Agency for Healthcare Research and Quality (1998b). *AHCPR's Evidence-Based Practice Centers,* Rockville, MD: Author.

Agency for Healthcare Research and Quality (1998c) *Clinician's Handbook of Preventive Services,* Rockville, MD: Author.

Agency for Healthcare Research and Quality (1998d). *Invitation To Submit Guidelines to the National Guideline Clearinghouse* (TM). Rockville, MD: Author.

Agency for Healthcare Research and Quality (1999a). *Evaluations of the put prevention into practice program.* Rockville, MD: Author.

Agency for Healthcare Research and Quality (1999b). *National Guideline Clearinghouse To Be Unveiled January, 14,* Press Release.

Agency for Healthcare Research and Quality (2002). *Guide to Clinical Preventive Services, 3*rd *Edition, 2000–2002.* Rockville, MD. Electronic, 7/02.

American Medical Association (1995). Put prevention into practice: More than an apple a day. Reprinted with permission of *American Medical News.* U.S. Department of Health and Human Services. Electronic, 9/97.

Atkins, D., Kamerow, D., & Eisenberg, J. M. (1998). *Evidence-based medicine at the Agency for Health Care Policy and Research.* Editorial in ACP Journal Club. March/April 1998.

Backer, T. E. (1991a). *Drug abuse technology transfer.* Rockville, MD: National Institute on Drug Abuse.

Backer, T. E. (1991b). Knowledge utilization: The third wave. *Knowledge: Creation, Diffusion, Utilization, 12*(3), 225–240.

Backer, T. E. (1995a). Assessing and enhancing readiness for change: Implications for technology transfer. In T. E. Backer, S. L. David, & G. Soucy (Eds.), *Reviewing the behavioral science knowledge base on technology transfer* [Research Monograph 155] (pp. 21–41). Rockville, MD: National Institute on Drug Abuse.

Backer, T. E. (1995b). Integrating behavioral and systems strategies to change clinical practice. *Joint Commission Journal on Quality Improvement, 21*(7), 351–353.

Backer, T. E. (1997). Managing the human side of change in VA's transformation. *Hospital & Health Services Administration, 42*(3), 433–459.

Backer, T. E. (2000). The future of success: Challenges of disseminating effective substance abuse prevention programs. *Journal of Community Psychology, 28,* 363–373.

Backer, T. E., & David, S. L. (1995). Synthesis of behavioral science learnings about technology transfer. In T. E. Backer, S. L. David, & G. Soucy (Eds.), *Reviewing the behavioral science knowledge base on technology transfer* [Research Monograph 155] (pp. 262–279). Rockville, MD: National Institute on Drug Abuse.

Backer, T. E., David, S. L., & Soucy, G. (1995). Introduction. In T. E. Backer, S. L. David, & G. Soucy (Eds.), *Reviewing the behavioral science knowledge base on technology transfer* [Research Monograph 155] (pp. 1–20). Rockville, MD: National Institute on Drug Abuse.

Backer, T. E., & Koon, S. L. (1995). Demonstrate, evaluate, disseminate. Repeat. *Foundation News & Commentary, 28,* 32–34.

Backer, T. E., & Newman, S. S. (1995). Organizational linkage and information dissemination 6+ strategies to integrate the substance abuse and disability fields. *Rehabilitation Counseling Bulletin, 38*(2), 93–107.

Biglan, A. (1993). A functional contextualist framework for community interventions. In S. C. Hayes, L. J. Hayes, H. W. Reese, & T. R. Sarbin (Eds.), *Varieties of scientific contextualism* (pp. 251–276). Reno, NV: Context Press.

Biglan, A. (1995). *Changing cultural practices: A contextualist framework for intervention research.* Reno, NV: Context Press.

Biglan, A., & Hayes, S. C. (1996). Should the behavioral sciences become more pragmatic? The case for functional contextualism in research on human behavior. *Applied and Preventive Psychology 5,* 47–57.

Brown, B. (1995). Reducing impediments to technology transfer in drug abuse programming. In T. E. Backer, S. L. David, & G. Soucy (Eds.), *Reviewing the behavioral science knowledge base on technology transfer* [Research Monograph 155] (pp. 169–185). Rockville, MD: National Institute on Drug Abuse.

Brown, A. (1997). Making the science and policy connection. Unpublished presentation materials. Phoenix, AZ: Author.

Center for Substance Abuse Prevention (1995). *Guidelines and benchmarks for prevention programming.* Rockville, MD: Author.

Center for Substance Abuse Prevention (2001a). *Closing the gap between research and practice: Lessons of the first three Years of CSAP's national CAPT system: 1997–2000.* Rockville, MD: Author.

Center for Substance Abuse Prevention (2001b). *Finding the balance: Program fidelity and adaptation in substance abuse prevention: Executive summary of a state-of-the-art review.* Rockville, MD: Author

Center for Substance Abuse Prevention (2001c). *Principles of ssubstance abuse prevention.* Rockville, MD: Author.

Center for Substance Abuse Prevention (2001d). *Promising and proven substance abuse prevention programs.* Rockville, MD: Author.

Center for Substance Abuse Prevention, (2001e). *Science-based substance abuse prevention: A guide.* Rockville, MD: Author.

Center for Substance Abuse Prevention (1997a). *Reducing tobacco use among youth: Community-based approaches.* Rockville, MD: Author.

Center for Substance Abuse Prevention (1997b). *Request for proposal for the CSAP cooperative agreements for centers for the application of prevention technologies (CAPT).* Rockville, MD: Author.

Center for Substance Abuse Prevention (1998a). *A catalog from CSAP's findings bank of science-based prevention practices.* Rockville, MD: Author. Conference edition.

Center for Substance Abuse Prevention (1998b). *Preventing substance abuse among children and adolescents: Family-centered approaches.* Rockville, MD: Author

Center for Substance Abuse Prevention (1999). *Understanding substance abuse prevention: Toward the 21st century: A primer on effective programs.* Rockville, MD: Author.

Center for Substance Abuse Prevention (2000a). *CSAP's decision support system for states and communities—Prototype 1.4.* Electronic, 3/01.

Center for Substance Abuse Prevention (2000 b). *CSAP's model programs.* Rockville, MD: Author.

Center for Substance Abuse Prevention (2000c). *Preventing problems related to alcohol availability: Environmental approaches.* Rockville, MD: Author.

Center for Substance Abuse Prevention (Undated a). *National Center for the Advancement of Prevention (NCAP) fact sheet.* Rockville, MD: Author.

Center for Substance Abuse Prevention (Undated b). *State prevention workforce development: A technical assistance support guide, draft 4.* Rockville, MD: Author.

Center for the Study and Prevention of Violence (2002). *Blueprints for violence prevention.* Boulder, CO: Institute for Behavioral Science. Electronic, 7/02.

Columbia Assessment Services, Inc. (1997, draft). *ICRC: Overview of educational objectives: Moving toward an ATOD prevention curriculum.* Raleigh, NC: Author.

Drug Strategies (1997). *Making the grade: A guide to school drug prevention programs.* Washington, DC: Author.

Drug Strategies (1998a). *Keeping score: We can Reduce Drug Abuse.* Washington, DC: Author.

Drug Strategies (1998b). *Safe schools, safe students: A guide to violence prevention strategies.* Washington, DC: Author.

Dunn, C. (1993). The role of law enforcement in school-linked drug prevention. In *Evaluating school-linked prevention strategies: Alcohol, tobacco, and other drugs,* (pp. 40–42) [conference proceedings]. San Diego: University of California, San Diego Extension.

Edwards, R. W., Jumper-Thurman, P., Plested, B. A., Oetting, E. R., & Swanson, L. (2000). Community readiness: Research to practice. *Journal of Community Psychology, 28,* 291–307.

Ellickson, P. L. (1995). Schools. In R. H. Coombs & D. M. Ziedonis (Eds.), *Handbook on drug abuse prevention: A comprehensive strategy to prevent the abuse of alcohol and other drugs* (pp. 93–119). Boston: Allyn and Bacon.

Ennett, S. T., Ringwalt, C., & Flewelling, R. L. (1993). How effective is Project DARE? Preliminary findings from a review and assessment of DARE evaluations. In *Evaluating school-linked prevention strategies: Alcohol, tobacco, and other drugs* (pp. 51–70) [conference proceedings]. San Diego: University of California, San Diego Extension.

Ennet, S. T., Tobler, N. S., Ringwalt, C. L., & Flewelling, R. L. (1994). How effective is drug abuse resistance education? A meta-analysis of project DARE outcome evaluations. *American Journal of Public Health, 84*(9), 1394–1401.

Glaser, E. M., Abelson, H. H., & Garrison, K. N. (1983). *Putting knowledge to use: Facilitating the diffusion of knowledge and the implementation of planned change.* San Francisco, CA: Jossey–Bass.

Griffith, H. M., & Dickey, L. (1997). *Put prevention into practice: A systematic approach.* U.S. Department of Health and Human Services. Electronic, 10/97.

Harachi, T. W., Ayers, C. D., Hawkins, J. D., Catalano, R. F., & Cushing. J. (1996). Empowering communities to prevent adolescent substance abuse: Process evaluation results from a risk- and protection-focused community mobilization effort. *The Journal of Primary Prevention, 16*(3), 233–254.

Hawkins, J. D. (1995). Controlling crime before it happens: Risk-focused prevention. *National Institute of Justice Journal,* 10–16.

Hawkins, J. D., Catalano, R. F., & Associates. (1992). *Communities that care: Action for drug abuse prevention.* San Francisco: Jossey–Bass.

Henderson, J. P., & Heavner, S. (Eds.) (1994). *Alcohol, tobacco, and other drug abuse prevention specialist: role delineation study.* Raleigh, NC: International Certification Reciprocity Consortium/Alcohol and Other Drug Abuse, Inc.

Holder, H. D. (1997). Need for a scientific basis for alcohol-involved problem prevention including a consideration of cost and effectiveness. *Substance Use & Misuse, 32*(2), 203–209.

Holder, H. D., Boyd, G., Howard, J., Flay, B., Voas, R., & Grossman, M. (1995). Alcohol-problem prevention policy: The need for a phases research model. *Journal of Public Health Policy, 16*(3), 324–346.

Kumpfer, K. L. (1993). *Strengthening America's families: Promising parenting strategies for delinquency prevention: User's guide.* Washington, DC: Office of Juvenile Justice and Delinquency Prevention.

Laflin, M., Edmundson, E. W., & Moore-Hirschl, S. (1995). Enhancing adoption of an alcohol abuse prevention program: an application of diffusion theory. *The Journal of Primary Prevention, 15*(1), 75–101.

Lipton, D. S. (1992). How to maximize utilization of evaluation research by policymakers. *The Annals of the American Academy of Political and Social Science, 522,* 175–188.

Mahoney, M. E. (1995). Make known what you know. *Foundation News & Commentary,* 29–31.

Mattick, R. P., & Ward, J. (1992). Drug and alcohol treatment research, policy and practice: an Australian perspective. *The Journal of Drug Issues, 22*(3), 625–640.

Minnesota Prevention Resource Center (1993). *Pulling it all together: prevention research in Minnesota.* Anoka, MN: Author.

Minnesota Institute of Public Health (1997). *Drug abuse resistance education (DARE) program evaluation: Final report.* Anoka, MN: Author.

Mitsubishi Electric America Foundation (1997). *Road map: Creating and sustaining project impact—Guidelines for evaluation and dissemination.* Washington, DC: Author.

National Institute on Drug Abuse (1997a). *Community readiness for drug abuse prevention: Issues, tips & tools.* Rockville, MD: Author.

National Institute on Drug Abuse (1997b). *Drug abuse prevention package.* Rockville, MD: Author.

National Institute on Drug Abuse (1997c). *NIDA capsules: NIDA technology transfer program.* Electronic, 9/97.

National Institute on Drug Abuse (1997d). *Preventing drug use among children and adolescents: A research-based guide.* Rockville, MD: Author.

National Institute on Drug Abuse (2001). *The next generation of drug abuse prevention research.* Electronic, 1/01.

Office of National Drug Control Policy (2000). *Evidence-based principles for substance abuse prevention.* Washington, DC: Author.

Planning and Evaluation Service (1997). *School-based drug prevention programs: A longitudinal study in selected school districts.* Washington, DC: U.S. Department of Education.

Research Institute on Addictions (Spring 1996). Twenty-five years of excellence at RIA. *RIA Report.* Electronic, 11/97.

Research Institute on Addictions (Summer 1997). Communicating findings to the public. *RIA Report.* Electronic, 11/97.

Robert Wood Johnson Foundation (2000). *Prevention 2000: Moving effective programs into practice.* Unpublished notes.

Rogers, E. M. (1995a). *Diffusion of innovations* (4th edition). New York: The Free Press.

Rogers, E. M. (1995b). Diffusion of drug abuse prevention programs: spontaneous diffusion, agenda setting, and reinvention. In T. E. Backer, S. L. David, & G. Soucy (Eds.), *Reviewing the behavioral science knowledge base on technology transfer* [Research Monograph 155] (pp. 90–105). Rockville, MD: National Institute on Drug Abuse.

Rohrbach, L. A., D'Onofrio, C. N., Backer, T. E., & Montgomery, S. B. (1996). Diffusion of school-based substance abuse prevention programs. *American Behavioral Scientist, 39*(7), 919–934.

Rohrbach, L. A., Graham, J. W., & Hansen, W. B. (1993). Diffusion of a school-based substance abuse prevention program: Predictors of program implementation. *Preventive Medicine, 22,* 237–260.

Scattergood, P., Dash, K., Epstein, J., & Adler, M. (1998). *Applying effective strategies to prevent or reduce substance abuse, violence, and disruptive behavior among youth.* Newton, MA: Education Development Center, Ind. (draft).

Schinke, S. P., & Orlandi, M. A. (1991). Technology transfer. In C. G. Leukefeld & W. J. Bukoski (Eds.), *Drug abuse prevention intervention research: Methodological issues.* [Research Monograph 107] (pp. 248–263). Rockville, MD: National Institute on Drug Abuse.

Shanley, C., Lodge, M., & Mattick, R. P. (March, 1996). Dissemination of research findings to alcohol and other drug practitioners. *Drug and Alcohol Review, 15*(1), 89–94.

Shaperman, J., & Backer, T. E. (Fall, 1995). The role of knowledge utilization in adopting innovations from academic medical centers. *Hospital & Health Services Administration, 40*(3), 401–412.

Social Development Research Group (1997). *Diffusion of state risk/protection-focused prevention.* Briefing paper. University of Washington: Author.

Tanglewood Research (2001). *Prevention Knowledge Base.* Electronic, 1/01.

Tobler, N. S. (1993). Updated meta-analysis of adolescent drug prevention programs. In *Evaluating school-linked prevention strategies: Alcohol, tobacco, and other drugs* (pp. 71–86) [conference proceedings]. San Diego: University of California, San Diego Extension.

U.S. Department of Education (1998). *Safe and drug-free schools and communities act: State grants for drug and violence prevention program: Nonregulatory guidance for implementing the SDFSCA principles of effectiveness.* Washington, DC: Author.

U.S. Department of Education (2001). *The expert panel on safe, disciplined and drug-free schools searching for best programs: Expert panel identifies nine exemplary and thirty-three promising programs.* Electronic, 1/01.

U.S. Department of Health and Human Services (1996). *Alcohol and other drug abuse prevention: The national structured evaluation.* Third Report to Congress. Washington, DC: Author.

U.S. Department of Health and Human Services (1997). *Guide to community preventive services.* Washington, DC: Author.

U.S. Department of Health and Human Services (1999). *Science-based substance abuse prevention.* Washington, DC: Author (working draft).

U.S. Preventive Services Task Force (1996). *Guide to clinical preventive services.* Washington, DC: U.S. Department of Health and Human Services.

Walsh, D. C., Rudd, R. E., Moeykens, B. A., & Moloney, T. W. (1993). Social marketing for public health. *Health Affairs, 12*(2), 104–119.

Index

671